Oral Anatomy, Histology and Embryology

Oral Anatomy, Histology and Embryology

Sixth Edition

B.K.B. Berkovitz BDS, MSc, PhD, FDSRCS (Eng)
Emeritus Reader, Anatomy and Human Sciences, Biomedical and Health Sciences, King's College, London, UK

G.R. Holland BSc, BDS, PhD, CERT ENDO
Emeritus Professor of Dentistry, Department of Cariology, Restorative Sciences and Endodontics, School of Dentistry and Department of Cell and Developmental Biology, University of Michigan, Ann Arbor, MI, USA

B.J. Moxham BSc, BDS, PhD, FHEA, FRSB, Hon FAS, FSAE
Emeritus Professor of Anatomy, Cardiff School of Biosciences, Cardiff University, Cardiff, UK

For contributions to Dental Radiology

J. Makdissi DDS, MMedSc, FDSRCS (Eng), DDRRCR, FHEA, PhD
Clinical Senior Lecturer/Honorary Consultant in Dental and Maxillofacial Radiology, Queen Mary School of Medicine and Dentistry and Barts Health NHS Trust, London, UK

Associate editor responsible for writing the chapter on Regenerative Dentistry and for updating the chapter on Early Tooth Development

Ana Angelova Volponi DDS, PhD, FHEA
Reader in Regenerative Dentistry Education, Faculty of Dentistry, Oral & Craniofacial Sciences, King's College, London, UK

For additional online content visit Elsevier eBooks+

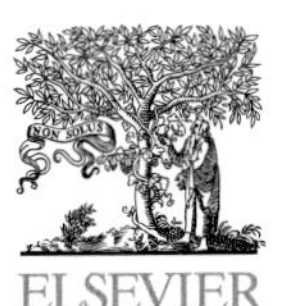

Publisher's note: *Elsevier* takes a neutral position with respect to territorial disputes or jurisdictional claims in its published content, including in maps and institutional affiliations.

First edition 1978
Second edition 2002
Third edition 2005
Fourth edition 2009
Fifth edition 2018
Sixth edition 2025

ISBN: 978-0-323-93521-0

Content Strategist: Alexandra Mortimer
Content Project Manager: Abdus Salam Mazumder
Design: Miles Hitchen
Marketing Manager: Deborah Watkins

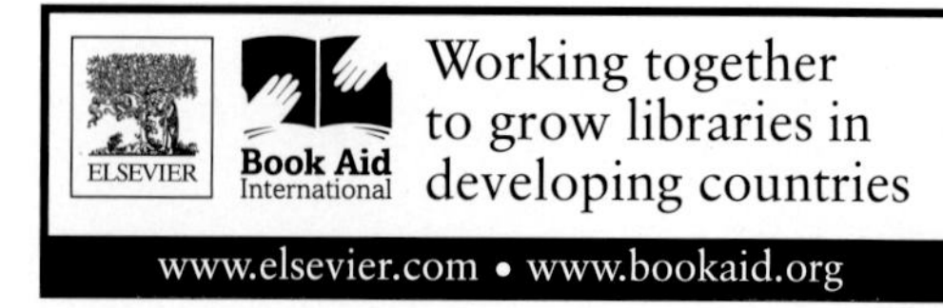

Printed in China by 1010 Printing International Ltd

Last digit is the print number: 9 8 7 6 5 4 3 2 1

Contents

Preface

The first edition of this book was written in the late 1970s and, although nearly half a century has now passed, we remain committed to the book's initial conception 'to gather together the diverse elements of oral anatomy which, in the past, have been scattered through many different textbooks, and to arrive at an integrated perspective of the subject'. We continue to be unafraid of being 'encyclopaedic' in our approach.

For this, the sixth edition of our book, we have revised most chapters, in particular the chapters on oral histology and development. A new chapter on repair and regeneration of the oro-dental tissues has been added, this being an area of intensive research and clinical promise. To aid student learning, this edition features 'mind maps' for each chapter to facilitate navigation through the text. Indeed, we believe that these maps aid how a subject's complexity can be organised and also facilitate an appreciation of how the progression of ideas have led to our present understandings. The maps have replaced the 'overviews' and 'learning outcomes' in the previous edition, these now seeming to be of more limited educational value. A 'mind map' can provide a better visual aid to learning that can be easily modified, or added to, as the reader grapples with the material.

A further area of difficulty relates to the importance of molecular biology in dental research and the plethora of terms and abbreviations that have appeared to identify signalling molecules, growth factors and genes. To aid the reader in understanding the abbreviations, a glossary has been provided at the end of the book.

As for the previous editions, we maintain that 'a picture is worth a thousand words'. We have therefore not only retained most of the previous images but have added nearly 70 new illustrations, many relating to clinical cases that add to the relevance of understanding 'normal' oro-dental anatomy and histology. Where possible, in the interests of equality and diversity, we have changed images to represent persons of different ancestral origins.

To encourage the deep learning necessary, in our opinion, for a learned profession, and to steer the student away from relying on superficial or strategic learning just for examinations, we have updated bibliographies and reference lists. These are included in a comprehensive online learning platform. This platform also has self-assessment questions to aid the reader's learning progress and revision and includes true/false questions, extended matching questions and picture tests.

It seems to us that dentistry is approaching a crossroads such that, while its past has been craft-based, relying upon the mechanical, its future could very well be biological. Indeed, recent advances into aspects of dental tissue regeneration emphasise how bioactive molecules trigger natural healing processes. It is for this reason that we have incorporated a chapter on the repair and regeneration of dental tissues. We are especially grateful that this chapter was written by a recognised authority on the subject who is also now the associate editor of this book (Dr. Ana Angelova Volponi). The implications of such developments should lead to the realisation that the future dental surgeon must not only be increasing conversant with oral biology to provide effective therapies, but also needs to educate patients who are often sceptical of therapies that 'tamper' with their biology. This will inevitably mean that students will once more have to pay increasing attention to advances in oral biology. To do this, they need to become less reliant on minimalistic 'core' syllabuses, or on mechanisms and strategies just to pass examinations, and become more willing to explore the 'details' of their discipline.

As stated in the prefaces of all previous editions of this book, we remain extremely grateful to all who have contributed to its production, either directly by providing invaluable material or indirectly through comments and criticisms. We welcome any further comments and suggestions and we still 'do not pretend to be infallible and would ask for indulgence if we have strayed from scientific rectitude'.

B.K.B. Berkovitz
B.J. Moxham
A. Angelova Volponi
April 2024

Acknowledgements

We are most grateful to the numerous colleagues who generously provided photographic material for our book and these have been acknowledged in the legends. We acknowledge photographic assistance from Mr. M. Simons. In addition, we owe a debt of thanks to the following researchers for their help and constructive criticisms of the text: Prof. T.R. Arnett, Dr. R.J. Cook, Prof. M.C. Dean, Dr. S. Elsharkawy, Dr. L. Feinberg, Dr. E. Gentleman, Prof. A. Grigoriadis, Dr. J.D. Harrison, Prof. A. Linde, Prof. R.W.A. Linden, Dr. A. Loughlin, Prof. P.R. Morgan, Prof. B.G. Proctor, Prof. A.J. Sloan, Prof. A.S. Tucker

The appearance of the oral cavity

1

The oral cavity (Fig. 1.1) extends from the lips and cheeks externally to the pillars of the fauces internally, where it continues into the oropharynx. It is subdivided into the vestibule external to the teeth and the oral cavity proper internal to the teeth. The palate forms the roof of the mouth and separates the oral and nasal cavities. The floor of the oral cavity consists of a mucous membrane covering the mylohyoid muscle and is occupied mainly by the tongue. The lateral walls of the oral cavity are defined by the cheeks and retromolar regions. The primary functions of the mouth are concerned with the ingestion (and selection) of food and with mastication and swallowing. Secondary functions include speech and ventilation (breathing).

Lips

The lips (Fig. 1.2) have a muscular and connective tissue skeleton. The muscle is the orbicularis oris muscle. Externally the lips are covered by skin and by a red zone that has been termed the vermilion. Internally the lips are covered by a non-keratinised labial mucosa. Where persons have an increased density of pigment (melanosomes), the red colour of the vermilion is masked and therefore the term may be deemed inappropriate. Although not yet approved by anatomical terminology, an alternative term might be external labial mucosa. The sharp junction of the vermilion and the skin has been termed the vermilion border but could also be called the labial mucocutaneous junction (Fig. 1.3).

In the upper lip there is a protrusion in the midline to form the tubercle. The lower lip shows a slight depression in the midline corresponding to the tubercle. From the midline to the corners of the mouth the lips widen and then narrow. Laterally the upper lip is separated from the cheeks by nasolabial grooves. Similar grooves appear with age at the corners of the mouth to delineate the lower lip from the cheeks (the labiomarginal sulci). The labiomental groove separates the lower lip from the chin. In the midline of the upper lip runs the philtrum. The corners of the lips (the labial commissures) are usually located adjacent to the maxillary canine and mandibular first premolar teeth. The lips exhibit sexual dimorphism; as a general rule, the skin of the male is thicker, firmer, hirsute and less mobile. The lips illustrated are lightly closed at rest and are described as being 'competent'. The lips provide an important aesthetic feature of the face, and psychologically the importance of the smile cannot be underestimated.

Lip posture varies from person to person and is dependent upon the soft tissues and musculature within the lips. At rest, the lips are separated normally by no more than 3–4 mm. At greater than this distance, the lips

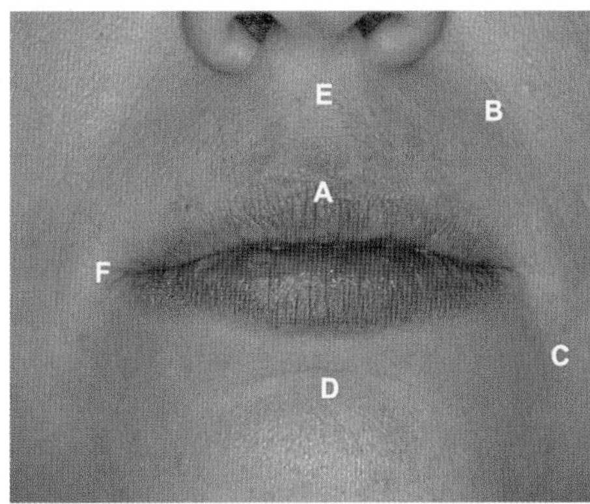

Fig. 1.2 The lips. A = tubercle; B = nasolabial groove; C = labiomarginal sulci; D = labiomental groove; E = philtrum; F = labial commissure.

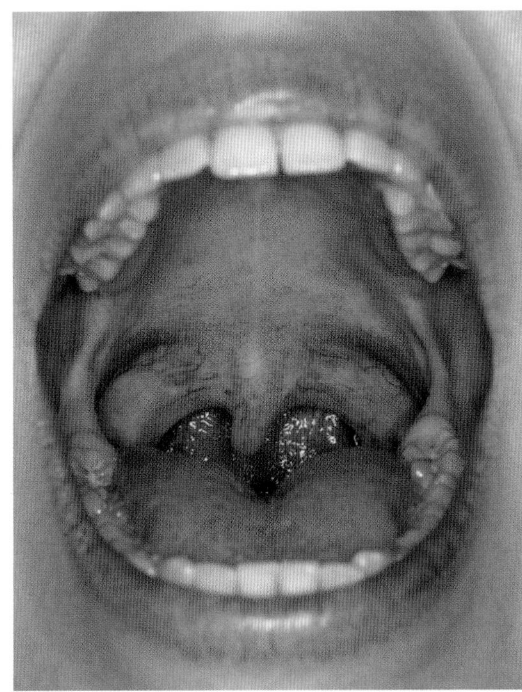

Fig. 1.1 The oral cavity.

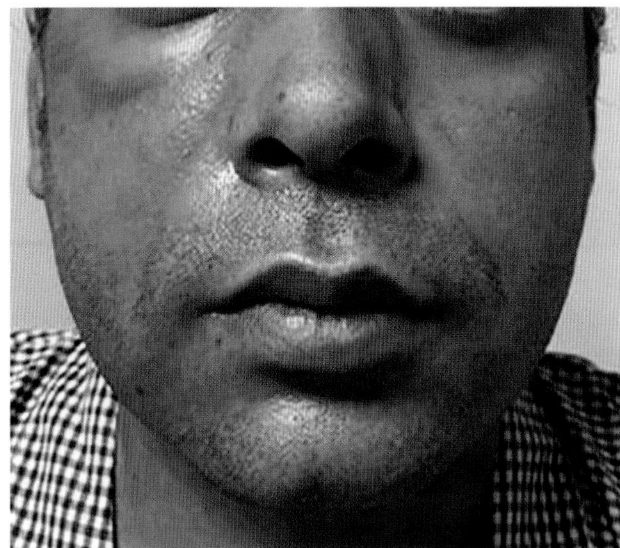

Fig. 1.3 Individual with increased melanin pigmentation, which reduces the red colouration of the external surface of the lips. From Dhingra, S., Dhingra, P.L., 2022. *Diseases of Ear, Nose and Throat & Head and Neck Surgery,* eighth ed. Elsevier.

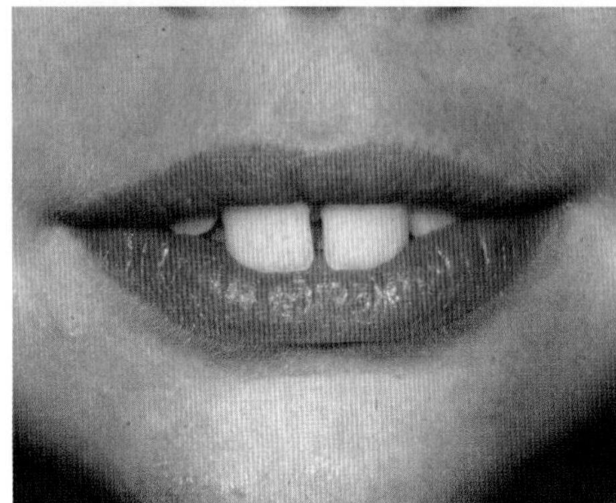

Fig. 1.4 Incompetent lips.

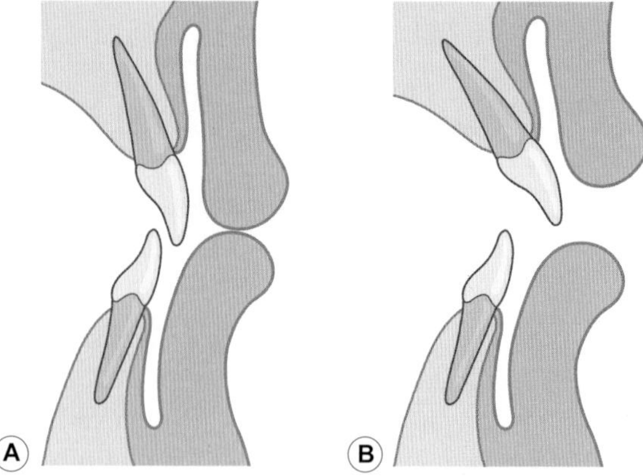

Fig. 1.5 (A) Competent lips maintaining normal inclination of the incisors. (B) Incompetent lips resulting in proclination of the upper incisors.

are said to be 'incompetent'. Thus, incompetent lips (Fig. 1.4) describe a situation where, at rest and with the facial muscles relaxed, a lip seal is not produced. It is of some importance that this is distinguished from conditions where the lips are merely held apart habitually (as often occurs with 'mouth breathers'). The lip posture illustrated in Fig. 1.4 can be described as being 'potentially competent', because the lips would be capable of producing a seal at rest if there was no interference caused by the protruding incisors. True lip incompetence is frequently seen alongside straining of the mentalis muscles in the lower lip and with lack of tonic activity (flaccidity) in other parts of the lip musculature. Another sign is eversion of the lower lip so that the vermilion is rolled forward.

Where the lips are incompetent, the pattern of swallowing sometimes needs to be modified to produce an anterior oral seal. Accordingly, an oral seal may be formed by contact between the lower lip (or the tongue) and the palatal mucosa, and there may even be a forcible tongue thrust. Furthermore, lip incompetence may be associated with problems of the alignment of the teeth (see later) and with speech defects.

It has been estimated that in the United Kingdom and the United States about 50% of children at the age of 11 years have some degree of lip incompetence because the lips are not fully developed until late adolescence. Studies suggest therefore that lip incompetence is often diminished by the age of 13 years. In addition, lip incompetence is commonly seen where persons suffer from air obstructions (e.g., from allergic rhinitis). An unfortunate effect occurs where, despite an ability to maintain an anterior oral seal, a person retains an habitual lip incompetence. Anecdotally, it is said that incompetent lips might be aesthetically pleasing, although this may relate to the gender of the individual.

The position and activity of the lips are important in controlling the degree of protrusion of the incisors. With competent lips (Fig. 1.5A) the tips of the maxillary incisors lie below the upper border of the lower lip; this arrangement helps to maintain the 'normal' inclination of the incisors (the upper incisors are 'normally' overlapped by the lower lip by 2–3 mm). With incompetent lips (Fig. 1.5B) the maxillary incisors may not be so controlled and the lower lip may even lie behind them, thus producing an exaggerated proclination of these teeth. If there is tongue thrusting to provide an anterior oral seal, further forces that tend to protrude the incisors are generated. A tight, or overactive, lip musculature may be associated with retroclined incisors.

Because in everyday English the term 'incompetent' often denotes inferiority or ineptitude, the terms 'competent' and 'incompetent' are perhaps inappropriate and could be replaced by 'complete' or 'incomplete' lip seal. However, these terms are not yet accepted in the dental clinic. Lip incompetence can be modified by orthodontic treatment and/or by exercising the lip musculature. It is of some importance that lip incompetence is distinguished from conditions where the lips are merely held apart habitually (as often occurs with mouth breathers). Mouth breathing often involves increased opening of the mandible at rest and this, with time, may lead to changes in dental alignment or even growth of the face.

To some extent, lip morphology contributes to facial attractiveness. Furthermore, in addition to often being associated with facial dysmorphology, it is important for many medical diagnoses and for facial and gender recognition, with lips being as unique as fingerprints.

The lips are frequently described as being full, wide, thin, heart-shaped, downward-turned or heavy upper or lower lips. In addition, the lines or grooves on the lips are sometimes used to distinguish different lip types:

- Type I: vertical lines that run across the entire lips or part of the lips
- Type II: branched, Y-shaped lines
- Type III: intersecting (crossed) lines
- Type IV: reticular (netlike) lines
- Type V: undetermined (mixed) lines

Lip morphology has also been classified according to a 'Wilson-Richmond' scale and, in the process of automating lip morphology, Davies, Richmond and Zhurov (2022) have provided a range of descriptive lip morphological traits and classes (Table 1.1).

Oral vestibule

The oral vestibule (Fig. 1.6) is a slit-like space between the lips and cheeks and the teeth and alveolus. At rest, or with the mouth open, the vestibule and oral cavity proper directly communicate between the teeth. When the teeth occlude, the vestibule is a closed space that communicates with the oral cavity proper only behind the last molars (the retromolar regions).

The mucosa covering the alveolus is reflected onto the lips and cheeks, forming a trough or sulcus called the vestibular fornix. In some regions of the sulcus the mucosa may show distinct sickle-shaped folds running from the cheeks and lips to the alveolus. The upper and lower labial frena or frenula are such folds in the midline. Other folds of variable dimensions may traverse the sulcus in the region of the canines or premolars. Such frena are said to be more pronounced in the lower sulcus. All folds contain loose connective tissue and are neither muscle attachments nor sites of large blood vessels.

The upper labial frenum should be attached well below the alveolar crest. A large frenum with an attachment near this crest may be associated with a midline diastema between the maxillary central incisors (Fig. 1.7). Prominent frena may also influence the stability of dentures.

Table 1.1 A range of descriptive lip morphological traits and classes

	1	2	3	4	5	6	7
Philtrum shape	Deep grove, narrow philtrum	Indentation near vermilion border, narrow philtrum	Indentation near vermilion border, wide philtrum	Deep groove, average philtrum width	No indentation wide philtrum	Indentation near nose, average philtrum width	Indentation in the middle, average philtrum width
Cupid's bow	Flat	U-shaped	V-shaped				
Upper lip contour	Concave	Straight	Pseudo convex	Convex			
Upper lip border	Full vermilion border and double border	Full border with clear border at cupid's bow	No vermilion border				
Lower lip contour	Narrow in the midline	Curved	Markedly curved	Straight			
Lower lip border	None	Full	Middle				
Lower lip-chin shape	Curved concavity	Marked angular concavity	Convex area	Angular concavity	Flat		
Lower lip tone	None	Central concavity	Marked lateral mounds and central concavity	Wide concavity	Bumped area		

From Davies, K.J.M., Richmond, S., Zhurov, A., 2022. Applying an automated method of classifying lip morphological traits. *Journal of Orthodontics* 49:412–419.

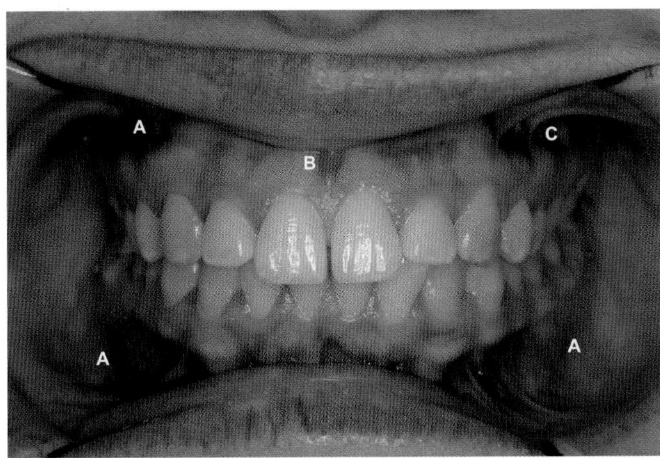

Fig. 1.6 The oral vestibule. A = vestibular fornix; B = upper labial frenum; C = frenum in the region of the upper premolar teeth. Courtesy Prof. P R Morgan.

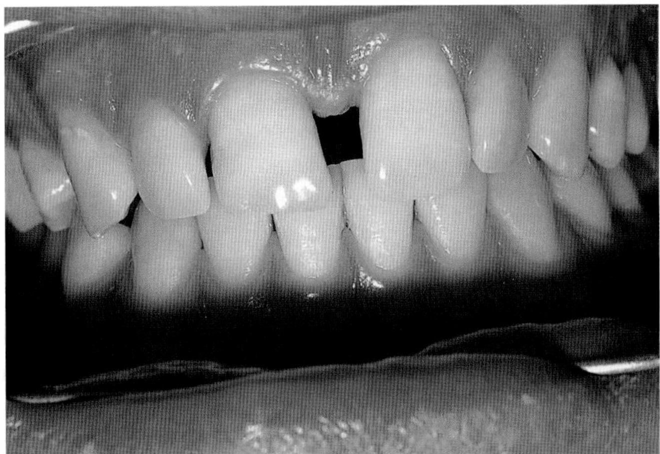

Fig. 1.7 Midline diastema between upper central incisor teeth, produced by an enlarged labial frenum.

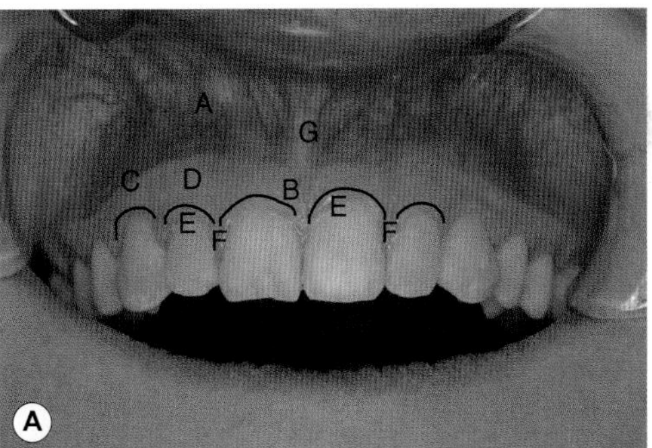

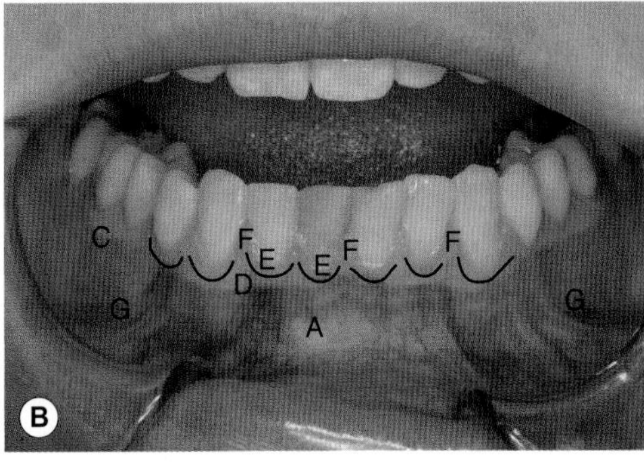

Fig. 1.8 Upper (A) and lower (B) gingivae. A = alveolar mucosa; B = free gingival groove indicated by curved black line; C = mucogingival junction; D = attached gingiva: E = free gingiva; F = interdental papilla; G = labial frenum. Courtesy Prof. P R Morgan.

Gingiva

The gums or gingivae, the oral mucosa covering the alveolar bone (which supports the roots of the teeth) and the necks (cervical regions) of the teeth, are divided into two main components (Fig. 1.8). The portion lining the lower part of the alveolus is loosely attached to the periosteum via a diffuse submucosa and is termed the alveolar mucosa. It is delineated from the gingiva (which covers the upper part of the alveolar bone and the necks of the teeth) by a well-defined junction, the mucogingival junction. The alveolar mucosa appears red and the gingiva appears pale pink. These colour differences relate to differences in the type of keratinisation and the proximity to the surface of underlying blood vessels. Indeed, small blood vessels may readily be seen coursing beneath the alveolar mucosa (Fig. 1.8B). The gingiva may be further subdivided into the attached gingiva and the free gingiva. The attached gingiva is firmly bound to the periosteum of the alveolus and to the teeth, and the free gingiva lies unattached around the cervical region of the tooth. A groove (the free gingival groove) may be seen between the free and attached gingivae. This groove corresponds

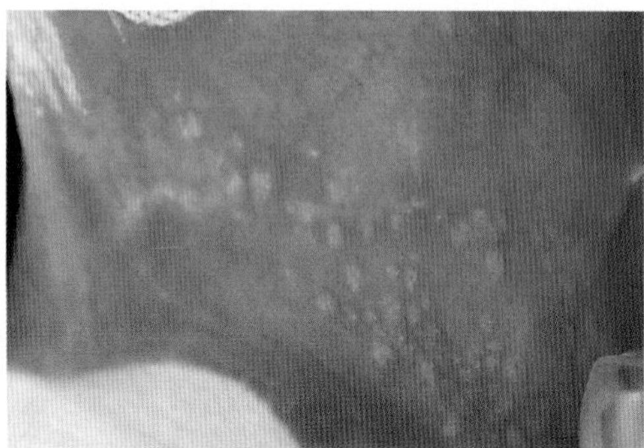

Fig. 1.9 Inner surface of the cheek, showing Fordyce spots as yellowish patches. From Cawson, R.A., Odell, E.W. (Eds.), 2008. *Cawson's Essentials of Oral Pathology and Oral Medicine,* eighth ed. Churchill Livingstone, Edinburgh, with permission.

approximately to the floor of the gingival sulcus that separates the inner surface of the attached gingiva from the enamel itself (Fig. 14.36). The interdental papilla is that part of the gingiva that fills the space between adjacent teeth. A feature of the attached gingiva is its surface stippling. The degree of stippling varies from individual to individual and according to age, sex and the health of the gingiva. Unlike the attached gingiva, the free gingiva is not stippled (see Fig. 1.19). On the lingual surface of the lower jaw the attached gingiva is sharply differentiated from the alveolar mucosa towards the floor of the mouth by a mucogingival line. On the palate, however, there is no obvious division between the attached gingiva and the rest of the palatal mucosa because this whole surface is keratinised masticatory mucosa.

Cheeks

The cheeks extend intraorally from the labial commissures anteriorly to the ridge of mucosa overlying the ascending ramus of the mandible posteriorly. They are bounded superiorly and inferiorly by the upper and lower vestibular fornices (Fig. 1.6). The mucosa is nonkeratinised and, being tightly adherent to the buccinator muscle, is stretched when the mouth is open and wrinkled when closed. Ectopic sebaceous glands without any associated hair follicles may be evident in the mucosa and are called Fordyce spots (Fig. 1.9). They are seen as small, yellowish-white spots, occurring singly or in clusters, and may also be seen on the margins of the lips (see Fig. 1.22). They can be seen in most patients and are said to increase with age.

Few structural landmarks are visible in the cheeks. The parotid duct drains into the cheek opposite the maxillary second molar tooth, and its opening may be covered by a small fold of mucosa termed the parotid papilla (see Fig. 1.25). In the retromolar region, in front of the pillars of the fauces, a fold of mucosa containing the pterygomandibular raphe extends from the upper to the lower alveolus (Fig. 1.10). The pterygomandibular space, in which the lingual and inferior alveolar nerves run, lies lateral to this fold and medial to a ridge produced by the mandibular ramus. The groove lying between the ridges produced by the raphe and the ramus of the mandible is an important landmark for insertion of a needle for local anaesthesia of the lingual and inferior alveolar nerves (see pages 109–110).

Palate

The palate forms the roof of the mouth and separates the oral and nasal cavities. It is divided into the immovable hard palate anteriorly and the movable soft palate posteriorly. As their names imply, the skeleton of the hard palate is bony, whereas that of the soft palate is fibrous.

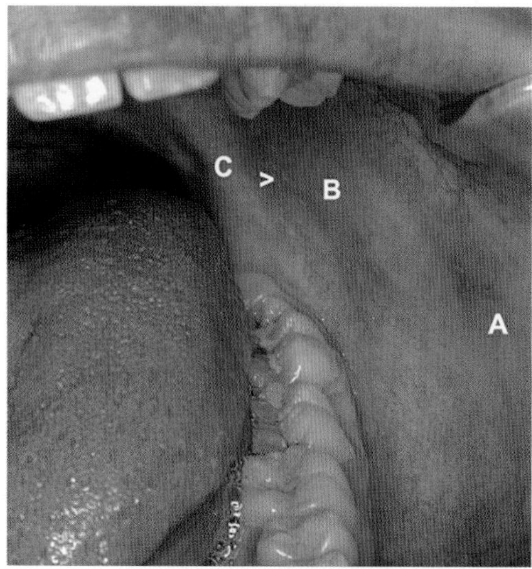

Fig. 1.10 Retromolar region. A = inner surface of cheek; B = ridge overlying ramus of mandible; C = ridge overlying the pterygomandibular raphe. The arrowhead indicates a landmark for the insertion of needle for local anaesthesia of the lingual and inferior alveolar nerves. Courtesy Prof. P R Morgan.

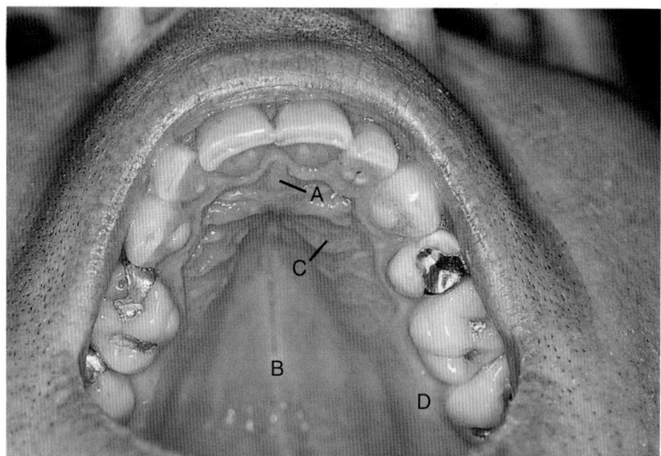

Fig. 1.11 The hard palate. A = incisive papilla; B = palatine raphe; C = palatine rugae; D = alveolus.

The hard palate is covered by a masticatory, keratinised mucosa that is firmly bound down to underlying bone and also contains some taste buds. It shows a distinct prominence immediately behind the maxillary central incisors, the incisive papilla (Fig. 1.11). This papilla overlies the incisive fossa through which the nasopalatine nerves enter onto the palate. Extending posteriorly in the midline from the papilla runs a ridge termed the palatine raphe. Here, the oral mucosa is attached directly to bone without the presence of a submucosal layer of tissue. Palatine rugae are elevated ridges in the anterior part of the hard palate that radiate transversely from the incisive papilla and the anterior part of the palatine raphe. Their pattern is unique to the individual and, like fingerprints, can be used for forensic purposes to help identify individuals. At the junction of the palate and the alveolus lies a mass of soft tissue (submucosa) in which the greater palatine nerves and vessels run. The shape and size of the dome of the palate vary considerably, being relatively shallow in some cases and having considerable depth in others.

The boundary between the soft palate and the hard palate is readily palpable and may be distinguished by a change in colour, with the soft palate having a yellowish tint. Extending laterally from the free border of the soft palate on each side are the palatoglossal and palatopharyngeal

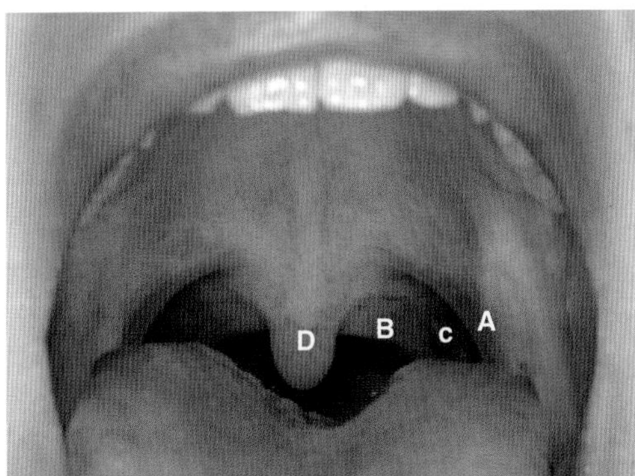

Fig. 1.12 The soft palate and oropharyngeal isthmus. A = palatoglossal fold; B = palatopharyngeal fold; C = palatine tonsil; D = uvula. Courtesy Prof. P R Morgan.

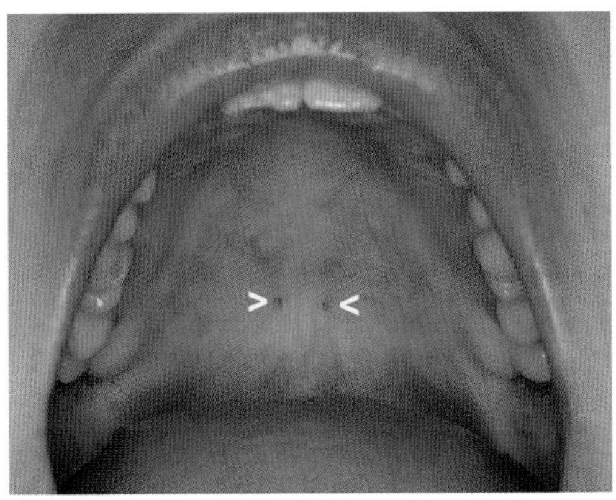

Fig. 1.13 Oral surface of the soft palate showing the fovea palatini (arrows). Courtesy Prof. P R Morgan.

folds (pillars of the fauces), with the palatoglossal fold being more anterior (Fig. 1.12). These folds cover the palatoglossus and palatopharyngeus muscles and between them lies the tonsillar fossa that houses the palatine tonsil. The palatine tonsil is a collection of lymphoid material of variable size that is likely to atrophy in the adult. It exhibits several slit-like invaginations (the tonsillar crypts), one of which is particularly deep and named the intratonsillar cleft. The free edge of the soft palate in the midline is termed the palatal uvula. The oropharyngeal isthmus is where the oral cavity and the oropharynx meet. It is delineated by the palatoglossal folds.

Knowledge of the anatomy of the palate has clinical relevance when siting the posterior border (postdam) of an upper denture. The denture needs to bed into the tissues at the anterior border of the soft palate (at a location sometimes referred to as the 'vibrating line' because the soft palate can be seen to move here on asking a patient to say 'ah'). In most individuals, two small pits, the fovea palatini, may be seen (Fig. 1.13) on either side of the midline; these represent the orifices of ducts from some of the minor mucous glands of the palate. The fovea palatini can also be seen on impressions of the palate, and a postdam may usually be safely placed a couple of millimetres behind the pits.

Floor of the mouth

The movable floor of the mouth is a small, horseshoe-shaped region above the mylohyoid muscle and beneath the movable part of the tongue (Fig. 1.14). It is covered by a lining of nonkeratinised mucosa. In the midline, near the base of the tongue, a fold of tissue called the lingual frenum extends onto the inferior surface of the tongue. The sublingual papilla, onto which the submandibular salivary ducts open into the mouth, is a large, centrally positioned protuberance at the base of the tongue. On either side of this papilla are the sublingual folds, beneath which lie the submandibular ducts and sublingual salivary glands.

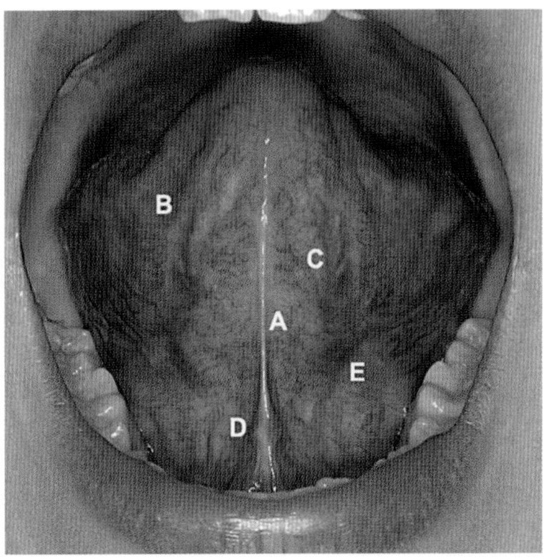

Fig. 1.14 Inferior surface of the tongue. A = lingual frenum; B = fimbriated fold; C = deep lingual vein; D = sublingual papilla; E = sublingual fold. Courtesy Prof. P R Morgan.

Tongue

The tongue is a muscular organ with its base attached to the floor of the mouth. It is attached to the inner surface of the mandible near the midline and gains support below from the hyoid bone. It functions in mastication, swallowing and speech, and carries out important sensory functions, particularly those of taste. The lymphoid material contained in its posterior third has a protective role.

The inferior (ventral) surface of the tongue, related to the floor of the mouth, is covered by a thin lining of nonkeratinised mucosa that is tightly bound down to the underlying muscles. In the midline, extending on to the floor of the mouth, lies the lingual frenum (Fig. 1.14). Occasionally this extends across the floor of the mouth to be attached to the mandibular alveolus. Such an overdeveloped lingual frenum (ankyloglossia) may restrict movements of the tongue. Lateral to the frenum lie irregular, fringed folds: the fimbriated folds. The deep lingual veins are also visible through the mucosa.

The upper (dorsal) surface of the tongue may be subdivided into an anterior two-thirds (palatal part) and a posterior one-third (pharyngeal part). The junction of the palatal and pharyngeal parts is marked by a shallow V-shaped groove, the sulcus terminalis (Fig. 1.15A). The angle (or V) of the sulcus terminalis is directed posteriorly. In the midline, near the angle, may be seen a small pit called the foramen caecum. This is the primordial site of development of the thyroid gland.

The mucosa of the palatal part of the dorsum of the tongue is mainly keratinised and is characterised by an abundance of projections (papillae) (Fig. 1.15B). The most numerous are the filiform papillae appearing as whitish, conical elevations (Fig. 1.16). Interspersed between the filiform papillae and readily seen at the tip of the tongue are isolated reddish prominences, the fungiform papillae. The largest papillae on the palatal surface of the tongue are the circumvallate papillae, which lie immediately in front of the sulcus terminalis. There are about 10 to 15 circumvallate papillae (Fig. 1.17). They do not project beyond the surface of the tongue and are surrounded by a circular 'trench'. Foliate papillae (Fig. 1.18) appear as a series of parallel, slit-like folds of mucosa on each lateral border of the

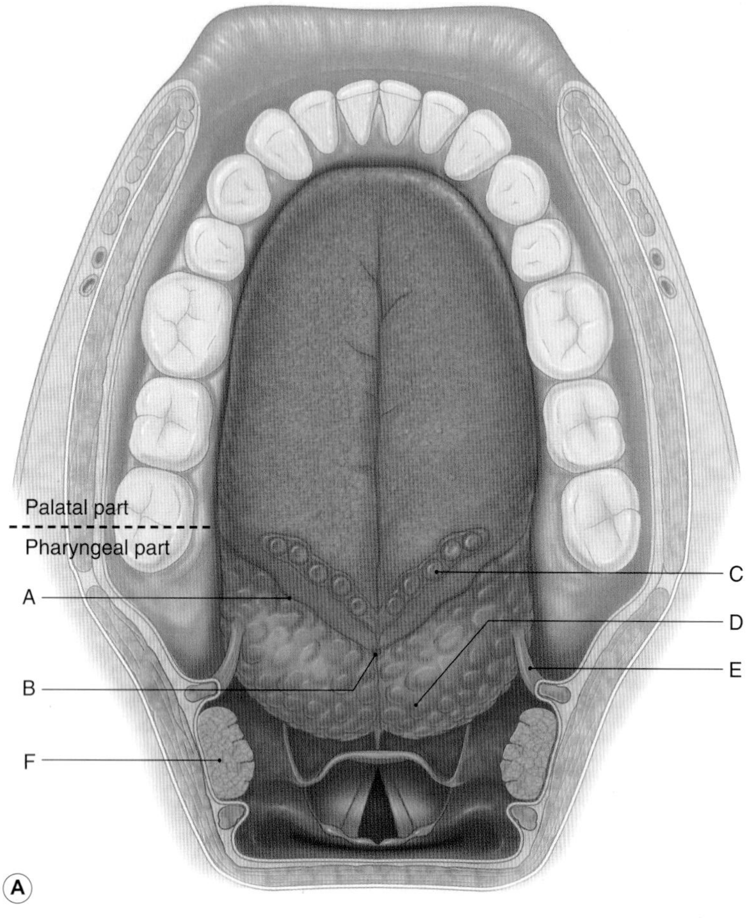

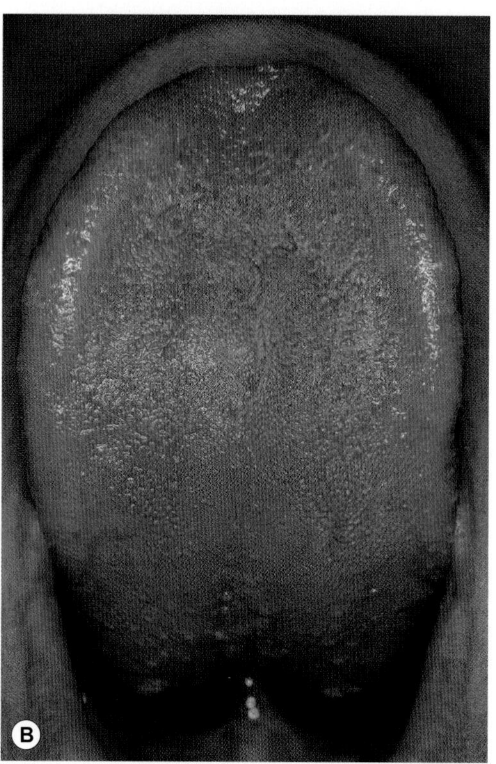

Fig. 1.15 (A) Dorsum of the tongue. A = sulcus terminalis; B = foramen caecum; C = circumvallate papillae; D = lingual follicles; E = palatoglossal arches; F = palatine tonsil. (B) Note the raised circumvallate papillae at the back of the tongue. (B). Courtesy Prof. P R Morgan.

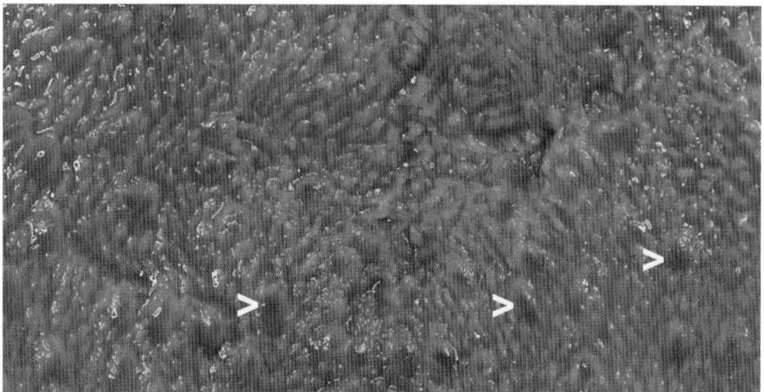

Fig. 1.16 Dorsum of the tongue, showing numerous keratinised, whitish filiform with fewer interspersed, reddish, nonkeratinised, fungiform papillae (arrowheads). Courtesy Prof. P R Morgan.

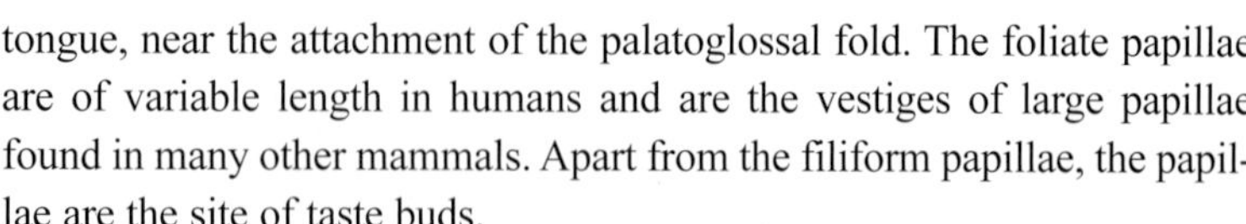

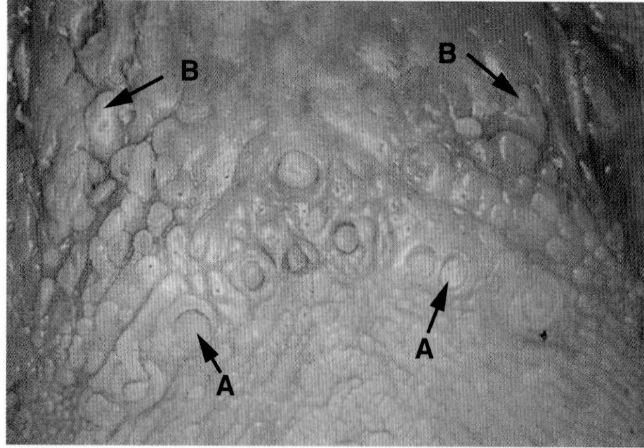

Fig. 1.17 Dorsum of the tongue, showing circumvallate papillae (A). B = lingual follicles.

tongue, near the attachment of the palatoglossal fold. The foliate papillae are of variable length in humans and are the vestiges of large papillae found in many other mammals. Apart from the filiform papillae, the papillae are the site of taste buds.

The pharyngeal surface of the dorsum of the tongue is nonkeratinised and is covered with large, rounded nodules termed the lingual follicles (Fig. 1.15). These follicles are composed of lymphoid tissue, collectively forming the lingual tonsil. The posterior part of the tongue slopes towards the epiglottis, where three folds of mucous membrane are seen: the median glossoepiglottic fold and two lateral glossoepiglottic folds. The anterior pillars of the fauces (the palatoglossal arches) extend from the soft palate to the sides of the tongue near the circumvallate papillae.

Clinical considerations

There are several conditions in the mouth that can be inspected in the nonclinical environment. They provide examples of 1) normal variation, 2) common benign disorders, and 3) disorders that may highlight normal features that may be otherwise inconspicuous.

Variation in pigmentation

As examples of normal variation, we can consider pigmentation, Fordyce spots and black hairy tongue. In dark-skinned patients, patches of melanin pigment may be seen in the mouth, particularly in the gingiva (Fig. 1.19).

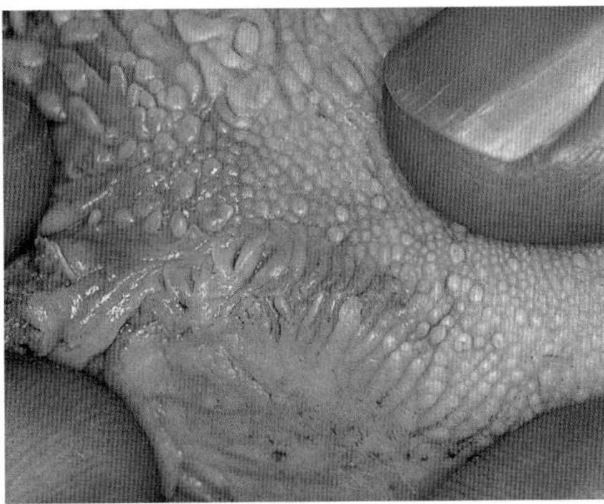

Fig. 1.18 Side of the tongue, showing slit-like appearance of foliate papillae.

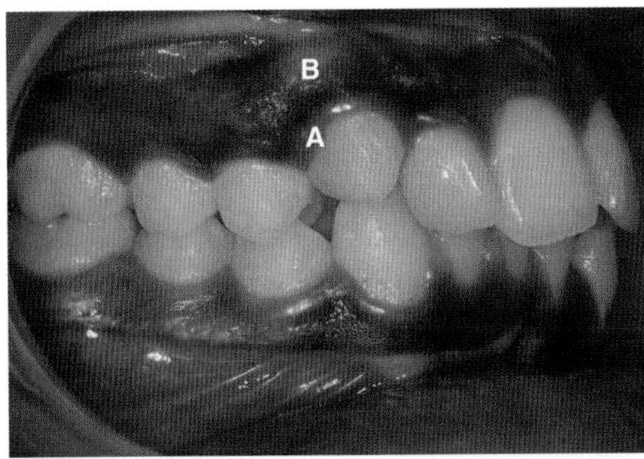

Fig. 1.19 Patches of dark melanin pigment appearing in the region of the attached gingiva. Note the free gingiva is not stippled (A), unlike the attached gingiva (B). Courtesy Drs P S Viswapurna and R Madan.

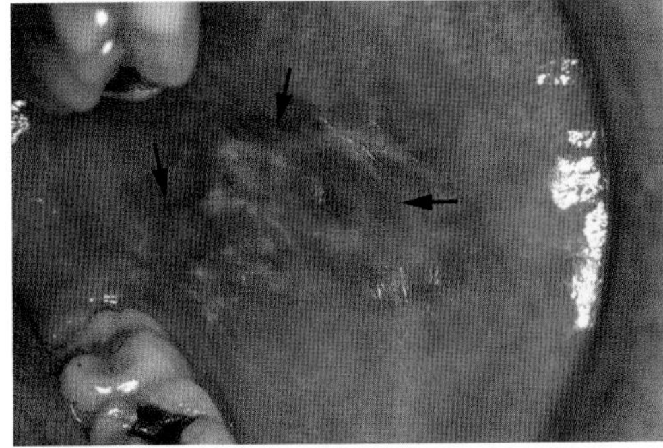

Fig. 1.20 Area of increased pigmentation (arrowed) associated with whitish patches caused by lichen planus. Courtesy Prof. P R Morgan.

This pigmentation is the result of the extra melanosome granules present within the oral epithelium (Fig. 14.22). Such pigmentation needs to be distinguished from other forms of mucosal pigmentation and from increased melanin pigmentation associated with a range of inflammatory conditions, such as lichen planus, where melanin pigment is held within macrophages in the lamina propria (Figs. 1.20, 1.21). Fordyce spots are seen to varying degrees as small, yellowish-white spots, occurring singly or in clusters on the margins of the lips (Fig. 1.22) or in the mucosa of the cheeks (see Fig. 1.9) (and other sites such as genital skin). They can be seen in most patients and are said to increase with age. They represent collections of sebaceous glands (Fig. 1.23) without any associated hair follicles. The range of variation in the filiform papillae on the dorsum of the tongue is well illustrated by black hairy tongue (lingua villosa nigra), a benign condition in which there is hypertrophy of these papillae (Fig. 1.24). Instead of being about 1 mm in length, the filiform papillae may reach up to 15 mm, giving the dorsum an appearance of being covered in fine hairs.

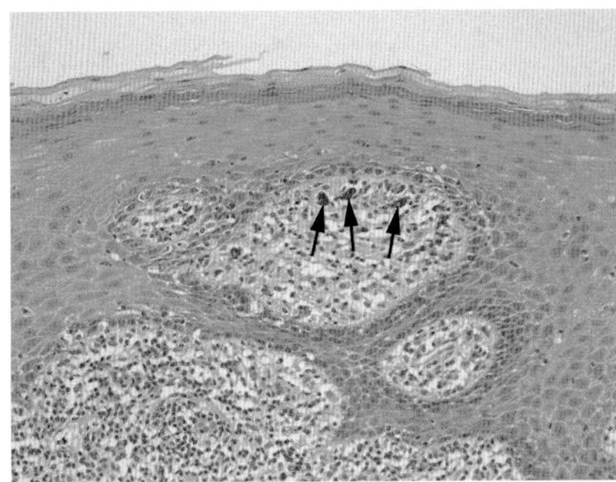

Fig. 1.21 Micrograph of biopsy taken from pigmented area shown in Fig. 1.20, showing melanin pigment within macrophages (arrows) lying within the lamina propria. The epithelium is parakeratinised, giving the whitish patches (H & E; ×80). Courtesy Prof. P R Morgan.

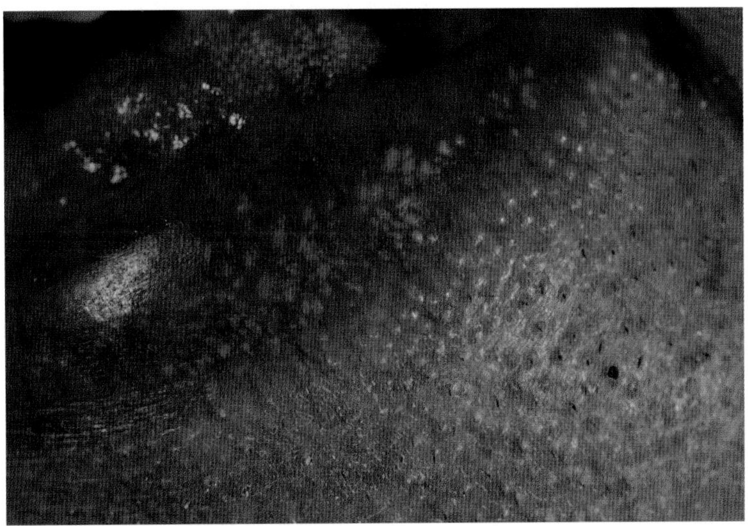

Fig. 1.22 Fordyce spots appearing as yellow spots on the vermilion (red zone) of the lip. The black spots below represent hair follicles on the surface of the adjacent skin of the chin. Courtesy Prof. P R Morgan.

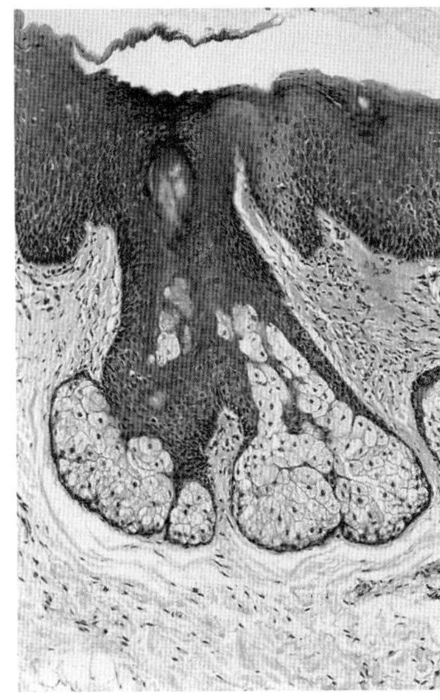

Fig. 1.23 Micrograph of a Fordyce spot, showing it to be a sebaceous gland (H & E; ×75). From Cawson, R.A., Odell, E.W. (Eds.), 2008. *Cawson's Essentials of Oral Pathology and Oral Medicine*, eighth ed. Churchill Livingstone, Edinburgh, with permission.)

This provides a suitable environment for bacteria (and sometimes fungi) to accumulate and, together with retained pigments of dietary or microbial origin, potentially to colour black the surface of the tongue black. The condition may also be associated with the administration of antibiotics or

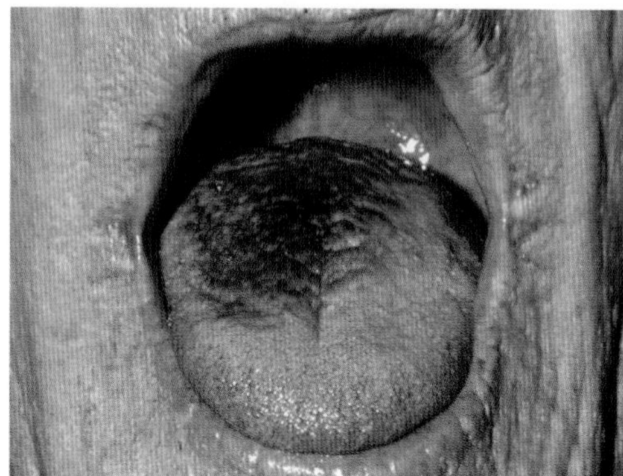

Fig. 1.24 Black hairy tongue. Courtesy Prof. P R Morgan.

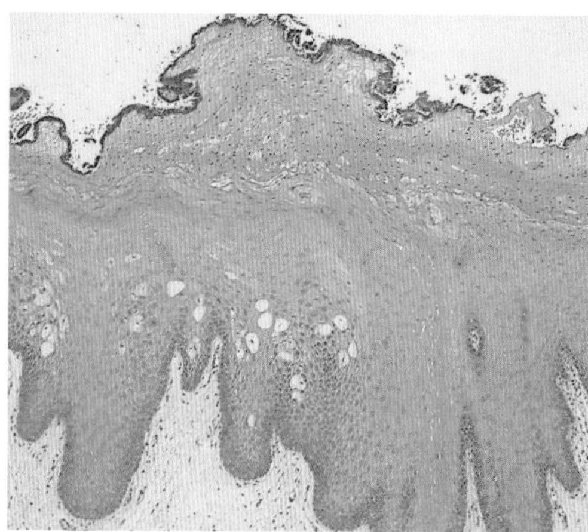

Fig. 1.26 Section of buccal mucosa showing the linea alba to be parakeratinised compared with the normal nonkeratinised state of the buccal mucosa (H & E; ×50). Courtesy Prof. P R Morgan.

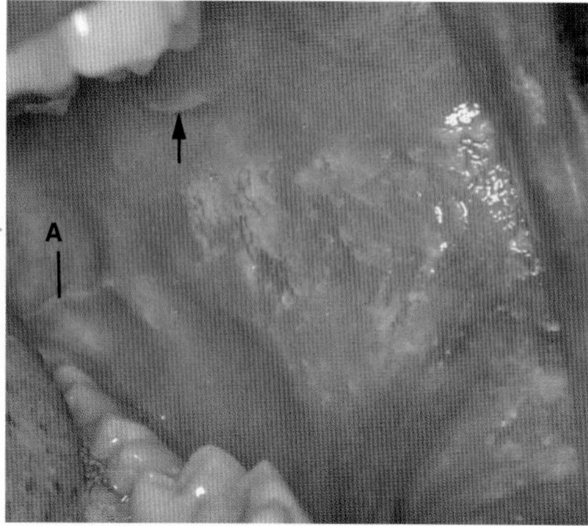

Fig. 1.25 View of buccal mucosa showing a linea alba adjacent to the molar teeth (A) at the level of the occlusal plane. In front of this line the white patches on the cheek represent more diverse cheek chewing. Arrow shows the parotid papilla. Courtesy Prof. P R Morgan.

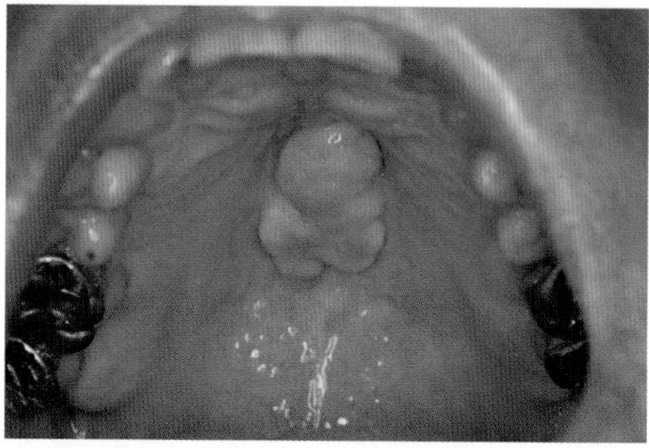

Fig. 1.27 Upper jaw showing a relatively small torus palatinus as an overgrowth of bone along the midline of the palate. Courtesy Dr C Dunlap.

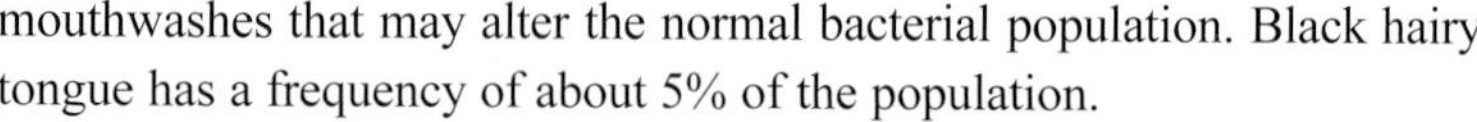

mouthwashes that may alter the normal bacterial population. Black hairy tongue has a frequency of about 5% of the population.

Benign disorders (linea alba, tori and smoker's keratosis)

Examples of common benign disorders are linea alba and tori. On the inside of the cheek and level with the occlusal plane, a linear, slightly raised whitish ridge may be seen, the linea alba (Fig. 1.25). It is commonly the result of low-grade, intermittent trauma owing to folds of cheek mucosa being trapped between the teeth. More active trauma associated with cheek chewing produces a much larger, irregular white patch (Fig. 1.25). The constant irritation converts the surface epithelium from its normal nonkeratinised state into a parakeratinised layer (Fig. 1.26).

Individual variation in the shape of the jaws is recognised by anatomists and pathologists. Such variations blend with benign conditions. As an example, tori are benign localised overgrowths of bone found in both the upper (torus palatinus) and lower (torus mandibularis) jaws, resulting in an increased radiopacity in the region. In the upper jaw, the enlargement is typically seen in the midline (Figs. 1.27–1.29), whereas in the lower jaw it is usually on the lingual aspect in the canine/premolar region and may be unilateral (Fig. 1.30) or bilateral (Fig. 1.31). However, a torus mandibularis may also affect the buccal surface of the mandible (Fig. 1.32). Torus palatinus is more common in females, whereas torus mandibularis is slightly more common in males. Tori vary in size from small to very large, and there is a tendency for them to increase in size with age. Tori may be related to functional adaptations, because there is some evidence that

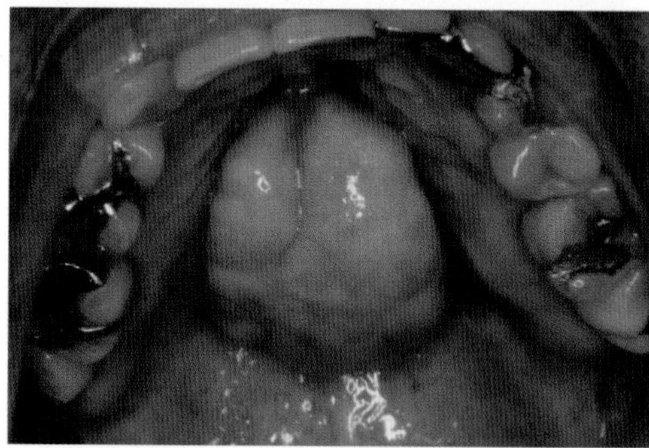

Fig. 1.28 Upper jaw showing a large torus palatinus as an overgrowth of bone along the midline of the palate. Courtesy Dr C Dunlap.

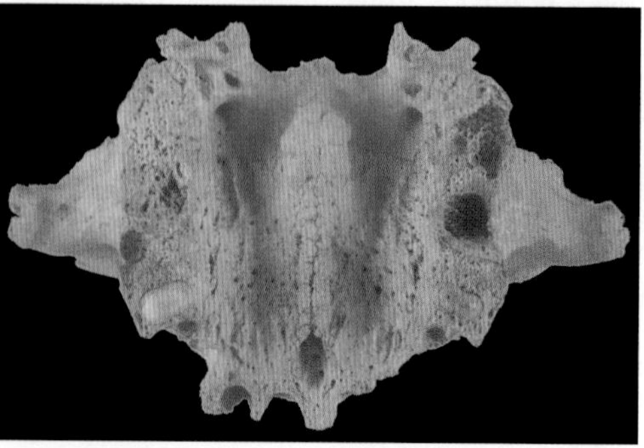

Fig. 1.29 Isolated palate showing torus palatinus as an overgrowth of bone along the midline. Copyright the Royal College of Surgeons of England.

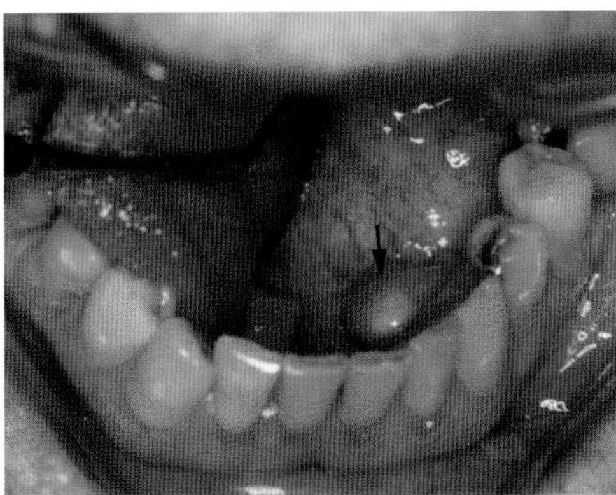

Fig. 1.30 Unilateral torus mandibularis (arrow) on the lingual surface of the mandible. Courtesy Prof. P R Morgan.

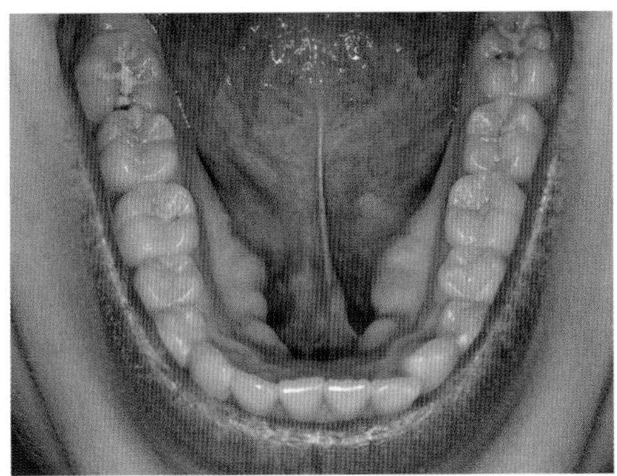

Fig. 1.31 Bilateral torus mandibularis on the lingual surface of the mandible. Courtesy Prof. P R Morgan.

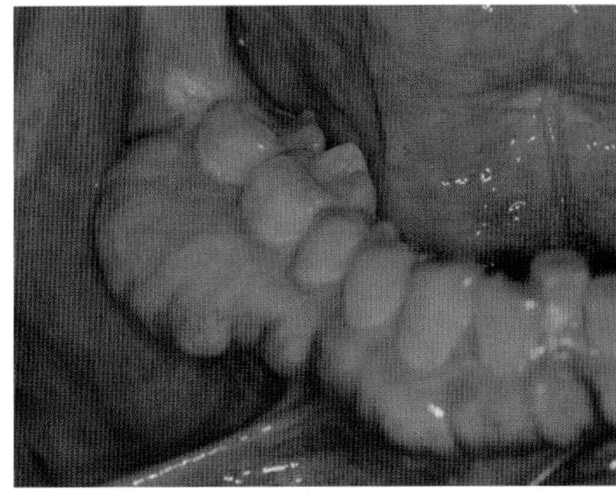

Fig. 1.32 Torus mandibularis on the buccal surface of the mandible. Courtesy Dr C Dunlap.

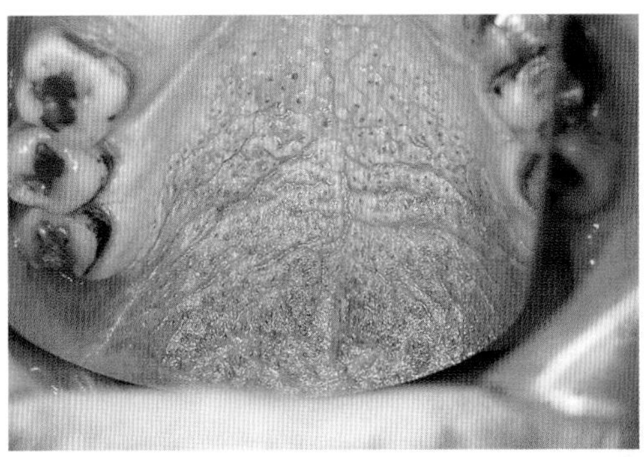

Fig. 1.33 The palate of a heavy smoker presenting with an overall whitish appearance to the mucosa that highlights the inflamed orifices of the mucous glands as red spots. From Cawson, R.A., Odell, E.W. (Eds.), 2008. *Cawson's Essentials of Oral Pathology and Oral Medicine,* eighth ed. Churchill Livingstone, Edinburgh, with permission.

their incidence is decreased in association with fewer teeth being present in the jaws. They require no treatment unless they interfere with the construction of satisfactory removable dentures. Their incidence varies from about 0.5% to more than 65%, being less frequent in Caucasians and more frequent in Eskimos, Mongoloids and other Asian groups. Torus palatinus has an hereditary basis to its aetiology (autosomal dominant).

As an example of a disorder that highlights normal features that may be otherwise inconspicuous, one can inspect the palate of a patient who smokes heavily, revealing a whitish appearance that highlights numerous reddish spots (Fig. 1.33). The white appearance is the result of a pronounced orthokeratinised layer being present as a result of chronic irritation, and this highlights the orifices of the ducts (as red spots) associated with the numerous mucous salivary glands present.

Explore online Self-assessment quiz to test and reinforce your understanding of the material in your free ebook. Follow instructions in the Inside Front Cover to unlock your access.

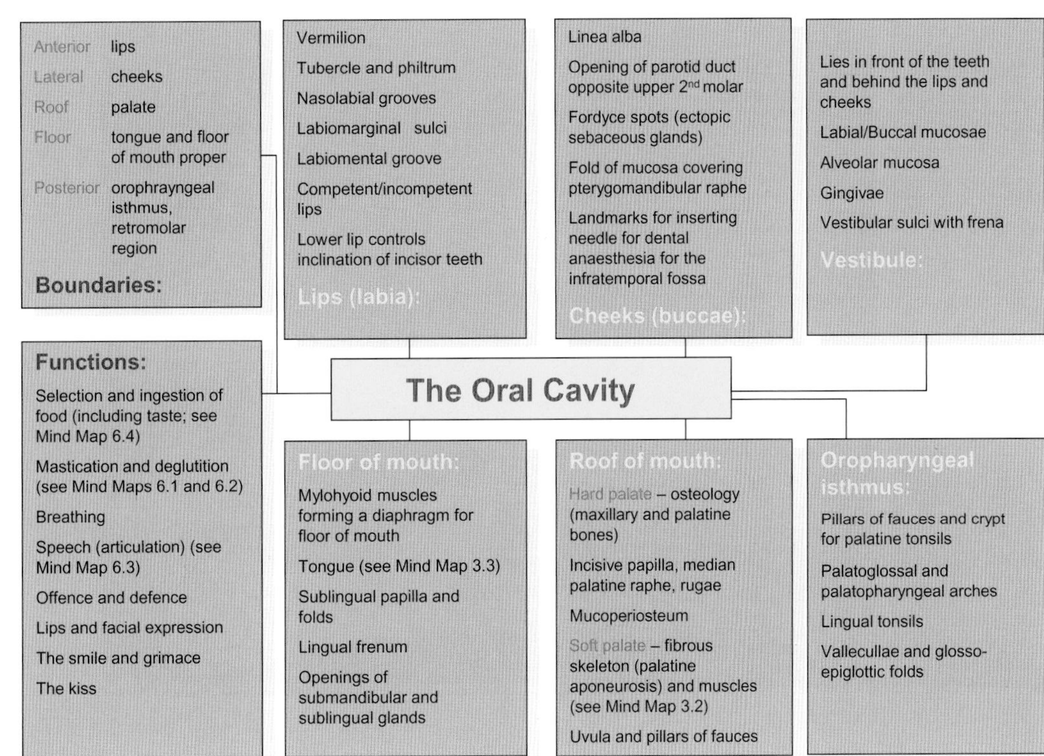

Mind Map 1.1 The oral cavity.

2 Dento-osseous structures

Jaws

The jaws are the tooth-bearing bones and comprise three bones. The two *maxillary bones* form the upper jaw, while the lower jaw is a single bone termed the mandible (Fig. 2.1).

The skull is the most complex osseous structure in the body. It protects the brain, the organs of special sense and the cranial parts of the respiratory and digestive systems. The skull is divided into the neurocranium (houses and protects the brain and the organs of special sense) and the viscerocranium (surrounds the upper parts of the respiratory and digestive tracts). The jaws contribute the major part of the viscerocranium, comprising about 25% of the skull. The jaws have evolved from the gill arch elements of early agnathan vertebrates. It is probable that one or two anterior gill arches gradually disappeared with the expansion of the mouth cavity, so that the gill arch that developed phylogenetically into the jaws of ancestral gnathostomes was not the first of the series. Note that the upper jaw not only contains teeth but also contributes to the skeleton of the nose, orbit, cheek and palate.

Maxilla

The maxilla consists of a body and four processes: the frontal, zygomatic, alveolar and palatine processes. Only the palatine process cannot be seen from the lateral aspect of the maxilla (Fig. 2.2). The anterolateral surface of the maxilla (the malar surface) forms the skeleton of the anterior part of the cheek. In the midline, the alveolar processes of the two maxillae meet at the intermaxillary suture, whence they diverge laterally to form the opening into the nasal fossae (the piriform aperture). At the lower border of the piriform aperture, in the midline, lies the bony projection termed the *anterior nasal spine*. The malar surface of the body of the maxilla is concave, forming the canine fossa. Superiorly, the malar surface is continuous with the orbital plate of the maxilla and forms the floor of the orbit. Anterior to the orbital plate, the frontal process extends above the piriform aperture to meet the nasal and frontal bones. Below the infraorbital rim lies the infraorbital foramen through which the infraorbital branch of the maxillary nerve and the infraorbital artery from the maxillary artery emerge onto the face. The posterolateral surface of the maxilla (the infratemporal surface) forms the anterior wall of the infratemporal fossa. The malar and infratemporal surfaces meet at a bony ridge extending from the zygomatic process to the alveolus adjacent to the first molar tooth. This ridge is called the *zygomatico-alveolar, or jugal, crest*. The posterior convexity of the infratemporal surface is termed the *maxillary tuberosity* and presents several small foramina associated with the posterior superior alveolar nerves (which supply the posterior maxillary teeth). The zygomatic process extends from both the malar and the infratemporal surfaces of the maxilla. From the entire lower surface of the body arises the alveolar process which supports the maxillary teeth.

The medial aspect of the maxilla forms the lateral wall of the nose (Fig. 2.3). In the specimen illustrated, the central hollow of the body of the maxilla (the maxillary air sinus or antrum) is divided by a bony septum. In front of the antrum lies a deep vertical groove called the *lacrimal groove*. This groove meets the lower edge of the lacrimal bone to form the

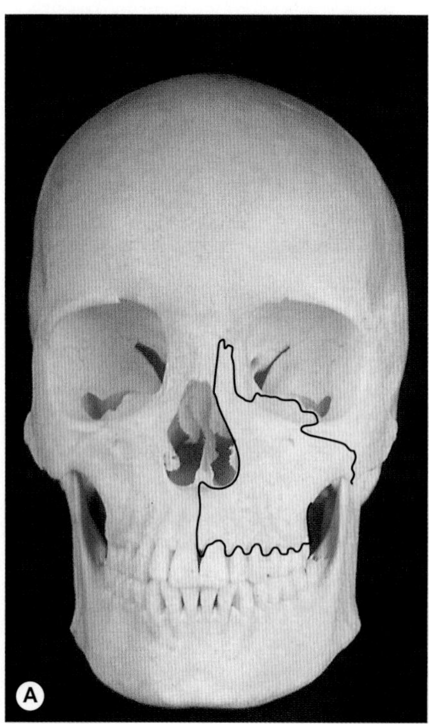

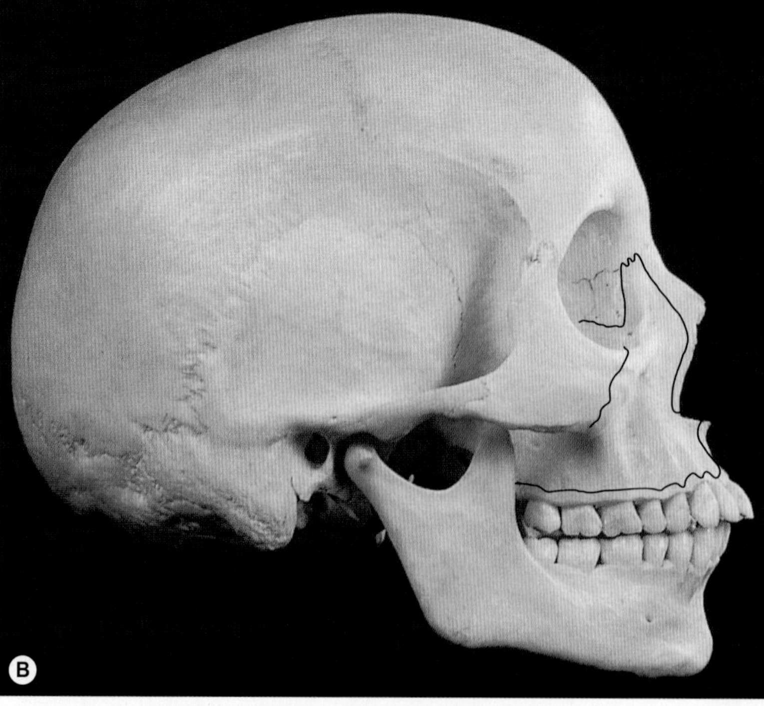

Fig. 2.1 Anterior (A) and lateral (B) views of the skull, showing the relationship between the jaws and the remainder of the skull. The black line describes the boundaries of a maxillary bone.

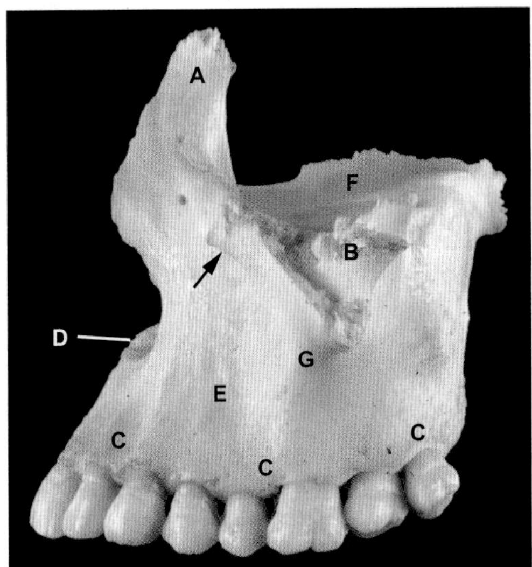

Fig. 2.2 Lateral aspect of the maxilla. A = frontal process; B = zygomatic process; C = alveolar process; D = site of anterior nasal spine; E = canine fossa; F = orbital plate; G = jugal crest. The infraorbital foramen is arrowed.

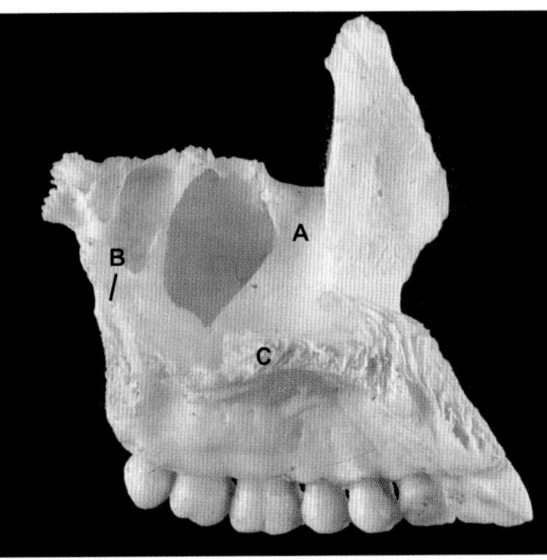

Fig. 2.3 Medial aspect of the maxilla. A = lacrimal groove; B = palatine groove; C = palatine process of maxilla. Note the large opening into the maxillary sinus.

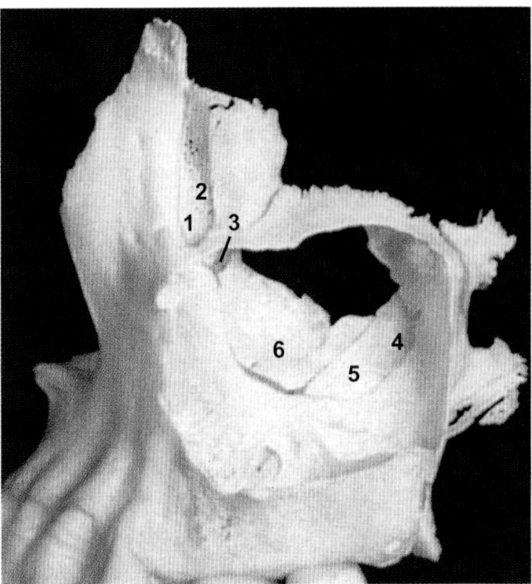

Fig. 2.4 Osteology of the maxillary air sinus showing adjacent bones reducing the size of the ostium. 1 = lacrimal groove of maxilla; 2 = lacrimal groove; 3 = lacrimal bone; 4 = ethmoid bone; 5 = palatine bone; 6 = inferior nasal concha. Courtesy Prof. R M H McMinn.

nasolacrimal canal. Behind the antrum lies the palatine groove, which is converted into a canal carrying the greater palatine nerve and artery by the perpendicular plate of the palatine bone. The maxillary palatine process extends horizontally from the medial surface of the maxilla where the body meets the alveolar process.

The lateral wall of the nasal fossa consists primarily of the medial surface of the maxilla and is occupied mainly by the large maxillary hiatus (Fig. 2.3). To reduce the size of this space *in vivo*, the hiatus is overlapped by the lacrimal bone and the ethmoid bone above, the palatine bone behind and the inferior concha below (Fig. 2.4).

Maxillary sinus

The maxillary sinus (antrum) is the largest of the paranasal sinuses and is situated in the body of the maxilla. It is pyramidal in shape. The base (medial wall) forms part of the lateral wall of the nose. The apex extends into the zygomatic process of the maxilla. The roof of the sinus is part of the floor of the orbit, and the floor of the sinus is formed by the alveolar process and part of the palatine process of the maxilla. The anterior wall of the sinus is the facial surface of the maxilla, and the posterior wall is the infratemporal surface of the maxilla. Running in the roof of the sinus are the infraorbital nerve and vessels. The anterior superior alveolar nerve and vessels run in the anterior wall of the sinus. The posterior superior alveolar nerve and vessels pass through canals in the posterior surface of the sinus. The medial wall of the maxillary sinus contains the opening (ostium) of the sinus that leads into the middle meatus of the nose. As this opening lies well above the floor of the sinus, its position is unfavourable for drainage (see Fig. 5.4A). Infections of the maxillary sinus may therefore require surgical intervention, creating a more favourable drainage channel closer to the floor of the sinus.

The roots of the cheek teeth are related to the floor of the maxillary sinus (Fig. 2.5). The most closely related are the roots of the second permanent maxillary molar, especially the apex of its palatal root; the roots of the first and third molars and the second premolar are only slightly farther away. Sometimes, only mucosa separates the roots from the sinus. Care must be taken (particularly when extracting fractured roots in this region) to avoid creating an oroantral fistula, when an epithelial-lined channel exists between the oral cavity and maxillary sinus.

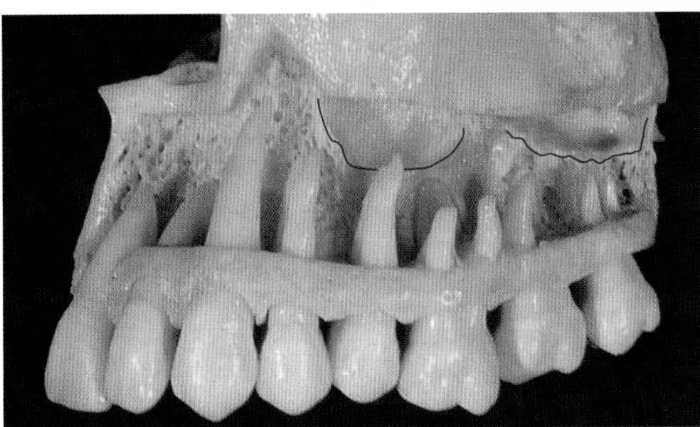

Fig. 2.5 Lateral view of the maxilla, showing close relationship of roots of the cheek teeth to the floor of the maxillary sinus (red outline).

The maxillary air sinus is lined by respiratory epithelium (a ciliated columnar epithelium), with numerous goblet cells. The sinus is innervated by the infraorbital nerve and superior alveolar branches of the maxillary nerve.

Osteology of the palate

An inferior view of the maxillae shows their important contributions to the hard palate (Fig. 2.6). The four major bones contributing to the hard palate are the palatine processes of the maxillae and the horizontal plates of the palatine bones. The maxillary palatine processes arise as horizontal plates at the junction of the bodies and alveolar processes of the maxillae. The boundary between the palatine and alveolar processes is well defined in its posterior aspect only; anteriorly, the angle between the two is less well defined. The junction between the palatine processes in the midline is termed the median palatine suture. Anteriorly, behind the central incisors, this junction is incomplete, thus forming the incisive fossa, through which pass the nasopalatine nerves. Unlike the nasal surface, the oral surface of the palatine process is rough and irregular. The posterior edges of the palatine processes articulate with the horizontal plates of the two palatine bones to form the transverse palatine suture. Laterally, this junction is incomplete, forming the greater palatine foramina through which pass the greater palatine nerves and vessels. Behind the greater palatine foramina

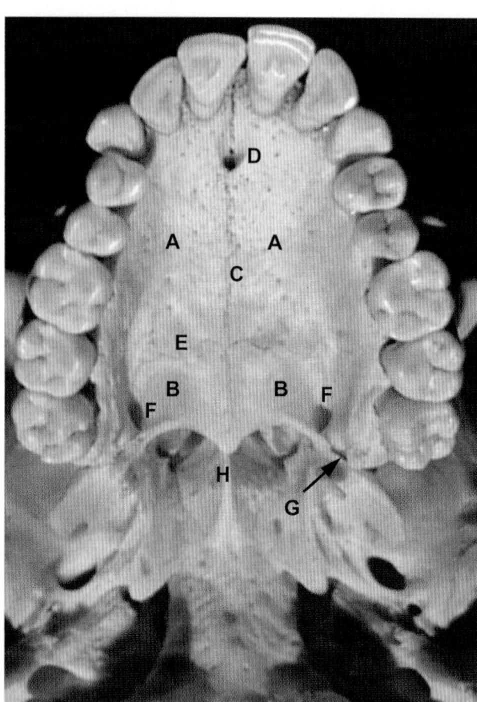

Fig. 2.6 Oral surface of the hard palate. A = palatine processes of maxillae; B = horizontal plates of the palatine bones; C = median palatine suture; D = incisive fossa; E = transverse palatine suture; F = greater palatine foramina; G = lesser palatine foramen; H = posterior nasal spine.

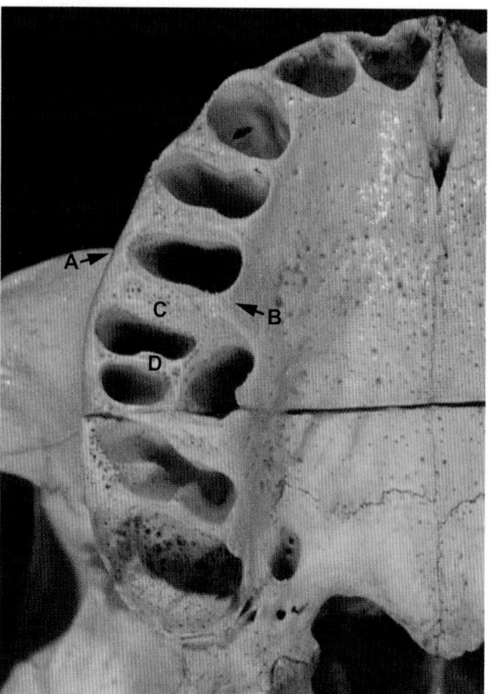

Fig. 2.7 View of the maxilla following removal of teeth to show the disposition of the roots in the alveolus. A = buccal alveolar plate; B = palatal alveolar plate; C = interdental bony septa between the second premolar and first permanent molar; D = interradicular septum between the buccal roots of first permanent molar.

lie the lesser palatine foramina through which pass the lesser palatine nerves and vessels. The junction of the two palatine bones in the midline completes the median palatine suture. The posterior borders of the horizontal palatine plates are concave and, in the midline, form a sharp ridge of bone called the posterior nasal spine. To the posterior edge of the hard palate is attached the fibrous palatine aponeurosis of the soft palate, which is formed by the tendons of the tensor veli palatini muscles.

Maxillary alveolus

The maxillary alveolar processes extend inferiorly from the bodies of the maxillae and support the teeth within bony sockets (Fig. 2.7). Each maxilla can contain a full quadrant of eight permanent teeth or five deciduous teeth. The form of the alveolus is related to the functional demands put on the teeth. When the teeth are lost, the alveolus resorbs.

The alveolar process consists of two parallel plates of cortical bone, the buccal and palatal alveolar plates, between which lie the sockets of individual teeth. Between each socket lie interalveolar or interdental septa. The floor of the socket has been termed the fundus; its rim the alveolar crest. The form and depth of each socket are defined by the form and length of the root it supports, and thus show considerable variation. In multirooted teeth, the sockets are divided by interradicular septa. The apical regions of the sockets of anterior teeth are closely related to the nasal fossae, while those of posterior teeth are closely related to the maxillary air sinuses. The positions of the sockets in relation to the buccal and palatal alveolar plates are shown in Fig. 2.12, page 14.

Mandible

The mandible consists of a horizontal, horseshoe-shaped component, the body of the mandible, and two vertical components, called the rami. The rami join the body posteriorly at obtuse angles. The body of the mandible carries the mandibular teeth and their associated alveolar processes. Before birth, the body consists of two lateral halves that meet in the midline at a symphysis. As viewed laterally (Fig. 2.8), on either side of the midline, close to the inferior margin of the body lies a distinct

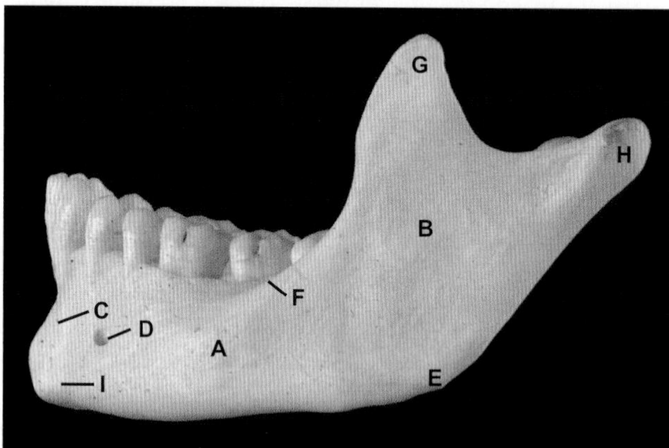

Fig. 2.8 Lateral aspect of the mandible. A = body; B = ramus; C = incisive fossa; D = mental foramen; E = angle; F = external oblique line; G = coronoid process; H = condyle; I = mental protuberance.

prominence called the *mental tubercle*. These tubercles constitute the mental protuberance, or chin. Above the mental protuberance lies a shallow depression termed the *incisive fossa*. Behind this fossa, the canine eminence overlies the root of the mandibular canine. Midway in the height of the body of the mandible, related to the premolar teeth, is the mental foramen. The mental branches of the inferior alveolar nerve and artery pass to the face through this foramen. The most common position for the mental foramen is a vertical line passing through the mandibular second premolar. During the first and second years of life, as the prominence of the chin develops, the direction of the opening of the mental foramen alters from facing forwards to facing upwards and backwards. Accessory mental foramina are found in approximately 14% of cases, although bilateral accessory foramina are only found in about 0.5% of mandibles. Unilateral foramina occur either singly or in double or triple forms. They are located usually at the same level or in a higher position as the mental foramen. However, large accessory foramina tend to be found close, or anterosuperiorly, to the mental foramen. In addition to nerves, arteries pass through the accessory mental foramina. Accessory mental foramina are clinically important in relation to periodontal, endodontic and implant surgery.

The inferior margin of the mandibular body meets the posterior margin of the ramus at the angle of the mandible. This area is irregular, being the site of insertion of the masseter muscle and stylomandibular ligament. The alveolus forms the superior margin of the mandibular body. The junction of the alveolus and ramus is demarcated by a ridge of bone, the external oblique line, which continues downwards and forwards across the body of the mandible to terminate below the mental foramen. As this line progresses upwards, it becomes the anterior margin of the ramus and ends as the tip of the coronoid process. The coronoid and condylar processes form the two processes of the superior border of the ramus. The coronoid process provides attachment for the temporalis muscle. The condylar process has a neck supporting an articular surface, which fits into the mandibular fossa of the temporal bone to form a moveable synovial joint (the temporomandibular joint [TMJ]). The concavity between the coronoid and condylar processes is called the *mandibular notch*.

Several important features are seen on the internal (medial) surface of the mandible (Fig. 2.9). Close to the midline, on the inferior surface of the mandibular body, lie two shallow depressions called the *digastric fossae*, into which are inserted the anterior bellies of the digastric muscles. Above the fossae, in the midline, are the genial spines or tubercles. There are generally two inferior and two superior spines, which serve as attachments for the geniohyoid muscles and the genioglossus muscles, respectively. Passing upwards and backwards across the medial surface of the body of the mandible is a prominent ridge. This is termed the *mylohyoid or internal oblique ridge*. From this ridge, the mylohyoid muscle takes its origin. The mylohyoid ridge arises between the genial spines and digastric fossa and increases in prominence as it passes backwards to end on the anterior surface of the ramus. Because the mylohyoid muscle forms the floor of the mouth, the bone above the mylohyoid ridge forms the anterior wall of the oral cavity proper, while that below the ridge forms the lateral wall of the submandibular space (see page 94). The following features may be seen on the medial surface of the ramus. Around the angle of the mandible, the bone is roughened for the attachment of the medial pterygoid muscle. Commencing at the tip of the coronoid process, a ridge of bone called the *temporal crest* runs down the anterior surface of the ramus to end behind the mandibular molars at the retromolar triangle. In the centre of the medial surface of the ramus lies the mandibular foramen, through which the inferior alveolar nerve and artery pass into the mandibular canal. A bony process, the lingula, extends from the anterosuperior surface of the foramen. The lingula is the site of attachment of the sphenomandibular ligament (see page 79). The mylohyoid groove may be seen running down from the posteroinferior surface of the foramen.

The mandibular canal, which transmits the inferior alveolar nerve, artery and veins, begins at the mandibular foramen and extends to the region of the premolar teeth, where it bifurcates into the mental and incisive canals (Fig. 2.10). The course of the mandibular canal and its relationship with the teeth are variable; this variation is illustrated in connection with the course of the inferior alveolar nerve (see Fig. 4.6).

Mandibular alveolus

As with the maxilla, the mandibular alveolus consists of buccal and lingual alveolar plates joined by interdental and interradicular septa (Fig. 2.11). In the region of the second and third molars, the external oblique line is superimposed upon the buccal alveolar plate. The form and depth of the tooth sockets are related to the morphology of the roots of the mandibular teeth and the functional demands placed upon them.

Fig. 2.12 illustrates buccolingual sections through the teeth and jaws, demonstrating the directional axes and bony relationships of the teeth and their alveoli and the relative thickness of the buccal and lingual alveolar plates. The relationships of the mandibular teeth to the mandibular canal and the maxillary teeth to the maxillary sinus have clinical significance. Thus, the thickness of bone may determine the direction in which teeth are levered during extractions and explains why local infiltration techniques can be used for anaesthetising anterior mandibular teeth but not mandibular molar teeth. The presence of the inferior alveolar nerve and its branches requires care when placing dental implants in the mandibular region.

Tooth morphology

Humans have two generations of teeth: the deciduous (or primary) dentition and the permanent (or secondary) dentition. No teeth are erupted into the mouth at birth. However, by the age of 3 years all the deciduous teeth have erupted. By 6 years the first permanent teeth appear, and thence the deciduous teeth are exfoliated and replaced by their permanent successors. A complete permanent dentition is present at or around the age of 18 years. Given the average life of 75 years, the functional lifespan of the deciduous dentition is only 5% of this total, while with care that of the permanent dentition can be over 90%. In the complete deciduous dentition there are 20 teeth – 10 in each jaw; in the complete permanent dentition there are 32 teeth – 16 in each jaw.

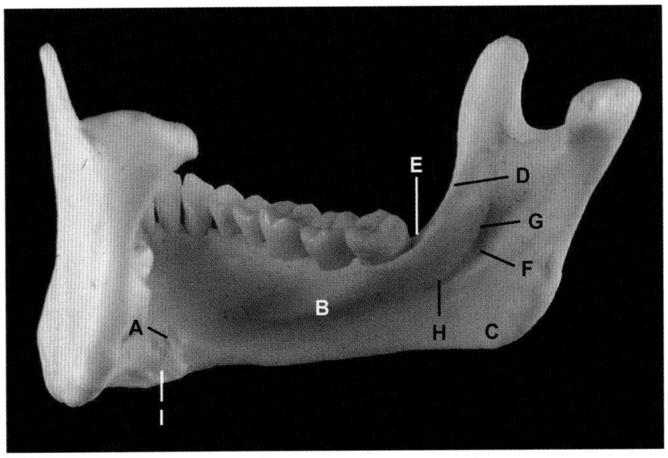

Fig. 2.9 Inner (medial) surface of the mandible. A = genial spines (tubercles); B = internal oblique ridge (mylohyoid ridge); C = attachment area for medial pterygoid muscle; D = temporal crest; E = retromolar triangle; F = mandibular foramen; G = lingula; H = mylohyoid groove; I = digastric fossa.

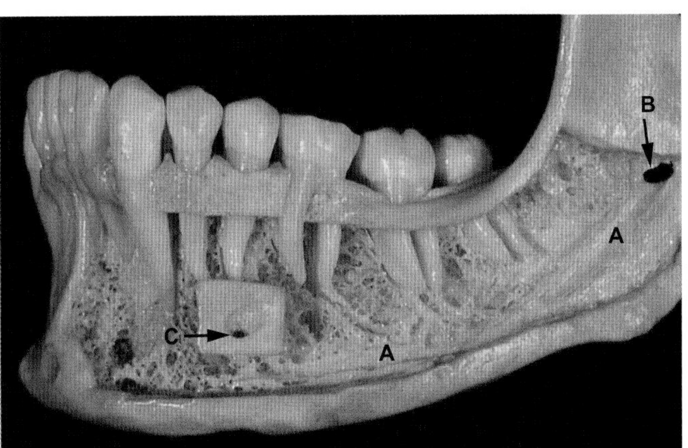

Fig. 2.10 Lateral view of the mandible, showing the roots of the teeth and the relationship to the mandibular canal (A). B = mandibular foramen; C= mental foramen.

In both dentitions there are three basic tooth forms: incisiform, caniniform and molariform. Incisiform teeth (incisors) are cutting teeth, with thin, bladelike crowns. Caniniform teeth (canines) are piercing or tearing teeth, having a single, stout, pointed, cone-shaped crown. Molariform teeth (molars and premolars) are grinding teeth possessing several cusps on an otherwise flattened biting surface. Premolars are bicuspid teeth; they are specific to the permanent dentition and replace the deciduous molars. Table 2.1 gives the definitions of terms used for the descriptions of tooth form.

Dental notation

The types and numbers of teeth in any mammalian dentition can be expressed using dental formulae. The type of tooth is represented by its initial letter – I for incisors, C for canines, P for premolars, M for molars. The deciduous dentition is indicated by the letter D. The formula for the deciduous human dentition is $DI\frac{2}{2}DC\frac{1}{1}DM\frac{2}{2} = 10$, and for the permanent dentition $I\frac{2}{2}C\frac{1}{1}PM\frac{2}{2}M\frac{3}{3}=16$, where the numbers following each letter refer to the number of teeth of each type in the upper and lower jaws on one side only. Identification of teeth is made not only according to the dentition to which they belong and to their basic tooth form but also according to their anatomical location within the jaws. The tooth-bearing region of the jaws can be divided into four quadrants: the right and left maxillary and mandibular quadrants. A tooth may thus be identified according to the quadrant in which it is located (e.g., a right maxillary deciduous incisor or a left mandibular permanent molar). In both the permanent and deciduous dentitions, the incisors may be distinguished according to their relationship to the midline. Thus, the incisor nearest the midline is the central (or first) incisor and the more laterally positioned incisor the lateral (or second) incisor. The permanent premolars and the permanent and deciduous molars can also be distinguished according to their mesiodistal relationships (Fig. 2.13). The molar most mesially positioned is designated the first molar, the one behind it being the second molar. In the permanent dentition, the tooth most distally positioned is the third molar. The mesial premolar is the first premolar, and the premolar behind it is the second premolar.

Dental shorthand may be used in the clinic to simplify tooth identification. The permanent teeth in each quadrant are numbered 1–8 and the deciduous teeth in each quadrant are lettered A–E. The symbols for the quadrants are derived from an imaginary cross, with the horizontal bar placed between the upper and lower jaws and the vertical bar running between the upper and lower central incisors in the midline. Thus, the maxillary right first permanent molar is allocated the symbol $\underline{6|}$ and the mandibular left deciduous canine $\overline{|C}$. This system of dental shorthand is termed the *Zsigmondy*

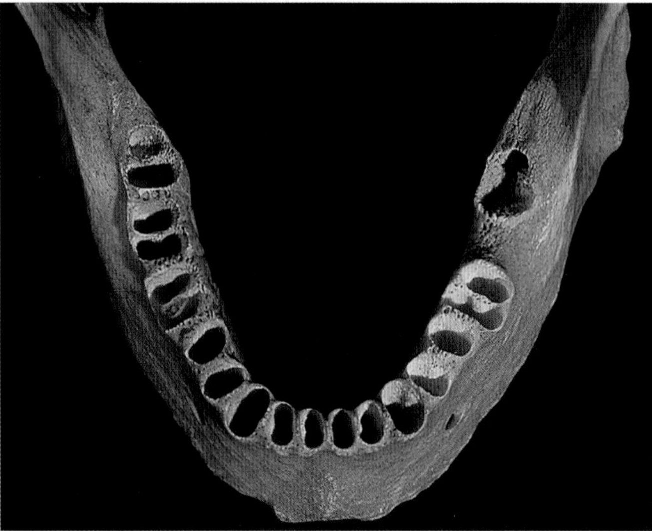

Fig. 2.11 The mandibular alveolus and the arrangement of the tooth sockets. Note that the left second permanent mandibular molar has previously been extracted and the socket has healed.

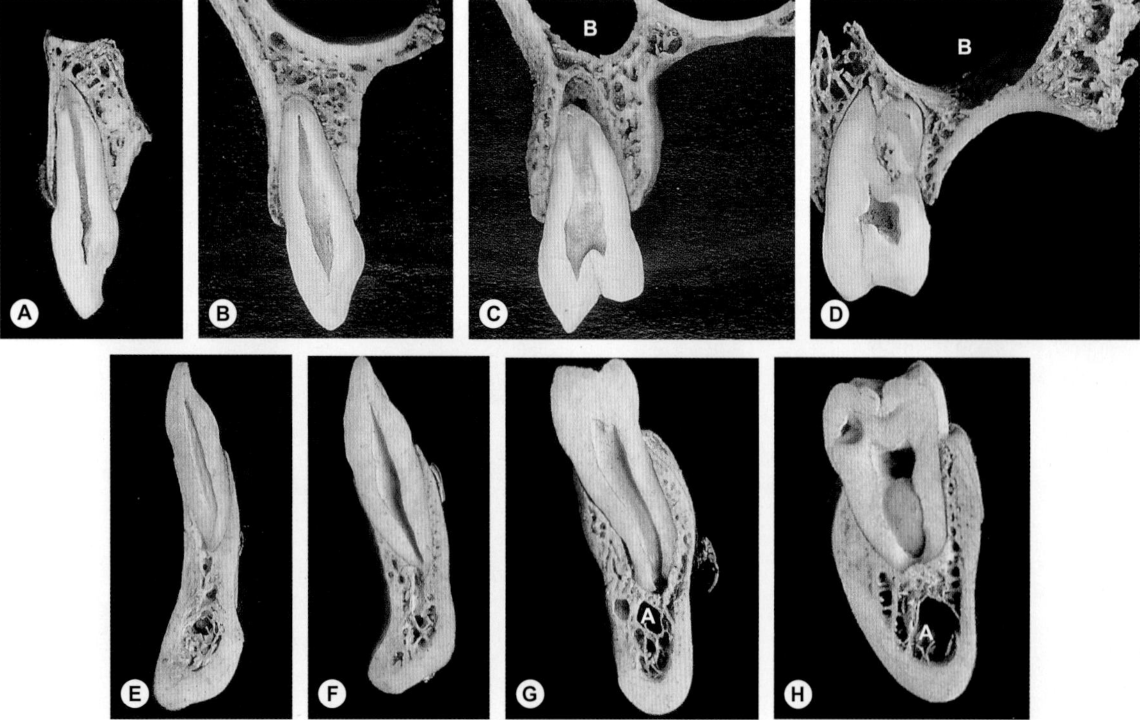

Fig. 2.12 Buccolingual sections through the maxilla and mandible demonstrating the distribution of alveolar bone in relation to the roots of the teeth. A = maxillary incisor region; B = maxillary canine region; C = maxillary premolar region; D = maxillary molar region; E = mandibular incisor region; F = mandibular canine region; G = mandibular premolar region; H = mandibular molar region. Note the relationship of the mandibular cheek teeth to the mandibular canal (A) and of the maxillary cheek teeth to the maxillary sinus (B). Copyright the Royal College of Surgeons of England.

Table 2.1 Terms for the description of tooth form

Crown	Clinical crown – portion of a tooth visible in the oral cavity.
	Anatomical crown – portion of a tooth covered with enamel.
Root	Clinical root – portion of a tooth which lies within the alveolus.
	Anatomical root – portion of a tooth covered by cementum.
Cervical margin	The junction of the anatomical crown and the anatomical root.
Occlusal surface	The biting surface of a posterior tooth (molar or premolar).
Cusp	A pronounced elevation on the occlusal surface of a tooth.
Incisal margin	The cutting edge of anterior teeth, analogous to the occlusal surface of the posterior teeth.
Tubercle	A small elevation on the crown.
Cingulum	A bulbous convexity near the cervical region of a tooth.
Ridge	A linear elevation on the surface of a tooth.
Marginal ridge	A ridge at the mesial or distal edge of the occlusal surface of posterior teeth. Some anterior teeth have equivalent ridges.
Fissure	A long cleft between cusps or ridges.
Fossa	A rounded depression in a surface of a tooth.
Buccal	Towards, or adjacent to, the cheek. The term buccal surface is reserved for that surface of a premolar or molar which is positioned immediately adjacent to the cheek.
Labial	Towards, or adjacent to, the lips. The term labial surface is reserved for that surface of an incisor or canine which is positioned immediately adjacent to the lips.
Palatal	Towards, or adjacent to, the palate. The term palatal surface is reserved for that surface of a maxillary tooth which is positioned immediately adjacent to the palate.
Lingual	Towards, or adjacent to, the tongue. The term lingual surface is reserved for that surface of a mandibular tooth which lies immediately adjacent to the tongue.
Mesial	Towards the median. The mesial surface is that surface which faces towards the median line following the curve of the dental arch.
Distal	Away from the median. The distal surface is that surface which faces away from the median line following the curve of the dental arch.

system. An alternative scheme has been devised by the Federation Dentaire Internationale in which the quadrant is represented by a number (see Table 2.15). In this system, the quadrant number prefixes a tooth number. Thus, the maxillary left first permanent molar is symbolised as 26 (see Fig. 2.13), and the mandibular left deciduous canine as 73.

Fig. 2.13 summarises some of the terminology employed for the identification of teeth according to their location in the jaws.

Differences between teeth of the deciduous and permanent dentitions

1) The dental formulae for the deciduous and permanent dentitions differ:

$$DI\frac{2}{2}DC\frac{1}{1}DM\frac{2}{2} = 10$$

Permanent maxillary arch

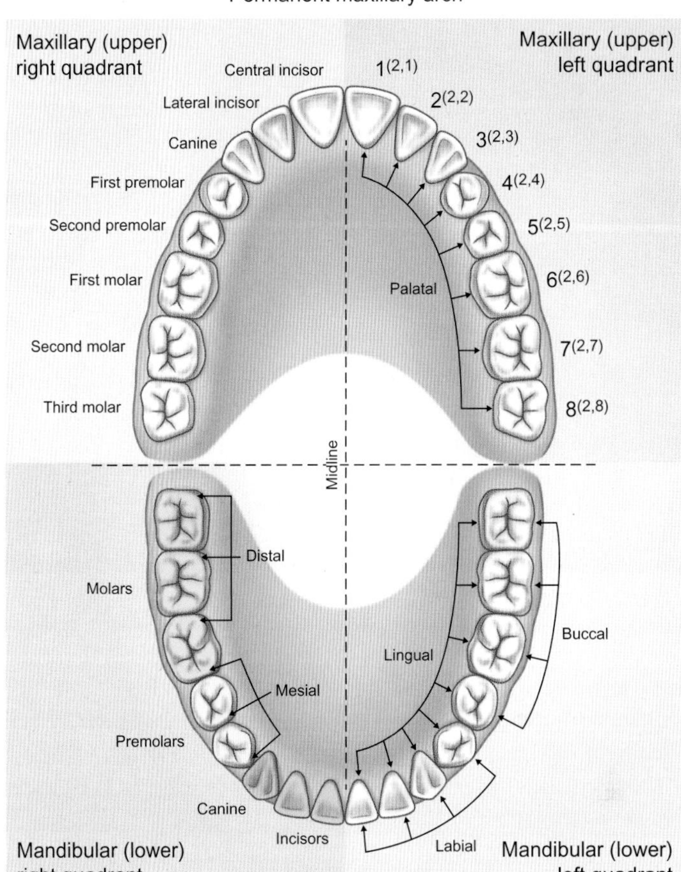

Permanent mandibular arch

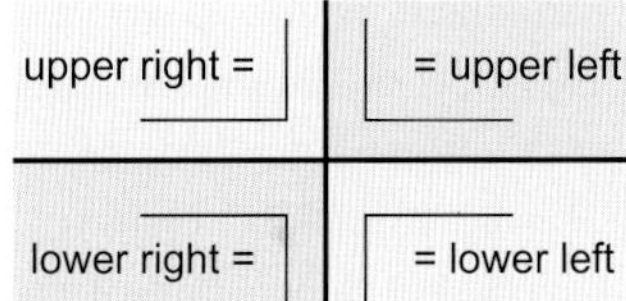

Fig. 2.13 Terminology employed for the identification of teeth according to their location in the jaws.

$$I\frac{2}{2}C\frac{1}{1}PM\frac{2}{2}M\frac{3}{3} = 16$$

2) The deciduous teeth are smaller than their corresponding permanent successors, although the mesiodistal dimensions of the permanent premolars are generally less than those for the deciduous molars.
3) Deciduous teeth have a greater constancy of shape than permanent teeth.
4) The crowns of deciduous teeth appear bulbous, often having pronounced labial or buccal cingula.
5) The cervical margins of deciduous teeth are more sharply demarcated and pronounced than those of the permanent teeth, with the enamel bulging at the cervical margins rather than gently tapering.
6) The cusps of newly erupted deciduous teeth are more pointed than those of the corresponding permanent teeth.
7) The crowns of deciduous teeth have a thinner covering of enamel (average width 0.5–1.0 mm) than the crowns of permanent teeth (average width 2.5 mm).
8) The enamel of deciduous teeth, being more opaque than that of permanent teeth, gives the crown a whiter appearance.
9) The enamel of deciduous teeth is softer than that of permanent teeth and is more easily worn.

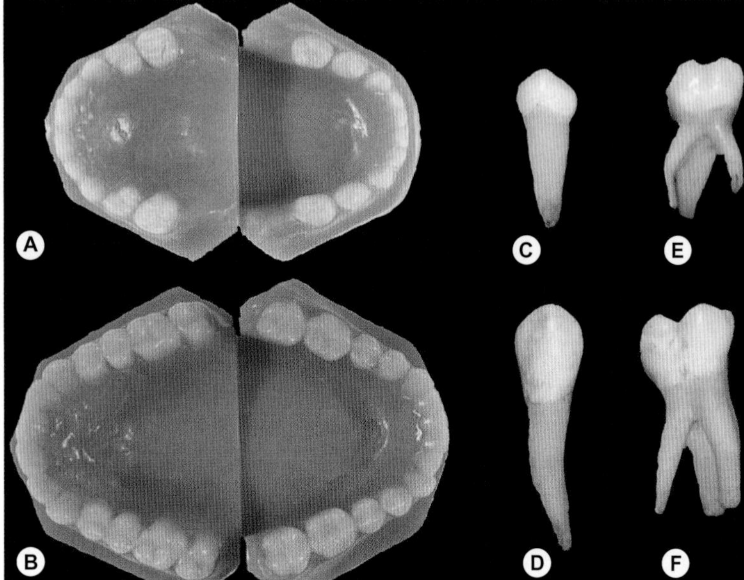

Fig. 2.14 Models of deciduous (A) and permanent (B) dental arches and some examples of deciduous and permanent teeth. C = deciduous canine; D = permanent canine; E = deciduous second molar; F = permanent first molar.

10) Enamel of deciduous teeth is more permeable than that of permanent teeth.
11) The aprismatic layer of surface enamel (see page 143) is wider in deciduous teeth.
12) The enamel and dentine of all deciduous teeth exhibit neonatal lines (see pages 152 and 179).
13) The roots of deciduous teeth are shorter and less robust than those of permanent teeth.
14) The roots of deciduous incisors and canines are longer in proportion to the crown than those of their permanent counterparts.
15) The roots of deciduous molars are widely divergent, extending beyond the dimensions of the crown.
16) The pulp chambers of deciduous teeth are proportionally larger in relation to the crowns than those of the permanent teeth. The pulp horns in deciduous teeth are more prominent.
17) The root canals of deciduous teeth are extremely fine.
18) The dental arches for the deciduous dentition are smaller.

Some of these differences are illustrated in Fig. 2.14.

The following descriptions of individual teeth will be considered according to tooth class (incisors, canines, premolars and molars) rather than by membership of the permanent or deciduous dentition. For each class, the permanent teeth will be described before the deciduous teeth. This arrangement allows emphasis of the basic features common to each class.

To help visualise the tooth as a three-dimensional object, the illustrations of each tooth are arranged according to the 'third angle projection technique', which aligns each side of a tooth to its occlusal or incisal aspect. The morphology of the pulp is treated independently of the morphology of the external surfaces of the teeth on pages 33–39. For the chronology of the developing dentitions, see page 463; for the average dimensions of the teeth, see Tables 2.2 and 2.3; and for ethnic variations in tooth morphology, see page 33.

Incisors

Human incisors have thin, bladelike crowns that are adapted for the cutting and shearing of food preparatory to grinding. Viewed mesially or distally, the crowns of the incisors are roughly triangular in shape, with the apex of the triangle at the incisal margin of the tooth (Fig. 2.15). This shape is thought to facilitate the penetration and cutting of food. Viewed buccally or lingually, the incisors are trapezoidal, the shortest of the uneven sides being the base of the crown cervically.

Table 2.2 Average dimensions of the permanent teeth

Tooth	Crown height (mm)	Length of root (mm)	Mediodistal crown diameter (mm)	Labiolingual crown diameter (mm)
Maxillary				
1	10.5	13.0	8.5	7.0
2	9.0	13.0	6.5	6.0
3	10.0	17.0	7.5	8.0
4	8.5	14.5	7.0	9.0
5	8.5	14.0	7.0	9.0
6	7.5	12.5	10.5	11.0
7	7.0	11.5	9.5	11.0
8	6.5	11.0	8.5	10.0
Mandibular				
1	9.0	12.5	5.0	6.0
2	9.5	14.0	5.5	6.5
3	11.0	15.5	7.0	7.5
4	8.5	14.0	7.0	7.5
5	8.0	14.5	7.0	8.0
6	7.5	14.0	11.0	10.0
7	7.0	12.0	10.5	10.0
8	7.0	11.0	10.0	9.5

Table 2.3 Average dimensions of the deciduous teeth

Tooth	Crown height (mm)	Length of root (mm)	Mediodistal crown diameter (mm)	Labiolingual crown diameter (mm)
Maxillary				
A	6.0	10.0	6.5	5.0
B	5.6	10.2	5.2	4.0
C	6.5	13.0	6.8	7.0
D	5.1	10.0	7.1	8.5
E	5.7	11.7	8.4	10.0
Mandibular				
A	5.0	9.0	4.0	4.0
B	5.2	9.8	4.5	4.0
C	6.0	11.2	5.5	4.9
D	6.0	9.8	7.7	7.0
E	5.5	12.5	9.7	8.7

Maxillary first (central) permanent incisor

This tooth (Fig. 2.16) is the widest mesiodistally of all the permanent incisors and canines, the crown being almost as wide as it is long. Like all incisors, it is basically wedge- or chisel-shaped and has a single conical root.

From the incisal view, the crown and incisal margin are centrally positioned over the root of the tooth. The incisal margin presents as a narrow, flattened ridge rather than as a fine, sharp edge. The incisal margin may be grooved by two troughs: the labial lobe grooves, which correspond to

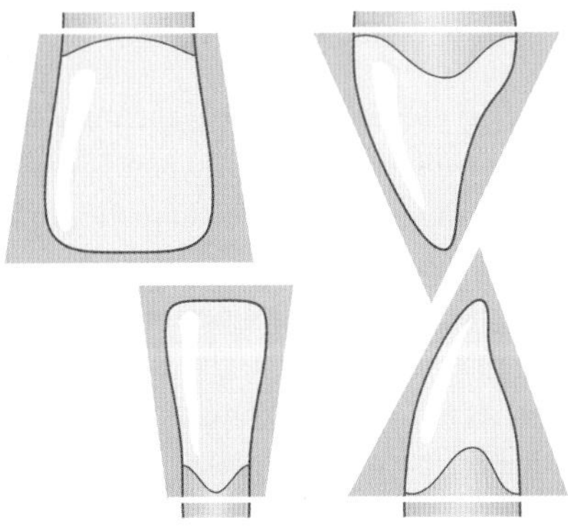

Fig. 2.15 Schematic drawings of incisor crown form, illustrating the relationship between the anatomical and geometrical forms. Redrawn after Dr. R C Wheeler.

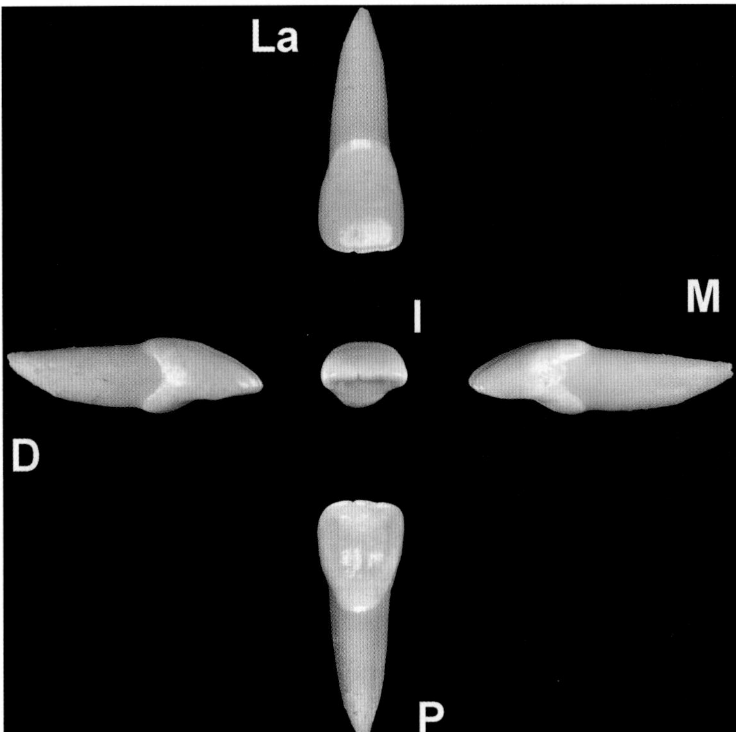

Fig. 2.16 Maxillary first (central) permanent incisor. I = incisal surface; La = labial surface; P = palatal surface; M = mesial surface; D = distal surface.

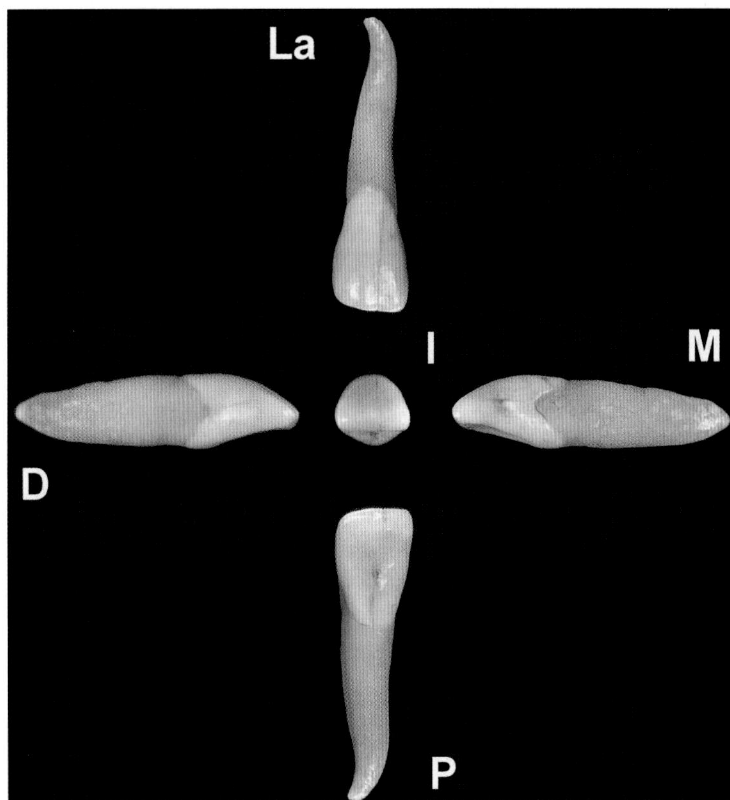

Fig. 2.17 Maxillary second (lateral) permanent incisor. I = incisal surface; La = labial surface; P = palatal surface; M = mesial surface; D = distal surface.

the divisions between three developmental lobes (or mamelons) seen on newly erupted incisors (Fig. 2.171). The mamelons are lost by attrition soon after eruption. From the incisal aspect, the crown outline is bilaterally symmetrical, being triangular. However, the mesial profile may appear slightly larger than the distal profile. From the labial view, the crown length can be seen to be almost as great as the root length. The crown has a smooth, convex labial surface. It may be marked by two faint grooves that run vertically towards the cervical margin and are extensions of the labial lobe grooves. The convexity of the labial surface is especially marked cervically, the labial surface sometimes being flat at its middle and incisal regions. The mesial surface is straight and approximately at right angles to the incisal margin, while the distoincisal angle is more rounded and the distal outline more convex. A line drawn through the axial centre of the tooth lies roughly parallel to the mesial outline of the crown and root. Viewed palatally, the crown is more irregular, its middle and incisal regions being concave, giving a slightly shovel-shaped appearance to the incisor. The palatal surface of the crown is bordered by mesial and distal marginal ridges. Near the cervical margin lies a prominent cingulum. The cingulum may be single, divided or replaced by prominent portions of the marginal ridges. Occasionally, a slight ridge of enamel may run towards the incisal margin, dividing the palatal surface into two shallow depressions. The mesial and distal views of the crown illustrate the fundamental wedge-shaped or triangular crown form of the incisor.

The sinuous cervical margin is concave towards the crown on the palatal and labial surfaces and convex towards the crown on the mesial and distal surfaces, with the curvature on the mesial surface being the most pronounced of any tooth in the dentition. The single root of the first incisor tapers towards the apex. The root is conical in cross-section and appears narrower from the palatal than from the labial aspect.

Maxillary second (lateral) permanent incisor

This is one of the most variable teeth in the dentition, although generally it is morphologically a diminutive form of the maxillary central incisor with slight modifications (Fig. 2.17). The crown is much narrower and shorter than that of the first incisor, although the crown–to–root length ratio is considerably decreased.

From the incisal aspect, the crown has a more rounded outline than the adjacent first incisor. Viewed labially, the mesioincisal and distoincisal angles and the mesial and distal crown margins are more rounded than those of the first incisor. The palatal aspect of the crown is similar to that of the first incisor, although the marginal ridges and cingulum are often more pronounced. Consequently, the palatal concavity appears deeper. Lying in front of the cingulum is a pit (foramen caecum) that may extend into the root. The mesial and distal aspects of the second incisor differ little from those of the first incisor. A common morphological variation is the so-called 'peg-shaped' lateral incisor, which has a thin root surmounted by a small conical crown (see Fig. 2.47).

The course of the cervical margin and the shape of the root are similar to those of the first incisor. However, the root is often slightly compressed and grooved on the mesial and distal surfaces.

The mandibular incisors have the smallest mesiodistal dimensions of any teeth in the permanent dentition. They can be distinguished from the maxillary incisors not only by their size but also by the marked lingual inclination of the crowns over the roots, the mesiodistal compression of their roots and the poor development of the marginal ridges and cingula.

Mandibular first (central) permanent incisor

Viewed incisally, this tooth has a bilaterally symmetrical triangular shape (Fig. 2.18). The incisal margin in the specimen shown in the figure has been worn and appears flat, although the newly erupted tooth has three mamelons (see Fig. 2.172). The incisal margin is at right angles to a line bisecting the tooth labiolingually. Viewed labially, the crown of the incisor is almost twice as long as it is wide. The unworn incisal margin is straight and approximately at right angles to the long axis of the tooth. The mesioincisal and distoincisal angles are sharp, and the mesial and distal surfaces are approximately at right angles to the incisal margin. The profiles of the mesial and distal surfaces appear similar, being convex in their incisal thirds and relatively flattened in the middle and cervical thirds. The lingual surface is smooth and slightly concave, while the lingual cingulum and mesial and distal marginal ridges appear less distinct than those of the maxillary incisors. The mesial and distal views show the characteristic wedge shape of the incisor and the inclination of the crown lingually over the root.

The cervical margins on the labial and lingual surfaces show their maximum convexities midway between the mesial and distal borders of the root. The cervical margin on the distal surface is said to be less curved than that on the mesial surface. The root is narrow and conical, although flattened mesiodistally. It is frequently grooved on the mesial and distal surfaces, the distal groove being more marked and deeper.

Mandibular second (lateral) permanent incisor

The mandibular second incisor (Fig. 2.19) closely resembles the mandibular first incisor. However, it is slightly wider mesiodistally and is more asymmetrical in shape. The distal surface diverges at a greater angle from the long axis of the tooth, giving it a fan-shaped appearance, and the distoincisal angle is more acute and rounded. Another distinguishing characteristic is the angulation of the incisal margin relative to the labiolingual axis of the root; in the first incisor the incisal margin forms a right angle with the labiolingual axis, whereas that of the second incisor is 'twisted' distally in a lingual direction.

Maxillary first (central) deciduous incisor

This is similar morphologically to the corresponding permanent tooth (Fig. 2.20). However, it appears plumper than its permanent successor because the width of the crown of the deciduous incisor nearly equals the length. From the incisal view, the straight incisal margin appears to be centred over the bulk of the crown. Unlike the permanent teeth, no mamelons are seen on the incisal margin of the newly erupted deciduous incisor. The labial surface is slightly convex in all planes and unmarked by grooves, lobes or depressions. The mesioincisal angle is sharp and acute, while the distoincisal angle is more rounded and obtuse. On the palatal surface, the cingulum is a prominent bulge that extends some way up the crown (sometimes to the incisal margin to form a ridge). Unlike those of its permanent successor, the marginal ridges are poorly defined and the concavity of the palatal surface is shallow. Mesial and distal views show the typical incisal form of the crown. There is a low, rounded cingulum at the margin of the labial surface.

As with all deciduous teeth, the cervical margins are more pronounced but less sinuous than those of their permanent successors. The fully

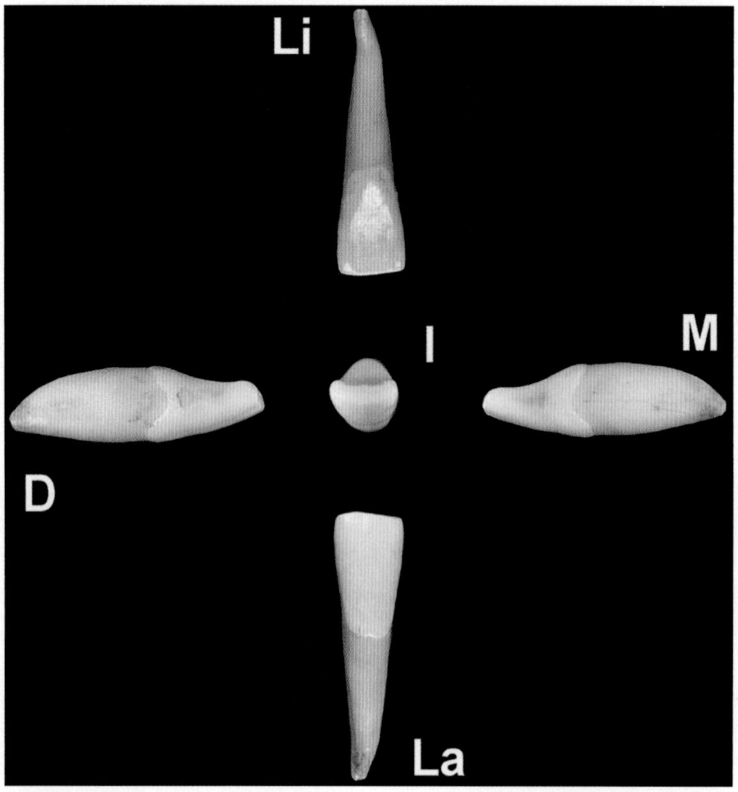

Fig. 2.18 Mandibular first (central) right permanent incisor. I = incisal surface; La = labial surface; Li = lingual surface; M = mesial surface; D = distal surface.

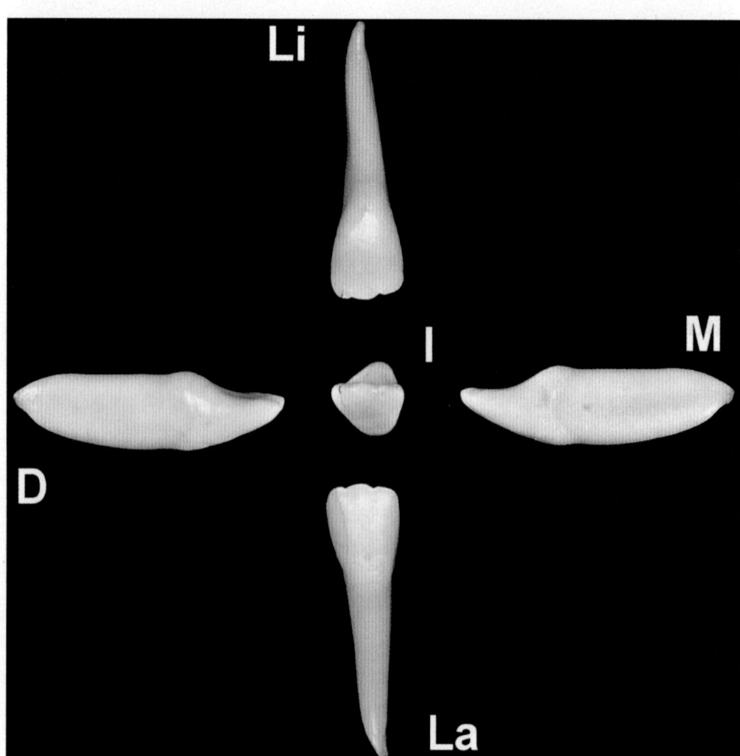

Fig. 2.19 Mandibular second (lateral) right permanent incisor. I = incisal surface; La = labial surface; Li = lingual surface; M = mesial surface; D = distal surface.

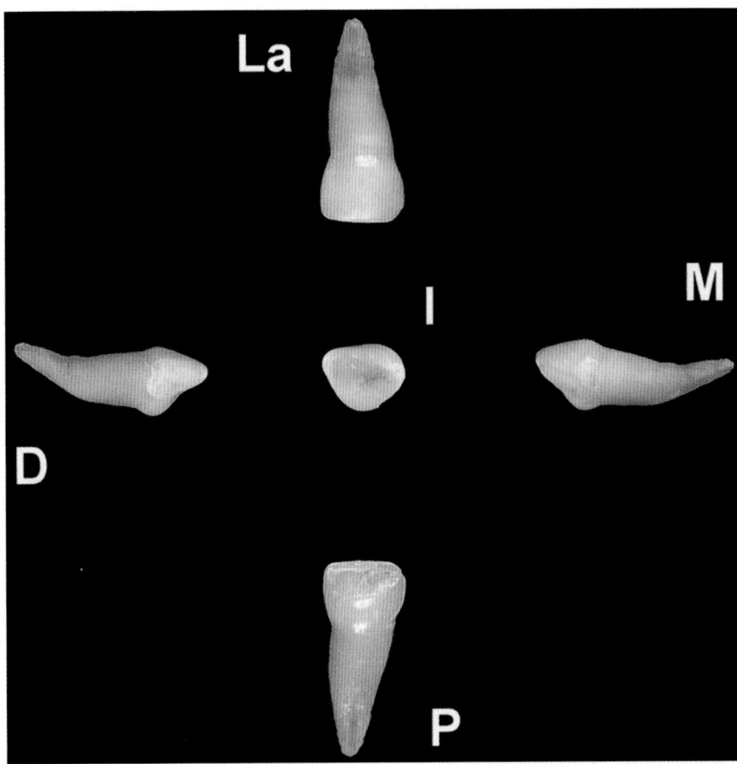

Fig. 2.20 Maxillary first (central) right deciduous incisor. I = incisal surface; La = labial surface; P = palatal surface; M = mesial surface; D = distal surface.

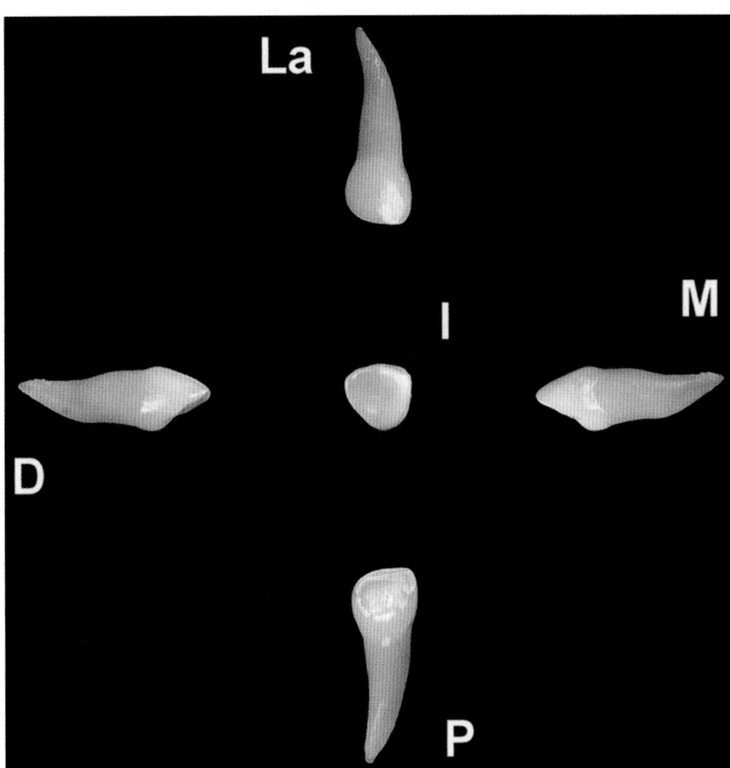

Fig. 2.21 Maxillary second (lateral) right deciduous incisor. I = incisal surface; La = labial surface; P = palatal surface; M = mesial surface; D = distal surface.

formed root is conical in shape, tapering apically to a rather blunt apex. Compared with the corresponding permanent tooth, the root is longer in proportion to the crown.

Maxillary second (lateral) deciduous incisor

This is similar in shape to the maxillary first deciduous incisor, although smaller (Fig. 2.21). One obvious difference is the more acute mesioincisal angle and the more rounded distoincisal angle. The palatal surface is more concave and the marginal ridges more pronounced. Viewed incisally, the crown appears almost circular (in contrast to the first incisor, which appears diamond-shaped). As with the first deciduous incisor, there is a rounded labial cingulum cervically. The palatal cingulum is generally lower than that of the first deciduous incisor.

The course of the cervical margin and the shape of the root are similar to those of the first deciduous incisor.

Mandibular first (central) deciduous incisor

The mandibular first deciduous incisor (Fig. 2.22) is morphologically similar to its permanent successor. However, it is much shorter and has a low labial cingulum. The mesioincisal and distoincisal angles are sharp right angles, and the incisal margin is straight in the horizontal plane. The lingual cingulum and the marginal ridges are poorly defined.

The single root is more rounded than that of the corresponding permanent tooth and, when complete, tapers and tends to incline distally.

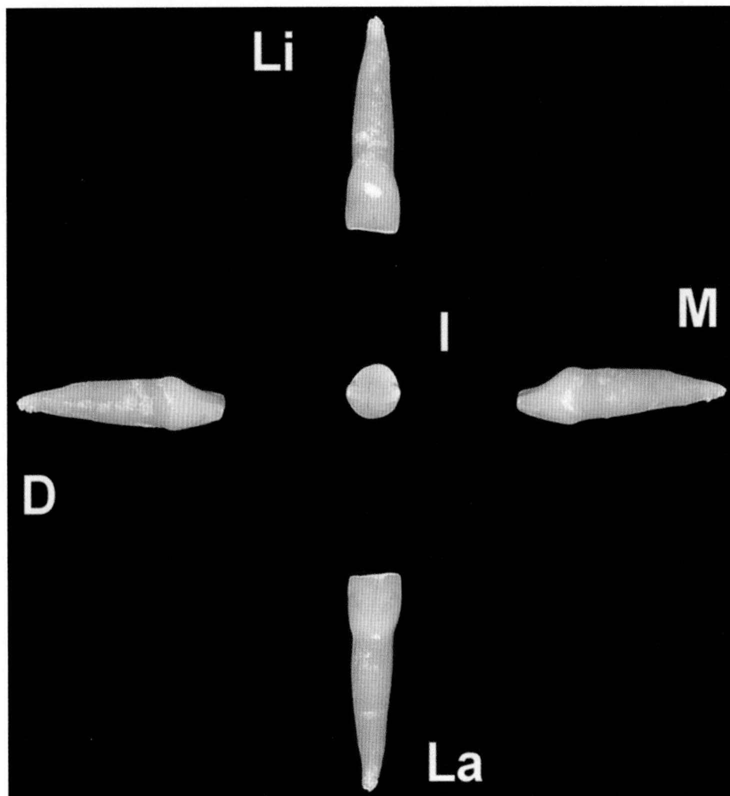

Fig. 2.22 Mandibular first (central) right deciduous incisor. I = incisal surface; La = labial surface; Li = lingual surface; M = mesial surface; D = distal surface.

Mandibular second (lateral) deciduous incisor

This is a bulbous tooth that resembles its permanent successor (Fig. 2.23). It is wider than the mandibular first deciduous incisor and is asymmetrical. The mesioincisal angle is more obtuse and rounded than that of the mandibular first deciduous incisor, and the incisal margin slopes downwards distally. Should the distoincisal angle be markedly rounded, the tooth may be difficult to distinguish from a maxillary second deciduous incisor.

Unlike the permanent tooth, the root is rounded. When complete, it is longer than the root of the mandibular first deciduous incisor.

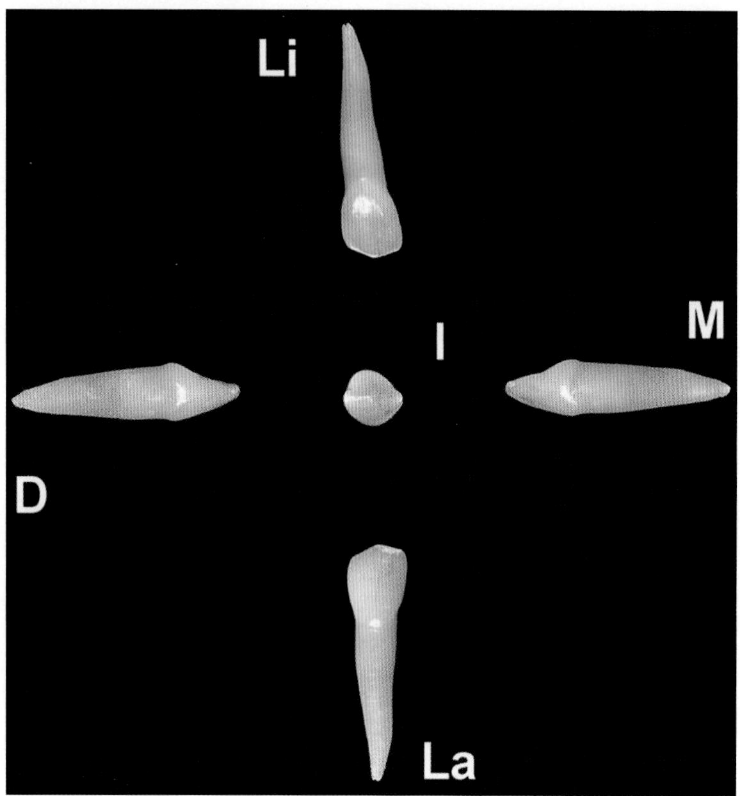

Fig. 2.23 Mandibular second (lateral) right deciduous incisor. I = incisal surface; La = labial surface; Li = lingual surface; M = mesial surface; D = distal surface.

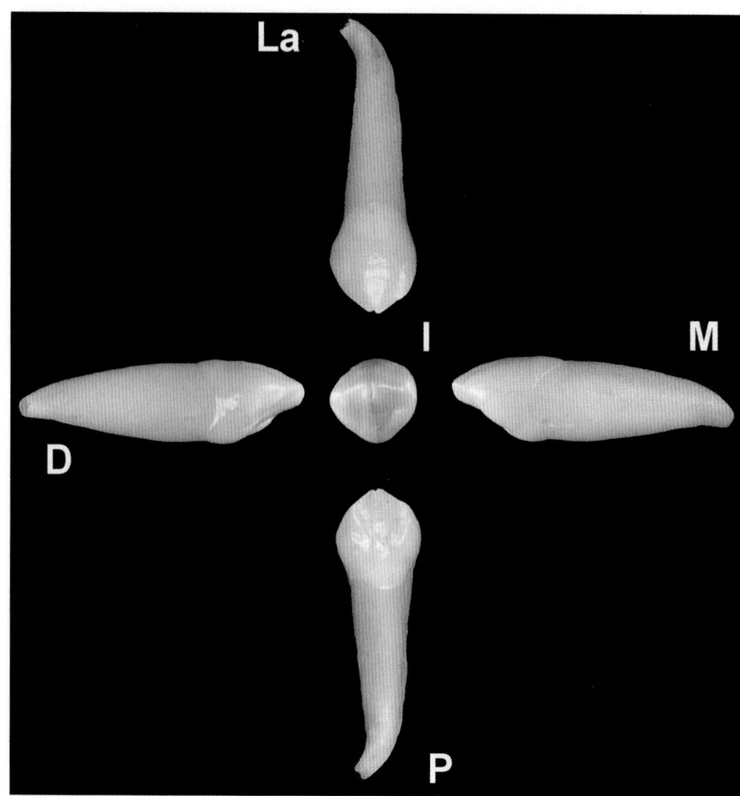

Fig. 2.25 Maxillary right permanent canine. I = incisal surface; La = labial surface; P = palatal surface; M = mesial surface; D = distal surface.

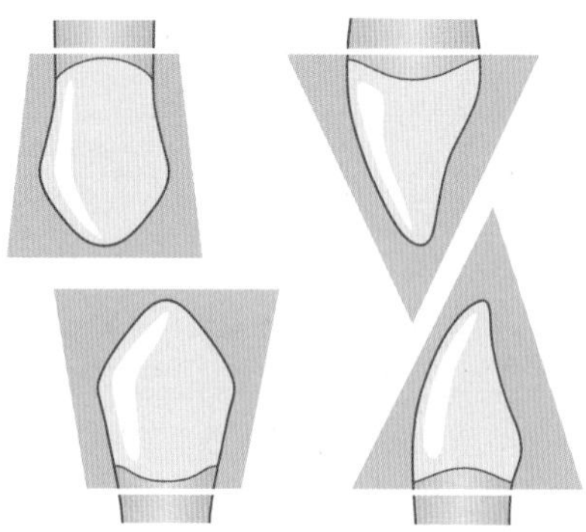

Fig. 2.24 Schematic drawings of canine crown form, illustrating the relationship between the anatomical and geometrical forms. Redrawn after Dr. R C Wheeler.

Canines

Canines are the only teeth in the dentition with a single cusp. Morphologically they can be considered transitional between incisors and premolars. As for the incisors, the crowns of canines are essentially triangular in shape when viewed mesially or distally and trapezoidal buccally and lingually (Fig. 2.24).

Maxillary permanent canine

This is a stout tooth (Fig. 2.25) with a well-developed cingulum and the longest root of any tooth. Viewed from its incisal aspect, it appears asymmetrical. If a plane is envisaged passing through the apex of the cusp to the cingulum on the palatal surface, then the distal portion of the crown is much wider than the mesial portion. It is thought that the pointed shape of the canine tooth is related to an increase in size of a central mamelon at the expense of mesial and distal mamelons. Prominent longitudinal ridges pass from the cusp tip down both the labial and the palatal surfaces. A relatively frequent variation in the morphology of the incisal ridge is the development of an accessory cusp on its distal arm. The labial surface of the canine is marked by the longitudinal ridge, which extends from the cusp towards the cervical margin. The incisal part of the crown occupies at least one-third of the crown height. Note that from this view the mesial arm of the incisal margin is shorter than the distal arm and the distoincisal angle is more rounded than the mesioincisal angle. The profiles of the mesial and distal surfaces converge markedly towards the cervix of the tooth. The mesial profile is slightly convex, while the distal profile is markedly convex. The mesial surface of the crown forms a straight line with the root, while the distal surface meets the root at an obtuse angle. The palatal surface shows distinct mesial and distal marginal ridges and a well-defined cingulum. The longitudinal ridge from the tip of the cusp meets the cingulum and is separated from the marginal ridges on either side by distinct grooves or fossae. Viewed mesially or distally, the distinctive feature is the stout character of the crown and the great width of the cervical third of both the crown and the root.

The cervical margin of this tooth follows a course similar to that of the incisors but the curves are less pronounced. The curvature of the cervical margin on the distal surface is less marked than that on the mesial surface. The root is the largest and stoutest in the dentition and is triangular in cross-section (its labial surface being wider than its palatal surface). The mesial and distal surfaces of the root are often grooved longitudinally.

Mandibular permanent canine

This is similar to the maxillary canine but smaller, more slender and more symmetrical (Fig. 2.26). The cusp is generally less well developed: indeed, with attrition the low cusp may be lost and the tooth may resemble a maxillary second permanent incisor.

From the incisal aspect, there are no distinct longitudinal ridges from the tip of the cusp on to the labial and lingual surfaces. Viewed labially, the

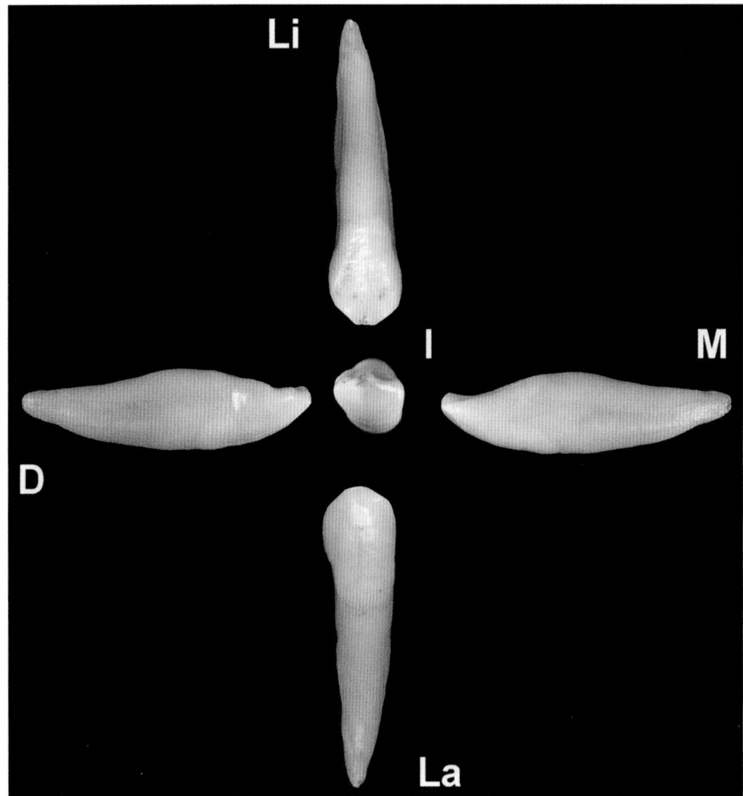

Fig. 2.26 Mandibular right permanent canine. I = incisal surface; La = labial surface; Li = lingual surface; M = mesial surface; D = distal surface.

incisal margin occupies only one-fifth of the crown height, and the cusp is less pointed than the maxillary canine. The crown is narrower mesiodistally than that of the maxillary canine, so it appears longer, narrower and more slender. The mesial and distal profiles tend to be parallel or only slightly convergent towards the cervix. The labial and mesial surfaces are clearly defined, being inclined acutely to each other, whereas the labial surface merges gradually into the distal surface. On the lingual surface, the cingulum, marginal ridges and fossae are indistinct. The lingual surface is flatter than the corresponding palatal surface of the maxillary permanent canine and simulates the lingual surface of the mandibular incisors. Viewed mesially and distally, the wedge-shaped appearance of the canine is clear. These proximal surfaces are longer than those of the maxillary canine. The labiolingual diameter of the crown near the cervix is less than the corresponding labiopalatal diameter of the maxillary canine.

The cervical margin of this tooth follows a course similar to that of the incisors. The crownward convexity on the mesial surface is generally more marked than that on the distal surface. The root is normally single, though occasionally it may bifurcate. In cross-section, the root is oval, being flattened mesially and distally. The root is grooved longitudinally on both its mesial and its distal surfaces.

Maxillary deciduous canine

This tooth has a fang-like appearance and is similar morphologically to its permanent successor, though more bulbous (Fig. 2.27). It is generally symmetrical; however, where there is asymmetry, it is usual for the mesial slope of the cusp to be longer than the distal slope. Bulging of the tooth gives the crown a diamond-shaped appearance when viewed labially or palatally, with the crown margins overhanging the root profiles. The width of the crown is greater than its length. On the labial surface, there is a low cingulum cervically, from which runs a longitudinal ridge up to the tip of

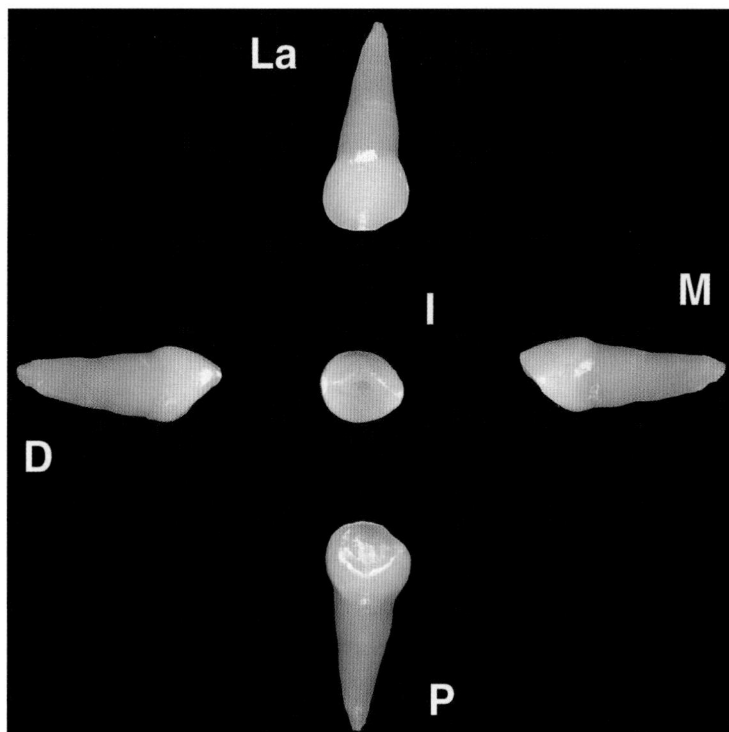

Fig. 2.27 Maxillary right deciduous canine. I = incisal surface; La = labial surface; P = palatal surface; M = mesial surface; D = distal surface.

the cusp. A similar longitudinal ridge also runs on the palatal surface. This ridge extends from the cusp apex to the palatal cingulum and divides the palatal surface into two shallow pits. The marginal ridges on the palatal surface are low and indistinct.

The root is long compared with the crown height and is triangular in cross-section.

Mandibular deciduous canine

This is more slender than the maxillary deciduous canine (Fig. 2.28). The crown is asymmetrical and the cusp tip displaced mesially. Consequently, the mesial arm is shorter and more vertical than the distal arm. On the labial surface there is a low, labial cingulum. On the lingual surface, the cingulum and marginal ridges are less pronounced than the corresponding structures on the palatal surface of the maxillary deciduous canine. The longitudinal ridges on both the labial and the lingual surfaces are poorly developed. The width of the crown is less than the length. The root is single and tends to be triangular in cross-section.

Premolars

Premolars are specific to the permanent dentition. They are sometimes referred to as 'bicuspids' because they have two main cusps – a buccal and a palatal (or lingual) cusp – separated by a mesiodistal occlusal fissure. The buccal surface of the buccal cusp is similar in shape to the cusp of a canine, to which it may be considered analogous, while the palatal or lingual cusp corresponds developmentally to the cingulum of the anterior teeth. Thus, premolars are considered to be transitional between canines and molars.

Viewed mesially or distally, the maxillary premolars are trapezoidal in shape, the longest side of the trapezoid being the base of the crown at the cervical margin (Fig. 2.29). Because the occlusal surface is not as wide as the base of the crown, it is thought that the tooth can penetrate food more

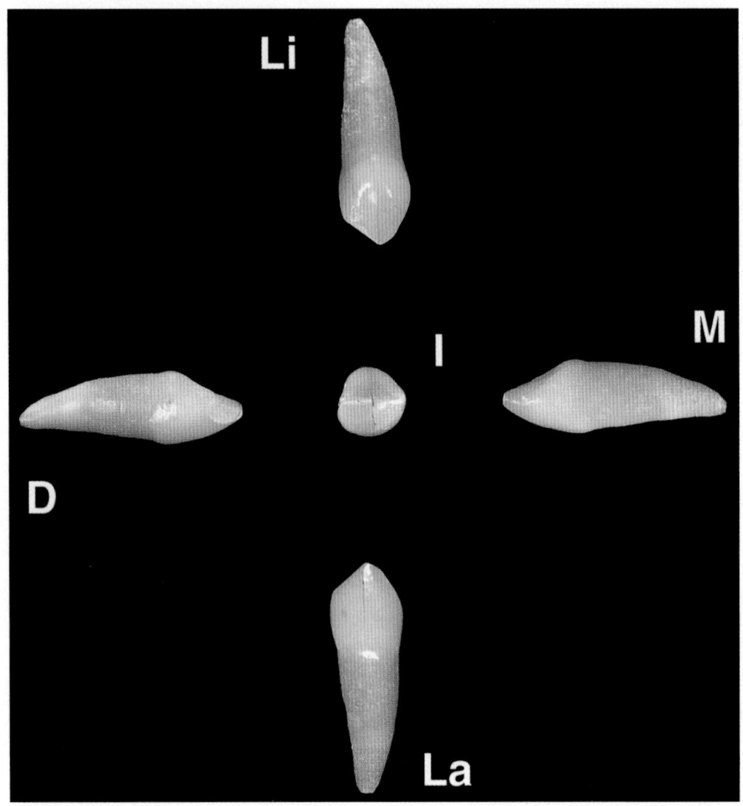

Fig. 2.28 Mandibular right deciduous canine. I = incisal surface; La = labial surface; Li = lingual surface; M = mesial surface; D = distal surface.

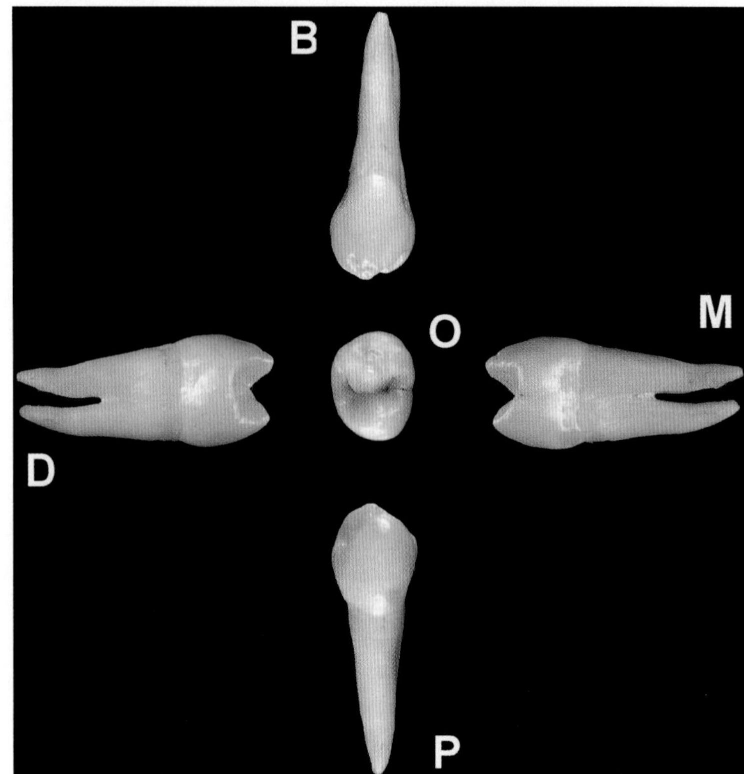

Fig. 2.30 Maxillary first right premolar. O = occlusal surface; B = buccal surface; P = palatal surface; M = mesial surface; D = distal surface.

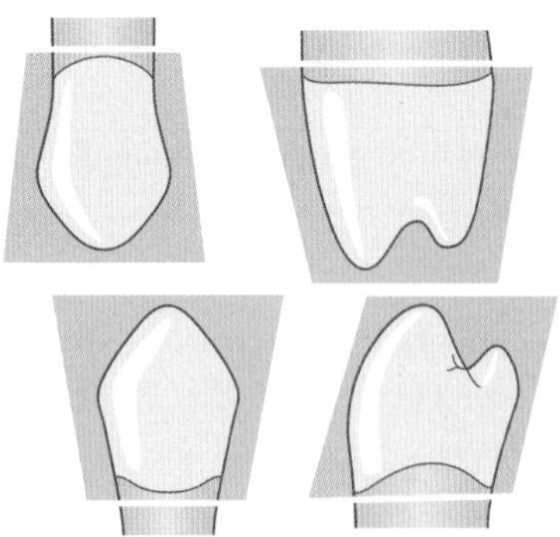

Fig. 2.29 Schematic drawings of premolar crown form, illustrating the relationship between the anatomical and geometrical forms. Redrawn after Dr. R C Wheeler.

easily while minimising the occlusal forces. The mandibular premolars, however, are essentially rhomboidal in shape. The rhomboidal outline is inclined lingually, thus allowing correct intercuspal contact with the maxillary antagonists. Viewed buccally or lingually, all the premolars are trapezoidal, the shortest of the uneven sides being the bases of the crowns cervically.

Maxillary first premolar

When viewed occlusally, this tooth has a crown that appears ovoid, being broader buccally than palatally (Fig. 2.30). Thus, the profiles of the mesial and distal surfaces converge palatally. The mesiobuccal and distobuccal corners are less rounded than the mesiopalatal and distopalatal corners. The mesial and distal borders of the occlusal surface are marked by distinct ridges: the mesial and distal marginal ridges. The buccal and palatal cusps are separated by a central occlusal fissure that runs in a mesiodistal direction. The occlusal fissure crosses the mesial marginal ridge on to the mesial surface. On the distal side, the fissure terminates in a fossa before the distal marginal ridge. Supplementary grooves from the central fissure are rare.

Viewed buccally, the first premolar bears a distinct resemblance to the adjacent canine. A longitudinal ridge may be seen passing down the buccal cusp. The mesial and distal ridges of the buccal cusp each form a 30-degree slope and the mesio- and disto-occlusal angles are prominent, giving the crown a 'bulging-shouldered' ovoid appearance. The mesial slope is generally longer than the distal slope.

Viewed palatally, the buccal part of the crown appears larger in all dimensions than the palatal part so that the entire buccal profile of the crown is visible from the palatal aspect. The palatal cusp is lower and its tip lies more mesially than the tip of the buccal cusp.

From the mesial aspect, the unequal height of the cusps is clearly seen. Note the canine groove extending across the marginal ridge from the occlusal surface. The cervical third of the mesial surface is marked by a distinct concavity, the canine fossa.

The distal aspect of the crown differs from the mesial aspect in that it lacks a canine groove and a canine fossa.

The cervical margin follows a level course around the crown, although deviating slightly towards the root on the buccal and palatal surfaces and away from the root on the mesial and distal surfaces. There are usually two roots, a buccal and palatal root, although sometimes there is only a single root that would then be deeply grooved on its mesial and distal surfaces.

Maxillary second premolar

This tooth (Fig. 2.31) is similar in shape to the maxillary first premolar, except for the following features. Viewed occlusally, the mesiobuccal and distobuccal corners are more rounded and the mesial and distal profiles do not converge lingually, being nearly parallel. The occlusal surface appears more compressed, with the mesiodistal dimension of the crown being smaller. The central fissure appears shorter and does not cross the mesial marginal ridge. From the buccal aspect, the mesio- and disto-occlusal

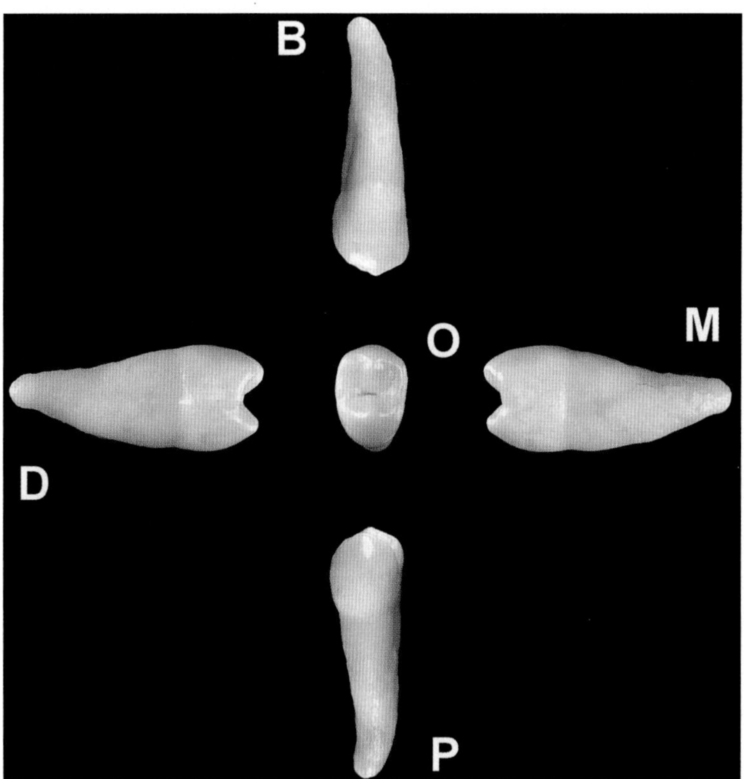

Fig. 2.31 Maxillary second right premolar. O = occlusal surface; B = buccal surface; P = palatal surface; M = mesial surface; D = distal surface.

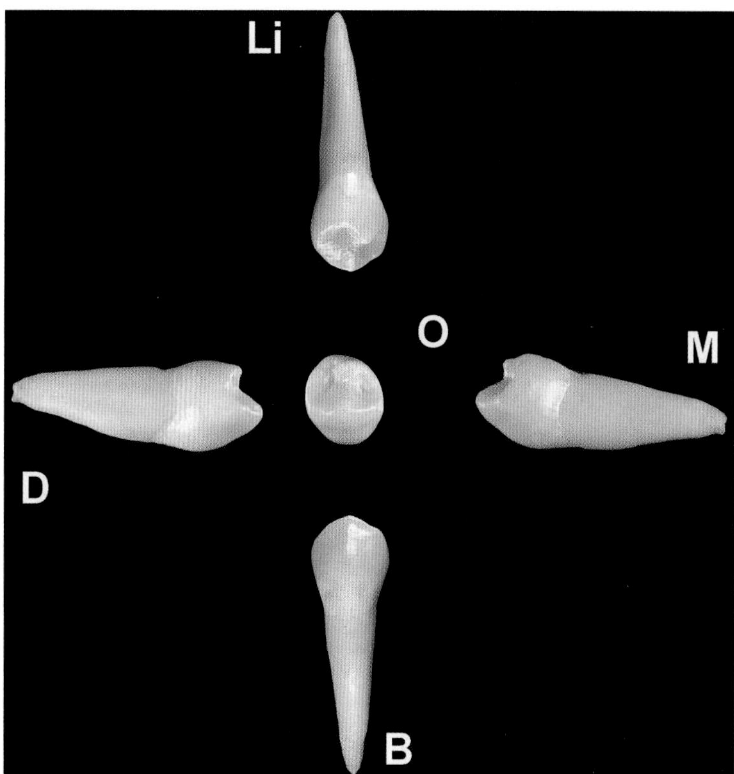

Fig. 2.32 Mandibular first right premolar. O = occlusal surface; B = buccal surface; Li = lingual surface; M = mesial surface; D = distal surface.

angles are less prominent. These features give the crown a 'narrow-shouldered' appearance. The two cusps are smaller and more equal in size than those of the first premolar. The height of the buccal cusp is one-quarter of the height of the crown measured from the base of the occlusal fissure, while the height of the buccal cusp of the first premolar is up to one-half the height of the crown. Viewed palatally, less of the buccal profile is visible. Mesially and distally, the tooth appears similar to the first premolar but there is no canine fossa or canine groove on the mesial surface.

The cervical margin appears similar to that of the maxillary first premolar but is slightly less undulating and the root is single.

The mandibular premolars differ from the maxillary premolars in that occlusally the crowns appear rounder and the cusps are of unequal size, the buccal cusp being the most prominent. Furthermore, the first and second premolars differ more from each other than do the maxillary premolars.

Mandibular first premolar

This is the smallest premolar (Fig. 2.32). As it comprises a dominant buccal cusp and a very small lingual cusp that appears not unlike a cingulum, it might be considered to be a modified canine. From the occlusal aspect, more than two-thirds of the buccal surface is visible, although only a small portion of the lingual surface can be seen. The occlusal outline is diamond-shaped and the occlusal table, outlined by the cusps and marginal ridges, is triangular. The buccal cusp is broad with its apex approximately overlying the midpoint of the crown. The lingual cusp is less than half the size of the buccal cusp. The buccal and lingual cusps are connected by a blunt, transverse ridge that divides the poorly developed mesiodistal occlusal fissure into mesial and distal fossae. The mesial fossa is generally smaller than the distal fossa. A canine groove often extends from the mesial fossa over the mesial marginal ridge on to the mesiolingual surface of the crown. Viewed buccally, the crown is nearly symmetrical, although the mesial profile is more curved than the distal. The buccal surface is markedly convex in all planes. From the lingual aspect, the entire buccal profile and the occlusal surface are visible. Thus, the mandibular first premolar differs from other premolars in that the occlusal plane does not lie perpendicular to the long axis of the tooth but is inclined lingually. The tilt of the occlusal plane can also be appreciated from the mesial and distal aspects.

The cervical line follows an almost level course around the tooth. The root is single, conical and oval to nearly round in cross-section. The root is grooved longitudinally both mesially and distally, the mesial groove being the more prominent.

Mandibular second premolar

The mandibular second premolar (Fig. 2.33) differs from the mandibular first premolar in several respects. Its crown is generally larger and the lingual cusp is better developed, although it is not quite as large as the buccal cusp. From the occlusal aspect, the tooth's outline appears round or square, the mesial and distal profiles being straight and parallel. The mesiodistal occlusal fissure between the cusps is well defined. However, like the first premolar, the fissure ends in mesial and distal fossae, the distal fossa being generally larger than the mesial. Unlike the first premolar, a transverse ridge does not usually join the apices of the cusps. Accessory cusplets are common on both buccal and lingual cusps. The lingual cusp is usually subdivided into mesiolingual and distolingual cusps, the mesiolingual cusp being wider and higher than the distolingual. The groove separating the mesiolingual and distolingual cusps lies opposite the tip of the buccal cusp. From the buccal aspect, the crown of the second premolar is symmetrical. From this view, the buccal cusp generally appears shorter and more rounded than that of the mandibular first premolar. Lingually, little, if any, of the occlusal surface and buccal profile is visible. From the mesial and distal aspects, the occlusal surface appears horizontal to the long axis of the tooth, unlike the mandibular first premolar. The crown is

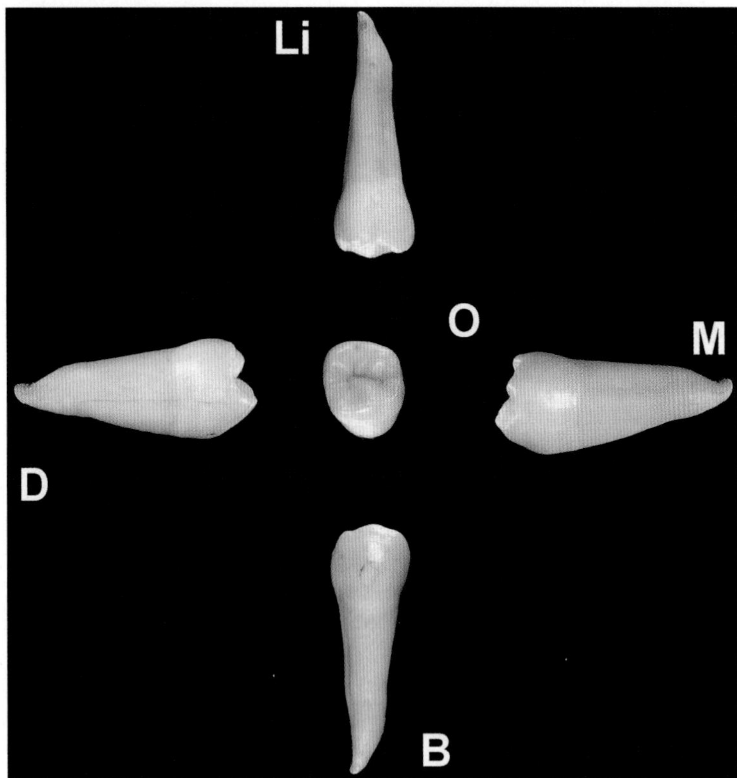

Fig. 2.33 Mandibular second right premolar. O = occlusal surface; B = buccal surface; Li = lingual surface; M = mesial surface; D = distal surface.

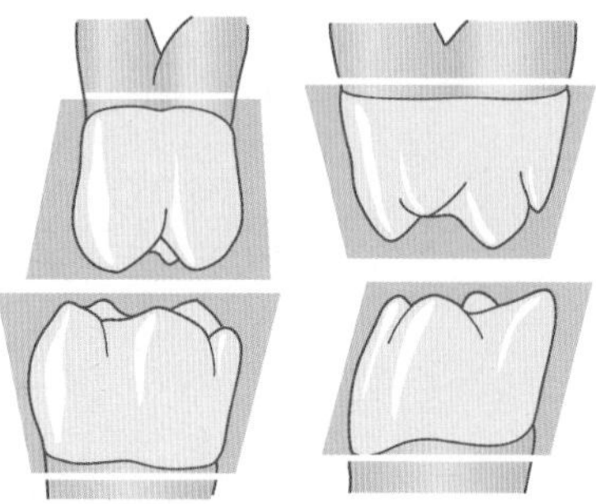

Fig. 2.34 Schematic drawings of molar crown form, illustrating the relationship between the anatomical and geometrical forms. Redrawn after Dr. R C Wheeler.

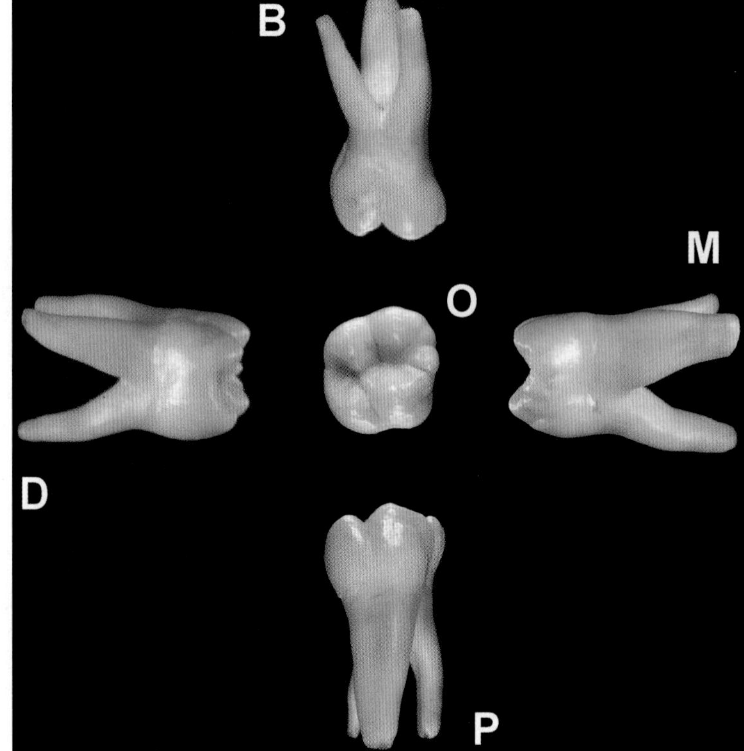

Fig. 2.35 Maxillary first right permanent molar. O = occlusal surface; B = buccal surface; P = palatal surface; M = mesial surface; D = distal surface.

wider buccolingually than that of the first premolar, and the buccal cusp does not incline as far over the root. The mesial marginal ridge is higher than the distal marginal ridge. The cervical margin follows an almost level course around the tooth. The root is single, conical and nearly round in cross-section.

Molars

Molars present the largest occlusal surfaces of all teeth. They have three to five major cusps (although the maxillary first deciduous molar has only two). Molars are the only teeth that have more than one buccal cusp. Generally, the lower molars have two roots while the upper have three. The permanent molars do not have deciduous predecessors.

As with the premolars, the maxillary molars are approximately trapezoidal when viewed mesially and distally, while the mandibular molars are rhomboidal. Viewed buccally or lingually, the molars are trapezoidal (Fig. 2.34).

Maxillary first permanent molar

This is usually the largest molar in each quadrant (Fig. 2.35). Viewed occlusally, the crown is rhomboid in outline. The mesiopalatal and distobuccal angles are obtuse. The longest diameter of the crown runs from the mesiobuccal to the distopalatal corners. It has four major cusps separated by an irregular H-shaped occlusal fissure. The occlusal table may be divided into two distinct components (the trigone and talon) by an oblique ridge that passes diagonally across the occlusal table from the mesiopalatal cusp to the distobuccal cusp. The trigone bears the mesiobuccal, mesiopalatal and distobuccal cusps, and the talon bears the distopalatal cusp. The trigone is characteristically triangular in shape, the apex of the triangle being directed palatally. The mesiopalatal cusp is the largest cusp. The buccal cusps form the base of the trigone and are approximately equal in size. The mesial marginal ridge forms the mesial side of the trigone, and its distal side is formed by the oblique ridge. An accessory cusplet of variable size may be seen on the palatal surface of the mesiopalatal cusp. This cusplet is termed the *tubercle of Carabelli* and is found on about 60% of maxillary first permanent molars. The trigone has a central fossa from which a fissure extends mesially to terminate in a mesial pit before the mesial marginal ridge. Another fissure extends buccally from the central fossa to pass to the buccal surface of the crown between the two buccal cusps. The distopalatal cusp of the talon is generally the smallest cusp of the tooth and is separated from the mesiopalatal cusp by a distopalatal fissure, which curves distally to end in a distal pit before the distal marginal ridge. The oblique ridge may be crossed by a shallow fissure that connects the central fossa of the trigone with the distopalatal fissure and distal pit of the talon, completing the H-shaped fissure pattern. Characteristic of the maxillary molars is that the tips of the palatal cusps are situated nearer the mid-mesiodistal diameter of the crown than those of the buccal cusps.

From the buccal aspect, the buccal cusps are seen to be approximately equal in height, although the mesiobuccal cusp is wider than the distobuccal cusp. The buccal surface is convex in its cervical third but relatively flat in its middle and occlusal thirds. The buccal groove extends from the occlusal table, passing between the cusps to end about halfway up the buccal surface. The mesial profile is convex in its occlusal and middle thirds but flat, or even concave, in the cervical third. The distal profile, on the other hand, is convex in all regions.

Viewed palatally, the disproportion in size between the mesiopalatal and distopalatal cusps is most evident. The mesiopalatal cusp is blunt and occupies approximately three-fifths of the mesiodistal width of the palatal surface. The palatal surface is more or less uniformly convex in all regions. A palatal groove extends from the distal pit to the occlusal surface between the palatal cusps to terminate approximately halfway up the palatal surface.

From the mesial and distal aspects, the maximum buccopalatal dimension is at the cervical margin, from which the buccal and palatal profiles converge occlusally. The mesial marginal ridge is more prominent than the distal ridge and may have a number of distinct tubercles, although such tubercles are rare on the distal marginal ridge.

The cervical margin follows a fairly even contour around the tooth. There are three roots, two buccal and one palatal, arising from a common root stalk. The palatal root is the longest and strongest and is circular in cross-section. The buccal roots are more slender and are flattened mesiodistally; the mesiobuccal root is usually the larger and wider of the two. At the root stalk, the palatal root is more commonly related to the distobuccal root than to the mesiobuccal root.

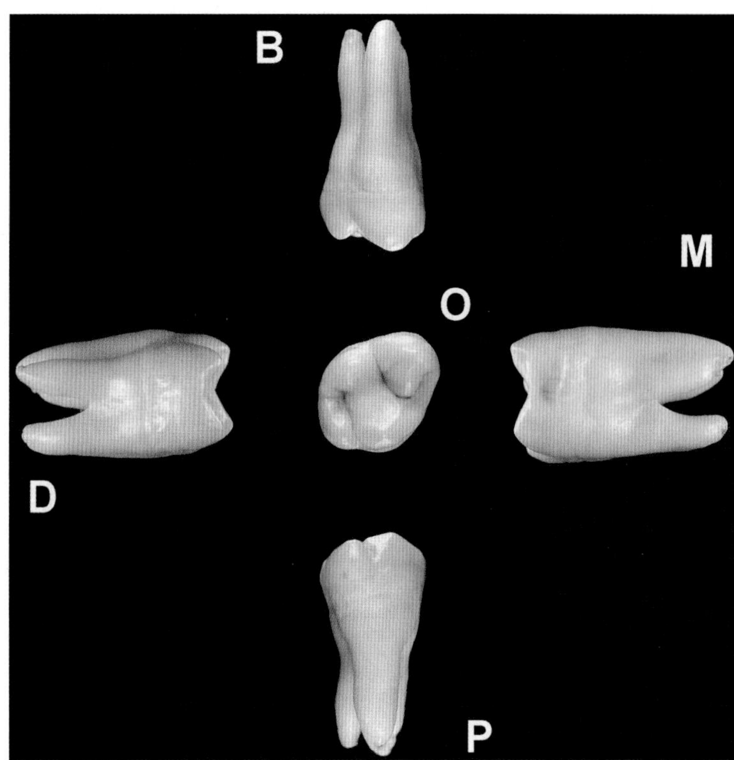

Fig. 2.36 Maxillary second right permanent molar. O = occlusal surface; B = buccal surface; P = palatal surface; M = mesial surface; D = distal surface.

Maxillary second permanent molar

This closely resembles the maxillary first permanent molar but shows some reduction in size and slightly different cusp relationships (Fig. 2.36). Viewed occlusally, the rhomboid form is more pronounced than in the first molar, and the oblique ridge is smaller. The talon (distopalatal fissure cusp) is considerably reduced. The occlusal fissure pattern is similar to that of the first molar but is more variable, and supplemental grooves are more frequent. Two features of the buccal surface differentiate the second molar: the smaller size of the crown and the distobuccal cusp. From the palatal view, the reduction in size of the distopalatal cusp is more visible. A tubercle of Carabelli is not usually found on the mesiopalatal cusp. The mesial and distal surfaces differ little from those of the first molar except that the tubercles on the mesial marginal ridge are less numerous and less pronounced.

As for the maxillary first molar, the second molar has three roots, two buccal and one palatal. However, they are shorter and less divergent than those of the first molar and may be partly fused. The apex of the mesiobuccal root is generally in line with the centre of the crown, unlike that of the first molar, which generally lies in line with the tip of the mesiobuccal cusp.

Variations in morphology of the maxillary second permanent molar are quite common. Total reduction of the distopalatal cusp such that only the trigone remains is frequent. Less frequently, the crown may appear compressed because of fusion of the mesiopalatal and distobuccal cusps, resulting in an oval crown possessing three cusps in a straight line.

Maxillary third permanent molar

Being the most variable in the dentition, this tooth is not illustrated. Its morphology may range from that characteristic of the adjacent maxillary permanent molars to a rounded, triangular crown with a deep central fossa from which numerous irregular fissures radiate outwards. Most commonly, the crown is triangular in shape, having the three cusps of the trigone but no talon. The roots are often fused and irregular in form. Third permanent molars are the teeth most often absent congenitally.

Differences between maxillary and mandibular molars

The mandibular molars differ from the maxillary molars in the following respects:

1) The mandibular molars have two roots, one mesial and one distal.
2) They are considered to be derived from a five-cusped form.
3) The crowns of the lower molars are oblong, being broader mesiodistally than buccolingually.
4) The fissure pattern is cross-shaped.
5) The lingual cusps are of more equal size.
6) The tips of the buccal cusps are shifted lingually so that, from the occlusal view, the whole of the buccal surface is visible.

Mandibular first permanent molar

The crown of this tooth, when viewed occlusally, is somewhat pentagonal in outline (Fig. 2.37). It is broader mesiodistally than buccolingually. The occlusal surface is divided into buccal and lingual parts by a mesiodistal occlusal fissure, which arises from a deep central fossa. The buccal side of the occlusal table has three distinct cusps: mesiobuccal, distobuccal and distal. Each cusp is separated by a groove, which joins the mesiodistal fissure. On the lingual side are two cusps: mesiolingual and distolingual. The fissure separating the lingual cusps joins the mesiodistal fissure in the region of the central fossa. The lingual cusps tend to be larger and more pointed, although they are not disproportionately larger than the mesiobuccal and distobuccal cusps. The tips of the buccal cusps are displaced lingually, are rounded and are lower than the lingual cusps. The smallest cusp is the distal cusp, which is displaced slightly towards the buccal surface. In 90% of cases, the mesiolingual cusp is joined to the distobuccal cusp across the floor of the central fossa. This feature, and the five-cusped

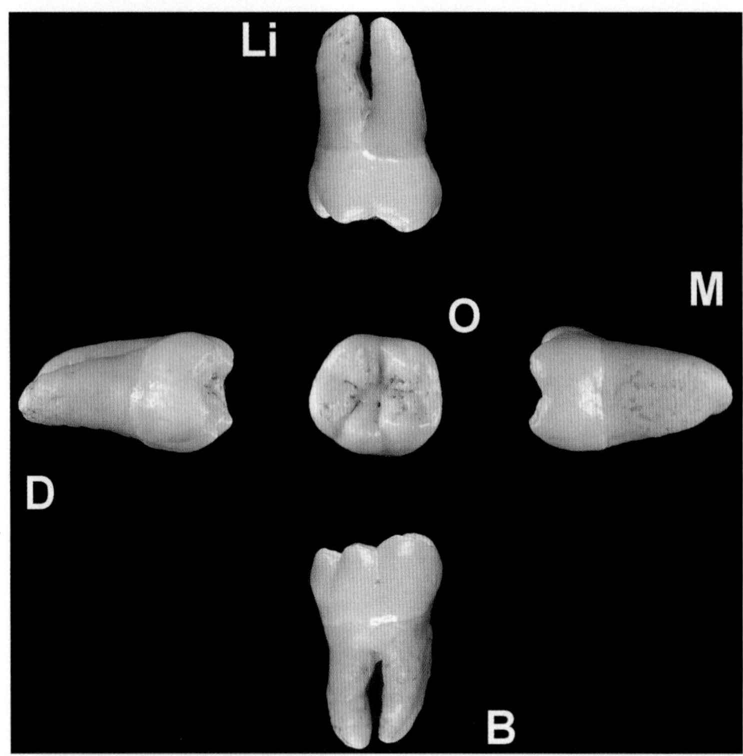

Fig. 2.37 Mandibular first right permanent molar. O = occlusal surface; B = buccal surface; Li = lingual surface; M = mesial surface; D = distal surface.

pattern, is termed the *Dryopithecus* pattern. This 'primitive' pattern is characteristic of all the lower molars of the anthropoid apes and their early ancestors, the dryopithecines. Because of the resulting Y-shaped fissure pattern and the five cusps, the *Dryopithecus* pattern is sometimes referred to as a 'Y5' pattern. In the 10% of cases where the mesiobuccal and distolingual cusps meet, a more cruciate system of fissures is produced: this is sometimes referred to as a '+5' pattern.

From the buccal aspect, three cusps are seen, the distal cusp being the smallest. The fissure separating the mesiobuccal and distobuccal cusps arises from the central fossa on the occlusal surface and terminates halfway up the buccal surface in a buccal pit. The buccal surface appears markedly convex, especially at the cervical third of the crown. This convexity is associated with the characteristic lingual inclination of the buccal cusps.

From the lingual aspect, although the two lingual cusps are nearly equal in size, the mesiolingual cusp appears slightly larger. The fissure between the lingual cusps arises from the central fossa on the occlusal surface but does not extend a significant way down the lingual surface. The lingual surface is convex in its occlusal and middle thirds but is flat or concave cervically. Part of the buccal profiles and proximal surfaces may be seen.

Viewed mesially, the mesial marginal ridge joining the mesiobuccal and mesiolingual cusps is V-shaped, being notched at its midpoint. The mesial surface is flat or concave cervically and convex in its middle and occlusal thirds.

From the distal aspect, the distal marginal ridge joining the distal and distolingual cusps also appears V-shaped. The cervical third of the distal surface is relatively flat, the middle and occlusal thirds highly convex. Thus, the distal surface is more convex than the mesial surface because of the distal cusp. The proximal views of the illustration highlight the greater convex slope of the buccal surface compared with the lingual surface.

The cervical margin follows a uniform contour around the tooth. The two roots, one mesial and one distal, arise from a common root stalk. They are both markedly flattened mesiodistally, and the mesial root is usually deeply grooved. Both roots usually curve distally.

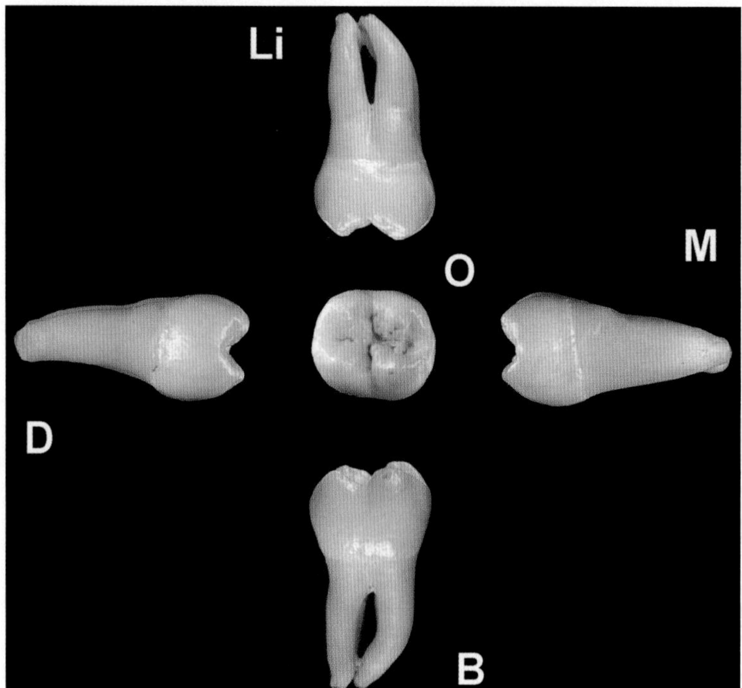

Fig. 2.38 Mandibular second right permanent molar. O = occlusal surface; B = buccal surface; Li = lingual surface; M = mesial surface; D = distal surface.

Mandibular second permanent molar

When viewed occlusally, the crown exhibits a regular, rectangular shape (Fig. 2.38); the buccal profile is thus nearly equal in length to the lingual profile, unlike the mandibular first permanent molar. There are four cusps, with the mesiobuccal and mesiolingual cusps being slightly larger than the distobuccal and distolingual cusps. The cusps are separated by a cross-shaped occlusal fissure pattern that may be complicated by numerous supplemental grooves. From the buccal aspect, the crown appears smaller than that of the first molar. A fissure extends between the buccal cusps from the occlusal surface and terminates approximately halfway up the buccal surface. As for the mandibular first molar, the buccal surface is highly convex. From the lingual aspect, the buccal profiles and proximal surfaces are not visible and the crown is noticeably shorter than the first molar. The mesial and distal aspects of the second molar resemble those of the first molar, although becausE there is no distal cusp the proximal surfaces are more equal in terms of their convexity. The mesial and distal marginal ridges do not converge and are not as markedly notched at their midpoint.

The mesial and distal roots are flattened mesiodistally and are smaller and less divergent than those of the first molar. They may be partly fused. The mesial root is not as broad as that of the first molar, and the distal inclination of the roots is usually more marked.

Mandibular third permanent molar

This has a variable morphology, although not as variable as that of the maxillary third permanent molar. Its clinical significance lies in the fact that it is commonly impacted. It is the smallest of the mandibular molars but can be as large as the mandibular first molar. The crown usually has four or five cusps. In shape, it is normally a rounded rectangle or is circular. Its occlusal fissure pattern is generally very irregular. As a rule, the

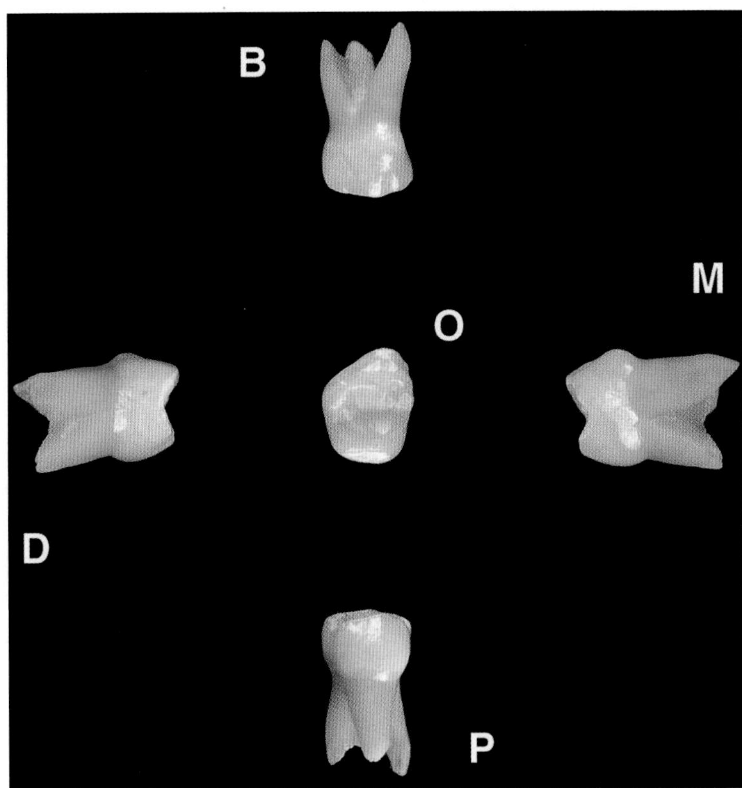

Fig. 2.39 Maxillary first right deciduous molar. O = occlusal surface; B = buccal surface; P = palatal surface; M = mesial surface; D = distal surface.

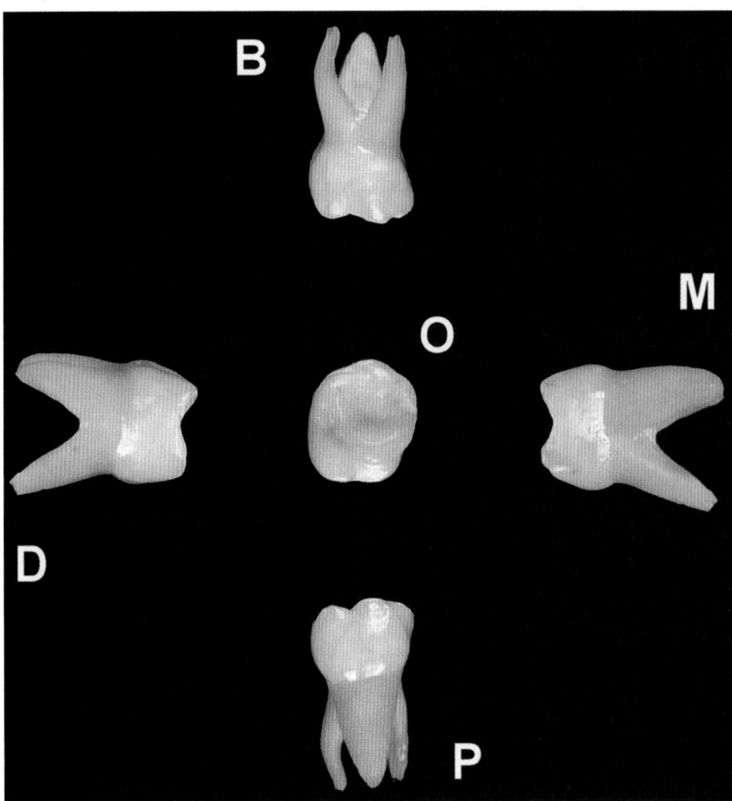

Fig. 2.40 Maxillary second right deciduous molar. O = occlusal surface; B = buccal surface; P = palatal surface; M = mesial surface; D = distal surface.

roots are greatly reduced in size and are fused. They show a marked distal inclination.

Maxillary first deciduous molar

This is the most atypical of all molars, deciduous or permanent (Fig. 2.39). In form it appears intermediate between a premolar and a molar. It is the smallest molar.

Viewed occlusally, the crown is an irregular quadrilateral, with the buccal and palatal surfaces lying parallel to one another. However, the mesiobuccal corner is extended to produce a prominent bulge, the molar tubercle. If crowns are to be fitted, this bulge may have to be smoothed over because of the undercut. The mesiopalatal angle is markedly obtuse. The tooth is generally bicuspid; the buccal (more pronounced) and palatal cusps are separated by an occlusal fissure that runs mesiodistally. A shallow buccal fissure may extend from the central mesiodistal fissure to divide the buccal cusp into two, the mesial part being the larger. The palatal cusp also may be subdivided into two. The tips of the cusps converge towards the midline, reducing the occlusal surface of the tooth. From the buccal aspect, the crown appears squat, its height being less than its width. On the mesial side lies the buccal cingulum, which extends to the molar tubercle. From the palatal aspect, the palatal surface appears shorter mesiodistally than the buccal surface, the profile of which can be seen from this view. The mesial and distal views show the cervical bulbosity of the buccal and palatal surfaces. Note the prominent molar tubercle mesially. Marginal ridges link the buccal and palatal cusps. No fissure crosses the marginal ridges.

The tooth has three roots (two buccal and one palatal), which arise from a common root stalk. The mesiobuccal root is flattened mesiodistally, the distobuccal root is smaller and more circular, and the palatal root is the largest and is round in cross-section. The distobuccal and palatal roots may be partly fused.

Maxillary second deciduous molar

The maxillary second deciduous molar (Fig. 2.40) closely resembles the maxillary first permanent molar (see Fig. 2.35), although its size, whiteness, widely diverging roots and low buccal cingulum distinguish it. A tubercle of Carabelli on the mesiopalatal cusp is often well developed.

Mandibular first deciduous molar

Unlike the maxillary first deciduous molar, this is molariform but has a number of unique features (Fig. 2.41). From the occlusal aspect the crown appears elongated mesiodistally and is an irregular quadrilateral with parallel buccal and lingual surfaces. The mesiobuccal corner is extended, forming a molar tubercle, and the mesiolingual angle is markedly obtuse. The occlusal table can be divided into buccal and lingual parts by a mesiodistal fissure. The buccal part consists of two cusps, the mesiobuccal cusp being larger than the distobuccal cusp. The lingual part of the tooth is narrower than the buccal part and has two cusps separated by a lingual fissure, with the mesiolingual cusp being larger than the distolingual cusp. The buccal cusps are larger than the lingual cusps. A transverse ridge may connect the mesial cusps, dividing the mesiodistal fissure into a distal fissure and a mesial pit. Often a distal pit is found just mesial to the distal marginal ridge. A supplemental groove from the mesial pit may extend over the mesial marginal ridge. From the buccal aspect, the mesiobuccal cusp occupies at least two-thirds of the crown area and projects higher occlusally than the distobuccal cusp. The distal slopes of the buccal cusps are longer than the mesial. The profile of the mesial surface appears flat, whereas that of the distal surface is convex. The molar tubercle on the mesial corner of the buccal surface can be seen in this view. From the lingual aspect, the cusps are conical in shape. The distolingual cusp appears only as a bulging protuberance on the distal margin. Mesially and distally,

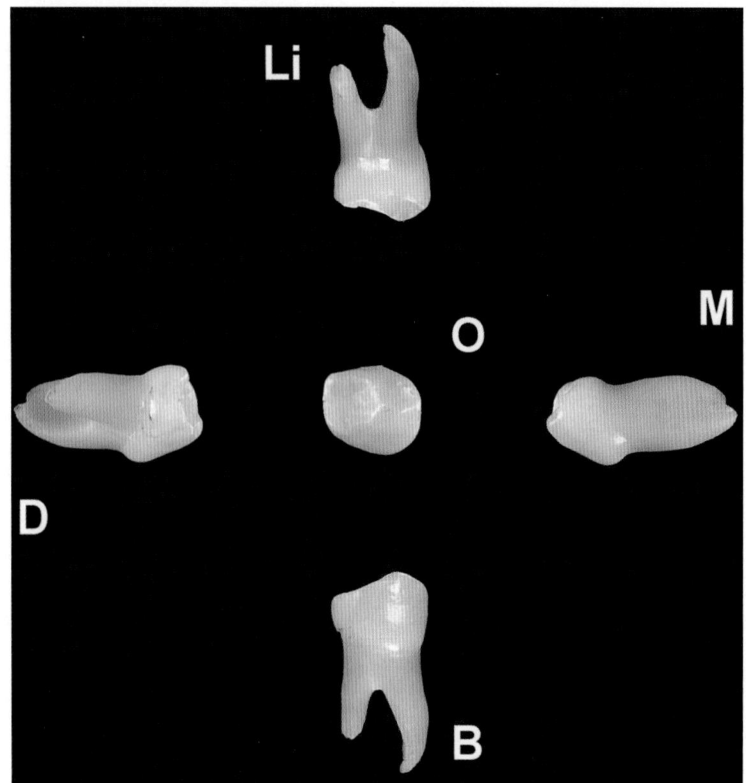

Fig. 2.41 Mandibular first right deciduous molar. O = occlusal surface; B = buccal surface; Li = lingual surface; M = mesial surface; D = distal surface.

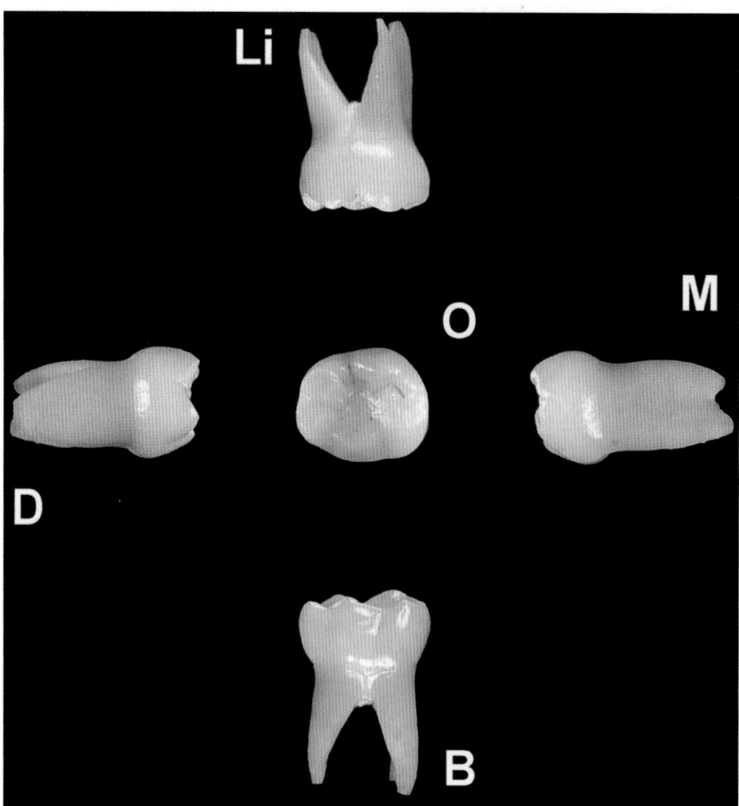

Fig. 2.42 Mandibular second right deciduous molar. O = occlusal surface; B = buccal surface; Li = lingual surface; M = mesial surface; D = distal surface.

the buccal and lingual aspects converge towards the midline of the crown. The mesial marginal ridge is more prominent than the distal marginal ridge. Note the bulge associated with the buccal cingulum near the cervical margin of the mesiobuccal cusp.

The mandibular first deciduous molar has two divergent roots, mesial and distal, which are flattened mesiodistally. The mesial root is often grooved.

Mandibular second deciduous molar

This is a smaller version of the mandibular first permanent molar (see Fig. 2.37), although it is narrower and whiter and has widely diverging roots (Fig. 2.42). Other distinguishing features are the cingulum on the mesiobuccal corner of the crown, with the greater convexity of the mesial and distal surfaces and the more extensive central fossa on the occlusal surface. The mesiolingual and distobuccal cusps are not usually joined to give the *Dryopithecus* pattern.

The average dimensions of the permanent and deciduous teeth are listed in Tables 2.2 and 2.3 (page 16), and the principal features of each tooth are summarised in Tables 2.4 and 2.5.

Some aspects of dental anthropology

Dental anthropology relates to the study of teeth and how such information can illuminate human development and relationships of both past and present populations. This topic involves detailed descriptions of the normal development and morphology of the crowns and their roots and the type of variation found. Additional important information may be gleaned about living conditions from features such as the presence of dental mutilations (altering tooth form for cultural purposes), the nature of tooth wear (both attrition and abrasion) and the types and degrees of pathologies such as periodontal disease and dental caries. Even more specialised information relating to diet and climate can be gleaned by the nature of radioisotopes in the enamel and dentine (see pages 482–486).

A particular aim of dental anthropology is to use the morphology of teeth as a means of determining the relationships between populations. Thus, if the same highly heritable dental variants occur with a similar frequency in two populations, then the populations are likely to have a high degree of affinity. These anthropological studies generally utilise complex statistical analyses on groups of traits rather than a single feature. Where frequencies of the features are low, a large sample size is necessary. This is particularly relevant when considering the evolution of early humans, when teeth may be the only physical traces that are preserved. Very few of the dental features to be discussed have a simple Mendelian type of inheritance (i.e., autosomal dominant, autosomal recessive, sex-linked conditions). Therefore, their inheritance depends on several genes (polygenic) but varies minimally in response to environmental factors. As an introduction to the topic, the following section will deal with aspects of tooth morphology.

Two broad divisions of dental features can be considered. *Metric features* are those considered to be readily amenable to direct quantification, such as crown length, breadth and height. Such measurements are uncomplicated in newly erupted and unworn teeth. However, when the teeth have been functioning in the mouth, allowance must be made for any loss of dental tissues owing to attrition and abrasion. The overall size of teeth in males is slightly greater (2–6%) than in females. This feature, especially in the case of lower canines, can be used in some circumstances to help separate dentitions according to sex. The teeth of females also erupt slightly earlier than their male counterparts. Using multivariate analysis, the size of teeth is also valuable in helping to distinguish different geographical populations, the largest crowns in living populations being found in Aboriginal Australians and the smallest among Asians and Europeans.

Table 2.4 The principal morphological features of the permanent teeth

Tooth	Cusps	Roots	Distinctive features
Permanent dentition			
Maxillary central (first) incisor	None	1	Widest crown of the incisors; root length and crown length similar; rounded distoincisal angle.
Maxillary lateral (second) incisor	None	1	Similar to adjacent first incisor, though not as wide; pit near palatal cingulum.
Mandibular central (first) incisor	None	1	Symmetrical crown, lingually inclined over root; indistinct lingual cingulum; distal groove on root more prominent.
Mandibular lateral (second) incisor	None	1	Similar to adjacent first incisor but is fan-shaped owing to distal extension of crown. Incisal edge twisted distally.
Maxillary canine	1	1	Stout tooth with cusp occupying one-third of crown height; distal surface more convex than mesial. Distal slope of cusp longer than mesial slope.
Mandibular canine	1	1	Crown height much greater than width with cusp occupying one-fifth of height; distal slope of cusp longer than mesial slope. Distal surface rounded when meeting labial surface.
Maxillary first premolar	2	2	Canine fossa on mesial side of crown and root; ovoid occlusal surface with buccal cusp taller and larger than palatal. Tip of palatal cusp lies more mesial.
Maxillary second premolar	2	1	Similar to adjacent first premolar but with no canine fossa and buccal and palatal cusps nearly equal in size. Tip of palatal cusp lies more mesial.
Mandibular first premolar	2	1	Round occlusal outline; very large buccal cusp, very small lingual cusp; transverse ridge joining cusps. Distal fossa on occlusal surface larger than mesial.
Mandibular second premolar	2/3	1	Square occlusal outline; buccal and lingual cusps more equal; lingual cusp often has two prominences (mesial larger).
Maxillary first molar	4 (+Carabelli trait)	3	Rhomboid occlusal outline; mesio-palatal cusp largest with Carabelli trait and joined by ridge to distobuccal cusp; tubercles on mesial marginal ridge.
Maxillary second molar	3/4	3	Similar to adjacent first molar but more rhomboid: distopalatal cusp smaller; Carabelli trait missing.
Maxillary third molar	Variable	Usually 3	Very variable morphology.
Mandibular first molar	5	2	Rectangular occlusal outline with three cusps buccally (distal smallest) and two cusps lingually. Buccal surface more convex.
Mandibular second molar	4	2	Square occlusal outline; occlusal fissure pattern; mesial cusps larger than distal.
Mandibular third molar	Variable	usually 2	Very variable morphology.

Table 2.5 The principal morphological features of the deciduous teeth

Tooth	Cusps	Roots	Distinctive features
Deciduous dentition			
Maxillary central (first) incisor	None	1	Similar to corresponding permanent tooth but smaller and more bulbous
Maxillary lateral (second) incisor	None	1	Similar to corresponding permanent tooth but smaller and more bulbous
Mandibular central (first) incisor	None	1	Similar to corresponding permanent tooth but smaller and more bulbous
Mandibular lateral (second) incisor	None	1	Similar to corresponding permanent tooth but smaller and more bulbous
Maxillary canine	1	1	Similar to corresponding permanent tooth but smaller and more bulbous
Mandibular canine	1	1	Similar to corresponding permanent tooth but smaller and more bulbous
Maxillary first molar	2	3	Unique shape resembling premolar but with three roots; buccal cusp (ridge) larger and wider than palatal cusp (ridge); mesial palatal corner obtuse: cervical margin with mesiobuccal tubercle
Maxillary second molar	4	3	Tooth resembles permanent maxillary first molar tooth but more bulbous; low buccal cingulum
Mandibular first molar	4 + Mesial tubercle	2	Rectangular occlusal outline with mesiobuccal corner extended to form molar tubercle; transverse ridge joins mesial cusps: mesiolingual corner obtuse; mesiobuccal cingulum
Mandibular second molar	5	2	Tooth resembles permanent maxillary first molar tooth but more bulbous; mesiobuccal cingulum

The preceding description of the morphology of teeth is, of necessity, only generalised and is related to that found in western Eurasia. However, superimposed on the basic shapes of teeth described are several morphological variations affecting both deciduous and permanent teeth. In any population, these may be absent or present and display a varying degree of penetrance ranging from barely perceptible to very prominent. Because of the present difficulty in accurately quantifying such features within a reasonable period of time, these traits are considered to be *nonmetric features*. However, to allow research scientists to attain some common agreement as to the degree of penetrance, a series of casts (plaques) for each feature with wide international acceptance have been produced by Arizona State University and disseminated to researchers in the field, three of which are illustrated in Figs 2.43–2.45.

Over 100 secondary dental traits have been described in the literature, but only the more common are indicated here.

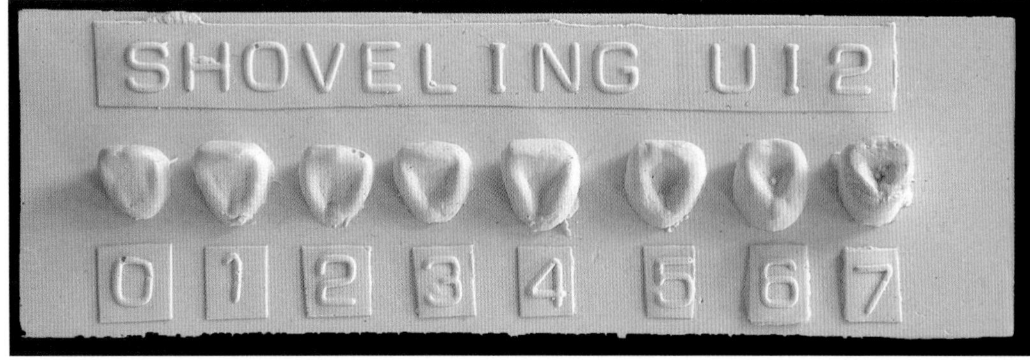

Fig. 2.43 Arizona State University reference plaque detailing scoring system for shovelling on the maxillary second incisor. 0 = *none*: lingual surface is essentially flat; 1 = *faint*: very slight elevations of mesial and distal aspects of lingual surface can be seen and palpated; 2 = *trace*: elevations are easily seen; 3 = *semishovel*: stronger ridging is present and there is a tendency for ridge convergence at the cingulum; 4 = *semishovel*: convergence and ridging are stronger than in grade 3; 5 = *shovel*: strong development of ridges, which almost contact at the cingulum; 6 = *marked shovel*: strongest development – mesial and distal lingual ridges are sometimes in contact at the cingulum; 7 = *barrel* (maxillary first and second incisors only): expression exceeds grade 6. From Turner, C.G. II, Nichol, C.R., Scott, G.R., 1991. Scoring procedures for key morphological traits of the permanent dentition: the Arizona State University dental anthropology system. In: Kelley, M.A., Larsen, C.S. (Eds.), *Advances in dental anthropology*. Wiley–Liss, New York, pp 13–31. Courtesy Dr. D Hawksey and Dr. S Haddow.

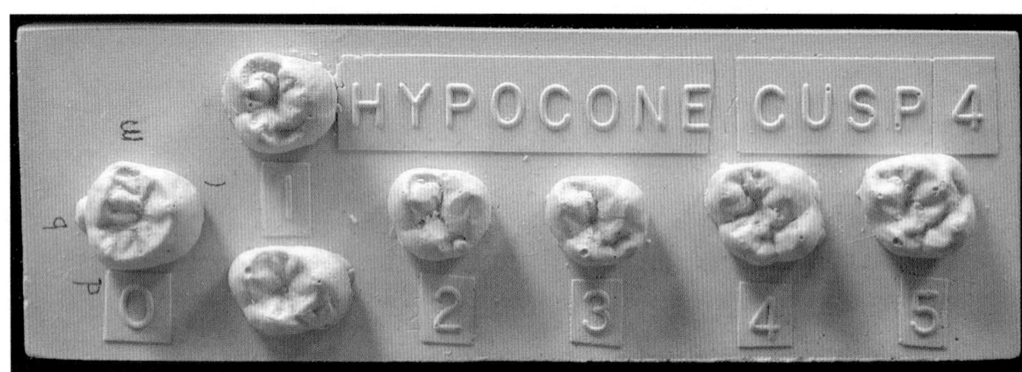

Fig. 2.44 Arizona State University reference plaque detailing scoring system for the distolingual cusp (hypocone) in maxillary molars. 0 = no hypocone – site is smooth; 1 = faint ridging present at the site; 2 = faint cuspule present; 3 = small cusp present but not shown; 3.5 = moderate-sized cusp present (not shown); 4 = large cusp present; 5 = very large cusp present. From Turner, C.G. II, Nichol, C.R., Scott, G.R., 1991. Scoring procedures for key morphological traits of the permanent dentition: the Arizona State University dental anthropology system. In: Kelley, M.A., Larsen, C.S. (Eds.), *Advances in dental anthropology.* Wiley–Liss, New York, pp 13–31.Courtesy Dr. D Hawksey and Dr. S Haddow.

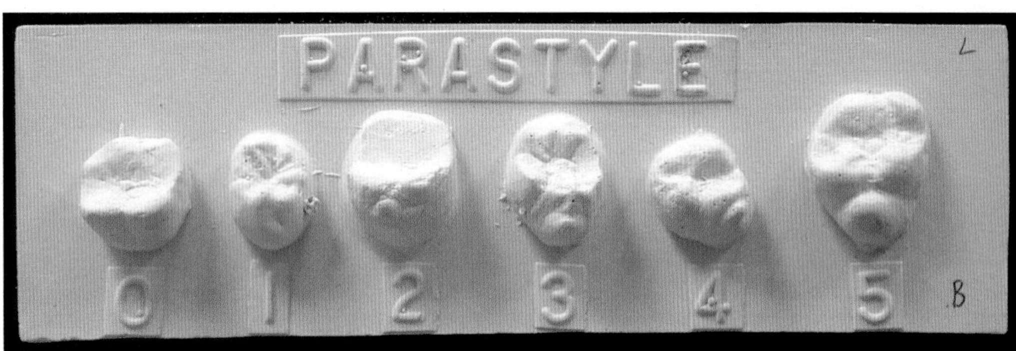

Fig. 2.45 Arizona State University reference plaque detailing scoring system for the parastyle, most commonly appearing on the buccal surface of the mesiobuccal cusp (the paracone) of the maxillary third molar. 0 = the buccal surfaces of the buccal cusps are smooth; 1 = a pit is present in or near the buccal groove between the buccal cusps; 2 = a small cusp with an attached apex is present; 3 = a medium-sized cusp with a free apex is present; 4 = a large cusp with a free apex is present; 5 = a very large cusp with a free apex is present – this form usually involves the buccal surface of both buccal cusps; 6 = an effectively free, peg-shaped crown attached to the root of the third molar is present – this condition is extremely rare, and is not shown on the plaque. From Turner, C.G. II, Nichol, C.R., Scott, G.R., 1991. Scoring procedures for key morphological traits of the permanent dentition: the Arizona State University dental anthropology system. In: Kelley, M.A., Larsen, C.S. (Eds.), *Advances in dental anthropology.* Wiley–Liss, New York, pp 13–31.Courtesy Dr D Hawksey and Dr S Haddow.

Traits found in incisors and canine teeth

Shovel-shaped incisors

Exaggerated and extensive mesial and distal marginal ridges combine to result in an exaggerated palatal concavity. This gives the crown a shovel shape (Fig. 2.46). The ridging may extend onto the labial surface, giving rise to a 'double-shovelled' appearance. While it may be present on all the anterior teeth, shovelling is predominantly found in the maxillary incisors.

Maxillary second incisor traits

This tooth has the most variable form in the dentition (apart from third molars), one common variant being 'peg-shaped' (Fig. 2.47).

Cingulum traits

These are found on the palatal surface of the maxillary teeth and are reflected as variations in the nature of the cingulum and associated ridges, fossae and grooves (e.g., interruption grooves), especially in relation to the second incisor and canine (Figs 2.48, 2.49).

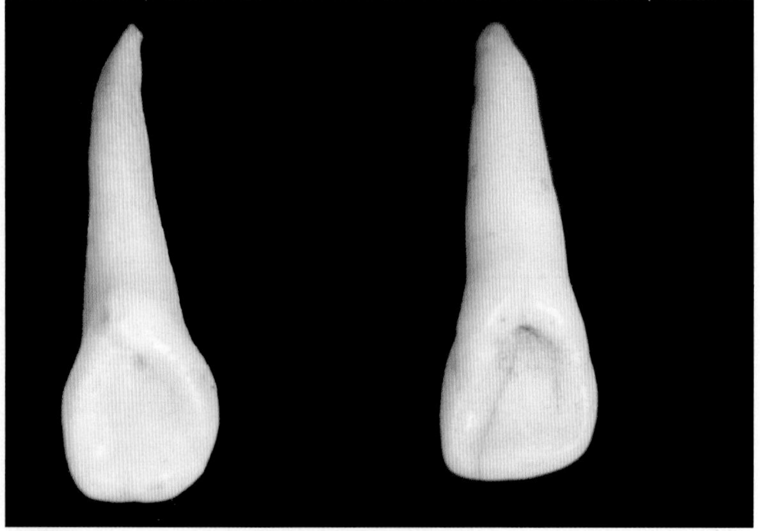

Fig. 2.46 Shovel-shaped maxillary permanent lateral incisors. Copyright the Royal College of Surgeons of England.

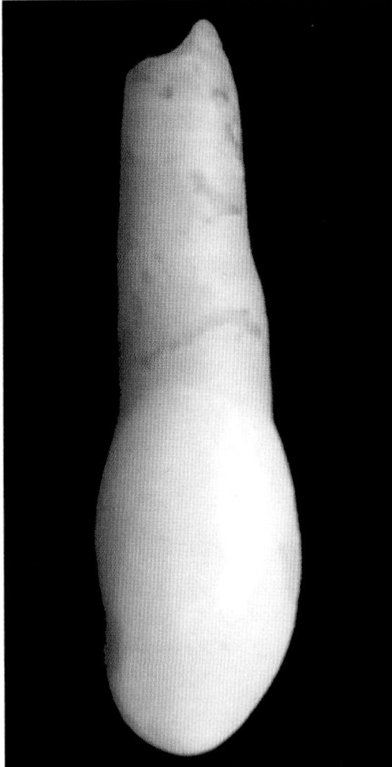

Fig. 2.47 Peg-shaped maxillary permanent second incisor.

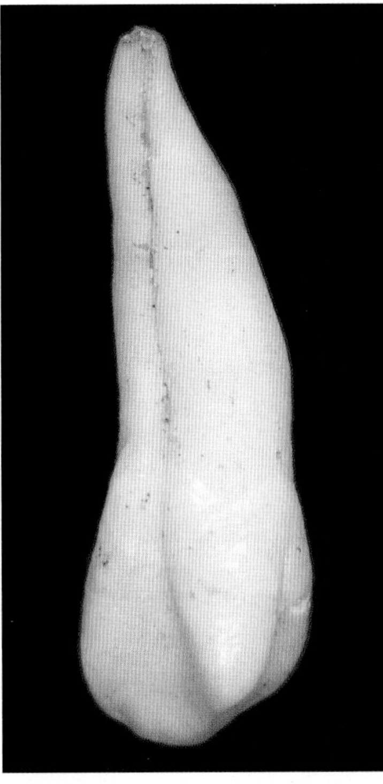

Fig. 2.48 Maxillary permanent second incisor exhibiting a prominent palatal tubercle and a deeply grooved root. Copyright the Royal College of Surgeons of England.

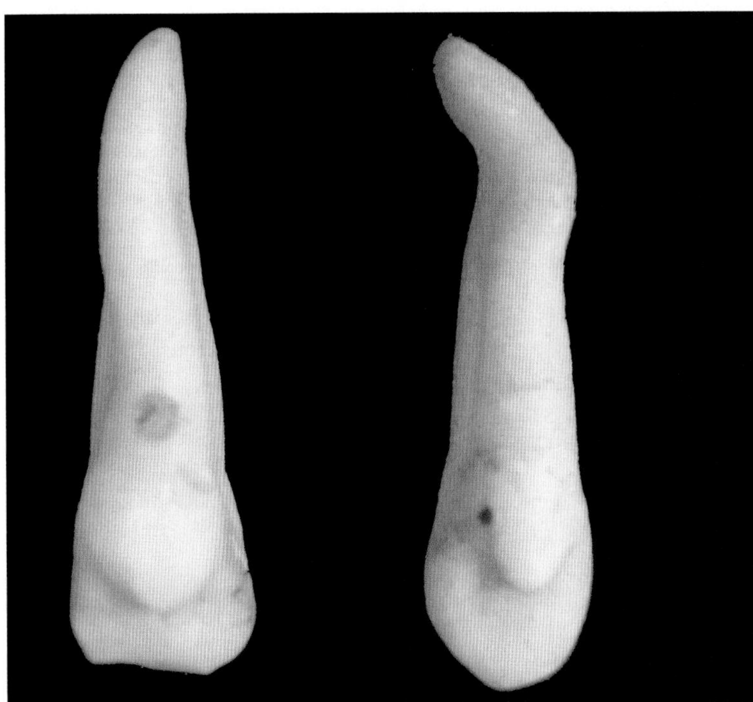

Fig. 2.49 Palatal surface of maxillary permanent canines showing prominent tubercles. Copyright the Royal College of Surgeons of England.

Canine ridges

This trait relates to extra ridging occurring on the mesial (Bushman canine) or distal slope of the cusp of the maxillary canine.

Winging of maxillary first incisors

Although not related to any variation in form, this trait concerns variation in the orientation of the teeth. Instead of the first incisors being straight and arranged along the dental arch, they are inclined mesially and their incisal edges form a V shape.

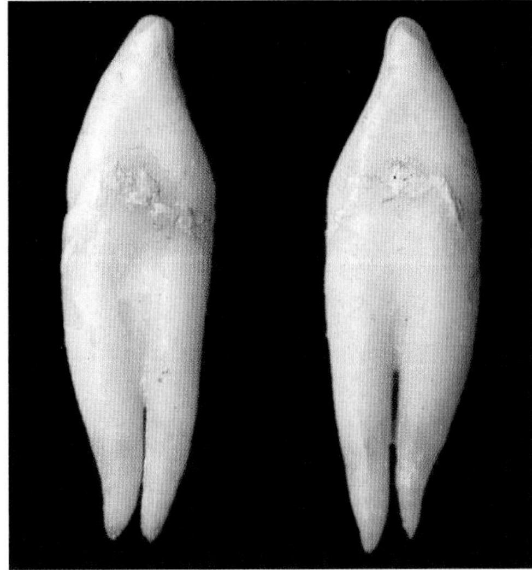

Fig. 2.50 Two-rooted mandibular permanent canines. Copyright the Royal College of Surgeons of England.

Root variation

Whereas the root in all anterior teeth is usually single, that of the mandibular canine in some populations may show evidence of bifurcation at the apex in 5% to 10% of cases (Fig. 2.50).

Traits found in premolar teeth

Accessory marginal tubercles

These tubercles are associated with the distal marginal ridge of maxillary premolars.

Odontome

This rare trait is a tubercle that can occur on the inner surface of the buccal cusp of premolars. It overlies a pulp horn in about half the cases.

Accessory buccal ridges

These lie within the normal mesial and distal marginal ridges associated with the buccal cusp and are more common in the maxillary premolars than the mandibular.

Disto-sagittal ridge (Uto-Aztecan premolar)

This trait, found in the maxillary first premolars of Native Americans, is characterised by distal displacement of the buccal cusp, associated with which is a distal fossa.

Additional lingual cusps

Instead of the typical single lingual cusp present in mandibular second premolars, this trait relates to the presence of up to three cusps (cusplets).

Root traits

Instead of the normal two roots (very rarely one), the first maxillary premolar tooth may have one or three roots (Fig. 2.51). Similarly, the normal single-rooted mandibular first premolar may present with two roots instead of one (Fig. 2.52).

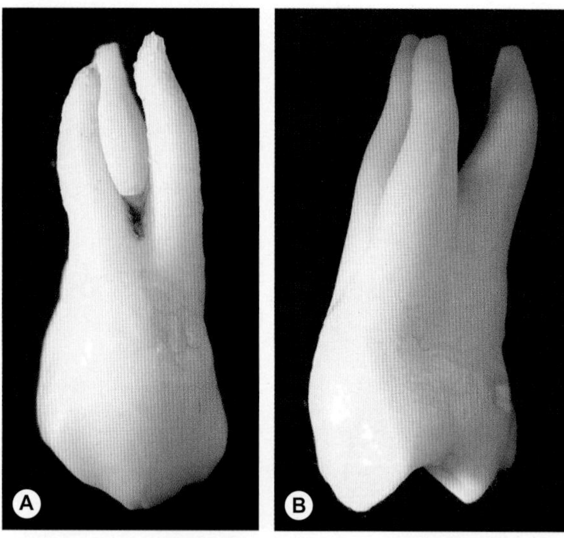

Fig. 2.51 Three rooted maxillary first premolar: (A) viewed from front; (B) viewed from side.

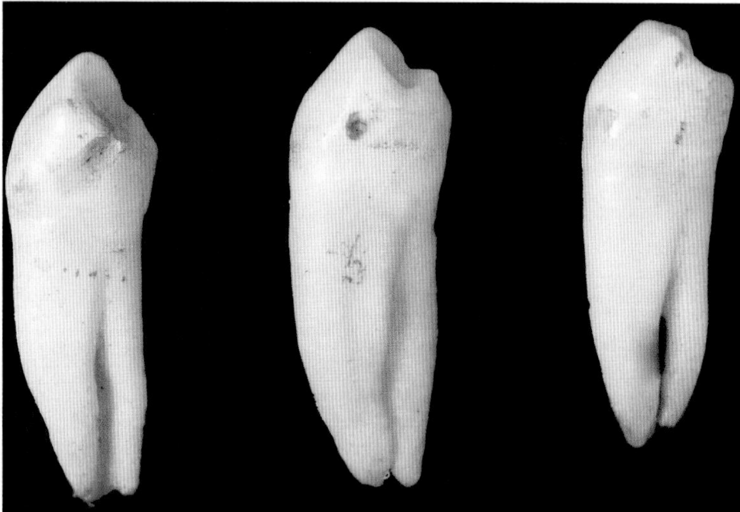

Fig. 2.52 Two-rooted mandibular first premolars. *Copyright the Royal College of Surgeons of England.*

Traits found in molar teeth

Maxillary molars

Cusplet (tubercle) of Carabelli

This cusplet is situated on the palatal surface of the mesiopalatal cusp and is primarily considered with respect to the first molar tooth. It may be absent or show varying degrees of penetrance (see page 24).

Distopalatal cusp

While this cusp is invariably present on the first molar, it may show variable degrees of reduction in the second molar tooth.

Accessory tubercles on the marginal ridge

This trait can occur on both the mesial and the distal marginal ridges, primarily involving the first molar. Generally single on the distal marginal ridge (where it has been referred to as cusp 5), it may be multiple on the mesial marginal ridge.

Paramolar tubercle (parastyle)

This trait is represented by the presence of a tubercle on the buccal side of the mesiobuccal cusp (Fig. 2.53).

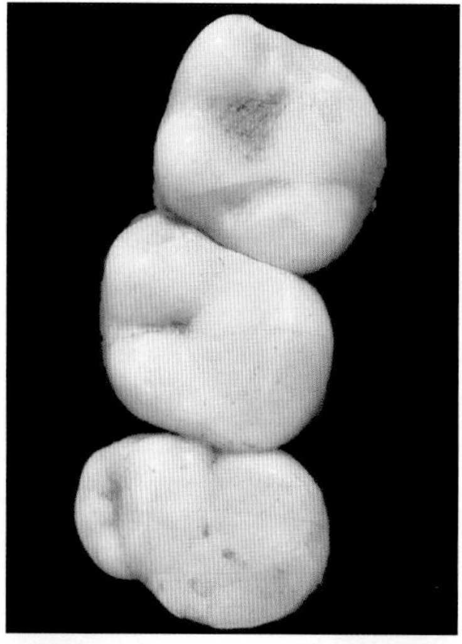

Fig. 2.53 Maxillary right permanent third molar exhibiting a parastyle. Copyright the Royal College of Surgeons of England.

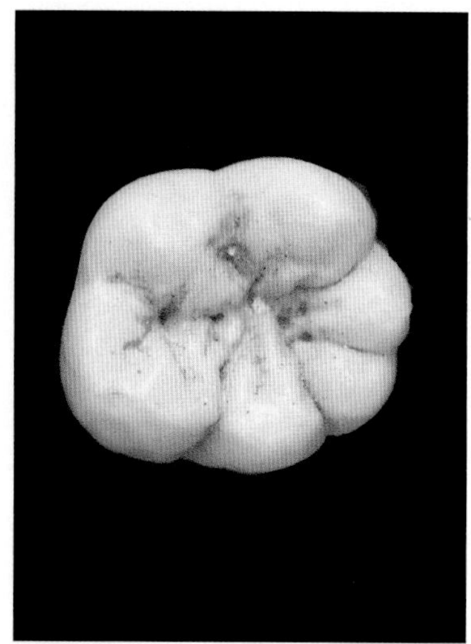

Fig. 2.54 Six-cusped mandibular permanent molar. Copyright the Royal College of Surgeons of England.

Enamel extensions

Thin extensions of enamel in the region of the root bifurcation, especially on the buccal surface, may occur in maxillary and mandibular molar teeth (as well as premolars).

Root traits

The typical number of three roots generally present on the first molar may be reduced to one or two in the second molar.

Mandibular molars

Four-cusp form

While the first molar generally has five cusps, it may be reduced to a four-cusp form because of loss of the distal cusp.

Six- or seven-cusp forms

An additional cusp (cusp 6) may occur on the first molar between the distolingual and distal cusps (Fig. 2.54). A further cusp (cusp 7) may occur between the mesiolingual and distolingual cusps.

Paramolar tubercle (protostylid)

As with the maxillary teeth, the mandibular molars may exhibit a tubercle on the buccal side of the mesiobuccal cusp.

Fissure pattern

The classification of the fissure pattern is primarily dependent on the type of contact between the cusps in the central fossa region. If the mesiolingual and distobuccal cusps contact to intervene between the mesiobuccal and distolingual cusps, then the fissure pattern is said to have a 'Y' configuration. If the reverse is the case, the configuration is said to be an 'X' pattern. If the four cusps meet equally at the base of the fissure, the pattern is described as a '+' (Fig. 2.55).

Ridges on the first molar

The presence of an accessory ridge parallel to the mesial marginal ridge isolates an anterior fossa (fovea or precuspidal fossa). Another ridge may connect the two mesial cusps (distal trigonid crest). The crest passing from the mesiolingual cusp to the central fossa may be angulated (deflecting wrinkle).

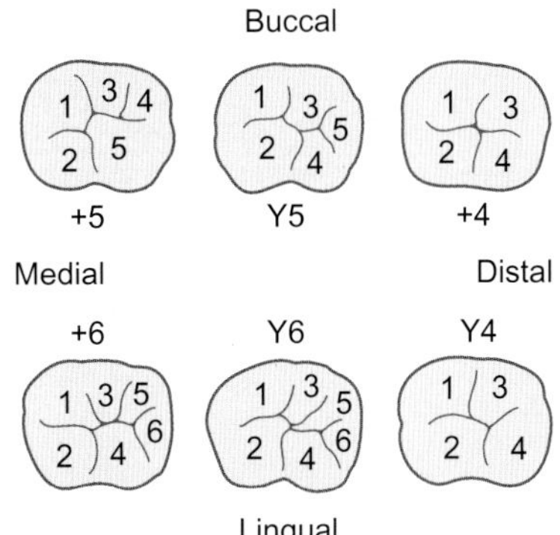

Fig. 2.55 Mandibular molars showing variation in fissure pattern and number of cusps.

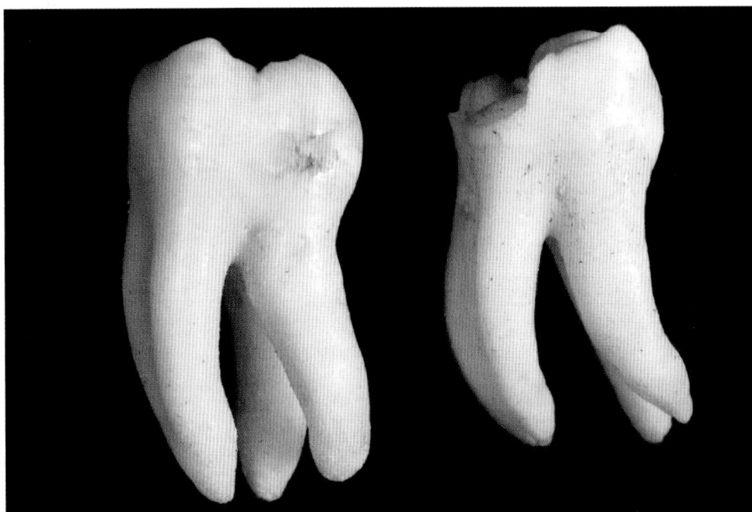

Fig. 2.56 Three-rooted mandibular permanent molar. Copyright the Royal College of Surgeons of England.

Root traits

Whereas the mandibular molars normally have two roots, three roots may be present (Fig. 2.56), a trait associated particularly with first molars. The second molar may possess only a single root.

Two additional features are often incorporated into anthropological investigations of dental variation, even though they are not strictly morphological features. These are hypodontia (the frequency of missing teeth) and hyperdontia (the frequency of supernumerary teeth).

Geographical variation in dentitions

It is possible to distinguish the dentitions of different geographical populations according to the distribution of the dental traits described earlier. Although individual dental traits may occur at high frequencies in selective populations, it is necessary to catalogue the distribution of many dental traits in helping to identify the population with more certainty. A population may be categorised by some traits occurring at high frequencies, some traits at low frequencies and others at intermediate frequencies. For example, shovel-shaped incisors have a mean frequency of about 3% in Eastern Europeans and about 85% in Native Americans. Six-cusped lower first molars have a mean frequency of about 4% in European populations compared with over 50% in Aboriginal Australian peoples. From detailed examination of the dentition, it is possible to construct a complex of dental traits that helps distinguish one geographical human population from another, allowing for the possibility of separating human populations into related groups.

A major classification of the geographical subdivisions of humanity considers it capable of being divided into five major groupings.

Western Eurasia/Caucasoids (to include Western Europe, Northern Europe and North Africa)

The dental traits that occur with the highest frequencies compared to other groups are two-rooted mandibular canines and four-cusped first and second mandibular molars. In many other respects, dental traits occur with an intermediate frequency, indicating that the group is defined more by a comparative absence of traits rather than by their presence.

Sub-Saharan Africa (to include West and South Africa)

Among the traits that occur with high frequency in this group are the presence of a mesial canine ridge on the maxillary canine, a cusp 7 on mandibular first molars and a ‘Y’ fissure pattern on the mandibular second molar. There is a low degree of root traits and four-cusped mandibular second molars.

Sinu-Americas (to include China–Mongolia, Japan, North and South America, Siberia and the Eskimo–Aleuts of the American Arctic)

This group is generally most easily recognised by the high frequency of many dental traits, such as shovelling of incisors, winging, enamel extensions, odontomes in premolars and the low frequency of two-rooted maxillary first premolars and three-rooted maxillary second molars.

Sunda–Pacific (to include Southeast Asia, Polynesia and Micronesia)

This group seems to have no characteristic dental trait occurring with a high frequency that might help characterise them, but shows intermediate frequency of many traits (e.g., shovelling, winging, odontomes) that help to characterise their dentitions.

Sahul–Pacific (to include Australia, New Guinea and Melanesia)

This group, like the Sunda–Pacific population, has few dental traits occurring at high frequency; the dentition is more characterised by a low frequency of many traits.

Pulp morphology

The dental pulp occupies the pulp chamber in the crown of the tooth and the root canal(s) in the root(s). The pulp chamber conforms, in basic shape, to the external form of the crown (Fig. 2.57). Root canal anatomy varies with tooth type and root morphology. At the apex of the root, the root canal becomes continuous with the periapical periodontal tissues through an apical foramen. Knowledge of the morphology of the pulp chamber and root canal is clinically significant: for example, when removing caries and restoring teeth, it is important to avoid exposing the pulp. Furthermore, when the pulp is diseased and must be removed and replaced with a filling material (root canal therapy), it is essential to remove and replace all the pulp tissue and avoid injuring the periapical supporting tissues.

In the general descriptions of the pulp morphology in teeth of the permanent dentition that follow, each tooth is illustrated from the labial (buccal) and distal surfaces. The red outline shows the pulp cavity in the young tooth;

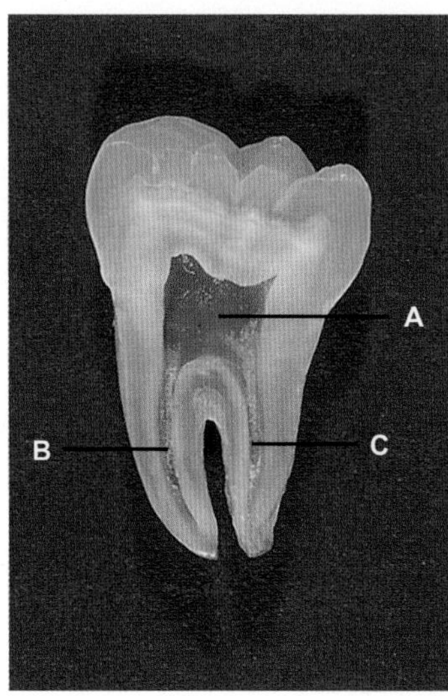

Fig. 2.57 Ground section of a molar tooth showing the pulp chamber (A) and root canals (B, C).

the blue outline shows the pulp in the old tooth. For anterior teeth, the pulp chambers merge almost imperceptibly into the root canals. For premolar and molar teeth, the pulp chambers and root canals are distinct. Pulp horns (or cornua) extend from the pulp chambers to the mesial and distal angles of the incisor tooth crowns and towards the cusps of posterior teeth.

A variety of root canal configurations exist (Fig. 2.58). Most commonly, each root contains one root canal (type I), but two separate root canals (type IV) are not unusual (mandibular molars, for example, commonly have two root canals in their mesial roots). When roots are fused, the tooth still maintains the usual number of root canals. Basically, single root canals may show varying degrees of branching that may end in single (types II and III), double (types V, VI, VII) or multiple openings (type VIII) at the root apex.

The size of the pulp chamber and the diameters of the root canals decrease significantly with age and in response to caries, attrition or other external stimuli. This is the result of the deposition of secondary (and sometimes tertiary) dentine (see pages 180–183). When the tooth first erupts into the oral cavity, root development is incomplete, being only about two-thirds complete, and the apical foramen is wide (see Fig. 25.2). It takes about another 3 years for the root to complete its growth, when the apical foramen narrows with subsequent development of the root.

Knowledge of the location of the narrowest part of the root canal, the apical foramen, is critical for successful root canal therapy, as the root canal filling material should neither end too short of this point nor overextend into the surrounding tissues. Studies indicate that the apical foramen rarely coincides with the anatomical apex, especially with the continued formation of cementum at the root apex. The mean distance between the apical foramen and the most apical part of the root is between 0.2 and 2 mm (Fig. 2.59). The apical constriction tends to occur about 0.5–1 mm from the apical foramen. Ideally, the root canal filling material should terminate at the apical constriction, and specialised electronic equipment is now available to help locate this feature.

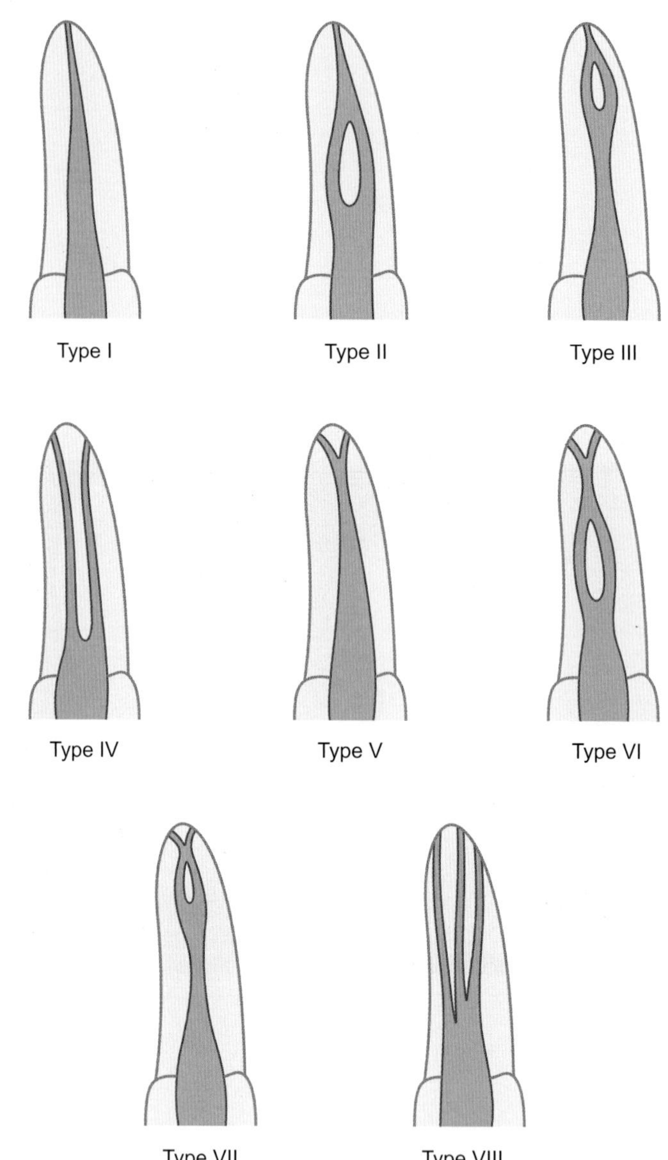

Fig. 2.58 Types of root canal configuration. From Chong, B.S. (Ed.), 2016. *Harty's endodontics in clinical practice, seventh ed.* Elsevier, with permission.

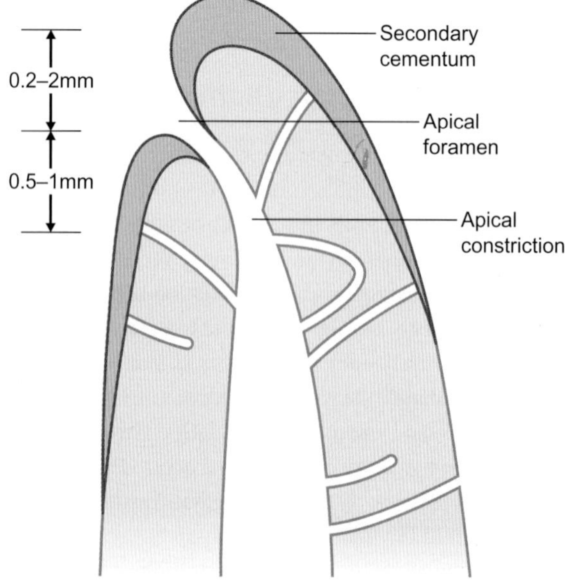

Fig. 2.59 Diagrammatic section through apical third of root showing position of apical constriction. From Chong, B.S. (Ed.), 2016. *Harty's endodontics in clinical practice,* seventh ed. Elsevier, with permission.

Incisors

Maxillary first (central) permanent incisor

Viewed from the labial aspect, the pulp chamber of the maxillary first permanent incisor (Figs 2.60, 2.61) follows the outline of the crown, being widest towards the incisal edge. In a young tooth, the pulp chamber has three

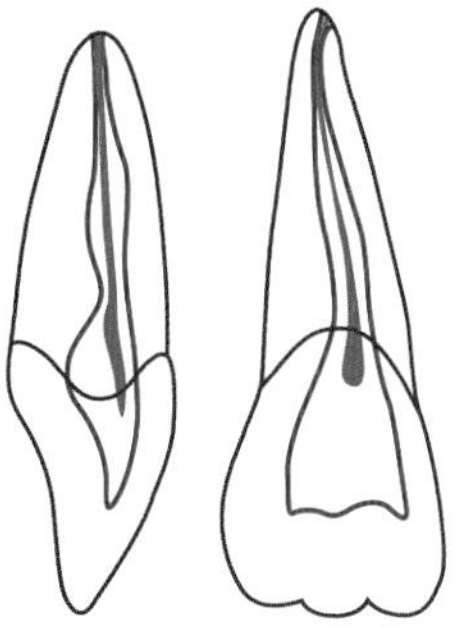

Fig. 2.60 Schematic representation of the pulp morphology of the maxillary first permanent incisor.

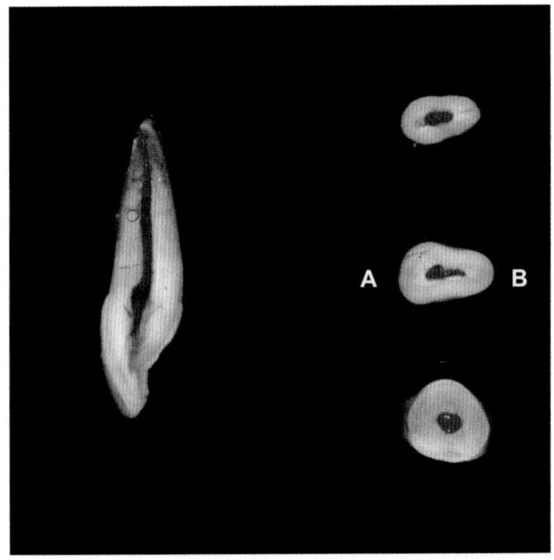

Fig. 2.61 Sectioned maxillary first permanent incisor demonstrating pulp morphology. A = labial; B = palatal.

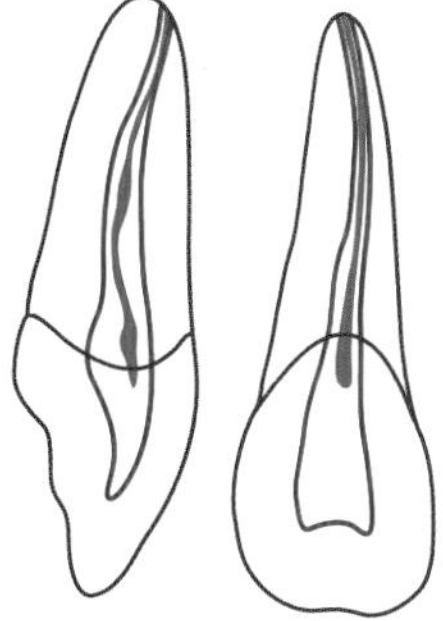

Fig. 2.62 Schematic representation of the pulp morphology of the maxillary second permanent incisor.

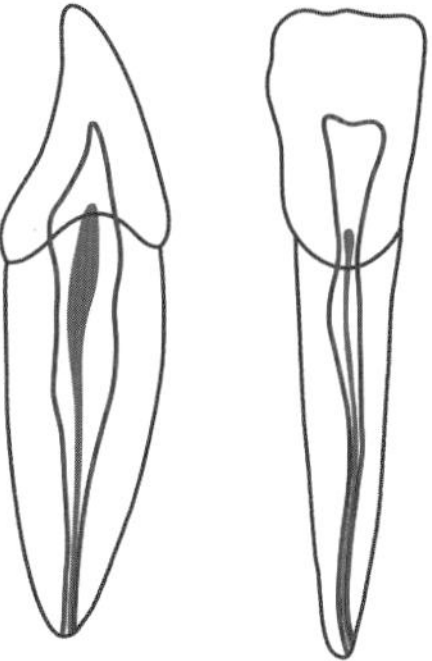

Fig. 2.63 Schematic representation of the pulp morphology of the mandibular first permanent incisor.

pulp horns that correspond to the mamelons present during development. Viewed distally, the pulp tapers towards the incisal edge and widens cervically. A constriction (the cervical bulge) separates the single and centrally placed root canal from the pulp chamber. The root canal tapers towards the apical foramen, where it may curve slightly either distally or labially. In cross-section, the root canal is ovoid for much of its extent but, in common with canals in other teeth, becomes round as it nears the apex. With age, the dimensions of the pulp chamber and root canal are reduced as secondary dentine is laid down. The pulp chamber recedes and may disappear completely. In conducting root canal therapy on older teeth, locating the root canal in the absence of a pulp chamber may be the major clinical challenge.

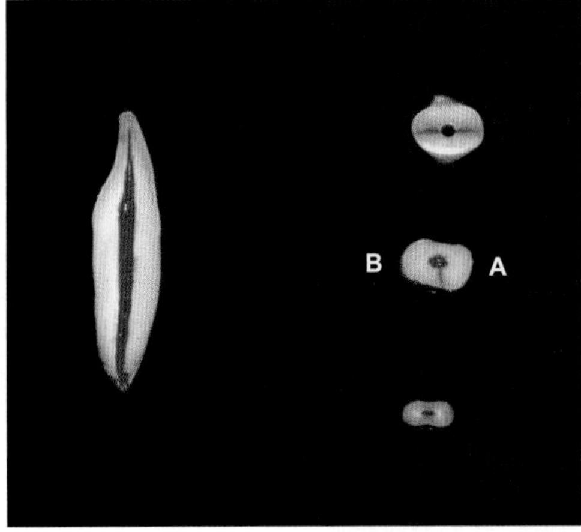

Fig. 2.64 Sectioned mandibular first permanent incisor demonstrating pulp morphology. A = labial; B = lingual.

Maxillary second (lateral) permanent incisor

The pulp chamber of this incisor (Fig. 2.62) is similar to, but smaller than, that of the maxillary central incisor. The root canal is single, slightly ovoid and commonly curves both distally and palatally.

Mandibular first (central) permanent incisor

The pulp chamber of the mandibular first permanent incisor is similar to that described for the maxillary first incisor, although, being in a much smaller tooth, it is smaller (Figs 2.63, 2.64). The pulp chamber is oval in cross-section, being wider labiolingually than mesiodistally, and is constricted at the cervical margin. The root canal is ovoid, becoming round in the apical third. As many as 30% of mandibular first incisors have two root canals, although most of these fuse near the apex and exit by a single foramen.

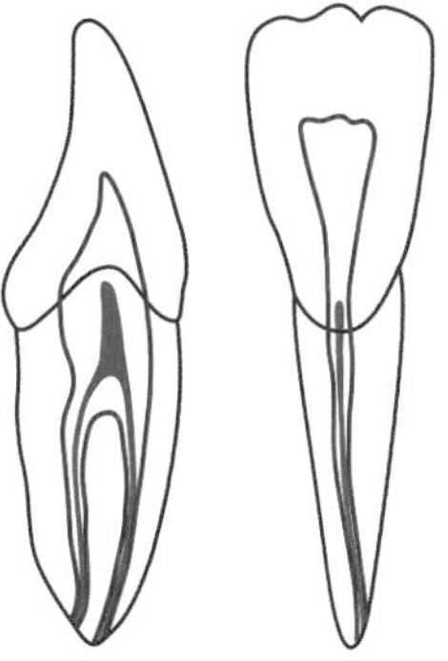

Fig. 2.65 Schematic representation of the pulp morphology of the mandibular second permanent incisor.

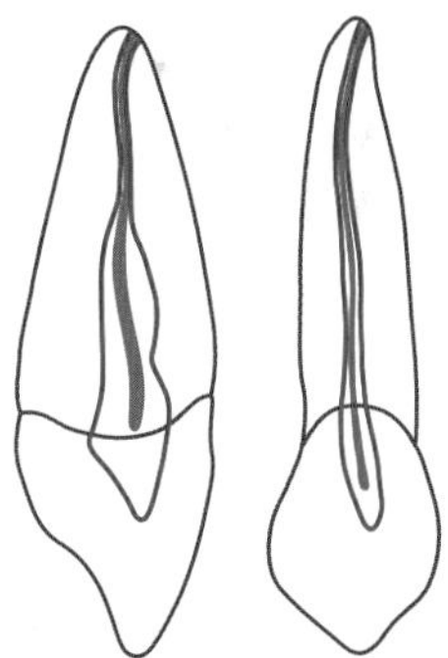

Fig. 2.66 Schematic representation of the pulp morphology of the maxillary permanent canine.

Mandibular second (lateral) permanent incisor

Both tooth and root canal systems are larger than those of the mandibular first incisor (Fig. 2.65). Two root canals are somewhat more common (43%). Most of these root canals exit by separate foramina.

Canines

Maxillary permanent canine

The pulp chamber of the maxillary permanent canine is narrow, with a single pulp horn that points cuspally (Figs 2.66, 2.67). Both the pulp chamber and the single root canal are wider labiopalatally than mesiodistally. The root canal does not constrict markedly until the apical third of the root is reached. The root canal, which is always single, is oval or triangular in cross-section except at its apical third, where it is round.

Mandibular permanent canine

The pulp cavity of the mandibular permanent canine (Figs 2.68, 2.69) resembles that of the maxillary permanent canine, although it is smaller in all dimensions. The root canal is oval in cross-section, being wider buccopalatally, but becomes round apically. About 6% of these teeth have two root canals, usually with separate foramina.

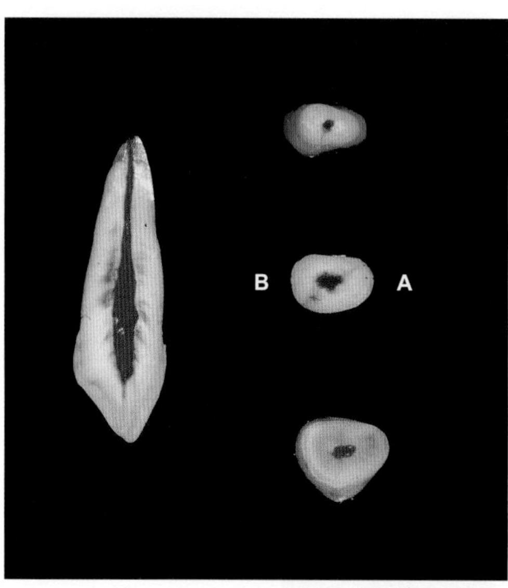

Fig. 2.67 Sectioned maxillary permanent canine demonstrating pulp morphology. A = labial; B = palatal.

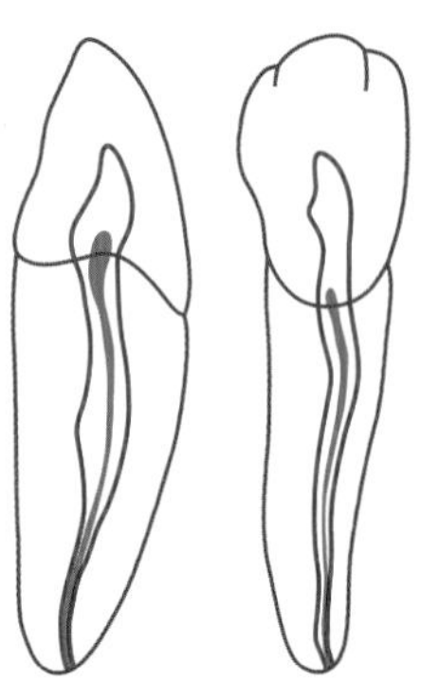

Fig. 2.68 Schematic representation of the pulp morphology of the mandibular permanent canine.

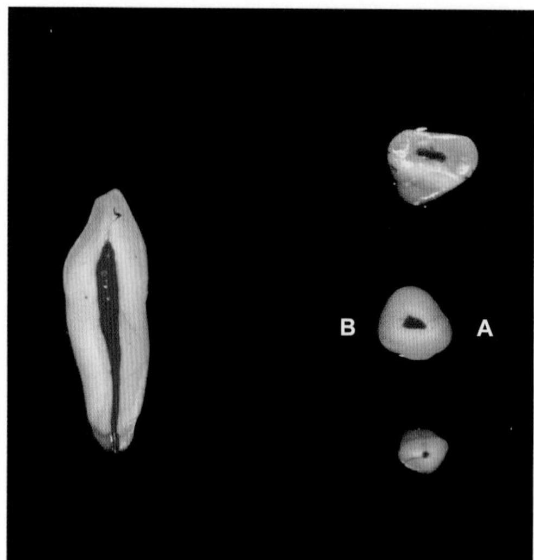

Fig. 2.69 Sectioned mandibular permanent canine tooth demonstrating pulp morphology. A = labial; B = lingual.

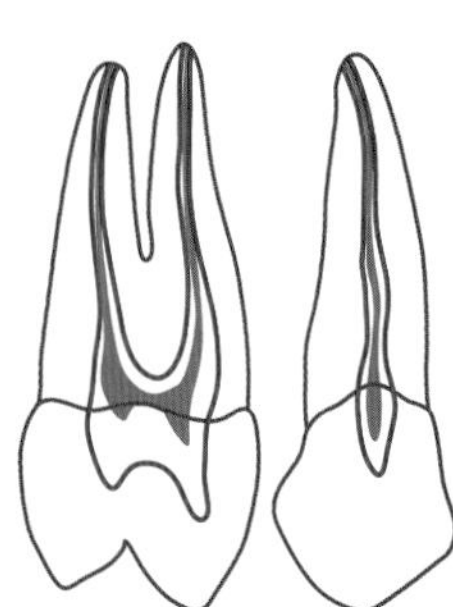

Fig. 2.70 Schematic representation of the pulp morphology of the maxillary first premolar.

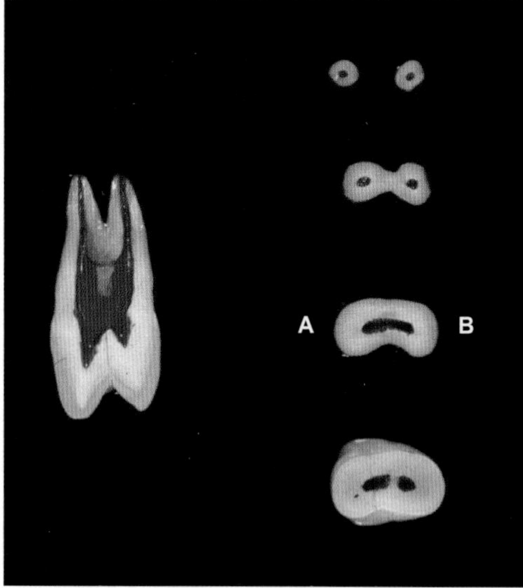

Fig. 2.71 Sectioned maxillary first premolar demonstrating pulp morphology. A = buccal; B = palatal.

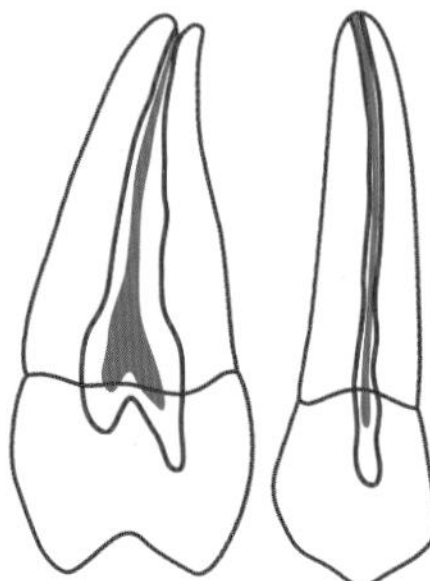

Fig. 2.72 Schematic representation of the pulp morphology of the maxillary second premolar.

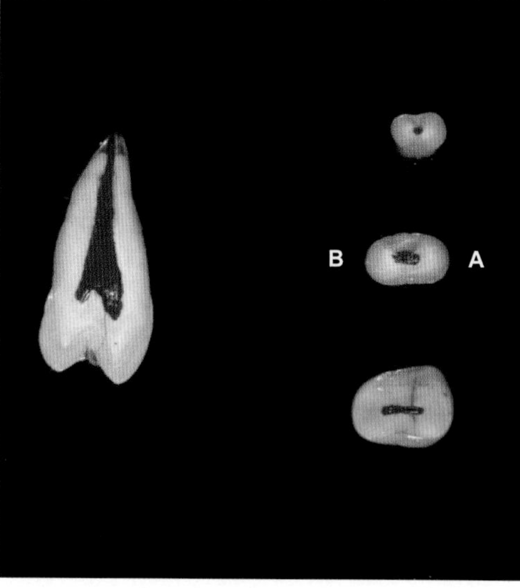

Fig. 2.73 Sectioned maxillary second premolar demonstrating pulp morphology. A = buccal; B = palatal.

Premolars

Maxillary first premolar

The maxillary first premolar usually has two roots (85% of cases), although they are sometimes fused (Figs 2.70, 2.71). The two canals generally exit by separate foramina. A single root and single canal are present in less than 10% of cases. A small number (5%) have three canals (sometimes in three roots). The pulp chamber is wide buccopalatally with two distinct pulp horns pointing towards the cusps. From the buccal view, the pulp chamber is much narrower. The floor of the pulp chamber is rounded, with the highest point in the centre. It usually lies within the root just apical to the cervix. Where the root canals arise from the pulp chamber, the orifices are funnel-shaped. The pulp chamber is closest to the surface mesially, where the shape of the crown is indented by the canine fossa. The dental pulp may be exposed in this area by caries or restorative cavities that are extended interproximally. The root canals diverge but are usually straight individually and taper evenly from their origin to the apical foramina. In cross-section, the root canals are generally round. With age, the general shape of the pulp cavity remains the same, but its dimensions, particularly the height of the pulp chamber, are reduced.

Maxillary second premolar

The maxillary second premolar has in most instances (75%) a single root with a single root canal (Figs 2.72, 2.73). Its pulp chamber extends apically well below the cervical margin. The appearance of the pulp cavity viewed from the buccal aspect is similar to that in the first premolar. When two canals are present, they most commonly have separate apical foramina. In cross-section the root canal is oval until the apical third of the root, where it becomes round.

Mandibular first premolar

The pulp chamber in the mandibular first premolar (Figs 2.74, 2.75), as for the maxillary premolars, is wider buccolingually than mesiodistally. Unlike the maxillary premolars, there is usually only one pulp horn, which

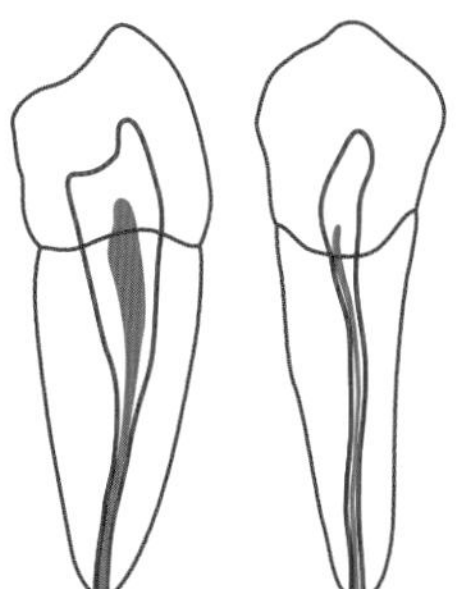

Fig. 2.74 Schematic representation of the pulp morphology of the mandibular first premolar.

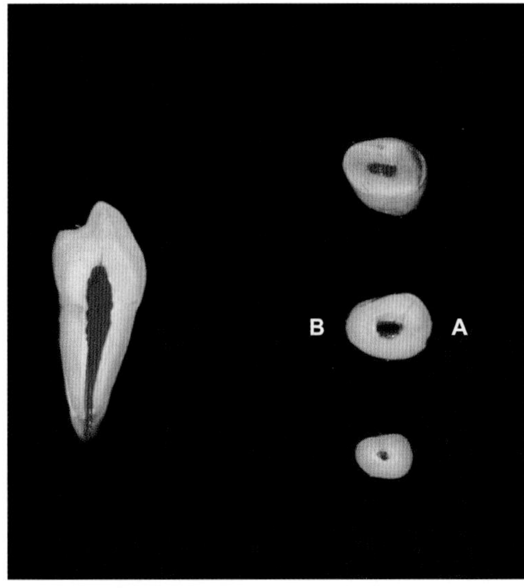

Fig. 2.75 Sectioned mandibular first premolar demonstrating pulp morphology. A = buccal; B = lingual.

extends into the buccal cusp. Occasionally, a small pulp horn may pass to the reduced lingual cusp. There is usually a single root canal (in 75% of cases) that becomes constricted towards the middle third of the root. Most teeth that have two canals have two apical foramina.

Mandibular second premolar

The pulp morphology of the mandibular second premolar differs little from that described for the mandibular first premolar, although a higher proportion (85%) have single canals, and there are usually two well-developed pulp horns projecting towards its cusps (Fig. 2.76).

Molars

Maxillary first permanent molar

The pulp chamber of the maxillary first permanent molar is rhomboidal in shape, being wider buccopalatally than mesiodistally (Figs 2.77, 2.78). Four pulp horns arise from the roof, one for each of the major cusps. The pulp horn to the mesiobuccal cusp is the longest. The floor of the pulp chamber generally lies below the cervical margin. Three root canals are present (or four in 60% of cases), their orifices being funnel-shaped. The root canal of the mesiobuccal root leaves the pulp chamber in a mesial direction and is often significantly curved. In cross-section, it appears as a narrow slit, being wider buccopalatally. Its anatomy may be complicated by irregular branching or bifurcation near the apical foramen. When a fourth canal is present, it is in the mesiobuccal root. Two-thirds of the fourth canals rejoin the main canal of the mesiobuccal root near the root apex. The palatal root canal is the widest and longest of the root canals. The floor of the pulp chamber is marked by a series of developmental grooves that join the orifices of the root canals.

Maxillary second permanent molar

The pulp cavity of the maxillary second permanent molar is similar to that of the first molar, but smaller with the rhomboidal shape more compressed (Fig. 2.79). The roots of this tooth are more convergent, bringing the root canal orifices closer together on the pulpal floor. The roots are commonly

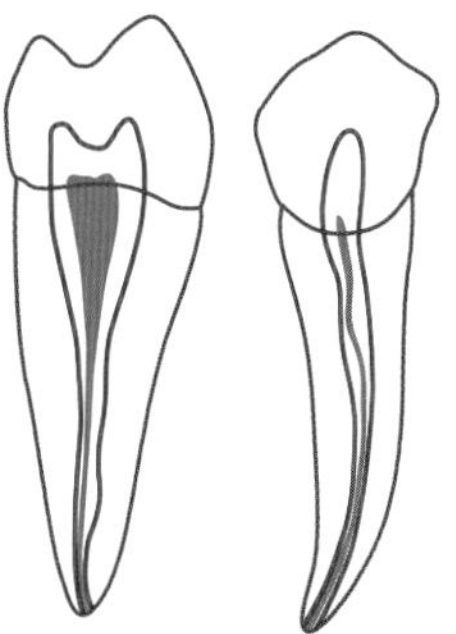

Fig. 2.76 Schematic representation of the pulp morphology of the mandibular second premolar.

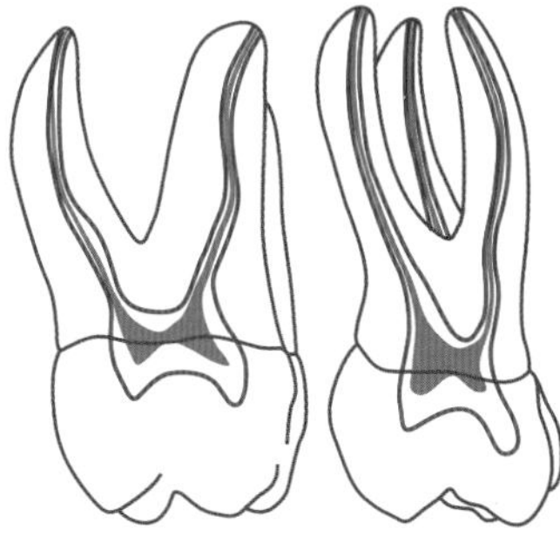

Fig. 2.77 Schematic representation of the pulp morphology of the maxillary first permanent molar.

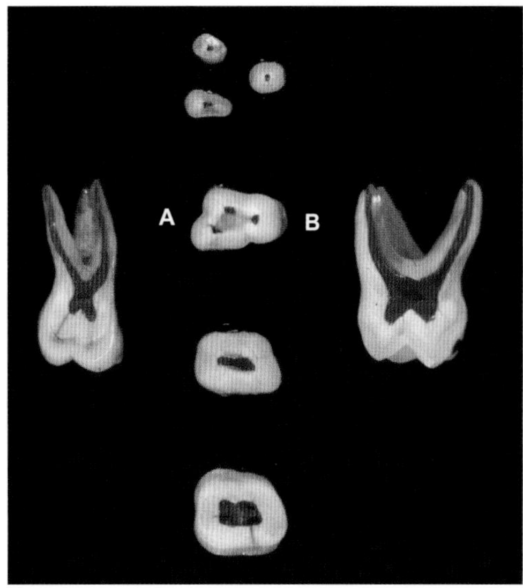

Fig. 2.78 Sectioned maxillary first permanent molar demonstrating pulp morphology. The tooth on the left shows the root canals of the mesiobuccal and palatal roots, while that on the right shows the two buccal root canals. A = buccal; B = palatal.

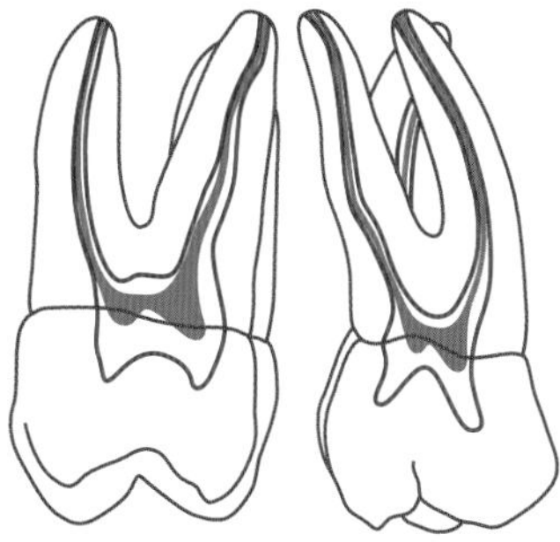

Fig. 2.79 Schematic representation of the pulp morphology of the maxillary second permanent molar.

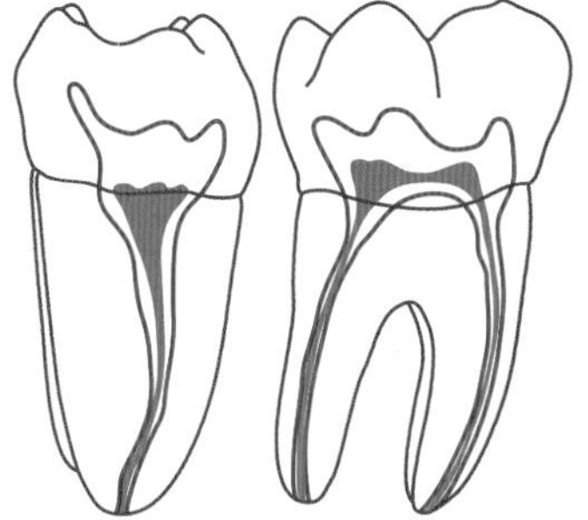

Fig. 2.80 Schematic representation of the pulp morphology of the mandibular first permanent molar.

fused. A second mesiobuccal canal is less common than in the first molar (40% of cases).

Mandibular first permanent molar

The pulp chamber in the mandibular first permanent molar is wider mesiodistally than buccolingually (Figs 2.80, 2.81). It is also wider mesially than distally. There are five pulp horns projecting to the cusps, the lingual pulp horns being longer and more pointed. The floor of the pulp chamber lies at, or just below, the level of the cervical margin. The root canals leave the pulp chamber through funnel-shaped orifices, of which the mesial are finer than the distal. The mesial root has two root canals, mesiobuccal and mesiolingual. The mesiobuccal root canal follows a curved path, while the mesiolingual canal is straighter; both are circular

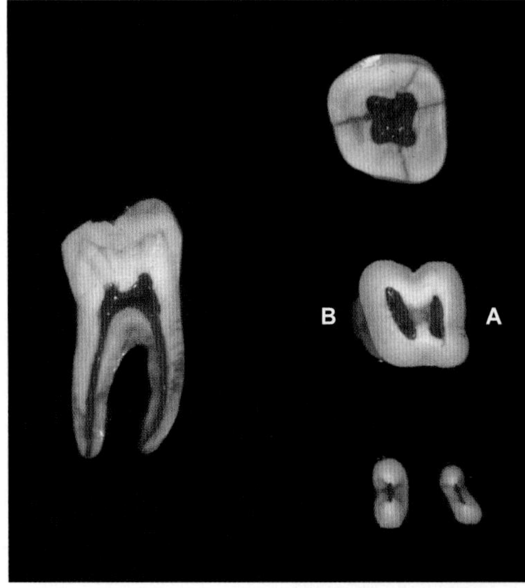

Fig. 2.81 Sectioned mandibular first permanent molar demonstrating pulp morphology. A = buccal; B = lingual.

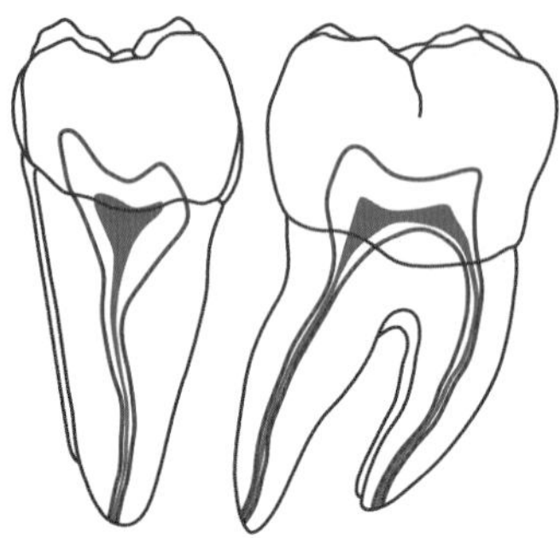

Fig. 2.82 Schematic representation of the pulp morphology of the mandibular second permanent molar.

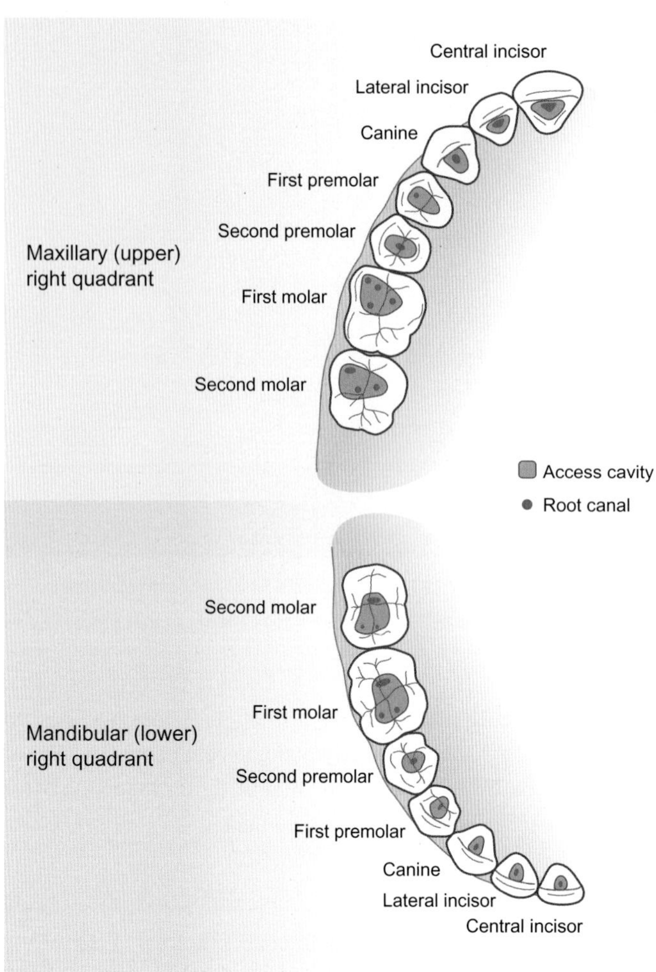

Fig. 2.83 Outline of access cavities (red) necessary to gain entrance into the root canals (blue) of the permanent dentition.

in cross-section. In 30% of teeth, the distal root has two canals. The distal canal, especially when single, is considerably larger and more oval in cross-section than the mesial root canals and follows a straighter course.

Mandibular second permanent molar

The pulp morphology of the mandibular second permanent molar closely resembles that of the adjacent first molar, although there are only four pulp horns and only rarely (8% of cases) two canals in the distal root (Fig. 2.82).

Knowledge of both tooth morphology and dental pulp anatomy is essential during endodontic therapy when, because of disease, the pulp is not able to repair itself. In this situation, it may be necessary to remove the contents of the pulp chamber and root canals and replace them with a suitable root canal filling. Access cavities must then first be cut into the crown to expose the pulp chamber. The cavity must allow for complete vision of the root canal openings and provide straight-line access into the root canals. The anatomy of the pulp reflects the general anatomy of the tooth, but, as previously mentioned, its dimensions decrease with age as secondary dentine is deposited. The general shapes and positions of access cavities are shown in Fig. 2.83. "Laws" have been devised to help the student learn the features of access cavities shown in Table 2.6.

Shape of the pulp chamber in deciduous teeth

As for permanent teeth, the shape of the deciduous pulp chamber reflects the shape of the crown, but, in the deciduous teeth, the chamber is relatively larger and the pulp horns longer and closer to the surface of the tooth. All incisors and canines have single canals that are either round or oval (being compressed mesiodistally). In 10% of deciduous mandibular incisors there are two root canals. The pulp chambers of deciduous mandibular molars are proportionately larger than those of the deciduous maxillary molars. The mesiobuccal pulp horn in deciduous molars is particularly near to the occlusal surface and thus highly vulnerable to exposure by dental caries, trauma or cavity preparation. Small canals running from the pulp chamber to the furcation region are common in deciduous molars. In the slender roots of deciduous molars, the root canals are narrower mesiodistally and more ribbon-shaped than those in permanent teeth. This, and the severe curvature of deciduous roots, makes complete debridement and obturation of the root canal system difficult. Although pulpotomy is the more common treatment for the diseased deciduous pulp, pulpectomy and canal obturation are feasible. When resorption of the deciduous root begins, it commences on the lingual surfaces of the anterior teeth and furcal surfaces of molars; this complicates root canal therapy, as the exit to the canal system becomes very wide and may be some distance from the root end as visualised radiographically. Other features to bear in mind are:

- The maxillary first deciduous molar has two to four root canals, with two canals in the mesiobuccal root in 75% of cases. The palatal and distobuccal roots are often fused (one-third of cases) but contain distinct canals.
- The maxillary second deciduous molar has two to five root canals (Fig. 2.84). The mesiobuccal root usually bifurcates or contains two canals (90% of cases). Palatal and distobuccal roots sometimes fuse and contain a single, common canal.

Table 2.6 Laws relating to pulp chamber anatomy

Law of centrality	The floor of the pulp chamber is always located in the centre of the tooth at the level of the cemento-enamel junction (CEJ).
Law of concentricity	At the level of the CEJ, the shape of the pulp chamber mimics the external anatomy of the tooth.
Law of the CEJ	The distance from the external surface of the tooth to the wall of the pulp chamber is the same throughout the circumference of the tooth at the level of the CEJ. The CEJ is the most reliable and consistent feature for ascertaining the position of the pulp chamber.
First law of symmetry	With the exception of the maxillary molar, the orifices of the canals are equidistant either side of a line drawn mesial to distal through the floor of the pulp chamber.
Second law of symmetry	With the exception of the maxillary molars, the orifices of the canals lie on a line perpendicular to the line drawn mesial to distal through the floor of the pulp chamber.
The law of colour change	The dentine of the floor of the pulp chamber is invariably a darker colour than the roof and walls. With good magnification and illumination, this allows the clinician to differentiate and selectively remove tissue.
First law of orifice location	The orifices of the root canals are located where the walls and the floor meet.
Second law of orifice location	The orifices of the root canals are located at the angles in the floor/wall junctions.
Third law of orifice location	The orifices of the root canals are located at the ends of the root developmental fusion lines.

Adapted from Krasner and Rankow and Peters. 2016. In: Chong, B.S. (Ed.), *Harty's endodontics in clinical practice*. seventh ed. Elsevier, London.

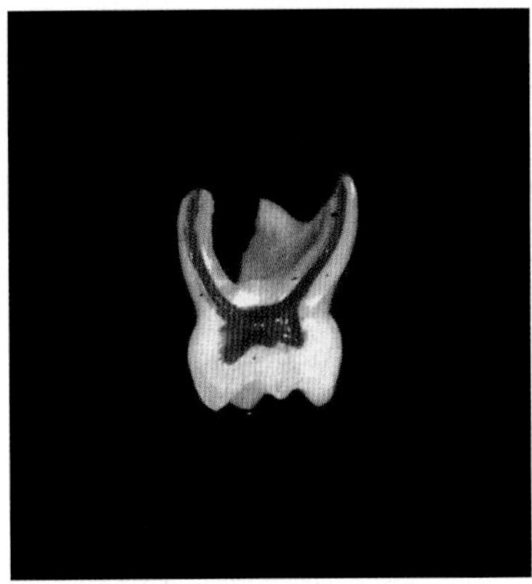

Fig. 2.84 Sectioned maxillary second deciduous molar demonstrating pulp morphology.

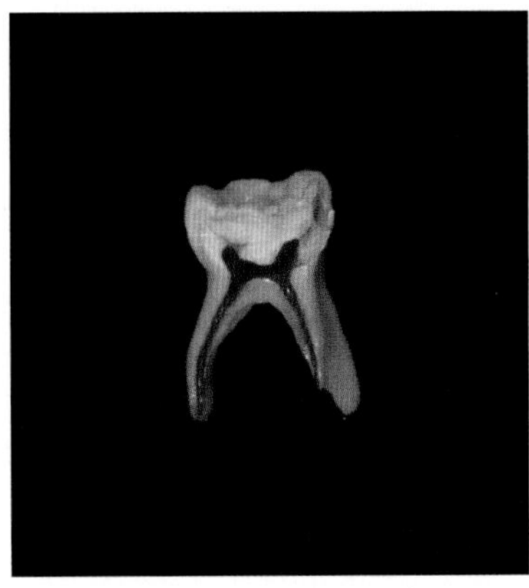

Fig. 2.85 Sectioned mandibular second deciduous molar demonstrating pulp morphology.

- The mandibular first deciduous molar may have two to four canals. Most mesial roots (75%) have two canals.
- The mandibular second deciduous molar usually has three canals but can vary from two to five (Fig. 2.85). Two canals are seen in 85% of mesial roots, but only 25% of distal roots have two canals.

Alignment and occlusion of the permanent teeth

The relationships of the teeth, both within and between the dental arches, are of fundamental importance to an understanding of mastication and for such clinical disciplines as orthodontics and restorative dentistry. *Tooth alignment* is the term that refers to the arrangement of the teeth within the dental arches; *occlusion* refers to the relationship of the dental arches when tooth contact is made.

Traditionally, textbooks describe a standard set of tooth relationships that is called 'normal' (i.e., normal alignment and normal occlusion). Normal is a term that is generally used to describe situations that are the ordinary or most frequent; alternatively, normal may define an authoritative standard or ideal that, in medical terms, is the healthy state. In these terms, malocclusions could be regarded as normal for they are more commonly found in the population than 'normal' occlusion (approximately 75% of the population of the United States has some degree of occlusal 'disharmony').

Malocclusions do not always predispose to dental disease and, in most cases, are not associated with masticatory dysfunction, speech defects, bruxism or pain in and around the temporomandibular joint. Furthermore, our knowledge of the association between the structure and function of the dental arches during mastication is not yet sufficient to provide an authoritative standard for tooth relationships; in structural terms, the ideal occlusion is a rather subjective concept. If there is an ideal occlusion, it can presently be defined only in broad functional terms. We believe therefore that the occlusion is 'ideal' when:

- The teeth are aligned such that the masticatory loads are within physiological range and act through the long axes of as many teeth in the arch as possible.
- Mastication involves alternating bilateral jaw movements (and not habitual, unilateral biting preferences as a result of adaptation to occlusal interference).
- Lateral jaw movements occur without undue mechanical interference.
- In the rest position of the jaw, the gap between teeth (the freeway space; see pages 46–47) is correct for the individual concerned.
- The tooth alignment is aesthetically pleasing to its possessor.

Despite our reservations, the traditional descriptions of 'normal' tooth relationships provide a convenient model for the classification of malocclusions in clinical situations. However, we have chosen to use the terms 'anatomical alignment' and 'anatomical occlusion' instead of 'normal alignment' and 'normal occlusion' in order to avoid the difficulties of defining normality with respect to tooth relationships. The occlusion of the deciduous dentition and the development of occlusion are considered in Chapter 26.

Anatomical alignment of teeth

Each dental arch (maxillary/upper and mandibular/lower) generally takes the form of a catenary curve (Fig. 2.86). Such a curve is described when a rope or chain is hung at both ends. There are no spacings or rotations of teeth within the arch, and therefore all teeth are in contact with neighbouring teeth along the arch.

Superimposed on the occlusal surfaces of the teeth shown in Fig. 2.86 are Angle's 'lines of occlusion'. Because the maxillary arch is broader than the mandibular arch, the line of occlusion for the maxillary arch passes through the cingula of the anterior teeth and through the central fossae of the posterior teeth. However, the line of occlusion for the mandibular arch runs along the incisal edges of the anterior teeth and along the buccal cusps of the posterior teeth.

The well-aligned dental arch may be divided into different segments. A curved line in the coronal plane describes the anterior segment. This segment extends across the midline from canine to canine. The middle

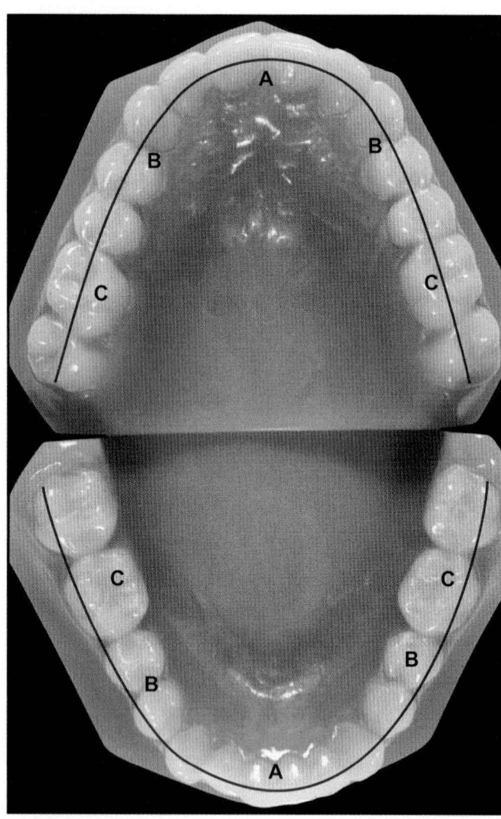

Fig. 2.86 The form of the maxillary and mandibular dental arches showing the anatomical alignment of the teeth and Angle's lines of occlusion. A = Anterior segment; B = Middle segment; C = Posterior segment.

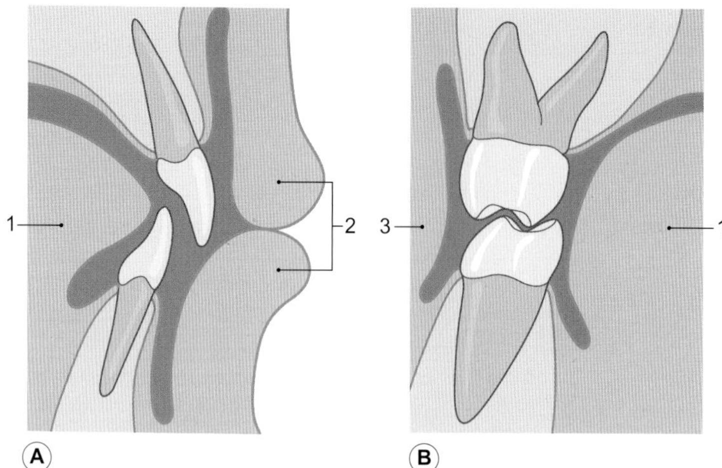

Fig. 2.87 The configuration of the neutral zone (the dark pink area) in the incisor region (A) and the molar region (B). 1 = tongue; 2 = lips; 3 = cheek. Redrawn after Jordan, R.E., 1992. Kraus' dental anatomy and occlusion. second ed. Mosby year Book, St Louis.

Table 2.7 Average widths of the dental arches (males)

Age (years)	Between maxillary canines (mm)	Between mandibular canines (mm)	Between maxillary first molars (mm)	Between mandibular first molars (mm)
6	28	23	42	40
18	32	25	47	43

segments are described by straight lines extending from the distal edges of the canines to the mesiobuccal cusps of the first molars. The posterior segments extend from the mesiobuccal cusps of the first molars backwards. Both the middle and posterior segments lie in the sagittal plane, the posterior segments being more nearly parallel to this plane than the middle segments.

The positions of the teeth within the dental arch are determined by numerous factors and forces. Indeed, the spatial configuration of the arches is dependent upon an interaction between the eruptive movements carrying the teeth into their functional positions and, once erupted, the forces brought to bear upon each tooth. The term 'neutral zone' is used to describe that space in which there is equilibrium of forces so that the teeth attain a position of relative stability (Fig. 2.87). A change in balance in this system, such as that produced by abnormal tongue-thrusting behaviour and abnormal lip posture, can result in malalignment of the teeth.

The size of the dental arches varies considerably between individuals. Table 2.7 provides the average widths of the dental arches for the completed deciduous dentition (6 years) and the completed permanent dentition (18 years) for males. Averages for females are usually 1 mm less.

Figs 2.88–2.95 describe the angulation or axial positioning of individual teeth within the alveolus relative to perpendiculars dropped from a hypothetically flat occlusal plane. In these diagrams, the angles quoted are average figures, although variation is considerable.

Viewed labially, the maxillary incisors have slight distal inclinations, whereas the canine has a distinct mesial angulation. When these teeth are viewed distally, all show pronounced proclinations into the lip (although the canine is slightly more vertical). For the mandibular incisors and canine, when viewed labially, the incisors are more or less vertical and the canine has a slight mesial inclination. When viewed distally, these anterior mandibular teeth, like the anterior maxillary teeth, are proclined.

When viewed buccally, the maxillary premolars and molars change from a slight mesial angulation (premolars) to a distal inclination (the third molar). This contrasts with the mandibular posterior teeth, which show increasing mesial inclination moving back through the arch. When the maxillary premolars and molars are viewed distally, the teeth change from being essentially vertical in the premolar region to being distinctly buccally inclined in the molars. This again contrasts with the mandibular premolars and molars, where the teeth become more lingually inclined moving through the arch.

Curvatures of the teeth and arches

The impression could readily be gained from Figs 2.88–2.95 that the axes of the teeth are straight and run perpendicular to a horizontal, flat, occlusal plane. However, neither the axes of the teeth nor the occlusal planes are straight, but are curved in all directions (Figs 2.96, 2.97). The curved axes of the teeth have a tendency to parallelism and are inclined mesially. It is often thought, mistakenly so, that the forces of mastication are at right angles to the occlusal surfaces of the teeth. If this were so, and if the occlusal planes and axes of the teeth were not curved, the arches might not be stable and the masticatory loads might be at an unfavourable angle to the teeth. It is thought that during mastication the loads strike the teeth such that there is a mesial component of force (see page 472). The occlusal plane shows two types of curvature – the curve of Spee and the curve of Wilson.

The teeth align themselves such that the occlusal plane is not flat but describes a relatively linear curve in the anteroposterior direction, the curve of Spee (Fig. 2.98). The mandibular curve of Spee is concave, whereas the maxillary curve is convex. An appreciation of the contribution of each tooth to the curve of Spee may be gained from analysis of the alignment

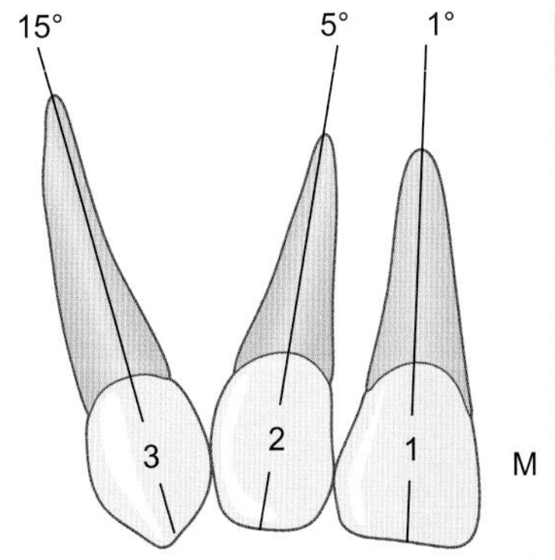

Fig. 2.88 The alignment of the maxillary incisors and canine viewed labially. The teeth are not drawn to scale, and the numerical dental shorthand is used to identify the tooth. All angles quoted are average figures. M = mesial.

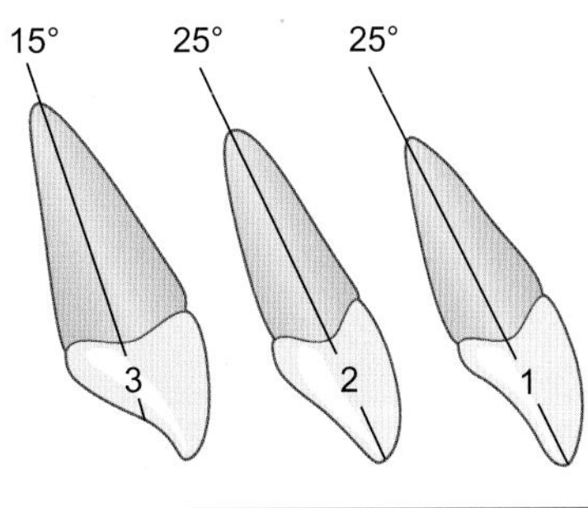

Fig. 2.89 The alignment of the maxillary incisors and canine viewed distally. The teeth are not drawn to scale, and the numerical dental shorthand is used to identify the tooth. All angles quoted are average figures.

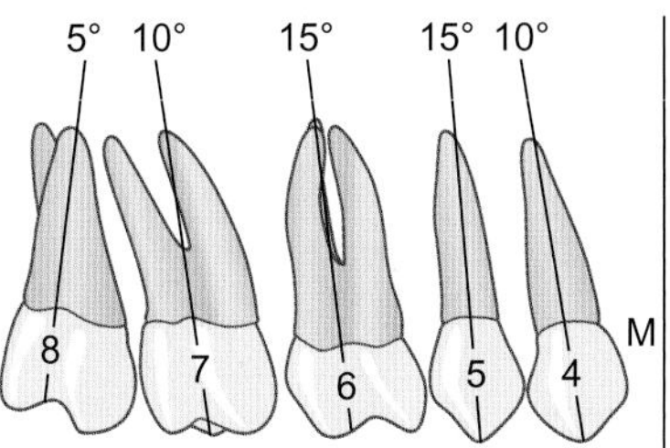

Fig. 2.90 The alignment of the maxillary premolars and molars viewed buccally. The teeth are not drawn to scale, and the numerical dental shorthand is used to identify the tooth. All angles quoted are average figures. M = mesial.

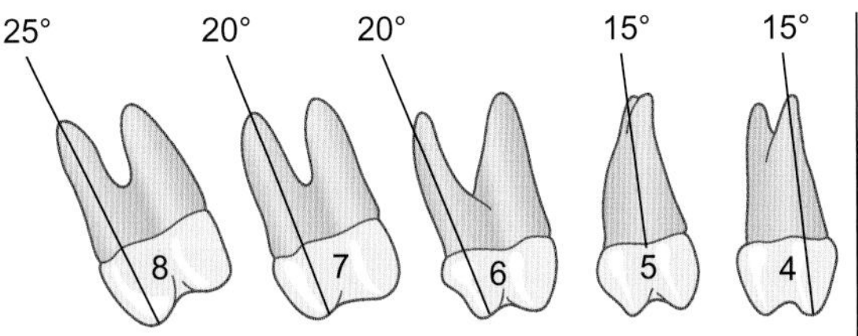

Fig. 2.91 The alignment of the maxillary premolars and molars viewed distally. The teeth are not drawn to scale, and the numerical dental shorthand is used to identify the tooth. All angles quoted are average figures.

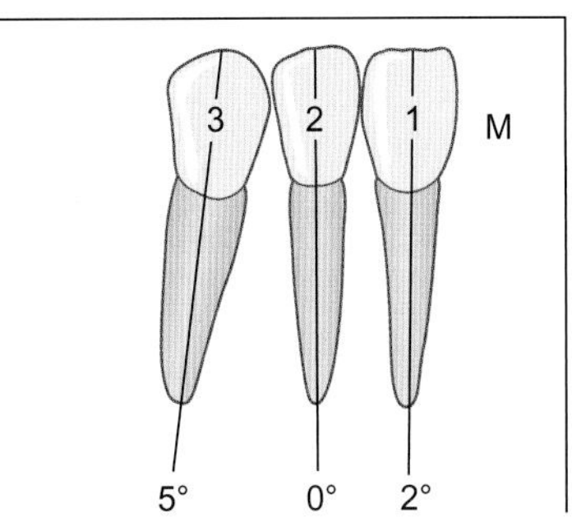

Fig. 2.92 The alignment of the mandibular incisors and canine viewed labially. The teeth are not drawn to scale, and the numerical dental shorthand is used to identify the tooth. All angles quoted are average figures. M = mesial.

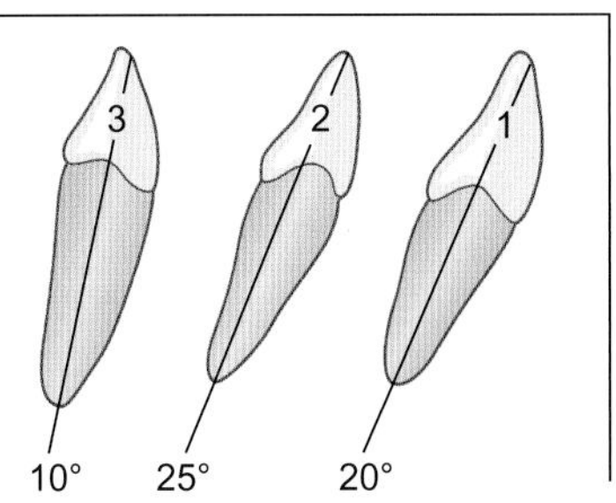

Fig. 2.93 The alignment of the mandibular incisors and canine viewed distally. The teeth are not drawn to scale, and the numerical dental shorthand is used to identify the tooth. All angles quoted are average figures.

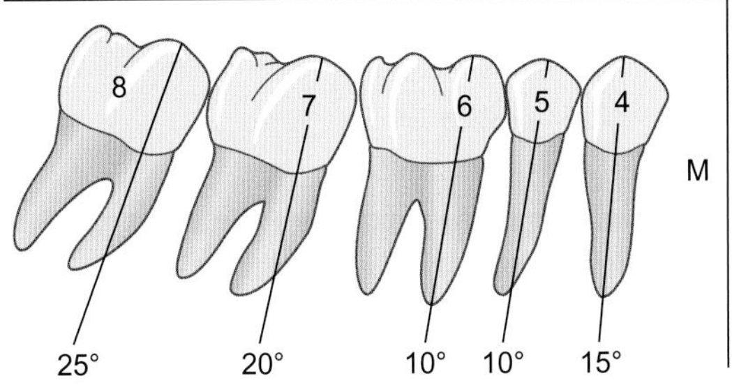

Fig. 2.94 The alignment of the mandibular premolars and molars viewed buccally. The teeth are not drawn to scale, and the numerical dental shorthand is used to identify the tooth. All angles quoted are average figures. M = mesial.

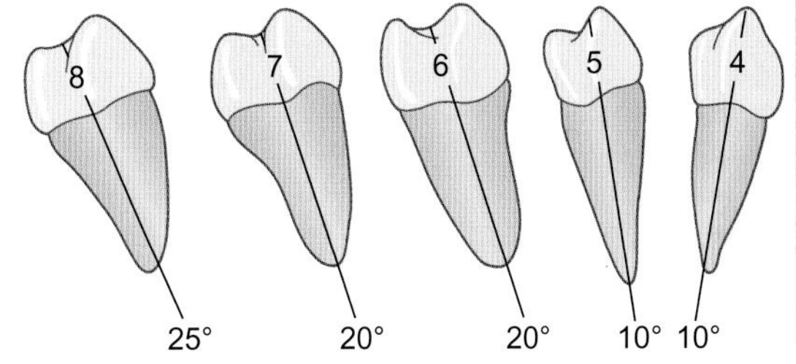

Fig. 2.95 The alignment of the mandibular premolars and molars viewed distally. The teeth are not drawn to scale, and the numerical dental shorthand is used to identify the tooth. All angles quoted are average figures.

of the long axes of the posterior teeth viewed buccally (Figs 2.90, 2.94) and from the axes of the anterior teeth viewed distally (Figs 2.89, 2.93). Although the maxillary and mandibular curves of Spee are different, they are complementary and thereby may help achieve occlusal balance during mastication by encouraging simultaneous contact in more than one area of the dental arches. If the curves are exaggerated, there will be crowding in the mandibular arch and increased spacing in the maxillary arch.

The occlusal curves of Wilson are aligned in the transverse plane (Fig. 2.99). Analysis of the alignment of the long axes of the posterior teeth shows that the curves of Wilson are such that the occlusal surfaces of the mandibular molars are directed lingually, while those of the maxillary molars are directed buccally (Figs 2.91, 2.95). As for the curves of Spee, the curves of Wilson for the maxillary and mandibular posterior teeth are opposite but complementary. The curves of Spee and Wilson were once thought to be related three-dimensionally, with the occlusal surfaces of the teeth being aligned on the curved surface of a segment of a sphere having a radius of about 10 cm. However, attempts to demonstrate, and then measure, the spherical curves (of Monson) have been unsuccessful.

With age, and as a result of wear (attrition), the cusps of the teeth are worn away so that the curvatures of the occlusal plane are lost and the plane becomes flat (Fig. 2.100). In addition, wear will affect the overjet and overbite for the anterior teeth (see pages 42–43) and the nature of the tooth contacts (see centric stops, page 43).

Anatomical occlusion of teeth

The relationships of the jaws in function are so variable that our understanding of the functional articulation of teeth remains poor. To simplify analysis, several occlusal positions have been strictly defined. These positions may be classified into those that are symmetrical and those that are asymmetrical. This corresponds with the classification of mandibular movements into symmetrical and asymmetrical movements. The symmetrical occlusal positions include centric occlusion and bilaterally protrusive position. The asymmetrical occlusal positions are those associated with lateral (side-to-side) movements. Within the clinic, centric occlusal position is regarded as the 'standard' or 'model' for orthodontic and prosthetic

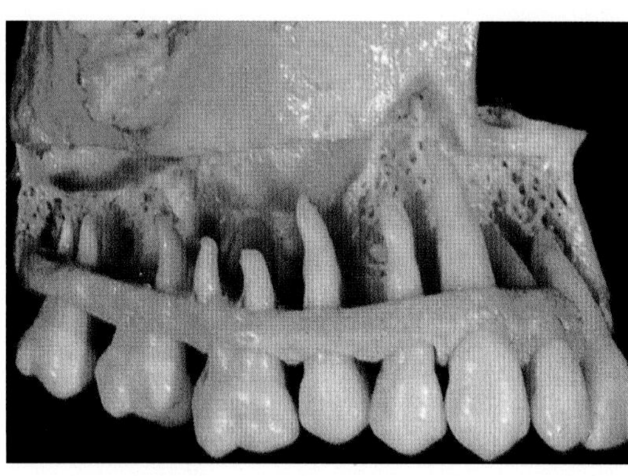

Fig. 2.96 The curvatures of the maxillary teeth within the alveolar bone of the maxilla.

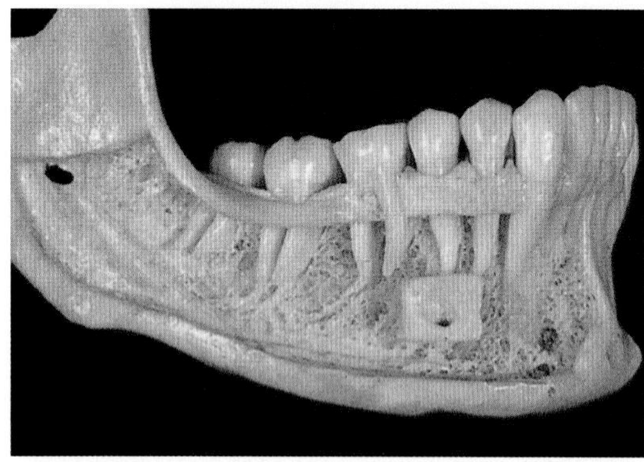

Fig. 2.97 The curvatures of the mandibular teeth within the alveolar bone of the mandible.

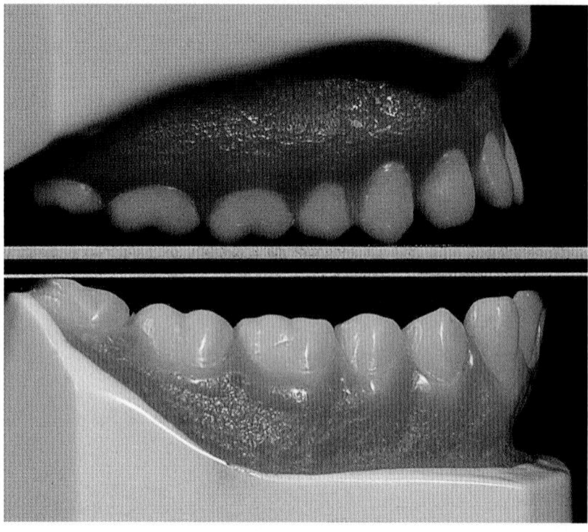

Fig. 2.98 Curvatures of the occlusal plane – the curves of Spee.

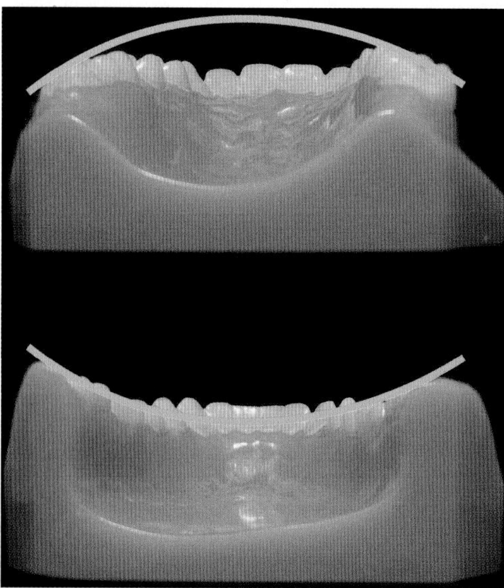

Fig. 2.99 Curvatures of the occlusal plane – the curves of Wilson.

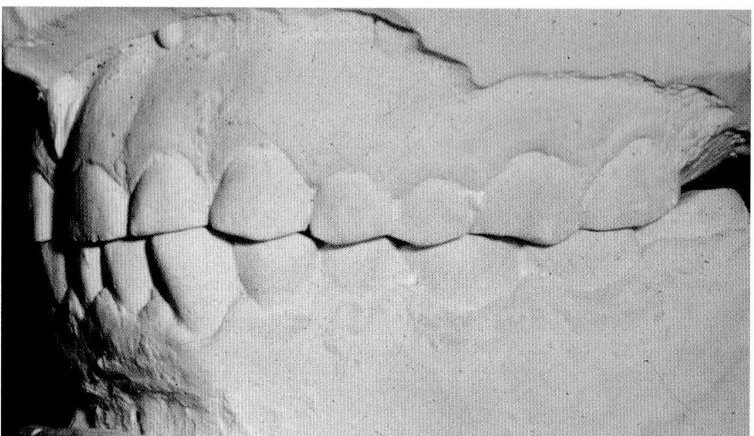

Fig. 2.100 Effects of wear on the curvatures of the occlusal plane, which becomes flat.

diagnoses and treatments. While it is important in the dental clinic to be confident that oral examinations are based upon an accurate recording of tooth relationships in centric occlusion, the consistent attainment of centric occlusal position for some patients is notoriously difficult. Clinicians have consequently developed a variety of strategies to attain this position, including palpating the mandibular condyles within the mandibular fossae; pronouncing certain sounds, words or phrases; fatiguing the mandible by asking the patient make rapid movements of the lower jaw; and even hypnosis.

Centric occlusal position

The centric occlusal position is defined as the terminal position of physiological jaw movements (Fig. 2.101). It is the relationship between the two arches when the teeth are brought into contact with the mandibular condyles centrally positioned at rest in the mandibular fossae.

According to the pioneer orthodontist Edward Angle, the key to the intercuspal relationships between the teeth in the centric occlusal position is to be found in the relative positions of the maxillary and mandibular first permanent molars. In the anatomical condition, each arch is bilaterally symmetrical. The anterior maxillary segment is slightly larger than the corresponding mandibular segment because of the unequal sizes of the maxillary and mandibular first incisors. Thus, each maxillary tooth will contact its corresponding mandibular antagonist and its distal neighbour. The maxillary first permanent molar will contact the distal part of the mandibular first permanent molar and the mesial part of the mandibular second permanent molar. The only exceptions are the mandibular first incisor and the maxillary third molar. The relationships between maxillary and mandibular permanent teeth in anatomical centric occlusal position are shown in Fig. 2.102.

Fig. 2.103 illustrates the relationships between the maxillary and mandibular permanent teeth in anatomical centric occlusion by superimposing the occlusal surfaces of the teeth in the maxillary arch on those of the mandibular arch. This diagram shows not only the general anteroposterior relationships of the maxillary teeth and their antagonists but also the buccolingual relationships of the arches. As the maxillary arch is a little larger and broader than the mandibular arch, there is a slight overlap of the mandibular arch by the maxillary arch such that the buccal cusps of the maxillary teeth extend a few millimetres beyond the buccal occlusal edges of the mandibular teeth. This overlap is termed *overjet*.

When the buccolingual incisor relationships in anatomical centric occlusion are considered, two types of 'overlap' of the mandibular incisors

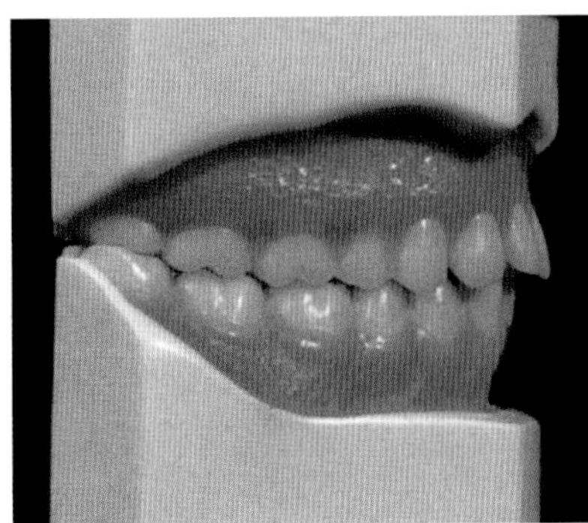

Fig. 2.101 Lateral view of the arrangement of teeth in anatomical centric occlusion.

Maxillary	8	7	6	5	4	3	2	1
Mandibular	8	7	6	5	4	3	2	1

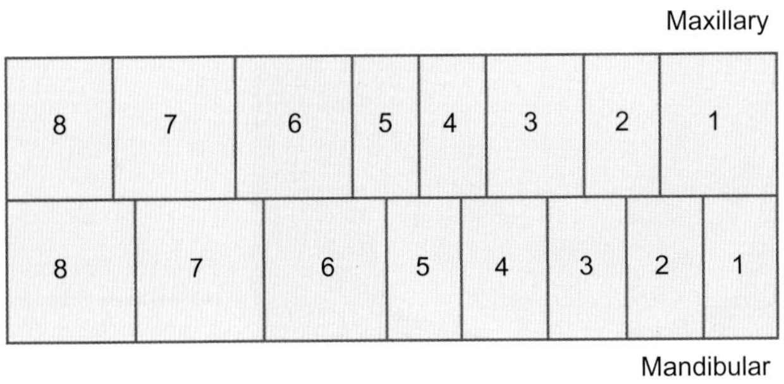

Fig. 2.102 Diagram illustrating the relationships between maxillary and mandibular permanent teeth in anatomical centric occlusal position. The teeth are identified according to the Palmer–Zsigmondy system.

by the maxillary incisors can be discerned (Figs 2.104, 2.105). The overlap in the horizontal plane (overjet) is approximately 2–3 mm. The vertical overlap, specific to the incisors and canines, is termed *overbite* (and is also approximately 2–3 mm). The overbite in anatomical centric occlusion is such that the palatal surfaces of the maxillary incisors on average overlap the incisal third of the labial surfaces of the mandibular incisors. Furthermore, the incisal edges of the mandibular incisors are related to the cingulum areas of the maxillary incisors. Fig. 2.106 provides a classification of overbite used in the orthodontic clinic. The dimensions of the overjet and overbite decrease with age and as a result of attrition.

Fig. 2.107 shows the occlusal surfaces of the permanent dentition marked with the positions of hard contact in anatomical centric occlusion. These contacts are termed 'centric stops' (also sometimes referred to as 'holding contacts') and represent the intercuspal contact positions. When the 32 teeth within the permanent dentition occlude, there are 138 centric stops, although this is seldom achieved during the normal bite. The major markings register on the occlusal surfaces of the posterior teeth (Fig. 2.107). The slopes of the maxillary palatal cusps make stops coincident with the stops within the central fossae of the mandibular posterior teeth. The stops in the central fossae of the maxillary teeth coincide with the stops on the slopes of the buccal cusps of the mandibular posterior teeth. The cusps seated in the central fossae are sometimes referred to as 'supporting cusps'. As befits the anatomical overjet relationships, the tips of the maxillary buccal cusps and the mandibular lingual cusps remain relatively unmarked. For the anterior teeth, the mandibular incisors have the centric stops on the incisal edges, whereas the stops on the maxillary incisors are positioned down their palatal surfaces.

Similar marks to centric stops can be made in the clinic by interposing articulating paper between the teeth and then instructing the patient to go into centric occlusal position. With age, and with attrition, the occlusal surfaces become flattened as the cusps are worn, and consequently the centric stops are significantly altered. Box 2.1 lists some of the main occlusal features of the dentition.

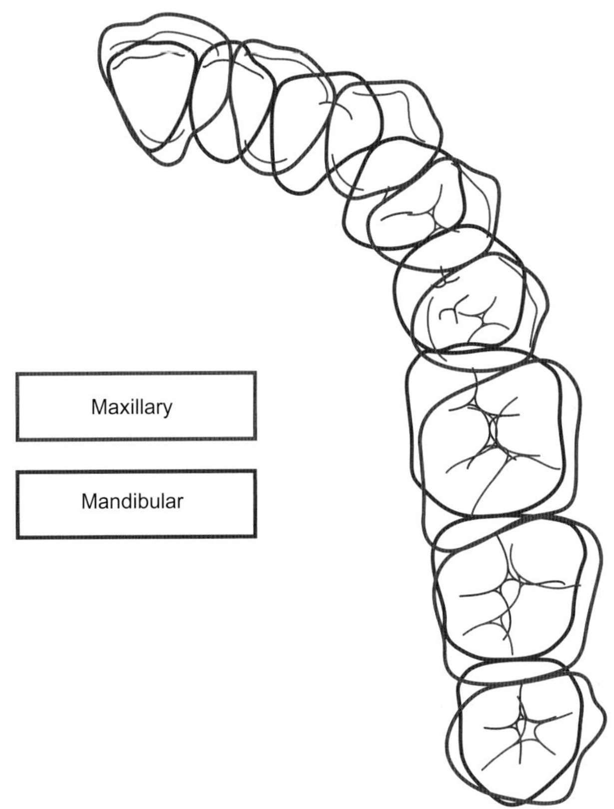

Fig. 2.103 The relationships between the occlusal surfaces of the maxillary (red) and mandibular (blue) permanent teeth in anatomical centric occlusion.

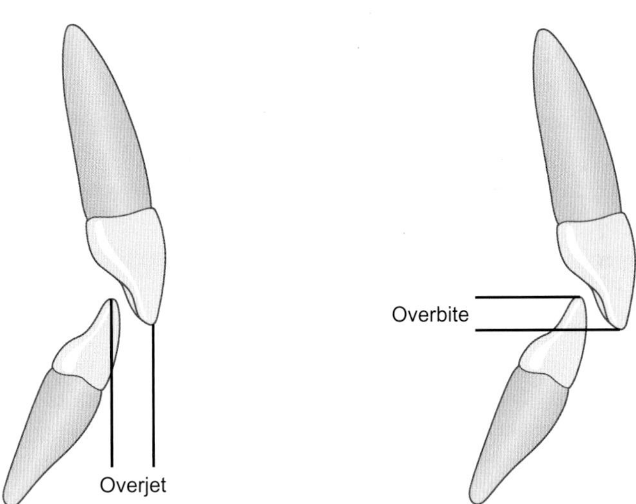

Fig. 2.104 The buccolingual incisor relationships in anatomical centric occlusion – overjet.

Fig. 2.105 The buccolingual incisor relationships in anatomical centric occlusion – overbite.

Variations in the relationships of the dental arches in centric position

Malocclusions should be regarded as anatomical variations rather than abnormalities for they are rarely involved in masticatory dysfunction. Our lack of understanding of the relationships between masticatory efficiency and tooth and arch form is responsible for the classification of malocclusion in terms of variations in the anatomical centric position and not in more functional terms.

Malocclusions result from malposition of individual teeth, malrelationship of the dental arches and/or variation in skeletal morphology of the jaws. Techniques for determining the skeletal relationships of the jaws are described on pages 48–52. Two classifications describing

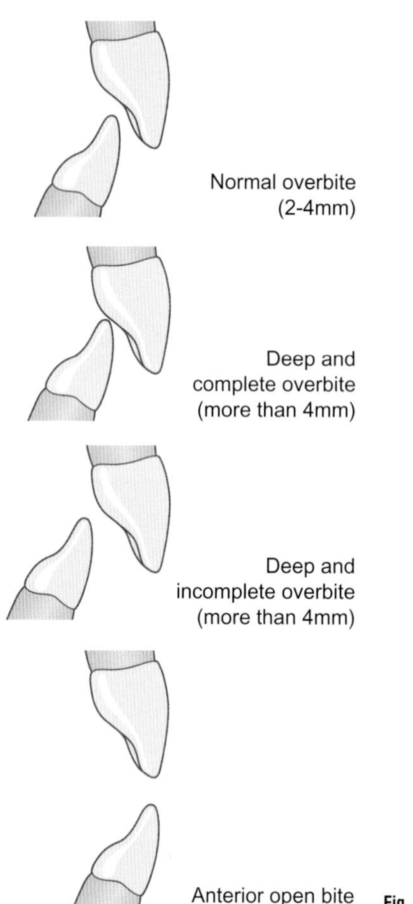

Fig. 2.106 Classification of overbite.

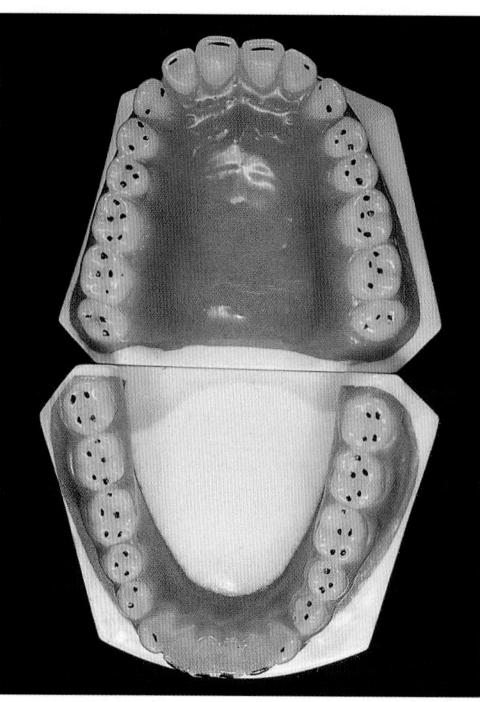

Fig. 2.107 The occlusal surfaces of the permanent dentition marked to show the position of centric stops in anatomical centric occlusion.

malposition of teeth and malrelationship of the arches are in general use – Angle's classification and a classification based upon the relationships of the incisors. A classification of malocclusion based upon canine relationships is also available for clinical use. However, this is much less employed than Angle's classification and the incisor relationship classification.

Angle's classification

Angle's classification of malocclusion was derived at the end of the 19th century. It relies upon the relationship of the arches in the anteroposterior plane using the maxillary and mandibular first permanent molars as key teeth (with some additional information regarding incisor positions). Nowadays, clinicians will consider the relationship of the molars, canines and incisors as three separate elements but, perhaps confusingly, still use Angle's original terminology.

Angle's class I malocclusion

Although one or more of the teeth are malpositioned, this does not affect the 'standard' anatomical relationship of the first permanent molars. Thus, the mesiobuccal cusp of the permanent maxillary first molar tooth occludes with the mid-buccal groove of the permanent mandibular first molar tooth. Recently, two further elements have been added:

1) The distal surface of the distal marginal ridge of the maxillary molar contacts, and occludes with, the mesial surface of the mesial marginal ridge of the mandibular second molar.
2) The mesiopalatal cusp of the maxillary molar sits in the central fossa of the mandibular molar.

In the models shown in Fig. 2.108, the maxillary canine is missing and the premolars are malaligned but the maxillary first molar tooth occludes correctly with the mandibular first and second molar teeth.

Box 2.1 **Basic features of occlusion**

1) The larger upper dental arch ensures an overjet on the maxillary teeth in relation to the mandibular teeth.
2) The majority of teeth occlude with two teeth in the opposing jaw, except for the mandibular first incisor and maxillary third molar.
3) The maxillary canine occludes between the mandibular canine and first premolar teeth.
4) In the molar teeth, each mandibular buccal cusp occludes in a groove between a maxillary buccal and palatal cusp.
5) The mesiopalatal cusp of the maxillary molars occludes in the centre of the basin of the corresponding mandibular molar.
6) The distobuccal cusp of the mandibular molars occludes in the centre of the basin between the two buccal cusps of the maxillary molar.
7) During lateral movement of the mandible, wear affects the upper palatal cusps and lower buccal cusps.

Angle's class II malocclusion

Angle's class II malocclusion is characterised by a 'prenormal' maxillary arch relationship, with the maxillary first permanent molars occluding at least half a cusp more mesial to the mandibular first permanent molars than the standard anatomical position. Thus, the mesiobuccal cusp of the permanent maxillary first molar tooth occludes mesial to the mid-buccal groove of the permanent mandibular first molar tooth.

Angle's class II malocclusion also takes into consideration incisor position.

Angle's class II malocclusion (division 1) indicates that the maxillary incisors are proclined (Fig. 2.109).

Angle's class II malocclusion (division 2) indicates that the maxillary incisors are retroclined (Fig. 2.110). Frequently only the first incisors are retroclined, with the second incisors being proclined. For this malocclusion, it is not uncommon to see increased overbite in the incisor region.

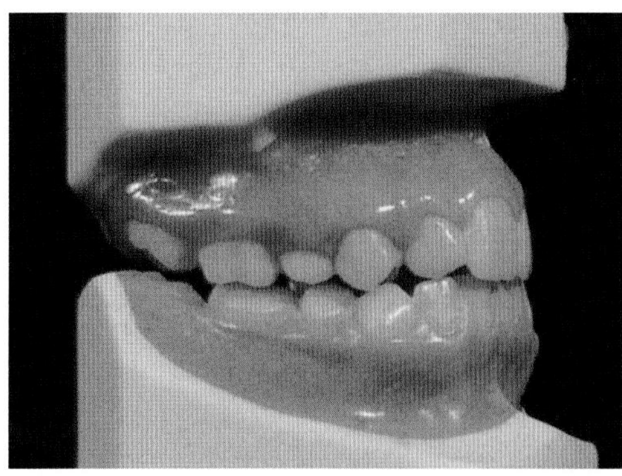

Fig. 2.108 Angle's class I malocclusion.

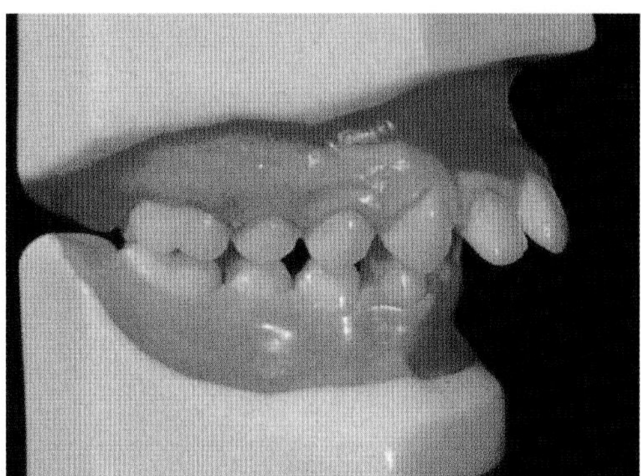

Fig. 2.109 Angle's class II malocclusion (division 1).

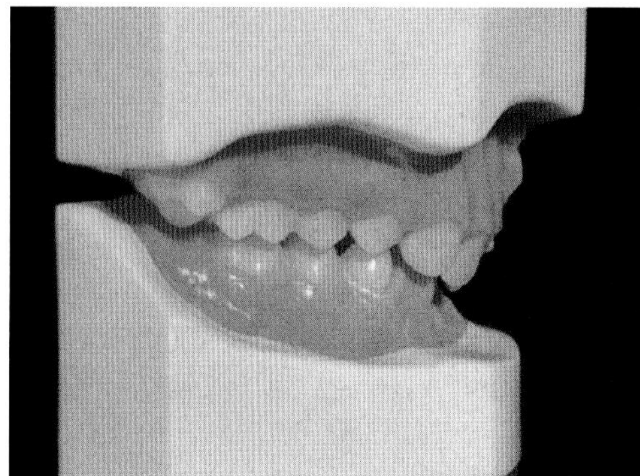

Fig. 2.110 Angle's class II malocclusion (division 2).

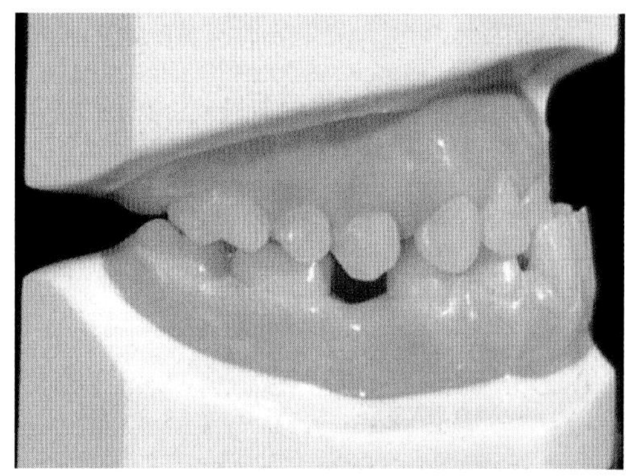

Fig. 2.111 Angle's class III malocclusion.

Angle's class III malocclusion

This malocclusion is characterised by a 'postnormal' maxillary arch relationship, with the maxillary first permanent molars occluding at least half a cusp more distal to the mandibular first permanent molars than the 'standard' anatomical position. Thus, the mesiobuccal cusp of the permanent maxillary first molar tooth occludes distal to the mid-buccal groove of the permanent mandibular first molar tooth. The incisor relationship varies from 'normal' overjet to an 'edge-to-edge' bite to reverse overjet (where the mandibular incisors lie labially to the maxillary incisors – as shown in Fig. 2.111).

Classification based on canine relationships

Class I

The cusp of the permanent maxillary canine tooth occludes in the embrasure between the permanent mandibular canine and first premolar teeth.

Class II

The permanent maxillary canine tooth occludes mesial to that in class I.

Class III

The permanent maxillary canine tooth occludes distal to that in class I.

Classification based on incisor relationships

As for Angle's classification, the classification of malocclusions based upon incisor relationships uses the categories class I, class II (division 1), class II (division 2) and class III. However, care must be taken not to confuse these classifications – for example, an Angle's class I molar relationship might exist alongside an incisor class III relationship in the same person.

As the permanent molars do not have a fixed relationship in the arch and may migrate following early loss of deciduous teeth, the classification of malocclusion based upon incisor relationships is often preferred to Angle's classification (Fig. 2.112). Furthermore, a classification of malocclusion related to the incisors is seen by many clinicians as being more appropriate because a major objective of orthodontic treatment is to establish an anatomical incisor relationship (patients being more concerned about, and aware of, the aesthetics of the incisor relationship than they are of the molar relationship). Thus, a classification based on incisor relationships is a much more informative method of describing the malocclusion. Furthermore, it avoids the confusion that can sometimes occur when trying to use Angle's original classification to describe a patient who presents with class I molars, class II canines and class III incisors (such as may occur in a patient with normal buccal segment relationships, missing maxillary second incisors and first incisors that are retroclined).

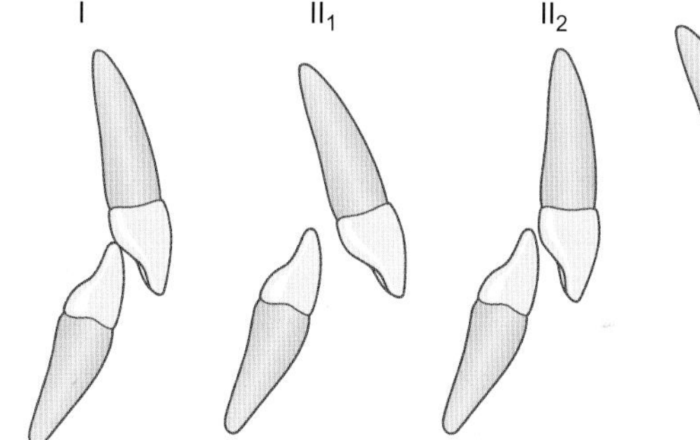

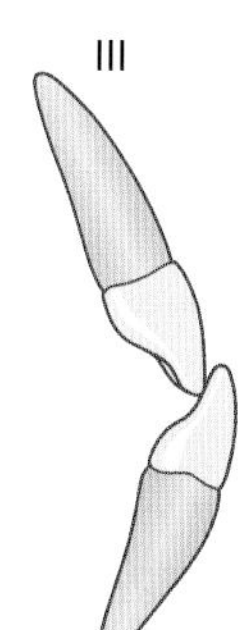

Fig. 2.112 Classification of malocclusion using incisor relationships.

The incisor relationship classification was devised by Ballard and Wayman in the 1960s and relies upon the relationship of incisors relative to a specific landmark – the cingulum plateau on the maxillary central incisor.

Class I incisor relationship

This represents the relationship where the incisors do not show any malposition. The incisal margins of the permanent mandibular incisors occlude with, or lie directly below, the middle third of the palatal surfaces of the permanent maxillary incisors (i.e., on or below the cingulum plateau area).

Class II incisor relationship

The incisal margins of the mandibular incisors lie behind the cingulum plateau area on the palatal surfaces of the maxillary incisors. Thus, the incisal margins of the mandibular incisors are related to the gingival third of the palatal surfaces of the maxillary incisors. Division 1 indicates that the maxillary central incisors are proclined with an increased overjet; division 2 indicates that the maxillary central incisors are retroclined and there is increased overbite.

Class III incisor relationship

The incisal margins of the permanent mandibular incisors lie in front of the cingulum plateau area on the palatal surfaces of the permanent maxillary incisors. Thus, the incisal margins of the mandibular incisors are related to the incisal third of the palatal surface of the maxillary incisors and there is a reduced, or even a reverse, overjet (the lower incisors lying anterior to the maxillary incisors).

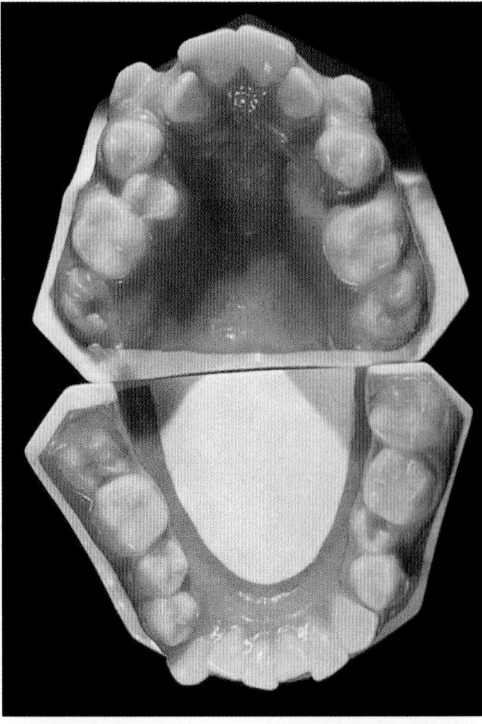

Fig. 2.113 Crowding within the dental arches.

Forms of malocclusion

Three common forms of malocclusion are crowding, anterior open bite and crossbite.

Crowding is the term used to describe the condition where teeth are markedly out of the line of the dental arch because there is disproportion between the size of the arch and the size of the teeth. The severe crowding illustrated in Fig. 2.113 reflects the developmental positions of the teeth before eruption (note that the second incisors develop inside the dental arch and the canines develop outside the arch). Spacing within an arch occurs where the teeth are small in relation to the size of the arch (or where there are missing teeth). The site of crowding also reflects the timing of eruption. The last teeth to erupt usually manifest the crowding – hence buccally displaced maxillary canines and impacted mandibular second premolars.

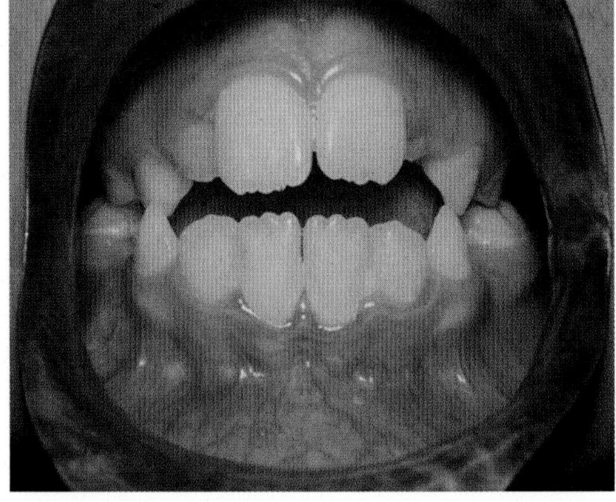

Fig. 2.114 Anterior open bite.

Anterior open bite occurs where there is no incisor contact and no incisor overbite (Fig. 2.114). It may be caused by thumb-sucking habits, abnormal swallowing patterns or skeletal anomalies. Skeletal anterior open bites sometimes result from lack of development of the anterior alveolar region but are more often associated with an increase in anterior intermaxillary height (i.e., the distance between the maxillary and mandibular dental bases; see Fig. 2.127). Anterior open bite may also be 'physiological' and related to the stage of eruption (incomplete eruption) of the incisors.

Crossbite is a transverse abnormality of the dental arches where there is an asymmetrical bite. It may affect just a single tooth (or part of) (Fig. 2.115A), a few teeth within an arch (Fig. 2.115B) or a whole quadrant. It may be unilateral or bilateral (Fig. 2.115C) and can affect the deciduous and/or the permanent dentition. Crossbites are frequently related to discrepancies in the widths of the dental bases and may involve the displacement of the mandible to one side to obtain maximal intercuspation.

Table 2.8 provides data indicating the severity and type of malocclusion in the population of the United States. Approximately 80% of children and adolescents in the United States thus show some degree of malocclusion. Most commonly there are problems of crowding (for about 40% of children and 80% of adolescents). The second most common type of malocclusion is excessive overjet of the maxillary incisors (about 15% of both children and adolescents).

Mandibular posture

When the mandible is at rest, a gap of a few millimetres remains between the occlusal surfaces of the teeth – the so-called 'freeway space'. The opinion has long been held that the position of rest is innate and unalterable throughout life. However, the concept of a fixed mandibular resting posture is an oversimplification. Indeed, psychological state, body posture and fatigue are well-known short-term influences that can change the resting interocclusal distance. Furthermore, research shows that following speech, mastication or swallowing, the mandible appears to return to whatever position of rest it can find. In the long term, ageing and the removal of occlusal contacts affect the resting position. Although the physiological mechanisms responsible for maintaining a rest position are not fully understood, evidence suggests that the physical properties of the soft tissues are responsible for the rest position and not the tonic activity of the elevator muscles of the jaw.

Several instruments and techniques have been devised to measure freeway space – some elaborate, some relatively simple. All suffer from inaccuracies produced by examiner bias and misconceptions about the nature of the mandibular resting posture. The use of measuring techniques relies upon the concept that the mandibular resting position is innate and

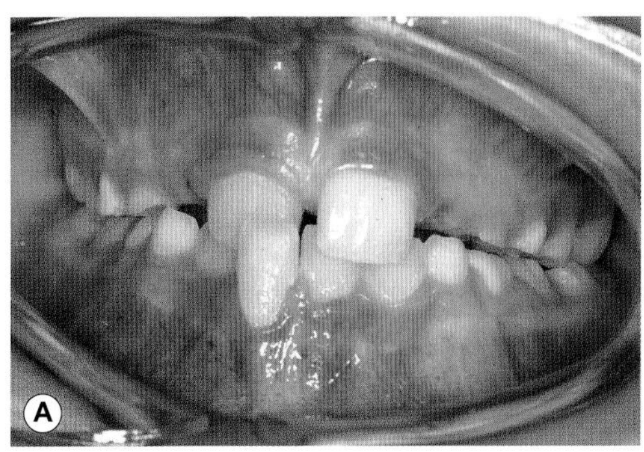
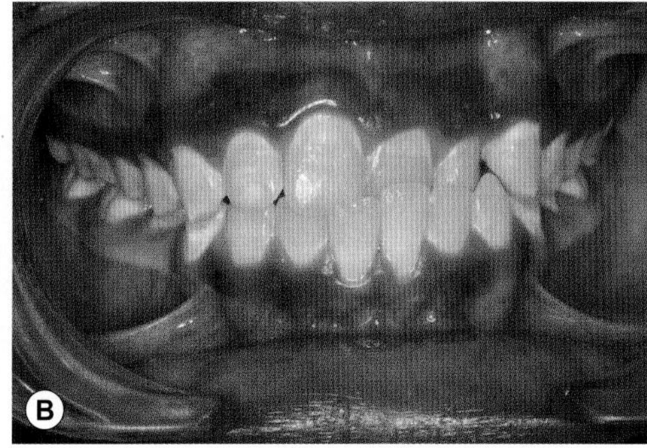
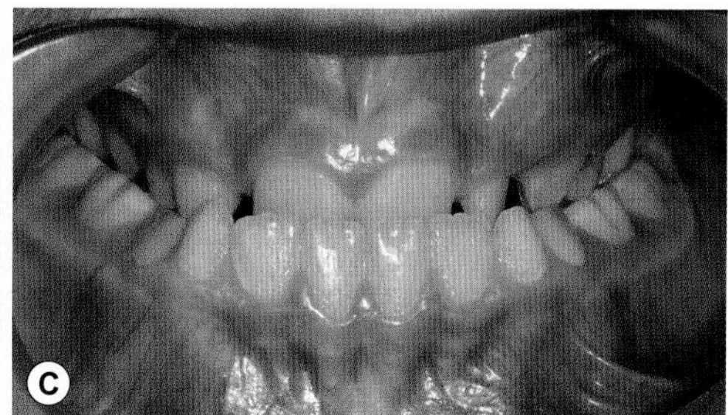

Fig. 2.115 (A) Crossbite affecting the mesial half of the permanent maxillary right central incisor. (B) Crossbite affecting the maxillary left permanent central and lateral incisors and the mesial half of the right central incisor. (C) Bilateral crossbite affecting the mixed dentition of a 9-year-old child. (A) Courtesy Dr. R Whatling. (B, C) Courtesy Drs. P S Viswapurna and R Madan.

Table 2.8 Severity and types of malocclusions in the general population of the United States

	Distribution (%)	
	Age 6–11 years	Age 12–17 years
Severity		
Near-ideal occlusion	23	10
Mild malocclusion	40	35
Moderate malocclusion	23	26
Severe or very severe malocclusion	14	29
Type		
Crowding/malalignment problems		
Ideal	57	13
Moderate	39	44
Severe	4	43
Anteroposterior problems		
Overjet (6 mm or more)	17	15
Reverse overjet (1 mm or more)	1	
Vertical problems		
Open bite (2 mm or more)	1	1
Overbite (6 mm or more)	8	12
Transverse problems		
Lingual crossbite (two or more teeth)	5	6
Buccal crossbite (two or more teeth)	1	2

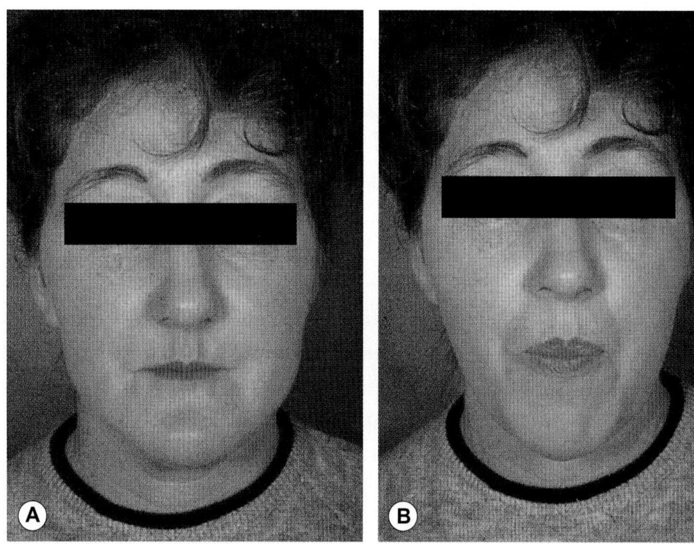

Fig. 2.116 The appearance produced as a result of over-opening. (A) Normal resting position and facial profile for a patient without dentures. (B) Over-opened appearance produced typically by wearing dentures without provision of adequate freeway space. Courtesy Prof. D C Berry.

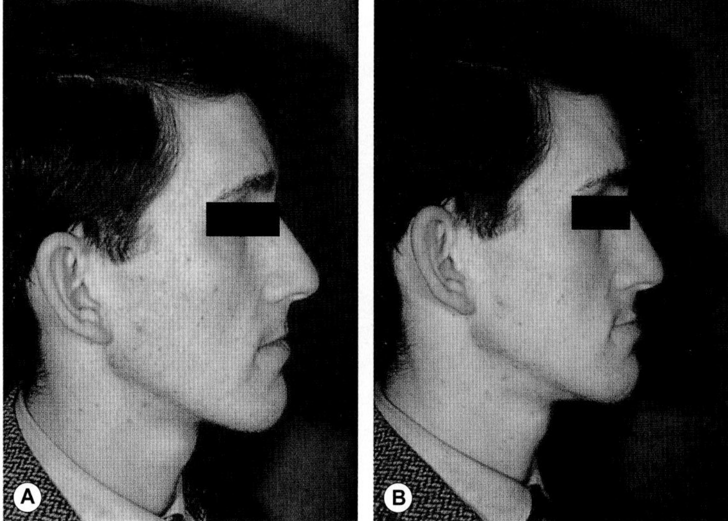

Fig. 2.117 The appearance produced by over-closure. (A) Normal resting position and facial profile of a patient who displays over-closure with an ill-fitting denture (B). Courtesy Prof. D C Berry.

unalterable. Consequently, the removal of teeth is deemed not to affect the rest position. Thus, when a patient has lost all natural occlusal contacts, it is considered necessary only to put a prosthesis into the mouth at a level which reproduces the freeway space to restore the original occlusal vertical dimension.

Although most clinicians would prefer objective criteria for determining vertical jaw relationships, many realise that because of the relative instability of such relationships, at best one has to rely upon such subjective assessments as overall facial appearance, mandibular position during deglutition, jaw posture giving greatest comfort, position allowing the development of maximum biting force and lip and tongue posture. Nevertheless, however one gauges the mandibular resting position, if prosthetic appliances are to be placed in the mouth, it is necessary to ensure that the vertical dimensions of the jaws are not adversely affected. The result of over-opening is an elongation of the face, a parting of the lips at rest and a 'strained' facial appearance (Fig. 2.116). The general effect of over-closure on facial appearance is to produce features of increased age (Fig. 2.117). There is a closer approximation of the nose and chin than normal. The greater the degree of over-closure, the more the soft tissues of the face appear to sag and fall in, and the more pronounced are the lines on the face.

Radiographic appearance of jaws and teeth

Dental radiography and radiology are concerned with the techniques of producing and interpreting photographic images of orodental tissues taken with X-rays. X-rays, being part of the spectrum of electromagnetic radiation, have a wavelength of approximately 10^{-8} cm (compared with wavelengths of around 10^{-4} cm for visible light). It is the short wavelength that allows X-rays to penetrate materials that would otherwise absorb or reflect light. However, X-rays do not pass through all matter with similar ease: materials composed of elements with low atomic numbers are readily penetrated and are described as being radiolucent, whereas elements with high atomic numbers absorb X-rays and are termed radio-opaque. Thus, gases and soft tissues are radiolucent, while calcified materials such as bone and teeth are radio-opaque. X-rays produce a photosensitisation reaction when they strike a silver–salt emulsion. When a radio-opaque structure is placed between a beam of X-rays and a photographic plate that is subsequently developed, the radio-opaque structure is 'mapped out' as a white area on the negative. It is because of the properties of tissue penetration and photosensitisation that X-rays can be used in dentistry to provide valuable information concerning underlying hard tissue structures not otherwise visible.

X-rays produce a shadow picture without a focus; therefore, the features of a large object such as a skull are not shown equally distinctly on a radiograph. As a general rule, structures nearest the photographic plate appear clearer than those some distance from it. Superimposition may also make interpretation of radiographs difficult because most radiographs are two-dimensional representations of three-dimensional objects. Care must be taken not to overinterpret radiographs by diagnosing pathological conditions without recourse to other diagnostic aids or clinical findings. The prime use of a radiograph is therefore to describe gross topographic features.

Extraoral radiographic projections of jaws and teeth

Table 2.9 outlines the major extraoral radiographic projections used to view the human jaws and dentition. In this context, 'extraoral' indicates that the radiographic plate is positioned outside the mouth.

Among the specialised techniques worthy of fuller description here, Figs 2.126–2.138 are concerned with cephalometric radiography, sialography and tomography.

Cephalometric analysis of lateral skull radiographs

Lateral skull radiographs are often used in dentistry to assess by measurement general skeletal morphology, particularly for recording relationships between the jaws and the cranial base (Fig. 2.126). They are also of use for the evaluation of the direction and the amount of growth, for determining dentoskeletal relationships and even for soft tissue analysis. In order to provide the most meaningful measurements, cephalometric radiographs are taken under standard conditions to enable comparisons between patients and for the same patient at different times. Thus, the position of the head must be standardised using a cephalostat (head holder) such that the beam of X-rays is shot in a predetermined plane to the head from a standard distance. This necessitates that the Frankfort plane (between the ear and orbit; see Fig. 2.128) is horizontal, that the dentition is in centric occlusion (see pages 42–43) and that the lips are in their habitual position.

Table 2.9 Extraoral radiographic projections describing jaws and teeth. Some of these projections are no longer used and are denoted 'historical'

Projection/technique	Purpose
Posteroanterior skull (PA) (Fig. 2.118)	Survey of facial bones and mandible (historical).
Anteroposterior skull (AP) (Fig. 2.119)	Survey of posterior part of cranium, mandible and temporomandibular articulation (historical).
Reverse Towne's (Fig. 2.120)	Anatomy of mandibular condyles and temporomandibular articulation (historical).
Occipitomental skull (Fig. 2.121)	Survey of facial bones and air sinuses.
Lateral skull (Fig. 2.122)	Survey of lateral regions of face, cranium and mandible. View of facial profile and covering soft tissues.
Lateral skull with cephalostat (Fig. 2.126)	Recording of relationships between teeth, jaws and cranial base.
Lateral oblique view of mandible (Fig. 2.123)	Survey of posterior regions of body and ramus of mandible.
Orthopantomogram (Fig. 2.124)	A tomogram to display both maxillae, the mandible and the dentition on a single film.
Transcranial temporomandibular joint (Fig. 2.125)	Movement of mandibular condyles in mandibular fossae (historical).
Sialography (Figs 2.136–2.137)	Infusion of radio-opaque material into the main salivary ducts to study their structure and distribution.
Tomography (Fig. 2.138)	Technique for the radiography of selected areas that, under standard radiographic technique, are obscured by superimposition of other structures (e.g., temporomandibular joint and air sinuses).

Lateral skull radiographs are preferred for dental cephalometry primarily because the facial variations of greatest importance are located in the sagittal plane. Normal values for cephalometric measurements are given in Table 2.10.

Fig. 2.127 shows a lateral view of a skull and tracing taken from a radiograph and illustrates the most common cephalometric landmarks used in dentistry (see also Table 2.11).

Cephalometric analysis of jaw relationships and facial form

The mandibular plane passes through the menton and gonion (Fig. 2.128). It is used in conjunction with the Frankfort, maxillary and Ba–N planes to assess the vertical development of the anterior part of the face (Table 2.11). The Frankfort plane extends from the orbitale to the porion. The Frankfort–mandibular angle in 'normal' subjects is said to be approximately 27 degrees. The maxillary plane extends through the anterior and posterior nasal spines (ANS, PNS) and is easier to identify on a lateral skull radiograph than the Frankfort plane. Both the maxillary–mandibular plane angle and the mandibular–cranial base (Ba–N) angle are of the same order as the Frankfort–mandibular plane angle. A plane termed the *facial line* can be drawn between the nasion and the pogonion. This plane aids in the assessment of facial profile, and the angle it makes with the Frankfort plane indicates whether the profile is orthognathic, prognathic or retrognathic.

Fig. 2.129 describes the use of SNA and SNB angles to record maxillary–mandibular skeletal relationships. SNA measures the degree of

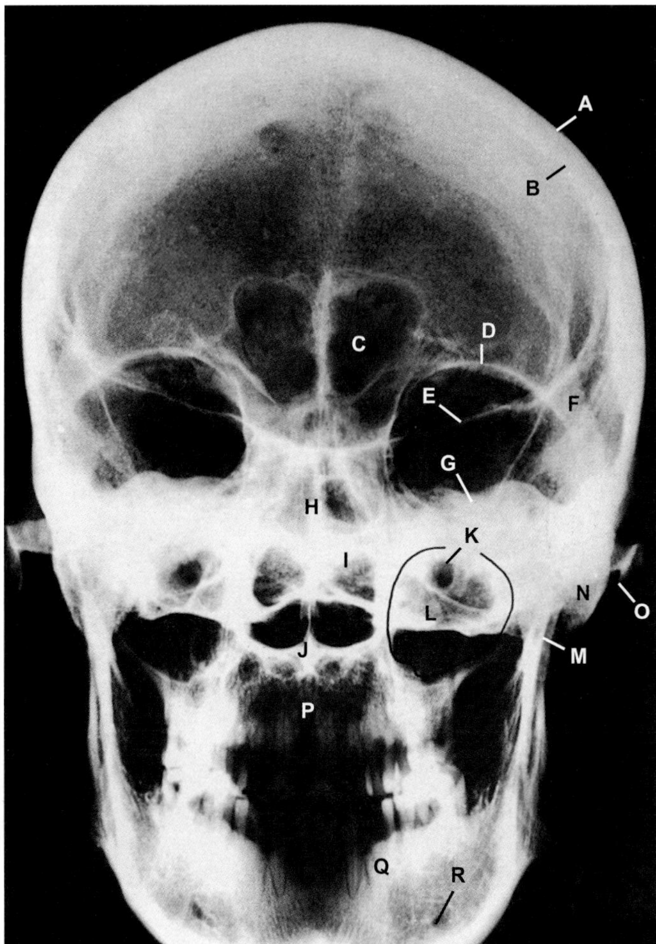

Fig. 2.118 Posteroanterior (PA) view of skull. A = outer table of cranium; B = inner table of cranium; C = frontal air sinus; D = superior rim of orbit; E = sphenoid ridge in middle cranial fossa; F = zygomatic process of frontal bone; G = petrous ridge; H = nasal septum; I = nasal fossa; J = anterior nasal spine; K = infraorbital foramen; L = maxillary air sinus; M = neck of mandibular condyle; N = mastoid process of temporal bone; O = zygomatic arch; P = maxilla and teeth; Q = body of mandible and teeth; R = mental foramen.

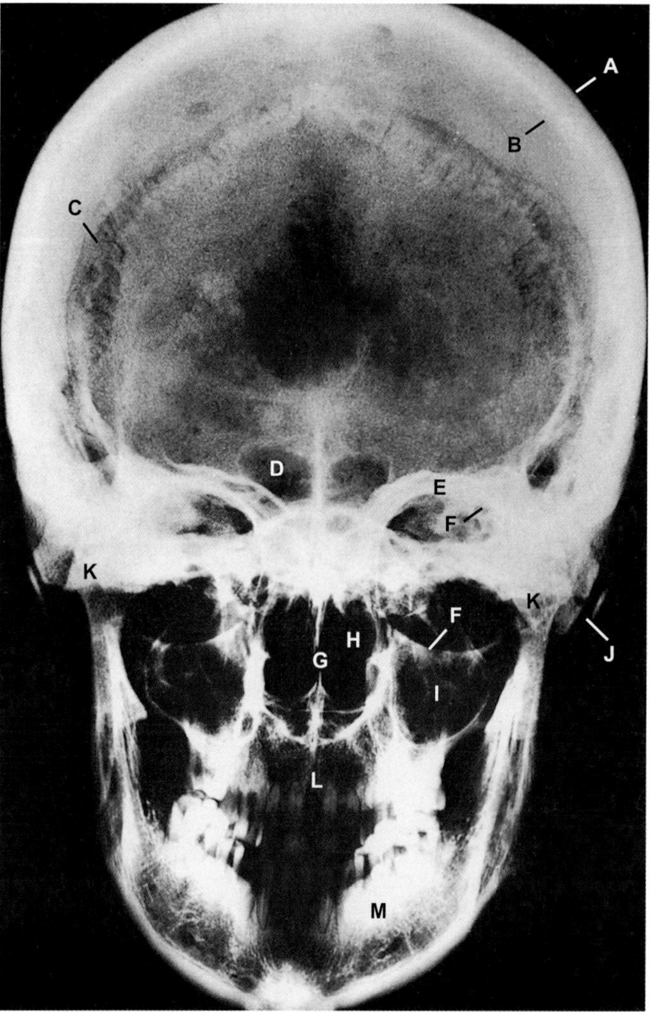

Fig. 2.119 Anteroposterior (AP) view of skull. A = outer table of cranium; B = inner table of cranium; C = lambdoid suture; D = frontal air sinus; E = superimposed sphenoid, petrous and supraorbital ridges; F = rim of orbit; G = nasal septum; H = nasal fossa; I = maxillary air sinus; J = zygoma; K = condyle of mandible; L = maxilla and teeth; M = body of mandible and teeth.

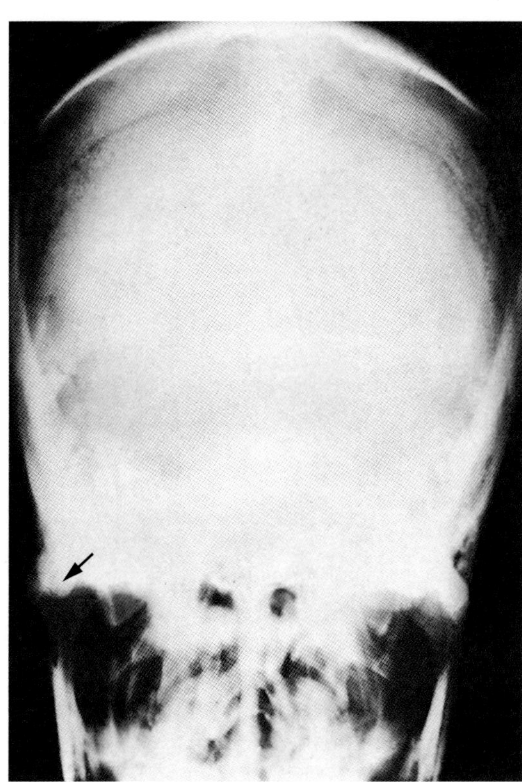

Fig. 2.120 Reverse Towne's view showing position of mandibular condyle (arrowed).

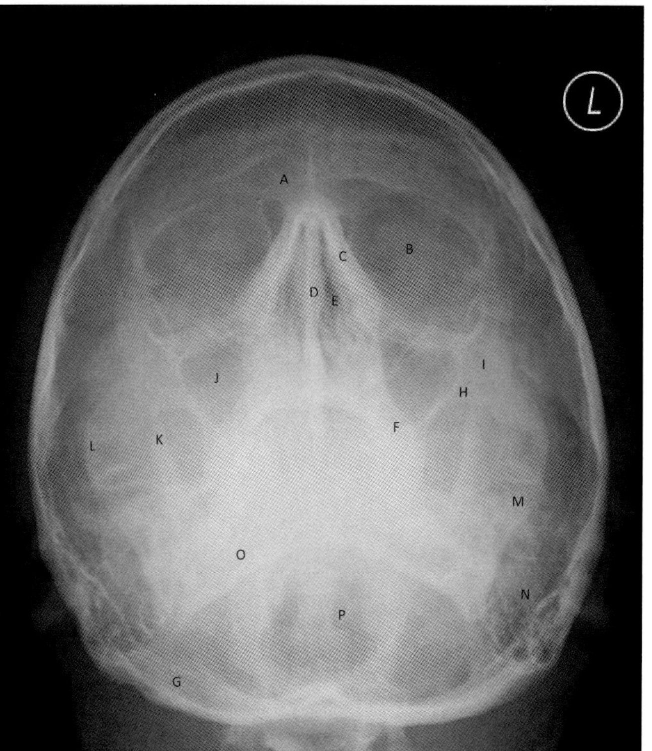

Fig. 2.121 Occipitomental view of skull (OM 30 degrees). A = frontal air sinus; B = orbit; C = nasal bones; D = nasal septum; E = nasal fossa with superimposed shadows of ethmoidal air cells; F = maxilla and teeth; G = lambdoid suture; H = malar (zygomatic) extension of maxillary sinus; I = zygoma; J = maxillary air sinus; K = coronoid process of mandible; L = zygomatic process of temporal bone; M = condyle of mandible; N = mastoid air cells; O = body of mandible and teeth; P = foramen magnum. Courtesy Dr. J Makdissi.

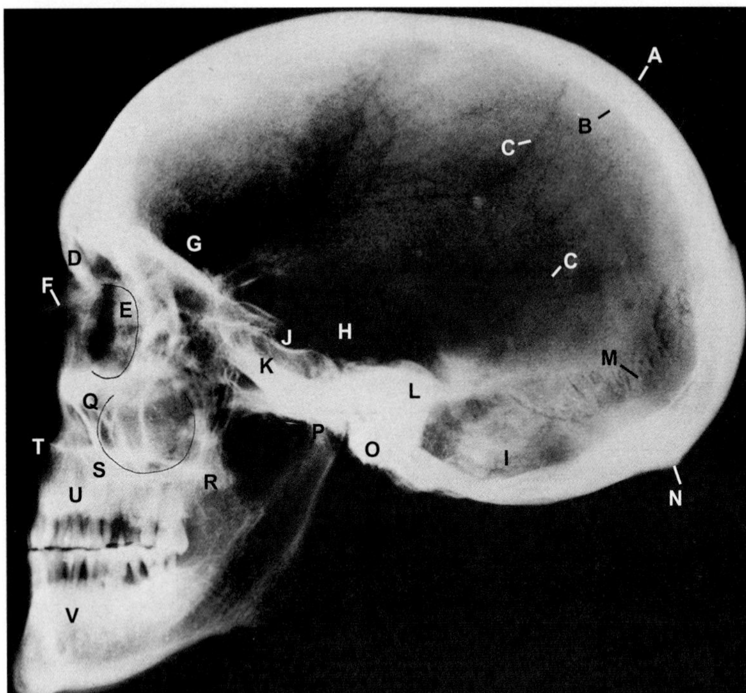

Fig. 2.122 Lateral skull radiograph. A = outer table of cranium; B = inner table of cranium; C = depressions in cranium related to middle meningeal vessels; D = frontal air sinus; E = margins of orbit; F = nasal bone; G = anterior cranial fossa; H = middle cranial fossa; I = posterior cranial fossa; J = hypophyseal (pituitary) fossa; K = sphenoid air sinus; L = petrous ridge; M = lambdoid suture; N = external occipital protuberance; O = mastoid process; P = condyle of mandible; Q = margin of maxillary air sinus; R = coronoid process of mandible; S = maxilla and teeth; T = anterior nasal spine; U = hard palate; V = body of mandible and teeth.

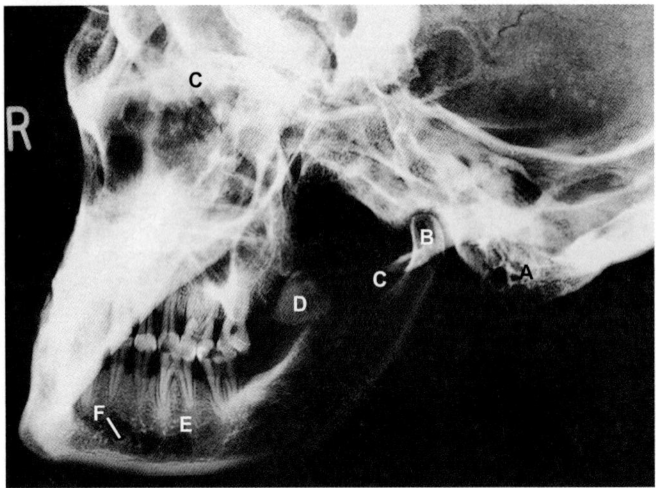

Fig. 2.123 Lateral oblique view of mandible. A = mastoid process of temporal bone; B = condyle of mandible lying in mandibular fossa of temporomandibular joint; C = zygomatic arch; D = shadow of mandibular coronoid process on maxillary tuberosity; E = body of mandible showing teeth posterior to premolars; F = mental foramen.

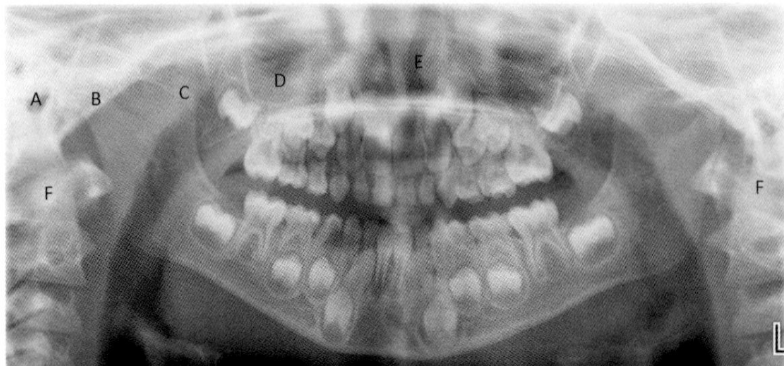

Fig. 2.124 Orthopantomogram (OPG). A panoramic radiographic survey of the jaws and teeth. Dentition is radiographed at 6 years of age. A = external acoustic meatus; B = mandibular condyle; C = coronoid process of mandible; D = maxillary air sinus; E = nasal cavity; F = vertebral column. Courtesy Dr. J Makdissi.

prognathism of the maxillary alveolar base: its average value is 82 degrees. SNB assesses the degree of prognathism of the mandibular alveolar base. The angle SNA–SNB (i.e., ANB) is frequently used to determine the skeletal pattern for the jaws because the cranial base (SN plane) is thought to undergo very little change from the later years of childhood. Where ANB is 2–5 degrees, the skeletal pattern is designated to be class I. Where ANB is greater than 5 degrees, the jaws show a class II relationship with maxillary prognathism. Where ANB is less than 2 degrees, the jaws show a class III relationship with mandibular prognathism. Should SNA be significantly different from its normal value, a correction must be made before assigning an ANB value to a specific skeletal class.

Fig. 2.130 and Table 2.12 provide the cephalometric landmarks used for assessing dentoskeletal relationships.

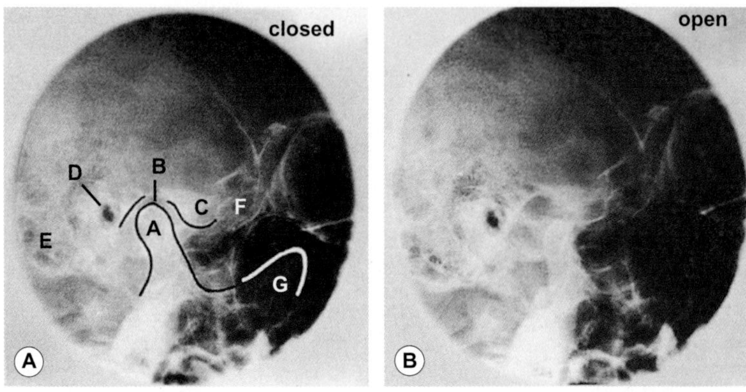

Fig. 2.125 Transcranial temporomandibular articulation (A, mouth closed; B, mouth open). A = mandibular condyle; B = temporomandibular joint cavity space; C = articular tubercle; D = external acoustic meatus; E = mastoid air cells; F = zygomatic arch; G = coronoid process.

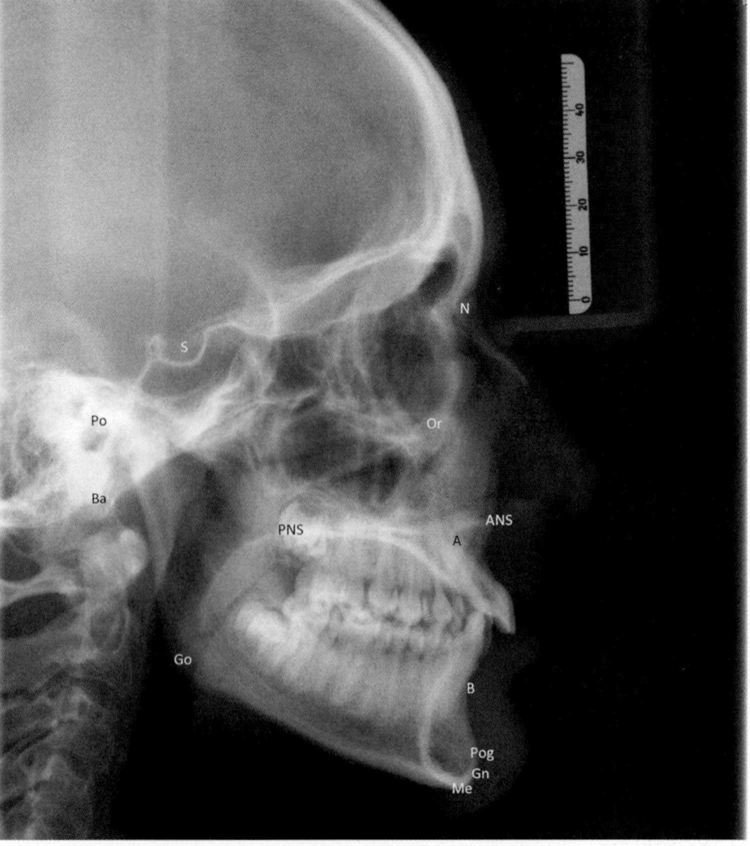

Fig. 2.126 Lateral cephalometric radiograph. For key to labelling, see Fig. 2.127. Courtesy Dr. J Mikdassi.

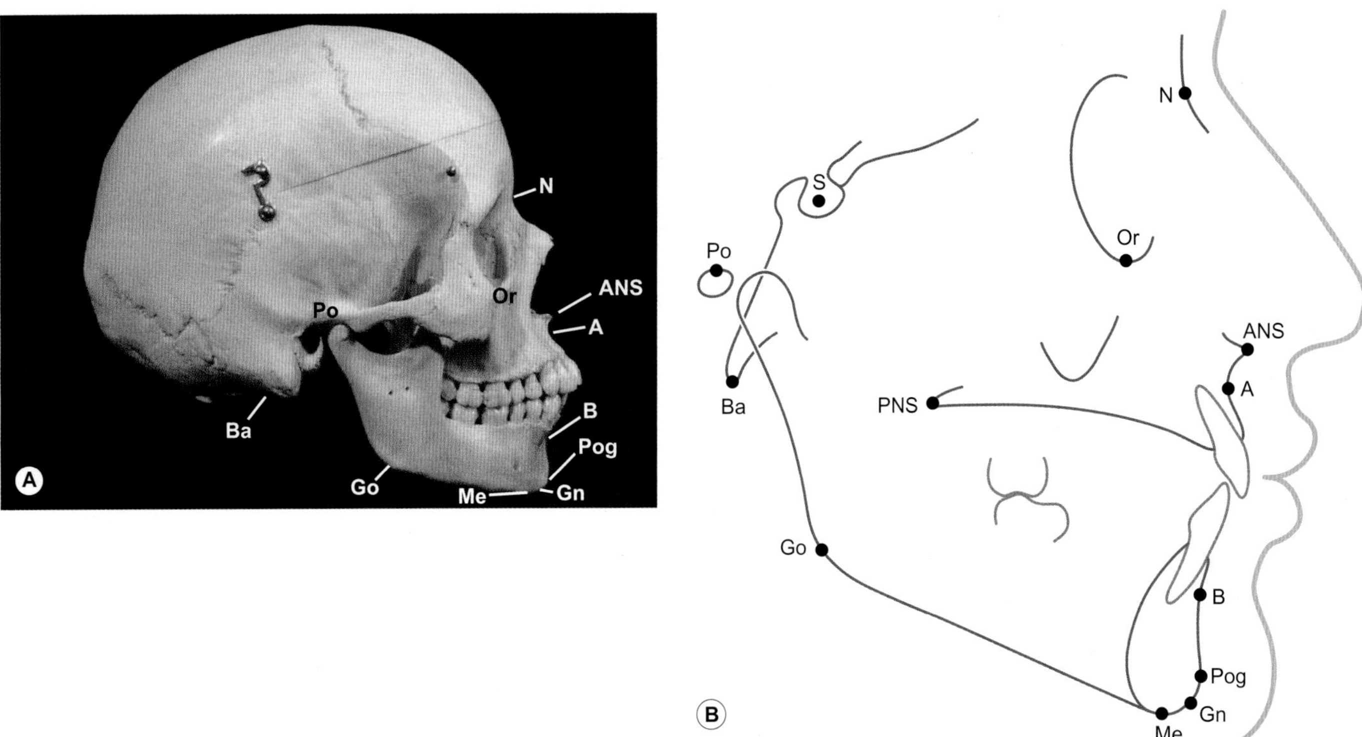

Fig. 2.127 Lateral view of skull (A) and tracing taken from a lateral skull radiograph (B), illustrating the most common cephalometric landmarks used in dentistry. A = subspinale (A point: position of greatest concavity of maxillary alveolus in the midline); ANS = anterior nasal spine; B = supramentale (B point: position of greatest concavity of mandibular alveolus in the midline); Ba = basion (the most inferior and posterior point on the basi-occiput, lying on the anterior margin of the foramen magnum); Gn = gnathion (point between the most anterior and inferior points of chin, established by bisecting the angle formed between the N–Pog and mandibular planes); Go = gonion (most inferior and posterior point at the angle of the mandible, established by bisecting the angle formed between the planes through the lower border of the mandible and posterior border of ramus); Me = menton (lowest point of the chin); N = nasion (junction between frontal and nasal bones in midline on the frontonasal suture); Or = orbitale (lowest point of the infraorbital margin); PNS = posterior nasal spine; Po = porion (highest bony point of margin of external acoustic meatus); Pog = pogonion (most anterior point on the chin); S = sella point (centre of shadow of sella turcica [pituitary fossa]).

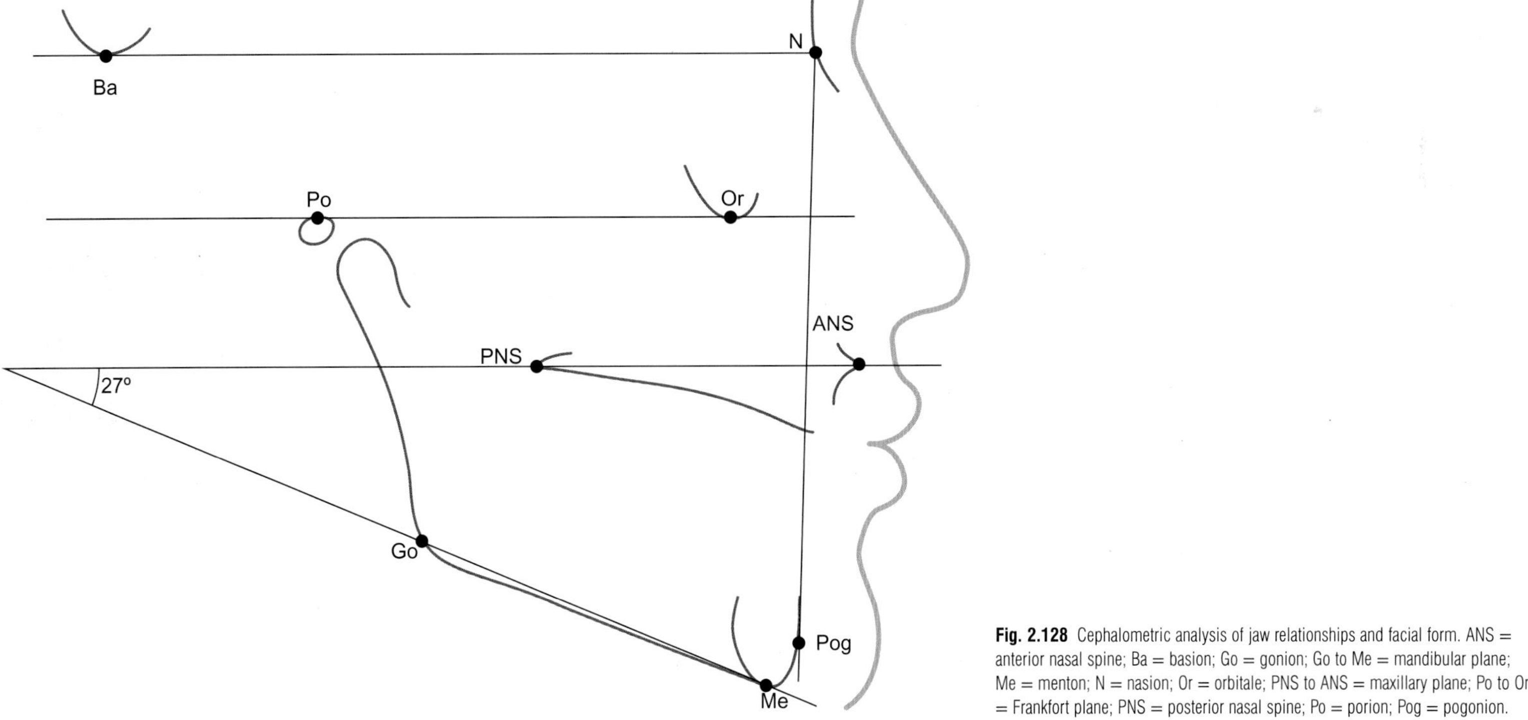

Fig. 2.128 Cephalometric analysis of jaw relationships and facial form. ANS = anterior nasal spine; Ba = basion; Go = gonion; Go to Me = mandibular plane; Me = menton; N = nasion; Or = orbitale; PNS to ANS = maxillary plane; Po to Or = Frankfort plane; PNS = posterior nasal spine; Po = porion; Pog = pogonion.

The inclinations of the incisors to the planes of the jaws are illustrated in Fig. 2.131. The inclination of the maxillary incisor can be determined by measuring the angle between a line drawn through its root axis and the Frankfort (or maxillary) plane. On average, this angle is 109 degrees. The inclination of the mandibular incisor is assessed by the angle formed between its root axis and the mandibular plane: it is approximately a right angle. Interincisor relationships are described in Fig. 2.132. The angle formed by the junction of the longitudinal axes of the maxillary and mandibular central incisors is of the order of 135 degrees; however, its clinical usefulness is limited because the antero-posterior relationship of the incisal edges is of greater importance. This is assessed by analysing the distance between the mandibular incisal

Table 2.10 Normal values for cephalometric measurements

Maxillary-mandibular plane angle	27 (±5) degrees
SNA angle	82 (±3) degrees
ANB angle	3 (±1) degrees
Maxillary incisor/maxillary plane angle	109 (±5) degrees
Mandibular incisor/mandibular plane angle	90 (±5) degrees
Maxillary incisor/mandibular incisor angle	135 (±9) degrees
N–S–Ba angle	130 degrees (150 degrees at birth)

For abbreviations see Table 2.12.

Table 2.11 The most common cephalometric landmarks used in dentistry

Basion (Ba)	The most inferior and posterior point on the basi-occiput, lying on the anterior margin of the foramen magnum
Sella point (S)	Centre of shadow of sella turcica (pituitary fossa)
Nasion (N)	Junction between frontal and nasal bones in the midline on the frontonasal suture
Porion (Po)	Highest bony point of the margin of the external acoustic meatus
Orbitale (Or)	Lowest point of the infraorbital margin
Anterior nasal spine (ANS)	
Posterior nasal spine (PNS)	
Subspinale (A point)	Position of greatest concavity of the maxillary alveolus in the midline
Supramentale (B point)	Position of greatest concavity of the mandibular alveolus in the midline
Pogonion (Pog)	Most anterior point on the chin
Menton (Me)	Lowest point of the chin
Gnathion (Gn)	Point between the most anterior and inferior points of chin established by bisecting the angle formed between the N–Pog and mandibular planes
Gonion (Go)	Most inferior and posterior point at the angle of the mandible established by bisecting the angle formed between the planes through the lower border of the mandible and posterior border of ramus

edge and the centroid of the maxillary incisor root. Two examples are shown in Fig. 2.132. In both, the maxillary and mandibular incisors meet at the same angle of approximately 135 degrees. However, they differ markedly in terms of the distances between the mandibular incisal edges and the centroids.

Cephalometric growth studies

Every bone of the skull in the growing child shows some degree of growth, and consequently no point can be considered ‘fixed’. For analytical convenience, however, several landmarks and strategies are defined and adopted to study the degree and direction of cranial growth. The Y-axis is a line from the sella point to the gnathion and is used to describe the general

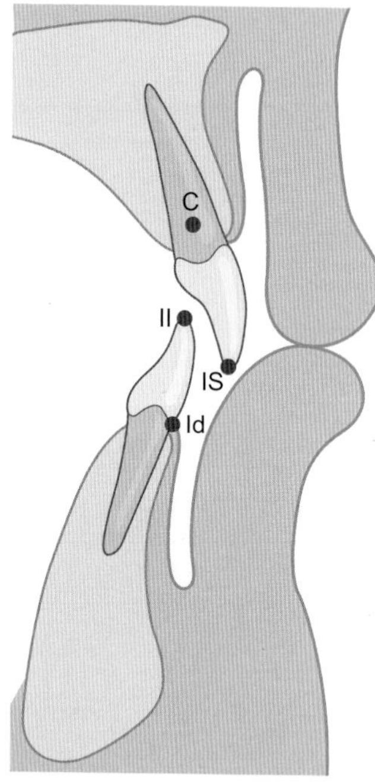

Fig. 2.130 Cephalometric landmarks used for assessing dentoskeletal relationships. C = centroid of the maxillary incisor root (the midpoint along the root axis of the most prominent maxillary incisor); II = incision inferius (the incisal tip of the most prominent mandibular incisor); IS = incision superius (the incisal tip of the most prominent maxillary incisor); Id = infradentale (the junction of alveolar crest with the outline of the most prominent mandibular incisor).

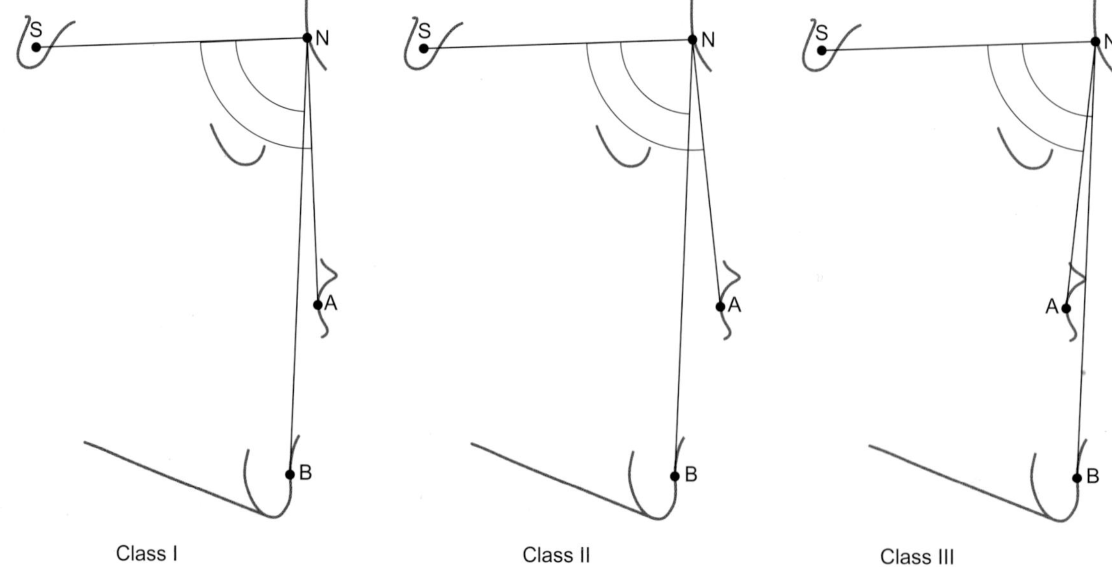

Fig. 2.129 The use of SNA and SNB angles to record maxillary–mandibular skeletal relationships. A = subspinale (A point); B = supramentale (B point); N = nasion; S = sella point.

Table 2.12 Cephalometric landmarks for assessing dentoskeletal relationships

Centroid of the maxillary incisor root (C)	The midpoint along the root axis of the most prominent maxillary incisor
Incision superius (IS)	The incisal tip of the most prominent maxillary incisor
Incision inferius (II)	The incisal tip of the most prominent mandibular incisor
Infradentale (Id)	The junction of the alveolar crest with the outline of the most prominent mandibular incisor

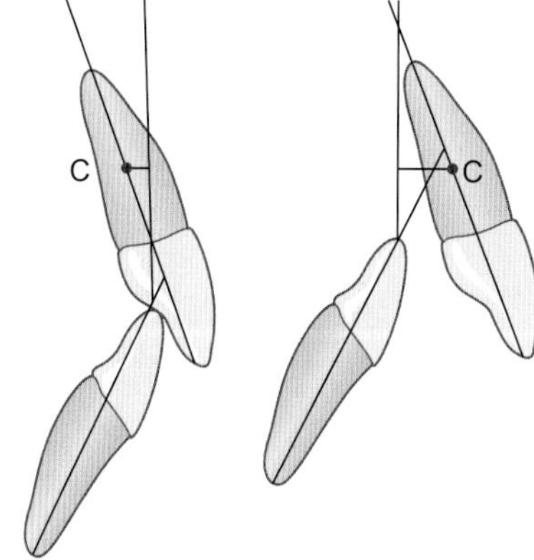

Fig. 2.132 Interincisor relationships. C = centroid of the maxillary incisor root. Redrawn after Prof. N J B Houston and Prof. W S Tulley.

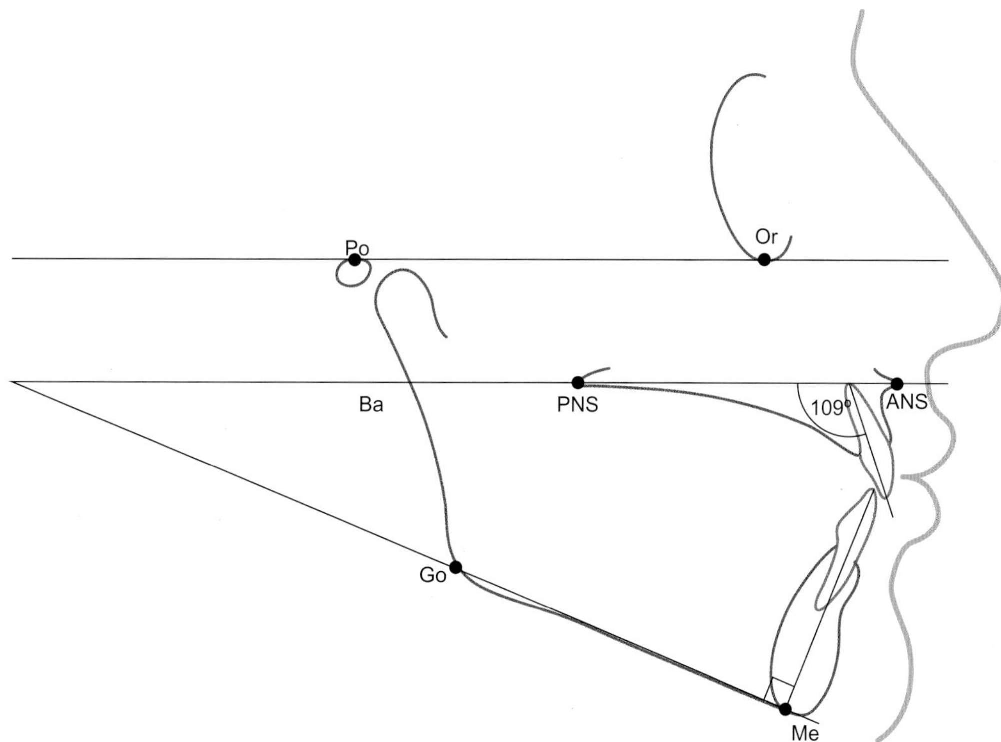

Fig. 2.131 The inclinations of the incisors to the planes of the jaws. Go to Me = Mandibular plane; PNS to ANS = Maxillary plane; Po to Or = Frankfort plane.

direction of facial growth relative to the cranial base (Fig. 2.133). The angle between the Y-axis and the Ba–N plane is used to assess changes in growth direction.

A frequently employed strategy to assess growth relies upon the superimposition of successive cephalometric tracings of the same individual at different ages (Fig. 2.134). A reasonably reliable picture of growth of the facial skeleton can be obtained by superimposition at the S–N planes with registration of the sella point. Growth at the maxillary region is notoriously difficult to assess but can be analysed by superimposition at the maxillary plane with registration of the anterior surface of the zygomatic process of the maxilla. For the mandibular region, it is necessary to superimpose at the mandibular canal and at the inner surface of the mandible behind the chin.

Soft tissue analysis

Soft tissue analysis is possible from cephalometric radiographs provided that the soft tissue outlines are sufficiently clear and that the lips are in their habitual posture (Fig. 2.135). To undertake such analysis, reference is often made to the following three planes:

- The H line (the Harmony line of Holdaway) is drawn between the chin and the vermilion border of the upper lip. It can be used to assess the degree of lower lip pout. The vermilion border of the lower lip should be within 1 mm of the H line.
- The upper lip tangent (ULT) describes the plane perpendicular to the Frankfort plane and tangential to the vermilion border of the upper lip. It is used to assess the amount of upper lip curl, the concavity of the upper lip profile normally being 1–4 mm behind the upper lip tangent.

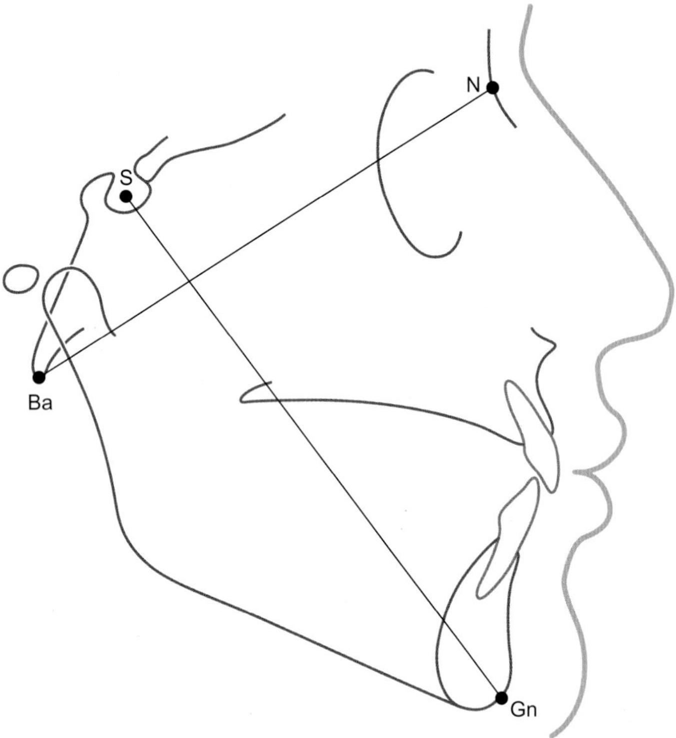

Fig. 2.133 Cephalometric growth studies – the Y-axis. Ba = basion; Gn = gnathion; N = nasion; S = sella point.

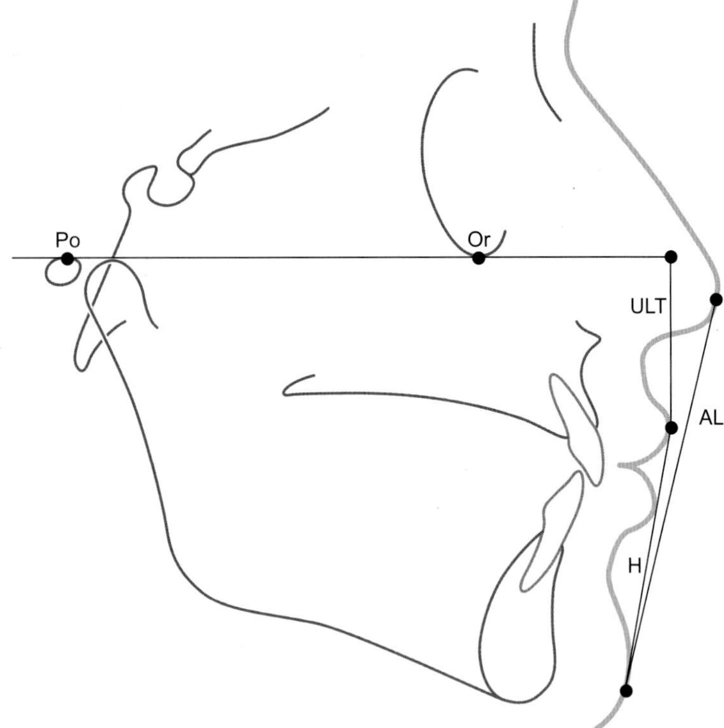

Fig. 2.135 Soft tissue analysis from cephalometric radiographs. AL = the aesthetic line; H = the harmony line of Holdaway (H line); Or = orbitale; Po = porion; ULT = the upper lip tangent.

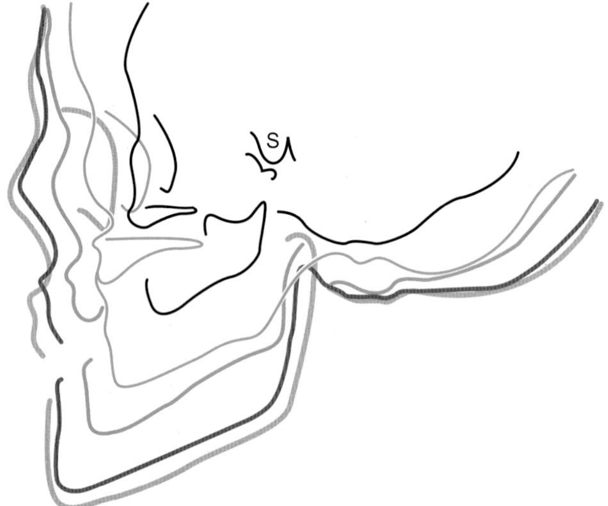

Fig. 2.134 Cephalometric growth studies – superimposition of tracings at different ages. S = sella point.

- The aesthetic line (AL) extends from the tip of the nose to the chin. The vermilion borders of both upper and lower lips usually lie close to the AL.

Sialography

Sialography is the technique whereby the duct systems of the major salivary glands are visualised by injecting an iodine-based contrast medium into the duct orifice (Fig. 2.136). This technique is used to identify obstructions (Fig. 2.137).

Tomographic examination of the temporomandibular joint

Tomography is a radiographic technique used to study layers within a volume of tissue, in a way analogous to the examination of a single portion

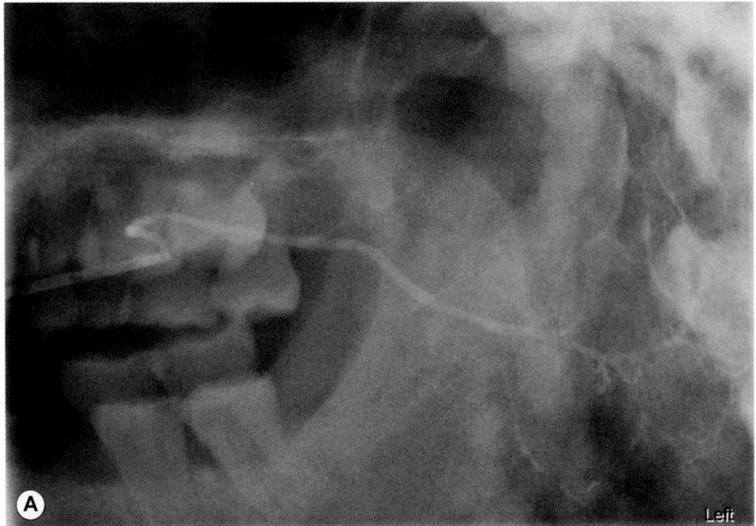

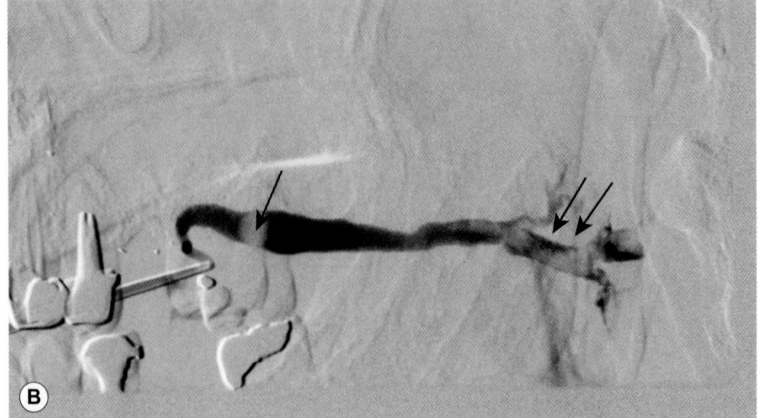

Fig. 2.136 (A) Sialogram showing normal parotid duct (B) Digital subtraction image showing a parotid duct with a stone (single arrow) and a mucus plug (2 arrows). Note that the main duct is dilated. (A) Courtesy Dr. N Drage. (B) Courtesy Dr. J Makdissi.

of bread within a whole loaf without physically slicing it. The two pictures of the TMJ illustrated here (Fig. 2.138) represent two layers in this region approximately 0.5 cm apart.

Intraoral radiographic projections of jaws and teeth

Table 2.13 outlines the major intraoral radiographic projections used to view the human jaws and dentition. In this context, 'intraoral' indicates that the radiographic plate is positioned inside the mouth.

There are two maxillary occlusal views – the vertex approach (Fig. 2.139) and the nasal approach (Fig. 2.140). As the names suggest, these views of the maxilla essentially differ in the positioning of the X-ray tube, which is either at the vertex of the skull or at the nasion. Differences in the radiographic pictures obtained relate to the degree of superimposition (greater in the vertex occlusal) and the direction and proportions of the longitudinal axes of the teeth (more vertical and less distorted roots with the vertex occlusal). In addition to surveying the maxillary dentition, the maxillary occlusal views may also be used to define the nasal fossae and maxillary air sinuses. Fig. 2.141 illustrates a mandibular occlusal view.

Anatomical features seen on intraoral radiographs

The importance of appreciating the radiographic appearance of the teeth and their supporting tissues need hardly be emphasised. However, equally essential for the interpretation of an apparent divergence from the normal is an awareness of non-dental anatomical structures, which, to the unwary, may simulate pathological lesions on intraoral radiographs. The radio-opacities of normal anatomical structures seen on intraoral radiographs are given in Table 2.14.

The radiographic image of a tooth is illustrated in Fig. 2.144. Tooth substance absorbs more X-rays than any other tissue of comparable size

Table 2.13 Intraoral radiographic projections describing jaws and teeth

Projection/technique	Purpose
Maxillary and mandibular occlusal views of teeth in buccolingual plane (Figs 2.139–2.141)	Relationships of structures.
Periapical view of teeth (Fig. 2.142)	Examination of apices of teeth. Relationships of structures in the mesiodistal plane.
Bitewing examination of teeth (Fig. 2.143)	Survey of crowns of teeth and the alveolar crests.

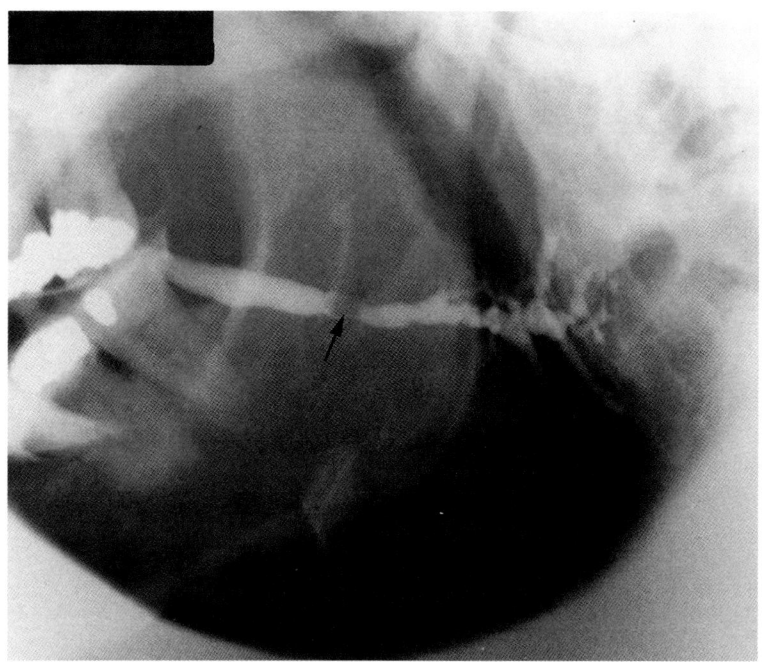

Fig. 2.137 Sialogram showing an obstruction in a dilated parotid duct (arrow). Courtesy Dr. N Drage.

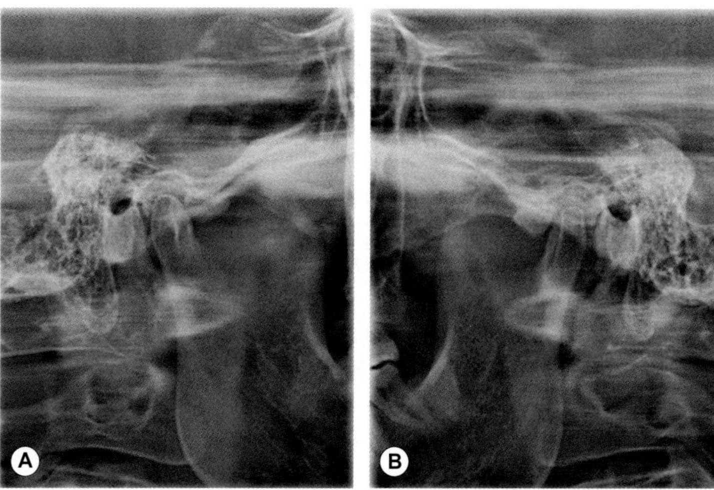

Fig. 2.138 Sectional panoramic radiographs of the right (A) and left (B) temporomandibular joints. The two images (A and B) are about 0.5 cm apart. Courtesy Dr. J Makdissi.

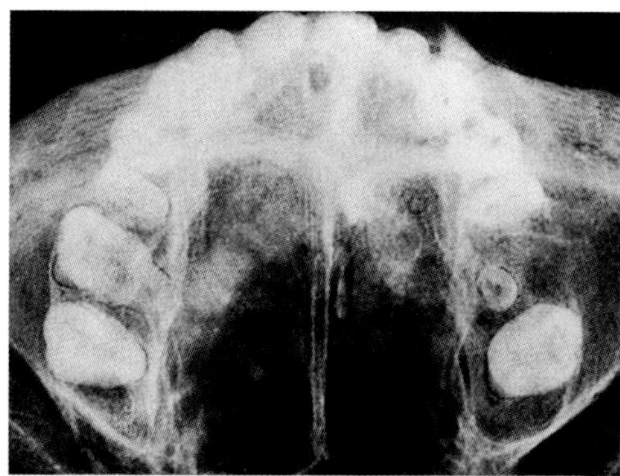

Fig. 2.139 Maxillary occlusal view – vertex approach. Historical view.

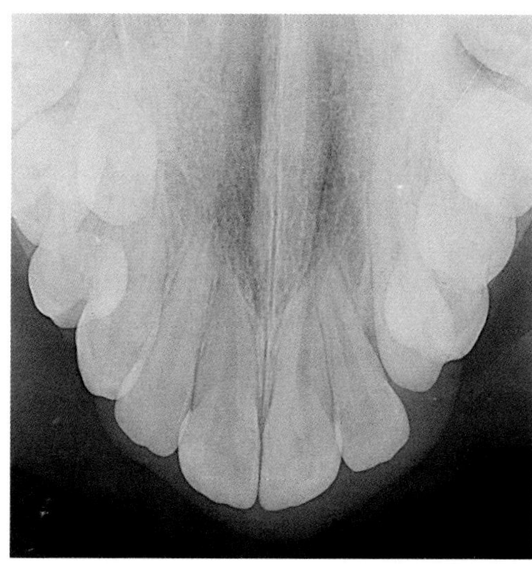

Fig. 2.140 Maxillary occlusal view – nasal approach. Courtesy Dr. J Makdissi.

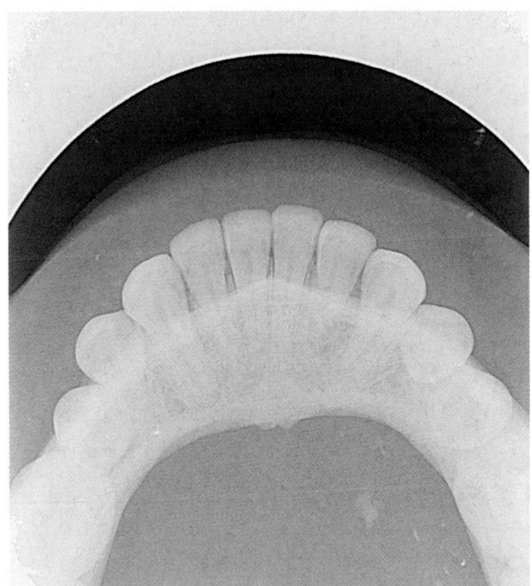

Fig. 2.141 Mandibular occlusal view. Courtesy Dr. J Makdissi.

Table 2.14 Radio-opacity of normal anatomical structures seen on intraoral radiographs

Radiolucent	Radio-opaque
Dental pulp	Enamel
Gingiva and periodontal ligament	Dentine
Bone marrow	Cementum
	Cortical bony plates
	Lamina dura
Maxillary sinus	Bony walls of maxillary sinus
Nasal cavity	Bony walls of nasal cavity
Incisive foramen	Nasal septum
Median palatine suture	Anterior nasal spine
Intermaxillary suture	Maxillary tuberosity
Nasolacrimal canal	Zygomatic arch
	Coronoid process
Mandibular canal	Pterygoid hamulus
	Internal and external oblique lines of mandible
Mental foramen	Borders of mandibular canal
Mandibular symphysis	Mental and canine prominences
	Genial spines
Bony depressions (e.g., mental and submandibular fossa)	
Nutrient canals	

and thickness. Enamel is the most radio-opaque and is easily distinguished covering the anatomical crown of the tooth. In normal teeth, the enamel is of uniform density, although in some areas where the enamel is thin (e.g., the cervical regions), it may appear relatively radiolucent. Such an appearance may easily be misinterpreted as dental caries. Dentine and cementum cannot be readily distinguished from each other radiographically because of their similar capacity to absorb X-rays. Owing to the lower radio-opacity of dentine, it appears comparatively 'greyer' than the enamel, and thus the enamel–dentine junction is clearly demarcated. The pulp of a tooth, being soft tissue, is readily penetrated by X-rays, and consequently on a radiograph the pulp cavity is clearly defined as the central radiolucent region of the tooth. However, because of distortion, foreshortening and superimposition, care should be taken in assessing the pulpal anatomy from radiographs. The tooth is supported in the bony alveolus. In this text, the alveolus refers to the whole of the bony supporting tissue of the tooth, and the lamina dura refers to the compact bone lining the tooth socket. The morphology of the margins of the alveolus (alveolar crest) is important in the diagnosis of periodontal disease. As a general rule, the width of the crest depends upon the distance the teeth are separated. Consequently, between the molars the crests are flat and horizontal, while between the incisors the crests rise only as points or spines. In the healthy situation, the crest rises to just below the level of the cementum–enamel junction. The lamina dura is considered to be a very important structure in the radiographic interpretation of periodontal and periapical pathologies. It appears as a continuous radio-opaque lining of the socket and usually is continuous over the alveolar crests. However, the radio-opacity of the lamina dura does not indicate any hypermineralisation, being a consequence of superimposition. Discontinuity of the lamina dura in the root region is usually indicative of abnormality or disease. Between the root of the tooth and the lamina dura of the socket is the connective tissue of the periodontal ligament, which appears as a thin radiolucent region. Fig. 2.145 shows the appearance of developing and erupting teeth (molars and premolars) where there are radiolucent regions around the emerging crowns and around the developing root apices.

With respect to anatomical structures that appear in association with the maxillary dentition, Fig. 2.146 describes some radiolucent anatomical features seen on an intraoral maxillary occlusal oblique view (i.e., the maxillary air sinus, the incisive foramen, the nasolacrimal canal and the nasal fossae). Fig. 2.147 shows how the incisive foramen and the nasal fossae can be seen on an intraoral periapical view of the maxillary first incisors. The medial palatine suture seen on an intraoral periapical view of the maxillary first incisors is illustrated in Fig. 2.148. The malar (zygomatic) shadow viewed on an intraoral periapical view of the maxillary molars seen in Figs 2.149 and 2.150 shows the radio-opaque shadow cast by a coronoid process of the mandible superimposed on a maxillary tuberosity.

Of particular importance in the upper jaw is the appearance of the maxillary air sinus or antrum. The floor of the sinus viewed on an intraoral periapical view of the maxillary premolars and molars is shown in Fig. 2.151. The maxillary air sinus is an air-filled cavity of varying dimensions; it appears radiographically as a dark, radiolucent shadow bounded by radio-opaque lines representing the lining layers of cortical bone. The radiolucency is not usually uniform because of superimposition of the zygomatic process and the soft tissues of the cheek. The air sinus often presents not as a single sinus but as several compartments because of bony septation. It is said that the cortical lining of the air sinus is not continuous, but exhibits numerous small, linear interruptions associated with nutrient canals. This radiographic characteristic may be important in avoiding misinterpretation of the sinus as a pathological lesion. The floor of the maxillary air sinus is closely related to the root apices of the maxillary teeth. Generally, the sinus extends from the premolars to the tuberosity, although variations are frequent. Because of the close relationship of the teeth to the maxillary air sinus, communication between the sinus and the oral cavity (oroantral fistula) following tooth extractions is unfortunately all too frequent. Because of the problems of interpreting three-dimensional situations on a two-dimensional radiograph, care must be taken to avoid misreading the relationship of the teeth to the sinus. Fig. 2.152 illustrates the configuration termed the 'Y of Ennis' that is formed by the abutment of the anterior wall of the maxillary air sinus and the floor of the nasal fossa.

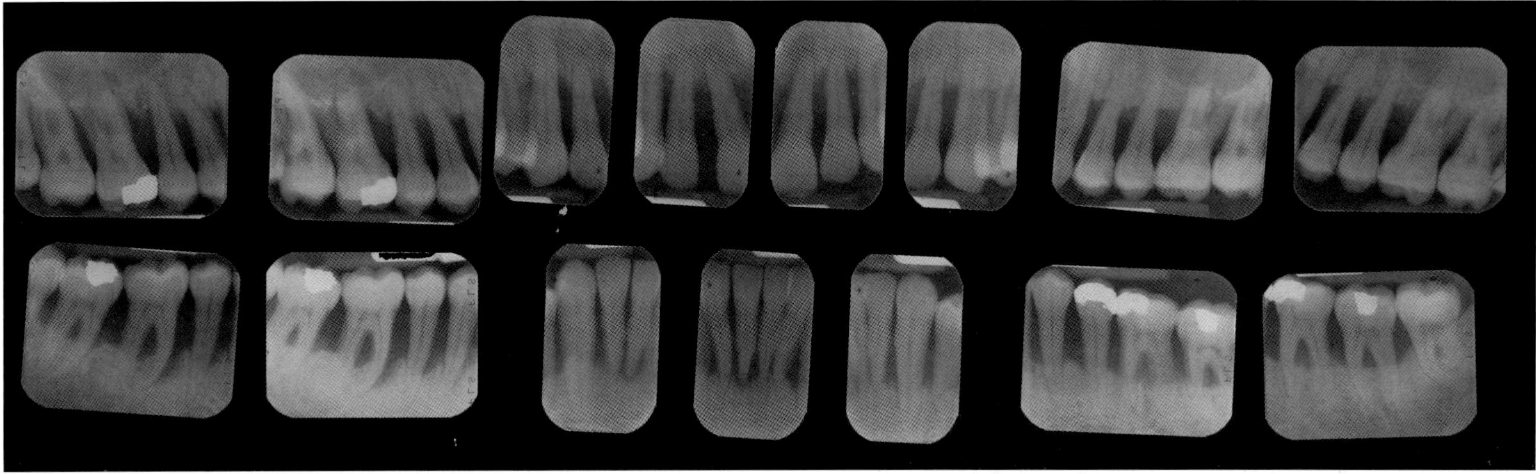

Fig. 2.142 Full mouth series of intraoral periapical views of the teeth. Courtesy Dr. J Makdissi.

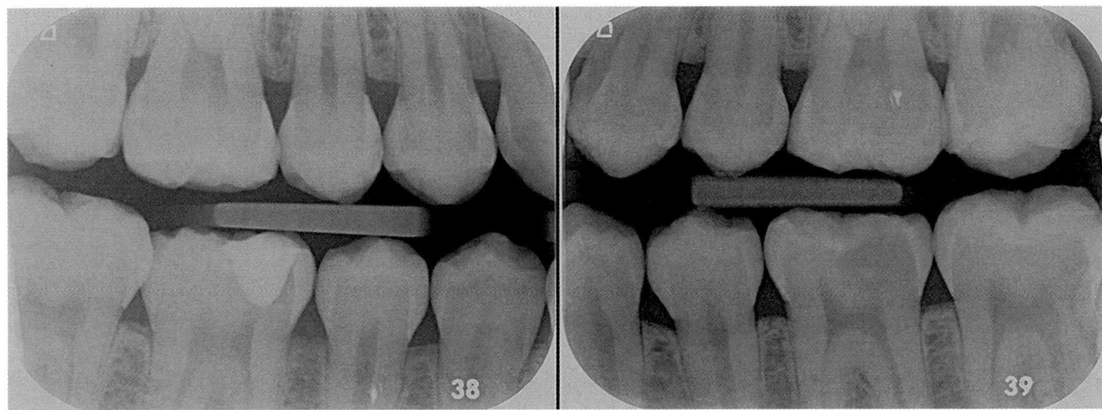

Fig. 2.143 Examination of the crowns of the permanent molars and associated alveolar crests using bitewing radiographs. Courtesy Dr. J Makdissi.

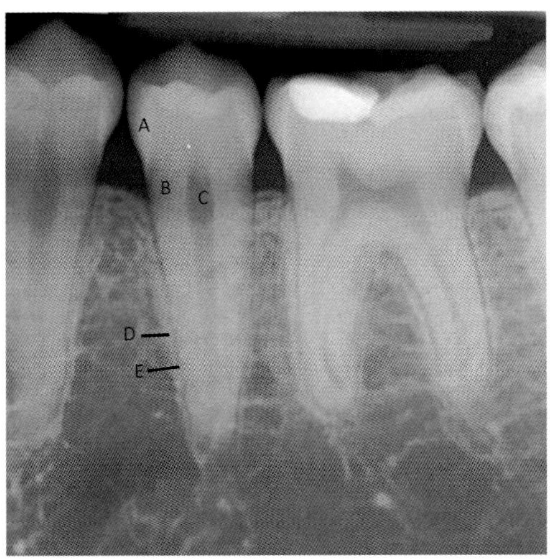

Fig. 2.144 Radiographic image of a tooth. A = enamel; B = dentine; C = dental pulp; D = lamina dura; E = periodontal space. Courtesy Dr. J Makdissi.

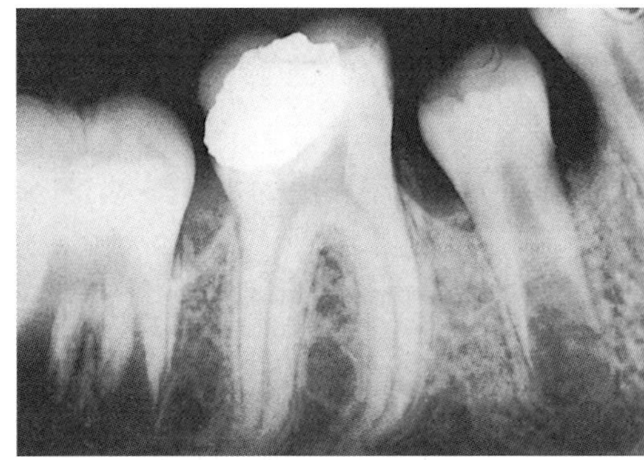

Fig. 2.145 Radiograph of developing and erupting molars and premolars.

With respect to anatomical structures that appear in association with the mandibular dentition, of particular importance is the radiographic appearance of the mandibular canal. The mandibular canal commences at the mandibular foramen and passes downwards and forwards from the ramus into the body of the mandible where, near the root apices of the premolars, it terminates by dividing into the mental and incisive canals (Fig. 2.153). The radiographic appearance of the mandibular canal is generally that of a radiolucent shadow bounded superiorly and inferiorly by radio-opaque lines. The width and position of the canal vary considerably. Most commonly, the canal is closely related to the roots of the molars, although it lies some distance from the roots of the premolars. Generally, the canal lies buccal to the root apices, a feature that should be remembered when interpreting the relationship of the root apices to the canal. The precise relationship of the teeth to the canal is difficult to determine from radiographs, although some hint of a very close relationship can be obtained by reference to the densities of shadows cast by the roots and canal, the

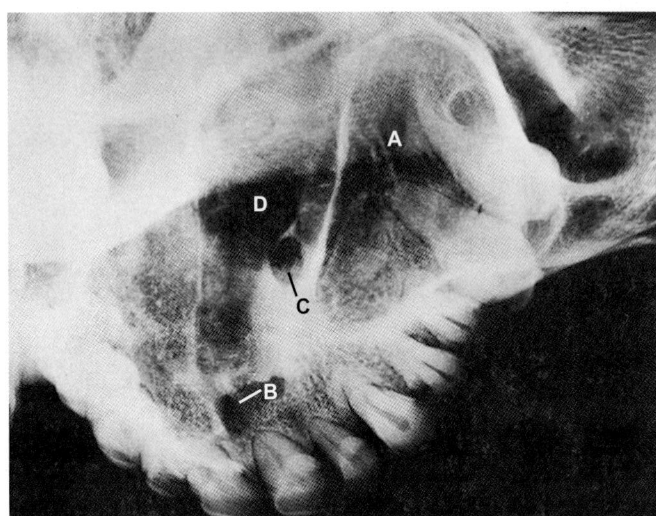

Fig. 2.146 Radiolucent, anatomical features seen on an intraoral maxillary occlusal oblique view. A = maxillary sinus (antrum); B = incisive foramen; C = nasolacrimal canal; D = nasal fossa. Historical view.

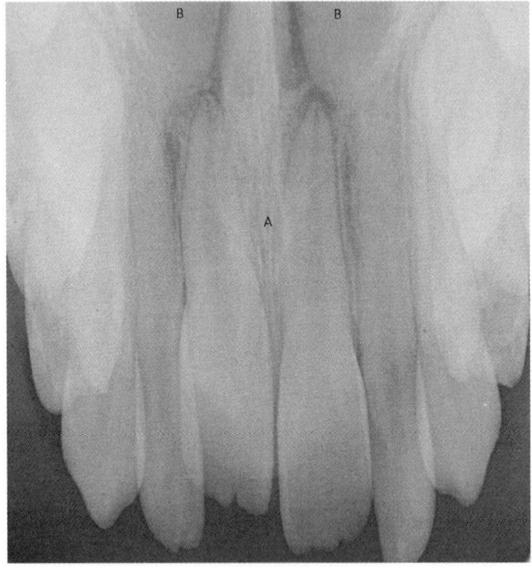

Fig. 2.147 The incisive foramen (A) and nasal fossae (B) seen on an upper occlusal radiograph. Courtesy Dr. J Makdissi.

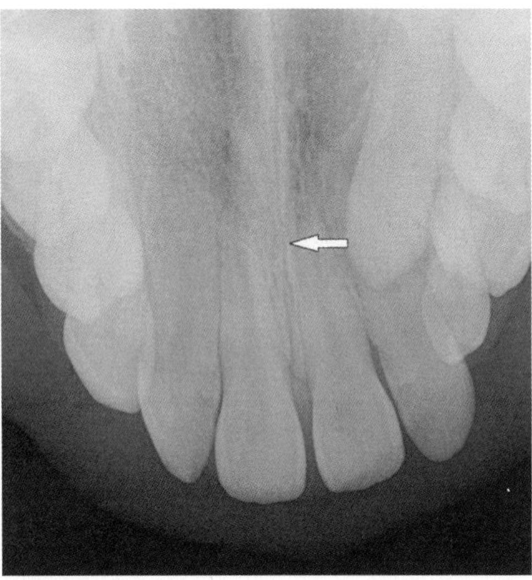

Fig. 2.148 The median palatine suture (arrowed) seen on an upper occlusal radiograph. Courtesy Dr. J Makdissi.

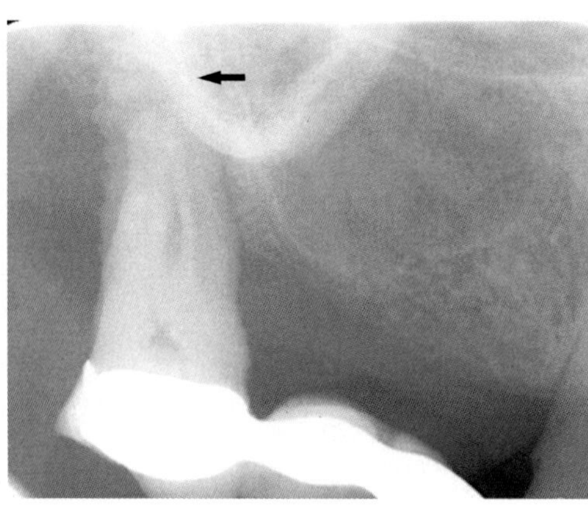

Fig. 2.149 Zygomatic buttress shadow (arrowed). Courtesy Dr. J Makdissi.

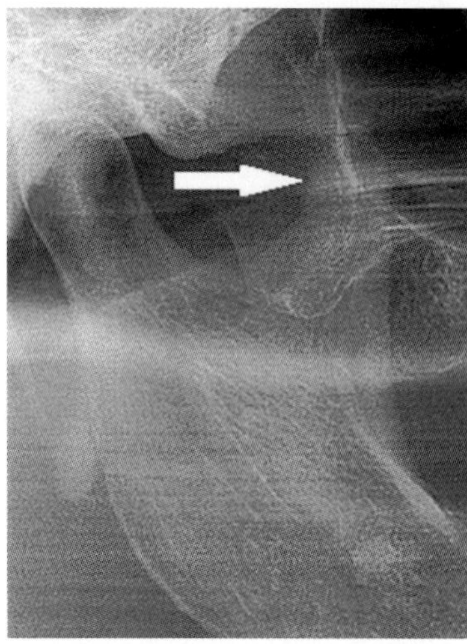

Fig. 2.150 Radio-opaque shadow cast by a coronoid process (arrowed). Courtesy Dr. J Makdissi.

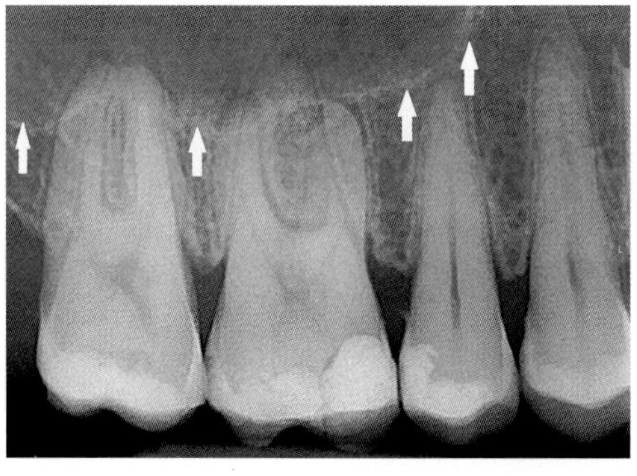

Fig. 2.151 The floor of the maxillary air sinus (arrows) seen on an intraoral periapical view of the maxillary premolars and molars. Courtesy Dr. J Makdissi.

position and densities of the lamina dura and the radio-opaque margins of the canal and the dimensions of the lumen of the canal.

The mandibular symphysis at birth is shown on an intraoral mandibular occlusal radiograph (Fig. 2.154). This symphysis closes by the age of 3 years. Fig. 2.155 illustrates the genial spines seen on an intraoral periapical view of the mandibular central incisors. Note the characteristic radiographic appearance of the genial spines (i.e., a radiolucent dot surrounded by a distinct radio-opaque region). The internal and external oblique lines of the mandible are seen in Fig. 2.156, where an occlusal view of an edentulous mandible demonstrates the prominent radio-opacities associated with these lines.

Clinical considerations

Facial fractures

Fractures of the facial skeleton (including the jaws) are very common, often as a result of road traffic accidents (RTAs), physical violence (i.e., interpersonal violence), work accidents and sports injuries. Fractures affecting the face are often complex, particularly for the middle third of

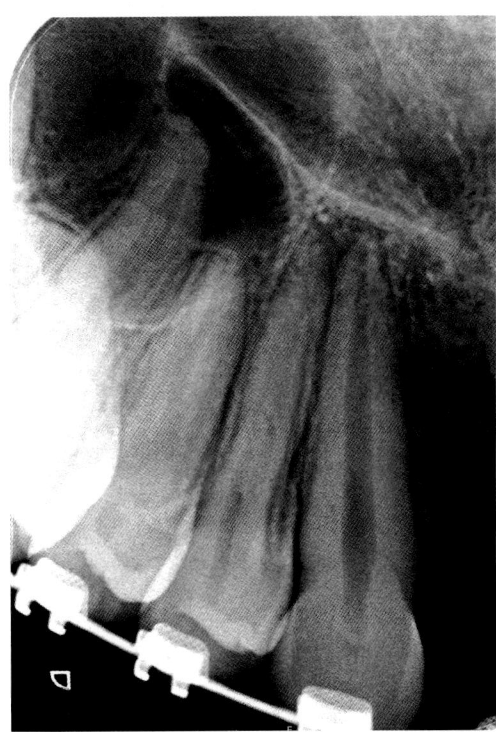

Fig. 2.152 The configuration termed the Y of Ennis. Courtesy Dr. J Makdissi.

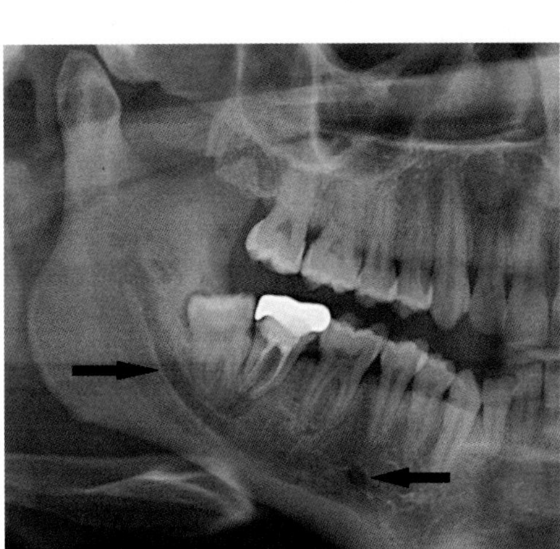

Fig. 2.153 Mandibular canal and mental foramen (arrows). Courtesy Dr J Makdissi.

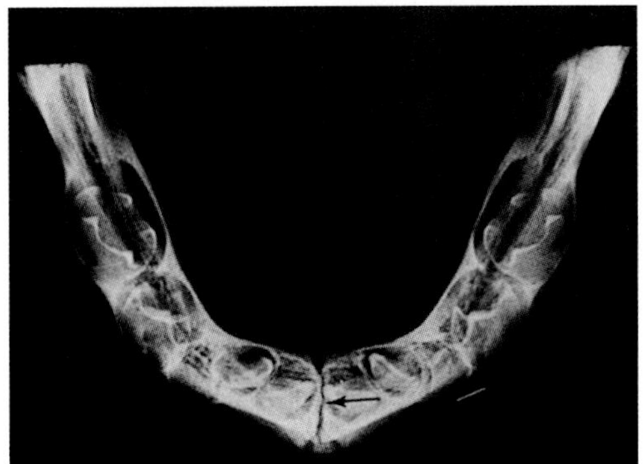

Fig. 2.154 The mandibular symphysis (arrowed) at birth.

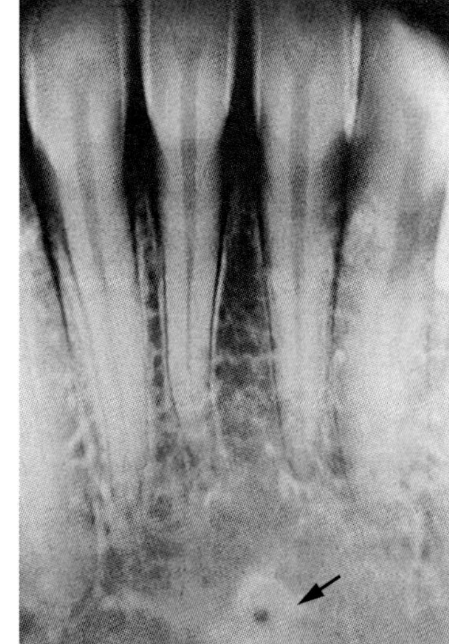

Fig. 2.155 The genial spines (arrowed).

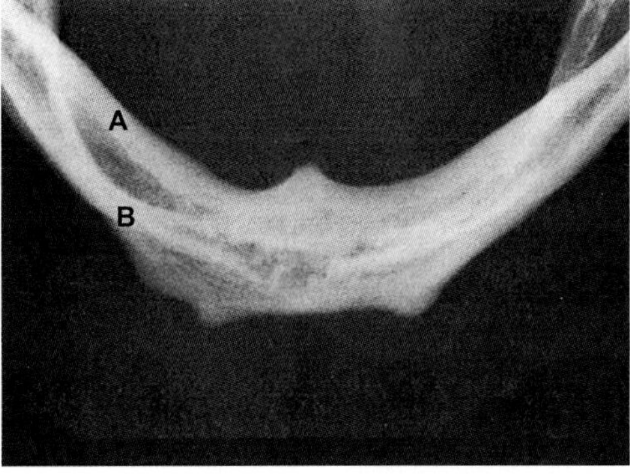

Fig. 2.156 Internal (A) and external (B) oblique lines of the mandible.

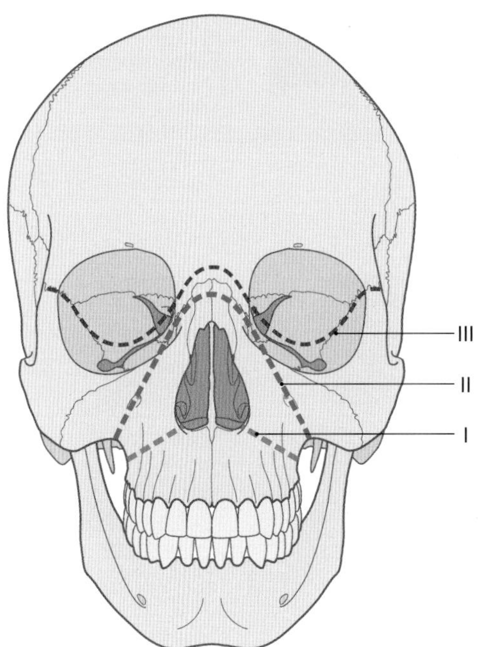

Fig. 2.157 Le Fort classification of fractures of the face I, II and III.

the face. In order to appreciate fractures of the central middle third of the face, it is necessary to understand the extent to which this region is supported by the maxillary bones. These bones not only form the alveolar processes (i.e., the upper jaws housing the maxillary dentition) but also contribute to the palate, the nasal aperture, the zygomatic complex (i.e., cheek bone region), the floor of the orbit and part of the bridge of the nose extending up to the forehead. Fractures of the central middle third of the face are categorised according to a Le Fort system of classification (Fig. 2.157). Le Fort I fractures have a fracture line running horizontally above the level of the floor of the nose and produce a mobile segment comprising the alveolar process, the palate and the lower region of the pterygoid plates. Le Fort II fractures have a more extensive involvement of the

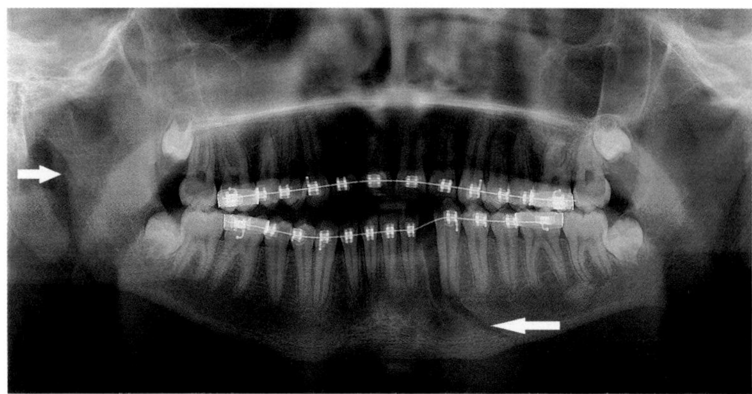

Fig. 2.158 Orthopantomogram of patient showing fracture of right condyle and left body of mandible *arrows. Courtesy Dr. J Makdissi.

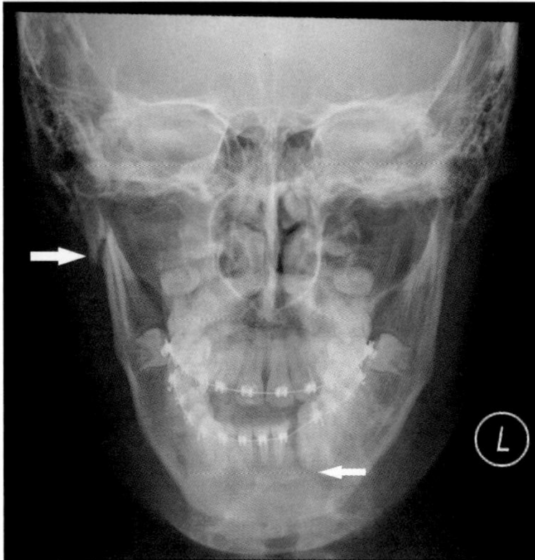

Fig. 2.159 Posteroanterior radiograph showing the fracture sites (arrows) from patient seen in Fig. 2.158. Courtesy Dr. J Makdissi.

maxillary bones. Le Fort III fractures separate the entire facial skeleton from the cranial base, with the fracture lines running parallel with the base of the skull.

It should be borne in mind that fractures of the central middle third of the face are not always bilaterally symmetrical, and separation of the fracture segments does not usually result from muscle pull. The fracture segments are generally displaced downwards and backwards, resulting in a 'dished-in' appearance of the face. Furthermore, the airway may become obstructed.

Fractures of the mandible, a bone that constitutes the lower third of the face, are also very common. In most instances, the mandible fractures at two (or more) sites, and consequently isolated fractures are unusual. In order of frequency, most fractures of the mandible occur at the neck of the condyle (Figs 2.158, 2.159), the angle (and ramus) of the mandible and the body of the mandible (Figs 2.158–2.161). Fractures at the neck of the condyle can occur when a patient receives a blow to the chin or to the body of the mandible on the contralateral side. When this occurs the condyle is usually displaced anteromedially as a result of the pull of the lateral pterygoid muscle. With a fracture of the angle of the mandible, the fracture line usually extends downwards and backwards from the alveolar bone and could involve the third molar tooth (and its socket). The posterior fragment would then be displaced upwards, inwards and forwards because of the pull of the masseter, temporalis and medial pterygoid muscles. Fractures of the body of the mandible are usually found in the canine or first molar regions as a result of a direct blow to these parts. Should the fracture line pass downwards and forwards, the fragments will not be greatly displaced because the upward pull of the masseter, temporalis and medial pterygoid muscles is counteracted by the downward and backward pull of the anterior belly of the digastric and geniohyoid muscles. However, if the fracture line runs downwards and backwards, the fragments may be considerably displaced, particularly if the patient is edentulous. It is important that several radiographic views are taken in different planes for a full appreciation of the nature of the fracture(s) and the degree of any displacement.

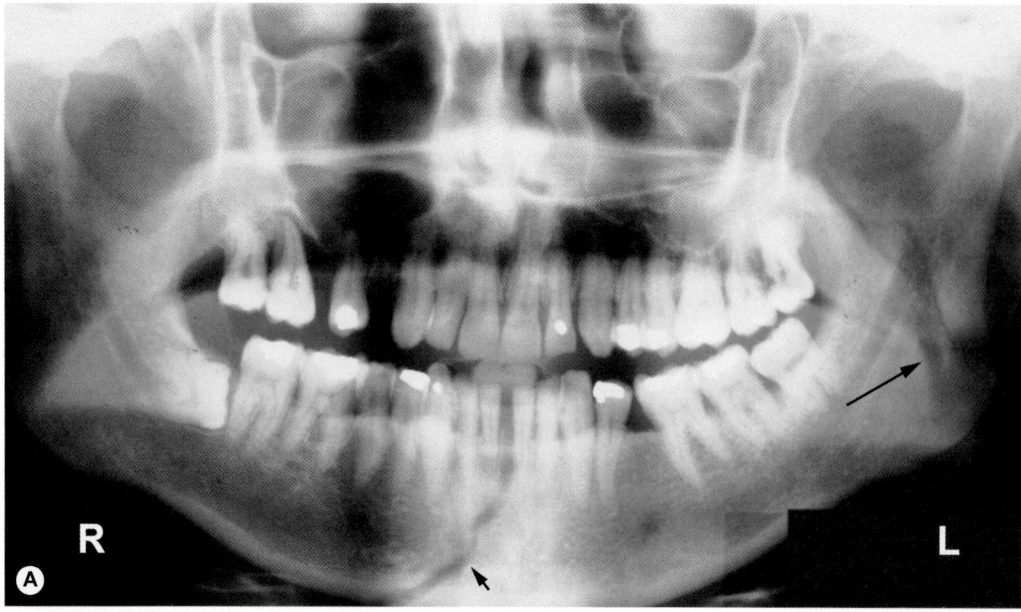

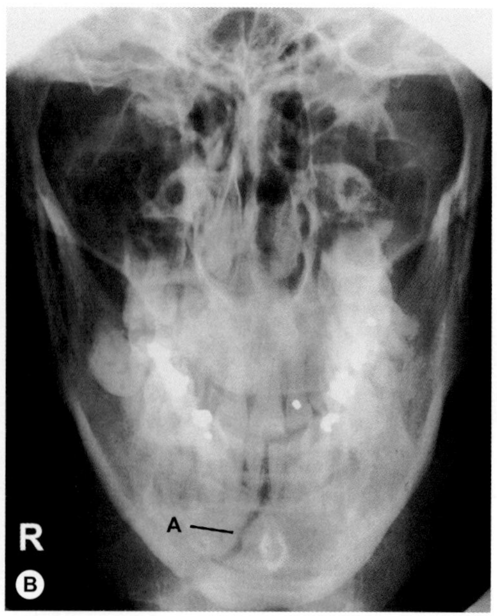

Fig. 2.160 (A) OPG of patient with a bilateral fracture of the body near the midline (small arrow) and angle and ramus (large arrow) of the left side of the mandible. (B) Posteroanterior radiograph showing favourable fracture line at angle of mandible with no displacement of left ramus. A = Line of fracture of body of mandible. Courtesy Dr. J Jones.

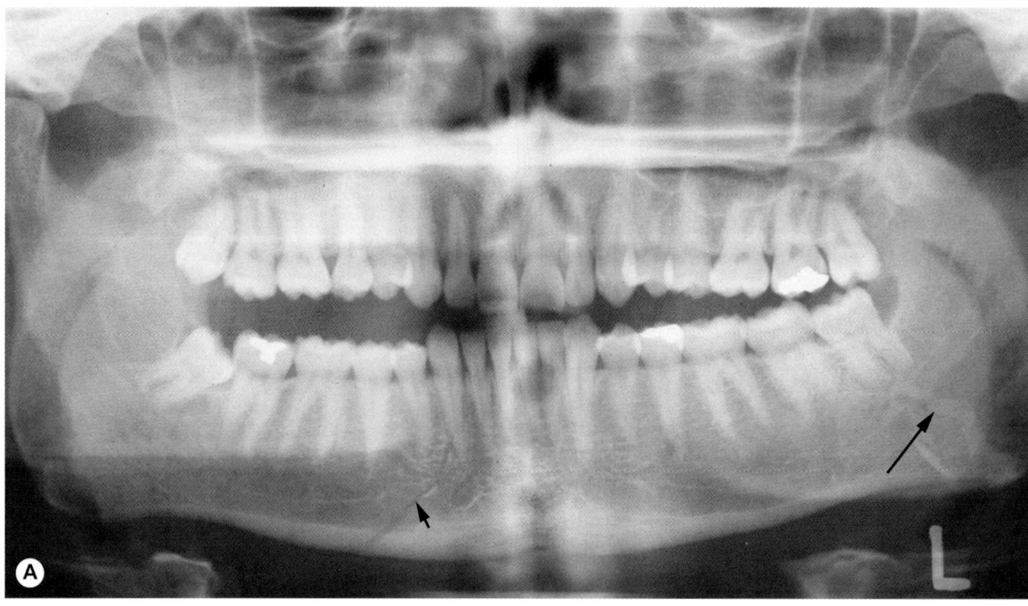

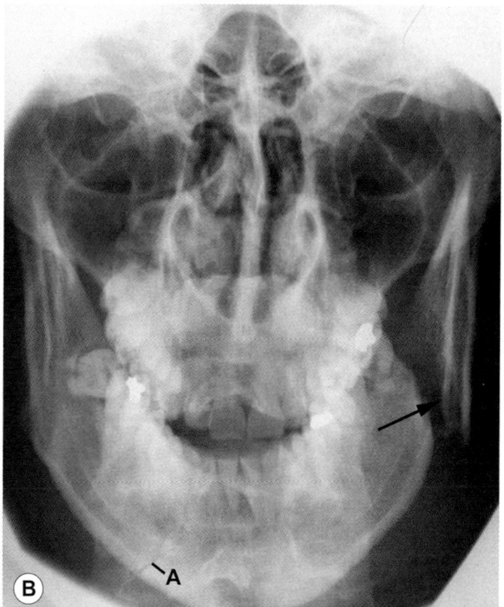

Fig. 2.161 (A) OPG of patient with a bilateral fracture of the right body (small arrow) and left angle (large arrow) of the mandible. (B) Posteroanterior radiograph showing unfavourable fracture line at angle of mandible with displacement of ramus (arrow). A = line of fracture of the body on the right side. Courtesy Dr. J Jones.

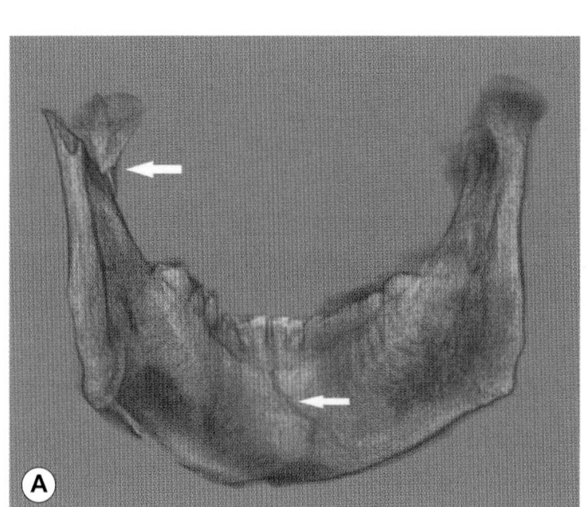

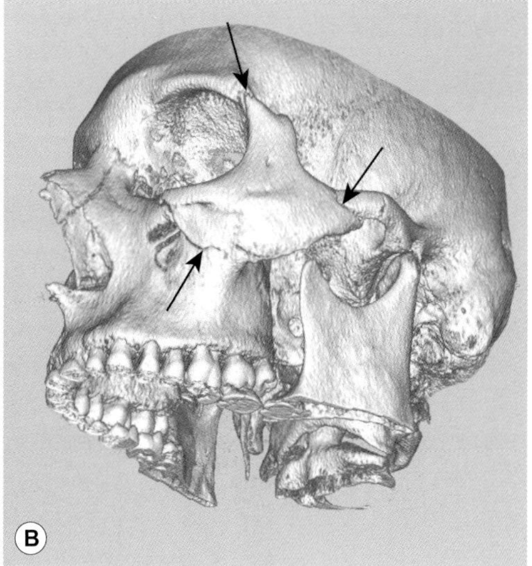

Fig. 2.162 Cone beam CT scan of (A) mandible showing a fractured left condyle and body of mandible near midline (arrows) and (B) showing fracture of zygoma at three sites (arrows). Courtesy Dr. J Makdissi.

Recent technical advances have led to cone beam computed tomography (CBCT) scans that allow three-dimensional reconstruction of the facial skeleton. This now aids surgeons with a complete picture of the operative site and allows them to rehearse their surgical procedures (Fig. 2.162).

Variation in tooth morphology

This topic is considered on pages 394–397.

Number of teeth

Although a full dentition numbers 32 teeth, a tooth may fail to develop, giving a reduced number. A complete absence of teeth is termed *anodontia* (see page 394). When a reduced number of teeth are present, this condition is commonly known as *hypodontia* (partial anodontia). The tooth most commonly absent (in about 25% of cases) is the third molar tooth, followed by the second premolar and the maxillary lateral incisor in about 2.5% of cases. The maxillary second incisor is also susceptible to a reduction in size in about another 2.5% of individuals, giving rise to the 'peg-shaped' incisor (see Fig. 2.47).

In rarer cases, more than one tooth type is missing. In rare congenital disorders, such as ectodermal dysplasia, all the teeth may be missing (anodontia). In ectodermal dysplasia, some teeth are generally present and may have a simplified morphology. Fig. 2.163 is a radiograph illustrating a patient in which the permanent dentition is entirely absent.

As well as teeth being reduced in number, there may be additional teeth present. These may be present in both the permanent and deciduous dentition, but are five times as common in the permanent dentition. Where they resemble the normal tooth morphology, they are referred to as *supplemental teeth*. These can represent any tooth type and can vary in number from a single tooth (Fig. 2.164) to, very occasionally, almost complete rows (Fig. 2.165). Most often, however, they have a simpler morphology and are termed *supernumerary teeth*. They are usually found in the midline between the maxillary central incisors and are called *mesiodens* (Fig. 2.166). Their presence may obstruct the eruption of the permanent central incisors, in which case they will need to be surgically removed (see Fig. 26.53).

Size of teeth

There is considerable variation in the size of the dentition in different individuals. Where a tooth (or teeth) is unusually small, the condition is referred to as *microdontia* (Fig. 2.167). Microdontia generally affects individual teeth, usually the maxillary second incisor and the third molar. Occasionally, many teeth in the same dentition may be affected, in which case the teeth may be spaced apart. Where a tooth is unusually large, the condition is referred to as *macrodontia* (megadontia) (Fig. 2.168). During early tooth development the enamel organ may partially divide resulting in the appearance of a large ‘double tooth’. This is known as a *geminated tooth* and can be found in most tooth positions (Figs 2.169, 2.170). The number of teeth present in these situations is normal. Fig. 2.171 illustrates an unusual example where a geminated maxillary left incisor is present, showing a single pulp cavity, while the maxillary right central and lateral incisors are fused (see next), showing two pulp cavities, as evidenced by the accompanying radiograph.

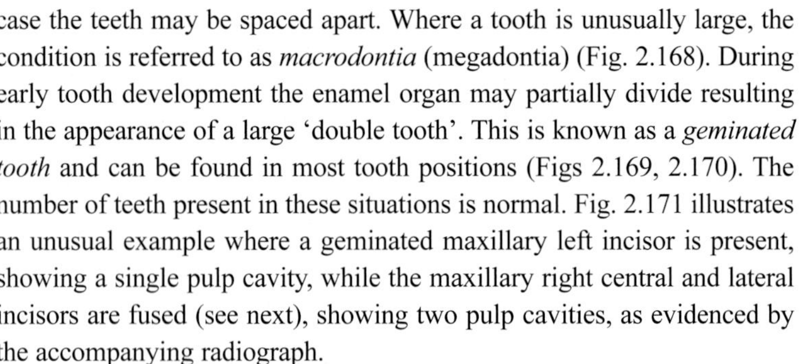

Fusion and transposition of teeth

Rarely, two adjacent teeth may be joined, giving rise to a fused tooth. In this situation, the total number of teeth would be one less than normal, distinguishing it from a geminated tooth (Fig. 2.172). Tooth transposition refers to the positional interchange of two adjacent teeth. The tooth most commonly involved is the permanent canine, with the maxillary being more frequently encountered than the mandibular. The maxillary canine is most frequently transposed with the first premolar rather than with the lateral incisor (Fig. 2.173). When the mandibular canine is involved, it is invariably transposed with the lateral incisor. Patients exhibiting transpositions also show a higher incidence of congenitally absent teeth, peg-shaped lateral incisors and/or supernumerary teeth.

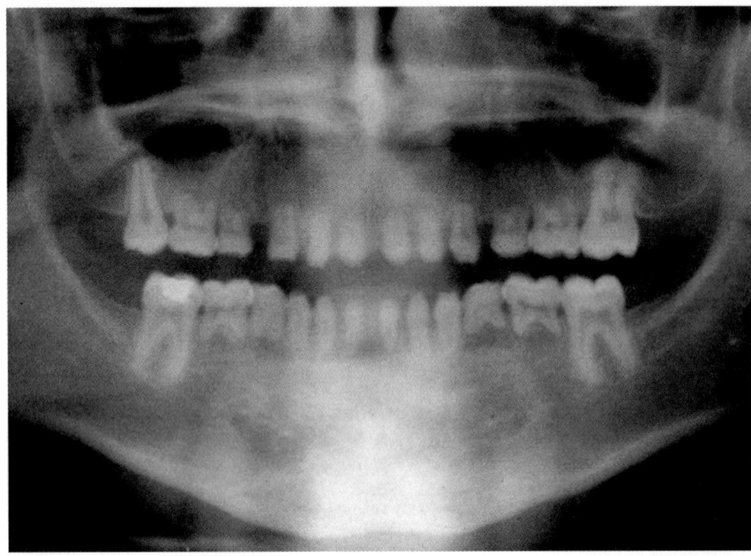

Fig. 2.163 Radiograph of patient with a complete deciduous dentition but with absence of the permanent dentition except for the first permanent molar. Courtesy Dr. P Smith.

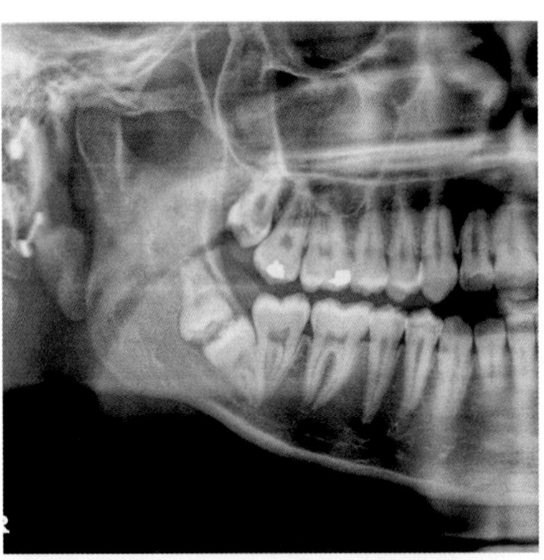

Fig. 2.164 Radiograph showing an inverted, supplemental (fourth), permanent molar, high up in the ramus of the mandible. Courtesy Dr. B J Doherty.

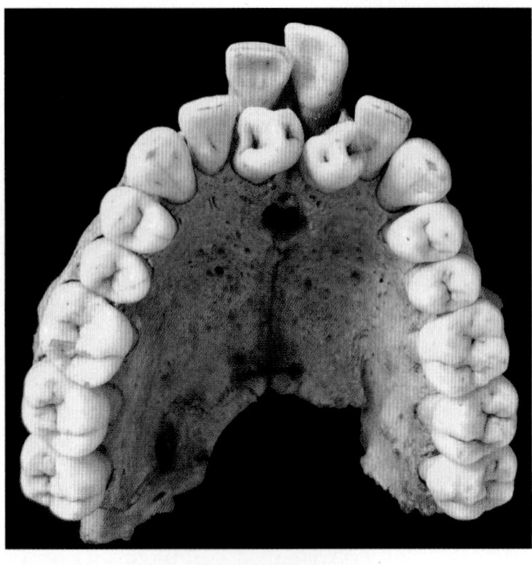

Fig. 2.166 Upper jaw showing the presence of two mesiodens. Copyright the Royal College of Surgeons of England.

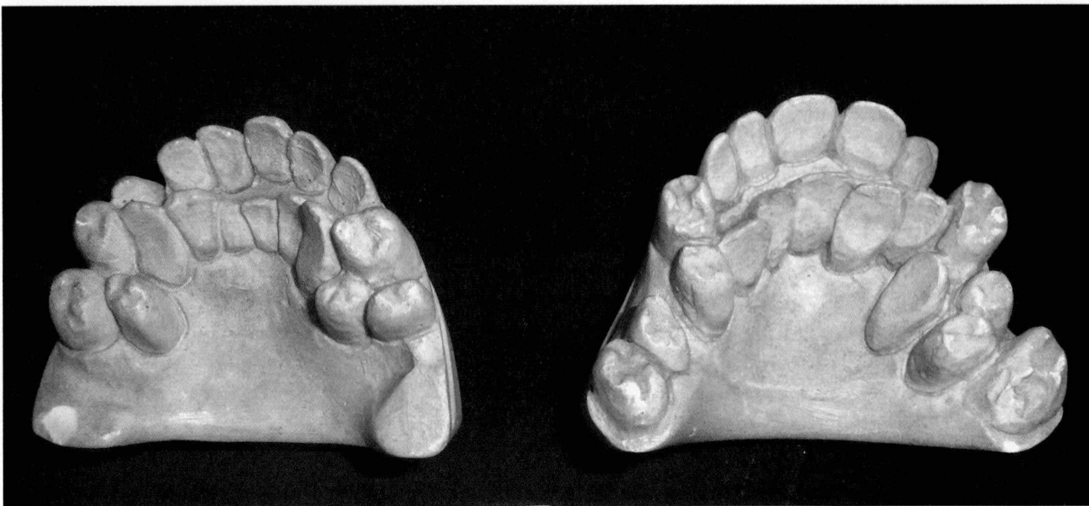

Fig. 2.165 Supplemental teeth forming almost complete second dental arches in both the lower (left image) and upper (right image) jaw of a patient. Copyright the Royal College of Surgeons of England.

Root and pulp morphology

There is extensive information available on root canal morphology obtained by examining and dissecting extracted teeth, making casts of the canal system and filling the system with fluids that can be visualised after clearing the teeth or that are radio-opaque. In the clinical setting the information available from an individual tooth is much more restricted. Radiographs are the main source, but are only two-dimensional shadows, suffering seriously from superimposition. This can be lessened somewhat by taking multiple radiographs at different angles. In the future, three-dimensional techniques such as computed tomography will reduce this limitation.

There is considerable variation in root morphology, but it is important to know the more common patterns, including the number of roots and root canals (see pages 34–38). Indeed, initial radiographs may alert the dental surgeon to the presence of extra roots and/or extra root canals (Figs 2.174–2.176).

Variation in root morphology will have clinical implications. The root may be unduly curved or show sudden bending (dilacerations), generally because of trauma encountered during development (Figs 2.177, 2.178), or present thickenings at the apex owing to hypercementosis (Figs 2.179A, 2.180 and see Fig. 11.35). Rarely, the roots of adjacent teeth may be joined by cementum (Fig. 2.179B). This is known as *concrescence* and usually

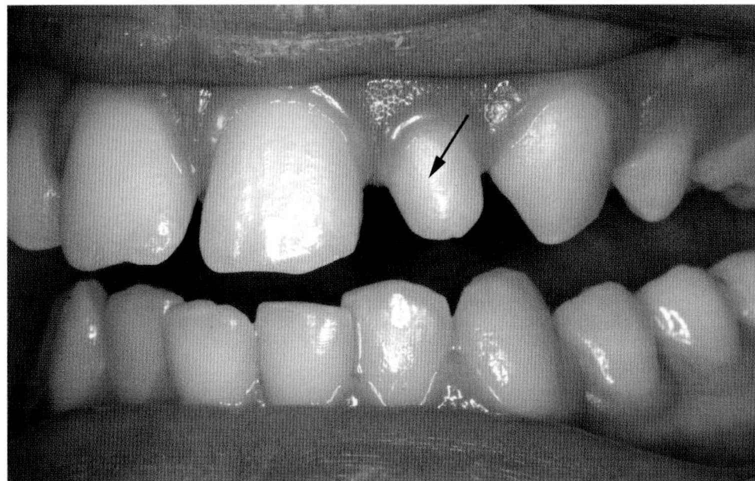

Fig. 2.167 An example of microdontia in the form of a 'peg' maxillary lateral incisor (arrow). Courtesy Dr. M Cobourne.

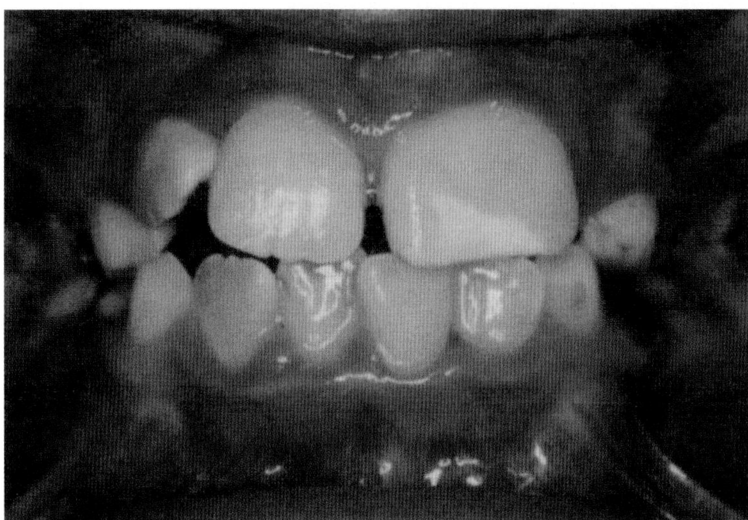

Fig. 2.168 An example of macrodontia affecting the maxillary left first incisor.

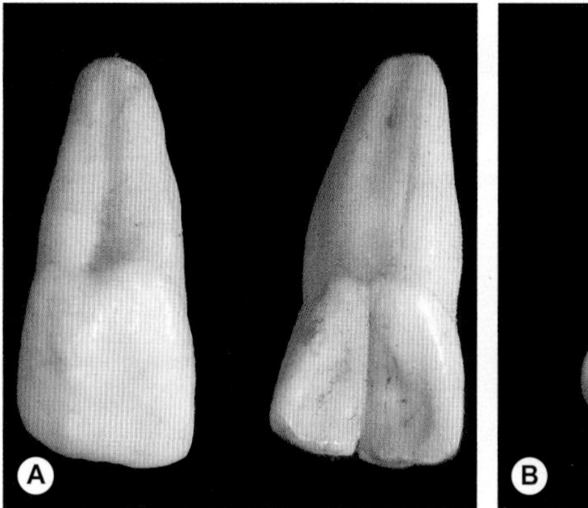

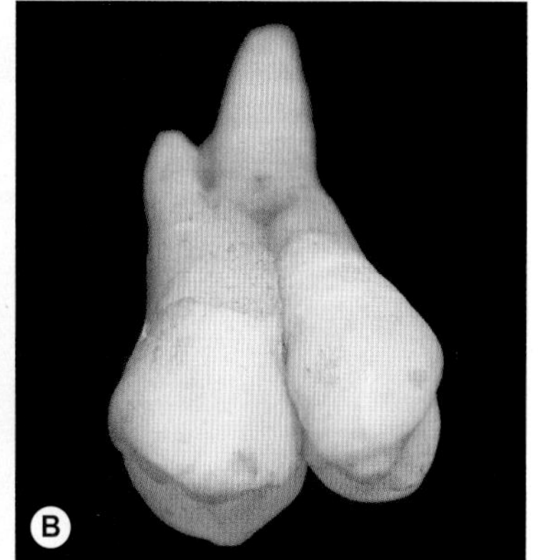

Fig. 2.169 (A) Geminated maxillary permanent incisor tooth. (B) Geminated maxillary premolar tooth. Copyright the Royal College of Surgeons of England.

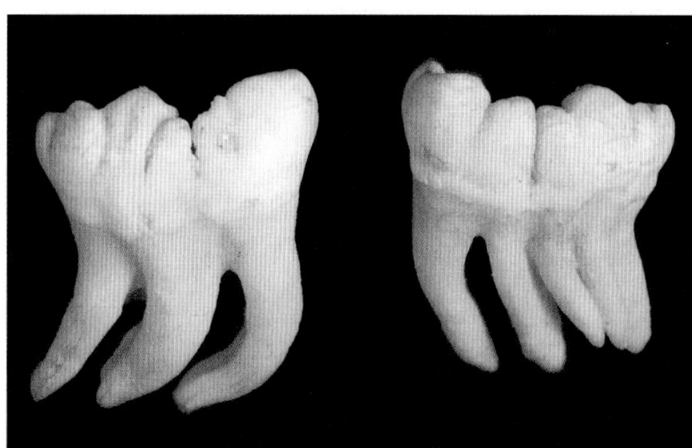

Fig. 2.170 Geminated mandibular permanent molar tooth. Copyright the Royal College of Surgeons of England.

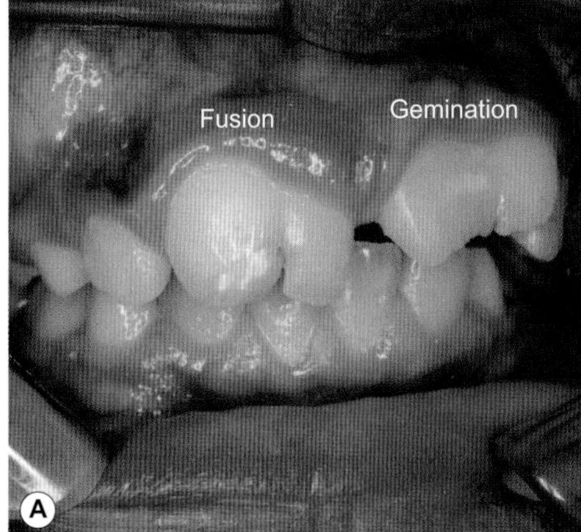

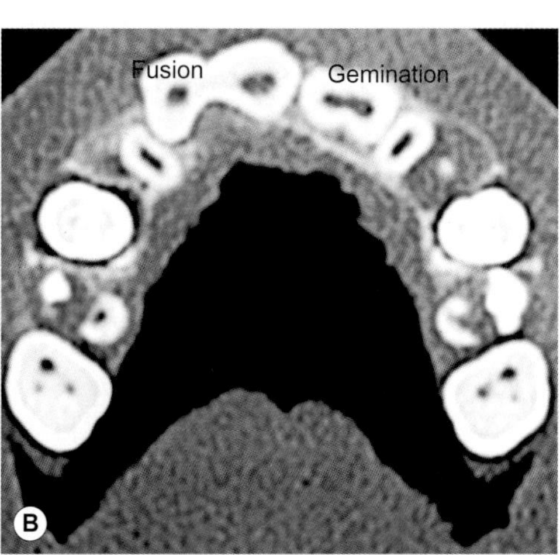

Fig. 2.171 An unusual example where a geminated maxillary left incisor is present, showing a single pulp cavity, while the maxillary right central and lateral incisors are fused, showing two pulp cavities, as evidenced by the accompanying radiograph. Courtesy Dr. Antonis Chaniotis.

affects second and third permanent molars. Such teeth will require special surgical treatment should tooth extraction be required.

The root apices of the upper cheek teeth are close to, and may even invaginate, the maxillary sinus (Figs 2.181, 2.182; see also Fig. 2.5). During removal of fractured root apices in this region, care must be taken to ensure that the root fragment is not pushed into the sinus. This may lead to the development of a patent oro-antral fistula, allowing food to enter the maxillary sinus (Fig. 2.183). A clear periapical radiograph is required before any tooth extraction is undertaken, as it may alert the dental surgeon to any problems that might be encountered. Thus, although normally lying beneath the roots of third permanent molar teeth, the inferior alveolar nerve and vessels lying in the mandibular canal may occupy a higher position and even run between the roots. Evidence of this close relationship may be seen in radiographs as a constriction of the mandibular canal or the radiolucent canal overlying the roots of the third molar (Fig. 2.184). In this situation, the neurovascular structures are at risk during extraction of third molars. The root of a mandibular premolar may occasionally be unusually long and can be in close relationship to the mental nerve and its parent branch, the inferior alveolar nerve, and these nerves are at risk during extraction of this tooth.

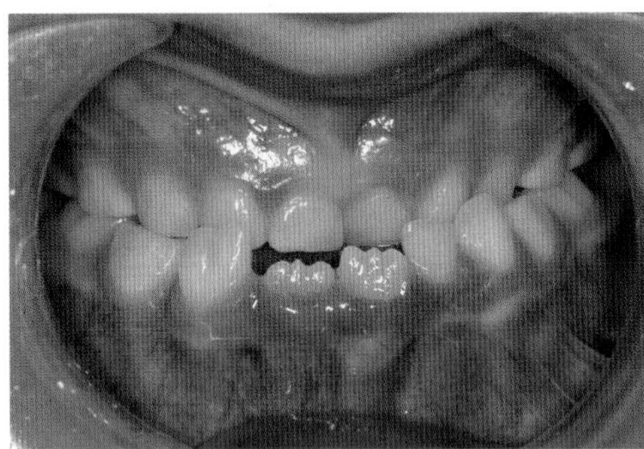

Fig. 2.172 Fusion affecting the mandibular right deciduous lateral incisor and canine in a 6-year-old child. Note the mamelons on the erupting mandibular deciduous central incisors and the bilateral crossbite. Courtesy Dr. R Whatling.

An understanding of the morphology of the pulp chamber and the root canal system is clearly essential in endodontic treatment (root canal therapy), in which a diseased pulp is removed and replaced with an inert filling material. As well as the number and shape of the root canals, it is important to know where the orifices of the root canals may be found on

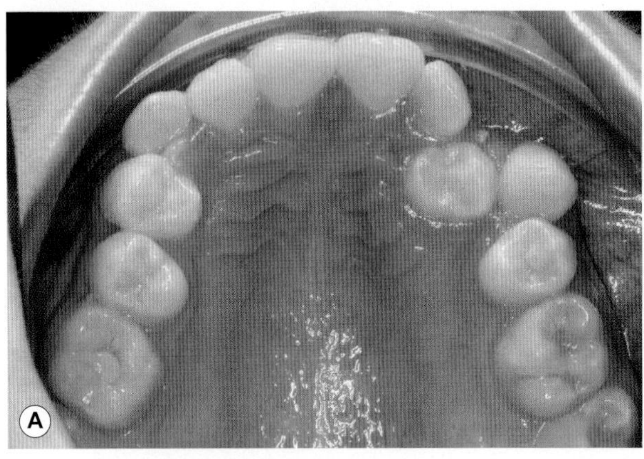

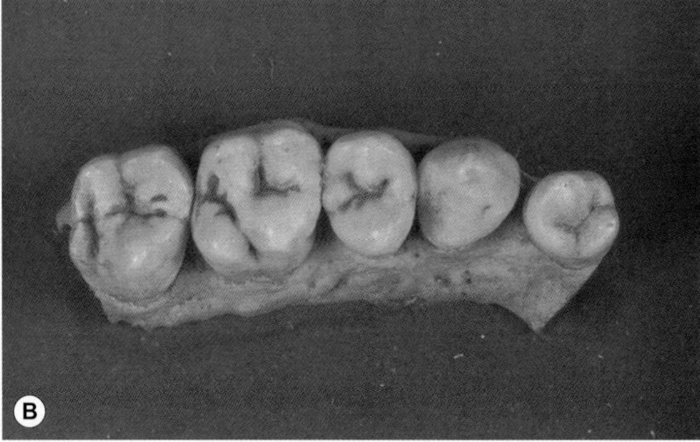

Fig. 2.173 (A) Transposition of a left maxillary canine with a first premolar. (B) Part of right maxilla showing transposition of left permanent canine with first premolar. (A) Courtesy Prof. F McDonald. (B) Copyright the Royal College of Surgeons of England.

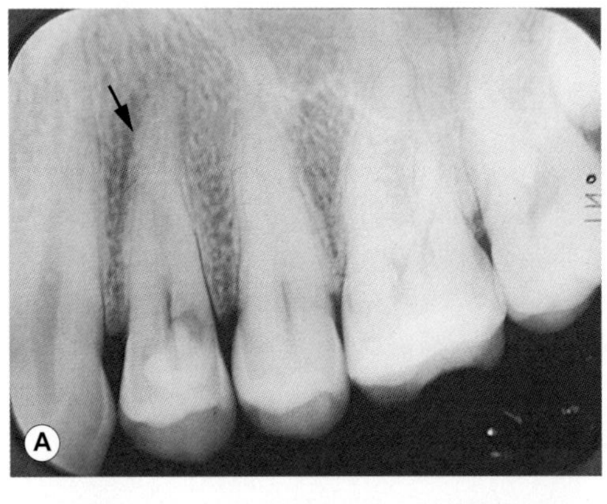

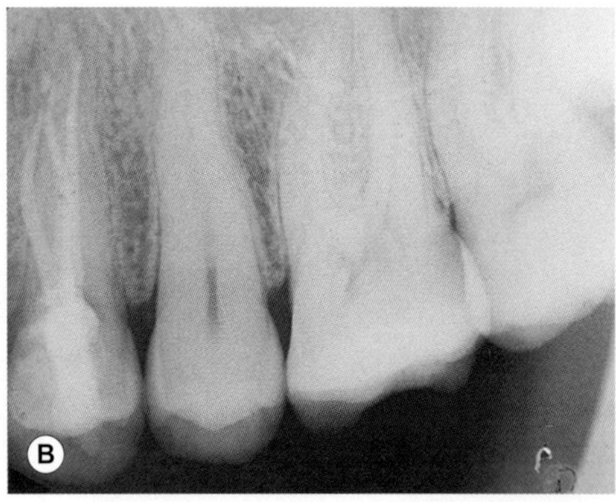

Fig. 2.174 (A) Radiograph showing evidence of three root canals (arrow) associated with a maxillary first premolar before endodontic treatment. (B) Same tooth after endodontic treatment. Courtesy Dr. S Patel.

A

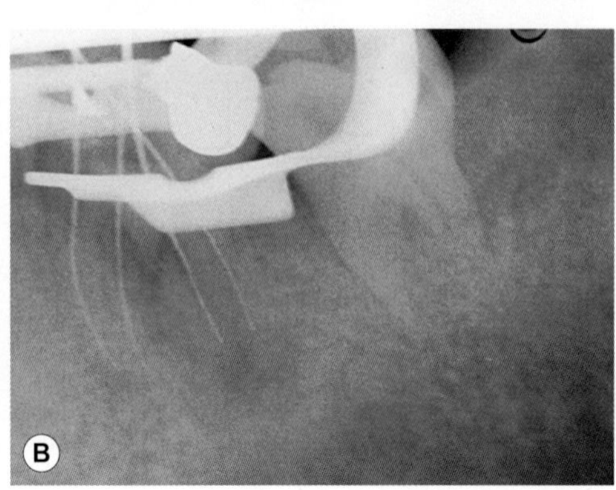

Fig. 2.175 (A) Radiograph showing evidence of an extra root on mandibular first permanent molar before endodontic treatment. (B) Same tooth during endodontic treatment.

the floor of the pulp chamber so that the correct cavity (access cavity) is cut on the crown to gain the best access (Fig. 2.185). With advancing age, the continued deposition of secondary, and perhaps tertiary, dentine leads to a reduction in size of the pulp chamber and root canals (Fig. 2.186).

The cementum–dentine junction at the root apex is a biologically significant point, as it marks the junction of the dental pulp and the periodontal tissues. As such, it is the level to which a filling replacing the dental pulp should extend. The cementum at the junction forms a constriction, the apical constriction (see Fig. 2.59), against which, in ideal circumstances, a filling material may be packed. This constriction is found a short but variable distance within the canal back from its exit on the root surface. The root canal exits on to the root surface a short distance below the anatomical apex of the root. Care must be taken to ensure that root filling material is not introduced into the tissues beyond the root apex, as in the case of the maxillary canine and the cheek teeth, where it may pass into the maxillary sinus (Fig. 2.187), and in the case of a mandibular molar into the mandibular canal (Fig. 2.188).

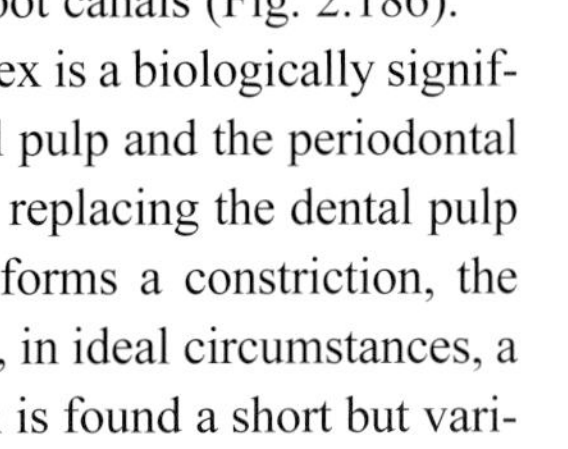

Occasionally a taurodont tooth may be evident on radiographs. In this type of tooth, the broad root only bifurcates near its apex, and therefore, the pulp chamber extends a significant distance into the root. The taurodont tooth will require a different mode of treatment from that for a tooth with normal root canals (Fig. 2.189).

Aesthetics, the smile and the alignment and occlusion of anterior teeth

The abnormalities described under malocclusion (see page 46) will probably require orthodontic treatment, with or without the necessity of tooth

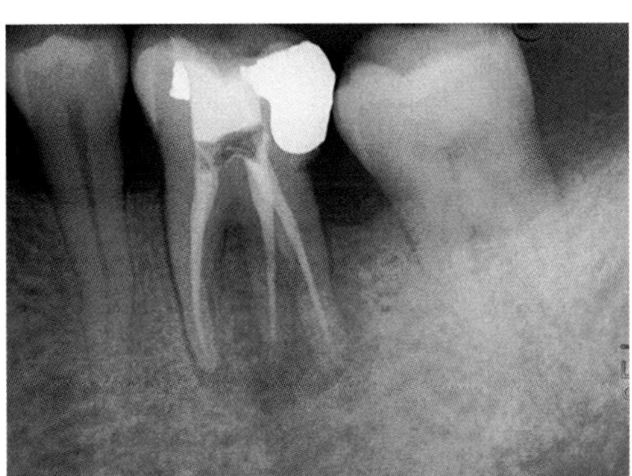

Fig. 2.176 Radiograph showing the presence of a three-rooted mandibular first permanent molar.

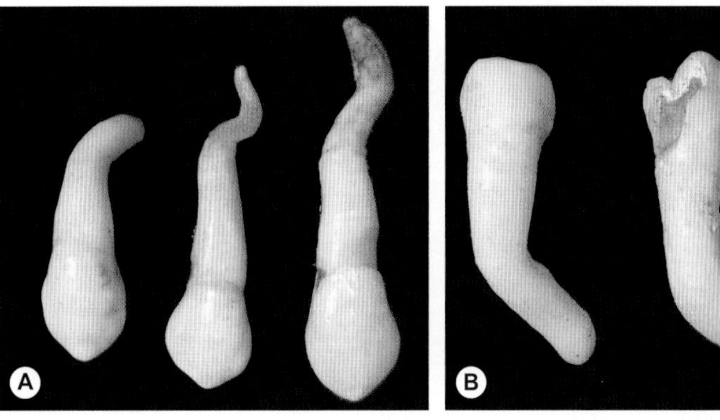

Fig. 2.177 Dilacerated roots in (A) permanent maxillary canine teeth; (B) mandibular premolars. Copyright the Royal College of Surgeons of England.

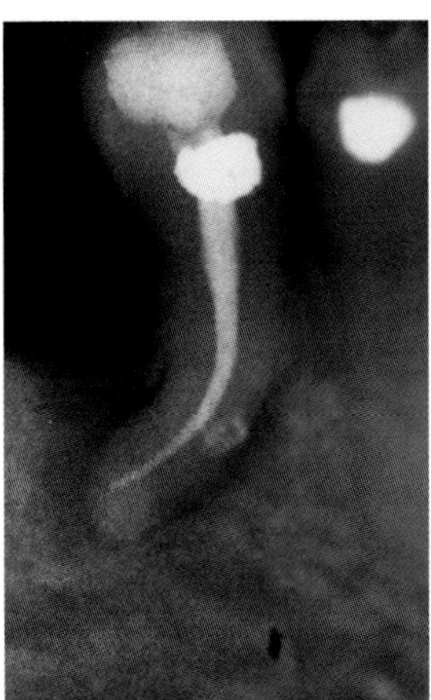

Fig. 2.178 A radiograph showing dilacerated mandibular premolar roots. Courtesy Dr. N McDonald.

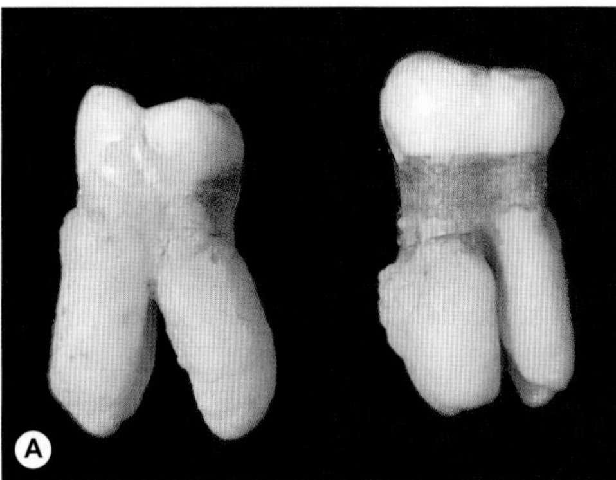

Fig. 2.179 (A) Hypercementosis along most of the roots of two mandibular molar teeth. (B) Second and third molar teeth fused at their roots via cementum (concrescence). (A) Copyright the Royal College of Surgeons of England. (B) Courtesy Prof. J Freher.

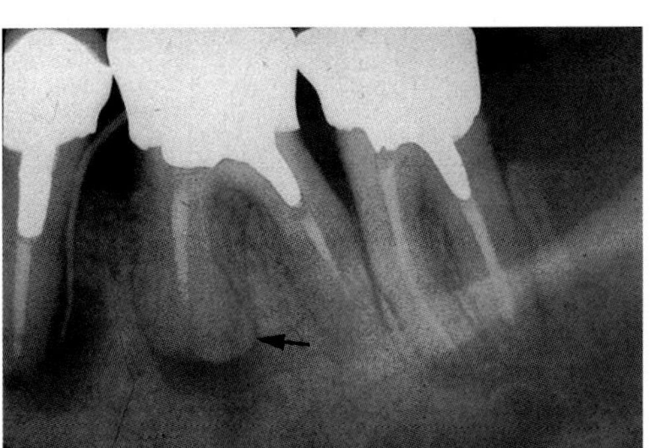

Fig. 2.180 Radiograph showing hypercementosis associated with the mesial root of a mandibular first permanent molar (arrow), which also shows evidence of periapical infection. Courtesy Dr. T Botero.

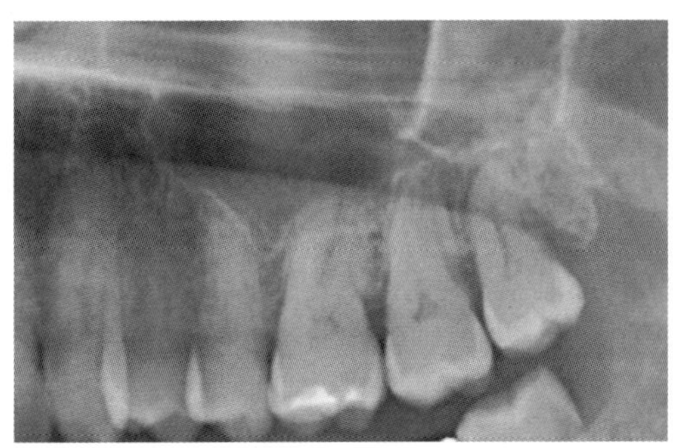

Fig. 2.181 Radiograph showing roots of premolar and molar teeth lying close to the floor of the maxillary sinus. Courtesy Dr. J Makdissi.

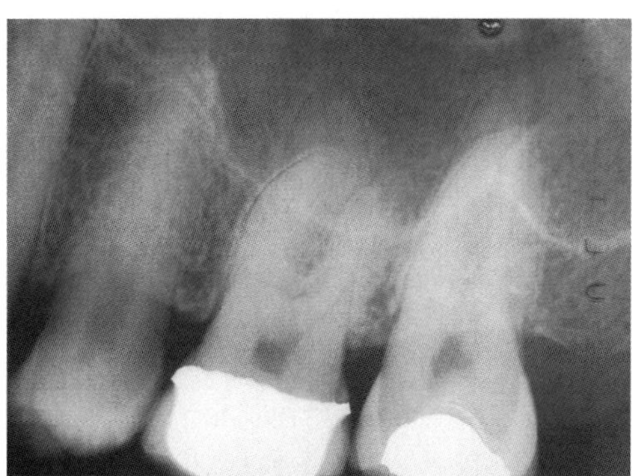

Fig. 2.182 Radiograph showing roots of the premolars and molars intimately related to the maxillary sinus.

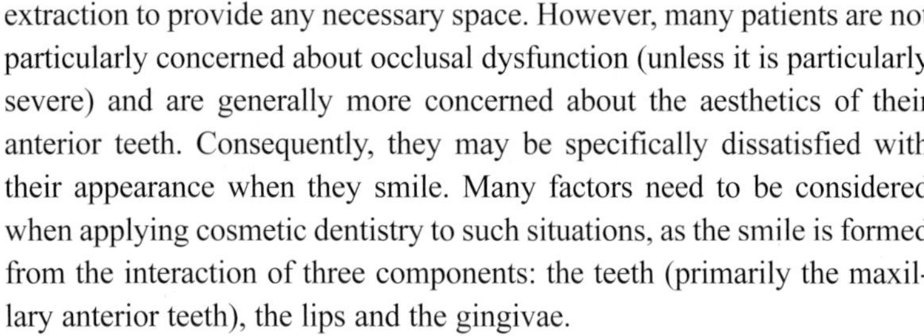

Fig. 2.183 Image of the palate region of a patient who had the maxillary first molar extracted 2 weeks previously. The wound has failed to heal, and two oro-antral fistulae are present at the wound site, connecting the mouth with the maxillary sinus. From Banerjee, A., Thavaraj, S. (Eds.), 2020. *Odell's clinical problem solving in dentistry*, fourth ed. Elsevier, London.

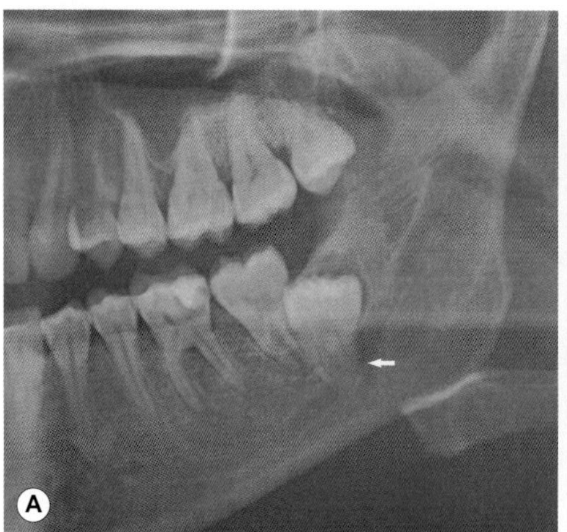

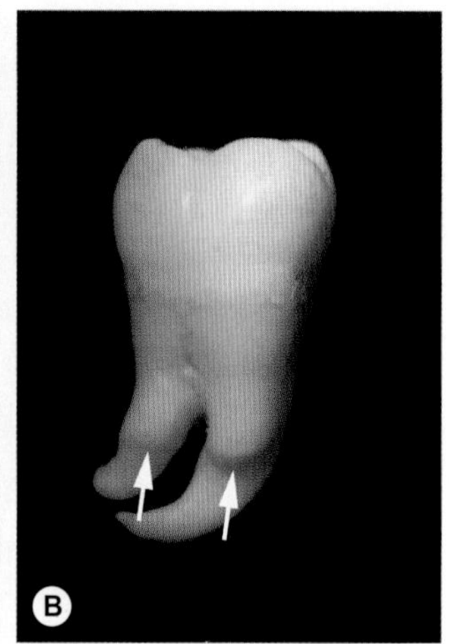

Fig. 2.184 (A) Radiograph indicating that the mandibular canal and its contents are closely related to the roots of the mandibular permanent third molar (arrow). (B) Grooves in apical part of the roots of the mandibular third molar (arrows) resulting from close association with inferior alveolar nerve and vessels. (A) Courtesy Dr. J Makdissi. (B) Courtesy Prof. J Freher.

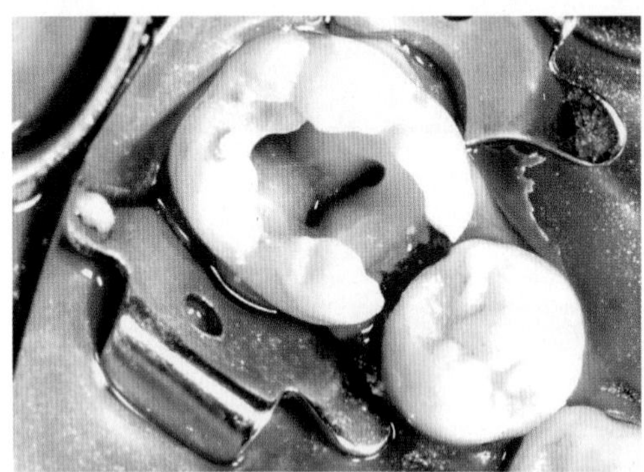

Fig. 2.185 Access cavity prepared on lower molar to provide good access to see the distal root canal.

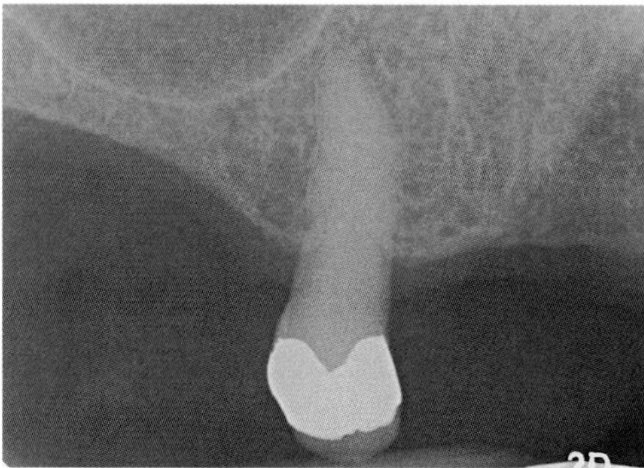

Fig. 2.186 Radiograph showing partial sclerosis of the root canal in a maxillary premolar owing to continued deposition of secondary dentine formation. Courtesy Dr. J Makdissi.

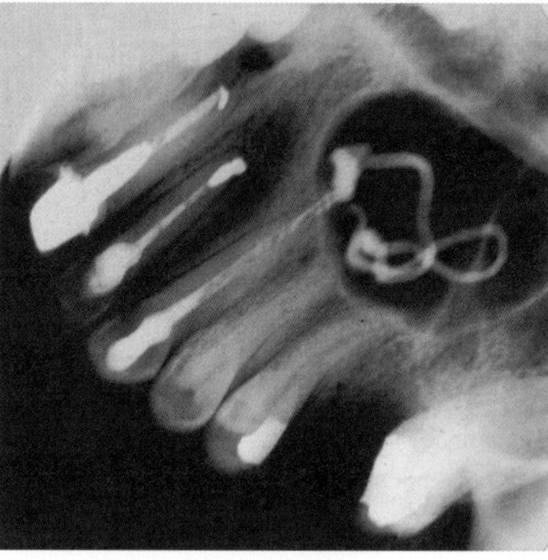

Fig. 2.187 Root filling material present in maxillary sinus because of overzealous force applied to upper permanent canine tooth. Courtesy Prof. J D Langdon.

extraction to provide any necessary space. However, many patients are not particularly concerned about occlusal dysfunction (unless it is particularly severe) and are generally more concerned about the aesthetics of their anterior teeth. Consequently, they may be specifically dissatisfied with their appearance when they smile. Many factors need to be considered when applying cosmetic dentistry to such situations, as the smile is formed from the interaction of three components: the teeth (primarily the maxillary anterior teeth), the lips and the gingivae.

Some dimensions of the teeth seen in a 'desirable' smile would be as follows:

- The height of the maxillary first (central) incisors would be approximately 11 mm, with the width being between 0.7 and 0.8 of the height. These first incisors need to be more than 2 mm shorter than normal before a difference is noticeable.
- The ratios of the width of the maxillary first (central) incisor, second (lateral) incisor and canine teeth as seen from the front would be 1.6:1.0:0.6, with each tooth's width being about two-thirds that of the tooth in front. (This rule also applies to the premolar teeth behind, which are also visible in the smile; Fig. 2.190.) The maxillary second incisors need to be about 3 mm narrower than the maxillary first incisors before a difference is noticeable.
- The long axes of the maxillary first (central) incisors should be parallel to the facial midline and to each other. The long axis of the second (lateral) incisor should slope about 5 degrees distal and the canine and premolars about 10–12 degrees distal to that of the first incisor (Fig. 2.191). Note that if the midline between the first incisors does not coincide with the facial midline, it needs to be more than about 4 mm off centre before this difference is noticeable.
- The visible areas of contact between the teeth (connectors) should be 50% of the height between the two maxillary first (central) incisors, 40% of the height of the first incisor between the first and second incisors and 30% of the height of the first incisor between the second incisor and canine (Fig. 2.192).

With regard to the lips, about 3–4 mm of the maxillary incisors should ideally be visible at rest, although this decreases with age. During smiling, a normal lip line (seen in about 45% of patients) is present when the upper lip is at the level of the gingival margins and the interdental gingivae are exposed. A low lip line (in about 45% of patients) is where the lip covers the interdental gingivae. A high lip line (in about 10% of patients) occurs when the lip exposes the gingivae above the gingival margin (Fig. 2.193). Figs 2.194 and 2.195 show examples of patients with unaesthetic smiles (before and after treatment).

Cone beam computed tomography (CBCT)

This is a cross-sectional imaging modality that utilises a rotating X-ray beam in relation to a cylindrical volume. It allows the acquisition of the data in an axial plane, which are then reconstructed in a multiplanar mode including panoramic view reconstruction. It is capable of providing three-dimensional data of the area of interest.

The volume size is adjustable, allowing the smallest volume to be acquired for the purpose of satisfying the clinical indication. This limits the radiation dose to the patient. Radiation dose ranges between 11 and 674 μSv for a dento-alveolar volume and 30 and 1076 μSv for a craniofacial volume. The radiation dose is, however, higher than conventional dental imaging.

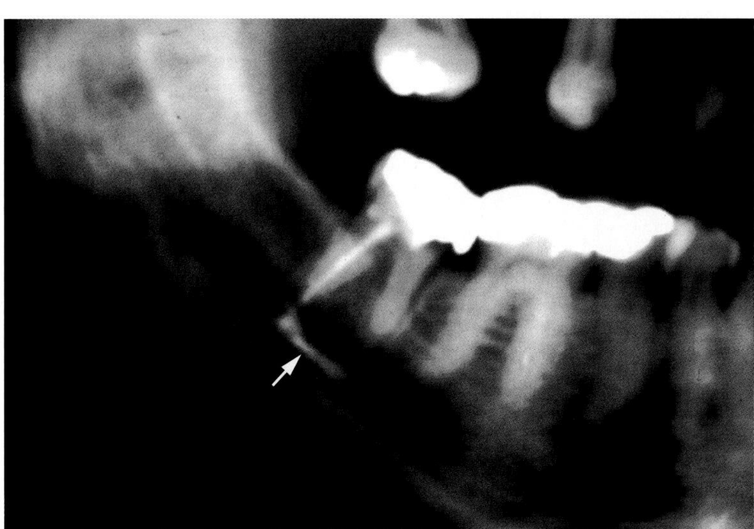

Fig. 2.188 Root filling material present in mandibular canal (arrow) due to overzealous force applied to mandibular second permanent molar. Courtesy Prof. J D Langdon.

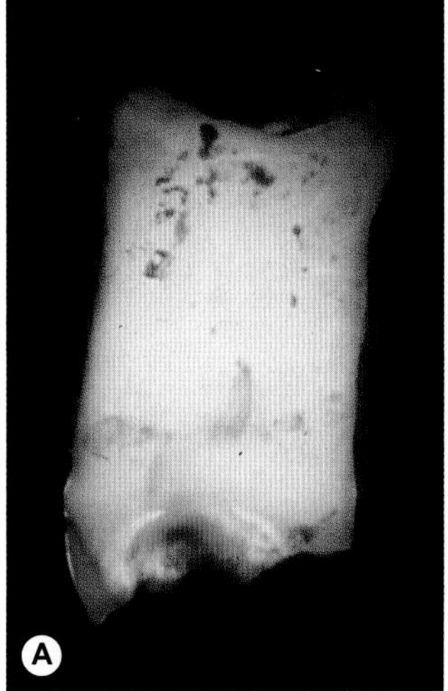

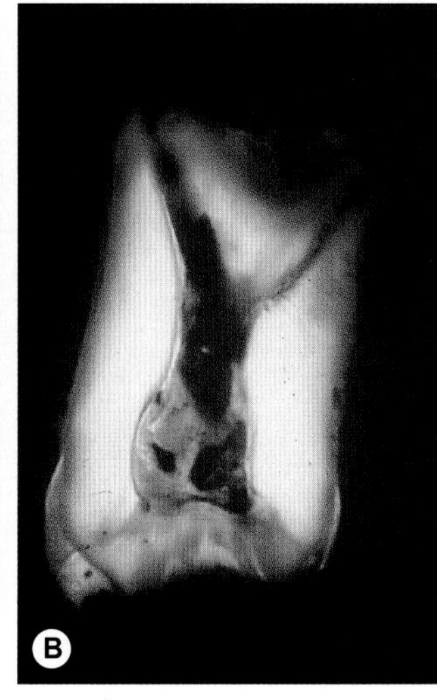

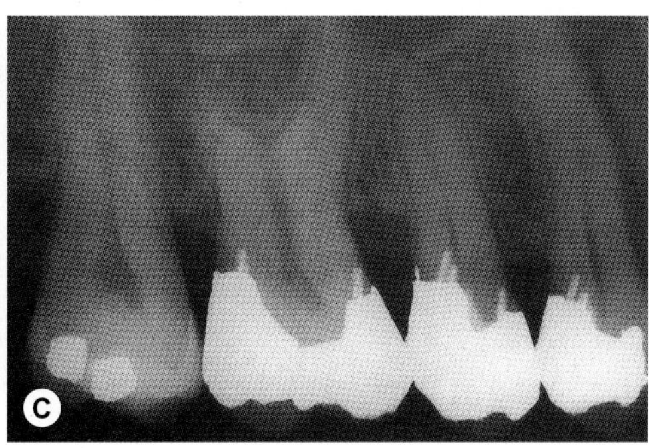

Fig. 2.189 (A) Taurodont molar tooth. Note lack of root bifurcation until near root apex. (B) Bisected taurodont tooth showing lack of division of pulp chamber until near root apex. (C) Radiograph of taurodont upper first permanent molar. (A, B) Courtesy Prof. C Franklin.

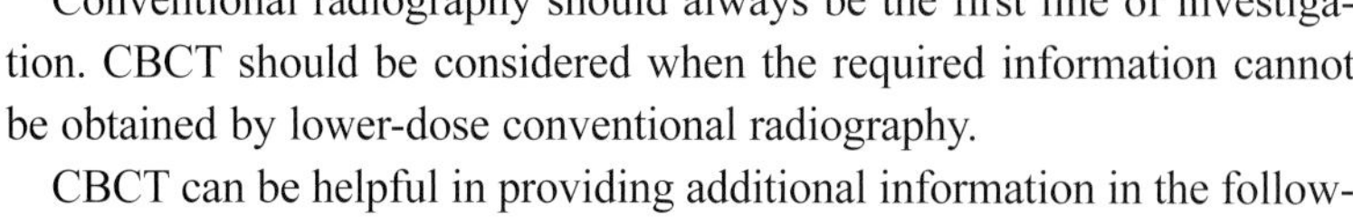

Conventional radiography should always be the first line of investigation. CBCT should be considered when the required information cannot be obtained by lower-dose conventional radiography.

CBCT can be helpful in providing additional information in the following clinical scenarios:

1) Assessment of lower third molars regarding the number and morphology of the roots and the position and relationship of the mandibular canal and its neurovascular bundle to the roots (Fig. 2.196).

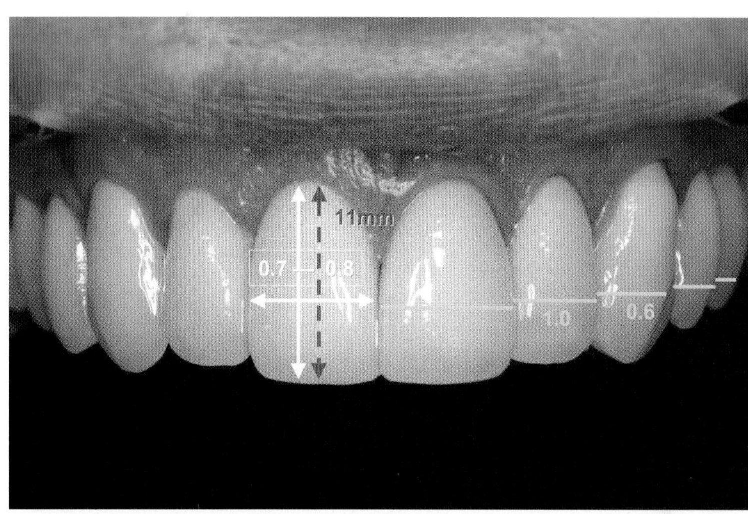

Fig. 2.190 Ideal length (red) and width:length ratio (white) for the maxillary first incisor and width proportions for the teeth as seen from the front (yellow). Courtesy Dr. C Orr.

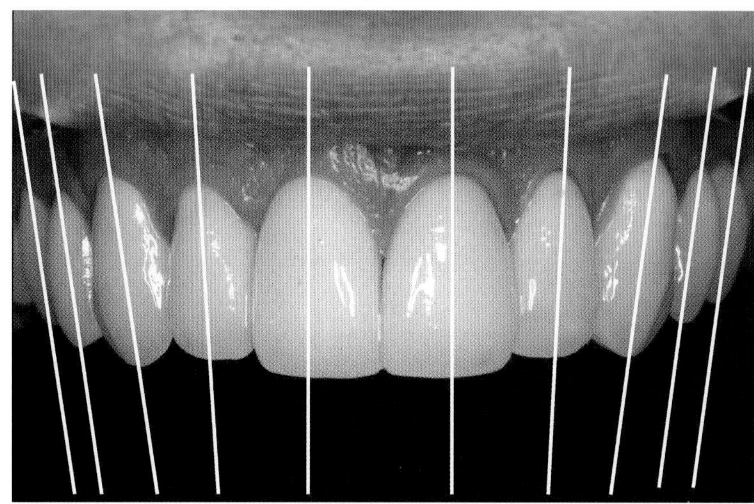

Fig. 2.191 Ideal arrangement of the long axis of the crowns of the maxillary teeth. Courtesy Dr. C Orr.

2) Assessment of ectopic teeth (including canines) and supernumerary teeth regarding the position and relationship of these teeth to the adjacent tissues and identifying resorption of the adjacent teeth (Figs. 2.197 and 2.198).
3) Endodontic planning in selected cases when conventional radiographs provide inadequate information about the number and position of root canals or the presence of root resorption or perforations (Figs. 2.199 and 2.200).

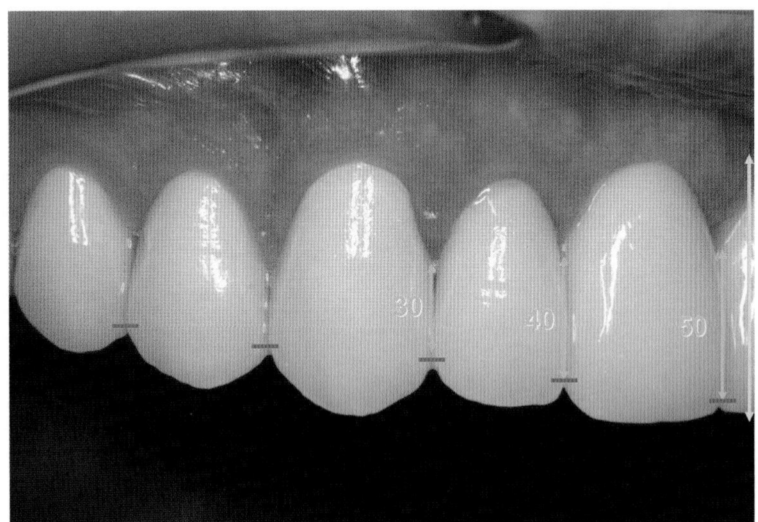

Fig. 2.192 Percentage comparisons of the contact lengths (connectors) of the anterior maxillary teeth (blue) compared with that between the two maxillary first incisors (yellow). Courtesy Dr. C Orr.

4) Revealing dento-alveolar and facial trauma (Fig. 2.201).
5) Use in implant dentistry to assess bone width and height in the region of interest, the relationship to the adjacent vital structures including virtual markings and the degree of healing of the socket (Figs 2.202–2.204).
6) Assessment of bony pathology, such as large cysts and odontogenic tumours (Fig. 2.205).

CBCT, however, is limited in assessing soft tissue, analysis of caries and bone density measurements. These limitations should be considered when interpreting CBCT images or choosing additional modalities.

Explore online Self-assessment quiz to test and reinforce your understanding of the material in your free ebook. Follow instructions in the Inside Front Cover to unlock your access.

Table 2.15 Federation Dentaire Internationale notation for tooth identification in which the jaw quadrant is represented by a number

Quadrant	Dentition
1 = maxillary right quadrant	Permanent
2 = maxillary left quadrant	
3 = mandibular left quadrant	
4 = mandibular right quadrant	
5 = maxillary right quadrant	Deciduous
6 = maxillary left quadrant	
7 = mandibular left quadrant	
8 = mandibular right quadrant	

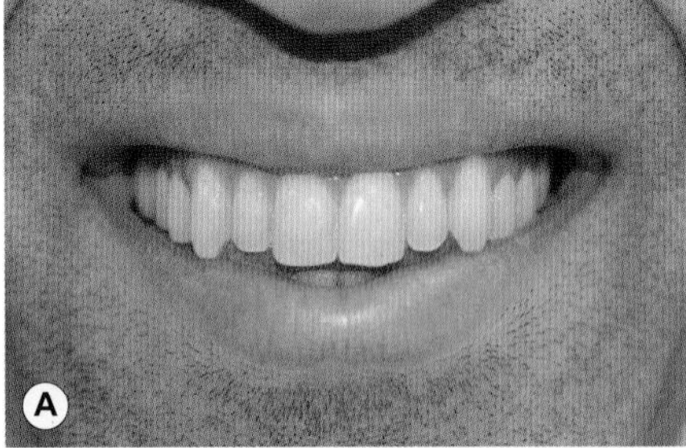

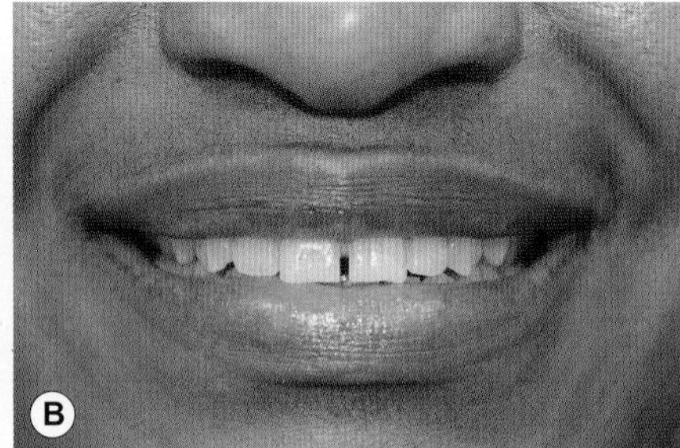

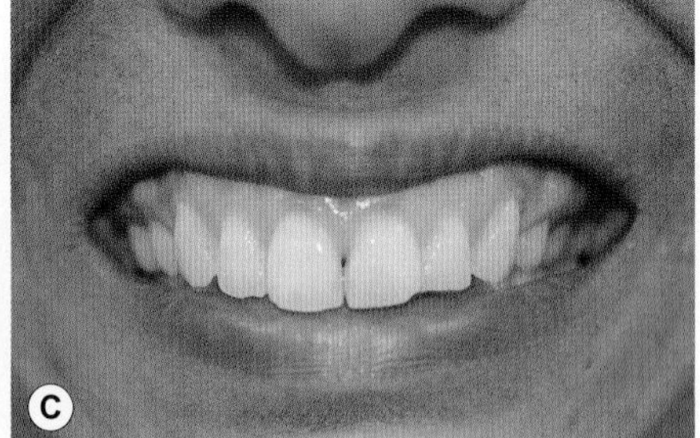

Fig. 2.193 (A) Normal lip line. (B) Low lip line. (C) High lip line. Courtesy Dr. M Seppala.

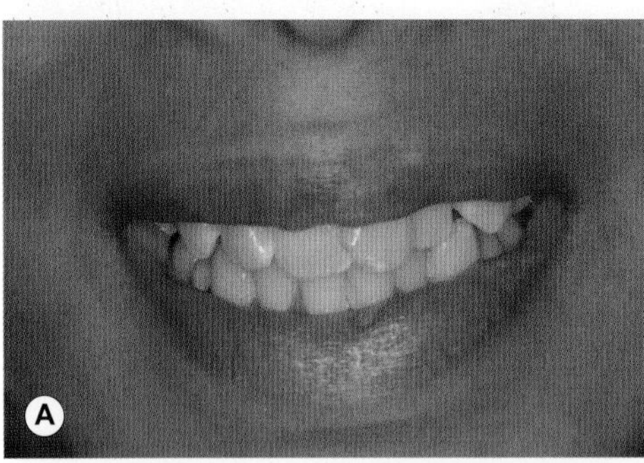

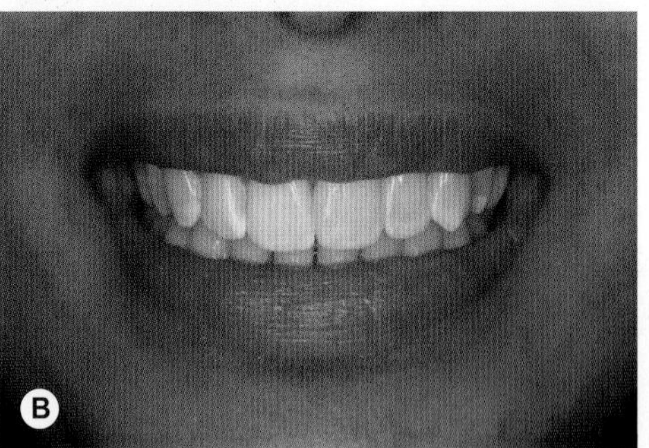

Fig. 2.194 (A) Patient before treatment, showing many irregularities of the anterior teeth when smiling. (B) Patient after treatment, showing a greatly improved appearance. Courtesy Dr. C Orr.

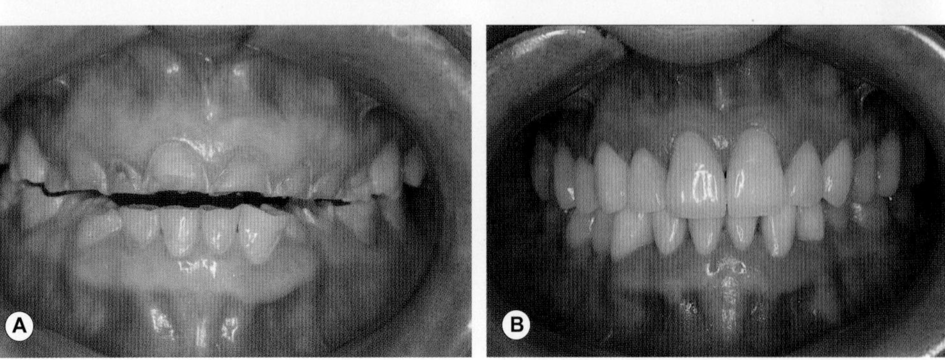

Fig. 2.195 (A) Patient before treatment showing severe loss of crown substance as a result of erosion. (B) Patient after treatment showing restoration of crown morphology. Courtesy Dr C Orr.

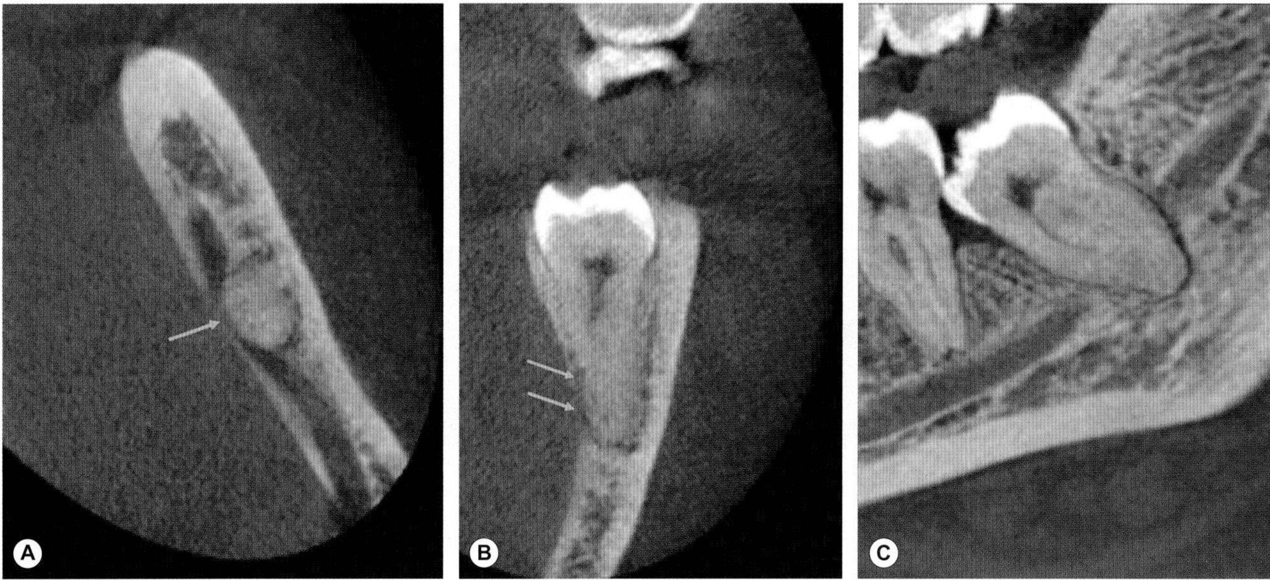

Fig. 2.196 Axial (A), coronal (B) and sagittal (C) images of the lower left third molar. Note the lingual position of the mandibular canal (arrows) in relation to the molar. There is significant narrowing, deviation and loss of the cortical outline of the canal at the point of contact with the molar. Courtesy Dr. J Makdissi.

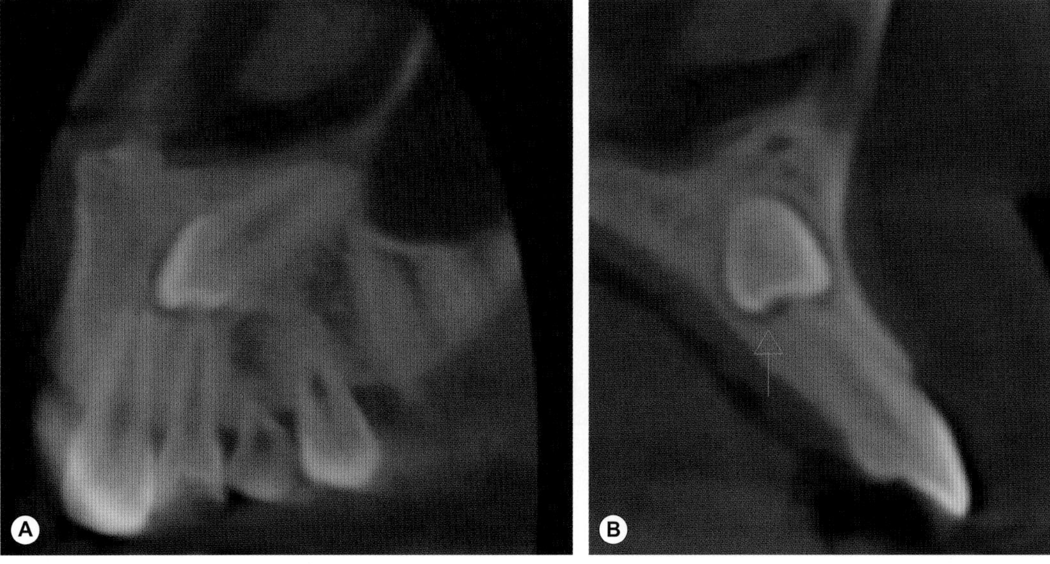

Fig. 2.197 Sagittal (A) and coronal (B) images of the upper left canine causing resorption of the apex of the upper left lateral incisor (arrow). Courtesy Dr. J Makdissi.

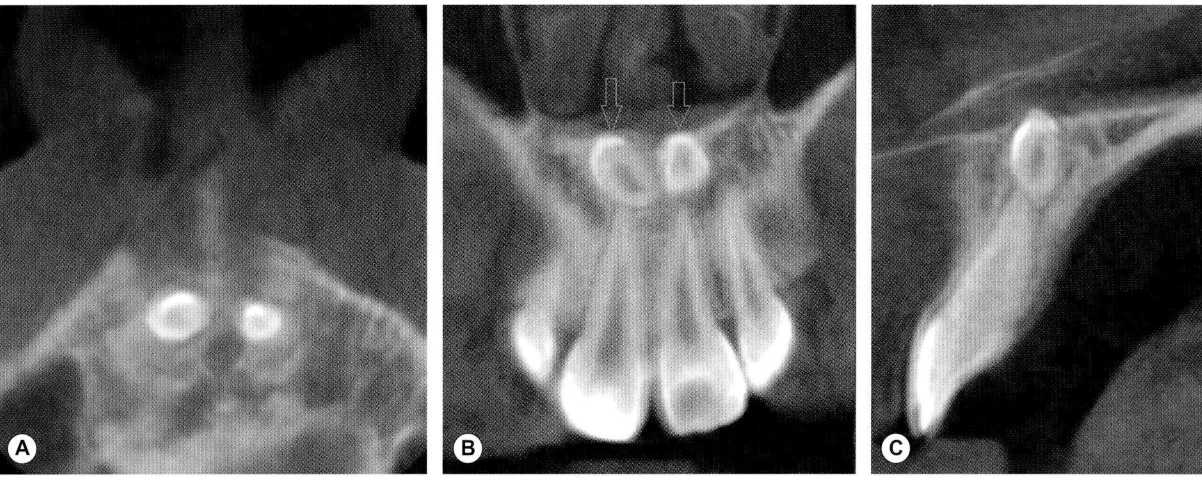

Fig. 2.198 Axial (A), coronal (B) and sagittal (C) images of the anterior maxilla showing two supernumerary teeth (arrows) apical to both upper left and right central incisors. Note the direct contact with the apex of the central incisor which shows minimal resorption. Courtesy Dr. J Makdissi.

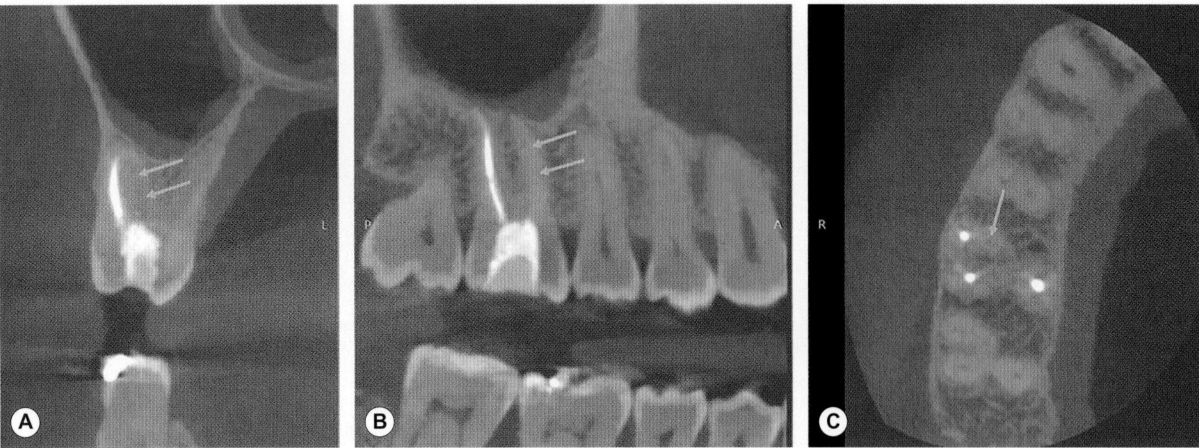

Fig. 2.199 Coronal (A), sagittal (B) and axial (C) images of the upper right first molar showing an unfilled mesio-buccal root canal (arrows). Courtesy Dr. J Makdissi.

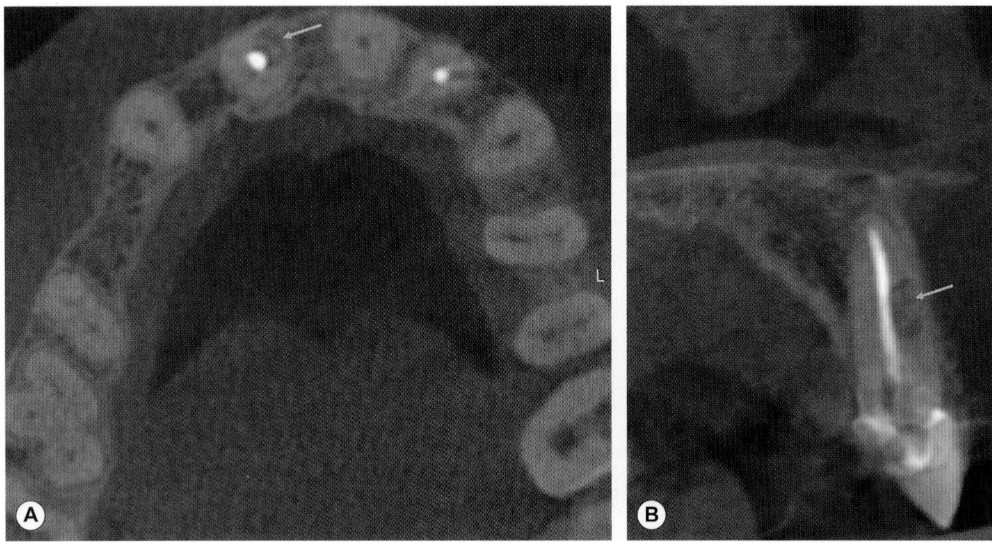

Fig. 2.200 Axial (A) and sagittal (B) images of the upper right central incisor showing an area of external resorption (arrows) affecting the mesio-buccal surface of the root at approximately mid root level. Courtesy Dr. J Makdissi.

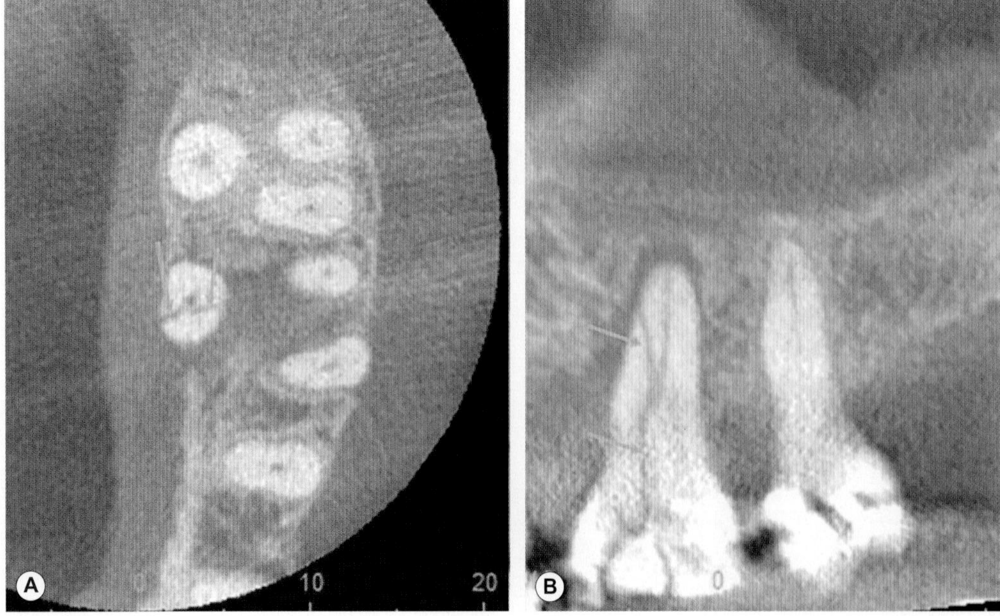

Fig. 2.201 Axial (A) and sagittal (B) images of the upper left first molar showing a vertical fracture through the palatal root (arrows). Courtesy Dr. J Makdissi.

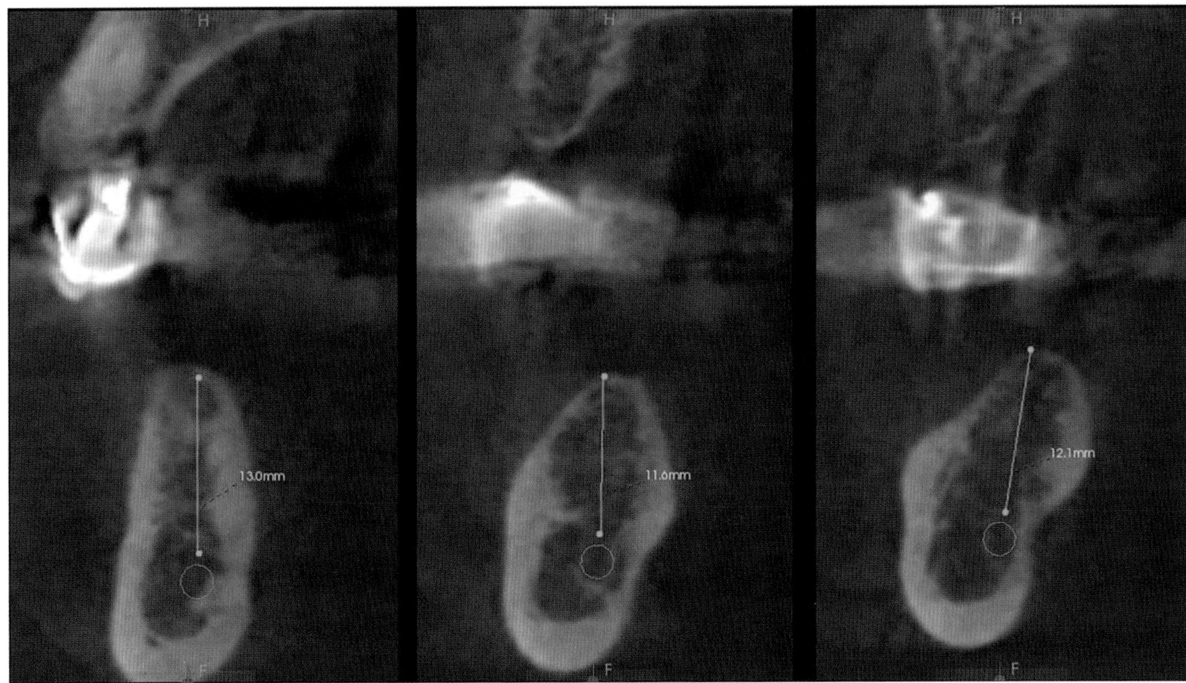

Fig. 2.202 Cross-sectional images through the mandible showing the available height of bone as part of an implant assessment. The measurements are made from the crest to the mandibular canal seen marked in orange circle. Courtesy Dr. J Makdissi.

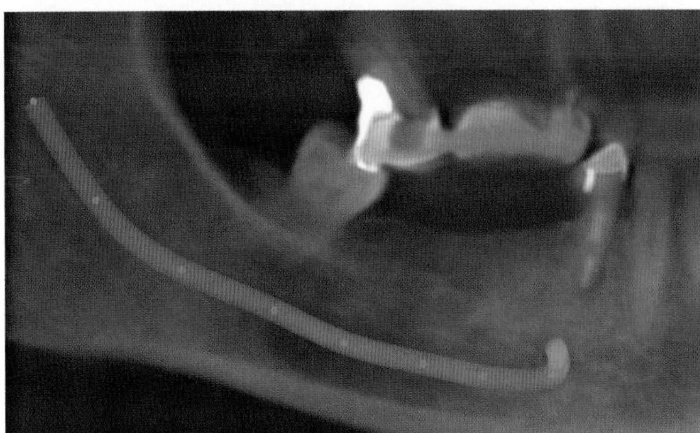

Fig. 2.203 Sagittal reconstruction of the mandible with the mandibular canal marked in orange. Courtesy Dr. J Makdissi.

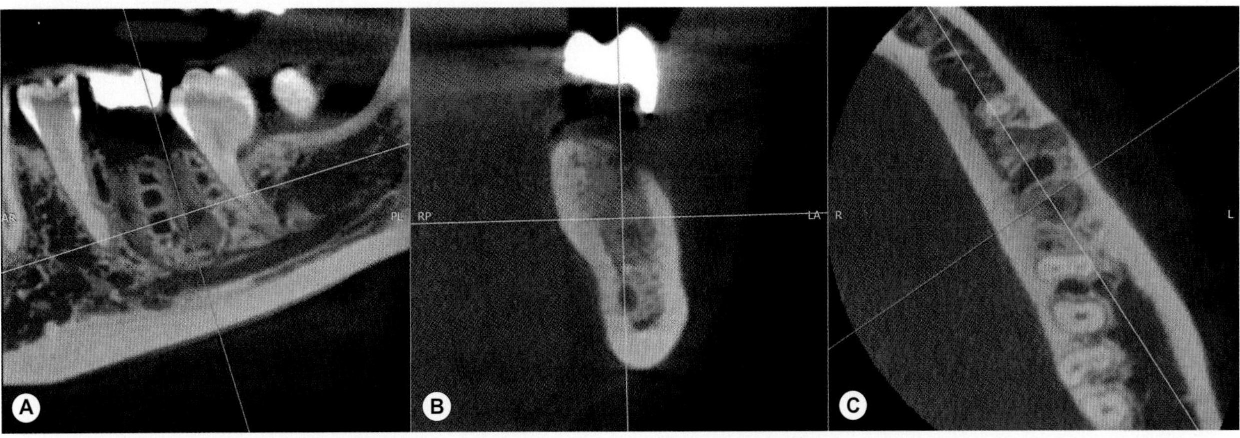

Fig. 2.204 Sagittal (A), coronal (B) and axial (C) images of the socket of lower left first molar showing partial bony remodelling. The position of the mandibular canal is identified. Courtesy Dr. J Makdissi.

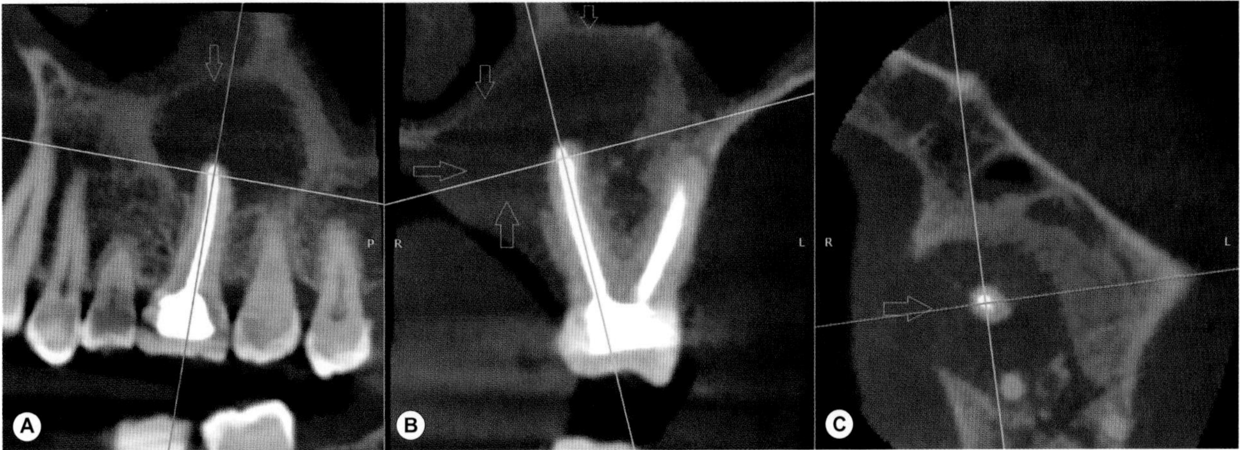

Fig. 2.205 Sagittal (A), coronal (B) and axial (C) showing a large cystic cavity associated with the palatal root of the root-filled upper left first molar. This is thinning of the floors of the nasal cavity and the maxillary sinus (orange arrows), causing dehiscence of the palatal cortex (blue arrows). The most likely diagnosis is a radicular cyst. Courtesy Dr. J Makdissi.

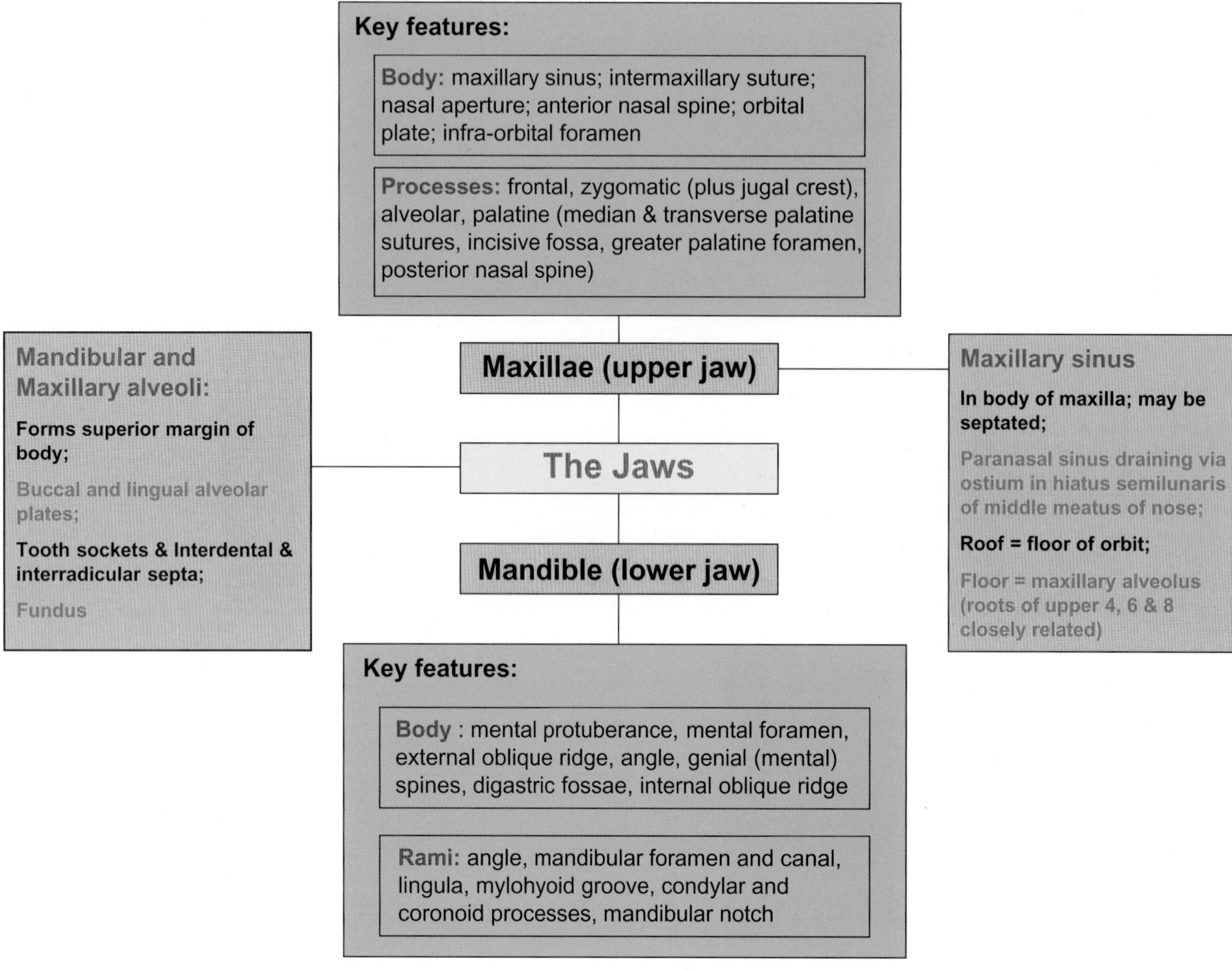
Key features:
Body: maxillary sinus; intermaxillary suture; nasal aperture; anterior nasal spine; orbital plate; infra-orbital foramen
Processes: frontal, zygomatic (plus jugal crest), alveolar, palatine (median & transverse palatine sutures, incisive fossa, greater palatine foramen, posterior nasal spine)
Maxillae (upper jaw)
Mandibular and Maxillary alveoli:
Forms superior margin of body;
Buccal and lingual alveolar plates;
Tooth sockets & Interdental & interradicular septa;
Fundus
The Jaws
Maxillary sinus
In body of maxilla; may be septated;
Paranasal sinus draining via ostium in hiatus semilunaris of middle meatus of nose;
Roof = floor of orbit;
Floor = maxillary alveolus (roots of upper 4, 6 & 8 closely related)
Mandible (lower jaw)
Key features:
Body : mental protuberance, mental foramen, external oblique ridge, angle, genial (mental) spines, digastric fossae, internal oblique ridge
Rami: angle, mandibular foramen and canal, lingula, mylohyoid groove, condylar and coronoid processes, mandibular notch

Mind Map 2.1 The jaw.

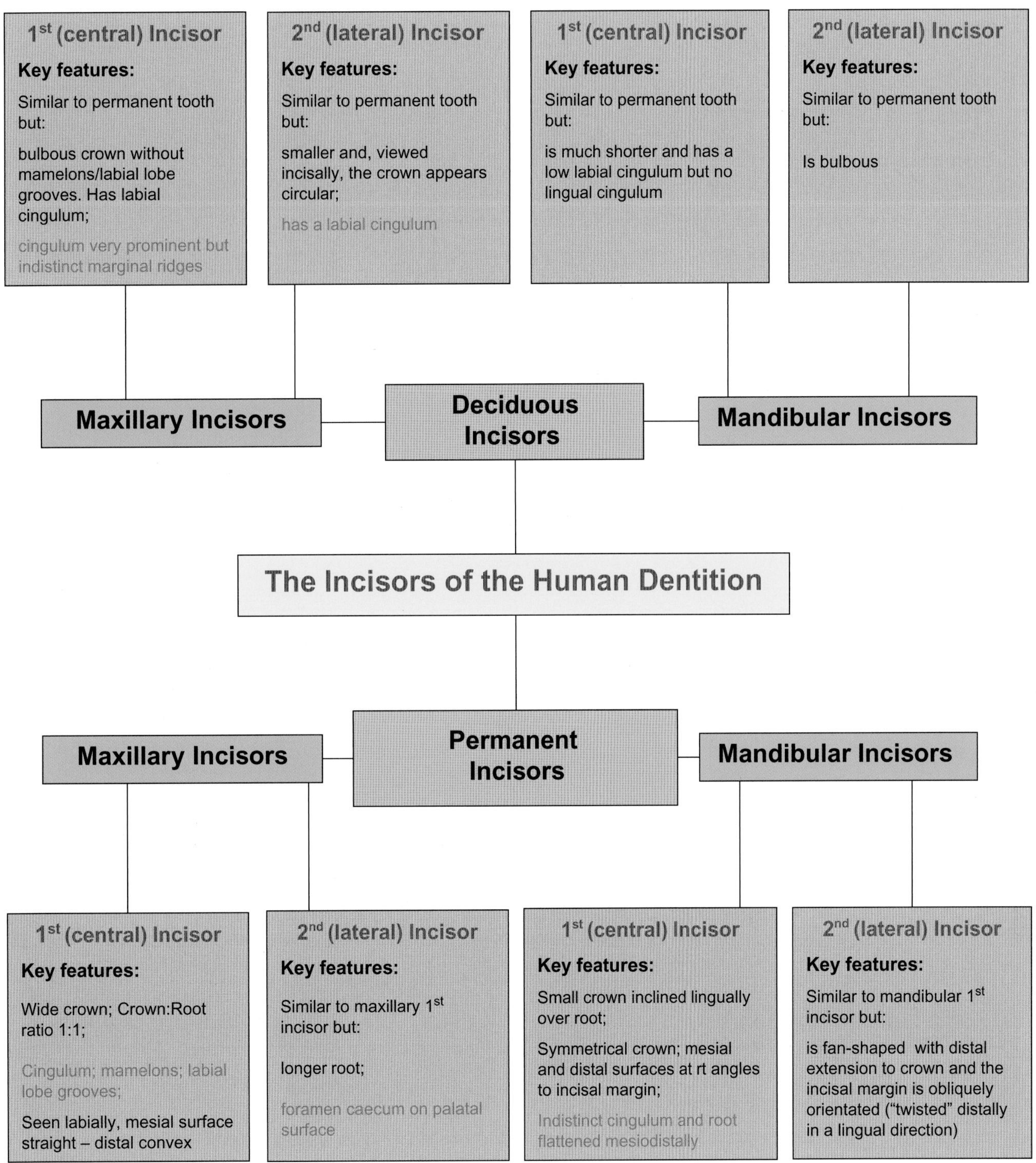

Mind Map 2.2 The incisors of the human dentition.

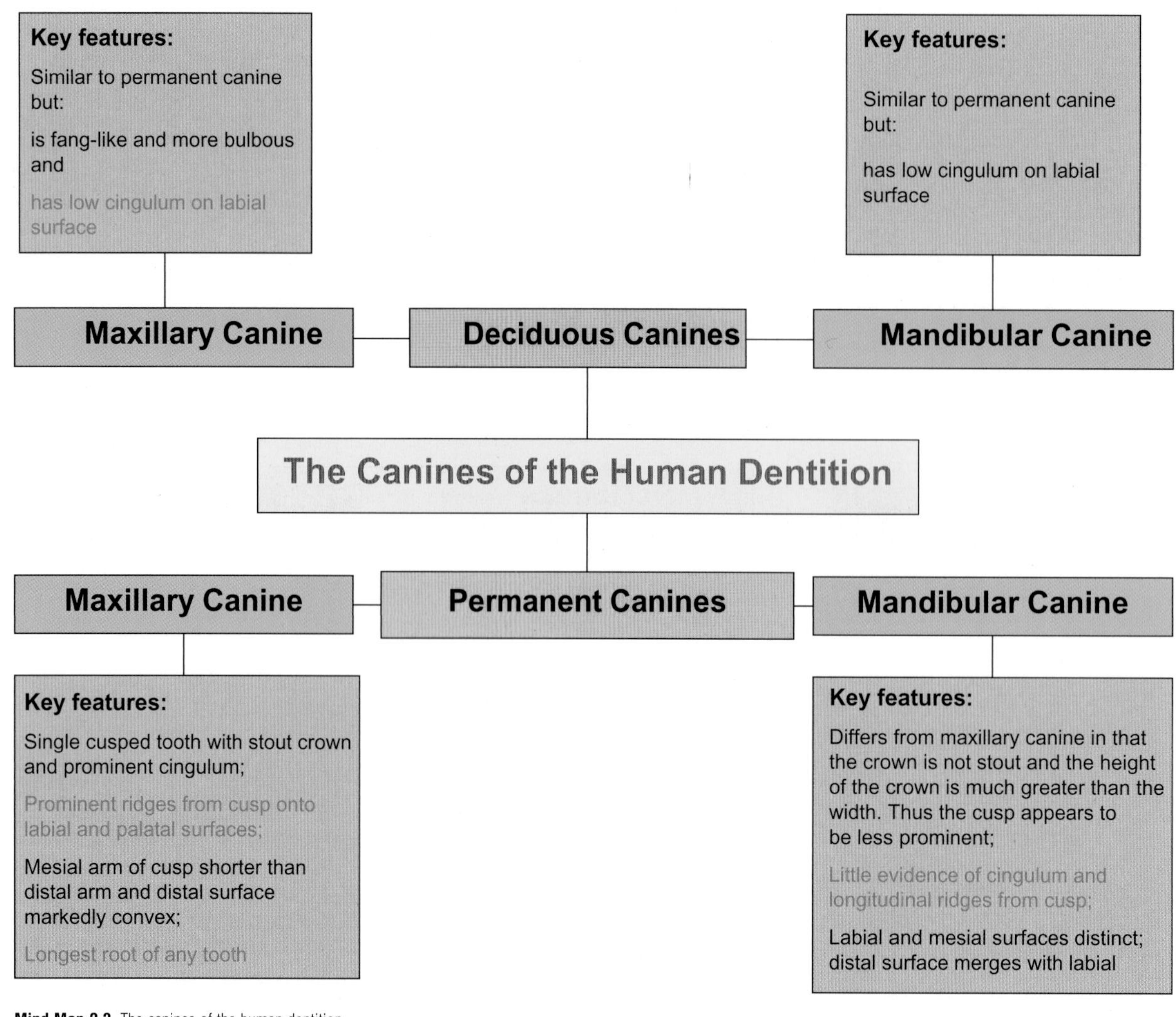

Similar to permanent canine but:
is fang-like and more bulbous and
has low cingulum on labial surface

Similar to permanent canine but:
has low cingulum on labial surface

Single cusped tooth with stout crown and prominent cingulum;
Prominent ridges from cusp onto labial and palatal surfaces;
Mesial arm of cusp shorter than distal arm and distal surface markedly convex;

Differs from maxillary canine in that the crown is not stout and the height of the crown is much greater than the width. Thus the cusp appears to be less prominent;

Labial and mesial surfaces distinct; distal surface merges with labial

Mind Map 2.3 The canines of the human dentition.

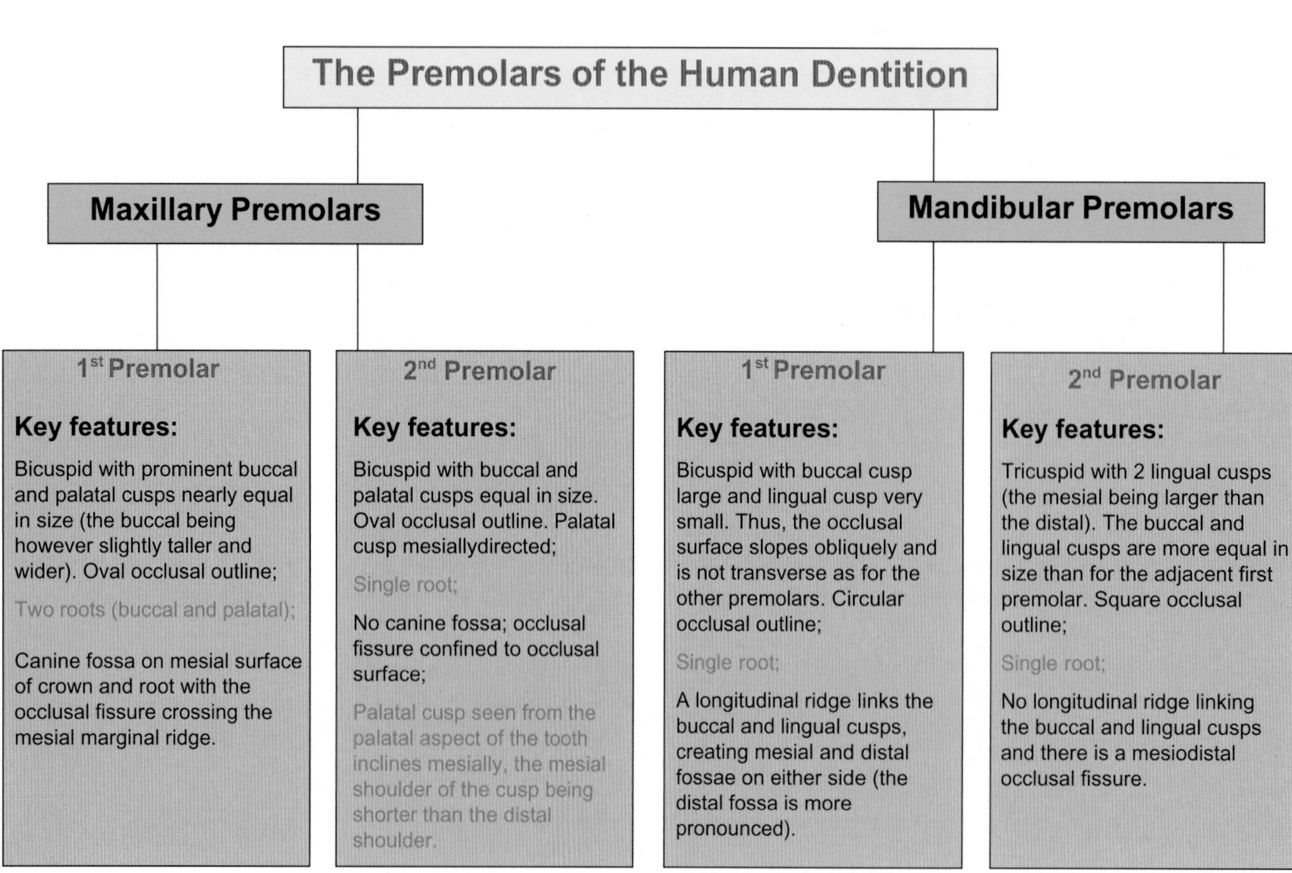

The Premolars of the Human Dentition
Maxillary Premolars
Mandibular Premolars
1st Premolar
Key features:
Bicuspid with prominent buccal and palatal cusps nearly equal in size (the buccal being however slightly taller and wider). Oval occlusal outline;
Two roots (buccal and palatal);
Canine fossa on mesial surface of crown and root with the occlusal fissure crossing the mesial marginal ridge.
2nd Premolar
Key features:
Bicuspid with buccal and palatal cusps equal in size. Oval occlusal outline. Palatal cusp mesiallydirected;
Single root;
No canine fossa; occlusal fissure confined to occlusal surface;
Palatal cusp seen from the palatal aspect of the tooth inclines mesially, the mesial shoulder of the cusp being shorter than the distal shoulder.
1st Premolar
Key features:
Bicuspid with buccal cusp large and lingual cusp very small. Thus, the occlusal surface slopes obliquely and is not transverse as for the other premolars. Circular occlusal outline;
Single root;
A longitudinal ridge links the buccal and lingual cusps, creating mesial and distal fossae on either side (the distal fossa is more pronounced).
2nd Premolar
Key features:
Tricuspid with 2 lingual cusps (the mesial being larger than the distal). The buccal and lingual cusps are more equal in size than for the adjacent first premolar. Square occlusal outline;
Single root;
No longitudinal ridge linking the buccal and lingual cusps and there is a mesiodistal occlusal fissure.

Mind Map 2.4 The premolars of the human dentition.

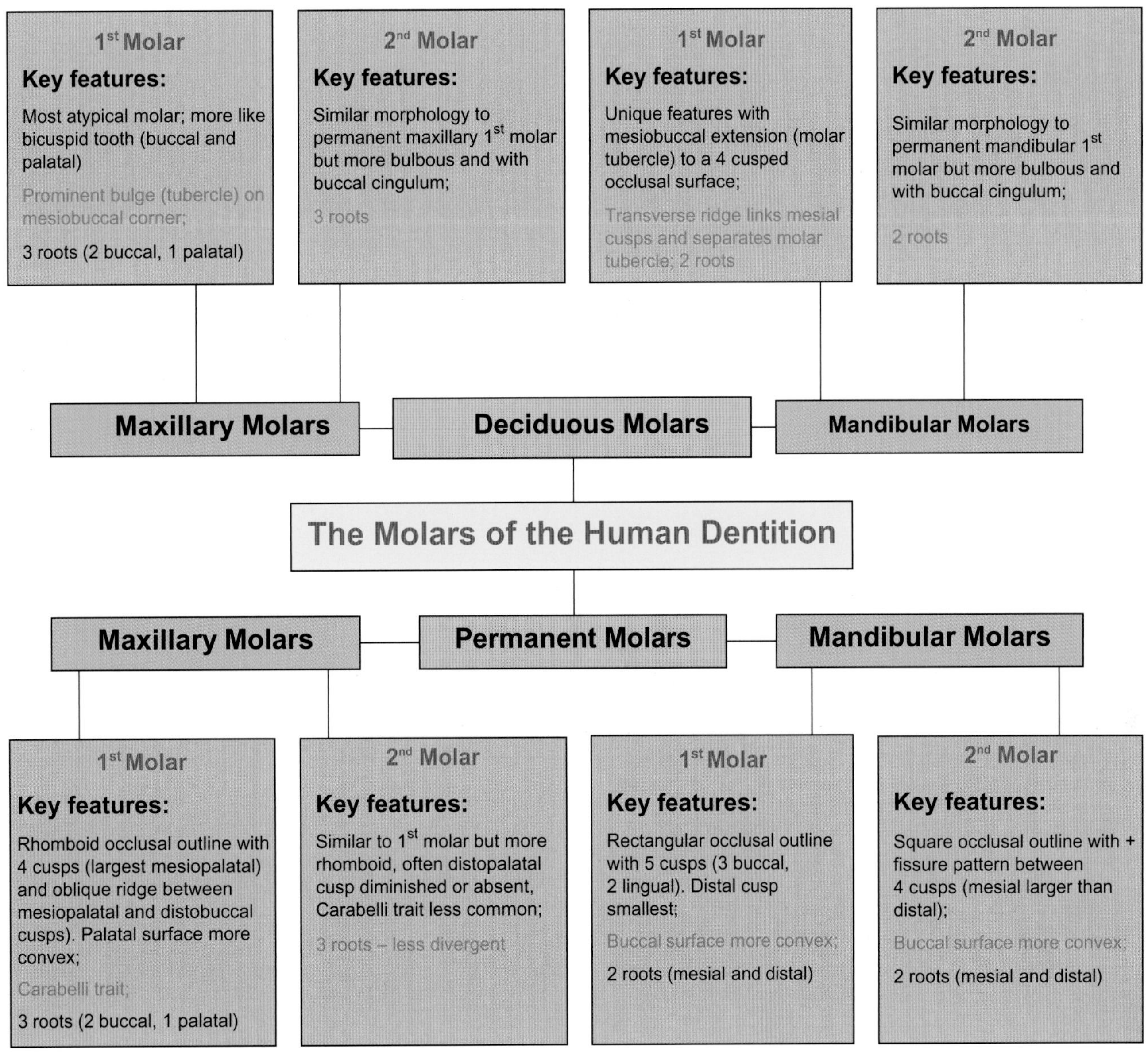
1st Molar
Key features:
Most atypical molar; more like bicuspid tooth (buccal and palatal)
Prominent bulge (tubercle) on mesiobuccal corner;
3 roots (2 buccal, 1 palatal)
2nd Molar
Key features:
Similar morphology to permanent maxillary 1st molar but more bulbous and with buccal cingulum;
3 roots
1st Molar
Key features:
Unique features with mesiobuccal extension (molar tubercle) to a 4 cusped occlusal surface;
Transverse ridge links mesial cusps and separates molar tubercle; 2 roots
2nd Molar
Key features:
Similar morphology to permanent mandibular 1st molar but more bulbous and with buccal cingulum;
2 roots
Maxillary Molars
Deciduous Molars
Mandibular Molars
The Molars of the Human Dentition
Maxillary Molars
Permanent Molars
Mandibular Molars
1st Molar
Key features:
Rhomboid occlusal outline with 4 cusps (largest mesiopalatal) and oblique ridge between mesiopalatal and distobuccal cusps). Palatal surface more convex;
Carabelli trait;
3 roots (2 buccal, 1 palatal)
2nd Molar
Key features:
Similar to 1st molar but more rhomboid, often distopalatal cusp diminished or absent, Carabelli trait less common;
3 roots – less divergent
1st Molar
Key features:
Rectangular occlusal outline with 5 cusps (3 buccal, 2 lingual). Distal cusp smallest;
Buccal surface more convex;
2 roots (mesial and distal)
2nd Molar
Key features:
Square occlusal outline with + fissure pattern between 4 cusps (mesial larger than distal);
Buccal surface more convex;
2 roots (mesial and distal)

Mind Map 2.5 The molars of the human dentition.

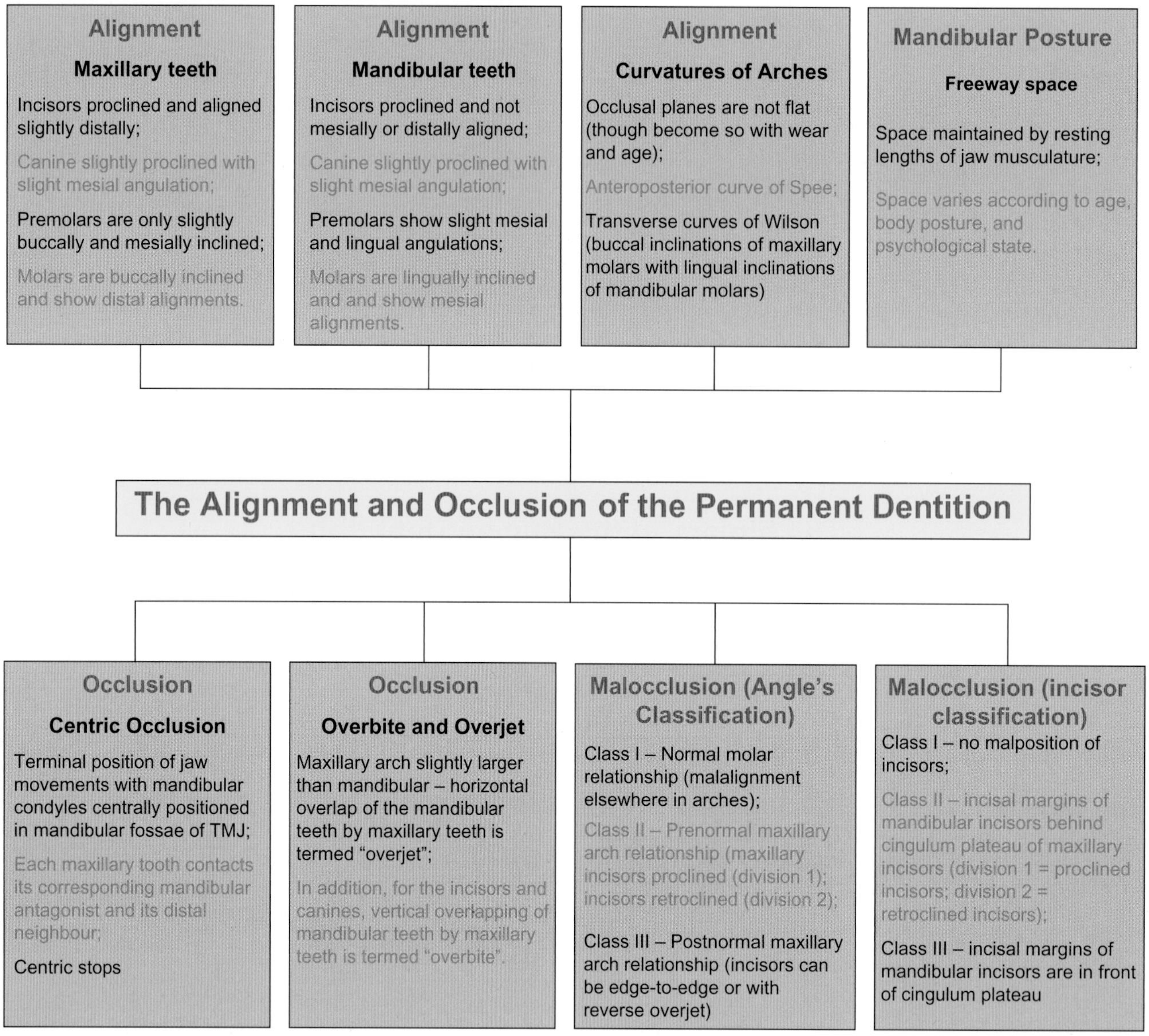

The Alignment and Occlusion of the Permanent Dentition

Alignment

Maxillary teeth

Incisors proclined and aligned slightly distally;

Canine slightly proclined with slight mesial angulation;

Premolars are only slightly buccally and mesially inclined;

Molars are buccally inclined and show distal alignments.

Alignment

Mandibular teeth

Incisors proclined and not mesially or distally aligned;

Canine slightly proclined with slight mesial angulation;

Premolars show slight mesial and lingual angulations;

Molars are lingually inclined and and show mesial alignments.

Alignment

Curvatures of Arches

Occlusal planes are not flat (though become so with wear and age);

Anteroposterior curve of Spee;

Transverse curves of Wilson (buccal inclinations of maxillary molars with lingual inclinations of mandibular molars)

Mandibular Posture

Freeway space

Space maintained by resting lengths of jaw musculature;

Space varies according to age, body posture, and psychological state.

Occlusion

Centric Occlusion

Terminal position of jaw movements with mandibular condyles centrally positioned in mandibular fossae of TMJ;

Each maxillary tooth contacts its corresponding mandibular antagonist and its distal neighbour;

Centric stops

Occlusion

Overbite and Overjet

Maxillary arch slightly larger than mandibular – horizontal overlap of the mandibular teeth by maxillary teeth is termed "overjet";

In addition, for the incisors and canines, vertical overlapping of mandibular teeth by maxillary teeth is termed "overbite".

Malocclusion (Angle's Classification)

Class I – Normal molar relationship (malalignment elsewhere in arches);

Class II – Prenormal maxillary arch relationship (maxillary incisors proclined (division 1); incisors retroclined (division 2);

Class III – Postnormal maxillary arch relationship (incisors can be edge-to-edge or with reverse overjet)

Malocclusion (incisor classification)

Class I – no malposition of incisors;

Class II – incisal margins of mandibular incisors behind cingulum plateau of maxillary incisors (division 1 = proclined incisors; division 2 = retroclined incisors);

Class III – incisal margins of mandibular incisors are in front of cingulum plateau

Mind Map 2.6 The alignment and occlusion of the permanent dentition.

Regional topography of the mouth and related areas

3

Temporomandibular joint (TMJ)

The TMJ is the synovial articulation between the mandible and the cranium. For this reason the joint is sometimes referred to as the craniomandibular joint. It is formed by the condylar process of the mandible articulating in the mandibular (glenoid) fossa of the temporal bone (Fig. 3.1). The TMJ, although basically a hinge joint, also allows for some gliding movements. Movement of the condylar head occurs within the mandibular fossa and down a bony prominence immediately anterior to the mandibular fossa, the articular eminence of the temporal bone.

Although having several features typical of synovial joints in other regions (e.g., a joint capsule, a synovial membrane secreting synovial fluid, ligaments to limit movement), the TMJ also has some specific features listed in Box 3.1. The histology of the TMJ is considered in Chapter 15.

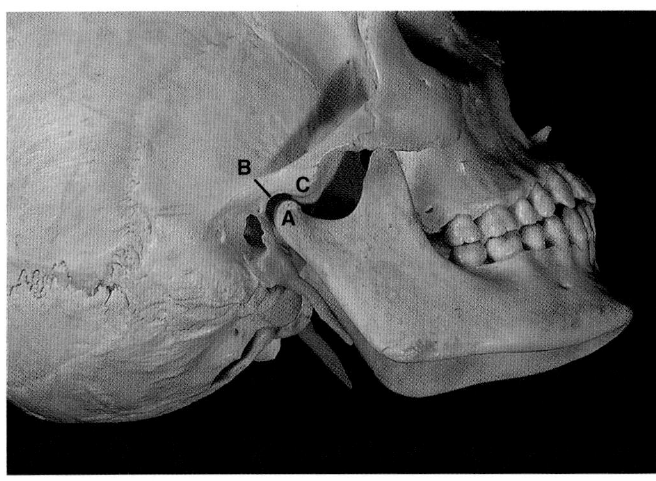

Fig. 3.1 The osteology of the temporomandibular joint. A = mandibular condyle; B = mandibular fossa of temporal bone; C = articular eminence of temporal bone.

Box 3.1 **Specific features of the temporomandibular joint**

- Intra-articular disc divides joint cavity into two joint spaces totalling 2 ml in volume
- Upper joint space allows translation movements (gliding-arthrodial)
- Lower joint space allows hinge movements (opening and closing gynglymus)
- Articular surfaces lined by fibrous tissue
- Secondary cartilage present
- Movements influenced by teeth
- The right and left joints cannot move independently

Mandibular fossa

The mandibular fossa (Fig. 3.2) is an oval depression in the temporal bone lying immediately anterior to the external acoustic meatus. Its mediolateral dimension is greater than its anteroposterior one to accommodate the mandibular condyle, and it is wider laterally than medially. The curvature of the mandibular fossa varies and may show some relationship to the nature of the occlusion. The mandibular fossa is bounded anteriorly by the articular eminence, laterally by the zygomatic process and posteriorly by the tympanic plate. The posterior margin is elevated to form the posterior auricular ridge, which may be enlarged laterally as the postglenoid tubercle just anterior to the external acoustic meatus. Medially the mandibular fossa may be defined by a ridge, the medial glenoid plane. The squamous and tympanic parts of the temporal bone are delineated laterally by the squamotympanic fissure. This fissure bifurcates medially because of the presence of a small component of the petrous portion, the tegmen tympani, giving rise to the petrosquamous fissure anteriorly and the petrotympanic fissure immediately behind. The petrotympanic fissure is the site at which the chorda tympani nerve exits from the cranium into the infratemporal fossa.

The shape of the mandibular fossa does not exactly conform to the shape of the mandibular condyle, the intra-articular disc moulding together the joint surfaces. The bone of the central part of the fossa is thin. This indicates that masticatory loads are not dissipated through the mandibular fossa but through the teeth and thence the facial bones and base of the cranium.

Mandibular condyle

The mandibular condyle varies considerably (Figs. 3.3, 3.4). When viewed from above, the condyle is roughly ovoid in outline, with the

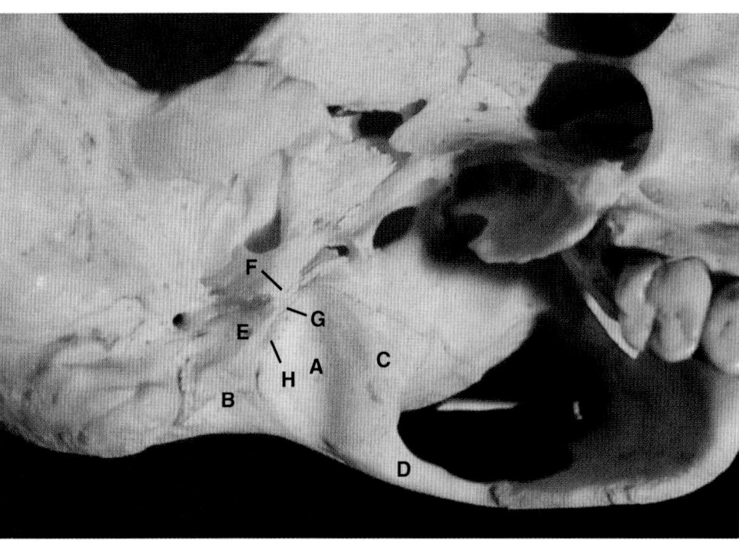

Fig. 3.2 The osteology of the mandibular fossa. A = mandibular fossa; B = external acoustic meatus; C = articular eminence; D = zygomatic process of temporal bone; E = tympanic plate; F = petrotympanic fissure; G = petrosquamous fissure; H = squamotympanic fissure.

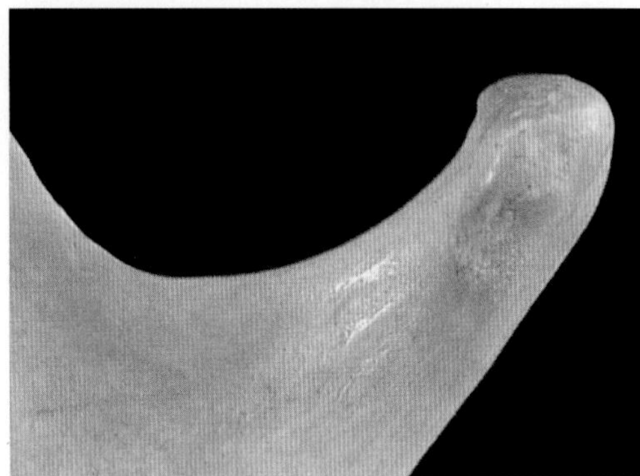

Fig. 3.3 The mandibular condyle viewed laterally.

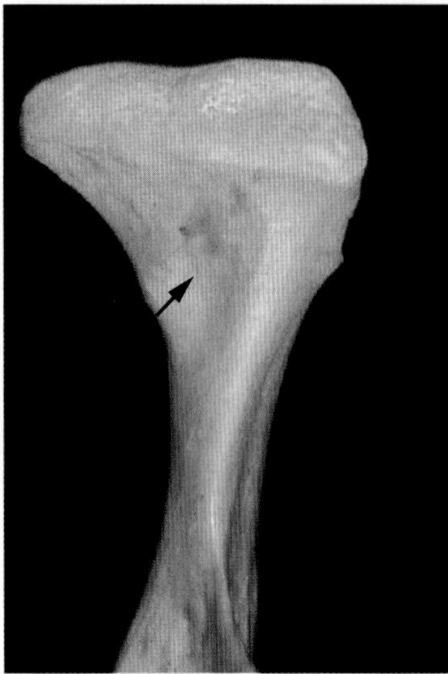

Fig. 3.4 The mandibular condyle viewed from above. The pterygoid fovea is arrowed.

anteroposterior dimension (approximately 1 cm) being about half the mediolateral dimension. The medial aspect is wider than the lateral. The long axis of the condyle is not, however, at right angles to the ramus, but diverges posteriorly from a strictly coronal plane. Thus the lateral pole of the condyle lies slightly anterior to the medial pole—if the long axes of the two condyles were extended, they would meet at an obtuse angle of approximately 145 degrees at the anterior border of the foramen magnum. The convex anterior and superior surfaces of the head of the condyle are the articular surfaces. The articular surface area of the condyle is of the order of 200 mm^2, which is about half that of the mandibular fossa. The non-articular posterior surface of the condyle is broad and flat. The articular surface may be separated from the non-articular surface by a slight ridge, indicating the site of attachment of the joint capsule. The broad articular head of the condyle joins the ramus through a thin, bony projection termed the neck of the condyle. A small depression, the pterygoid fovea, marks part of the attachment of the inferior head of the lateral pterygoid muscle and is situated on the anterior part of the neck below the articular surface of the condyle.

Joint capsule

The capsule of the TMJ is a thin, slack cuff that does not limit mandibular movements and is too weak to provide much support for the joint (Fig. 3.5). Above, it is attached to the mandibular fossa, extending anteriorly to just in front of the crest of the articular eminence, posteriorly to the squamotympanic and petrotympanic fissures, medially to the medial glenoid plane and laterally between the lateral margin of the articular eminence and the postglenoid process. Below, it is attached to the neck

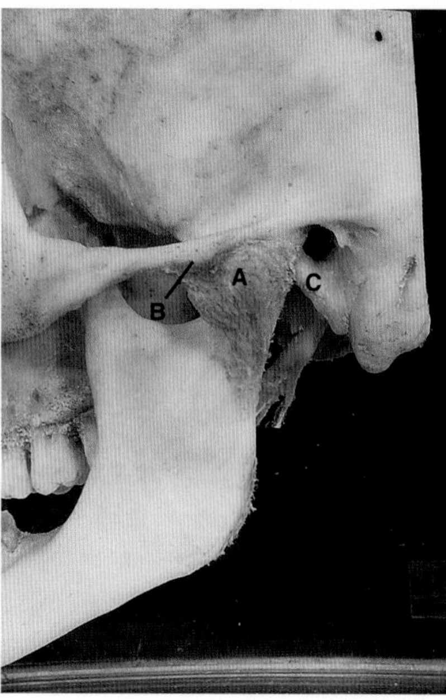

Fig. 3.5 The capsule of the temporomandibular joint (A). B = articular eminence; C = tympanic plate. Courtesy Prof. C Dean.

of the condyle of the mandible. The upper fibres of the capsule are more loosely arranged than the lower. Posteriorly the capsule is associated with the thick, vascular, but loosely arranged connective tissue of the bilaminar zone of the intra-articular disc (the retrodiscal pad). Internally, it is attached to the intra-articular disc and is lined by synovial membrane. The collagen fibres of the capsule run predominantly in a vertical direction. The capsule is richly innervated. There is debate as to whether muscle fibres of the superior head of the lateral pterygoid insert into the capsule or whether they also pass through to attach to the medial aspect of the anterior border of the intra-articular disc itself.

Synovial membrane

The synovial membrane lines the inner surface of the fibrous capsule and the margins of the intra-articular disc but does not cover the articular surfaces of the joint. The synovial membrane secretes the synovial fluid that occupies the joint cavities, lubricates the joint and presumably also has nutritive functions. Important components of the synovial fluid are the proteoglycans, which aid lubrication. At rest, the hydrostatic pressure of the synovial fluid has been reported to be subatmospheric, but this is greatly elevated during mastication.

Temporomandibular ligament

The joint capsule is strengthened by the temporomandibular (lateral) ligament. This ligament cannot be readily separated from the capsule. It takes origin from the lateral surface of the articular eminence of the temporal bone at the site of a small, bony protrusion, the articular tubercle. The temporomandibular ligament inserts onto the posterior surface of the condyle. This ligament provides the main means of support for the joint, restricting backward and inferior movements of the mandible and resisting dislocation during functional movements. The temporomandibular ligament is reinforced by a horizontal band of fibres running from the articular tubercle to the lateral surface of the condyle. These horizontal fibres restrict posterior movement of the condyle. The temporomandibular ligament is believed also to convert the potentially separating forces generated by the muscles opening the jaws into a force that compresses the condyle of the mandible onto the articular eminence. There is little evidence of any comparable ligament on the medial aspect of the joint capsule, so medial displacement is likely to be prevented by the temporomandibular ligament of the opposite side.

Accessory ligaments

The accessory ligaments of the TMJ traditionally described are the stylomandibular ligament, the sphenomandibular ligament, the discomalleolar ligament and the pterygomandibular raphe (Figs. 3.6, 3.7). However, only the sphenomandibular ligament is likely to have any significant influence on mandibular movements.

The *sphenomandibular ligament* is a remnant of the perichondrium of Meckel's cartilage (the cartilage of the embryonic first pharyngeal arch; see page 371) and extends from the spine of the sphenoid bone to the lingula near the mandibular foramen. The sphenomandibular ligament is slack when the jaws are closed but becomes tense at about the time when the condyle has passed in front of the temporomandibular ligament.

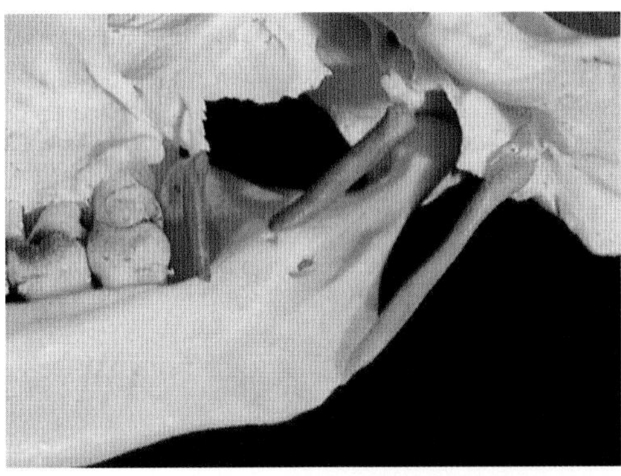

Fig. 3.6 Model showing accessory ligaments associated with the temporomandibular joint. Yellow = stylomandibular ligament; red = pterygomandibular raphe; green = sphenomandibular ligament.

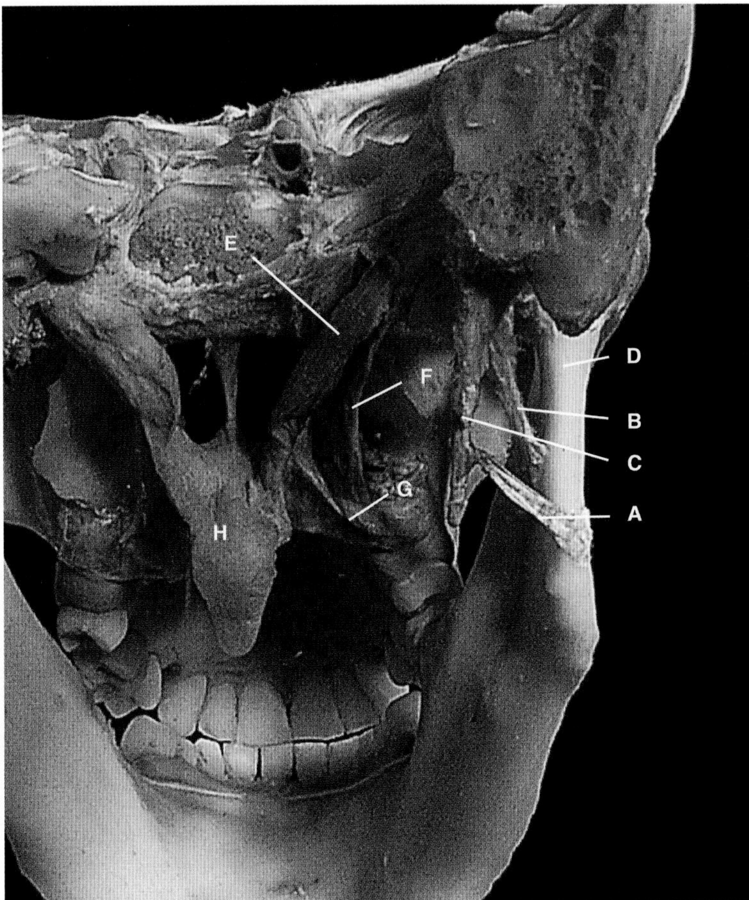

Fig. 3.7 Posterior view of the jaw apparatus showing the stylomandibular (A) and sphenomandibular (B) ligaments. C = styloid process; D = posterior border of ramus of mandible; E = levator veli palati muscle; F = tensor veli palati muscle; G = pterygoid hamulus; H = soft palate. Copyright the Museums of the Royal College of Surgeons of England.

The *stylomandibular ligament* is a reinforced lamina of the deep cervical fascia as it passes medially to the parotid salivary gland. It extends from the top of the styloid process of the temporal bone and from the stylohyoid ligament to the angle of the mandible.

The *discomalleolar ligament* passes from the medial aspect of the posterosuperior part of the articular disc and capsule to the neck and anterior process of the malleus ear ossicle. It therefore passes through the petrotympanic fissure in close relationship to the anterior ligament of the malleus and chorda tympani nerve. In addition to collagen, the ligament contains elastin fibres. Although some have suggested that tension within the ligament may cause movement of the malleus, others suggest that this is unlikely because of the attachment of part of the ligament to the margins of the petrotympanic fissure. The discomalleolar ligament may tense the synovial membrane during movements of the TMJ.

The *pterygomandibular raphe* (from which the buccinator and superior constrictor muscles arise) extends from the pterygoid hamulus to the posterior end of the mylohyoid line in the retromolar region of the mandible.

An additional ligament, the retinacular ligament, has been described in association with the temporomandibular ligament. This arises from the articular eminence, descends along the ramus of the mandible and inserts into the fascia overlying the masseter muscle at the angle of the mandible. Because this ligament is connected with the posterolateral aspect of the retrodiscal tissues and contains an accompanying vein, it may function in maintaining blood circulation during masticatory movements.

Intra-articular disc

The intra-articular disc (meniscus) is of a dense, fibrous consistency and is moulded to the bony joint surfaces above and below (Figs. 3.8–3.10). Blood vessels are evident only at the periphery of the intra-articular disc, the bulk of it being avascular. Above, the disc covers the slope of the articular eminence in front, while below it covers the condyle. When viewed in sagittal section, the upper surface of the disc is concavo-convex from front to back and the lower surface is concave (see Figs. 3.8 and 3.10). Viewed superiorly, the disc is somewhat rectangular or oval in outline. The disc is of variable thickness, being thinnest in its central part. It can be divided into three components: an anterior band, an intermediate zone and a posterior band. The intermediate zone is the thinnest (1 mm), and the posterior band the thickest (3 mm). The anterior band is about 2 mm thick. Both the intermediate zone and the posterior band are thicker medially than laterally. In the centric occlusal position the articular surface of the condyle lies against the thinner intermediate part of the intra-articular disc and faces the posterior slope of the articular eminence (see Fig. 3.8).

In the intermediate part of the intra-articular disc the collagen bundles have been described as running preferentially in an anteroposterior direction, whereas in the anterior and posterior bands they run both anteroposterior and mediolaterally. The overall shape of the intra-articular disc is thought to provide a self-centring mechanism, which automatically acts to maintain its correct relationship to the articular surface of the mandibular condyle during mandibular movements.

The margin of the intra-articular disc merges peripherally with the joint capsule. Anteriorly, fibrous bands connect the disc to the anterior margin of the articular eminence above and to the anterior margin of the condyle below. Issuing from the lateral and medial surfaces of the articular disc are

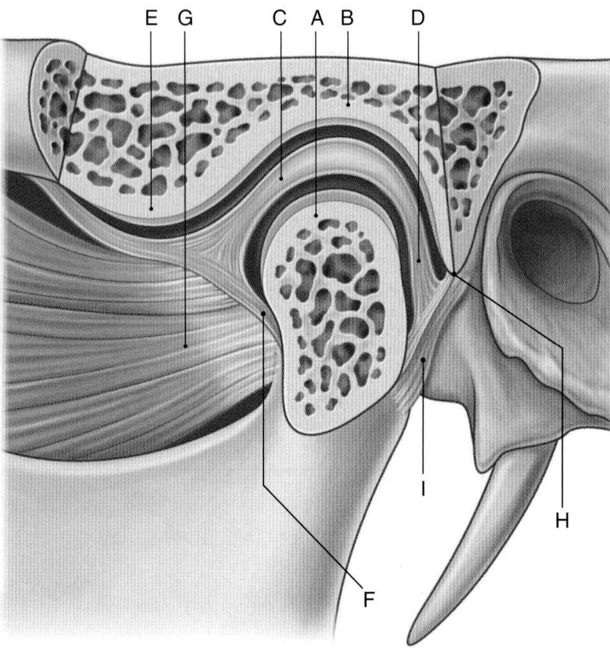

Fig. 3.8 Diagrammatic representation of the intra-articular disc. A = mandibular condyle; B = mandibular fossa; C = central part of intra-articular disc; D = posterior part of intra-articular disc; E = articular eminence; F = attachment of anterior part of intra-articular disc to anterior margin of mandibular condyle; G = lateral pterygoid muscle; H = attachment of upper part of bilaminar zone; I = attachment of the lower part of bilaminar zone.

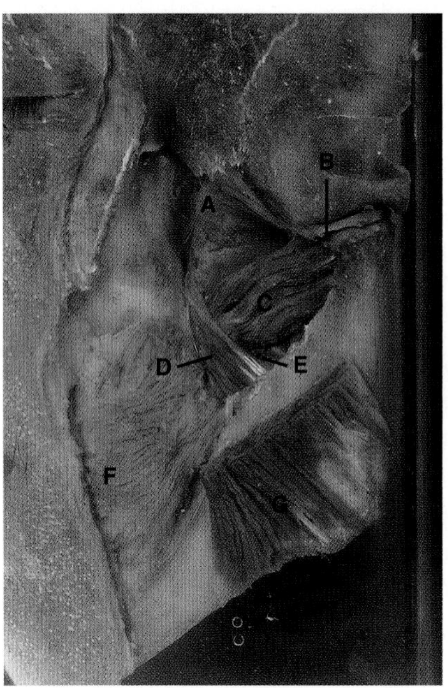

Fig. 3.9 Dissection showing the fibres of the upper head of the lateral pterygoid muscle (A) attaching to the intra-articular disc (B) of the temporomandibular joint. C = fibres of the inferior head of the lateral pterygoid muscle inserting into the pterygoid fovea of the mandibular condyle; D = superficial head of medial pterygoid muscle; E = deep head of medial pterygoid muscle; F = buccinator muscle; G = cut edge of masseter muscle. Courtesy Prof. L Garey.

lateral and medial collateral ligaments. The former divides, with the upper arm running upwards to insert into the capsule and the lower arm running downwards to insert onto the superficial layer of the articular cartilage of the condyle. A less conspicuous medial collateral ligament issuing from the medial surface of the articular disc has a similar insertion.

Posteriorly the disc is attached to the capsule by a bilaminar zone (retrodiscal tissue/pad). The superior lamina is loose and possesses numerous vascular elements and elastin fibres. It attaches to the anterior margin of the squamotympanic fissure. The inferior lamina is relatively avascular and less extensible (because it has few elastin fibres), and is attached to the posterior margin of the condyle. The volume of the retrodiscal tissue appears to increase about five times during jaw opening as a result of venous engorgement, because of its continuity with the pterygoid venous plexus lying medial to the condyle. This activity fills the vacated space in

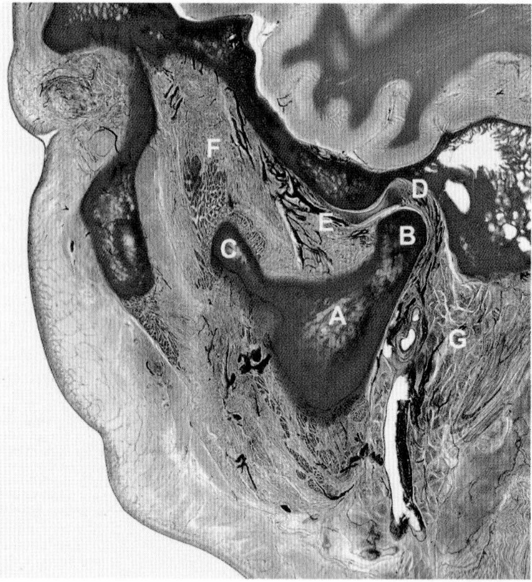

Fig. 3.10 Plastinated parasagittal section of head showing the intra-articular disc and its relations. A = ramus of mandible; B = condyle of mandible; C = coronoid process of mandible; D = mandibular fossa; E = lateral pterygoid muscle; F = temporalis muscle; G = parotid gland. Copyright the Royal College of Surgeons of England.

the mandibular fossa and rapidly equilibrates any changes in intracapsular pressures that may hinder jaw movement. Changes in tissue fluid pressure during mandibular movements could also help regulate the flow of blood in the retrodiscal pad. As the mandibular condyle moves backwards during jaw closure, blood leaves the retrodiscal tissues. The close relationship of elastin fibres to the walls of blood vessels in the retrodiscal tissues has led to the view that the fibres function as a pump, facilitating blood flow during venous dilatation and compression.

The return of the intra-articular disc to its original position may be aided by the elastic recoil of the superior lamella. The return could be passive, because of the shape of the disc and its firm insertion to the lateral and medial poles of the condyle of the mandible.

The intra-articular disc divides the TMJ cavity into superior and inferior joint cavities. About 1 ml of synovial fluid occupies the inferior joint cavity, while a little more occupies the superior joint cavity.

During jaw opening, two types of movement occur at the joint. The first is a hinge movement in the lower joint cavity of the head of the mandibular condyle around a horizontal axis. The second movement involves the upper joint cavity and is a forward or translatory movement of the condyle and the intra-articular disc. During opening and closing of the jaws, a combination of rotation and translation occurs: during wide opening, about 75% of the movement can be explained by rotation in the lower compartment. The condyle and disc move together anteriorly beneath the articular eminence. With the mouth closed, the condyle is in contact with the posterior band immediately above. As the condyle translates forward, it contacts the thinner intermediate zone of the intra-articular disc that separates it from the articular eminence. With the mouth fully opened, the condyle may lie beneath the anterior band of the disc.

Magnetic resonance images with the intra-articular disc highlighted in a normal patient with the jaw open and closed are illustrated in Fig. 3.11A. The TMJ is affected in the condition referred to as internal derangement. In internal derangement the posterior band of the intra-articular disc comes to lie in front of the condyle (see Fig. 3.11B). This is associated with stretching of the bilaminar zone. The intra-articular disc may return to its correct relationship to the condyle. This is referred to as anterior disc displacement with reduction (Fig. 3.12) and may be associated with a clicking joint. However, the intra-articular disc may remain anteriorly displaced. This is referred to as anterior disc displacement without reduction

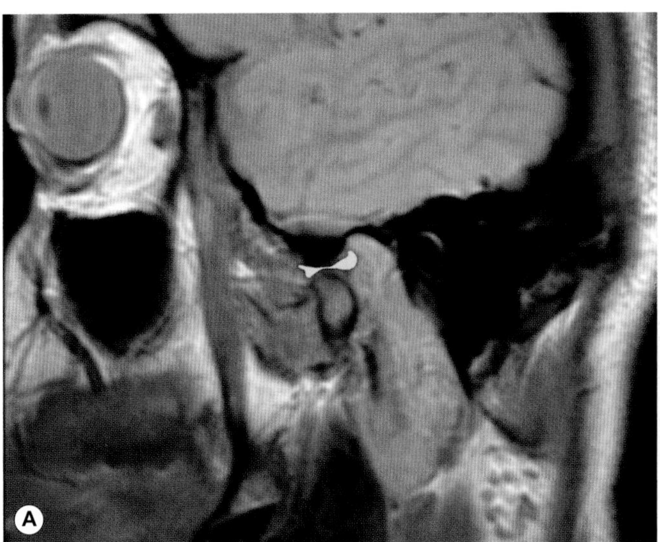

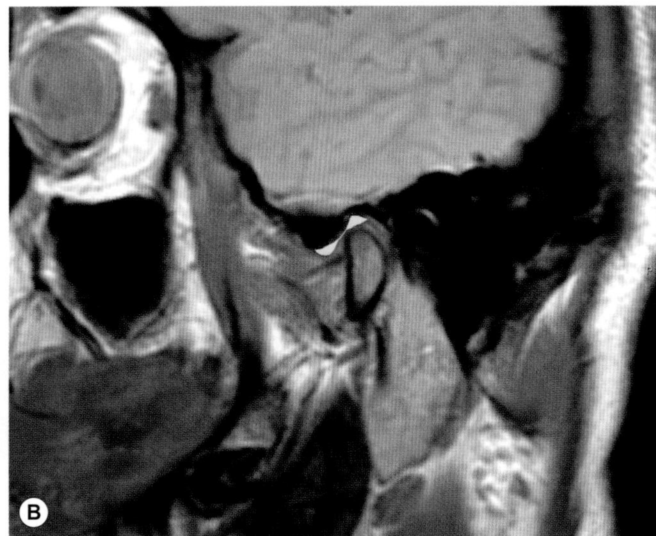

Fig. 3.11 Magnetic resonance images showing normal position of intra-articular disc (highlighted) with jaw open (A) and closed (B). Courtesy Dr J Makdissi.

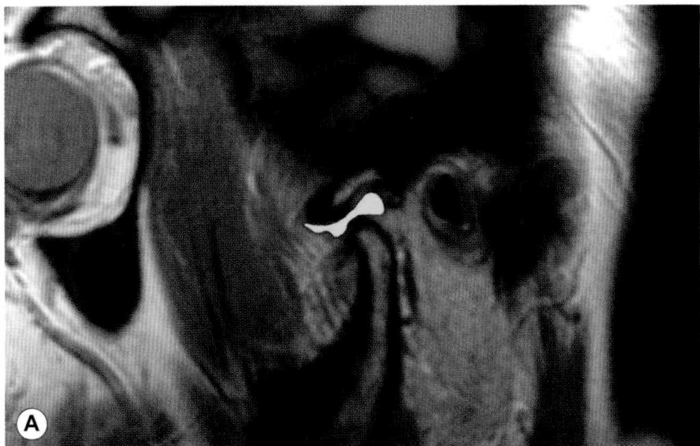

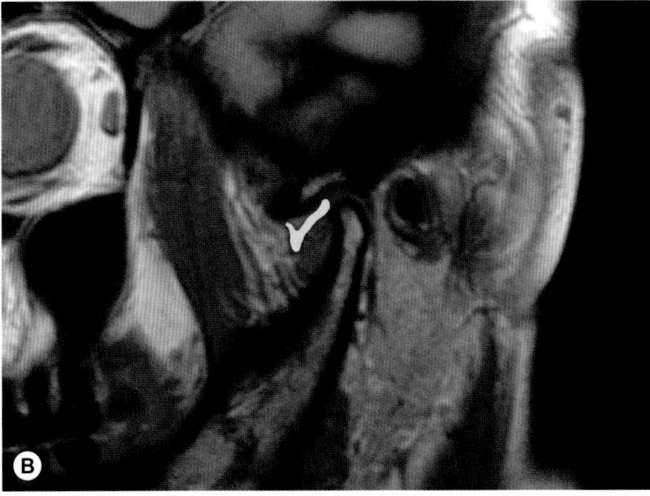

Fig. 3.12 Magnetic resonance images showing position of intra-articular disc (highlighted) in patient with anterior disc displacement with reduction with jaw open (A) and closed (B). Courtesy Dr J Makdissi.

(Fig. 3.13). Degenerative changes in the disc may lead to its perforation, and there may be a limitation of jaw movements.

The precise function(s) of the articular disc has not been identified, but some of these functions are listed in Box 3.2.

Nerves and vessels of the temporomandibular joint

The TMJ is richly innervated. Innervation for the joint is provided by the auriculotemporal, masseteric and deep temporal nerves of the mandibular division of the trigeminal nerve. The largest is the auriculotemporal nerve, supplying the medial, lateral and posterior parts of the joint. The remaining two nerves supply the anterior parts of the joint. Although free nerve endings associated with nociception are found everywhere in the joint capsule, of particular functional importance are more complex endings (e.g., Ruffini-like, Golgi tendon organs) associated with proprioception and important in the reflex control of mastication. The blood supply to the joint is mainly from the superficial temporal and maxillary arteries.

Muscles of mastication

Although many muscles, both in the head and the neck, are involved in the process of mastication, 'the muscles of mastication' is a collective term reserved for the masseter, temporalis and medial and lateral pterygoid muscles. All the muscles of mastication develop from the mesenchyme of the embryonic first pharyngeal arch. They therefore receive their innervation from the mandibular branch of the trigeminal nerve. The digastric muscle is closely associated, functionally and developmentally, with the muscles of mastication. The masseter and temporalis muscles lie on the superficial face, while the lateral and medial pterygoid muscles lie deeper within the infratemporal fossa.

Masseter

The masseter muscle consists of two overlapping heads (Fig. 3.14). The superficial head arises from the zygomatic process of the maxilla and from the anterior two-thirds of the lower border of the zygomatic arch. The deep head arises from the deep surface of the zygomatic arch. Internally the muscle has many tendinous septa that greatly increase the area for muscle attachment and provide a multipennate arrangement, thereby increasing its power. The superficial head passes downwards and backwards to insert into the lower half of the lateral surface of the mandibular ramus. The deep head, whose posterior fibres are more vertically oriented, inserts into the upper half of the lateral surface of the ramus, particularly over the coronoid process. The muscle elevates the mandible and is primarily active when grinding tough food. Indeed, the muscle exerts considerable power when the mandible is close to the centric occlusal position. On the basis of its fibre orientation, the posterior fibres of the deep head may have some retrusive capability for the mandible.

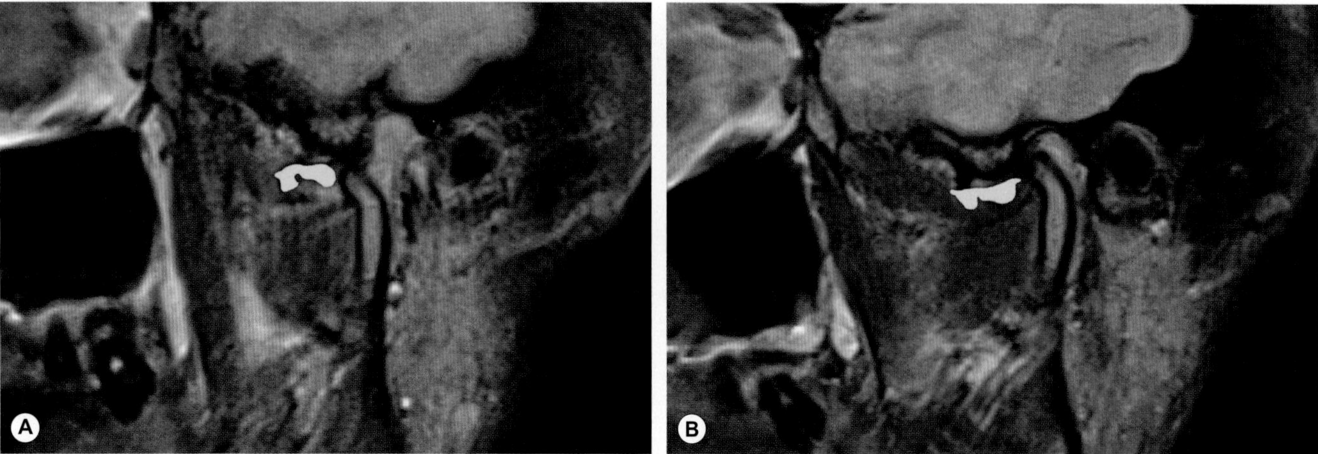

Fig. 3.13 Magnetic resonance images showing position of intra-articular disc in patient with anterior disc displacement without reduction with jaw open (A) and closed (B). Courtesy Dr J Makdissi.

Box 3.2 **Functions ascribed to the intra-articular disc**

- Improve the fit between the bony surfaces.
- Act as a shock absorber.
- Spread synovial fluid.
- Distribute load over a larger area.
- Protect the articular surfaces against shearing forces during jaw movement.
- Whereas some suggest the disc provides stability during movement, others claim it is associated with instability.

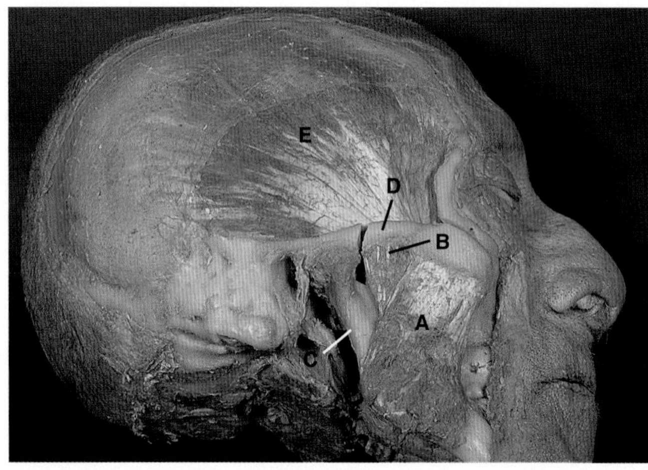

Fig. 3.14 The masseter muscle showing superficial (A) and deep (B) heads. C = posterior border of ramus of mandible; D = zygomatic arch; E = temporalis muscle.

Temporalis

The temporalis muscle is the largest muscle of mastication. It takes origin from the floor of the temporal fossa on the lateral surface of the skull and from the overlying temporal fascia. The muscle is considered a bipennate muscle. The attachment is limited above by the inferior temporal line. From this wide origin, the fibres of the temporalis muscle converge towards their insertion on the apex, the anterior and posterior borders and the medial surface of the coronoid process of the mandible (Fig. 3.15). Indeed, the insertion extends down the anterior border of the mandibular ramus almost as far as the third molar tooth. The posterior fibres of the muscle pass horizontally forwards, whereas the anterior fibres pass vertically downwards onto the coronoid process. To reach the coronoid process,

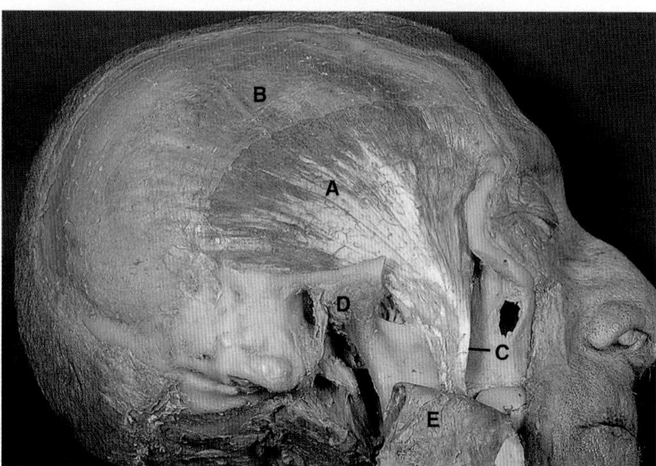

Fig. 3.15 The temporalis muscle (A) arising in part from the overlying temporal fascia (B) and inserting into the coronoid process (C) of the mandible. D = mandibular condyle; E = deep surface of masseter muscle revealed after reflection of the zygomatic arch.

the muscle runs beneath the zygomatic arch. The anterior (vertical) part elevates the mandible, whereas the posterior (horizontal) part retracts the protruded mandible. In certain sites the masseter and temporalis muscles are joined. This is particularly so for the deep fibres of the deep head of the masseter and the overlying temporalis muscle. The functional significance of this 'zygomatico-mandibular mass' is unclear.

Both the masseter and the temporalis muscles are innervated by branches of the anterior division of the mandibular nerve (see pages 106–108). Both receive their blood supply from the maxillary artery (masseteric and deep temporal branches), the superficial temporal artery (transverse facial and middle temporal branches) and, for the masseter muscle, the facial artery.

Pterygoids

To fully appreciate the anatomy of the pterygoid muscles, an understanding of the osteology of the infratemporal fossa is required because both muscles arise from bony landmarks within this fossa. The reader is therefore referred to page 91 and Fig. 3.35.

Lateral pterygoid

The lateral pterygoid muscle lies in the roof of the infratemporal fossa and has essentially a horizontal alignment. It has two heads, superior and inferior (Figs. 3.16–3.18). The superior (upper) head is the smaller and arises from the infratemporal surface of the greater wing of the sphenoid bone

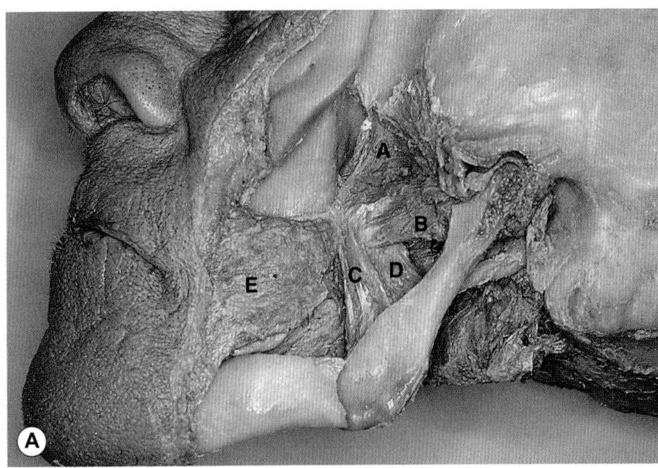

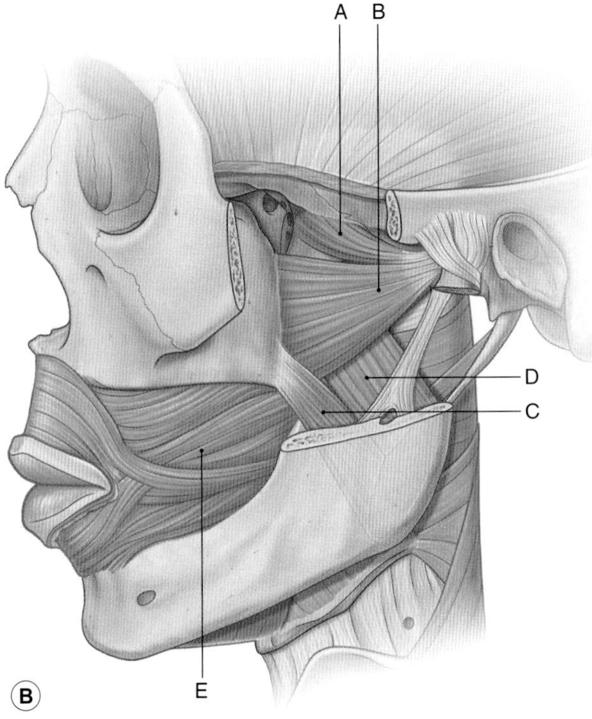

Fig. 3.16 Lateral view of the pterygoid muscles. A = superior head of lateral pterygoid; B = inferior head of lateral pterygoid; C = superficial head of medial pterygoid; D = deep head of lateral pterygoid; E = buccinator muscle.

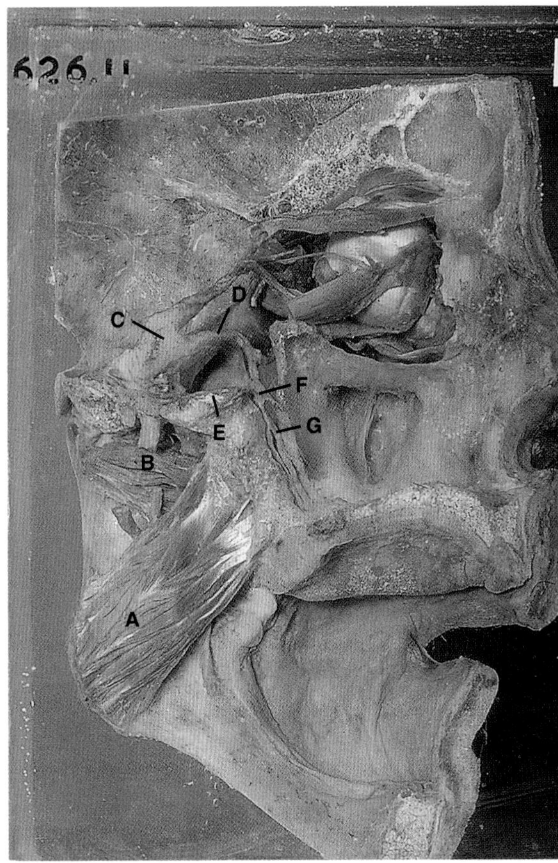

Fig. 3.17 Medial view of pterygoid muscles (A) in the infratemporal fossa. B = lateral pterygoid muscle; C = trigeminal ganglion; D = maxillary nerve; E = nerve of pterygoid canal; F = pterygopalatine ganglion; G = greater and lesser palatine nerves. Courtesy Prof. L Garey.

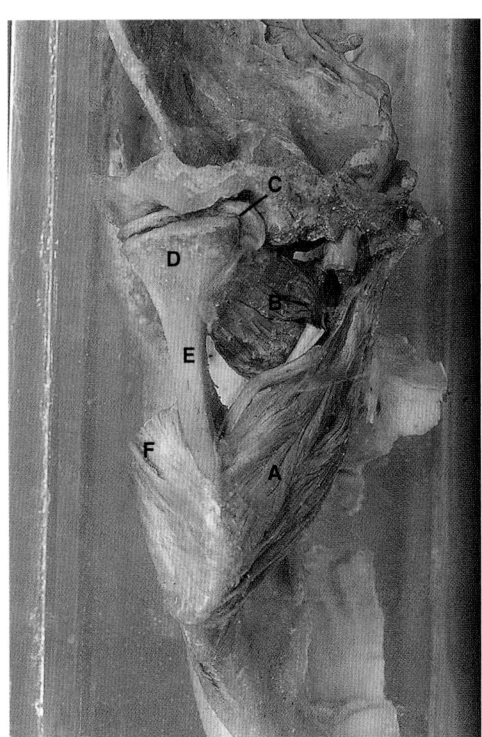

Fig. 3.18 Posterior view of the medial (A) and lateral (B) pterygoid muscles. C = intra-articular disc of temporomandibular joint; D = mandibular condyle; E = posterior border of ramus of mandible; F = cut edge of masseter muscle. Courtesy Prof. L Garey.

(see Fig. 3.35). The inferior (lower) head forms the bulk of the muscle and takes origin from the lateral surface of the lateral pterygoid plate of the sphenoid bone (see Fig. 3.35). Both heads pass backwards and outwards and appear to merge before their areas of insertion. The inferior head of the lateral pterygoid muscle inserts into the neck of the mandibular condyle at the fovea and into the capsule of the joint. The attachment of the superior head of lateral pterygoid has been a matter of controversy, but it appears to insert into the disc/capsule complex, as well as the condyle.

Concerning the function of the lateral pterygoid, it was generally thought that the inferior head of the lateral pterygoid was active during jaw opening, jaw protrusion, and contralateral jaw movements, whereas the superior head was active during jaw closing, jaw retrusion, and ipsilateral jaw movements. Both heads were therefore said to have a reciprocal pattern of activity. However, this interpretation was based on studies of electromyographic activity, where the precise position of the electrodes could not be fully determined. More recent studies in which the position of the electrodes was verified by computer tomography have provided a new interpretation of the actions of the lateral pterygoid muscle. Although the activity of the inferior head fit the classical view that the muscle is active during jaw opening, jaw protrusion and contralateral jaw movements (as well as protrusive or contralateral horizontal forces), the superior head was not seen to be active during jaw closure. Indeed, its activity was similar to

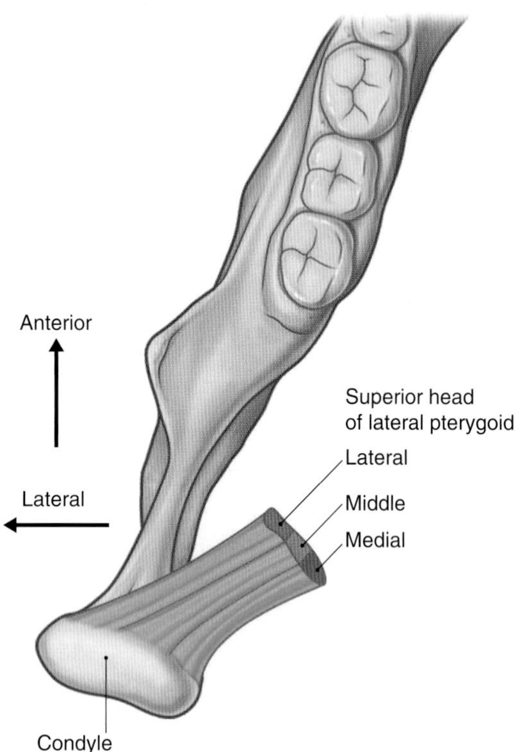

Fig. 3.19 Division of superior head of the lateral pterygoid muscle into three functional zones. The view is of the left condyle, anterior ramus and the lower molar teeth from the anterior and from a slightly superior and medial aspect. From Murray GM, Phanachet I, Uchida S, et al: The human lateral pterygoid muscle: a review of some experimental aspects and possible clinical relevance. *Aust Dent J* 49: 2–8, 2004, with permission.

that seen for the inferior head, namely, during contralateral, protrusive and jaw-opening movements.

As for the temporalis muscle, the lateral pterygoid muscle is fan shaped, with a broad origin but a narrow insertion. This means that there is a marked change in the alignment of muscle fibres from the uppermost to the lowermost muscle fibres and from the medial to the lateral side of the muscle. Selective activation of parts of each head of the muscle provides the opportunity for a range of jaw movements (Fig. 3.19). For the superior head the medial zone is active during jaw opening, jaw protrusion and contralateral jaw movements; the lateral zone is active during closing, retrusion and ipsilateral movements and retrusion; and the middle zone exhibits an intermediate range of patterns.

The superomedial part of the inferior head of the lateral pterygoid contains muscle fibres that are optimally orientated for contralateral and protrusive jaw movements. The superolateral and inferomedial parts of the inferior head contain muscle fibres that are optimally oriented to control contralateral and protrusive movements.

The lateral pterygoid should therefore be regarded as a single muscle whose fibres exhibit varying amounts of evenly graded activity throughout its entire range, with the distribution shaded according to the biomechanical demands of the task.

The precise insertions of the muscle are still controversial and may have clinical relevance with regard to TMJ disorders, particularly internal derangement where the disc is displaced, usually in an anteromedial position, and the jaw may become locked (see Fig. 3.13). Such conditions may be associated with clicking joints, limited jaw movements and pain, and some have attributed variations in the attachment, and therefore the function, of the superior head as an aetiological factor in the condition.

Medial pterygoid

The medial pterygoid muscle consists of two heads (see Figs. 3.16–3.18). The bulk of the muscle arises as a deep head from the medial surface of the lateral pterygoid plate of the sphenoid bone (see Fig. 3.35). The smaller superficial head arises from the maxillary tuberosity and the neighbouring part of the palatine bone (pyramidal process). From these sites of origin the fibres of the medial pterygoid pass downwards, backwards and laterally to insert into the roughened surface of the medial aspect of the angle of the mandible. Tendinous septa within the muscle increase the surface area for muscle attachment, providing a multipennate arrangement and therefore increasing the power the muscle can exert. The main action of the muscle is to elevate the mandible, but it also assists in lateral and protrusive movements. An accessory medial pterygoid muscle has been described as a separate slip of muscle close to the deep surface of the medial pterygoid. This takes origin from the base of the skull close to the foramen ovale and merges with the deep head of the medial pterygoid. Its function is unknown. The masseter and medial pterygoid muscles together form a muscular sling that supports the mandible on the cranium.

The medial pterygoid muscle is innervated by a branch of the mandibular nerve that arises proximal to the division of the mandibular nerve into anterior and posterior trunks (see Fig. 4.17 and page 106). The lateral pterygoid receives its nerve supply from the anterior trunk. Both muscles receive their blood supply as muscular branches from the maxillary artery.

Sphenomandibular

A fifth muscle of mastication has recently been described. It appears to take origin from the greater wing of the sphenoid bone (at the base of the temporal fossa) and extends downwards and backwards to be inserted onto the inner and anterior aspect of the mandibular coronoid process and the anterior edge of the mandibular ramus. From its orientation the muscle would aid elevation (and perhaps protrusion) of the mandible. An alternative explanation for the muscle is that it is a previously 'unidentified' component of a known muscle. Indeed, it may therefore be linked to the medial pterygoid muscle or be considered part of the temporalis muscle.

Digastric

Because of its functional associations, the digastric muscle is described here, although it is not usually strictly classified as a 'muscle of mastication'. This muscle is located below the inferior border of the mandible and consists of anterior and posterior bellies connected by an intermediate tendon (Fig. 3.20). The posterior belly arises from the mastoid notch immediately behind the mastoid process of the temporal bone; it passes downwards and forwards towards the hyoid bone, where it becomes the digastric tendon. The digastric muscle passes through the insertion of the stylohyoid muscle and is attached to the greater horn of the hyoid bone by a fibrous loop. The anterior belly of the digastric muscle is attached to the digastric fossa on the inferior border of the mandible and runs downwards and backwards to the digastric tendon. The digastric muscle depresses and retrudes the mandible and is involved in stabilising the position of the hyoid bone and in elevation of the hyoid during swallowing.

The anterior belly of the digastric muscle is innervated by the mylohyoid branch of the mandibular division of the trigeminal nerve, and the

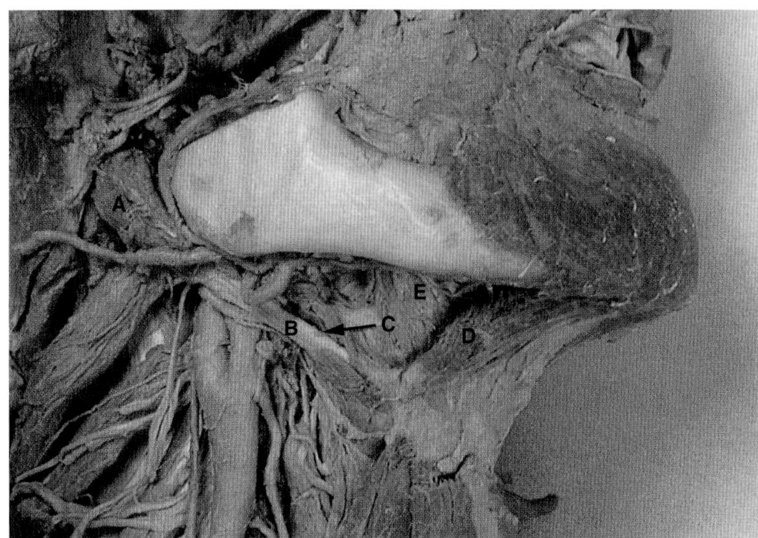

Fig. 3.20 The digastric muscle. A = posterior belly; B = tendon of digastric; C = stylohyoid muscle splitting around digastric tendon; D = anterior belly of digastric; E = mylohyoid muscle.

posterior belly by the digastric branch of the facial nerve. This reflects different embryological origins, from first and second pharyngeal arch mesenchyme, respectively. The anterior belly receives its blood supply from the facial artery, and the posterior belly from the posterior auricular and occipital arteries.

Muscles of the soft palate

The soft palate is supported by the fibrous palatine aponeurosis, the shape and position of which is altered by the activity of four pairs of muscles: the tensor veli palatini, the levator veli palatini, the palatoglossus and the palatopharyngeus muscles. In addition, there is the musculus uvulae.

Tensor veli palatini

The tensor veli palatini muscle (Figs. 3.21–3.23) arises from the scaphoid fossa of the sphenoid bone at the root of the pterygoid plates and from the lateral side of the cartilaginous part of the auditory (pharyngotympanic) tube. From its origin, the fibres converge towards the pterygoid hamulus, whence the muscle becomes tendinous (the tendon bending at right angles around the hamulus to become the palatine aponeurosis). The anterior border of the aponeurosis is attached to the posterior border of the hard palate. Medially, it merges with the aponeurosis of the other side. Posteriorly, it becomes indistinct, merging with submucosa at the posterior edge of the soft palate. When the tensor veli palatini muscle contracts, the aponeurosis becomes a taut, horizontal plate of tissue upon which other palatine muscles may act to change the position of the soft palate.

The motor innervation of the tensor veli palatini is derived from the mandibular branch of the trigeminal nerve (via the nerve to the medial pterygoid muscle and the otic ganglion).

Levator veli palatini

The levator veli palatini muscle (see Figs. 3.21–3.23) originates from the base of the skull at the apex of the petrous part of the temporal bone, anterior to the opening of the carotid canal, and from the medial side of the cartilaginous part of the auditory tube. The muscle curves downwards,

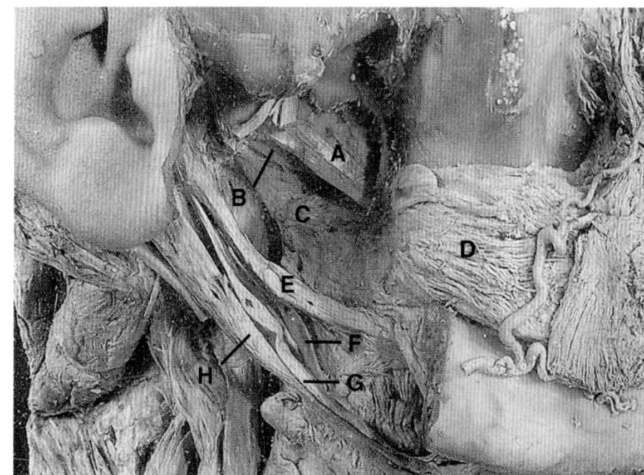

Fig. 3.21 Deep dissection of the infratemporal fossa to reveal tensor veli palatini muscle (A). B = partially obscured levator veli palatini muscle; C = superior constrictor muscle; D = buccinator muscle; E = styloglossus muscle; F = stylopharyngeus muscle; G = stylohyoid muscle; H = posterior belly of digastric muscle. Courtesy Prof. C Dean.

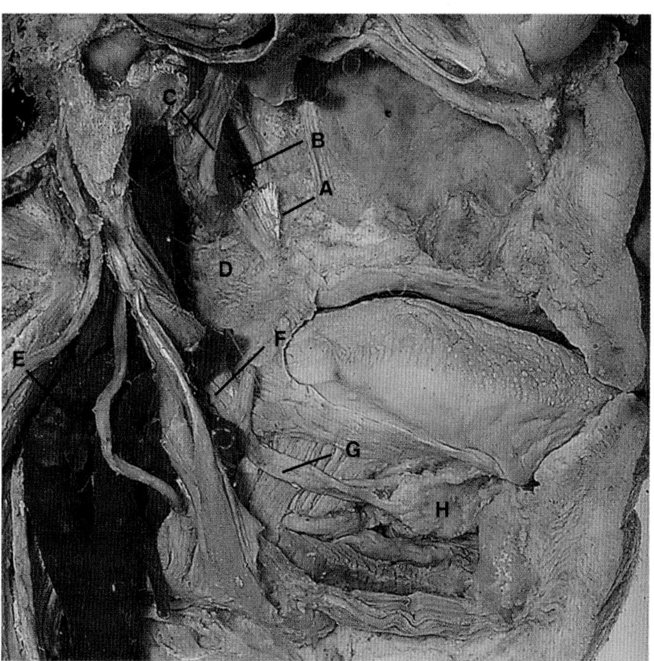

Fig. 3.22 Deep dissection of the infratemporal fossa with the tensor palati muscle (A) cut to reveal the levator palati muscle (B); C = mandibular nerve; D = superior constrictor; E = internal carotid artery; F = styloglossus muscle; G = lingual nerve on hyoglossus muscle; H = sublingual gland. Courtesy Prof. L Garey.

medially and forwards, to enter the palate immediately below the opening of the auditory tube.

The levator muscles of the palate form a U-shaped muscular sling (see Fig. 3.23). When the palatine aponeurosis is stiffened by the tensor muscles, contraction of the levator muscles produces an upwards and backwards movement of the soft palate. In this way the nasopharynx is shut off from the oropharynx by the apposition of the soft palate onto the posterior wall of the pharynx.

Palatopharyngeus

The palatopharyngeus muscle arises from two heads: one from the posterior border of the hard palate, the other from the upper surface of the palatine aponeurosis (see Fig. 3.23). The two heads unite after arching over the lateral edge of the palatine aponeurosis, where the muscle passes downwards beneath the mucous membrane of the lateral wall of the oropharynx as the palatopharyngeal fold (see Fig. 1.12). The muscle is inserted into the posterior border of the thyroid cartilage of the larynx.

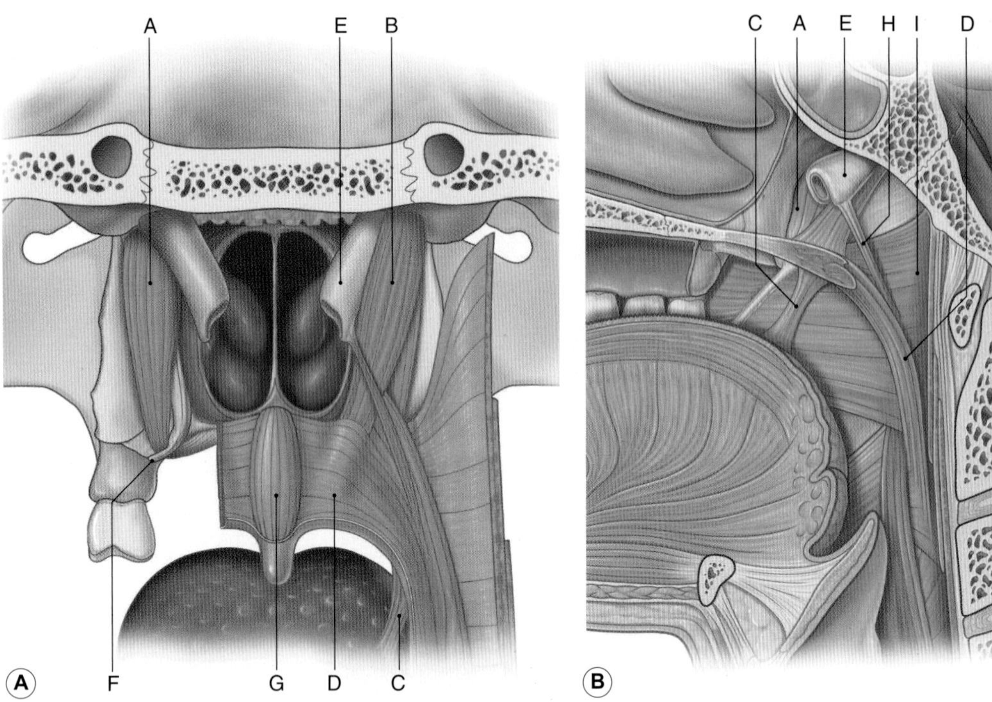

Fig. 3.23 Diagrammatic representation of palatal and pharyngeal muscles. (A) Posterior view. (B) Medial view. A = tensor veli palatini; B = levator veli palatini; C = palatoglossus; D = palatopharyngeus; E = auditory (pharyngotympanic or Eustachian) tube; F = pterygoid hamulus; G = musculus uvulae; H = salpingopharyngeus muscle; I = superior constrictor muscle.

The main action of the palatopharyngeus muscle is to elevate the larynx and pharynx, but it may also arch the relaxed palate and depress the tensed palate.

Palatoglossus

The palatoglossus muscle (see Fig. 3.23) arises from the aponeurosis of the soft palate and descends to the tongue in the palatoglossal fold (see Fig. 1.12), whence its fibres intercalate with the transverse fibres of the tongue. The action of the palatoglossus is to raise the tongue to narrow the transverse diameter of the oropharyngeal isthmus.

Musculus uvulae

The musculus uvulae (see Fig. 3.23) arises from the posterior nasal spine at the back of the hard palate and from the palatine aponeurosis. It passes backwards and downwards to insert into the mucosa of the uvula. It moves the uvula upwards and laterally and helps to complete the seal between the soft palate and pharynx in the midline region when the palate is elevated.

Nerve and blood supply

With the exception of the tensor veli palatini muscle, the nerve supply to the muscles of the palate is derived from the cranial part of the accessory nerve via the pharyngeal plexus. The arterial supply to the muscles of the soft palate is derived from the facial artery (ascending palatine branch), the ascending pharyngeal artery and the maxillary artery (palatine branches).

Passavant's muscle

Passavant's muscle is a sphincter-like muscle that encircles the pharynx at the level of the palate, inside the fibres of the superior constrictor muscles. It is formed by fibres arising from the anterior and lateral part of the upper surface of the palatine aponeurosis. Contraction of this muscle forms a ridge (Passavant's ridge), against which the soft palate is elevated.

Muscles of the tongue

The tongue is composed of intrinsic and extrinsic muscles. The intrinsic muscles are restricted to the substance of the tongue and change its shape, whereas the extrinsic muscles arise outside the tongue and are responsible for bodily movement of the tongue.

Intrinsic muscles

The intrinsic muscles of the tongue can be divided into three fibre groups: transverse, longitudinal and vertical. Rarely can these three groups be distinguished in dissections, but their interlacing gives the tongue its characteristic appearance in cross section (Fig. 3.24). The transverse fibres arise from a sheet of connective tissue called the lingual septum, running longitudinally through the midline of the tongue. These transverse fibres pass laterally from the septum to intercalate with fibres of the other groups of intrinsic muscles. The longitudinal fibres may be subdivided into upper and lower groups, the superior and inferior longitudinal muscles of the tongue. The vertical fibres pass directly between the upper and lower surfaces, particularly at the lateral borders of the tongue. Contraction of the vertical fibres would make the tongue thinner (and wider). Contraction of the longitudinal fibres would shorten (and thicken) the tongue. Contraction of the transverse fibres would narrow (and widen) the tongue. The intrinsic muscles receive their motor innervation from the hypoglossal cranial nerve.

Extrinsic muscles

The extrinsic muscles of the tongue arise from the skull and hyoid bone and thence spread into the body of the tongue. The extrinsic musculature is composed of four groups of muscles: genioglossus, hyoglossus, styloglossus and palatoglossus.

Genioglossus

The genioglossus muscle (Figs. 3.24–3.28) arises from the superior genial spine on the medial surface of the body of the mandible. At this level the

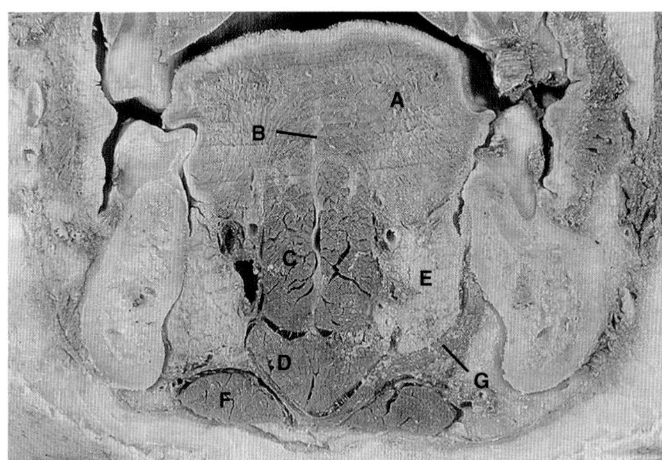

Fig. 3.24 Coronal section through the tongue and floor of the mouth. Note the interlacing of the intrinsic muscles in the body of the tongue (A). B = lingual septum; C = genioglossus muscle; D = geniohyoid muscle; E = sublingual gland above mylohyoid; F = anterior belly of digastric muscle; G = mylohyoid muscle.

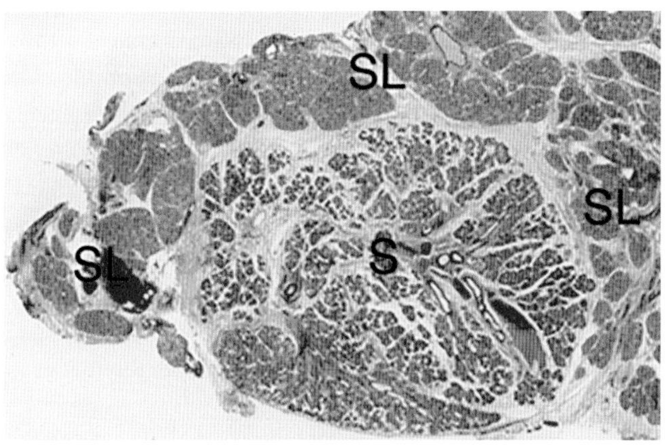

Fig. 3.25 A rounded lobule of submandibular gland (S) is enclosed by sublingual gland (SL) above and to both sides in the photomicrograph (hematoxylin and eosin stain; ×4). From Harrison, J. D. 2020. Salivary gland histology. From: Surgery of the salivary glands. Edited by Witt, R. L. Elsevier: Edinburgh. Pp 37–42.

two genioglossus muscles cannot readily be separated. As the muscles enter the tongue, a thin strip of connective tissue intervenes between the right and left genioglossus muscles. The bulk of the fibres fan out into the body of the tongue, but the superior fibres pass upwards and anteriorly to the tip of the tongue, and some of its inferior fibres insert onto the body of the hyoid bone. The genioglossus muscle is mainly a protractor and depressor of the tongue.

Hyoglossus

The hyoglossus muscle (see Figs. 3.26, 3.28) originates from the superior border of the greater horn of the hyoid bone and passes vertically upwards into the tongue. Its function is to depress the tongue. At its origin, the hyoglossus muscle is separated from the attachment of the middle constrictor muscle of the pharynx beneath by the lingual artery.

Styloglossus

The styloglossus muscle (see Figs. 3.21, 3.22, 3.26, 3.28) arises from the anterior surface of the styloid process of the temporal bone, from which the muscle runs downwards and forwards to enter the tongue below the insertion of the palatoglossus muscle. At this point, its fibres intercalate with the fibres of the hyoglossus before continuing forwards towards the tip of the tongue. The styloglossus muscle is a retractor of the tongue.

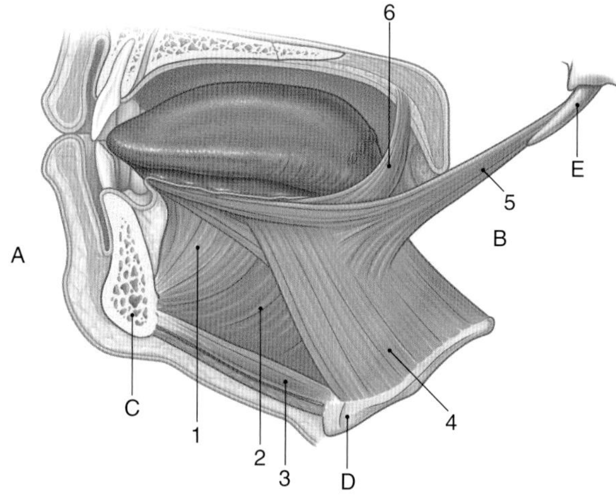

Fig. 3.26 Diagrammatic representation of the extrinsic muscles of the tongue. A = anterior; B = posterior; C = mandible; D = hyoid bone; E = styloid process; 1 = genioglossus; 2 = mylohyoid; 3 = geniohyoid; 4 = hyoglossus; 5 = styloglossus; 6 = palatoglossus.

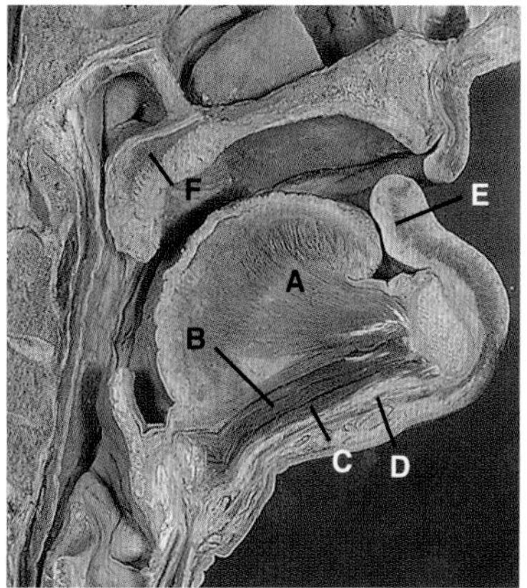

Fig. 3.27 Sagittal section of head showing genioglossus muscle (A). B = geniohyoid muscle; C = mylohyoid muscle; D = platysma muscle; E = orbicularis oris muscle; F = levator veli palatini muscle.

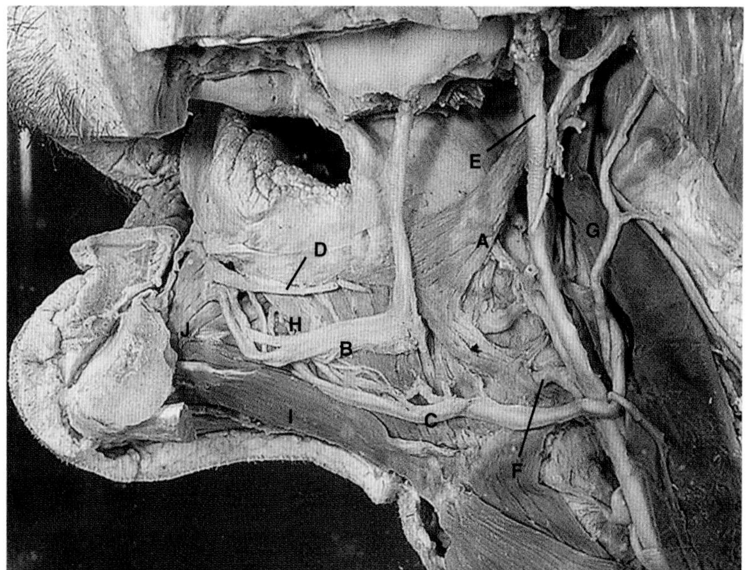

Fig. 3.28 Lateral view of tongue showing styloglossus muscle (A). B = lingual nerve; C = hypoglossal nerve; D = submandibular duct (cut); E = external carotid artery; F = lingual artery; G = glossopharyngeal nerve; H = hyoglossus muscle; I = geniohyoid muscle; J = genioglossus muscle. Courtesy Prof. C Dean.

Palatoglossus

The palatoglossus muscle (see Figs. 3.23, 3.26) arises from the aponeurosis of the soft palate and descends to the tongue in the anterior pillar of the fauces, whence its fibres intercalate with the transverse fibres of the tongue. The action of the palatoglossus muscles is to raise the tongue to narrow the transverse diameter of the oropharyngeal isthmus.

The extrinsic muscles of the tongue are innervated by the hypoglossal nerve (except for the palatoglossus, which is innervated by the cranial part of the accessory nerve via the pharyngeal plexus). The main source of the blood supply to the tongue is the lingual artery.

Muscles in the floor of the mouth

The floor of the mouth is the region located between the medial surface of the mandible, the inferior surface of the tongue and the mylohyoid muscles. The mylohyoid muscles are attached to the mylohyoid lines of the mandible, and consequently structures above these lines are related to the floor of the mouth, whereas structures below the lines are related to the upper part of the neck (suprahyoid region). This concept is of considerable clinical importance with respect to the spread of inflammation from infected teeth within the mandible (see pages 92–96). The two mylohyoid muscles form a muscular diaphragm for the floor of the mouth (see Figs. 3.20, 3.24, 3.27). Above this diaphragm are found the genioglossus and geniohyoid muscles medially and the hyoglossus muscles laterally. Below the diaphragm lie the digastric and stylohyoid muscles.

Mylohyoid

The mylohyoid muscle (Figs. 3.24, 3.27, 3.29) arises from the mylohyoid line on the inner surface of the body of the mandible. Its fibres slope downwards, forwards and inwards. The anterior fibres of the mylohyoid muscle interdigitate with the corresponding fibres on the opposite side to form a median raphe. This raphe is attached above to the chin and below to the hyoid bone. The posterior fibres are inserted onto the anterior surface of the body of the hyoid bone. The muscle raises the floor of the mouth during the early stages of swallowing. It also helps to depress the mandible when the hyoid bone is fixed. The mylohyoid muscle is supplied by the mylohyoid branch of the inferior alveolar branch of the mandibular division of the trigeminal nerve. Its blood supply is derived from the lingual artery (sublingual branch), the maxillary artery (mylohyoid branch of the inferior alveolar artery) and the facial artery (submental branch).

One or more mylohyoid hiatuses are found in almost half of the population. They are mainly present anteriorly or in the middle part. Hernias protrude through the hiatuses and consist of part of the sublingual gland or fat (see Fig. 3.29). This is of clinical significance when occasionally the entire sublingual gland herniates through and produces submandibular swelling. Furthermore, extravasated mucus from a damaged sublingual gland can reach the neck via a hiatus to produce a cervical or plunging ranula (see Fig. 16.52, page 350).

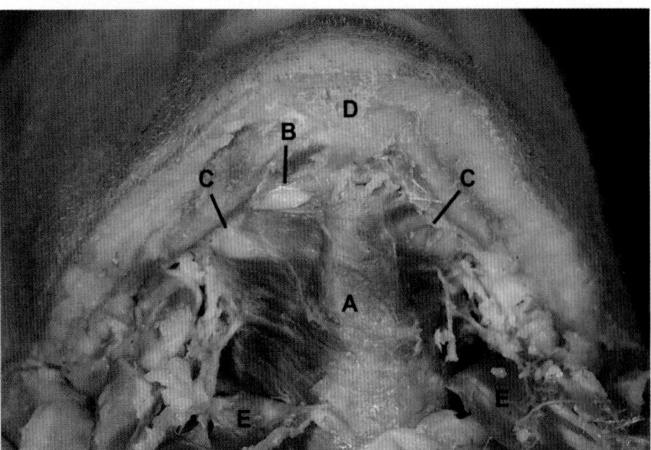

Fig. 3.29 Dissection showing mylohyoid hiatuses. Anteroinferior view of submandibular region shows three hernias protruding through hiatuses in the mylohyoid muscle (A). The most anterior hernia (B) is polypoid and consists of fat. The other two hernias (C) consist of sublingual gland. The inferior surface of the mandible (D) is seen anteriorly and laterally to the mylohyoid muscle, and the divided anterior bellies of the digastric muscles (E) are seen at the posterior margin of the mylohyoid muscle. Courtesy Prof. R P Morton and the editor of *Clinical Anatomy.* From Harrison, J.D., Kim, A., Al Ali, S., Morton, R.P., 2013. Postmortem investigation of mylohyoid hiatus and hernia: Aetiological factors of plunging ranula. *Clinical Anatomy* 26: 693–699.

Geniohyoid

The geniohyoid muscle (see Figs. 3.24, 3.27, 3.28) originates from the inferior genial spine. It passes backwards and slightly downwards onto the anterior surface of the body of the hyoid bone. The geniohyoid muscle elevates the hyoid bone and is a weak depressor of the mandible. Its innervation is from the first cervical spinal nerve travelling with the hypoglossal nerve. Its blood supply is derived from the lingual artery (sublingual branch).

Superficial muscles of the face

The muscles of facial expression (Figs. 3.30, 3.31) are characterised by their superficial arrangement in the face, by their activities on the skin (brought about directly by their attachment to the facial integument) and by their common motor innervation, the facial nerve. They are all derived embryologically from mesenchyme of the second pharyngeal arch. Functionally the muscles of facial expression are grouped around the orifices of the face (the orbit, nose, ear and mouth) and should be considered primarily as muscles controlling the degree of opening and closing of these apertures: the expressive functions of the muscles have developed secondarily. The muscles of facial expression vary considerably between individuals in terms of size, shape and strength.

The superficial muscles around the lips and cheeks may be subdivided into two groups: the various parts of the orbicularis oris muscle and muscles that are radially arranged from the orbicularis oris muscle. The fibres

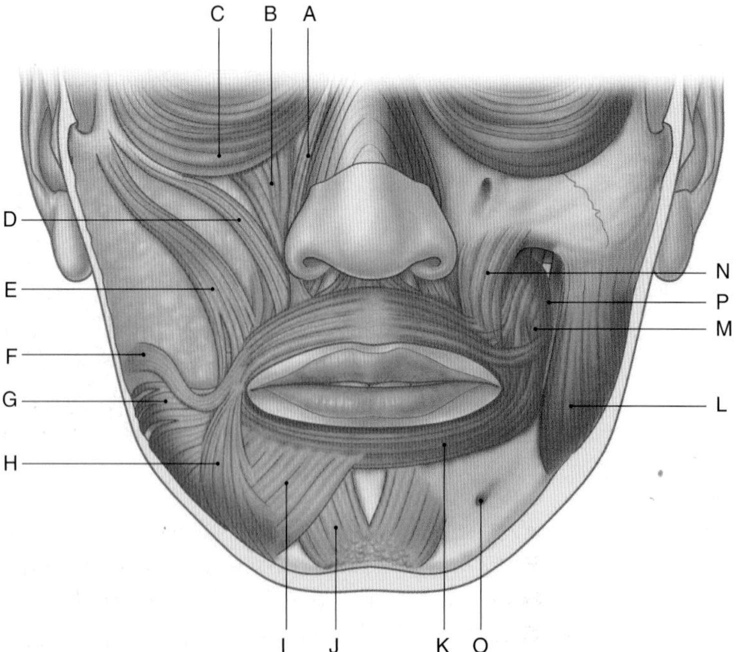

Fig. 3.30 Schematic diagram of the muscles of facial expression. A = levator labii superioris alaeque nasi; B = levator labii superioris; C = orbicularis oculi; D = zygomaticus minor; E = zygomaticus major; F = risorius; G = platysma; H = depressor anguli oris; I = depressor labii inferioris; J = mentalis; K = orbicularis oris; L = masseter; M = buccinator; N = levator anguli oris; O = mental foramen; P = position of opening for the parotid duct.

of orbicularis oris pass around the lips. The muscle is divided into four parts, each part corresponding to a quadrant of the lips. Its muscle fibres do not gain attachment directly to bone but occupy a central part of the lip. Muscle fibres in the philtrum insert onto the nasal septum. The range of movement produced by orbicularis oris includes lip closure, protrusion and pursing. The radial muscles can be divided into superficial and deep muscles of the upper and lower lips. The levator labii superioris, levator labii superioris alaeque nasi and zygomaticus major and minor are superficial muscle of the upper lip. The levator anguli oris is a deep muscle of the upper lip. The depressor anguli oris is a superficial muscle of the lower lip, and the depressor labii inferioris and mentalis muscles are deep muscles of the lower lip. As their names suggest, the levator labii superioris elevates the upper lip, the depressor labii inferioris depresses the lower lip and the corners of the mouth are raised and lowered by the levator and depressor anguli oris muscles, respectively.

Two muscles extend to the corner of the mouth: the risorius and buccinator muscles, with risorius lying superficial to buccinator. The risorius muscle stretches the angles of the mouth laterally. The buccinator muscle (see Fig. 3.9) arises from the pterygomandibular raphe and from the buccal side of the maxillary and mandibular alveoli above the molar teeth. Most of its fibres insert into mucous membrane covering the cheek; other fibres intercalate with orbicularis oris in the lips. As the fibres of buccinator converge towards the angle of the mouth, the central fibres decussate. The main function of the buccinator muscle is to maintain the tension of the cheek against the teeth during mastication.

Salivary glands

Parotid gland

The parotid gland (Fig. 3.32) is the largest of the major salivary glands and secretes a serous saliva. It occupies the region between the ramus of the mandible and the mastoid process. The parotid is pyramidal in shape; its apex extends beyond the angle of the mandible, and the base is closely related to the external acoustic meatus. A deep surface of the gland rests anteriorly on the mandibular ramus and masseter muscle and extends around the posterior border of the mandible, where it can reach the pharynx. The gland is surrounded by an unyielding tough fibrous capsule (the parotid capsule). The parotid duct (Stensen's duct) appears at the anterior border of the gland and passes horizontally across the masseter muscle before piercing the buccinator to terminate in the oral cavity opposite the maxillary second molar. Lying with the duct on the masseter may be an accessory parotid gland.

Within the parotid gland are found the external carotid artery, retromandibular veins and the facial nerve. Branches of the facial nerve are seen emerging from the anterior and inferior margins of the gland. Appearing

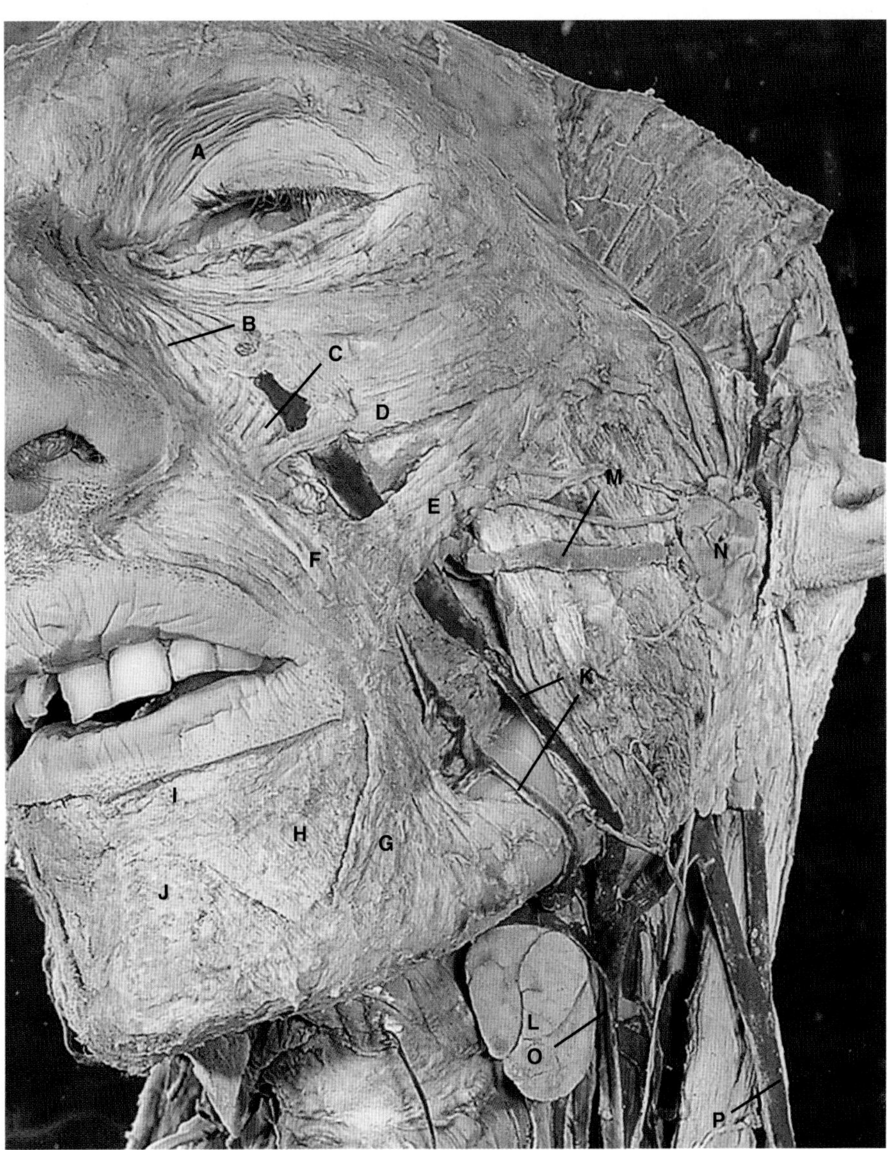

Fig. 3.31 The muscles of facial expression. A = orbicularis oculi; B = levator labii superioris alaeque nasi; C = levator labii superioris; D = zygomaticus minor; E = zygomaticus major; F = levator anguli oris; G = depressor anguli oris; H = depressor labii inferioris; I = orbicularis oris; J = mentalis; K = facial vessels; L = submandibular gland; M = parotid duct; N = parotid gland with facial nerve branches; O = facial vein receiving the anterior retromandibular vein; P = external jugular vein formed by the anterior branch of the retromandibular and the posterior auricular vein. Courtesy Prof. C Dean.

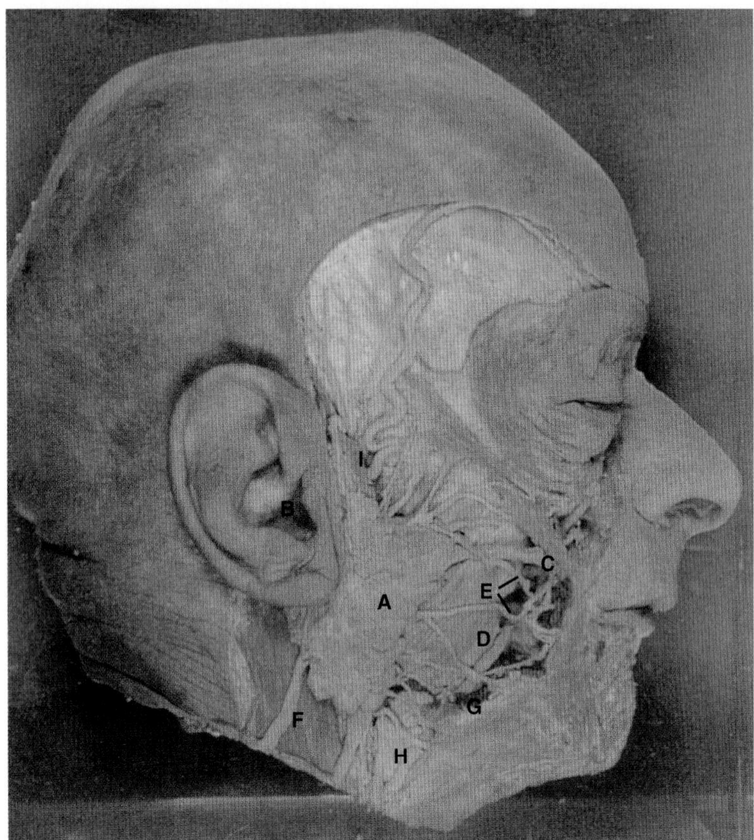

Fig. 3.32 The shape and relations of the parotid gland (A). B = external acoustic meatus; C = parotid duct; D = masseter muscle; E = branches of facial nerve; F = great auricular nerve; G = facial vessels coursing through muscles of facial expression; H = superficial part of submandibular gland; I = superficial temporal vessels and auriculotemporal nerve.

at the superior border of the gland are the superficial temporal vessels and the auriculotemporal nerve. From the inferior border of the gland may be seen the anterior and posterior retromandibular veins. The former joins the facial vein, with the latter joining the posterior auricular to form the external jugular vein (see Fig. 3.31). Lymph nodes are also associated with the parotid gland.

The parasympathetic innervation of the parotid gland is from the lesser petrosal branch of the glossopharyngeal nerve (see Fig. 4.13). The preganglionic fibres synapse in the otic ganglion, and postganglionic fibres reach the gland by travelling with the auriculotemporal branch of the mandibular nerve. The sensory innervation of the parotid capsule is by the great auricular nerve, a branch of the cervical plexus (see Fig. 3.32). The roots of this nerve are formed from the anterior primary rami of the second and third cervical nerves. The sensation of pain in mumps caused by enlargement of the gland (with subsequent tension on the unyielding parotid capsule) is mediated by the great auricular nerve.

Submandibular gland

The submandibular gland produces both serous and mucous saliva (in a 3:2 ratio). It is found in the floor of the mouth and in the suprahyoid region of the neck. A large part of the gland (the superficial part) is visible just beneath the inferior border of the mandible (Figs. 3.31–3.33). The gland has an important relationship with the mylohyoid muscle, wrapping around the free posterior border (not unlike the letter C). This gives rise to the smaller deep portion of the gland (Fig. 3.34). Posteriorly the submandibular gland comes close to the apex of the parotid gland, with only the stylomandibular ligament intervening. The submandibular duct (Wharton's duct) appears from the deep part of the gland and wraps

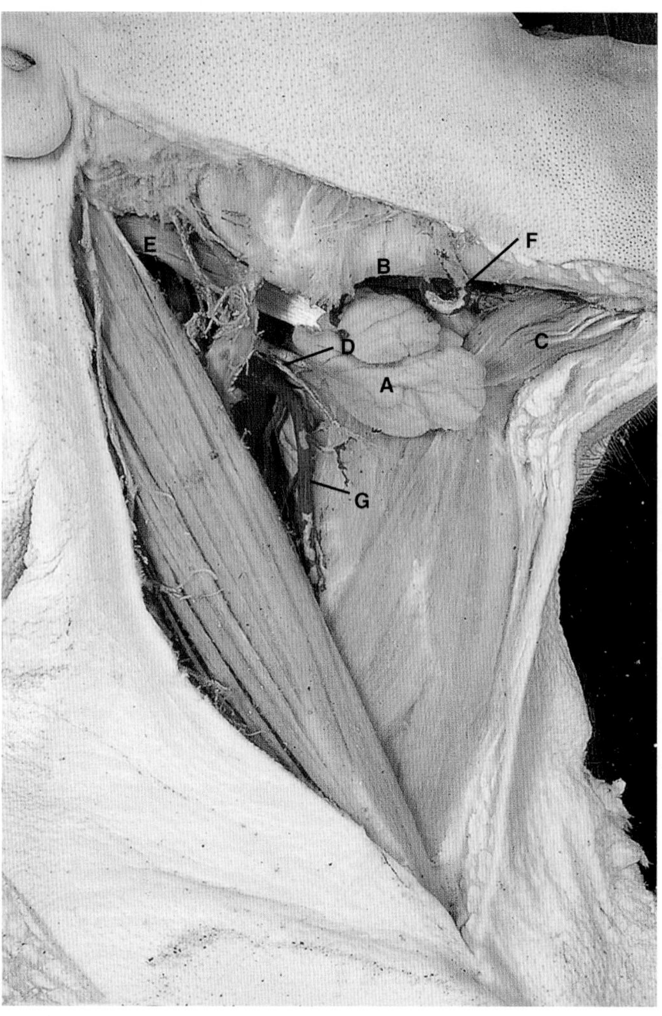

Fig. 3.33 The superficial part of the submandibular gland (A) seen in the upper part of the neck; B = inferior border of mandible; C = anterior belly of the digastric muscle; D = hypoglossal nerve; E = posterior belly of the digastric muscle; F = facial artery on the mylohyoid muscle; G = superior thyroid artery. Courtesy Prof. C Dean.

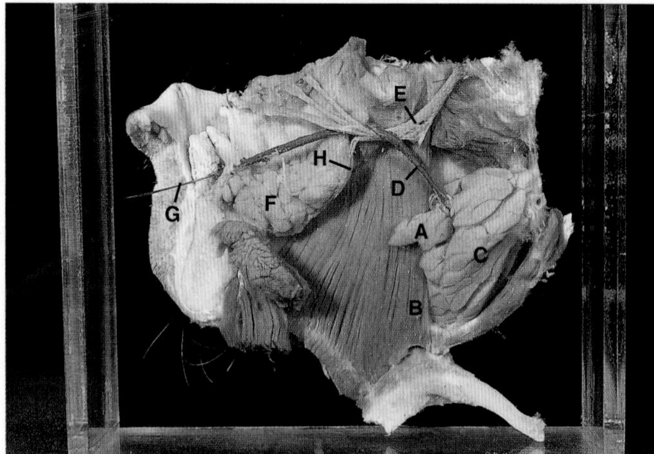

Fig. 3.34 Medial view of the floor of mouth showing the deep part of the submandibular gland (A) passing around the free posterior border of the mylohyoid muscle (B). C = superficial part of submandibular gland; D = submandibular duct wrapping around lingual nerve (E); F = sublingual gland; G = bristle in opening of the submandibular duct at the sublingual papilla; H = branches of the lingual nerve to the sublingual gland carrying parasympathetic fibres. Courtesy Prof. C Dean.

around the lingual nerve, as it crosses the hyoglossus muscle, to terminate on the sublingual papilla in the floor of the mouth (see Fig. 3.34).

Sublingual gland

The sublingual gland is the smallest of the three major pairs of salivary glands, and although it is commonly stated that it produces serous and mucous saliva, it has now been established that it produces only a mucous secretion (see page 345). It is located on the hyoglossus muscle in the floor of the mouth (see Fig. 3.22), adjacent to the sublingual fossa of the mandible. The gland is associated with the sublingual folds beneath the tongue. In coronal section, the gland rests on the mylohyoid muscle (see Fig. 3.24). The posterior part of the sublingual gland may be joined to the deep part of the submandibular gland to form a single sublingual–submandibular complex (see Fig. 3.25). The sublingual gland is subdivided into two parts. A lesser sublingual gland is always present and consists of a mass of small glands, which number from 7 to 15, and from every one of which a short main duct (a Rivinus duct) passes to drain onto the sublingual fold. A greater sublingual gland lies posterior to the lesser sublingual gland (only sometimes present), and a main duct (Bartholin's duct) leads from it to either join the submandibular duct or to drain directly onto the sublingual papilla.

The parasympathetic innervation of both the submandibular and sublingual glands is the chorda tympani branch of the facial nerve. Preganglionic fibres are carried with this nerve (via the lingual nerve) to the submandibular ganglion. Postganglionic fibres pass from this ganglion to the submandibular and sublingual glands (see Fig. 4.14).

Infratemporal fossa

The infratemporal fossa is the space located deep to the ramus of the mandible. Together with the temporal fossa, pterygoid processes and maxillary tuberosity, the infratemporal fossa has been thought of by some anatomists as part of a 'masticatory muscle compartment' or 'masticatory space'.

The infratemporal fossa (Fig. 3.35) is bounded anteriorly by the posterior surface of the maxilla, posteriorly by the styloid apparatus, carotid sheath and deep part of the parotid gland. Medially lie the lateral pterygoid plate and the superior constrictor of the pharynx. The roof is formed by the infratemporal surface of the greater wing of the sphenoid. The infratemporal fossa has no floor, being continuous with the neck. It communicates with the temporal fossa deep to the zygomatic arch and also with the pterygopalatine fossa through the pterygomaxillary fissure. At the base of the cranium the foramen ovale and foramen spinosum enter the fossa through the sphenoid bone. The foramen lacerum and the petrotympanic, squamotympanic and petrosquamous fissures are also found close to the infratemporal fossa. On the medial surface of the ramus of the mandible is the mandibular foramen.

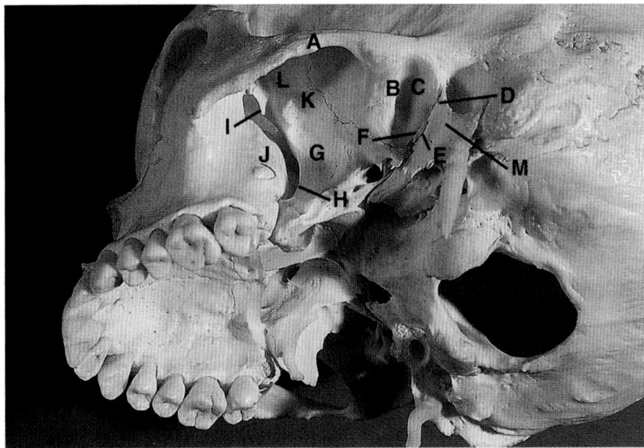

Fig. 3.35 The osteology of the infratemporal fossa. A = zygomatic arch; B = articular eminence; C = mandibular fossa; D = squamotympanic fissure; E = petrotympanic fissure; F = petrosquamous fissure; G = lateral pterygoid plate; H = pterygomaxillary fissure leading into the pterygopalatine fossa; I = inferior orbital fissure; J = posterior border of maxilla; K = infratemporal crest of sphenoid bone; L = infratemporal surface of greater wing of sphenoid bone; M = tympanic plate.

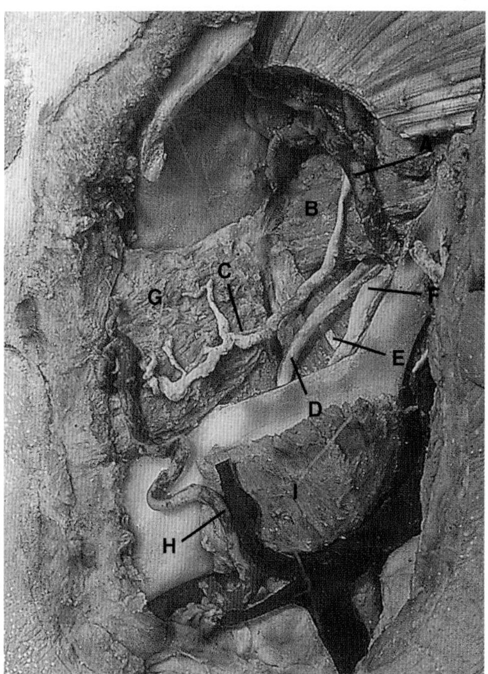

Fig. 3.36 Contents of the infratemporal fossa. A = maxillary artery; B = lateral pterygoid (lower head); C = buccal branch of mandibular division of trigeminal nerve; D = lingual nerve; E = medial pterygoid muscle; F = inferior alveolar nerve; G = buccinator muscle; H = facial blood vessels; I = masseter muscle. Courtesy Prof. L Garey.

The major structures within the infratemporal fossa (Fig. 3.36) are the lateral pterygoid and medial pterygoid muscles (see pages 82–84 for details), branches of the mandibular nerve (including the inferior alveolar, buccal and lingual nerves; see pages 106–108), the chorda tympani branch of the facial nerve, the otic ganglion, the maxillary artery and the pterygoid venous plexus.

Pterygopalatine fossa

The pterygopalatine fossa lies between the infratemporal (posterior) surface of the maxilla and the pterygoid process of the sphenoid bone. The pterygopalatine fossa contains three major structures: the maxillary nerve, the maxillary artery (third part) and the pterygopalatine parasympathetic ganglion.

The elongated cleft between the posterior surface of the maxilla and the pterygoid process of the sphenoid bone is the pterygomaxillary fissure (see Fig. 3.35), which forms the lateral aspect of the pterygopalatine fossa. The anterior wall of the fossa is the infratemporal surface of the maxilla. The posterior wall of the fossa is the pterygoid process below and the greater wing of the sphenoid above. The medial wall is formed by the perpendicular plate of the palatine bone (Fig. 3.37). The pyramidal process of the palatine bone is situated inferiorly and articulates with the tuberosity of the maxilla. It fills the triangular gap between the lower ends of the medial and lateral pterygoid plates.

Laterally the pterygopalatine fossa communicates with the infratemporal fossa through the pterygomaxillary fissure. The fissure continues above with the posterior end of the inferior orbital fissure in the floor of the orbit (see Fig. 3.35).

The pterygomaxillary fissure transmits the maxillary artery from the infratemporal fossa, the posterior superior alveolar branches of the maxillary division of the trigeminal nerve and the sphenopalatine veins.

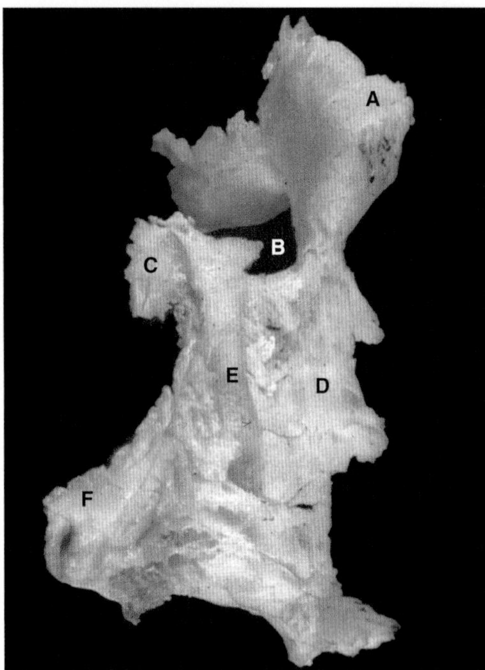

Fig. 3.37 Lateral view of palatine bone forming the medial wall of the pterygopalatine fossa. A = orbital process; B = sphenopalatine notch; C = sphenoidal process; D = perpendicular plate; E = greater palatine groove; F = pyramidal process.

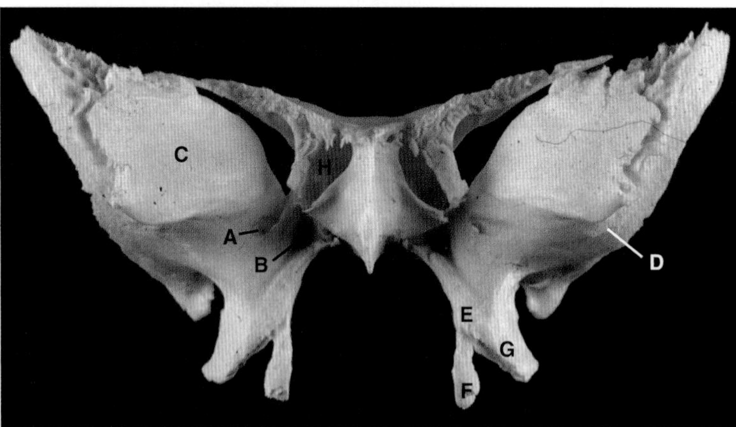

Fig. 3.38 Anterior surface of the sphenoid bone showing the foramen rotundum (A) and pterygoid canal (B). C = orbital surface of greater wing; D = infratemporal crest of greater wing; E = pterygoid process; F = pterygoid hamulus surmounting the medial pterygoid plate; G = lateral pterygoid plate; H = sphenoidal air sinus.

Passing through the inferior orbital fissure from the pterygopalatine fossa are the infraorbital and zygomatic branches of the maxillary nerve, the orbital branches of the pterygopalatine ganglion and the infraorbital vessels.

Entering the pterygopalatine fossa posteriorly are the foramen rotundum from the middle cranial fossa and the pterygoid canal from the region of the foramen lacerum at the base of the skull (Fig. 3.38). The foramen rotundum occupying the greater wing of the sphenoid bone lies above and lateral to the pterygoid canal. The maxillary division of the trigeminal nerve passes through the foramen rotundum. The pterygoid canal transmits the greater petrosal and deep petrosal nerves (which combine to form the nerve of the pterygoid canal) and an accompanying artery derived from the maxillary artery.

High up on the medial wall of the pterygopalatine fossa lies the sphenopalatine foramen. It is formed by the notch between the orbital and sphenoid processes of the perpendicular plate of the palatine bone (see Fig. 3.37) articulating with the body of the sphenoid bone. This foramen communicates with the lateral wall of the nasal cavity. It transmits the nasopalatine and posterior superior nasal nerves (from the pterygopalatine ganglion) and the sphenopalatine vessels.

At the base of the pterygopalatine fossa is found the opening of the anterior (greater) palatine canal. This canal is formed when the greater palatine groove running down the posterior margin of the lateral surface of the perpendicular plate of the palatine bone articulates with the posterior surface of the maxillary bone (see Fig. 2.3) and the medial pterygoid plate. In the lower part of the anterior palatine canal a smaller canal, the posterior palatine canal, is given off to run backwards in the pyramidal process of the palatine bone. The anterior palatine canal enters the hard palate at the anterior (greater) palatine foramen in the region of the transverse palatine suture (see Fig. 2.6). The posterior palatine canal enters the hard palate at the posterior (lesser) palatine foramen (foramina) (see Fig. 2.6). The anterior palatine canal transmits the greater and lesser palatine nerves (and the posterior inferior nasal branches from the pterygopalatine ganglion) together with accompanying vessels, and these pass to the hard palate to emerge at the anterior and posterior palatine foramina.

Tissue spaces around the jaws

Knowledge of the tissue spaces around the jaws is necessary to understand the possible spread of infections (including oedema and pus) from a dental site into the rest of the head and neck.

Most structures in the body are ensheathed by a connective tissue covering of varying thickness. If thin and delicate, this connective tissue presents little resistance to the spread of infection; if the connective tissue layer is thick, tendinous or membranous, it resists the spread of infection (particularly over certain muscles). Such thick connective tissues, capable of holding surgical sutures, are sometimes referred to as 'true fascia'. From clinical experience, it is evident that certain predictable pathways exist along which infection may spread. The loose connective tissue uniting fascial planes may be destroyed and the potential space delineated by adjacent structures considerably enlarged as inflammatory exudate accumulates. Such potential spaces are referred to as 'tissue spaces'.

The dissemination of infection in soft tissues is influenced by the natural barriers presented by bone, muscle and fascia. Around the jaws are body compartments, the so-called tissue spaces, the boundaries of which are primarily defined by the mylohyoid, buccinator, masseter, medial pterygoid, superior constrictor and orbicularis oris muscles. The fascial layers of the neck are less important in influencing the spread of infection around the jaws. None of the 'spaces' are actually empty; they are potential spaces normally occupied by loose connective tissue. It is only when inflammatory products (or bleeding or tumours) destroy the loose connective tissue that an anatomically defined space is produced.

Infection may spread from one tissue space to another where the spaces are in direct communication or along the side of structures that pass from one tissue space to another (such as blood vessels or nerves). Infection can also invade tissue spaces by directly eroding the intervening fascia. In addition to such direct pathways, infection may also spread through the lymphatics and the blood vessels.

The most important potential tissue spaces around the jaws are shown in Box 3.3. With the exception of the submental, submandibular and palatal spaces, all the tissue spaces listed in the box are paired.

Fig. 3.39 shows the relationships of tissue spaces around the mandibular ramus. Because of the occurrence of inflammation in the soft tissues

Box 3.3 **The most important tissue spaces around the jaws**

Lower jaw

1) Submental
2) Submandibular
3) Sublingual
4) Buccal
5) Submasseteric
6) Parotid
7) Pterygomandibular
8) Parapharyngeal
9) Peritonsillar

Upper jaw

10) Palatal
11) Canine fossa
12) Infratemporal

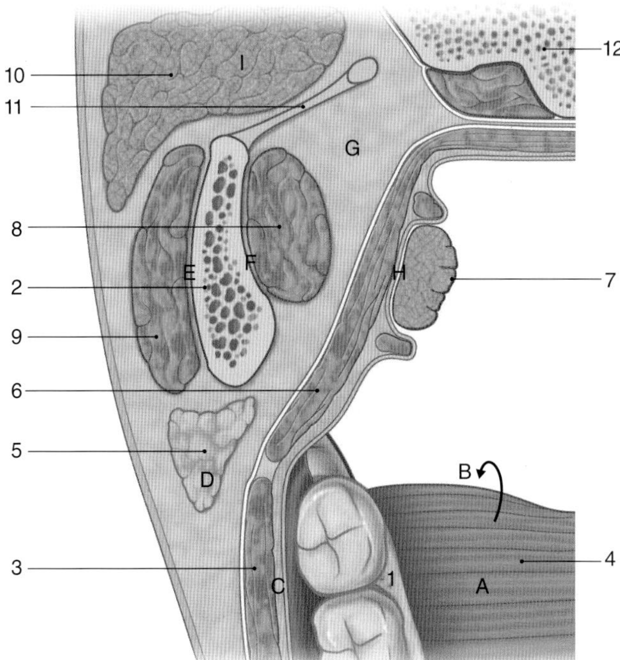

Fig. 3.39 The relationships of tissue spaces around the mandibular ramus. 1 = body of mandible bearing the molar teeth; 2 = ramus of mandible; 3 = buccinator muscle; 4 = mylohyoid muscle; 5 = buccal pad of fat; 6 = superior constrictor muscle; 7 = mucosa overlying palatal tonsil; 8 = medial pterygoid muscle; 9 = masseter muscle; 10 = parotid gland; 11 = stylomandibular ligament; 12 = base of skull; A = sublingual space in the floor of the mouth above the mylohyoid muscle, which, over its posterior margin, leads to B = submandibular space; C = buccal vestibule, delineated by the buccinator from D = buccal space; E = submasseteric spaces formed by the multiple insertion of the masseter muscle on the lateral surface of the ramus; F = pterygomandibular space bounded by the lateral surface of the medial pterygoid muscle and the medial surface of the ramus; G = parapharyngeal space bounded by the superior constrictor of the pharynx and the medial surface of the medial pterygoid muscle; H = peritonsillar space bounded by the medial surface of the superior constrictor of the pharynx and its mucosa; I = parotid space (in and around the parotid gland).

associated with partially impacted mandibular third molars (pericoronitis) and, less commonly, of dental abscesses of these teeth, the infratemporal fossa region is significant in terms of tissue spaces. This is due to the fact that the infratemporal fossa lies in a pivotal position, being intermediate between the tissue spaces of the face above and the tissue spaces of the neck below. The term *masticator tissue space* is sometimes used to describe the space enclosed by the investing layer of fascia ensheathing the muscles of mastication and the ramus of the mandible. The submasseteric, pterygomandibular, infratemporal and temporal tissue spaces are all part of this masticator tissue space.

Submasseteric space

The submasseteric space(s) may take the form of a series of spaces between the lateral surface of the ramus of the mandible and the masseter muscle. These spaces may form because the fibres of the masseter muscle have multiple insertions onto most of the lateral surface of the ramus, and spaces may be found between the attachments of the superficial and deep parts of the muscle. Alternatively, they may relate to the passage of the neurovascular bundles. Whatever the true explanation, abscesses may develop between the masseter and the ramus of the mandible.

Pterygomandibular space

The pterygomandibular space lies between the ramus of the mandible laterally and the medial pterygoid muscle medially. Above lies the inferior head of the lateral pterygoid muscle. Anteriorly, beneath the overlying oral mucosa, lie fibres of the buccinator muscle, which arise from the pterygomandibular raphe. Immediately beneath the buccinator lies the tendon of the temporalis muscle. Posteriorly the investing layer of deep cervical fascia covering the masseter and medial pterygoid muscles merges with the posterior border of the ramus, behind which lies the parotid gland. The pterygomandibular space is a prominent component of the infratemporal fossa. Between the ramus of the mandible and the medial pterygoid muscle lie the inferior alveolar and lingual nerves: the pterygomandibular space is therefore the site of injection for an inferior alveolar nerve block. It also contains the maxillary artery and pterygoid venous plexus.

Infratemporal space

The infratemporal space is the upper extremity of the pterygomandibular space. It lies behind the maxilla and is bounded medially by the lateral pterygoid plate and above by the base of the skull. It is in continuity with the deep temporal space laterally.

Temporal space

The temporal space consists of superficial and deep components that are found in relation to the temporalis muscle. The superficial temporal space lies on the lateral surface of the muscle, beneath the skin and the superficial (temporal) fascia. The deep temporal space lies between the medial (deep) surface of the muscle and the adjacent temporal bone.

Unlike infections involving odontogenic tissues that drain directly into the oral cavity (via the buccal or lingual sulci), those involving the tissue spaces around the infratemporal fossa do not drain directly into the oral cavity and have the potential to spread some distance through the head and neck. Of particular relevance in this regard are the tissue spaces around the pharynx, because involvement of these spaces may affect the larynx and thus compromise the airway. Symptoms associated with such conditions may include trismus, fever, dysphagia (difficulty in swallowing) and dyspnoea (difficulty in breathing), and patients must be treated quickly because of the potential development of life-threatening situations. In the most extreme situation, inflammation will eventually spread to involve the thorax.

Pharyngeal space

The pharyngeal tissue spaces can be subdivided into the peripharyngeal spaces around, and external to, the pharynx and the intrapharyngeal space within it. With regard to the peripharyngeal spaces, there is the parapharyngeal space laterally and the retropharyngeal space posteriorly. Some anatomists also include the submental and submandibular spaces as pharyngeal tissue spaces because they lie immediately anteriorly.

Each parapharyngeal space (or lateral pharyngeal space) passes laterally around the pharynx and is continuous posteriorly with the retropharyngeal space. Unlike the retropharyngeal space, however, it is a space that is restricted to the suprahyoid region. It contains loose connective tissue and is bounded medially by the pharynx (superior constrictor muscle) and laterally by the pterygoid muscles and the parotid gland. Superiorly, it is bounded by the base of the skull. Inferiorly, it does not extend right down the neck but is limited by the suprahyoid structures, such as the fascia associated with the styloid group of muscles and the submandibular gland. Behind is situated the carotid sheath. The lateral pharyngeal space is partly divided by the styloid process and associated group of muscles into an anterior compartment containing muscle and a posterior compartment containing the carotid sheath and cranial nerves IX–XII.

The retropharyngeal space is the area of loose connective tissue lying behind the pharynx and in front of the prevertebral fascia. It extends upwards to the base of the skull and downwards to the retrovisceral space in the infrahyoid part of the neck.

An intrapharyngeal space potentially exists between the inner surface of the constrictor muscles of the pharynx and the pharyngeal mucosa. Infections at this site are either restricted locally or spread through the pharynx into the retropharyngeal or parapharyngeal spaces. An important part of the intrapharyngeal space is the peritonsillar space. This lies around the palatine tonsil, between the pillars of the fauces. Infections here (quinsy) usually spread up or down the intrapharyngeal space, or through the pharynx into the parapharyngeal space.

The parapharyngeal space is particularly prone to infections from the jaws and teeth. This space is restricted to the suprahyoid region of the neck and the infratemporal region. For infection to spread inferiorly from the parapharyngeal space, it must first pass into the retropharyngeal region because suprahyoid structures (particularly the sheath around the submandibular gland formed by the investing layer of deep cervical fascia) provide a restrictive inferior boundary.

The tissue spaces below the inferior border of the mandible and in the suprahyoid region of the neck (i.e., the submental and submandibular tissue spaces) are illustrated in Fig. 3.40.

Submental space

The submental space lies beneath the chin in the midline, between the mylohyoid muscles below and the investing layer of deep cervical fascia and platysma muscle superficially. It is bounded laterally by the two anterior bellies of the digastric muscles. The submental space communicates posteriorly over the anterior bellies of the digastric muscles with the two submandibular spaces.

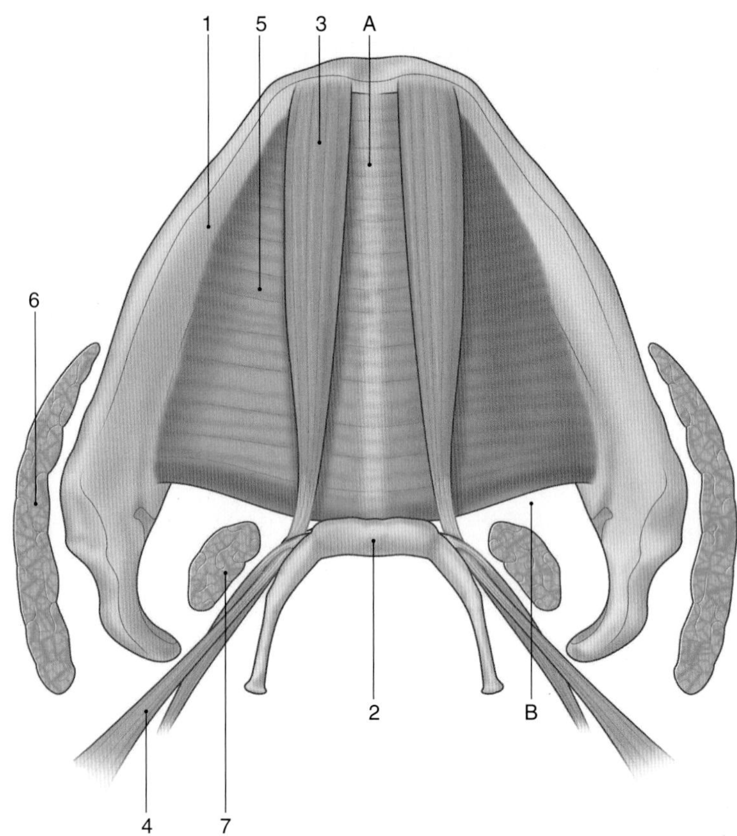

Fig. 3.40 Inferior view of the submental and submandibular tissue spaces. 1 = body of mandible; 2 = hyoid bone; 3 = anterior belly of digastric muscle; 4 = posterior belly of digastric muscle; 5 = mylohyoid muscle; 6 = masseter muscle; 7 = medial pterygoid muscle; A = submental space lying between the mylohyoid muscle and the investing layer of deep cervical fascia. Laterally, it is bound by the two anterior bellies of the digastric muscles. B = submandibular space. The submental space communicates posteriorly with the submandibular space, and the submandibular spaces communicate with the sublingual tissue space around the posterior borders of the mylohyoid muscles.

Submandibular space

The submandibular space is situated between the anterior and posterior bellies of the digastric muscle and is bounded above and laterally by the body of the mandible. It lies superficial to (below) the mylohyoid muscle (and more posteriorly the hyoglossus and styloglossus muscles) and is covered by the platysma muscle and by the investing layer of deep cervical fascia, which explains why abscesses in this region do not readily drain through the skin. The submandibular space communicates with the sublingual space around the posterior free border of the mylohyoid muscle and via small deficiencies within the muscular tissue of the mylohyoid muscle. The submandibular space contains the submandibular gland, facial vessels and submandibular lymph nodes. A submandibular abscess is commonly caused by spread of infection from the second or third mandibular molar tooth (see Fig. 3.44).

The suprahyoid spaces (submental and submandibular spaces) are bounded inferiorly by the attachment of the investing layer of deep cervical fascia to the hyoid bone. Consequently, if oedema or pus accumulates in the suprahyoid region, there will be a restriction in the spread into the rest of the neck. This is potentially very dangerous because the suprahyoid region will swell markedly and restrict the airway (Ludwig's angina).

Sublingual space

Fig. 3.41 illustrates the relationships of tissue spaces to the tongue. The sublingual space lies in the floor of the mouth, above the mylohyoid muscles and below the oral mucosa. It is delineated in front, and at the sides,

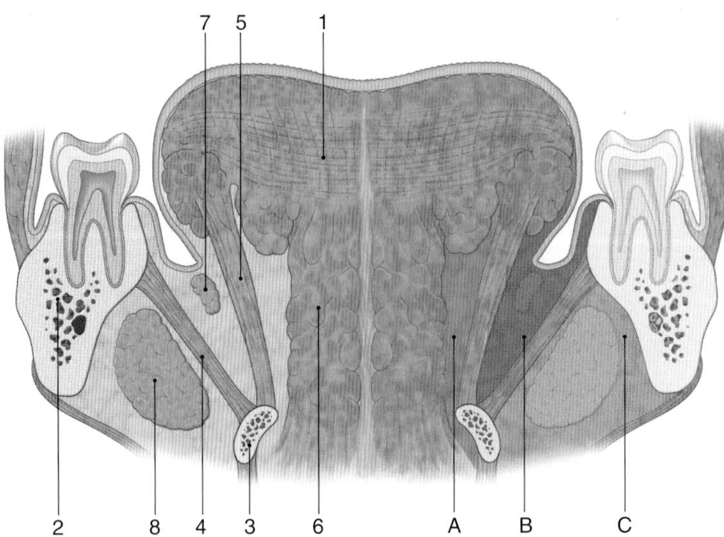

Fig. 3.41 The relationships of a number of tissue spaces to the tongue. 1 = tongue; 2 = body of mandible; 3 = hyoid bone; 4 = mylohyoid muscle; 5 = hyoglossus; 6 = genioglossus; 7 = sublingual salivary gland; 8 = submandibular salivary gland; A = cleft between genioglossus and hyoglossus muscles that communicates directly with the parapharyngeal space; B = sublingual space between the mylohyoid and hyoglossus muscles; C = submandibular space below the mylohyoid muscle.

by the body of the mandible and behind (and below) by the attachment of the mylohyoid muscle to the hyoid bone. The sublingual space contains the sublingual gland and the submandibular duct.

In the anterior region of both the upper and lower jaws, the orbicularis oris muscle presents a barrier to pus between the vestibule on the oral side and the skin of the lip on the facial side. In the upper jaw, pus may accumulate between the muscles of facial expression, particularly in the canine fossa between the levator labii superioris and zygomaticus muscles.

Other tissue spaces around the mouth

Other spaces around the mouth that need to be described are the buccal, parotid and palatal tissue spaces.

Buccal space

The buccal space is located in the cheek. It has the buccinator muscle (covered by a delicate connective tissue layer called the buccopharyngeal fascia) medially, the skin of the cheek laterally, the pterygomandibular raphe (giving origin to the buccinator muscle) posteriorly and some muscles of the orbicularis oris anteriorly. The buccal space contains the parotid duct accompanied by blood vessels and branches of the facial nerve, as well as the buccal pad of fat.

Parotid space

The parotid space surrounds the parotid gland and its contents. It is defined by the parotid capsule. The superficial layer of the parotid capsule is of variable thickness and is not a typical fascia because it contains muscle fibres that parallel those of the platysma muscle. It appears to be continuous with the fascia associated with the platysma muscle. The deep surface of the parotid capsule is derived from the investing layer of deep cervical fascia. Above the level of the stylomandibular ligament, the deep surface of the parotid capsule may be thin and may serve as a communicating pathway into the lateral pharyngeal space.

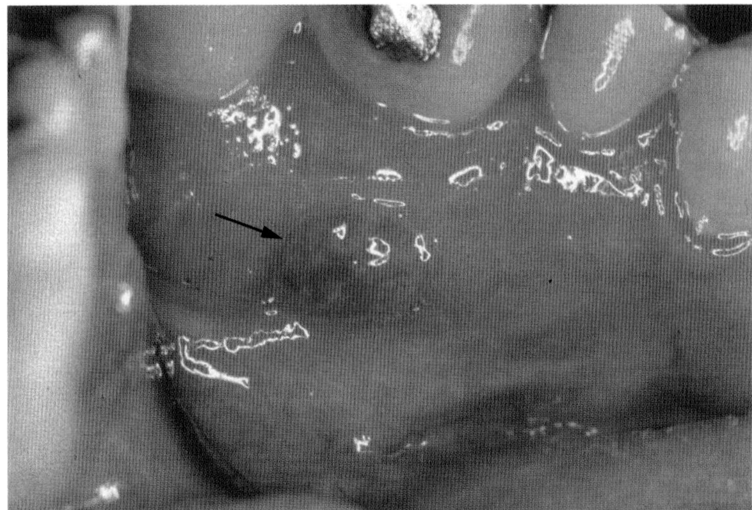

Fig. 3.42 A gingival abscess (arrowed), originating from a heavily filled mandibular first permanent molar, which will discharge into the vestibular sulcus. Courtesy Dr J Potts.

Palatal space

The palatal space in the hard palate exists only when pus strips the mucoperiosteum from the underlying bone of the hard palate.

The way in which infections of dental origin spread through the bone of the jaws into the tissue spaces naturally depends on the site at which the pus escapes the bone. Thus, pus from a periapical abscess in a mandibular incisor that escapes inferior to the mylohyoid muscle will enter the submental space, while pus escaping superior to this muscle will enter the sublingual space. It should also be borne in mind that the tissue spaces are not discrete regions; they intercommunicate. Thus, a sublingual abscess may spread from the sublingual space over the posterior margin of the mylohyoid muscle into the submandibular space (see Figs. 3.39, 3.40). Furthermore, none of the muscle or fascial barriers defining the spaces is impenetrable.

Clinical aspects

Spread of infection through tissue spaces

Infection of the infratemporal fossa is commonly met in dental practice and, because of the associated tissue spaces, is potentially dangerous. It is most commonly associated with a pericoronitis affecting a partially impacted mandibular third molar tooth. It may also be associated with a dental abscess of this tooth or occur as a result of infection following tooth extraction (dry socket). Rarely, it may result from an infected needle used during an inferior alveolar nerve block. Infection of the infratemporal region may be secondary because of spread from an adjacent infected tissue space. An important determinant of the subsequent spread of infection from teeth depends on the relationship of the root apices to muscle. For example, if the discharge of a dental abscess from a cheek tooth is below the attachment of the buccinator muscle, it will enter into the vestibule and drain harmlessly (Fig. 3.42). If, however, it drains above the attachment and into the buccal space, it will produce a fluctuant swelling over the cheek that will need surgical drainage (Fig. 3.43). Similarly, if an infected mandibular tooth drains above the attachment of the mylohyoid muscle, the infection would drain favourably into the oral cavity. If it drains below the attachment of mylohyoid, especially in the case of second and third mandibular molars, it may enter the submandibular tissue space and

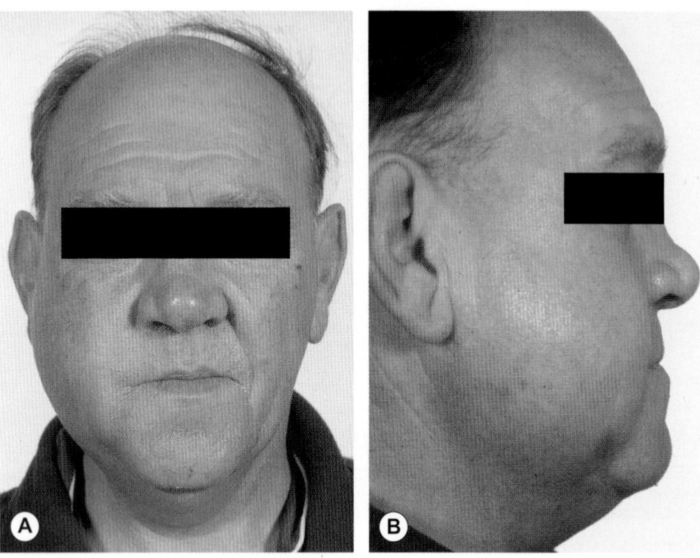

Fig. 3.43 Buccal space infection on the right side. (A) Front view. (B) View from right side. Courtesy Prof. J Langdon.

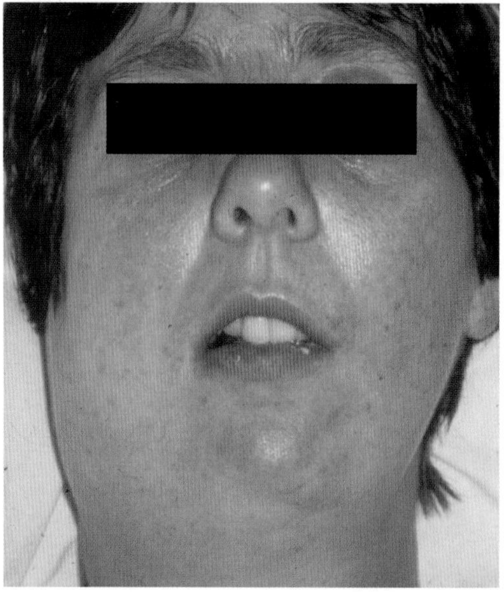

Fig. 3.45 Patient with Ludwig's angina. There are sublingual and submandibular cellulites, with a painful swelling of the upper part of the neck and the floor of the mouth on both sides. Courtesy Prof. J Langdon.

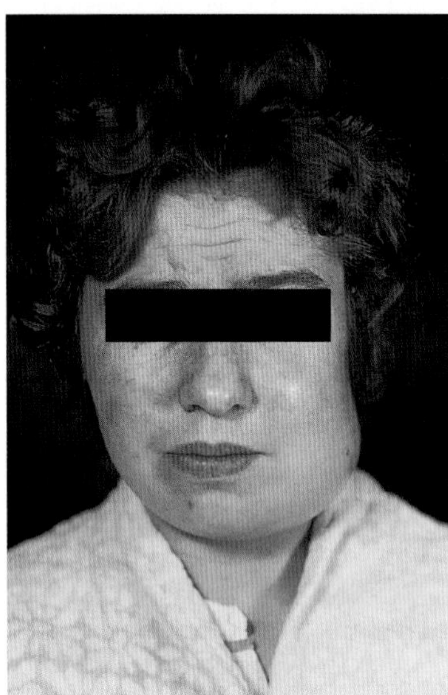

Fig. 3.44 Abscess within the submandibular tissue space. Courtesy Prof. J Langdon.

produce a swelling centred upon the upper part of the neck, mainly along the lower border of the mandible (Fig. 3.44).

Because the tissue spaces are interconnected, infection may spread from the submandibular space into the sublingual or parapharyngeal spaces. Ludwig's angina is characterised by rapid development of sublingual and submandibular cellulitis with a painful, brawny swelling of the upper part of the neck and the floor of the mouth on both sides (Fig. 3.45). When the parapharyngeal tissue space becomes involved, the swelling tracks down the neck and oedema readily spreads into the loose connective tissue around the glottis. There is difficulty in swallowing, opening the mouth may be limited and the tongue may be pushed up against the soft palate. Oedema of the glottis can cause increasing respiratory obstruction. The patient soon becomes seriously ill, with fever, headache and malaise.

Cavernous sinus thrombosis

Cavernous sinus thrombosis is a serious complication that can also arise from spread of infection from a maxillary anterior tooth. Infected thrombi in the anterior facial vein communicate with the cavernous sinus via the ophthalmic veins (a less common spread is through infection in the pterygoid plexus of veins reaching the cavernous sinus via emissary veins). Infection may also spread via the facial vein from infected spots or boils on the upper lip or in the anterior nares. In a cavernous sinus thrombosis, there is gross oedema of the eyelids together with pulsatile exophthalmos caused by venous obstruction. The venous stasis also leads to cyanosis. The patient is seriously ill with rigors and a high, swinging pyrexia. Initially one side of the face is affected, but, without treatment, both sides quickly become affected.

Spread of infection to lymphatics

Lymphatic drainage of the infratemporal fossa region is into the submandibular and upper deep cervical group of nodes, so enlargement of the nodes in this region should alert the clinician to the possibility of infection arising in the infratemporal fossa.

Paralysis of the hypoglossal nerve

Paralysis of the hypoglossal nerve, the XIIth cranial nerve, affects both the extrinsic and the intrinsic muscles of the tongue on the affected side. When this occurs, and on asking a patient to protrude his/her tongue, the tongue deviates to the affected side (because the muscles on the unaffected side are still active; analogous to a ship turning in water as a result of the propeller functioning on one side only) (Fig. 3.46). With time, there may be wasting of the tongue musculature on the paralysed side. The most common complaint is difficulty with speech, particularly for lingual sounds. With an upper motor neurone lesion, the tongue becomes spastic but does not waste. Thus, wasting is associated with a lower motor neurone lesion. The causes of hypoglossal nerve paralysis are many and may be associated with the course of the nerve either intracranially or extracranially. Tumours near the anterior condylar canal may be responsible, as may Paget's disease, where the foramen is severely reduced in size. Hypoglossal nerve paralysis can also arise with trauma, with excessive stretching of the neck, with intradural synovial cysts, after tonsillectomy, with trauma and even as an unusual result of receiving an influenza vaccine!

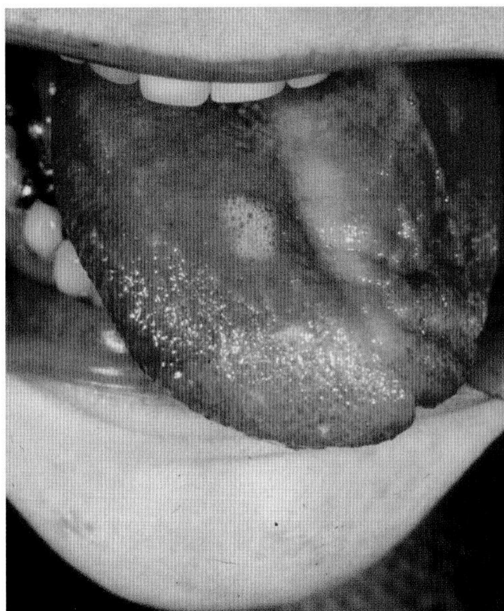

Fig. 3.46 Patient with damage to the left hypoglossal nerve after removal of a malignant tumour associated with the submandibular gland. There has been wasting of muscles on the left side of the tongue. On protrusion of the tongue, there is deviation to the affected side caused by unopposed activity of the unaffected musculature on the right side. Courtesy Prof. J Langdon.

Clinical aspects of the muscles of mastication

The muscles of mastication may be damaged or become nonfunctional under some situations as a result of otherwise normal clinical procedures. For example, following 'blocking' of the inferior alveolar nerve with local anaesthetic solution injected into the infratemporal fossa, there may be a painful reflex muscle spasm associated with the lateral and medial pterygoid muscles. This is termed 'trismus' and can result from bleeding into the muscles (haematoma) or from infection in the pterygomandibular space between the ramus of the mandible and the medial pterygoid muscle as a result of pericoronitis around an erupting third molar tooth. Externally, there may be little evidence of tissue swelling. Trismus may also result from TMJ dysfunction, tetanus, fracture of the mandibular condyle, or after a course of radiotherapy. Trismus nowadays is often used to describe any restriction to opening of the mouth. The inability to open the mouth can affect a patient's oral hygiene and ability to eat and chew. Furthermore, there may be problems with swallowing (particularly where there has been radiotherapy in the head and neck region). Additionally, and not surprisingly, a patient may have difficulty in speaking.

A pain reflex is elicited when a muscle is damaged; this is termed 'muscle guarding'. This pain results in muscle contraction and a restriction of the range of movements for the damaged muscle. This, being a reflex, cannot readily be controlled by the patient. Should the trismus persist, there may be signs of atrophy of the muscles involved. Treatment should involve gentle passive movements of the jaw.

In some cases, because of masseter muscle hypertrophy, prominent exostoses may be seen at the angles of the mandible. This is termed benign masseteric hypertrophy and can be either bilateral or unilateral. The patient with this condition most frequently complains of an unsightly appearance. It is relatively uncommon and is of unknown aetiology. Tension, fatigue or spasm of the muscles of mastication can be the cause of a condition known as myofascial pain syndrome. The symptoms of this syndrome include pain and tenderness, not just in the masticatory apparatus but generally in the head and neck region, and abnormal jaw movements. It may also be the cause of bruxism. The condition is most commonly seen in young females and those at menopause.

Explore online Self-assessment quiz to test and reinforce your understanding of the material in your free ebook. Follow instructions in the Inside Front Cover to unlock your access.

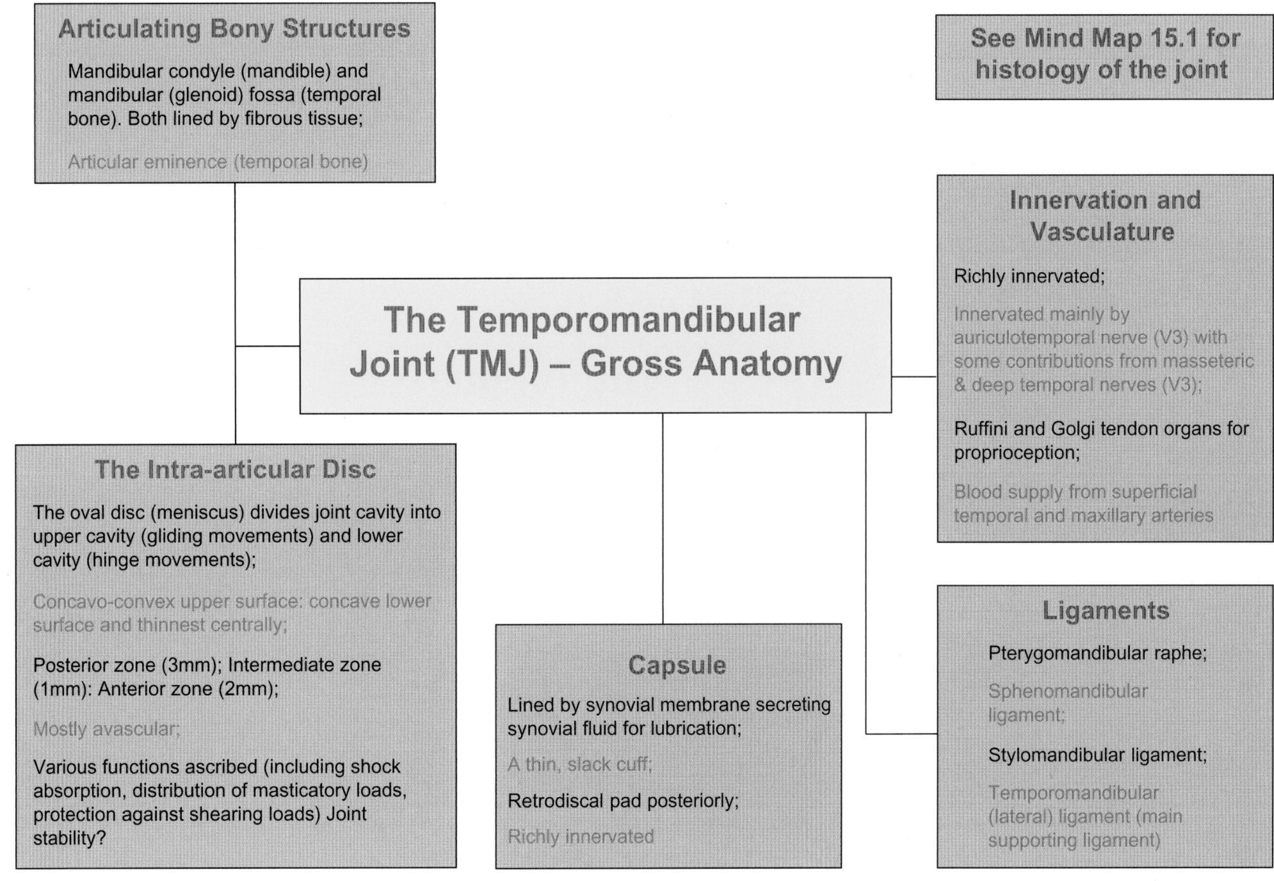

Mind Map 3.1 The temporomandibular joint (TMJ) – gross anatomy.

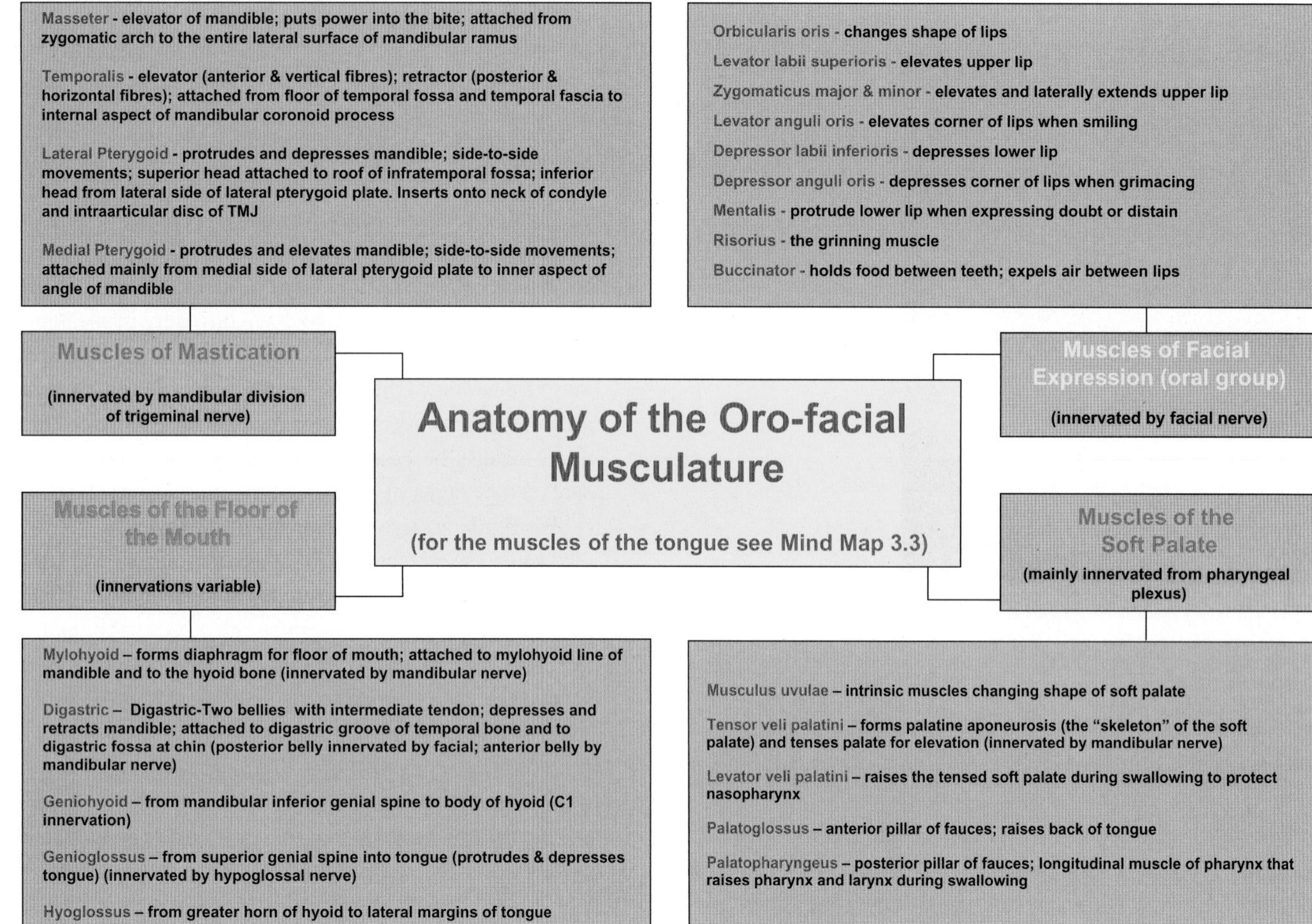

Anatomy of the Oro-facial Musculature
(for the muscles of the tongue see Mind Map 3.3)
Muscles of Mastication
(innervated by mandibular division of trigeminal nerve)
Masseter - elevator of mandible; puts power into the bite; attached from zygomatic arch to the entire lateral surface of mandibular ramus
Temporalis - elevator (anterior & vertical fibres); retractor (posterior & horizontal fibres); attached from floor of temporal fossa and temporal fascia to internal aspect of mandibular coronoid process
Lateral Pterygoid - protrudes and depresses mandible; side-to-side movements; superior head attached to roof of infratemporal fossa; inferior head from lateral side of lateral pterygoid plate. Inserts onto neck of condyle and intraarticular disc of TMJ
Medial Pterygoid - protrudes and elevates mandible; side-to-side movements; attached mainly from medial side of lateral pterygoid plate to inner aspect of angle of mandible
Muscles of Facial Expression (oral group)
(innervated by facial nerve)
Orbicularis oris - changes shape of lips
Levator labii superioris - elevates upper lip
Zygomaticus major & minor - elevates and laterally extends upper lip
Levator anguli oris - elevates corner of lips when smiling
Depressor labii inferioris - depresses lower lip
Depressor anguli oris - depresses corner of lips when grimacing
Mentalis - protrude lower lip when expressing doubt or distain
Risorius - the grinning muscle
Buccinator - holds food between teeth; expels air between lips
Muscles of the Floor of the Mouth
(innervations variable)
Mylohyoid – forms diaphragm for floor of mouth; attached to mylohyoid line of mandible and to the hyoid bone (innervated by mandibular nerve)
Digastric – Digastric-Two bellies with intermediate tendon; depresses and retracts mandible; attached to digastric groove of temporal bone and to digastric fossa at chin (posterior belly innervated by facial; anterior belly by mandibular nerve)
Geniohyoid – from mandibular inferior genial spine to body of hyoid (C1 innervation)
Genioglossus – from superior genial spine into tongue (protrudes & depresses tongue) (innervated by hypoglossal nerve)
Hyoglossus – from greater horn of hyoid to lateral margins of tongue
Muscles of the Soft Palate
(mainly innervated from pharyngeal plexus)
Musculus uvulae – intrinsic muscles changing shape of soft palate
Tensor veli palatini – forms palatine aponeurosis (the "skeleton" of the soft palate) and tenses palate for elevation (innervated by mandibular nerve)
Levator veli palatini – raises the tensed soft palate during swallowing to protect nasopharynx
Palatoglossus – anterior pillar of fauces; raises back of tongue
Palatopharyngeus – posterior pillar of fauces; longitudinal muscle of pharynx that raises pharynx and larynx during swallowing

Mind Map 3.2 Anatomy of the oro-facial musculature.

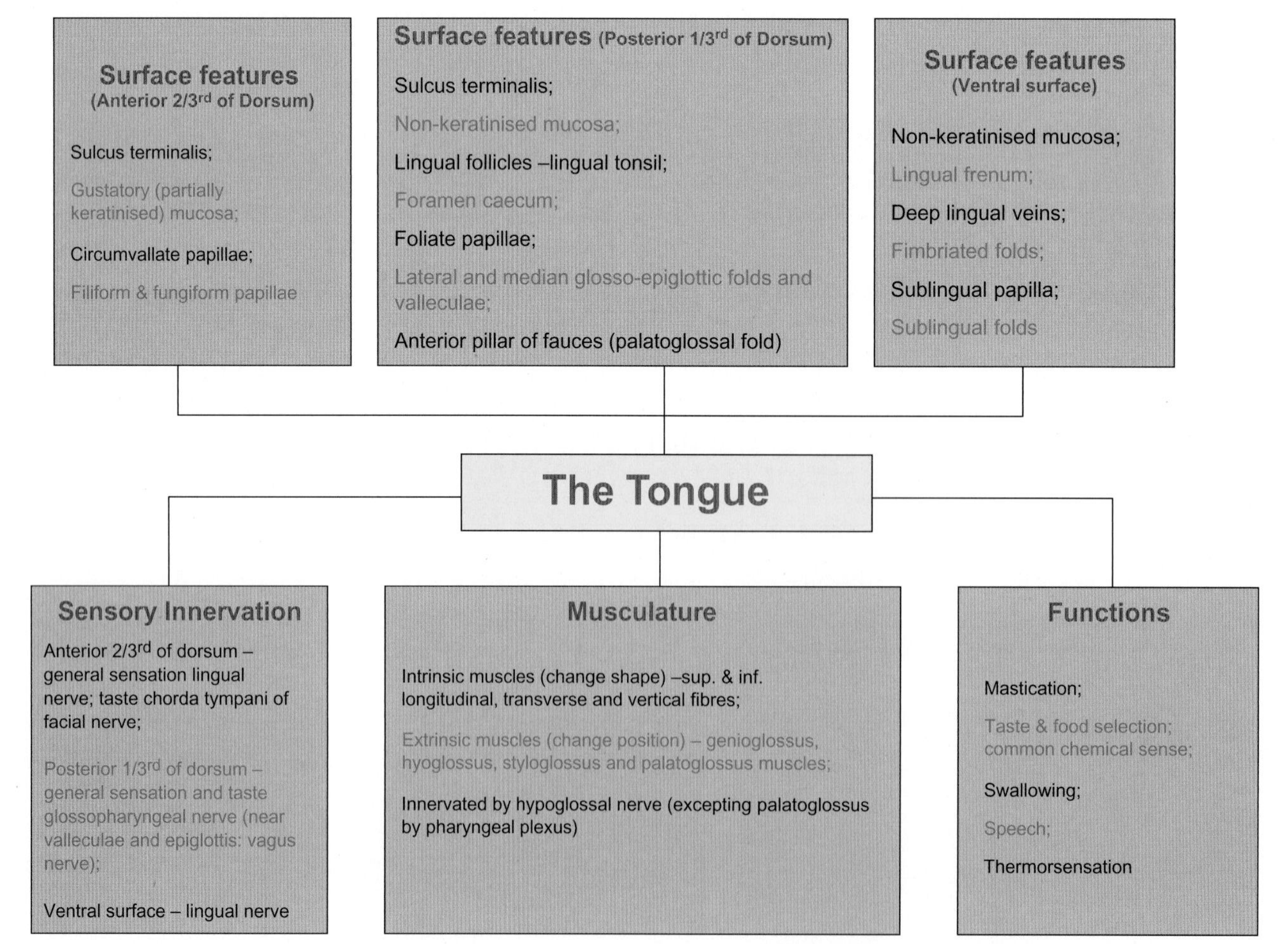

Mind Map 3.3 The tongue.

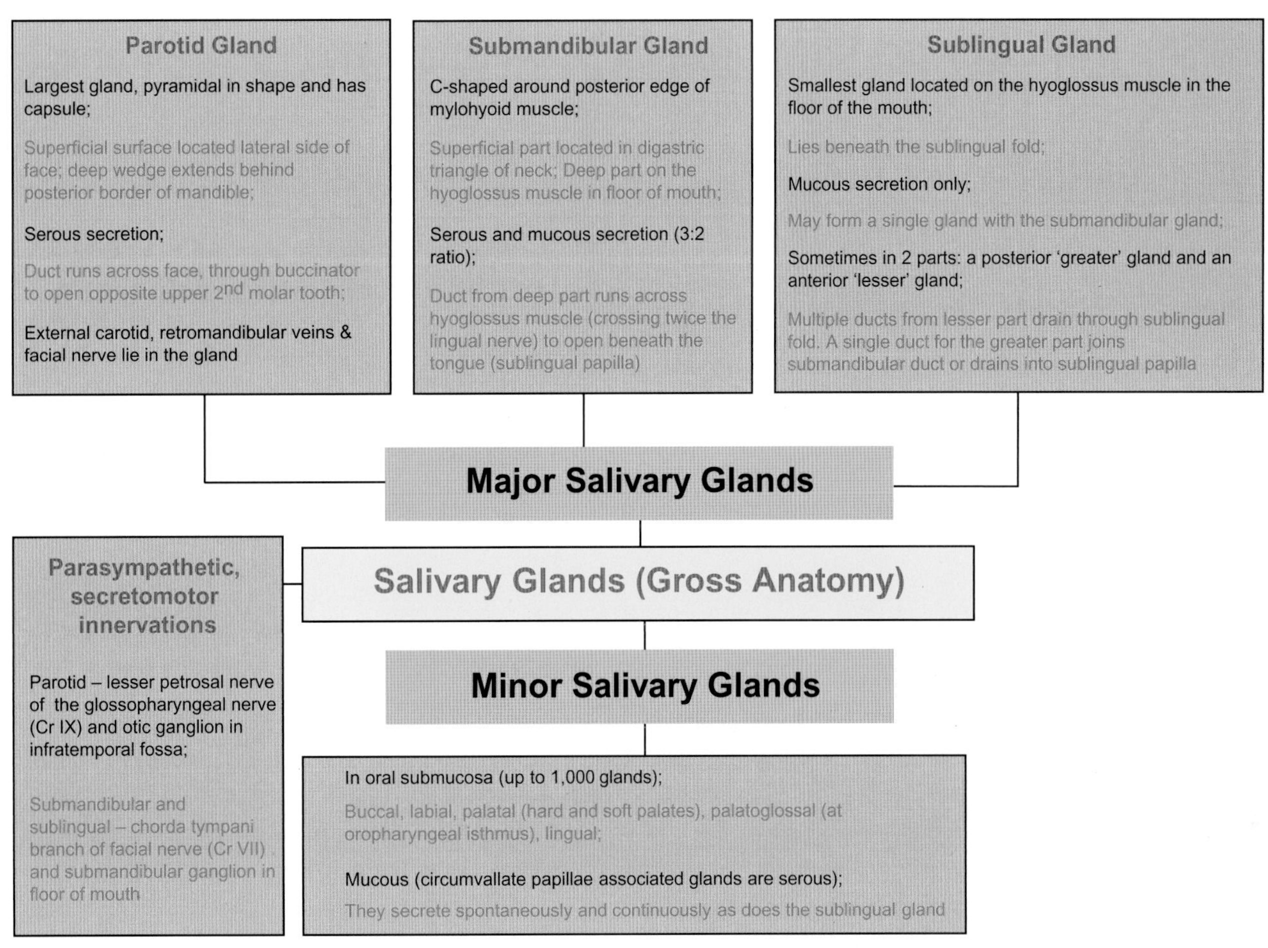

Mind Map 3.4 Salivary glands (gross anatomy).

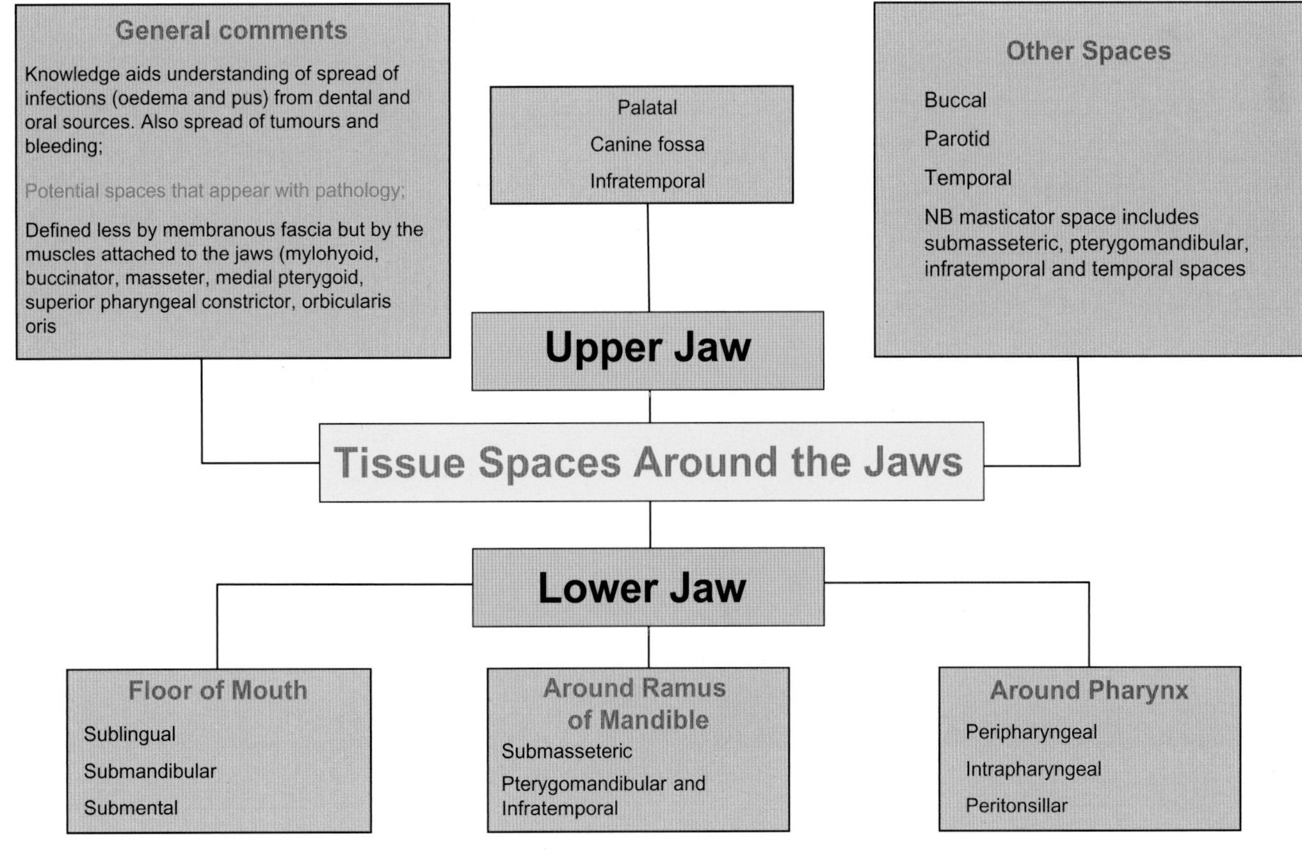

Mind Map 3.5 Tissue spaces around the jaws.

4 Vasculature and innervation of the mouth

Blood supply to orodental tissues

The face is supplied with blood mainly through the facial artery, a branch of the external carotid artery in the neck (Figs. 4.1, 4.2; see also Fig. 3.33). The facial artery first appears on the face as it hooks round the lower border of the mandible at the anterior edge of the masseter. It then runs a tortuous course between the facial muscles towards the medial angle of the eye. There is a rich anastomosis between the artery of the opposite side and additional vessels supplying the face (transverse facial branch of the superficial temporal artery; infraorbital and mental branches of the maxillary artery; dorsal nasal branch of the ophthalmic artery).

The main arteries to the teeth and jaws are derived from the maxillary artery, a terminal branch of the external carotid, which runs in the infratemporal fossa (see Fig. 4.2). The alveolar arteries follow essentially the same course as the alveolar nerves.

Mandibular teeth and periodontium

The inferior alveolar artery, which supplies the mandibular teeth, is derived from the maxillary artery before it crosses the lateral pterygoid muscle in the infratemporal fossa (Fig. 4.2). A mylohyoid branch is given off before the inferior alveolar artery enters the mandibular foramen in the ramus of the mandible. The inferior alveolar artery passes through the mandibular foramen to enter the mandibular canal and terminates as the mental and incisive arteries.

Posteriorly the buccal gingiva is supplied by the buccal artery (a branch of the maxillary artery as it crosses the lateral pterygoid muscle) and by perforating branches from the inferior alveolar artery. Anteriorly the labial gingiva is supplied by the mental artery and by perforating branches of the incisive artery. The lingual gingiva is supplied by perforating branches from the inferior alveolar artery and by the lingual artery, a branch of the external carotid artery.

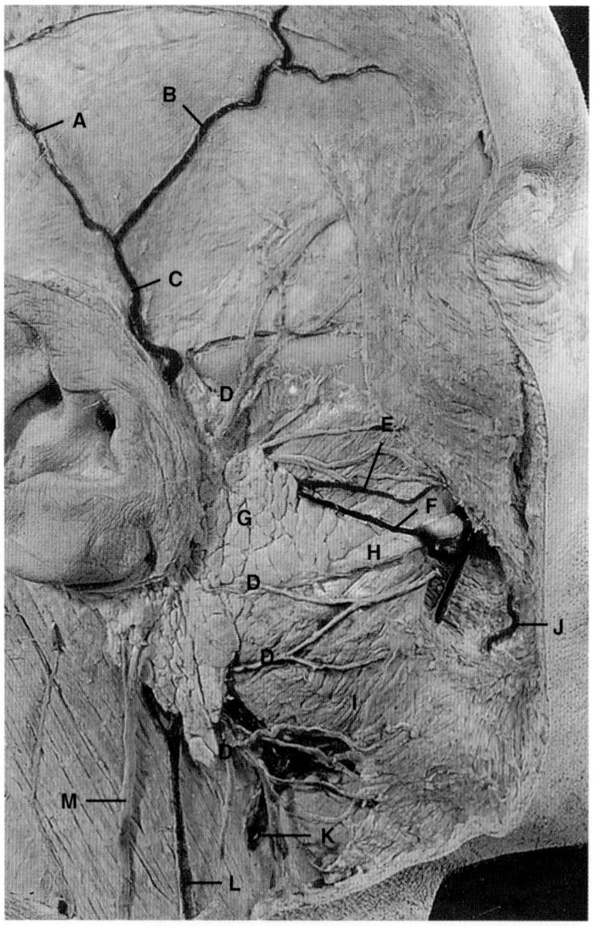

Fig. 4.1 Blood supply to the face. A = parietal branch of superficial temporal artery; B = frontal branch of superficial temporal artery; C = superficial temporal artery; D = branches of facial nerve; E = transverse facial branch of superficial temporal artery; F = transverse facial vein; G = parotid gland; H = parotid duct; I = masseter muscle; J = facial artery; K = facial vein formed by anterior branch of the retromandibular vein and facial veins; L = external jugular vein formed by posterior branch of the retromandibular and posterior auricular veins; M = great auricular nerve on sternocleidomastoid muscle. Courtesy Prof. C Dean.

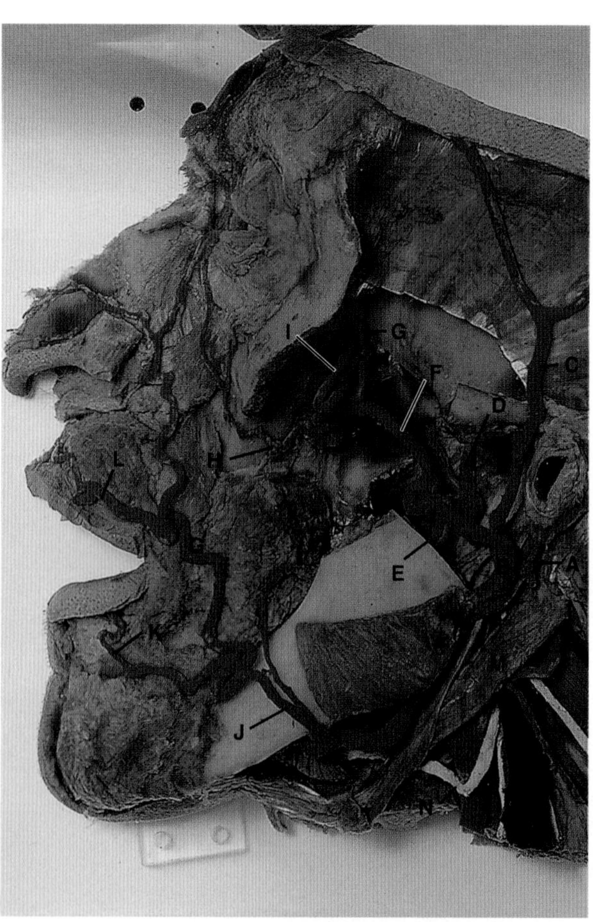

Fig. 4.2 Dissection showing the facial and maxillary arteries. A = posterior auricular artery; B = external carotid artery; C = superficial temporal artery; D = middle meningeal artery; E = inferior alveolar artery; F = maxillary artery; G = deep temporal artery; H = posterior superior alveolar artery; I = third part of maxillary artery entering the pterygopalatine fossa; J = facial artery; K = inferior labial artery; L = superior labial artery; M = posterior belly of the digastric muscle; N = hypoglossal nerve. Courtesy Prof. L Garey.

Maxillary teeth and periodontium

The posterior superior alveolar artery arises from the maxillary artery in the pterygopalatine fossa. Occasionally the posterior superior alveolar artery is derived from the buccal artery. It courses tortuously over the maxillary tuberosity before entering bony canals to supply molar and premolar teeth. The artery also gives off branches to the adjacent buccal gingiva, maxillary sinus and cheek.

The middle superior alveolar artery, when present, arises from the infraorbital artery (which is itself a branch of the third part of the maxillary artery in the pterygopalatine fossa). The middle superior alveolar artery runs in the lateral wall of the maxillary sinus, terminating near the canine tooth, where it anastomoses with the anterior and posterior superior alveolar arteries. The anterior superior alveolar artery also arises from the infraorbital artery and runs downwards in the anterior wall of the maxillary sinus to supply the anterior teeth. As for the superior alveolar nerves, the superior alveolar arteries form plexuses above the root apices.

The buccal gingiva around the posterior maxillary teeth is supplied by gingival and perforating branches from the posterior superior alveolar artery and by the buccal artery. The labial gingiva of anterior teeth is supplied by labial branches of the infraorbital artery and by perforating branches of the anterior superior alveolar artery.

The palatal gingiva around the maxillary teeth is supplied primarily by branches of the greater palatine artery, a branch of the third part of the maxillary artery in the pterygopalatine fossa.

Palate, cheek, tongue and lips

The palate derives its blood supply from the greater and lesser palatine branches of the maxillary artery. The greater palatine artery passes through the incisive fossa, where it anastomoses with the nasopalatine artery. The cheek is supplied by the buccal branch of the maxillary artery. The floor of the mouth and the tongue are supplied by the lingual arteries. The lips are mainly supplied by the superior and inferior labial branches of the facial arteries.

Venous drainage of orodental tissues

The venous drainage of this region is extremely variable. The facial vein is the main vein draining the face (see Figs 4.1 and 3.31). It begins at the medial corner of the eye by confluence of the supraorbital and supratrochlear veins and passes across the face behind the facial artery. Below the mandible, it receives the anterior branch of the retromandibular vein before draining into the internal jugular vein.

Teeth and periodontium

Small veins from the teeth and alveolar bone pass into larger veins surrounding the apex of each tooth, or into veins running in the interdental septa. In the mandible the veins are then collected into one or more inferior alveolar veins, which themselves may drain anteriorly through the mental foramen to join the facial vein or posteriorly through the mandibular foramen to join the pterygoid plexus of veins in the infratemporal fossa. In the maxilla the veins may drain anteriorly into the facial vein or posteriorly into the pterygoid plexus. No accurate description is available concerning the venous drainage of the gingiva, although it may be assumed that the buccal, lingual, greater palatine and nasopalatine veins are involved; apart from the lingual veins (which pass directly into the internal jugular veins), these veins run into the pterygoid plexuses.

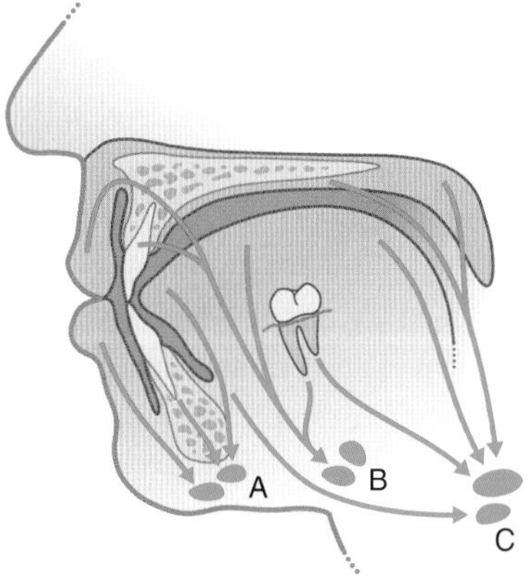

Fig. 4.3 Lymphatic drainage of oral structures. A = submental nodes; B = submandibular nodes; C = jugulodigastric nodes.

Palate, cheek, tongue and lips

The veins of the palate are diffuse and variable. However, those of the hard palate generally pass into the pterygoid venous plexus and those of the soft palate into the pharyngeal venous plexus. The buccal vein of the cheek drains into the pterygoid plexus. Venous blood from the lips drains into the facial veins via the superior and inferior labial veins. The veins of the tongue follow two different routes: those of the dorsum and sides of the tongue form the lingual veins, which, accompanying the lingual arteries, empty into the internal jugular veins; and those of the ventral surface form the deep lingual veins (see Fig. 1.14), which ultimately join the facial, internal jugular or lingual veins.

Lymphatic drainage of orodental tissues

As with the venous system, the lymphatic drainage is very variable: Fig. 4.3 provides a 'consensus' view of the lymphatic drainage of the oral structures.

Lymphatics from the lower part of the face generally pass through or around the buccal lymph nodes to reach the submandibular lymph nodes. However, lymphatics from the medial portion of the lower lip drain into the submental nodes.

The lymph vessels from the teeth usually run directly into the submandibular nodes on the same side. However, lymph from the mandibular incisors drains into the submental nodes. Occasionally lymph from the molars passes directly into the jugulodigastric group of nodes.

The lymph vessels of the labial and buccal gingivae of the maxillary and mandibular teeth unite to drain into the submandibular nodes, although in the labial region of the mandibular incisors they may drain into the submental nodes. The lingual and palatal gingivae drain into the jugulodigastric group of nodes, either directly or indirectly through the submandibular nodes.

Lymphatics from most areas of the palate terminate in the jugulodigastric group of nodes. Vessels from the posterior part of the soft palate terminate in pharyngeal lymph nodes. Lymph from the floor of the mouth region can drain directly to the jugulodigastric nodes.

Lymphatics from the anterior two-thirds of the tongue may be subdivided into two groups: marginal and central vessels. The marginal lymphatic vessels drain the lateral third of the dorsum of the tongue and the lateral margin of its ventral surface. The remaining regions drain into the central vessels. The marginal vessels pass to the submandibular lymph nodes of the same side. The central vessels at the tip of the tongue pass to the submental lymph nodes. Central vessels behind the tip drain into ipsilateral and contralateral submandibular lymph nodes. Some marginal and central lymph vessels pass directly to the jugulodigastric group of nodes (or even the jugulo-omohyoid nodes). Lymphatics from the posterior third of the tongue drain into the deep cervical group of nodes, vessels centrally draining both ipsilaterally and contralaterally. Knowledge of the ipsilateral and contralateral drainage from the tongue is important clinically, where, for example, a tumour near the central part of the tongue may be associated with spread into lymph nodes on both sides.

At the oropharyngeal isthmus lie the palatine tonsils between the pillars of the fauces (see Fig. 1.12) and the lingual tonsils on the pharyngeal surface of the tongue (see Fig. 1.15). These tonsils form part of a ring of lymphoid tissue known as Waldeyer's tonsillar ring. The other components are the tubal tonsils and adenoid tissue (pharyngeal tonsils) located in the nasopharynx.

Innervation of orodental tissues

Excluding regions around the oropharyngeal isthmus, the oral mucosa receives sensory innervation from the maxillary and mandibular divisions of the trigeminal nerve. The trigeminal nerve also supplies the teeth and their supporting tissues (Table 4.1). Both the major and minor salivary glands are supplied by secretomotor parasympathetic fibres from the facial and glossopharyngeal nerves. The motor innervation of the muscles of the jaws and oral cavity is from the trigeminal, facial, accessory and hypoglossal nerves.

Fig. 4.4 illustrates the cutaneous innervation of the face. All three divisions of the trigeminal nerve are involved: the ophthalmic division supplying the upper part of the face, forehead and scalp; and the maxillary and mandibular divisions essentially supplying the upper and lower jaw regions, respectively. Knowledge of these areas, and of the specific branches involved, is important clinically for assessing the effects of nerve damage and for an understanding of the successful anaesthetising of the buccal, infraorbital and inferior alveolar (mental) nerves during dental treatment. The areas supplied by the three divisions of the trigeminal nerve also relate to aspects of the development of the face (see page 356).

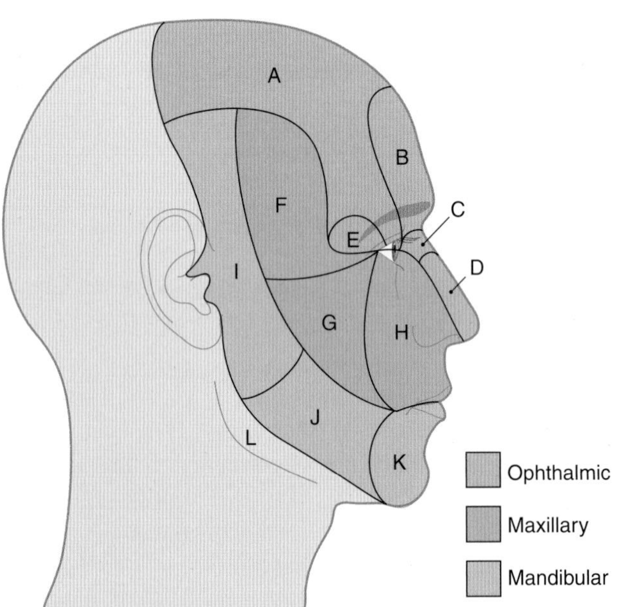

Fig. 4.4 Schematic diagram showing cutaneous innervation of the face by the trigeminal cranial nerve. A = supraorbital nerve; B = supratrochlear nerve; C = infratrochlear nerve; D = external nasal nerve; E = lacrimal nerve; F = zygomaticotemporal nerve; G = zygomaticofacial nerve; H = infraorbital nerve; I = auriculotemporal nerve; J = buccal nerve; K = mental nerve; L = great auricular nerve (from the second and third cervical spinal nerves).

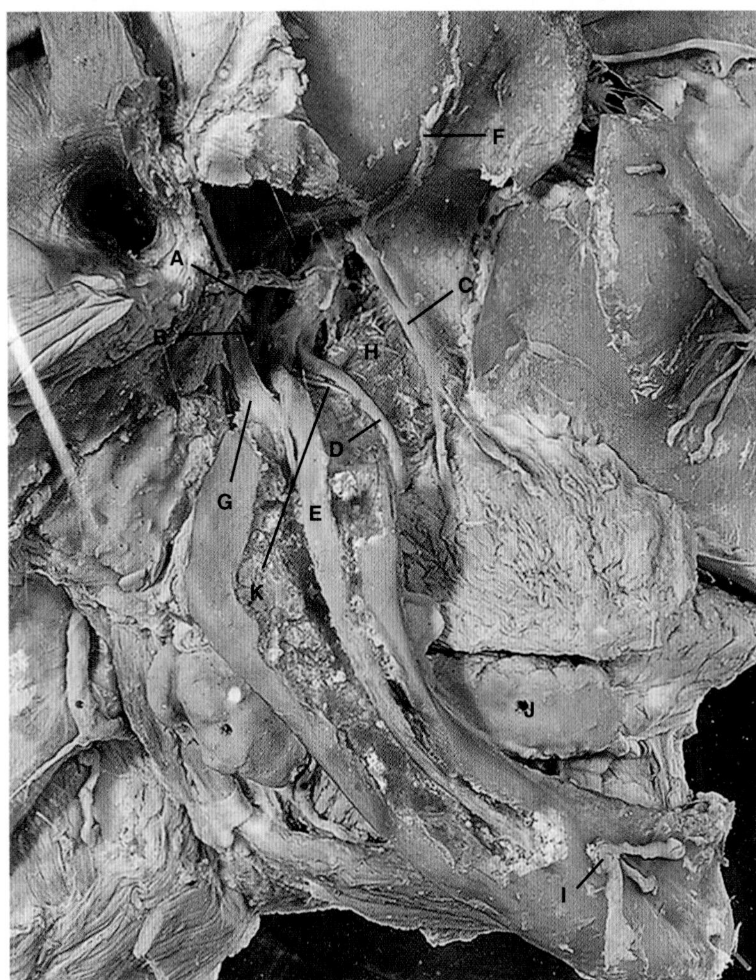

Fig. 4.5 Infratemporal fossa showing distribution of the mandibular nerve and the course of its inferior alveolar branch. A = auriculotemporal nerve; B = middle meningeal artery; C = buccal branch; D = lingual nerve; E = inferior alveolar nerve with mylohyoid branch; F = deep temporal nerve; G = sphenomandibular ligament; H = medial pterygoid muscle; I = mental nerve; J = sublingual gland; K = chorda tympani. Courtesy Prof. C Dean.

Table 4.1 Nerve supply to the teeth and gingivae

	Nasopalatine nerve			Greater palatine nerve					Palatal gingiva
Maxilla	Anterior superior alveolar nerve			Middle superior alveolar nerve		Posterior superior alveolar nerve			**Teeth**
	Infraorbital nerve			Posterior superior alveolar nerve and buccal nerve					**Buccal gingiva**
	1	2	3	4	5	6	7	8	**Tooth position (Palmer-Zsigmondy system)**
	Mental nerve			Buccal nerve and perforating branches of inferior alveolar nerve					**Buccal gingiva**
Mandible	Incisive nerve			Inferior alveolar nerve					**Teeth**
	Lingual nerve and perforating branches of inferior alveolar nerve								**Lingual gingiva**

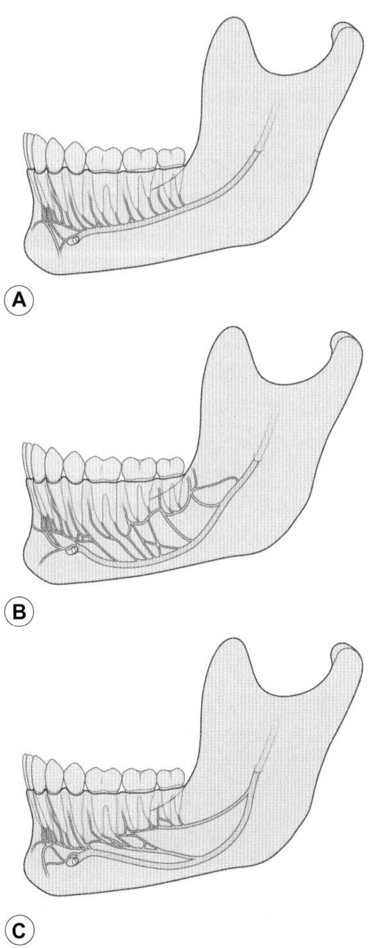

Fig. 4.6 Schematic diagram showing variation in the course of the inferior alveolar nerve through the mandible. See text for explanation. Redrawn after Dr R B Carter and Dr E N Keen.

Inferior alveolar nerve

The course of the inferior alveolar nerve through the mandible is illustrated in Figs. 4.5 and 4.6. The distribution of nerves to the mandibular premolars and molars is variable, with dental branches coming either directly from the inferior alveolar nerve by short (Fig. 4.6A) or long (Fig. 4.6B) branches or indirectly through several alveolar branches (Fig. 4.6C). In rare instances the nerve to the mandibular third molar may arise from the inferior alveolar nerve before it enters the mandibular canal. Communications between the inferior alveolar nerve and nerves from the temporalis and lateral pterygoid muscles have been described, with the nerves penetrating the mandible through foramina in the region of muscle attachments. It has been suggested that such nerve connections might explain why, in approximately 5% of patients, the teeth may not be anaesthetised after the main trunk of the inferior alveolar nerve has been blocked at the mandibular foramen by the injection of local anaesthetic solution.

It is said that in any one individual, the mandibular canal remains in a relatively fixed position with respect to the lower border of the mandible. The canal is often closely related to the roots of the mandibular molars (see fig. 2.182). Indeed, the roots of the lower third molars may even be perforated by the mandibular canal.

In the premolar region the main trunk of the inferior alveolar nerve divides into mental and incisive nerves. The mental nerve runs for a short distance in a mental canal before leaving the body of the mandible at the mental foramen to emerge onto the face. In about 50% of cases the mental foramen lies on a vertical line passing through the mandibular second premolar. However, in some ethnic groups the mental foramen may be situated slightly more posteriorly, midway between the roots of the second premolar and first permanent molar. In an adult with a full dentition the mental foramen usually lies midway between the upper and lower borders of the mandible. During the first and second years of life, as the prominence of the chin develops, the opening of the mental foramen alters in direction, from facing forwards to facing upwards and backwards. As well as supplying the skin of the lower lip, the mental nerve provides fibres to an incisor plexus that innervates the labial periodontium of the mandibular incisors. The incisive nerve runs forwards in an intraosseous incisive canal. This nerve primarily supplies the incisors and canines but may also supply the first premolar. In some instances the canine may be supplied directly from the inferior alveolar nerve.

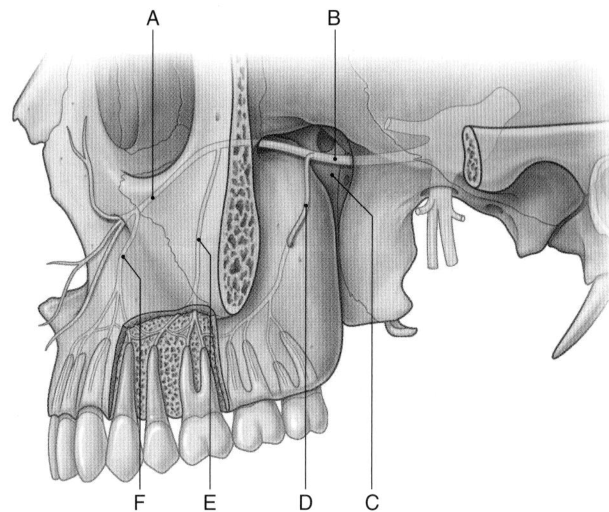

Fig. 4.7 The superior alveolar nerves and associated dental plexuses. A = infraorbital nerve; B = trunk of the maxillary division of the trigeminal nerve; C = pterygopalatine fossa; D = posterior superior alveolar nerves; E = middle superior alveolar nerve; F = anterior superior alveolar nerve.

Superior alveolar nerve

The superior alveolar nerves and associated dental plexuses are shown in Fig. 4.7. The posterior superior alveolar nerve arises from the maxillary nerve in the pterygopalatine fossa, whence it passes through the pterygomaxillary fissure to descend on the posterior wall (tuberosity) of the maxilla (Fig. 4.8). The dental branches of the nerve enter the maxilla and run in narrow posterior superior alveolar canals above the roots of the molar teeth. A gingival branch does not enter the bone but runs downwards and forwards along the outer surface of the maxillary tuberosity. The dental branches of the posterior superior alveolar nerve may arise from a common nerve trunk within the bone (Fig. 4.9B) or on the tuberosity before entering bone (Fig. 4.9A). Alternatively, they may appear as separate nerve trunks from the main trunk of the maxillary nerve in the pterygopalatine fossa (Fig. 4.9C). The middle superior alveolar nerve is found in about 70% of subjects. The nerve generally arises from the infraorbital nerve in the floor of the orbit/roof of the maxillary air sinus, although it may arise from the maxillary nerve in the pterygopalatine fossa. The nerve may run in the posterior, lateral or anterior walls of the maxillary sinus. It terminates above the roots of the premolar teeth. In the absence of a middle superior alveolar nerve, fibres from the anterior superior alveolar nerve supply the maxillary premolar region. The anterior superior alveolar nerve arises from the infraorbital nerve within the infraorbital canal, generally as a single nerve but occasionally as two or three small branches. The nerve leaves the infraorbital canal near its termination and then, diverging laterally from the infraorbital nerve, runs in the anterior wall of the maxillary sinus. It terminates near the anterior nasal spine after giving off a small nasal branch. Note that the posterior superior alveolar nerve has an extra-bony course that permits anaesthesia of the nerve trunk(s) as it passes across the maxillary tuberosity. The middle and anterior superior alveolar nerves, however, are entirely intrabony in their course and cannot be 'blocked' with an anaesthetic injection.

The superior alveolar nerve forms a plexus above the root apices of the maxillary teeth (Fig. 4.7). From this plexus, nerves pass to the teeth, although it is difficult to trace the precise innervation of the teeth from specific superior alveolar nerves. As a general rule, the incisors and canines are supplied by the anterior nerve, the molars by the posterior nerve and intermediate areas by the middle nerve.

Sensory nerves to oral cavity

The sensory nerve supply to the palate is described in Figs. 4.10 and 4.11. The nerve supply is derived from the maxillary division of the trigeminal nerve via branches of the pterygopalatine ganglion. A small area behind the maxillary incisor teeth is supplied by terminal branches of the nasopalatine nerves. These nerves emerge from the incisive fossa onto the palate. The remainder of the hard palate is supplied by the greater palatine nerves emerging from the greater palatine foramina onto the palate. The soft palate is supplied by the lesser palatine nerves emerging from the lesser palatine foramina onto the palate. Although the maxillary division of the trigeminal nerve supplies most of the palate, there is evidence to suggest that some areas supplied by the lesser palatine nerves may also be innervated by fibres from the facial nerve. The posterior part of the soft palate and the uvula may be supplied by the glossopharyngeal nerve.

The sensory innervation of the tongue is illustrated in Fig. 4.12. Three distinct nerve fields can be recognised on the dorsum of the tongue. The anterior part of the tongue, in front of the circumvallate papillae, is supplied by the lingual branch of the mandibular division of the trigeminal nerve (Fig. 4.5). However, the accompanying chorda tympani fibres from the nervus intermedius part of the facial nerve are those associated with the perception of taste. Fig. 4.5 shows the chorda tympani joining the lingual nerve in the infratemporal fossa. Behind, and including the circumvallate

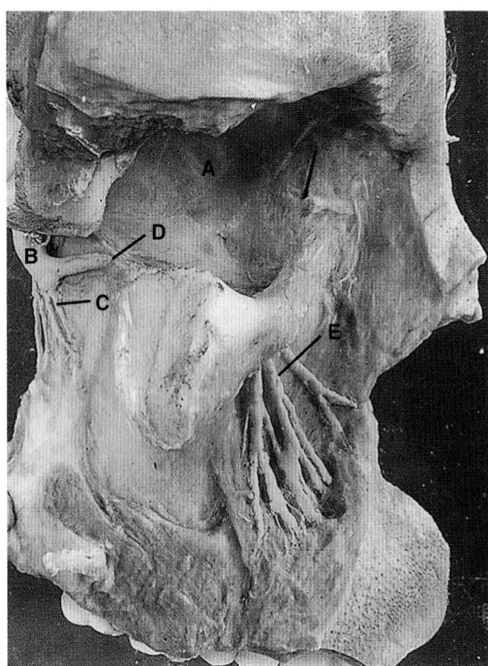

Fig. 4.8 Frontal aspect of face showing the maxillary nerve. A = orbit; B = maxillary nerve; C = posterior superior alveolar nerve; D = infraorbital nerve in floor of orbit; E = infraorbital nerve entering the face at the infraorbital foramen.

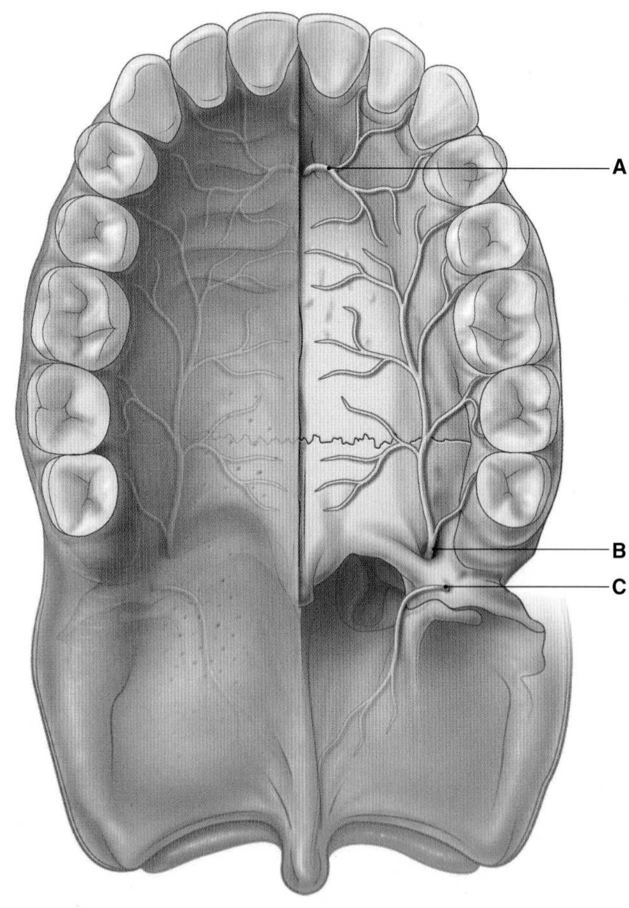

Fig. 4.10 The sensory nerve supply to the palate. A = nasopalatine nerves; B = greater palatine nerve; C = lesser palatine nerve.

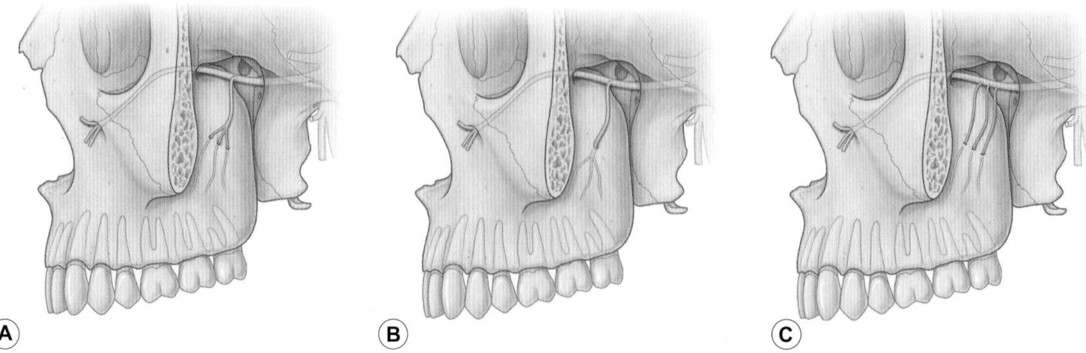

Fig. 4.9 Three different patterns for the posterior superior alveolar nerves on the tuberosity of the maxilla See text for explanation.

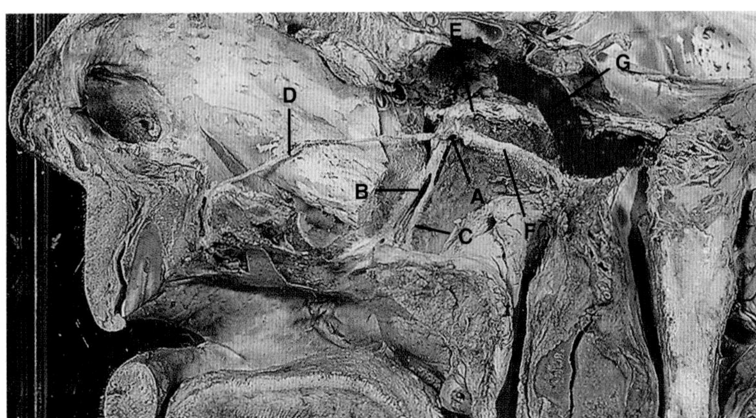

Fig. 4.11 The pterygopalatine ganglion (A) giving rise to the greater (B) and lesser (C) palatine nerves and the nasopalatine nerve (D). E = maxillary nerve; F = nerve of pterygoid canal; G = internal carotid artery.

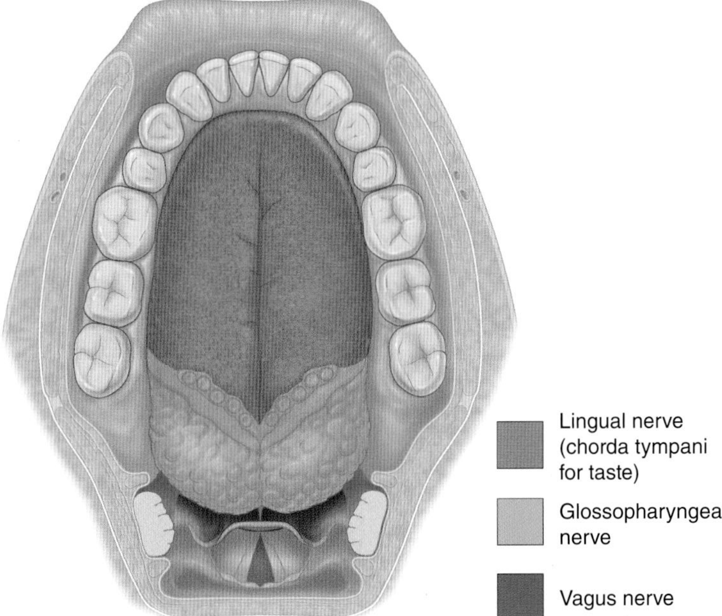

Fig. 4.12 Schematic representation of the sensory innervation of the tongue.

papillae, the tongue is supplied primarily by the glossopharyngeal nerve (providing both general sensation and taste). A small area on the posterior part of the tongue around the epiglottis is supplied by the vagus nerve (via its superior laryngeal branch). The mucosa on the ventral surface of the tongue is supplied by the lingual nerve.

The mucosa of the upper lip is supplied by the infraorbital branch of the maxillary division of the trigeminal nerve. That of the lower lip is supplied by the mental branch of the mandibular division of the trigeminal nerve (Fig. 4.5). The mucosa of the cheeks is supplied by the buccal branch of the mandibular division of the trigeminal nerve. The mucosa on the floor of the mouth is innervated by the lingual branch of the mandibular division of the trigeminal nerve. The mucosa over the pillars of the fauces (the oropharyngeal isthmus) is supplied by the glossopharyngeal nerve.

Secretomotor innervation of the salivary glands

Parotid gland

The secretomotor supply of the parotid gland is derived from the otic parasympathetic ganglion (Fig. 4.13). This ganglion is situated in the roof of the infratemporal fossa, close to the foramen ovale and the mandibular division of the trigeminal nerve. Like other parasympathetic ganglia in the head, three types of nerve fibre are associated with it: parasympathetic, sympathetic and sensory. However, only the parasympathetic fibres synapse in the ganglion. The preganglionic parasympathetic fibres of the otic ganglion originate from the inferior salivatory nucleus in the brainstem and pass with the glossopharyngeal nerve via its lesser petrosal branch. The sympathetic root of the otic ganglion is derived from postganglionic fibres from the superior cervical ganglion and reaches the otic ganglion via the plexus around the middle meningeal artery in the infratemporal fossa. The sensory root is derived from the auriculotemporal branch of the mandibular division of the trigeminal nerve. The postganglionic parasympathetic fibres (with sensory and sympathetic fibres) reach the parotid gland through the auriculotemporal branch of the mandibular nerve.

Submandibular and sublingual glands

The secretomotor supply of the submandibular and sublingual glands is derived from the submandibular parasympathetic ganglion (Fig. 4.14). This ganglion is situated with the lingual nerve on the hyoglossus muscle in the floor of the mouth above the deep part of the submandibular gland. The preganglionic parasympathetic fibres of the ganglion originate from the superior salivatory nucleus in the brainstem and pass with the nervus intermedius of the facial nerve, and subsequently its chorda tympani branch, to reach the lingual nerve in the infratemporal fossa (Fig. 4.5). It is via the lingual nerve that the preganglionic fibres are conveyed to the submandibular ganglion. The sympathetic root of the ganglion is derived from postganglionic fibres from the superior cervical ganglion and reaches the submandibular ganglion via the plexus around the facial artery. The sensory root is derived from the lingual nerve. The postganglionic parasympathetic fibres (with sensory and sympathetic fibres) pass directly to the adjacent submandibular gland but reach the sublingual gland after re-entering the lingual nerve.

Innervation of the oral musculature

The functions of mastication, swallowing and speech are among the most complex in the body. This is reflected in the number and variety of muscles found around the mouth and by the range of cranial nerves that innervate them. Table 4.2 summarises the innervation of the oral musculature.

Trigeminal nerve (maxillary and mandibular divisions)

Maxillary division

The maxillary division of the trigeminal nerve contains only sensory fibres (Figs. 4.15, 4.16; see also Figs. 4.8 and 4.11). It supplies the maxillary teeth and their supporting structures, the palate, the maxillary air sinus, much of the nasal cavity and the skin overlying the middle part of the face. The nerve emerges into the pterygopalatine fossa through the foramen rotundum of the sphenoid bone. Its subsequent branches can be subdivided into branches from the main nerve trunk (Fig. 4.15) and branches from the pterygopalatine ganglion (Fig. 4.16). From the main trunk are the meningeal, ganglionic, zygomatic, posterior superior alveolar and infraorbital nerves. The infraorbital nerve gives rise to the middle

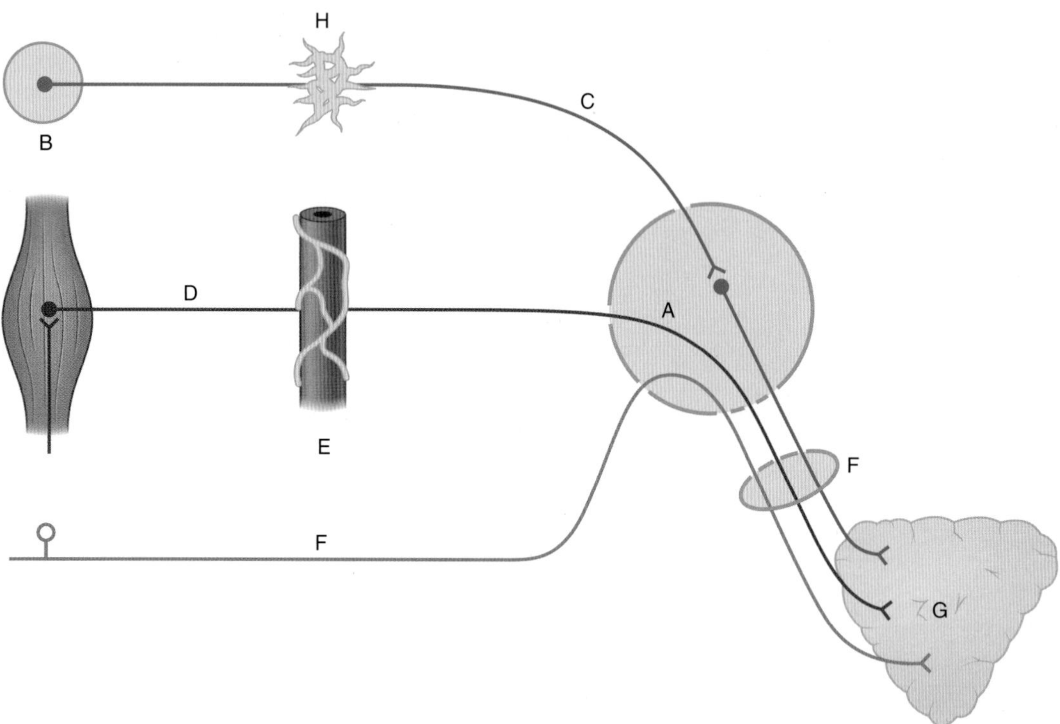

Fig. 4.13 The secretomotor supply to the parotid salivary gland. A = otic parasympathetic ganglion; B = inferior salivatory nucleus; C = lesser petrosal branch of the glossopharyngeal nerve; D = postganglionic fibres from the superior cervical ganglion; E = sympathetic plexus around the middle meningeal artery; F = auriculotemporal branch of mandibular division of trigeminal nerve; G = parotid gland; H = tympanic plexus.

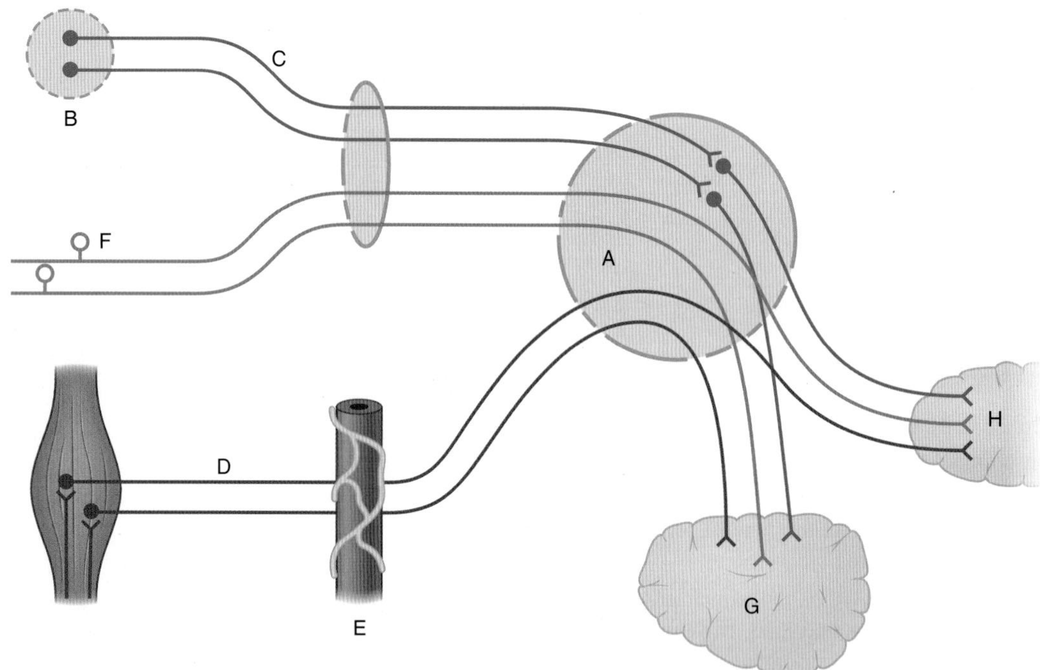

Fig. 4.14 The secretomotor supply to the submandibular and sublingual salivary glands. A = submandibular parasympathetic ganglion; B = superior salivatory nucleus; C = chorda tympani branch of facial nerve; D = postganglionic fibres from the superior cervical ganglion; E = sympathetic plexus around the facial artery; F = lingual nerve; G = submandibular gland; H = sublingual gland.

and anterior superior alveolar nerves. The branches of the maxillary nerve that arise via the pterygopalatine ganglion contain a mixture of sensory, parasympathetic (secretomotor) and sympathetic (vasomotor) fibres. The branches arising from the ganglion are the orbital, nasopalatine, posterior superior nasal, greater and lesser palatine and pharyngeal nerves. Thus the branches supplying the teeth and their supporting structures and the palate and the upper lip are the posterior, middle and anterior superior alveolar nerves, the nasopalatine and the greater and lesser palatine nerves, and the infraorbital nerve.

Mandibular division

The mandibular division of the trigeminal nerve is the largest division of the trigeminal nerve (Fig. 4.17; see also Figs 3.34 and 4.5). It is the only division that contains motor fibres and sensory fibres. Its sensory fibres supply the mandibular teeth (and their supporting structures), the mucosa of the anterior two-thirds of the tongue and the floor of the mouth, the skin of the lower part of the face, and parts of the temple and auricle. Its motor fibres supply the muscles of mastication, the mylohyoid, the

Table 4.2 Innervation of the oral musculature. C1 = first cervical spinal nerve

Region	Muscle	Nerve
Lips	Orbicularis oris	Facial
Cheeks	Buccinator	Facial
Tongue (intrinsic musculature)	Transverse Longitudinal Vertical	Hypoglossal
Tongue (extrinsic musculature)	Genioglossus Hyoglossus Styloglossus	Hypoglossal
	Palatoglossus	Accessory (cranial part)
Floor of mouth	Mylohyoid	Mandibular division of trigeminal
	Geniohyoid	Hypoglossal (C1 fibres)
Palate	Tensor veli palatini	Mandibular division of trigeminal
	Levator veli palatini Palatoglossus Palatopharyngeus Musculus uvulae	Accessory (cranial part)

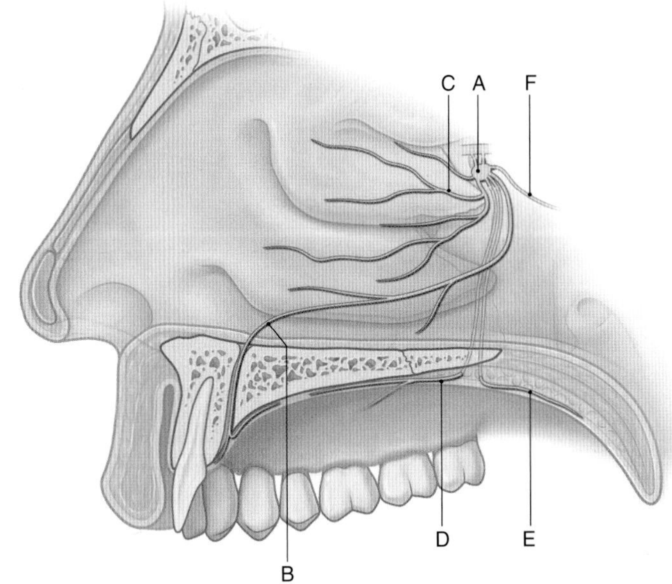

Fig. 4.16 Diagrammatic representation of the maxillary division of the trigeminal nerve and the branches that are derived via the pterygopalatine ganglion. A = pterygopalatine ganglion; B = nasopalatine nerve; C = posterior superior nasal nerve; D = greater palatine nerve; E = lesser palatine nerve; F = pharyngeal nerve.

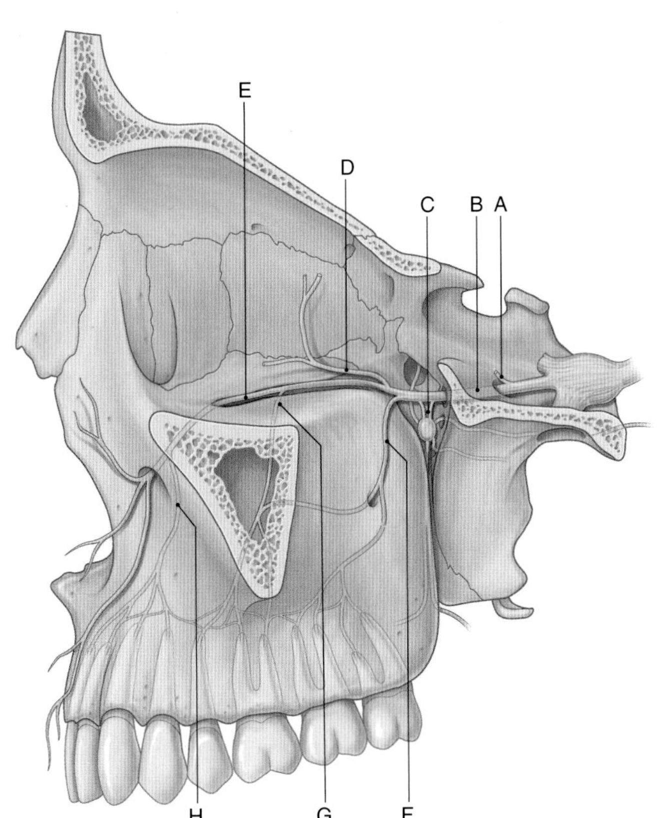

Fig. 4.15 Diagrammatic representation of the maxillary division of the trigeminal nerve and the branches that are derived directly from the nerve trunk. A = meningeal branch; B = maxillary nerve trunk passing through the foramen rotundum into the pterygopalatine fossa; C = ganglionic branch; D = main zygomatic nerve; E = infraorbital nerve; F = posterior superior alveolar nerve; G = middle superior alveolar nerve; H = anterior superior alveolar nerve.

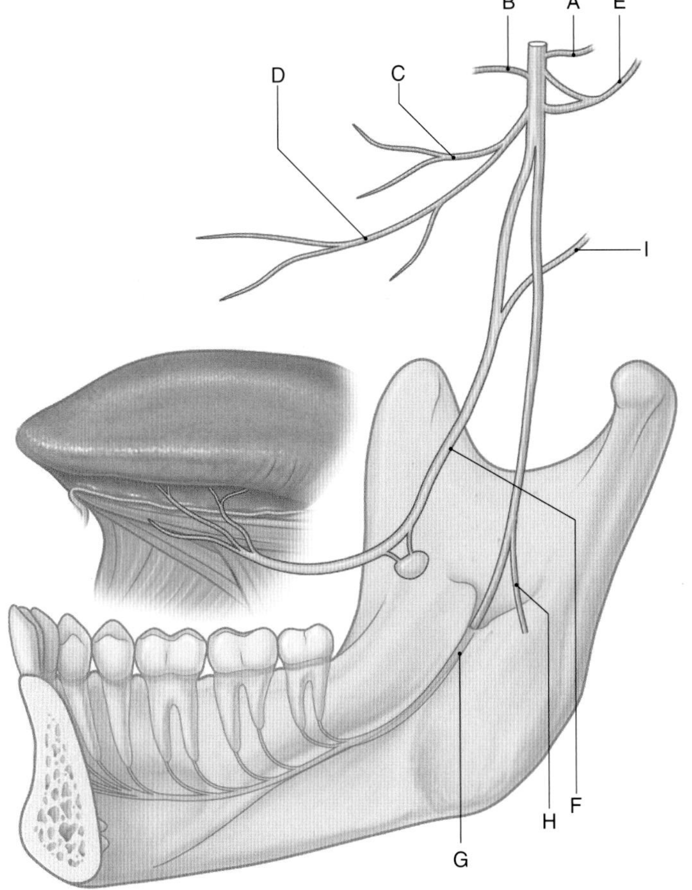

Fig. 4.17 Schematic diagram of the mandibular division of the trigeminal nerve. A = meningeal branch; B = nerve to medial pterygoid; C = anterior trunk giving motor branches to masseter, temporalis and lateral pterygoid muscles; D = buccal nerve; E = auriculotemporal nerve; F = lingual nerve; G = inferior alveolar nerve; H = mylohyoid nerve; I = chorda tympani branch of facial nerve joining the lingual nerve.

anterior belly of the digastric, and the tensor veli palatini and tensor tympani muscles. The mandibular nerve emerges into the infratemporal fossa through the foramen ovale of the sphenoid bone. It lies deep to the lateral pterygoid muscle, where it gives off all its branches, dividing into anterior (mainly motor) and posterior (mainly sensory) trunks. Proximal to this division, it gives off the meningeal branch and the nerve to the medial pterygoid.

The meningeal branch passes back into the middle cranial fossa through the foramen spinosum of the sphenoid bone (accompanied by the middle meningeal artery). The nerve to the medial pterygoid muscle passes through the otic ganglion (without synapsing) and, after supplying the muscle, continues on to supply the tensor veli palatini and tensor tympani muscles. The anterior trunk gives motor branches to the masseter, temporalis and lateral pterygoid, and the sensory buccal nerve. The posterior trunk gives off the sensory auriculotemporal, lingual and inferior alveolar nerves, and the motor mylohyoid nerve. Note that the chorda tympani branch of the facial nerve joins the lingual nerve, and that postganglionic fibres from the otic parasympathetic ganglion run with the auriculotemporal nerve to provide secretomotor fibres to the parotid gland.

Central connections

Central connections of the trigeminal nerve are summarised in Fig. 4.18. The trigeminal nerve conveys discriminative tactile information from the ipsilateral half of the face and the top of the head; the axons of the trigeminal ganglion cells pass to the principal sensory nucleus and to the pars oralis of the spinal tract of the trigeminal nerve. Proprioceptive information from the ipsilateral muscles of mastication and the temporomandibular joint reaches the mesencephalic nucleus of the trigeminal nerve. However, evidence suggests that proprioceptive information from the teeth also passes to the principal sensory nucleus. Direct and indirect connections of these nuclei form the basis of cranial nerve reflexes. Signals from the principal sensory and mesencephalic nuclei are transmitted mainly via the contralateral ventral trigeminothalamic tract (trigeminal lemniscus) and the ipsilateral dorsal trigeminothalamic tract to the nucleus ventralis posterior medialis of the thalamus. Axons from this nucleus pass through the posterior limb of the internal capsule to the inferior part of the postcentral gyrus and frontoparietal operculum. The nucleus of the spinal tract of the trigeminal nerve is subdivided into the pars oralis, pars interpolaris and pars caudalis. The pars oralis deals mainly with tactile signals. The pars interpolaris receives cutaneous and proprioceptive information and sends fibres to the cerebellum. The pars caudalis deals primarily with nociceptive signals but also with tactile and thermal information. Fibres from the nucleus of the spinal tract pass to the reticular formation (for cranial nerve reflexes). Some fibres run near the medial lemniscus in the contralateral ventral trigeminothalamic tract to reach the various thalamic nuclei. The motor nucleus of the trigeminal nerve lies close to the principal central nucleus in the central part of the pons. It receives fibres from the other sensory trigeminal nuclei, the reticular formation, the cerebellum and the cerebral cortex via bilateral corticonuclear fibres.

Clinical considerations of the innervation and vasculature of the mouth

We have already seen on page 101 how spread of infection from teeth via the lymphatics can cause swellings of the neck. Such infectious swellings can be painful and be associated with fever. However, enlargements of the lymphatics glands in the neck can also be related to metastases from a carcinoma of the tongue, which may be unilateral or bilateral (Fig. 4.19). These swellings are usually not painful themselves. Swellings of the lymph glands in the neck may be completely unrelated to pathologies in the mouth. Fig. 4.20 shows a patient with a firm, painless swelling on the left side of the neck, which caused discomfort on swallowing. It had been slowly enlarging for some months. A biopsy revealed that the swelling

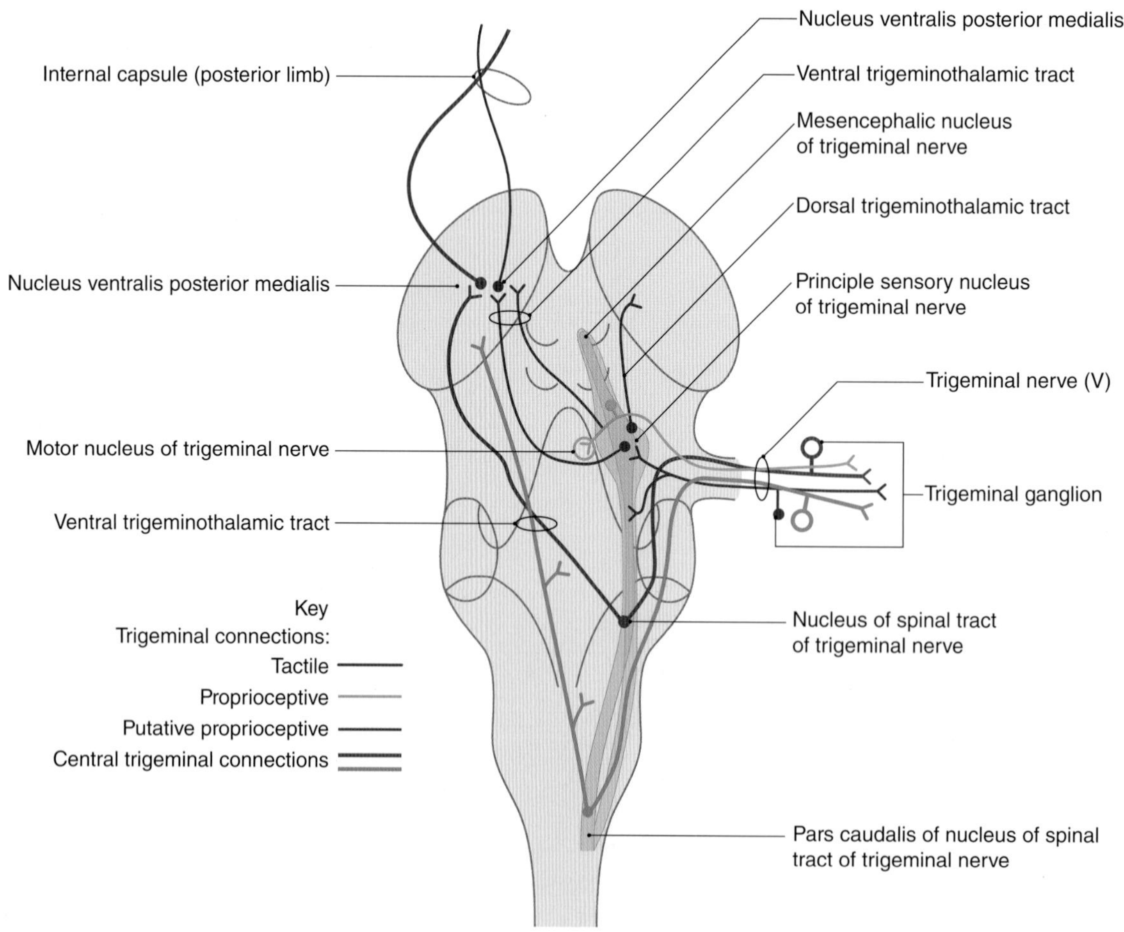

Fig. 4.18 The central connections of the trigeminal nerve.

was a squamous cell carcinoma and had metastasised to the lymph glands of the neck. There was no evidence on the tongue of any disease, and the primary lesion was traced to the oropharynx. Other sites for the primary lesion could be the maxillary sinus, larynx and even the lung. Other factors causing swellings of the neck include cysts, salivary gland tumours and tuberculosis.

Dental anaesthesia

To anaesthetise the teeth during various dental procedures, local infiltration techniques are usually adequate where the surrounding alveolar bone is thin (such as in the maxilla and anterior region of the mandible). However, when treating the mandibular cheek teeth, which are surrounded by thicker bone, it is necessary to anaesthetise the inferior alveolar nerve in the infratemporal fossa before it enters the mandibular canal. This involves placing the needle in the pterygomandibular space in a procedure known as an inferior alveolar nerve block (Fig. 4.21). In the routine open-mouth direct method, the patient is asked to open their mouth widely and, with the syringe held over the opposite mandibular first premolar tooth, the needle is inserted into the triangular fossa. This is situated between the ridges overlying the base of the pterygomandibular raphe medially and the internal oblique ridge of the ramus of the mandible laterally (see Fig. 1.9). The needle is advanced about 1 cm, where it comes close to the ramus and the inferior alveolar (and lingual) nerve. The needle should lie about 1 cm above the occlusal surface of the mandibular teeth. An alternative method intended to anaesthetise the whole of the mandibular nerve seeks to inject the anaesthetic solution at a higher level within the pterygomandibular space and is known as the intraoral 'high condyle' (Gow-Gates) technique.

From a knowledge of the anatomy of the infratemporal fossa (Fig. 4.21), the following common complications may arise after an inferior alveolar nerve block:

- If the needle (and anaesthetic solution) is injected too far medially, it may penetrate the medial pterygoid muscle; if placed too far laterally, it may penetrate the temporalis muscle. In either case, there will be an absence of anaesthesia that may be followed by trismus (painful spasm of the muscle).
- If the needle is advanced too deeply, the facial nerve may be affected, and a temporary unilateral facial palsy may result.
- The needle may rupture a vein(s) associated with the pterygoid venous plexus resulting in a haematoma.
- If the needle directly encounters the inferior alveolar nerve, the patient may experience the sensation of an 'electric shock'. The needle must be withdrawn before injecting the anaesthetic solution.
- Local anaesthetic solution may pass into the pterygomandibular space and thence into the inferior orbital fissure. The closest nerve is the abducens nerve, which may be temporarily anaesthetised, resulting in diplopia (double vision) due to paralysis of the lateral rectus muscle.
- The needle may penetrate the inferior alveolar artery, but to prevent the dire consequences of injecting anaesthetic solution directly into the artery, the needle should always be aspirated first.

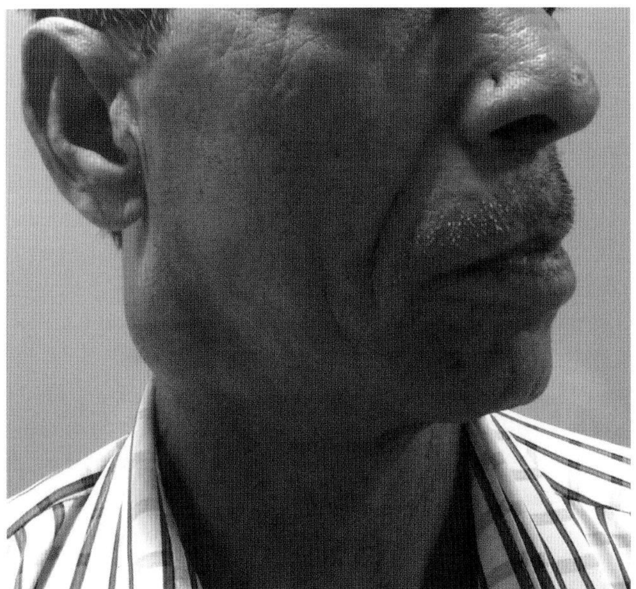

Fig. 4.19 Enlargement of the jugulodigastric nodes of the neck due to spread from a carcinoma of the base of the tongue on the right side. From Dhingra, S., Dhingra, P.L., 2022. *Diseases of Ear, Nose and Throat & Head and Neck Surgery*, eighth ed. Elsevier

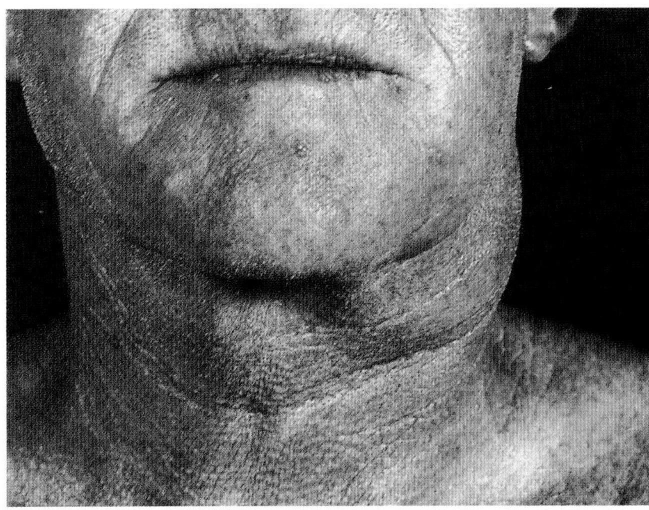

Fig. 4.20 Patient presenting with swelling on the left side of the neck. From Banerjee, A., Thavaraj, S. (Eds.), 2020. *Odell's Clinical Problem Solving in Dentistry*, fourth ed. Elsevier India.

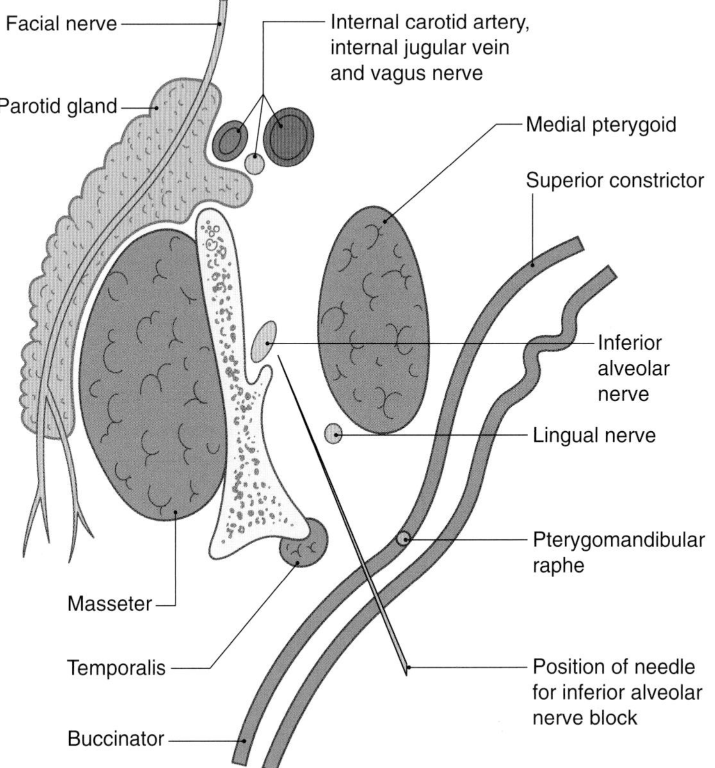

Fig. 4.21 Diagram showing position of needle in an inferior alveolar nerve block.

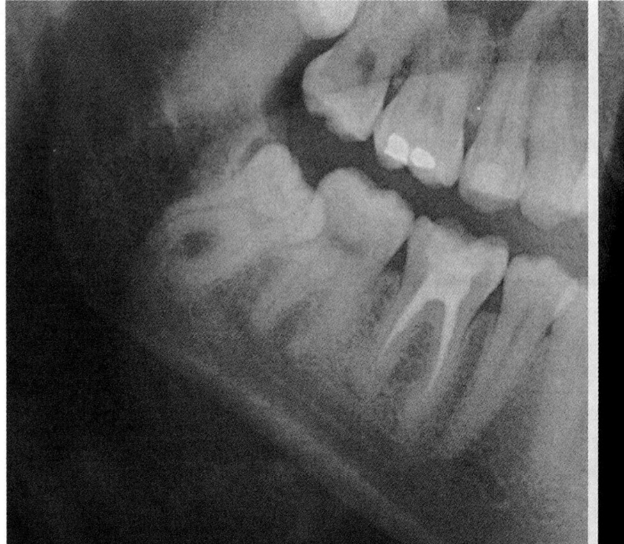

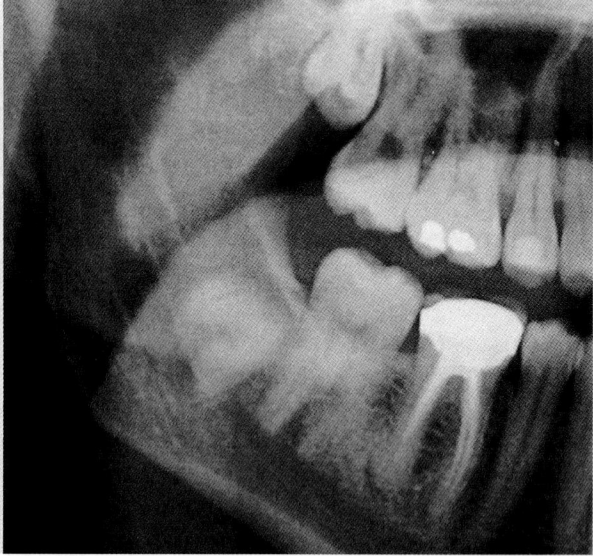

Fig. 4.22 (A) Radiograph showing an impacted right mandibular third permanent molar with roots close to the inferior mandibular canal. (B) Same patient as in (A) 9 years later after successful coronectomy without root filling. From Banerjee, A., Thavaraj, S. (Eds.), 2020. *Odell's Clinical Problem Solving in Dentistry,* fourth ed. Elsevier.

If a careful aseptic technique is not attained during anaesthesia, the possibility arises of introducing infective agents into the pterygomandibular space. From here, infection may spread to adjacent tissue spaces (see pages 92–96). Infection may spread via emissary veins from the pterygoid venous plexus to the cavernous sinus.

Even if a correct inferior alveolar nerve block is administered to anaesthetise a mandibular cheek tooth, pain may still be felt by a patient undergoing a clinical procedure. This 'escape from anaesthesia' may be related to anatomical variation. For example, a nerve branch supplying the tooth may be unaffected by the normal nerve block injection that is given lower down than the nerve branch high up from the parent inferior alveolar nerve in the infratemporal fossa. Occasionally additional branches supplying the tooth pass with the buccal or temporal branches of the mandibular nerve. Mandibular premolars also can receive sensory branches from the mylohyoid branch of the mandibular nerve, which is principally a motor nerve supplying the anterior belly of the digastric and mylohyoid muscles. Additional local infiltration of anaesthetic solution around the tooth may solve the problem.

Iatrogenic damage to the inferior alveolar nerve

Knowledge of the anatomy of the inferior alveolar nerve is important because dental treatment can adversely affect this nerve as it traverses the mandibular canal within the body of the mandible. The potential causes of inferior alveolar nerve injury include local anaesthetic injections, endodontic treatment, implants and oral surgery (particularly surgical removal of mandibular third molars). Injury due to local anaesthetic blocks of the inferior alveolar nerve within the infratemporal fossa are rare (between approximately 1 in 25,000 and 1 in 80,000 cases), and fortunately recovery takes place in about 90% of cases by the end of 2 months. The cause may be physical and related to the needle or chemical (with high concentrations of the local anaesthetic agent), and some have proposed that, instead of using a block technique within the infratemporal fossa, it is preferable to treat infiltrations around the tooth with high-concentration agents. For endodontics, any treatment for a tooth near the mandibular canal requires special attention, and injury to the inferior alveolar nerve may be caused by physical trauma or the use of chemical agents. Indeed, the effects of chemical injury are often permanent. Injury to the inferior alveolar nerve with surgical removal of mandibular third molars occurs in approximately 20% of cases where it is deemed radiologically that the tooth is close to the mandibular canal. This close relationship may be evident in radiographs, with the radiolucent nerve canal being superimposed on roots or being constricted as one of the warning signs (see Fig. 2.184). The age of the patient is a significant factor, as well as proximity of the mandibular canal and the assumed difficulty of the operative procedures. Such are the problems of extracting third molars that it is nowadays recommended that the whole tooth is not removed, just the crown with retention of the roots. This procedure is called a coronectomy (Fig. 4.22) and may require the retained roots to be root filled. Implant injuries to the inferior alveolar nerve have been reported to vary from 0% to 40%, with 25% of edentulous patients being affected. The recommendation is to leave a 4-mm safety zone away from the mandibular canal. Whatever the cause, iatrogenic injury of the inferior alveolar nerve can interfere markedly with normal function (e.g., eating and drinking, speaking, kissing, applying cosmetics and shaving) and also has repercussions socially and with the patient's quality of life.

The mental nerve exits the mental foramen, which lies close to the root apices of the mandibular premolar teeth and may be at risk when surgically removing the roots of such teeth (see Fig. 2.153). A clear radiograph of the region must be available to alert the operator of any problems, such as the presence of an abnormally long root. Damage to the mental nerve will manifest itself as paraesthesia in the lower lip of the affected side.

Iatrogenic damage to the lingual nerve

The close relationship of the lingual nerve to the alveolar process of the third molar tooth makes the nerve susceptible to damage during removal of the tooth. This may be more likely if the procedure is carried out with a lingual rather than a buccal approach. In addition, in about one in seven cases, the lingual nerve is located above the lingual bony plate in the third molar region and may be more at risk for damage during surgery. The symptoms of lingual nerve damage are paraesthesia in the distribution of the nerve (i.e., tongue, floor of mouth and gingiva). Injury of the lingual nerve is usually less problematic than injury to the inferior alveolar nerve with recovery without treatment in the first 10 weeks in 88% of cases.

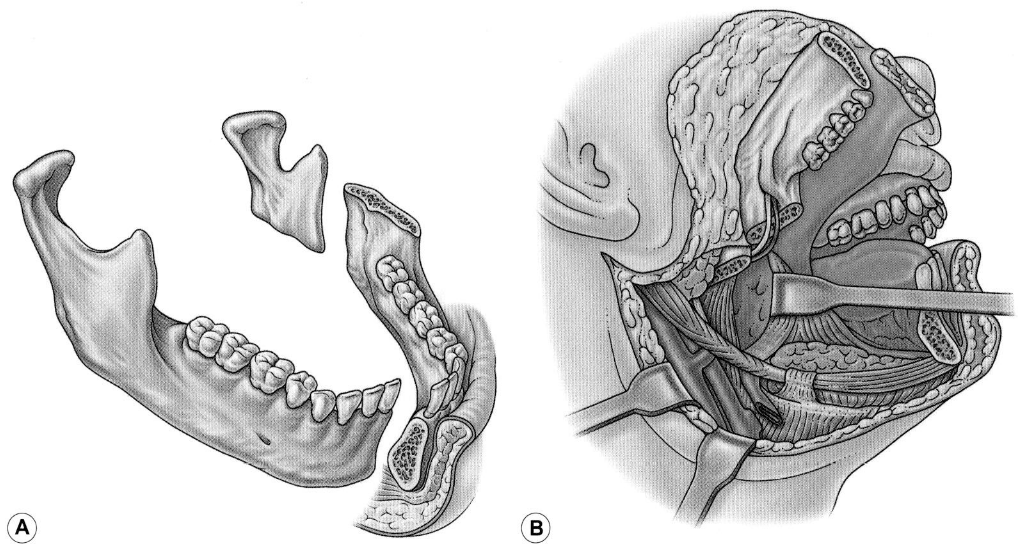

Fig. 4.23 The transmandibular surgical approach to the infratemporal fossa. (A) The sites for mandibular osteotomies. (B) The medial and lateral pterygoid muscles and the sphenomandibular ligament are detached, allowing the mandibular segment to be reflected superiorly to expose the infratemporal fossa while preserving the inferior alveolar nerve and vessels. Redrawn from Tiwari, R.M., 2002. Tumours and tumour-like disorders of the infratemporal fossa. In: Langdon, J.D., Berkovitz, B.K.B., Moxham, B.J. (Eds.), *Surgical Anatomy of the Infratemporal Fossa.* Dunitz, London, pp. 125–140.

Surgical approaches to the infratemporal and pterygopalatine fossae

A detailed knowledge of the infratemporal and pterygopalatine fossae is important in understanding and treating the damage that may occur from bony disruptions after maxillofacial trauma and orthognathic surgery. Of particular importance is consideration of the sphenoid bone that contributes to the roof and medial wall. Knowledge of the region is essential in gaining sufficient and clear surgical access to remove tumours and other pathologies from the region (the majority of tumours being contiguous or metastatic rather than primary). Neurosurgery may also require an approach to the cranial base via the infratemporal fossa.

Several surgical approaches are now available to expose the infratemporal fossa. These new approaches are possible because of advances in imaging and surgical techniques, including the development of rigid fixation systems that enable accurate replacement and retention of mobilised skull bones. Each surgical technique will involve the detachment and reflection of various skeletal elements (osteotomies). Two techniques are as follows:

- In the transmandibular approach the mandible is divided in the midline and along the ramus and is then reflected to expose the infratemporal fossa (Fig. 4.23).
- In the (subcranial) lateral transzygomatic approach the zygomatic arch is reflected inferiorly, after which a coronoidectomy is undertaken and the temporalis muscle is reflected superiorly (Fig. 4.24).

Explore online Self-assessment quiz to test and reinforce your understanding of the material in your free ebook. Follow instructions in the Inside Front Cover to unlock your access.

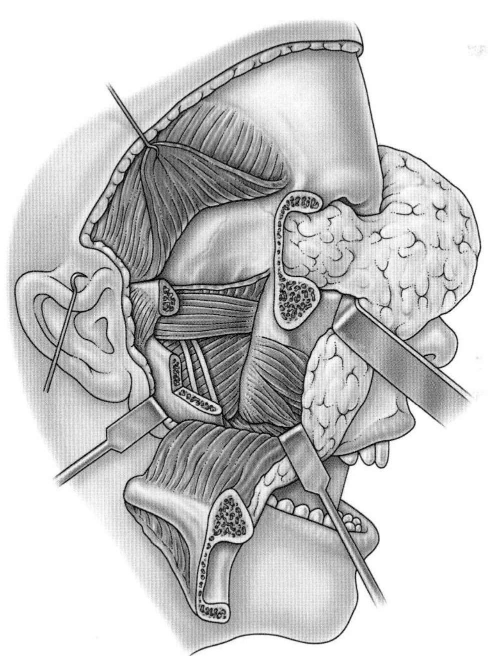

Fig. 4.24 The lateral transzygomatic surgical approach to the infratemporal fossa. This follows the reflection of the zygomatic arch inferiorly, coronoidectomy and the superior reflection of the temporalis muscle. Redrawn from Evans, B.T., Wiesenfeld, D., Clauser, L., Curioni, C., 2002. Surgical approaches to the infratemporal fossa. In: Langdon, J.D., Berkovitz, B.K.B., Moxham, B.J. (Eds.), *Surgical anatomy of the infratemporal fossa*. Dunitz, London, pp. 141–180.

Innervation of Oro-Dental Structures

Cutaneous innervation

(relating only to nerves supplying oro-dental tissues);

Infra-orbital branch of maxillary nerve – upper lip;

Buccal branch of mandibular nerve – cheeks ;

Mental branch of interior alveolar nerve (mandibular nerve) – lower lip

Innervation of oral cavity

Inferior alveolar nerve (mandibular nerve) for mandibular teeth and posterior, middle, anterior superior alveolar nerves (maxillary nerve) for maxillary teeth;

Tongue (see Mind Map 3.3);

Nasopalatine and greater & lesser palatine nerves (maxillary nerve) for palate;

Buccal nerve (mandibular nerve) for buccal mucosa and glossopharyngeal nerve at oroharyngeal isthmus. Labial mucosa infra-orbital and mental nerves.

Innervation of salivary glands

Parotid – lesser petrosal branch of glossopharyngeal via otic ganglion (postganglionic fibres with auriculotemporal nerve);

Submandibular and sublingual – chorda tympani branch of facial (travelling with lingual nerve) via submandibular ganglion

Motor innervation

Tongue muscles – hypoglossal nerve;

Muscles of lips and cheeks – facial nerve;

Floor of mouth (mylohyoid) – mandibular nerve;

Soft palate and oropharyngeal isthmus – mainly pharyngeal plexus

Mind Map 4.1 Innervation of oro-dental structures. n, nerve.

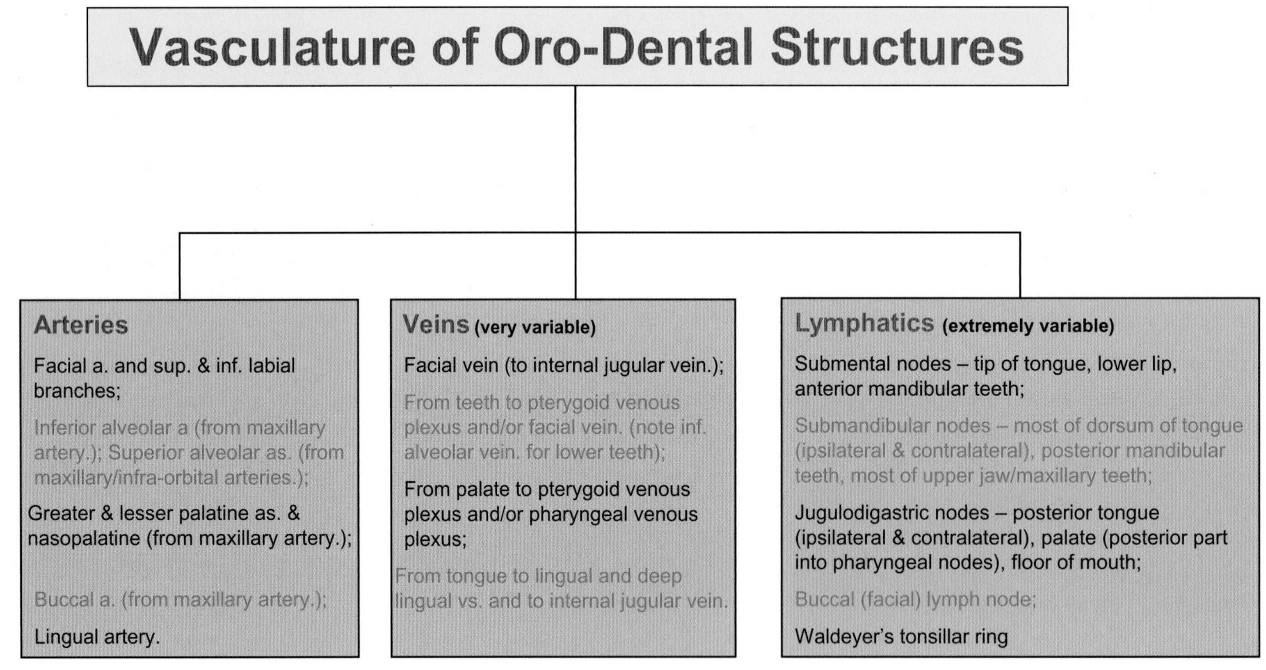

Mind Map 4.2 Vasculature of oro-dental structures. a, artery; as, arteries; v, vein.

5 Sectional anatomy of the oral cavity and related areas

The study of anatomical sections has become increasingly important in medicine with the advent of imaging techniques such as computed tomography (CT) and magnetic resonance imaging (MRI). Although these specialised techniques are available for some disciplines in dentistry, knowledge of sectional anatomy is important for all dentists because many of the procedures (surgical and anaesthetic) require good knowledge of the relationships of structures around the mouth. Thus the illustrations in this chapter (Figs. 5.1–5.7) provide sections through the head at various levels relative to the oral cavity and alongside corresponding magnetic resonance images.

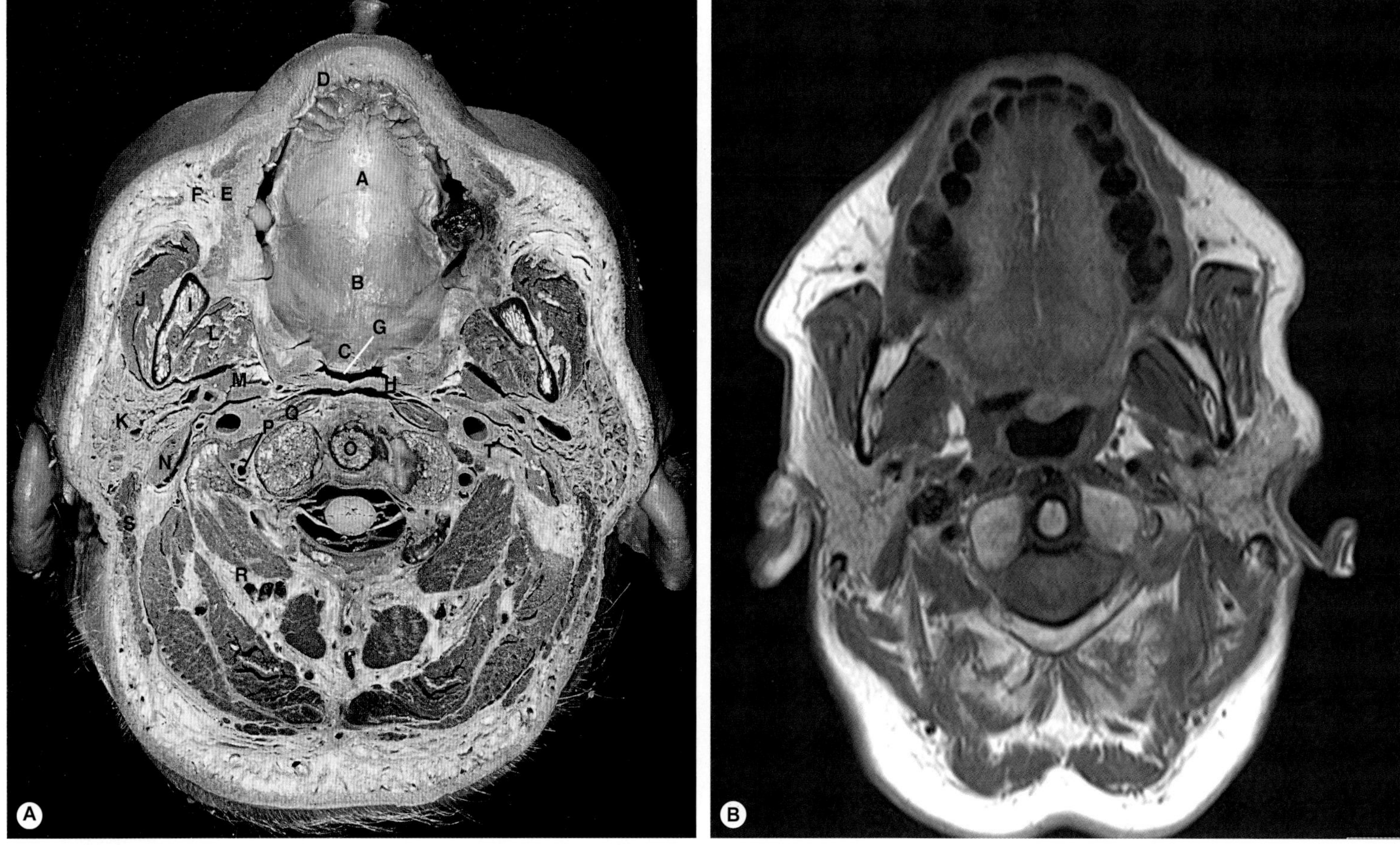

Fig. 5.1 (A) Transverse section through the head to show the palate and its topographic relationships. A = hard palate; B = soft palate; C = uvula; D = upper lip; E = buccinator muscle; F = buccal pad of fat; G = nasopharynx; H = superior constrictor muscle of pharynx; I = ramus of mandible; J = masseter muscle; K = parotid gland; L = medial pterygoid muscle; M = styloid group of muscles: stylopharyngeus, stylohyoid, styloglossus; N = posterior belly of digastric muscle; O = axis (second cervical vertebra); P = vertebral artery; Q = prevertebral muscles; R = postvertebral muscles; S = sternocleidomastoid muscle; T = internal carotid artery and internal jugular vein. (B) MRI scan of the head at the level of the palate. Courtesy Dr J Makdissi.

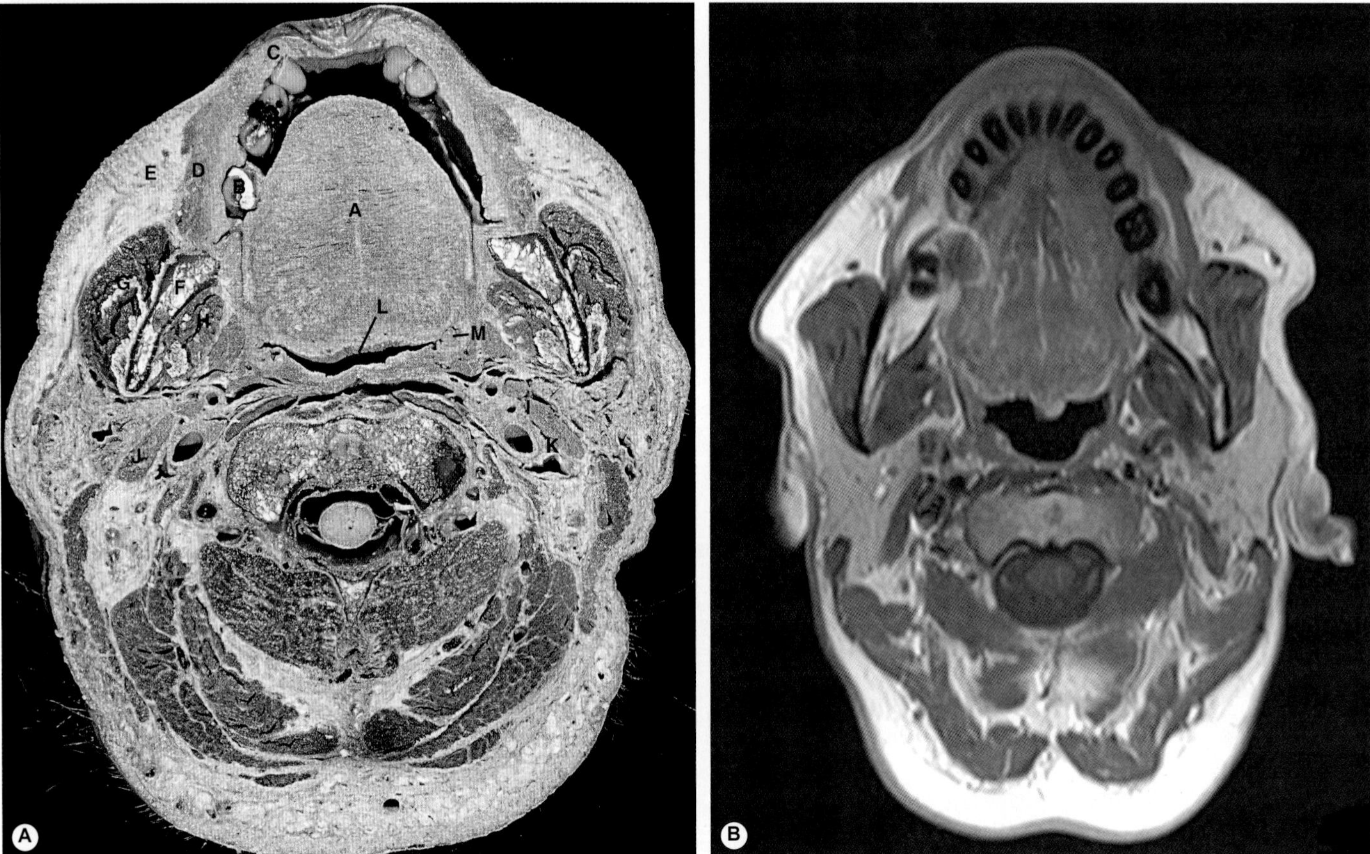

Fig. 5.2 (A) Transverse section through the head at the level of the palatine tonsil to show the tongue and its topographic relationships. A = tongue; B = mandibular molar; C = lower lip; D = buccinator muscle; E = buccal pad of fat; F = ramus of mandible; G = masseter muscle; H = medial pterygoid muscle; I = styloid group of muscles; J = posterior belly of digastric muscle; K = carotid sheath containing internal carotid artery, internal jugular vein and vagus nerve; L = oropharynx; M = palatopharyngeus muscle. (B) MRI scan of the head at the level of the tongue and palatine tonsil. Courtesy Dr J Makdissi.

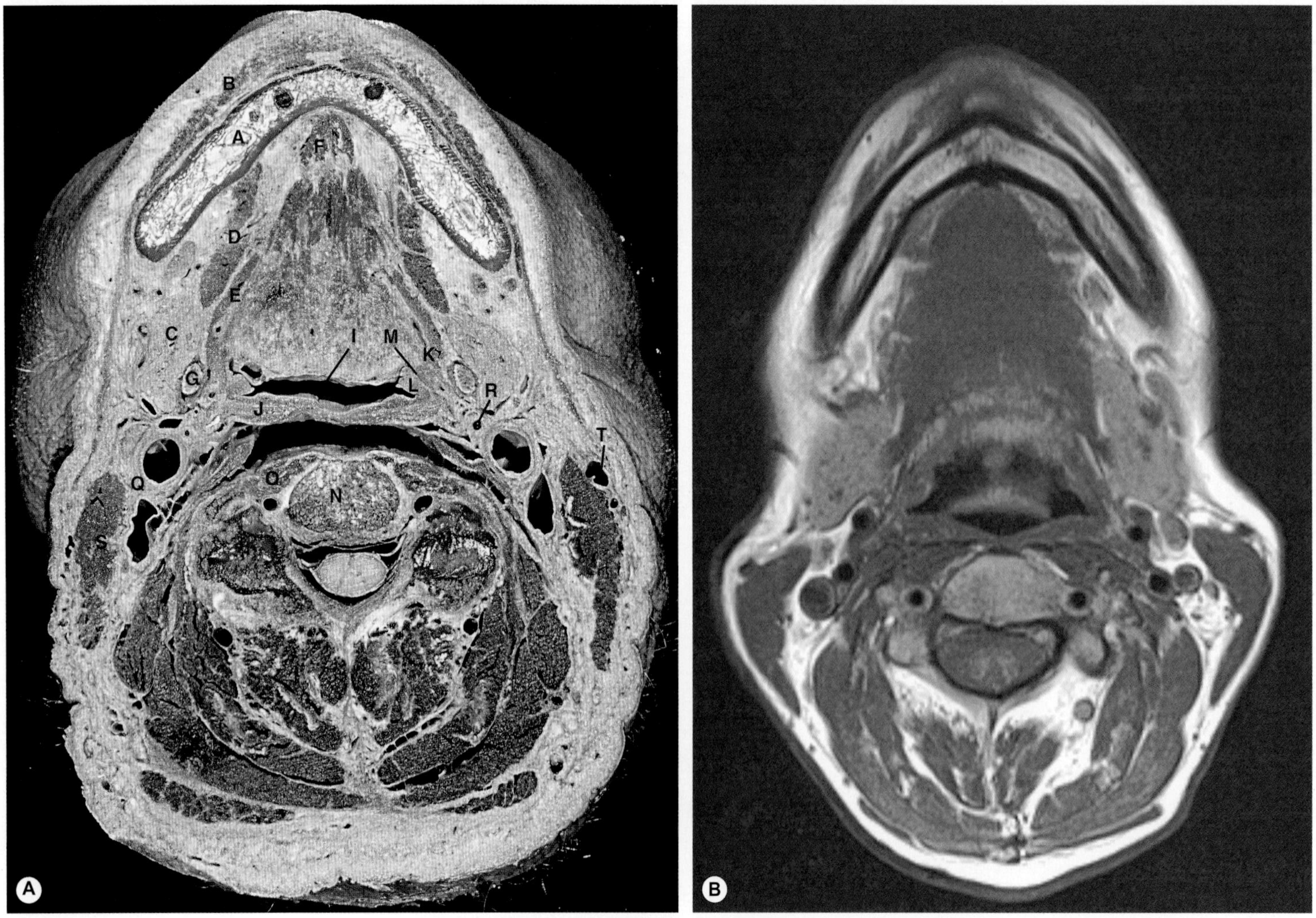

Fig. 5.3 (A) Transverse section through the head to show the floor of the mouth and its topographic relationships. A = body of mandible; B = depressor labii superioris and depressor anguli oris muscles; C = submandibular gland; D = mylohyoid muscle; E = hyoglossus muscle; F = genioglossus muscle; G = tendon of digastric muscle; I = oropharynx; J = middle constrictor muscle of pharynx; K = palatoglossal fold – anterior pillar of the fauces; L = palatopharyngeal fold – posterior pillars of the fauces; M = tonsillar crypt; N = cervical vertebra; O = prevertebral group of muscles; Q = carotid sheath containing internal carotid artery, internal jugular vein and vagus nerve; R = external carotid artery; S = sternocleidomastoid muscle; T = external jugular vein. (B) MRI scan of the head at the level of the floor of the mouth. Courtesy Dr J Makdissi.

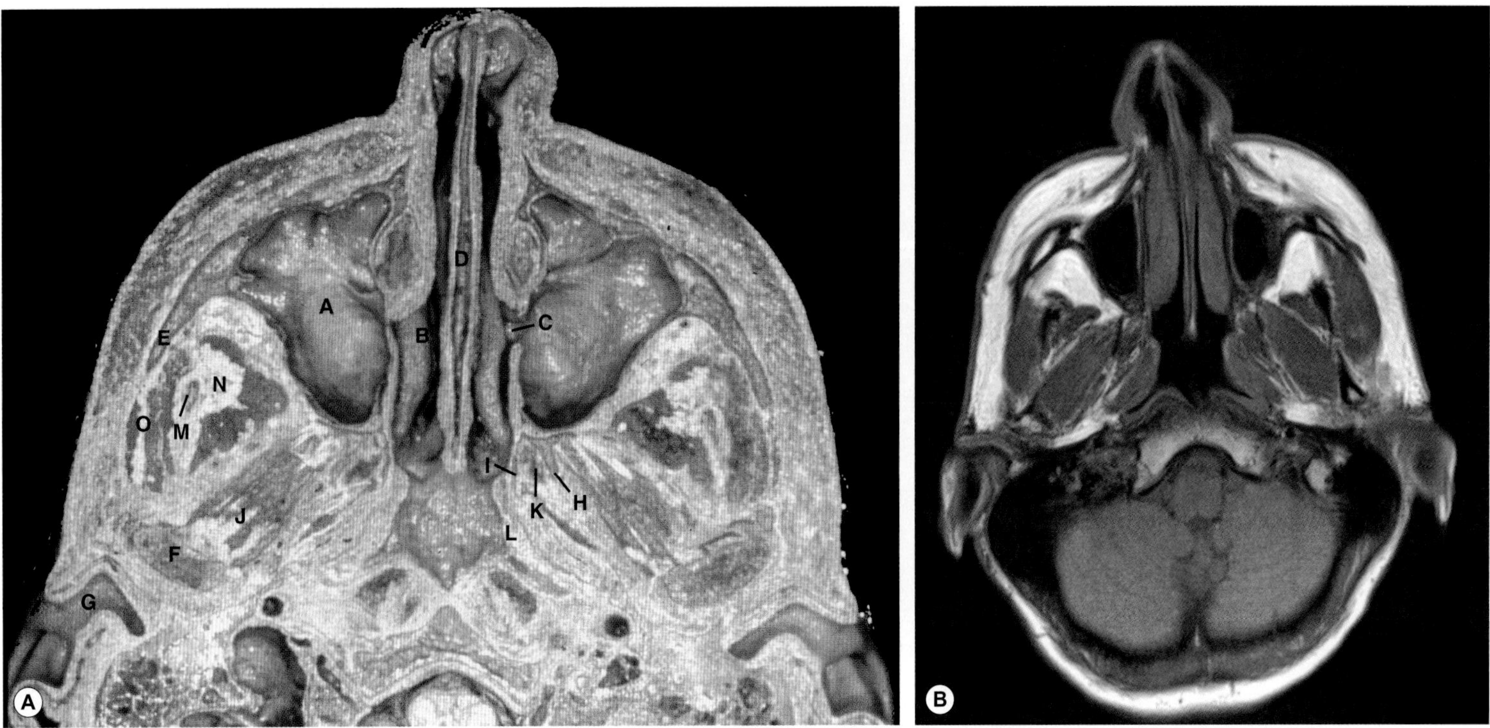

Fig. 5.4 (A) Transverse section through head to show the maxillary air sinuses and their topographic relationships. A = floor of maxillary air sinus; B = nasal fossa; C = ostium – opening of maxillary sinus into middle meatus on the lateral wall of the nose; D = nasal septum; E = zygomatic arch; F = condyle of mandible; G = external acoustic meatus; H = lateral pterygoid plate of sphenoid bone; I = medial pterygoid plate of sphenoid bone; J = lateral pterygoid muscle; K = medial pterygoid muscle; L = superior constrictor of pharynx; M = coronoid process of mandible; N = temporalis muscle; O = masseter muscle. (B) MRI scan of the head to show maxillary air sinuses. Courtesy Dr J Makdissi.

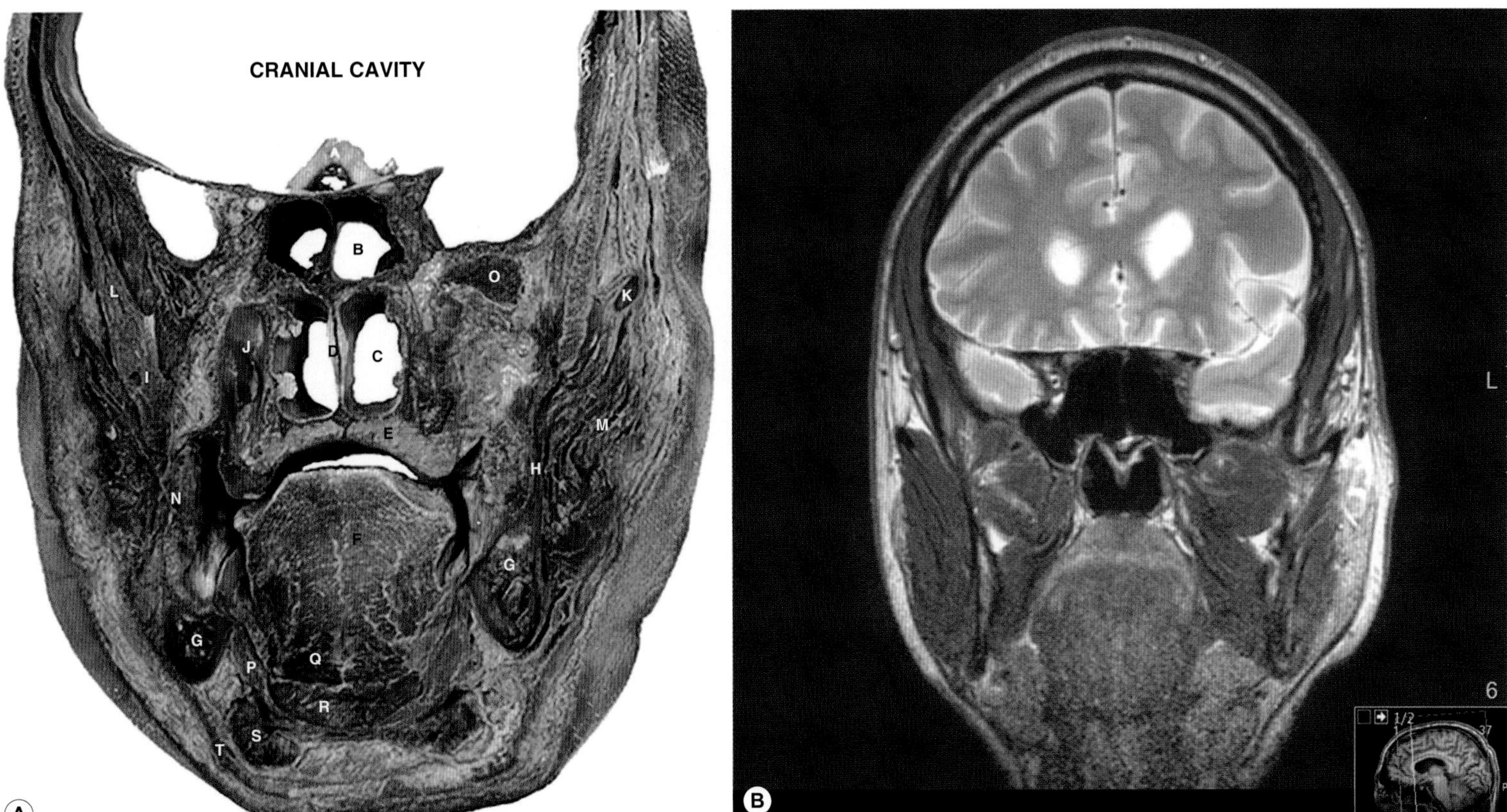

Fig. 5.5 (A) Coronal section of head to show structures at the level of the hard palate. A = optic chiasma; B = sphenoidal air sinus; C = nasal fossa; D = nasal septum; E = hard palate; F = tongue; G = body of mandible; H = ramus of mandible; I = tip of coronoid process of mandible; J = back of maxillary air sinus; K = zygomatic arch; L = temporalis muscle; M = masseter muscle; N = buccinator muscle; O = lateral pterygoid muscle; P = mylohyoid muscle; Q = genioglossus muscle; R = geniohyoid muscle; S = anterior belly of the digastric muscle; T = platysma muscle. (B) Coronal MRI of head to show structures at the level of the hard palate. Courtesy Dr J Makdissi.

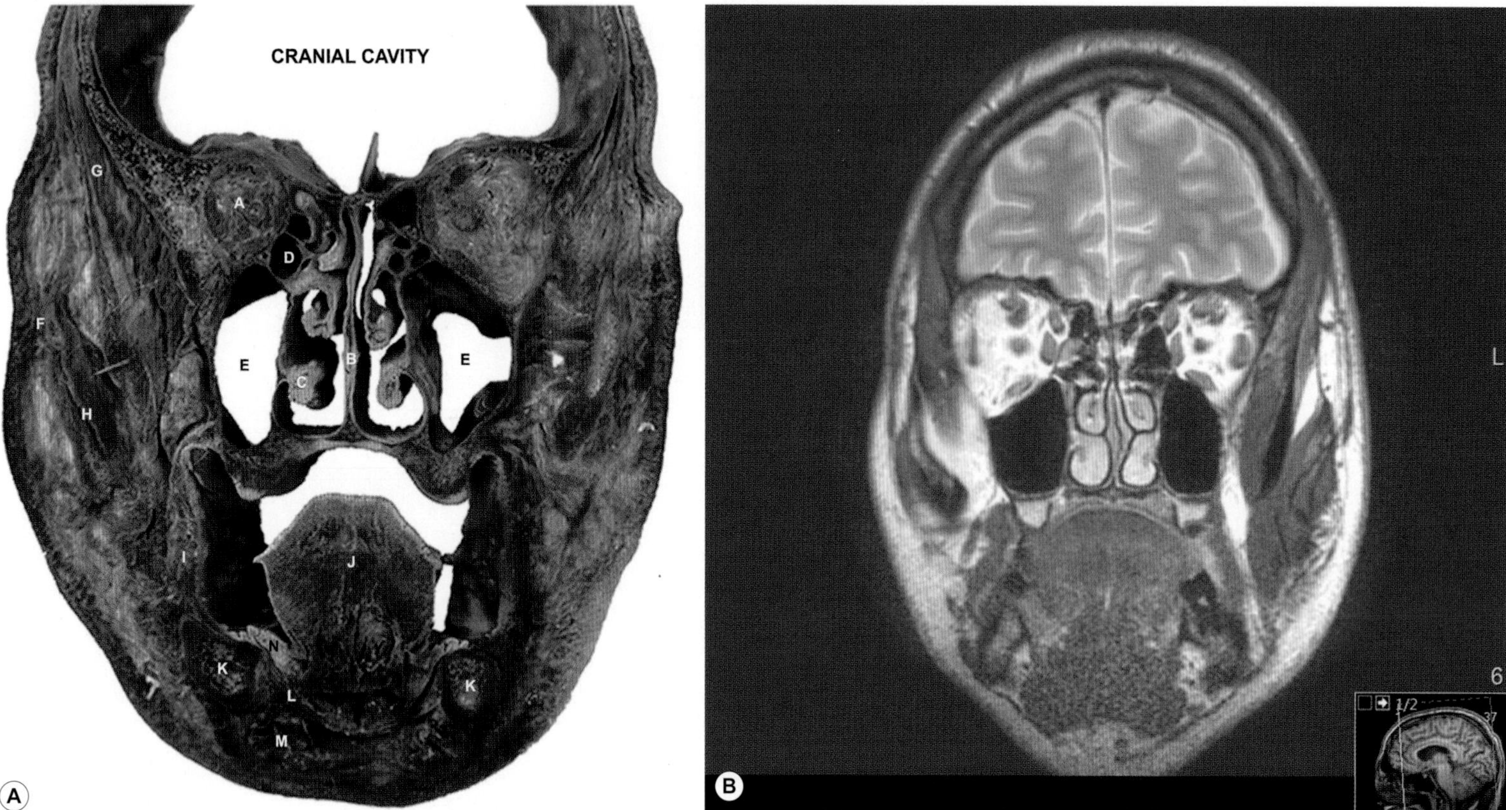

Fig. 5.6 (A) Coronal section of head to show structures at the level of the anterior region of the mouth. A = orbital structures; B = nasal septum; C = inferior concha on lateral wall of the nose; D = ethmoidal air cells; E = maxillary air sinus; F = zygomatic arch; G = temporalis muscle; H = masseter muscle; I = buccinator muscle; J = anterior part of tongue; K = body of mandible; L = mylohyoid muscle; M = anterior belly of digastric muscle; N = sublingual salivary gland. (B) Coronal MRI of head to show structures at the level of the anterior region of the mouth. Courtesy Dr J Makdissi.

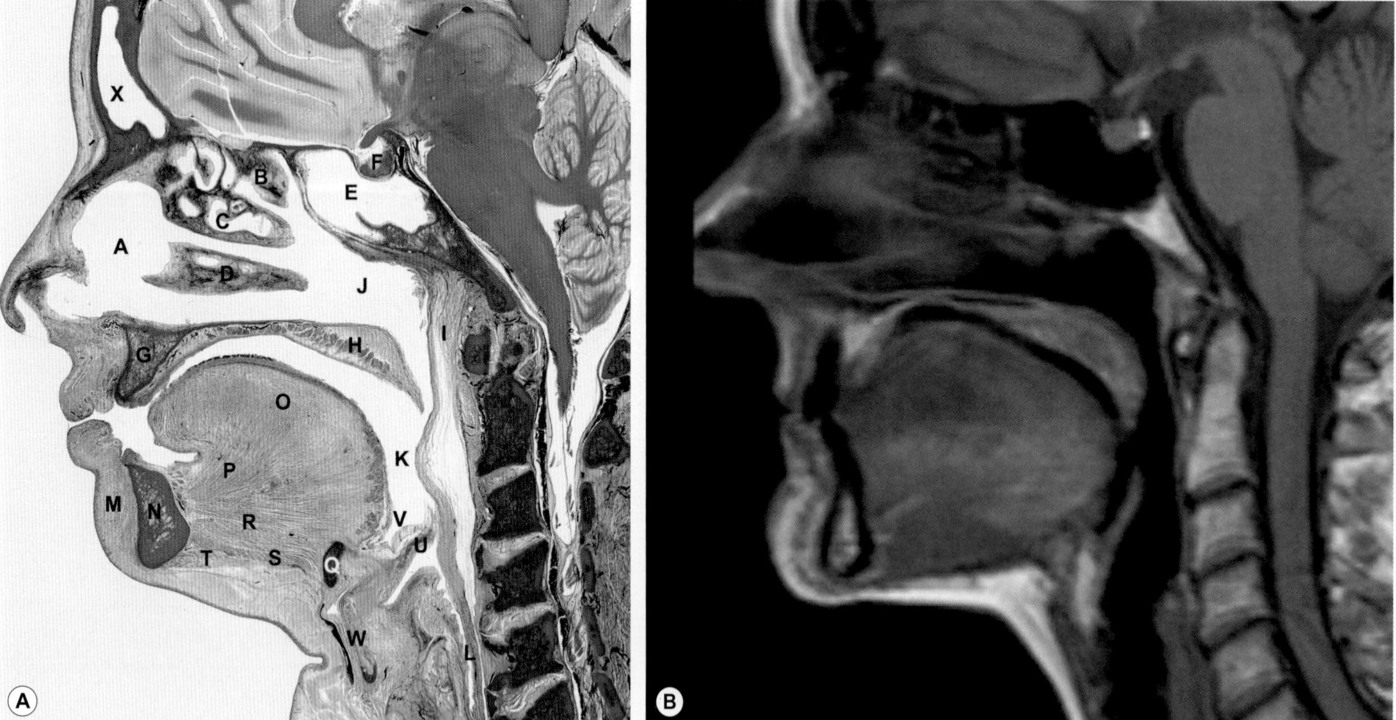

Fig. 5.7 (A) Medial sagittal section of head (plastinated specimen). A = nasal cavity; B = superior concha from the lateral wall of the nasal fossa; C = middle concha from the lateral wall of the nasal fossa; D = inferior concha from the lateral wall of the nasal fossa; E = sphenoidal air sinus; F = pituitary gland; G = hard palate; H = soft palate; I = superior constrictor of the pharynx; J = nasopharynx; K = oropharynx; L = laryngopharynx; M = lower lip and musculature; N = body of the mandible; O = intrinsic musculature of the tongue; P = genioglossus muscle; Q = hyoid bone; R = geniohyoid muscle; S = mylohyoid muscle; T = anterior belly of the digastric muscle; U = epiglottis of larynx; V = valleculae at back of tongue; W = thyroid cartilage of the larynx. Copyright the Royal College of Surgeons of England. (B) MRI of medial sagittal section of head. Courtesy Dr J Makdissi.

Functional anatomy

6

Mastication

Although it was once thought that all events that occur from the ingestion of food to the beginning of the swallow can be termed mastication, it is now thought that mastication is a term that should be confined to the act of chewing. Thus, mastication is the process whereby ingested food is cut or crushed into small pieces, mixed with saliva and formed into a bolus in preparation for swallowing. It is characteristic of mammals that possess teeth of different forms (heterodonty) adapted to the comminution of food. In non-mammalians the teeth are used mainly for prehension, the prey generally being seized headfirst and swallowed whole.

Various functions have been ascribed to mastication in humans:

1) It enables the food bolus to be easily swallowed.
2) It mixes the food with saliva, initiating digestion by the activity of salivary amylase.
3) It enhances the digestibility of food by:
   a) decreasing the size of particles to increase the surface area for enzyme activity and
   b) reflexively stimulating the secretion of digestive juices (e.g., saliva and gastric juice).
4) It prevents irritation of the gastrointestinal system by large food masses.
5) It ensures healthy growth and development of the oral tissues.
6) It releases particles that contribute to the senses of taste and smell.

Of all these, the increase in digestive efficiency is usually considered to be the primary purpose of mastication. Indeed, it has been suggested that there is an enormous gain in digestive efficiency without which the high rate of metabolism associated with homeothermy in mammals could not be sustained. However, the amount of mastication depends on the nature of the food ingested; solid substances are subjected to vigorous chewing before they are swallowed, whereas softer substances require less chewing, and liquids require no chewing at all and are simply transported to the back of the mouth for swallowing. Furthermore, some experimental evidence indicates that mastication produces little gain in digestive efficiency in humans. Table 6.1 classifies different foods according to the value of mastication in their digestion. The information in the table was obtained by research in which 1 g of either premasticated or unmasticated food was placed in cotton net bags, swallowed and subsequently collected from the faeces. Category 1 foods were those that left some large residues if swallowed with or without premastication. Category 2 foods left some residues when unchewed but were usually completely digested when chewed. Category 3 foods were likely to be fully digested with or without premastication. Thus, it is only for the few types of food in category 2 that mastication improves digestion. Because mastication produces little gain in digestive efficiency, this may simply be a reflection of the Western ability to select, grow and prepare foods so that all socially acceptable items of diet are inherently easily digestible.

Humans are omnivorous, being both meat and vegetation eaters, and human teeth are heterodont in that they have different anatomical forms and functions in different parts of the dental arch. The anterior teeth have sharp edges for grasping, incising and tearing foods; the posterior teeth are specialised for cutting flesh and grinding fibrous plant material. The teeth in humans are relatively unspecialised, in contrast with the specialised dentitions of carnivorous mammals, such as cats and dogs, or herbivorous mammals, such as horses and cattle. Nevertheless, studies of the cusps of posterior teeth in hominids and early humans have shown that they are worn down early in life, and that the occlusal surfaces are then flat and lack distinctive cuspal features. This suggests that the cusps of human posterior teeth may be more important in establishing tooth position and relationships during growth and eruption rather than having a dietary role.

Mastication occurs by the convergent movements of maxillary and mandibular teeth. In humans, most foods are first crushed by vertical movements of the mandible before being sheared by lateral to medial movements of the mandible. Indeed, the vertical and lateral jaw movements are similar to those of most herbivores but unlike pure carnivores that have only vertical movements. The initial crushing of the food does not require full occlusion of the teeth, and it is often only after the food has been well softened that the maxillary and mandibular teeth eventually contact. Once the cusps can interdigitate, the ridges on the slopes of the cusps shear the food as the mandibular teeth move across the maxillary teeth. As the cusps cross the depressions within the opposing occlusal surfaces, there is grinding of food, which has been likened to the action of a pestle and mortar. The food particles are progressively formed into a bolus by the tongue. Mastication does not, however, involve both sides of the jaws, there being a working side and a non-working side, with each individual person having preferred working sides.

Fig. 6.1 relates the morphology of the cheek teeth to the displacement of food during mastication. Several features common to all the cheek teeth provide protection for the adjacent gingiva during chewing. The marginal ridges bounding the interproximal edges of the occlusal surfaces of the teeth are important protective features. These ridges deflect most of the food, potentially driven between adjacent teeth by their opponents, onto the occlusal surfaces. The contact points beneath the marginal ridges

Table 6.1 Classification of different foods according to the importance of mastication in their digestion

Category 1	Category 2	Category 3
Roast and fried pork	Roast chicken	Fried and stewed beef fat
Fried bacon	Stewed lamb	Fried and boiled cod
Roast, fried and stewed beef		Fried kipper
Roast and stewed mutton		Hard-boiled egg
Roast and fried lamb		Boiled rice
Fried and boiled potatoes		White and wholemeal bread
Boiled garden peas		Cheddar cheese
Boiled carrots		

Modified after J.H. Farrell.

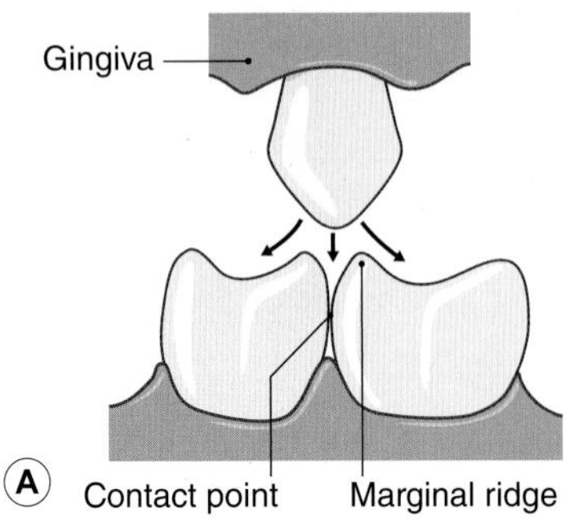

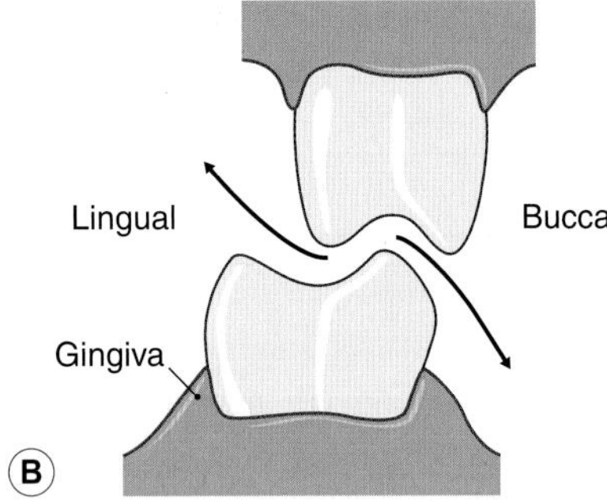

Fig. 6.1 Morphology of the cheek teeth in relation to the displacement of food (arrows). (A) Buccal view. (B) Interproximal view.

should abut firmly to prevent food being wedged between the teeth and above the interdental papillae. These contacts are maintained by the process of mesial drift (page 472), despite the constant attrition of interproximal dental tissue. The buccal cusps of the mandibular cheek teeth bite between the buccal and palatal cusps of the maxillary cheek teeth, with the result that food trapped between them is forced up over the palatal sides of the maxillary teeth and down over the buccal sides of the mandibular teeth. The palatal gingiva for the maxillary teeth is thus protected by the marked curvature of these teeth. In addition, it is the buccal surfaces of the mandibular cheek teeth that are the most curved.

Mastication is not simply a result of rhythmically closing teeth of a particular form on a piece of food. This would simply produce random breakage of food. Two other functions are essential: firstly, the placement of food between the occluding surfaces of the teeth by the tongue; secondly, the selection by the tongue of those pieces of food in the mouth that require further physical reduction. Other structural features associated with mastication that are peculiar to mammals include:

- temporomandibular joint (TMJ) jaw articulation
- serous salivary glands
- prismatic enamel
- secondary palate
- significant muscle development associated with lips, cheeks, tongue and muscles of mastication
- diphyodonty
- gomphosis type of tooth attachment

The evolution of an increased mass of the muscles of mastication allows the force of the bite to be increased, while the development of the TMJ articulation is associated with increased precision of more complex movements. Saliva adds to the moistening and lubrication of food during mastication, and its enzymes allow some carbohydrate digestion to commence at an early stage in the mouth. The prismatic arrangement of dental enamel (pages 139–143) and its greater thickness in mammals are said to be more efficient in resisting both masticatory loads and attrition than nonprismatic enamel. The development of a secondary palate is thought to be related to the necessity of maintaining ventilation during prolonged masticatory periods. The development of muscles within the lips, cheeks and tongue is associated with manipulation of the bolus within the mouth. The change from polyphyodonty (i.e., continuous tooth succession) to diphyodonty (two dentitions: deciduous and permanent) may be related to two factors: 1) a 'grinding-in' period necessary to produce an efficient cutting or grinding tooth surface, or possibly 2) the formation of a particular pattern of jaw movement by conditioned reflexes originating from stimulation of the periodontal receptors; it seems inefficient to replace such teeth too frequently. The gomphosis type of attachment (with a periodontal ligament; see Chapter 12) may be associated with the increased stresses and strains brought to bear on the tooth during mastication; it also allows for tooth movement. Such movement stimulates sensory receptors in the periodontal ligament, thus providing information on the loading and movement of individual teeth.

The forces that are exerted on the teeth and jaws are very large and physiologically significant. Normal maximum conscious, biting forces in humans, measured with a gnathodynamometer, have been recorded to be from 500 to 700 N between the molar teeth and 100 N between the incisors. However, forces of more than 1500 N have been reported, with as much as 4345 N recorded in a 37-year-old bruxist with hypertrophy of the masseter and temporalis muscles. It has been shown that the maximum molar force is achieved when the mouth is open and at approximately 50% of the maximum gape. However, experiments involving the implantation of force transducers into the occlusal surfaces of teeth have shown that the bite forces exerted during human mastication are considerably smaller, with a range between 70 and 150 N. The higher forces are achieved when eating harder foods (such as peanuts), and the lower forces achieved when eating softer foods (such as cheeses).

Rhythmic jaw movements (Fig. 6.2) are now generally accepted as being generated by a centre within the brainstem. This is referred to as an oral rhythm/pattern generator and is activated both by drive from the higher centres in the brain and by peripheral sensory input. The pattern of activity is distributed to the motor neurone pools, which also receive excitatory or inhibitory sensory inputs from a variety of peripheral structures. The hypothesis is that the sensory input generated by closing on hard food supports the generation of rhythmic jaw activity, whereas closure on a softened bolus promotes tongue movement and food transport, eliciting a swallow: the effect is to terminate the rhythmic jaw activity.

Chewing cycle

Mastication is dependent upon a complex chain of events that produce the rhythmic opening and closing movements of the jaws and correlated tongue movements. Mammals generally chew on one side at a time (there being working and non-working sides). Note that some foods do not require chewing and are soft and small enough to be reduced by squashing them between the tongue and hard palate. Two methods of chewing have been distinguished, depending upon the initial texture of the food and the stage in its breakdown:

- **Puncture/crushing**. Hard food is first crushed and pierced between the teeth without direct tooth-to-tooth contact. This results in wear (attrition) of the teeth, especially at the tips of the cusps.
- **Shearing stroke**. This method involves tooth contact that takes place only after the food has been sufficiently reduced. This type of movement produces attrition facets with characteristic directional scratch lines on the faces of the cusps.

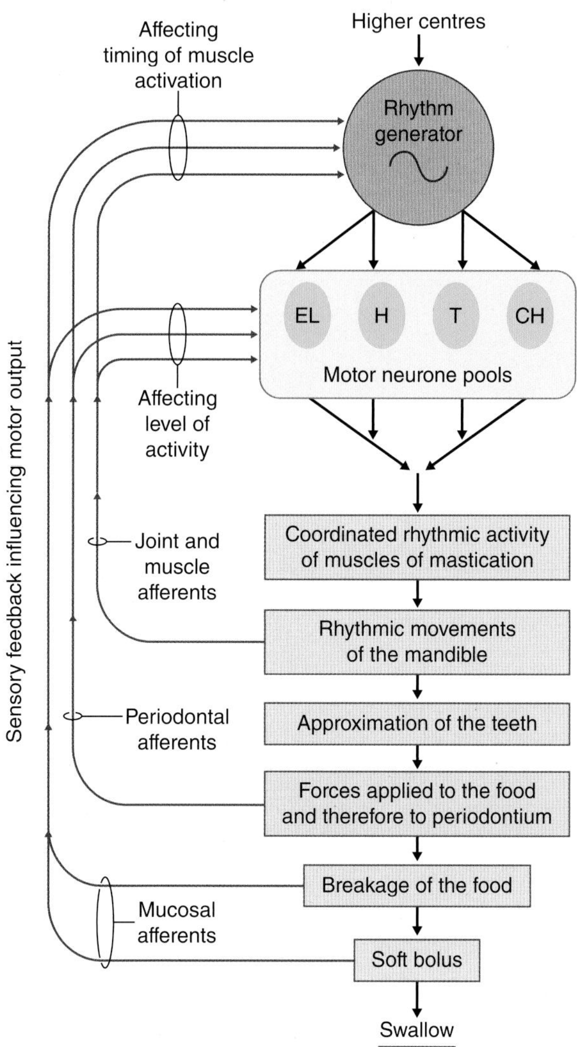

Fig. 6.2 A diagrammatic representation of the way jaw movements are thought to operate. CH = cheek and associated musculature; EL = jaw elevator musculature; H = hyoid and associated musculature; T = tongue and associated musculature. Courtesy Dr A Thexton.

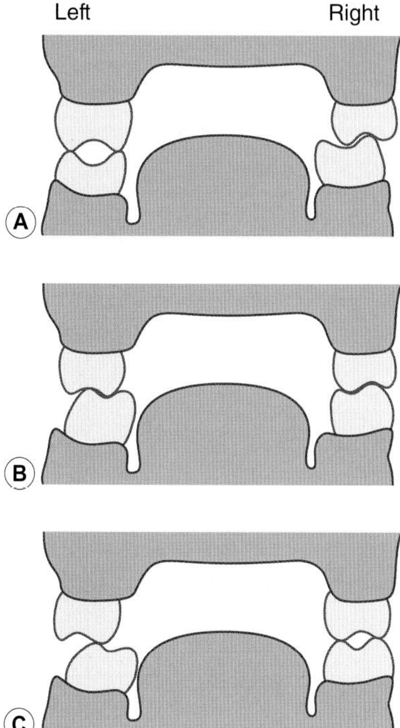

Fig. 6.3 Occlusal relationships of the cheek teeth during chewing on the left side. (A) Buccal phase on working (left) side. (B) Intercuspal position. (C) Lingual phase. Note the positions of the teeth on the balancing side (right).

The action of the teeth during mastication depends on their morphology, the movements of the mandible and the nature of the forces generated by the muscles of mastication. The chewing cycle involves three basic phases (or strokes) of the mandible in relation to the maxilla. From a position in which the jaw is open, the closing stroke results in the teeth being brought into initial contact with the food; the work done in this phase is really against gravity. This is followed by the power stroke, when the food undergoes reduction. Movement of the mandible in this phase is slower than in the closing stroke because of the resistance caused by the food, even though there may be vastly greater masseter and temporalis muscle activity during this time. Finally, there is the opening stroke, when the mandible is lowered, with an initial slower stage followed by a faster stage.

Fig. 6.3 shows the occlusal relationships of the cheek teeth during chewing (shearing) on the left side. From an open position the mandible is moved upwards and outwards, bringing the buccal cusps of the maxillary and mandibular teeth on the working (left) side in contact (Fig. 6.3A). As mentioned previously, the teeth may not contact each other during the initial masticatory cycle. In the power stroke, the mandibular teeth then slide upwards and medially against the maxillary teeth to momentarily attain intercuspal position (Fig. 6.3B). Following attainment of the intercuspal position, the mandibular teeth continue downwards and inwards against the maxillary teeth (the lingual phase, Fig. 6.3C). The opening stroke then follows and the cycle is repeated. The relationships of the teeth on the balancing side are also illustrated. Note that, while the teeth on the working side are moving through the buccal phase, those on the balancing (right) side are in the lingual phase but in the reverse direction. Although the diagrams show tooth contact, it is probable that any contact on the balancing side is only transient.

In primates (including humans), the chewing cycle differs depending upon whether the food is solid or soft (Fig. 6.4), and the number of chewing cycles also depends on the consistency of the food. Note that the vertical component of condylar movement results from its movement up and down the slope of the articular eminence (page 77). The first cycle has a profile that is commonly found when solid food is chewed. After a previous opening, the jaw accelerates into relatively fast closing (phase labelled 'FC'). At this stage, the food is being accelerated only against gravity, and the electromyographic activity in the jaw-closing muscles is of low amplitude. As tooth–food–tooth (TFT) contact is made, activity in the jaw-closing muscles increases and force is exerted on the food. The food resistance slows the jaw closing (SC). As the cusps continue to interdigitate, closing velocity slows to zero. The duration of this stationary phase is a matter of dispute. Because of uncertainty, the intercuspal phase (ICP) is shown as a dashed line. The jaw subsequently opens with a relatively constant velocity. There is relatively little movement of the tongue producing food transport towards the pharynx. The second cycle shown in Fig. 6.4 is characteristic of the ingestion of soft food. The closing phase consists largely of fast closing because the food offers little resistance to jaw closure. Opening now consists of two phases: slow opening followed by fast opening. The duration of the first phase of opening (slow opening) correlates with the amplitude of tongue movement and with food transport towards the pharynx.

A main feature of the chewing cycle described earlier is that its form is variable, depending upon the sensory feedback (see pages 121–123).

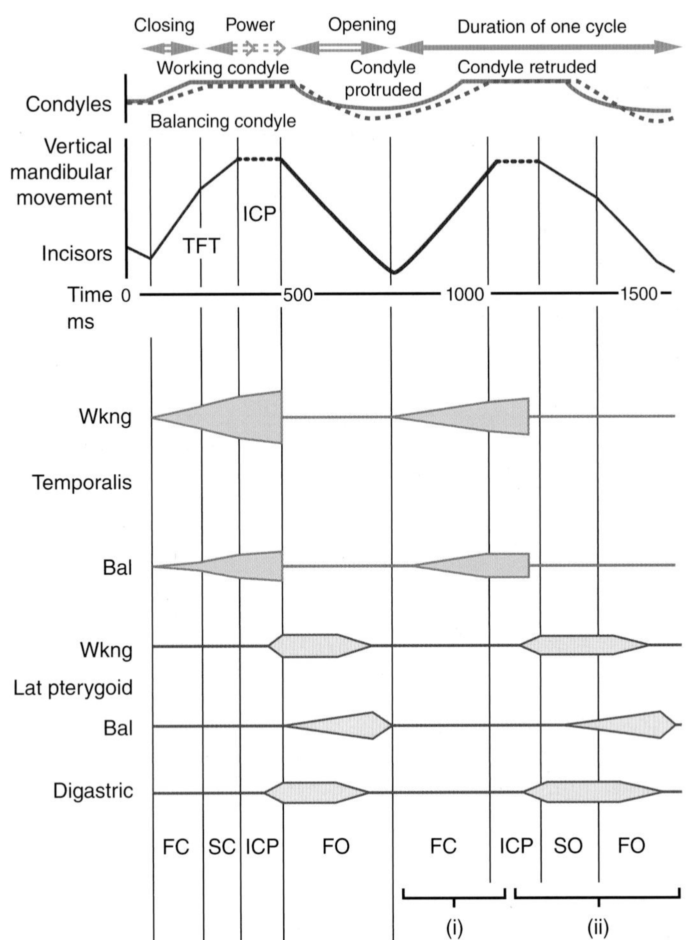

Fig. 6.4 Patterns of chewing cycle. Bal = balancing side; FC = fast-closing phase; FO = fast-opening phase; ICP = intercuspal phase; SC = slow-closing phase; SO = slow-opening phase; TFT = tooth–food–tooth contact; Wkng = working side. Courtesy Dr. A Thexton.

During the three phases of the chewing cycle, the lips remain closed together, providing an anterior oral seal (see pages 1–2), and although the main movements described earlier are vertical and horizontal in buccal-lingual directions, there are also possible movements in horizontal anterior-posterior and medial-lateral directions.

The chewing cycle usually follows immediately from what has been defined as 'stage I transport of food' in the mouth. When a piece of food is placed in the mouth or bitten off by the anterior teeth, the lips confine the piece of food and prevent it leaving the mouth by creating an anterior oral seal. The food is then transported by the tongue to the posterior teeth by a mechanism described as the 'pull-back' process. This takes about a second and is associated with retraction of the hyoid bone and narrowing of the oropharynx. If the food needs to be chewed, then a series of chewing cycles occurs as described earlier. The action of the tongue and other soft tissues in the mouth helps to control the bolus of food. At the end of the 'stage I transport of food', the tongue places the bolus on the working side of the mouth, and during the chewing process the bolus is kept on that side by the combination of rhythmic tongue and cheek movements. Sometimes the tongue will move the bolus from one side of the mouth to the other, thereby switching the working side. In each chewing cycle the tongue moves forwards and downwards to carry food onto its surface. This activity leads to a buildup of food at the front of the mouth and, after a time, this swallowable material is then moved towards the oropharynx by a process called 'squeeze-back'. In this process the tongue moves upwards and backwards against the hard palate, being accompanied by movement of the hyoid bone. The final movement of the food distally to the posterior

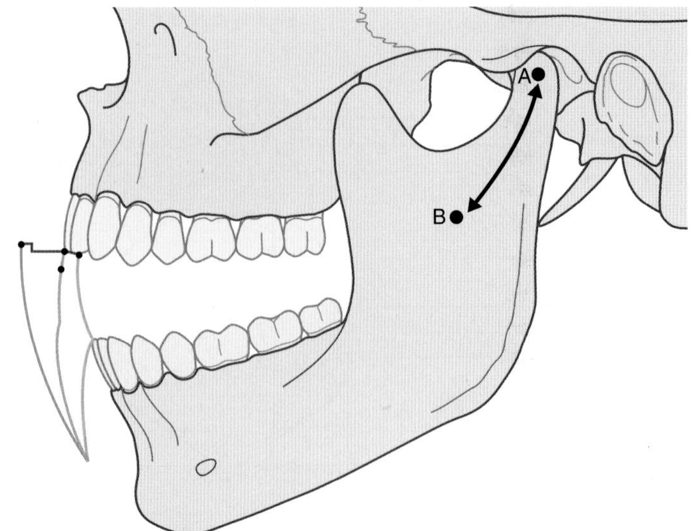

Fig. 6.5 The envelope of motion of the contact point between the mandibular incisors when viewed from the side (laterally and in the sagittal plane). See text for explanation of coloured trajectories and for the change in the fulcrum of movements from point A to point B.

surface of the tongue is called 'stage II transport of food' and is preparatory to swallowing (see pages 123–126).

Envelope of motion

The pathway followed by the mandible during chewing is termed 'the envelope of motion' (Fig. 6.5). This demonstrates the symmetrical mandibular movements produced during opening and closing of the jaw.

The envelope of motion is the volume of space within which all movements of a specified point on the mandible occur. The envelope is limited by anatomical considerations such as ligaments and tooth contacts. Most natural movements do not utilise this maximum volume but occur well within the 'envelope'. The yellow trajectory shown in Fig. 6.5 depicts a two-phased, conscious movement from the rest position to the fully opened position. The first phase is a hinge-like movement during which the condyles remain retruded within the mandibular fossae. When the teeth become separated by approximately 25 mm, the second phase of opening occurs and involves anterior movement or protrusion of the condyles down the articular eminences. The blue and red trajectories shown in Fig. 6.5 describe a biphasic path of closure from the fully opened mandibular position, which can be performed only with conscious effort. The first phase (the blue trajectory) takes the mandible up to a protruded closed position, while the second phase (the red trajectory) takes the mandible from this protruded contact position to a retruded contact position. The green trajectory describes the free, habitual, unconscious movement during both mandibular opening and closing. The points on the ramus of the mandible in Fig. 6.5 represent the centres of rotation during opening and closure. Point A is the fulcrum associated with simple hinge-like movements. The path described between points A and B represents the shift of the centre of rotation of the mandible; this shift occurs because of the transition from a pure hinge movement at the condyle to protrusion and rotation during opening (with the reverse during closing). Point B has been described as representing the point of rotation around the attachment of the sphenomandibular ligament at the lingula.

A 'profile' or 'envelope of motion' showing the average incisal movements in the frontal plane during a masticatory cycle is shown in Fig. 6.6. In this coronal plane (i.e., viewed from in front) the opening movement rarely goes straight down but deviates to one side. There is a wide variation in profiles between individuals and also continuous variation between

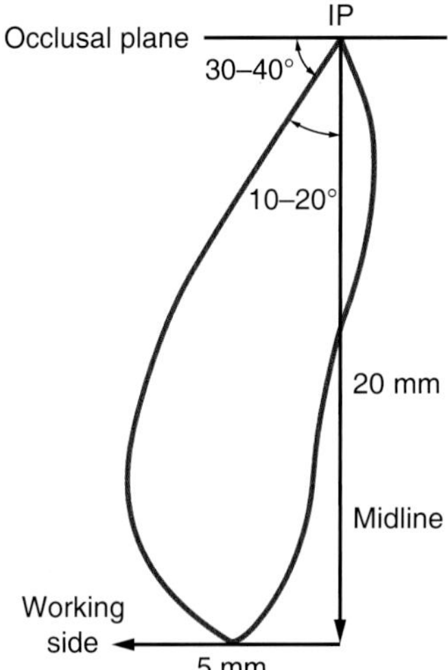

Fig. 6.6 Profile/envelope of motion showing the average incisal movements in the frontal plane during a masticatory cycle. Redrawn after Prof. J Ahlgren.

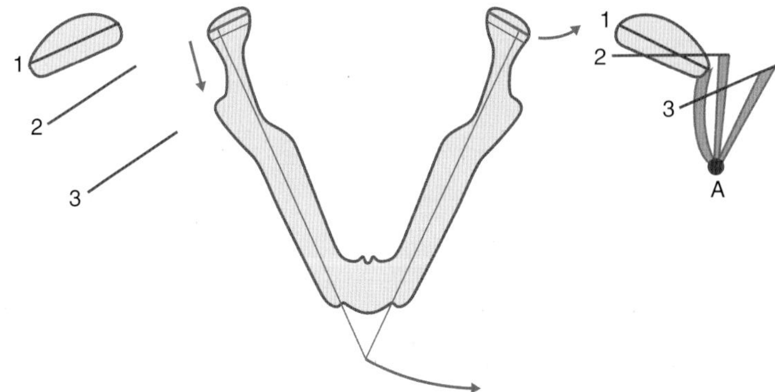

Fig. 6.7 Transverse movements of the lower jaw (lateral excursions or side-to-side movements). The thick blue lines represent the horizontal band of the TMJ ligament, and the red lines represent the mediolateral axes of the condyles. Movements of the condyles are shown for the working side (right) and the balancing side (left). The labels 1–3 show the beginning (1), middle (2) and end (3) of the lateral excursion. A = articular eminence. Redrawn after Prof. H Sicher and E L Dubrul:

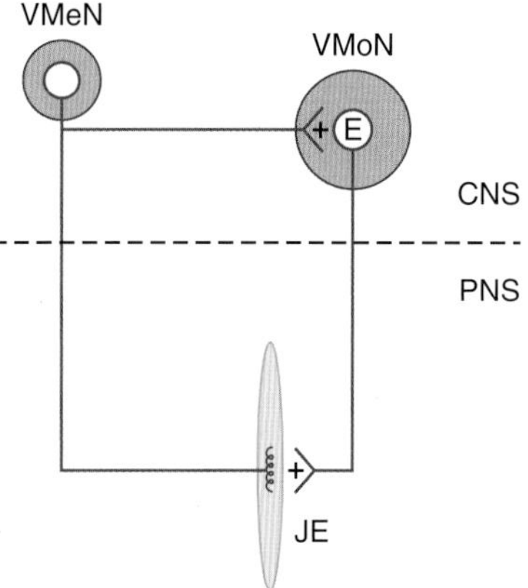

Fig. 6.8 Schematic representation of pathway of the jaw-jerk reflex. There are monosynaptic connections between afferent nerves and from spindles in the jaw elevator (JE) muscles and the motor neurones to these same muscles. Shaded areas represent brainstem nuclei. + = excitatory synapse; CNS = central nervous system; E = jaw elevator motor neurone; PNS = peripheral nervous system; VMeN = trigeminal mesencephalic nucleus; VMoN = trigeminal motor nucleus.

consecutive chewing cycles in the same individual: for example, the initial deviation may be towards the chewing side or away from it, as shown. Furthermore, the profiles differ according to the type of occlusion and the texture of the food.

The transverse movements of the lower jaw (i.e., lateral excursions or side-to-side movements as viewed from above) are illustrated in Fig. 6.7. These movements involve bilaterally asymmetric movements of the mandible. They are produced by protrusion of the mandibular condyle down the articular eminence of the temporal bone on one side with reactive movements of the other condyle (rotation around a laterally shifting axis). The illustration describes the changing positions of the long axes of the mandibular condyles during lateral movements of the mandible to the left. Fig. 6.7 also shows the change in the horizontal band of the TMJ ligament passing from the articular tubercle to the lateral surface of the condyle during lateral movements. A slight lateral shift in the condyle (Bennett shift) produces tension in the horizontal band.

Control of mastication

Mastication is regarded as a voluntary process involving the cerebral cortex and motor neurone areas in the trigeminal motor nucleus. However, little conscious effort is involved, and mastication is principally an automatic process very similar to breathing and walking. Mastication, breathing and walking are all now known to be controlled by 'neural pattern generators'. In the past, much controversy existed concerning the origin and control of the rhythmic activity of the jaws during mastication. One older view, the cerebral hemispheres theory, held that mastication was a conscious act, a patterned set of instructions originating in the higher centres of the central nervous system (in particular the motor cortex) and descending to directly drive the motor neurones within the brainstem (trigeminal, facial and hypoglossal motor neurones). Another older idea, the reflex-chain theory, held that mastication involved a series of interacting chains of reflexes. Accordingly, sensory input from the region of the mouth (e.g., pressure on the teeth) triggered the motor neurones in the brainstem to elicit a jaw-opening movement. In turn, this movement produced another sensory input (e.g., from stretch receptors in the jaw muscles), which resulted in a jaw-closing reflex. Although there are several well-recognised types of jaw reflex (Figs. 6.8–6.10), objections to the reflex-chain theory have been raised on the basis that mastication involves prolonged bursts of muscle activity and not the brief and abrupt behaviour usually associated with reflex activation of muscle.

Central pattern generator

The rhythm (pattern) generator theory has been proposed to explain rhythmic jaw functioning. This theory is based upon the proposition that there are central pattern generators (CPGs) within the brainstem that can be stimulated from either higher centres or sensory inputs in the region of the mouth, so that they are driven into rhythmic activity. This idea could account for rhythmic activity obtained by stimulating either the motor cortex or, in decerebrate animals and anencephalics (where the cerebral hemispheres are congenitally absent), the oral cavity.

A CPG is a set of closely interconnected neurones that generates a series of rhythmic outputs passing to the different groups of motor neurones involved in a particular movement (e.g., suckling, chewing). Consequently, each motor neurone group, and therefore each muscle, is activated at the correct time for that rhythmic movement. The exact location of the CPG for mastication is not known, but it is thought to lie in the pons, close to the trigeminal motor nucleus, maybe either in the medial reticular formation or within the trigeminal main sensory nucleus itself. The role of the CPG is to send out a sequence of appropriate signals to the motor neurones involved in directing the various muscles of

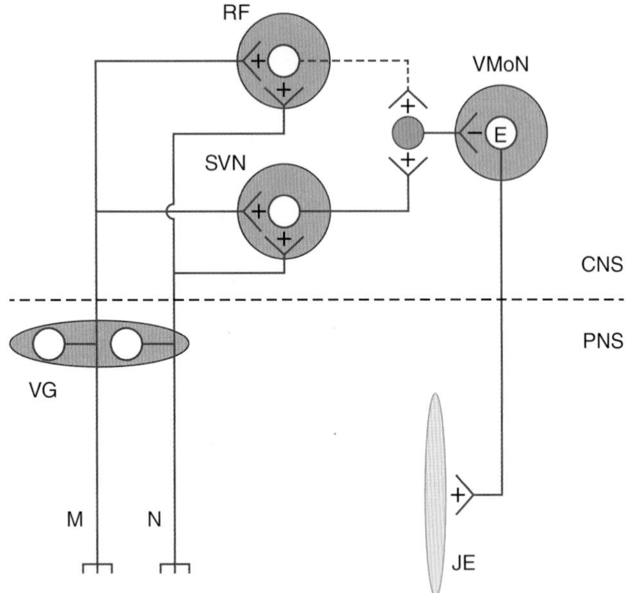

Fig. 6.9 Inhibitory exteroceptive jaw reflexes: schematic representation of probable pathways. These reflexes can be produced most effectively by stimulation of mechanoreceptors (M) or nociceptors (N) from the mouth and face. Two responses can be identified: a short-latency one mediated by a disynaptic or trisynaptic pathway through the supratrigeminal nucleus and a long-latency one mediated by a polysynaptic pathway through the reticular formation. Shaded areas represent ganglia or nuclei. Broken line represents uncertainty about the number of synapses involved in that pathway. + = excitatory synapse; − = inhibitory synapse; CNS = central nervous system; E = jaw elevator motor neurone; JE = jaw elevator muscle; PNS = peripheral nervous system; RF = reticular formation; SVN = supratrigeminal nucleus; VG = trigeminal ganglion; VMoN = trigeminal motor nucleus.

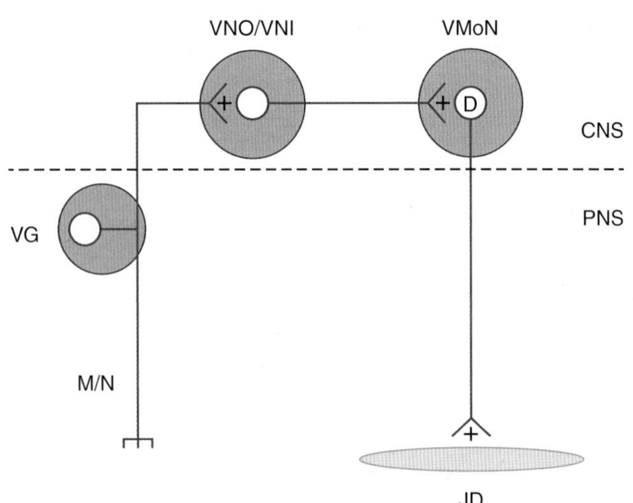

Fig. 6.10 Schematic representation of pathway of jaw opening reflex involving the digastric muscle. There are disynaptic connections between afferent nerves from orofacial mechanoreceptors and nociceptors (M/N) through the trigeminal sensory nuclei oralis (VNO) and/or interpolaris (VNI) to jaw depressor motor neurones (D). Shaded areas represent ganglia or brainstem nuclei. + = excitatory synapse; CNS = central nervous system; JD = jaw depressor muscle; PNS = peripheral nervous system; VG = trigeminal ganglion; VMoN = trigeminal motor nucleus.

mastication. This CPG determines the sequence of muscle actions, the order, the duration and the rhythm of the contractions and relaxations. These basic patterns, and in particular the strength and duration of the phases of movement, can be modulated by inputs from the mouth (such as the hardness or softness of the food and the size of the bolus), thereby slowing the frequency of chewing when encountering hard or tough foods or larger boluses. The masticatory rhythm can also be overridden or modulated by voluntary control. Descending pathways from the motor cortex may influence the CPG by switching on or off the process or by altering the duration of the chewing cycle themselves. There is also evidence that signals from higher centres may directly influence the trigeminal motor neurones to achieve a special effect, such as biting hard into food as a purely voluntary act. There is strong evidence that the CPG is also affected by signals from sensory receptors, particularly mechanoreceptors, in and around the mouth. These receptors not only provide feedback to the CPG but also provide sensory information to the somatosensory cortex regarding the physical state of the food in the mouth. This provides direct input into the reflex control of motor neurone activity during chewing. Mechanoreceptors within the periodontal ligament are particularly important in providing sensory feedback relative to biting forces. For example, if the periodontal ligaments of the premolars are anaesthetised, the maximum biting force for their subjects decreased by approximately 40%. Furthermore, anaesthetisation of the maxillary and mandibular incisors resulted in the ability to discriminate between differences in biting force to be significantly impaired.

The relative importance of the two sources of excitation of the CPG (i.e., conscious drive and the presence of food in the mouth) seems to vary with age. The human adult may be unable to feed at all after damage to the cerebral cortex, while in the anencephalic infant, suckling movements can be elicited simply by stimulating the lips.

While the cyclic activity generated by the CPG is subject to modification by sensory input from the mouth, if equivalent types of sensory input are generated experimentally by controlled stimuli applied to oral sites, then reflex responses can be generated quite independently of any pre-existing rhythmic activity. Whether a particular sensory input elicits a reflex, fails to elicit a reflex or modifies ongoing activity simply depends upon what else is going into the central nervous system.

In the last 100 years, at least a dozen oral reflexes have been described, forgotten and redescribed. In humans, the main jaw reflexes are those involving the jaw-elevator muscles, namely, the jaw-jerk reflex and the so-called jaw-opening reflexes.

Jaw-jerk

The jaw-jerk reflex (Fig. 6.8) is similar to the knee-jerk or stretch reflex seen when a tap is made on the patella tendon. This is the simplest reflex seen in the human body and is a so-called monosynaptic reflex because it involves only two neurones (an afferent and an efferent) and one central synapse. The jaw-jerk reflex can be elicited by a downwards tap to the chin, thus causing a stretch of the jaw-elevator muscle spindles (specialised stretch mechanoreceptors that lie in parallel with the extrafusal muscle fibres), which in turn produces a reflex activation of the same muscle in which they lie via their α-motor neurone. Although a tap on the chin is not a normal physiological stimulus, there is evidence that the jaw-jerk reflex pathways are present continuously to a greater or lesser extent during normal chewing. When the teeth are farther apart because of a large bolus or more solid food between the teeth, the jaw-elevator muscles and their muscle spindles will also be more stretched during the closing phase of the chewing cycle, thereby producing a greater excitatory input onto the motor neurone pool. This will in turn assist in the generation of a greater force in order to crush the food. The jaw-jerk reflex has been shown to be strongest during the closing phase of the chewing cycle or when there is resistance to jaw closing.

Jaw-opening reflexes

The jaw-opening reflexes are more complex (polysynaptic) and can be produced by applying mechanical or electrical stimuli to oral mucosa, periodontal ligament or teeth; the stimuli do not have to be painful to elicit the reflex, but stronger stimuli do produce correspondingly more

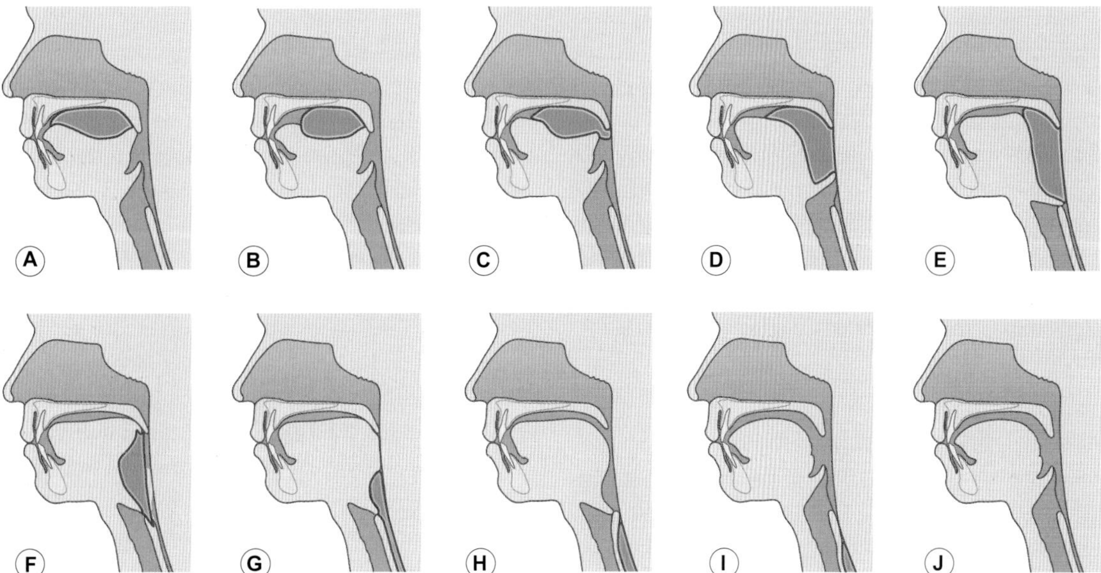

Fig. 6.11 The stages of swallowing: (A–C) oral stage, (D–F) pharyngeal stage, and (G–J) oesophageal stage.

vigorous responses. In humans the reflex is characterised by a brief period of inhibition of activity in the motor neurones of the jaw-closing muscles (Fig. 6.9). However, in other mammals (and in some neurological disorders in humans), there is also a simultaneous activation of the jaw-opening muscles (e.g., digastric and infrahyoid muscles) (Fig. 6.10). It is generally agreed that the inhibitory jaw-opening reflexes involve three or more synapses and thus have been termed polysynaptic reflexes. Inhibition of jaw-elevator muscles can have the effect of stopping jaw closing and can even produce a reflex jaw opening. Their importance in human beings is that they are thought to help prevent overloading of the teeth and muscles during chewing. They may also reduce the likelihood of injury from extremely hard or sharp objects within the food whilst eating.

There is some evidence that the same sort of stimulation, both mechanical and noxious, may, besides producing an inhibitory response, produce an excitatory response in the same muscle. It has been suggested that they may, like the jaw-jerk reflex, provide a feedback mechanism to the CPG during mastication to allow for different consistencies of food. It has been postulated that these inhibitory or excitatory influences depend on the phase of the chewing cycle (opening, closing or occlusal) at which the stimulus occurs, but so far no clear explanation has been given.

Jaw-unloading reflex

The jaw-unloading reflex is not a true masticatory reflex because it occurs during static biting on a hard object. However, it involves an act commonly experienced during the process of eating. This reflex occurs when a hard object is held between the maxillary and mandibular teeth, bitten upon and then suddenly breaks, thereby 'unloading' the jaw elevator muscles of the resistance against which they were biting. There is a cessation of muscle activity (relaxation) in the jaw-elevator muscles together with an activation (excitation) of the jaw-depressor muscles. One result of this is that the opposing teeth do not come clashing together and damage one another. Whether this is as a result of the reflex or because of the physical properties of the jaw-elevator muscles is not known. The exact mechanism is not clear, but it is known that we prepare our jaw-opening muscles for activation when we bite on something we know will eventually break, whereas we activate our jaw-closing muscles during biting. This leads to an active priming of the depressor muscles during the biting phase of this reflex.

Swallowing

Swallowing (deglutition) involves an ordered sequence of events that carry food (or saliva) from the mouth into the stomach. Although a continuous activity, swallowing is subdivided into stages for descriptive convenience. Humans swallow approximately 600 times every 24 hours, but only about 150 of these are concerned with food and drink; the rest simply clear saliva from the mouth. It is important to appreciate that, alongside muscle activity required to move the bolus, there must be mechanisms to protect the airway (e.g., closure of the nasopharynx by the soft palate, elevation of the larynx, closure of the laryngeal inlet by the epiglottis).

The size of the food particles alone does not determine whether a bolus is swallowed: it appears to be more dependent on the physical consistency of the food and whether it is well lubricated by saliva or other fluids.

The stages of swallowing

Although the act of swallowing is not discontinuous, classically it has been divided into three stages for descriptive convenience: the oral stage, the pharyngeal stage and the oesophageal stage (Fig. 6.11). At each stage it is necessary to consider not only the movement of the bolus but also how the airway is isolated from the food.

Stage I: Oral stage (the 'stage II transport of food' in the mouth preparatory to swallowing)

The jaw is elevated by the actions of the masseter and temporalis muscles, and the lips are approximated by the circumoral muscles to form the anterior oral seal. A longitudinal midline furrow is produced in the dorsum of the tongue by the bilateral actions of the styloglossus muscles inserted into the lateral edges of the tongue, by the vertical fibres of the intrinsic musculature and by the genioglossus muscles inserted close to the midline. The tongue is then elevated against the palate by the actions of the mylohyoid muscles, and the groove in the tongue is progressively emptied from front to back, moving the bolus rapidly towards the pharynx. The kinetic energy imparted to the bolus moves it towards the oropharyngeal isthmus. Here, the food accumulates on the pharyngeal surface of the tongue and in the valleculae waiting to be swallowed.

The airway remains open at this stage, with the soft palate lying away from the posterior wall of the pharynx. It is often suggested that, because the soft palate contacts the back of the tongue, a posterior oral seal is produced. During the processing of solid foods, however, the mouth is continuous with the oropharynx, and there is no evidence of a posterior oral seal caused by the lowering of the soft palate onto the posterior surface of the tongue. However, this posterior oral seal may be produced during the ingestion of liquids to confine the fluid to the mouth before swallowing. Liquids are swallowed from the mouth without 'stage II transport', in contrast with solids, which are swallowed both from the mouth and the oropharynx.

Stage II: Pharyngeal stage

During the pharyngeal stage the food is squeezed through the pillars of the fauces at the oropharyngeal isthmus by the so-called squeeze back mechanism. Within the pharynx, contractions of the circularly arranged pharyngeal constrictor muscles complete the movement of the bolus down towards the oesophagus. As the bolus leaves the oral cavity, the palatoglossal folds at the oropharyngeal isthmus contract behind the bolus. The tensor veli palatini and levator veli palatini muscles are activated so that the soft palate elevates to contact the posterior wall of the pharynx, closing the nasopharynx. The larynx is elevated and its opening is protected by the bulge of the back of the tongue and by being covered by the epiglottis, which is flexed mainly by the drag of the bolus (the actions of aryepiglottic muscles are weak in humans). The laryngeal inlet is also protected by closure of the glottis (although if food enters the larynx, then little protection from death by asphyxiation occurs because of closure of the vocal cords; viz. 'café coronary' syndrome).

Stage III: Oesophageal stage

Relaxation of the cricopharyngeal part of the inferior constrictor muscle allows the food into the oesophagus, where a peristaltic wave moves the bolus on towards the stomach. Once the bolus is in the oesophagus, the cricopharyngeal sphincter closes to prevent reflux. The passage of the bolus into the stomach requires relaxation of the lower oesophageal (or cardiac) sphincter. The airway is re-established during the oesophageal phase; that is, the soft palate, tongue and epiglottis return to their normal positions and the glottis opens.

The human swallow has traditionally been studied as a single, isolated event involving a voluntary swallow of a liquid on demand. This involves holding the liquid bolus in the mouth, contained between an anterior oral seal and a posterior oral seal, and then swallowing on command whilst measurements are taken. It is as a result of such studies that the three phases of swallowing have been described. However, swallowing is now regarded as a more complex process and comprises a subset of a continuous series of automatic events that transport food from the level of the incisor teeth to the stomach and involves, when necessary, a period of chewing of the food between the transportation of the food from incisor to stomach. The swallowing of liquids, in which no chewing takes place, is more like the traditional three-phase account. However, the swallowing of solids or solids mixed with liquids is more complex.

Solids or solids mixed with liquids are often chewed and can be transported through the oropharyngeal isthmus to the posterior part of the tongue before they are swallowed. The food bolus is often not a neat single piece of food but can be smeared over a large area of the mouth and oropharynx at any moment of time during eating. Food collects on the pharyngeal surface of the tongue and accumulates at the back of the tongue. The bolus of food that is eventually to be swallowed collects in the lower oropharynx and is in turn propelled through the laryngopharynx, past the laryngeal inlet and the relaxed upper oesophageal sphincter and thus into the oesophagus. The main difference between swallowing liquids or solids is that liquids are swallowed from the mouth and there is a true oral phase, but when solids or solids mixed with liquids are swallowed, they are swallowed both from the mouth and/or from the oropharynx in what would best be described as an oral and oropharyngeal phase. During the so-called pharyngeal phase, liquids are pushed through the oropharynx and laryngopharynx into the oesophagus, and solids and solids mixed with liquids are collected in the oropharynx and pushed through the laryngopharynx into the oesophagus. The so-called hypopharyngeal (laryngopharyngeal) transit time is normally less than 0.5 second; this is a critical time because this is when the food is passing the laryngeal inlet. During this time, breathing is inhibited, the hyoid laryngeal complex is raised and moves forward, the glottis is closed and the bolus pushes the tip of the epiglottis over the tracheal opening, and there is adduction of the vocal folds. All of these actions prevent food from entering the trachea. As the bolus enters the oesophagus, these changes reverse, and the larynx opens and breathing restarts.

During the oesophageal phase of swallowing, once the bolus has passed through the relaxed upper oesophageal sphincter, it then closes and the bolus is propelled the 25 cm (approximately) to the stomach by a process called peristalsis, a coordinated series of waves of contractions behind the bolus of the circular and longitudinal muscle layers of the oesophagus. This series of waves forces the food into the stomach through another relaxed sphincter called the lower oesophageal sphincter. This can take all of 5 seconds to complete.

Swallowing in the neonate and the 'vallecular space'

In contrast to the adult human, where swallowing and breathing cannot safely occur at the same time, in the human newborn and generally in other mammals (both infant and adult), the larynx occupies a relatively higher position (Fig. 6.12). In these cases the laryngeal opening is usually above the level of the soft palate, the lateral part of which extends around the larynx. In this situation, there is a degree of anatomical separation of the respiratory tract and the alimentary tract (in some animals the high larynx completely divides the pharynx into two passages, which pass laterally on either side of the larynx, rejoining behind and below it). The timed separation of swallowing and breathing is consequently less critical in this situation than it is in adult humans.

The anatomical differences between adults and neonates also produce differences in the way that the swallow is executed. In the case of the high larynx in the infant, the epiglottis contacts the posterior edge of the U-shaped soft palate, so that a potential space is formed, bounded above by the soft palate, behind by the anterior surface of the epiglottis/larynx, and in front and below by the dorsum of the tongue. During feeding, this space accumulates food before its onward passage via the pharynx and oesophagus to the stomach. The potential space (filled by the posterior part of the tongue; Fig. 6.12) includes the valleculae (the pockets formed between the epiglottal base and the surface of the back of the tongue). For convenience, this storage area will be referred to as the 'vallecular space'.

Growth in length of the human pharynx (starting a few months after birth) causes the larynx to take up a relatively lower position in the pharynx so that its contact with the soft palate is lost (Fig. 6.13). There is consequently no longer an enclosed space in which food can be stored or

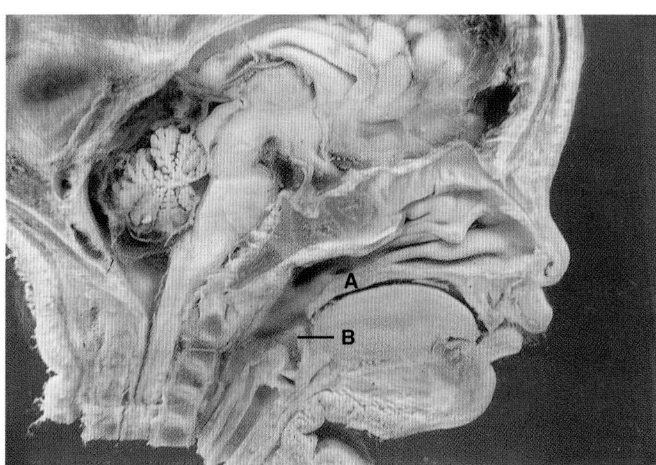

Fig. 6.12 Sagittal section of the head of a neonate. Note the relatively high position of the larynx, the opening being at the level of the soft palate (A). B = epiglottis.

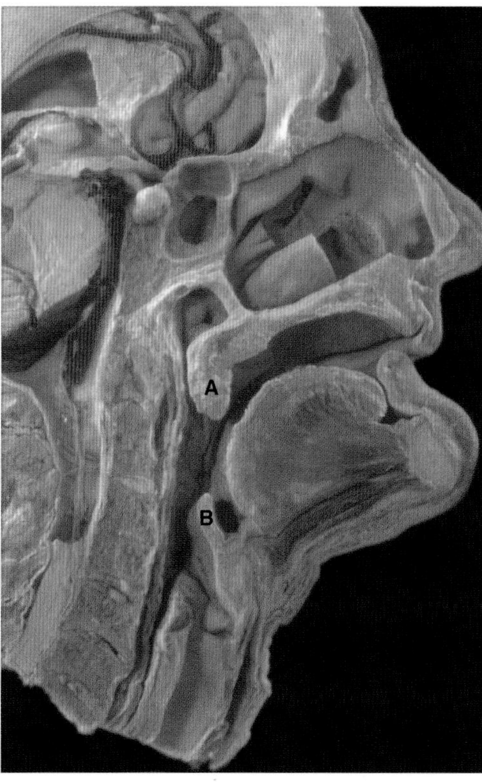

Fig. 6.13 Sagittal section of an adult head. Compared with Fig. 6.12, the opening of the larynx lies well below the level of the soft palate (A). B = epiglottis.

accumulated, and the airway is no longer anatomically separated from the food passage. A variety of measures operate to protect the airway during swallowing in this situation, including interruption of breathing, closure of the glottis, tipping the larynx forward so that the back of the tongue bulges over it during swallowing, plus bending of the epiglottis back and down over the laryngeal opening. At the same time the nasal airway is closed by elevation of the soft palate against an upper pharynx narrowed by the pharyngeal constrictor muscles. Because of the low position of the larynx, the pattern of swallowing in the adult human is the exception to the general pattern in mammals (at least in non-primate mammals).

For most mammalian (and human infant) feeding the 'vallecular space' is gradually filled during the course of a number of food transport cycles (which may include mastication where appropriate). Adequate filling of the 'vallecular space' appears to be the trigger for its periodic emptying. The contents then pass down the pharynx and oesophagus. Unless one includes all of the tongue and jaw movements involved in suckling, lapping or chewing that are associated with filling the 'vallecular space', the true swallow consists only of emptying that space and the subsequent movement of the bolus down the pharynx and oesophagus. In animals, the ratio of the number of cycles filling the 'vallecular space' to the number of cycles in which swallowing (vallecular emptying) occurs varies from about 2:1 to 14:1. The situation is different in the human adult where the descent of the larynx means that the 'vallecular space' no longer exists as a potentially closed cavity and storage area. In this situation, a swallow is initiated immediately as the first trace of food material or saliva enters the true valleculae. The question then becomes one of how vallecular emptying is triggered so readily in the adult human when (unlike other mammals where a significant amount of food is transported into the 'vallecular space' over a number of cycles) only a trace of food or liquid may have reached the region. Furthermore, in humans the movement of the bolus backwards from the mouth to the valleculae is followed by vallecular emptying generally on a 1:1 basis. Consequently, the transport of the bolus into the valleculae is regarded as part of the swallow and is classically described as the first (oral) phase of the swallow in adult humans.

Control of swallowing

In mammals generally, the neural mechanisms involved in swallowing depend upon sensory input from branches of the glossopharyngeal and vagus nerves that supply the mucous membrane of the 'vallecular space'. Through its internal laryngeal branch, the superior laryngeal nerve (a branch of the vagus) carries important sensory inputs from the larynx, epiglottis and valleculae; this is one of the most powerful sensory pathways involved in eliciting a swallow. In the case of the high larynx, swallowing can be elicited reflexly by fluid in the 'vallecular space' even when the brainstem has no connections with higher centres (as in decerebrate animals and in infants with anencephaly). It can therefore be assumed, firstly, that all the necessary neural components for swallowing are located in the brainstem. Secondly, it can be assumed that sensory input from the surface of the palate, epiglottis and tongue (the walls of the 'vallecular space' of animals and human infants) is alone sufficient to elicit a swallow. The generally accepted view is that the peripheral sensory input activates a set of neural circuits within the brainstem that collectively produce the pattern of motor activity constituting a swallow. These circuits constitute a CPG for the activity involving the 30 or so muscles that take part in a swallow. The relevant network of brainstem neurones receives not only peripheral sensory input but also excitatory fibres descending from the cerebral cortex, in this way being similar to the CPG for mastication.

In the adult human, where there is no longer an enclosed 'vallecular space' and no possibility of significant storage of food, the level of sensory input from the periphery must be less than that arising in other mammals. The initiation of swallowing in adult humans can, however, be explained on the basis of high levels of activity in the excitatory pathway descending from the cerebral cortex exciting the swallowing CPG, so that it requires only a trace more sensory input from the peripheral nerves to trigger the swallow. In other words, the descending drive lowers the threshold for reflex emptying of the valleculae. Because only a weak sensory input is necessary, only a trace of material has to reach the vallecula to elicit its emptying and all the subsequent components of the swallow. The lower threshold does, however, mean that other sensory inputs (e.g., glossopharyngeal) play a larger role in eliciting the swallow.

The CPG within the brainstem for swallowing is located in the medulla and consists of two parts, one located dorsally in the medulla (mostly in the nucleus of the solitary tract) and the other more ventrally in the medulla. The dorsal medullary pattern generator is largely responsible for receiving inputs which trigger the swallowing process and is responsible for generating the patterns of neuronal activity necessary for the contraction and relaxation of the muscles involved in swallowing. The more ventral medullary pattern generator is responsible for the inputs from the dorsal pattern generator and then relaying them to the appropriate motor neurones involved in swallowing (motor neurones of cranial nerves V, VII, IX, X, XI and XII, as well as motor neurones in the first three cervical segments of the spinal cord).

Swallowing can be inhibited by a voluntary mechanism which originates from the higher centres of the brain, most probably from the cerebral cortex. However, subcortical areas such as the internal capsule, the hypothalamus and the mesencephalic reticular formation have also been implicated in what has been termed voluntary swallowing.

Swallowing can also be initiated by a series of reflexes, by the stimulation of mechanoreceptors and chemoreceptors at the back of the mouth. These receptors are innervated by cranial nerves V, IX and X. The most important of these seems to be those innervated by the superior laryngeal branch of the vagus nerve (cranial nerve X), it being the only one that appears to initiate a swallow if it alone is stimulated. All the others appear to need facilitatory inputs from either higher centres or other peripheral nerves.

Speech

The acquisition of language, together with its associated processes of writing and reading, is probably the most complex sensorimotor developmental process in a person's life. Indeed, individuals can be readily recognised and distinguished by the distinctive features of their voice, which, in turn, relate to the special anatomical and functional characteristics of that person's 'vocal tract' (the region from the larynx to the mouth).

Speech is initiated voluntarily and involves a complex set of muscles around the mouth, the larynx and the throat. It also involves the interruption of breathing and the many muscles of expiration. Sounds are produced during exhalation and initially within the larynx ('voice box'), a structure that has evolved from its original purpose of protecting the trachea from inhaling food substances to enable the production of very complex sound patterns. This process is called phonation and involves the coordinated movements of abdominal, thoracic and laryngeal muscles. The major way of producing sounds involves using the air pressure provided by the lungs to cause the vocal folds of the larynx to vibrate, and the resulting sound is then altered by the variety of constrictions and openings in parts of the vocal tract. The process of speech production, speech transmission and speech perception is referred to as the 'speech chain', and it is the configuration of the human vocal tract that gives rise to the acoustic properties of speech.

Modification of this laryngeal sound to generate meaningful speech occurs principally within the resonating chambers of the pharyngeal, oral and nasal cavities (a process termed articulation). This section primarily describes the role of oral structures in speech, and the reader is referred elsewhere for detailed accounts of the role of the larynx.

The fundamental laryngeal note has a thin and reedy quality. This sound therefore contains a limited amount of speech information and thus is modified within resonating chambers (Box 6.1) acting as acoustic filters (amplifying selected frequencies and attenuating others by a process of sympathetic vibration) and by the activity of organs such as the lips, cheeks, teeth, tongue and palate. In addition, the relative positions of the maxillary and mandibular teeth (and therefore the position of the mandible) have important effects.

Classification of sounds

Phonetics is the linguistic science dealing with pronunciation and features the way in which phonemes are produced by the vocal apparatus. Phonemes are defined as the essential sequential contrastive units within a language and they therefore vary considerably between languages.

Sounds may be voiced (i.e., the vocal folds in the larynx vibrate for sound production) or breathed (i.e., the vocal folds do not vibrate). The two main groups of speech sounds are vowels and consonants.

Vowel sounds are modified by resonance, and all vowel sounds are voiced. They are produced without interruption of the air flow, the air being channelled or restricted by the position of the tongue and lips (Fig. 6.14). The range of higher harmonics defines or characterises the vowel sound. Closed vowels are those produced when the tongue is positioned high in the mouth, and open vowels result when the tongue is low in the mouth. Furthermore, front and back vowels are generated when the tongue is located forwards or backwards in the mouth.

A consonant is produced when the air flow is impeded before it is released. Consonants may be voiced (e.g., b, d, z) or breathed (e.g., p, t, s). Consonant sounds are of low amplitude (vowels are created by high-amplitude waves) and are classified in two ways: according to the place of articulation or according to the manner of articulation.

For the classification based upon the place of articulation (Table 6.2), consonants are categorised into bilabial, labiodental, linguodental, linguopalatal and glottal sounds. In bilabial sounds (e.g., b, p, m) the two lips are used. In labiodental sounds the lower lip meets the maxillary incisors (e.g., f, v). Linguodental sounds (e.g., d, t) involve the tip of the tongue contacting the maxillary incisors and the adjacent hard palate; for linguopalatal sounds the tongue meets the palate away from the region of the maxillary incisors (e.g., g, k).

For the classification of consonant sounds based upon the manner of articulation (Table 6.3), the degree of stoppage of the air flow is an important criterion. For example, a plosive consonant (e.g., b, p) requires sudden release of air. Note that, although one may describe the position

Box 6.1 **The vocal resonators**

The following spaces are present in the vocal apparatus, any or all of which might be available as variable resonating chambers:

1) Between the true and false vocal cords
2) Between the larynx and the root of the tongue, possibly involving the epiglottis
3) Between the pharyngeal wall and the soft palate and uvula
4) Between the dorsum of the tongue and the posterior surface of the hard palate
5) Between the dorsum of the tongue and the anterior surface of the hard palate
6) Between the tip of the tongue and the teeth
7) Between the teeth and the lips
8) The nasal passages.

of articulators for a particular vowel or consonant, there are no fixed positions during speech, only continuous movement. Both systems for classifying consonant sounds can be linked, as in Table 6.2. The configuration of the oral structures during consonant articulations is illustrated in Fig. 6.15. From this it can be seen that the tongue has a significant role during speech, although all oral structures (including the soft palate) are important.

Control of speech

Fig. 6.16 summarises the principal sensory and motor mechanisms in speech. As for other patterns of voluntary movement, speech originates in the cerebral cortex. However, several other parts of the brain, such as the cerebellum and the brainstem, together with sensory feedback, can modify and regulate the descending nerve impulses to the motor neurones that activate the various muscles involved in speech. The motor neurones involved are to be found in the brainstem, and their axons travel to the muscles of the vocal apparatus. Speech also depends on the coordination of the motor neurones in the cervical and thoracic parts of the spinal cord that innervate the muscles that are involved in breathing.

The main speech area of the brain is located within the temporoparietal region of the dominant cerebral hemisphere (i.e., the left cerebral hemisphere for a right-handed person) (Fig. 6.17). Fig. 6.16 indicates the many monitoring systems involved in the control of speech (such as hearing and proprioceptive information from the various muscles involved). Note that there has to be coordinated activity of respiration, laryngeal behaviour and oral structures to produce effective speech.

The first stages of speech (the formation in the mind of thoughts that need to be expressed, as well as the choice of words to be used) involve the functions of the sensory association area of the brain and, in particular, an area called Wernicke's area in the posterior part of the superior temporal gyrus. If Wernicke's area in the dominant hemisphere (the left hemisphere for a right-handed person) is damaged or destroyed, the person has what is termed Wernicke's aphasia, in which they are capable of understanding the spoken or written word but are unable to interpret the thought that it expresses or formulate the thoughts that are to be communicated. Another area of the cortex called Broca's area is involved in speech. Broca's area lies in the prefrontal and premotor facial regions of the cortex, about 95% of the time in the left hemisphere. Skilled motor patterns for the control of the larynx, lips, mouth, respiratory system and other accessory muscles involved in speech are all initiated from

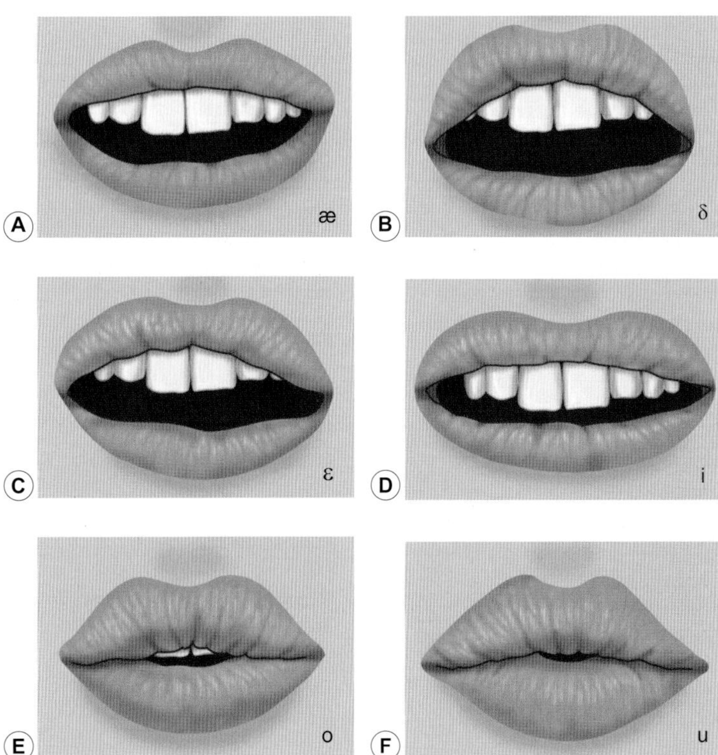

Fig. 6.14 Lip postures during the production of vowel sounds. (A, C, E) The short vowel sounds are shown. (B, D, F) The long vowel sounds are shown.

Table 6.3 Classification of consonant sounds based upon manner of articulation

Plosives	(p, b, t, d, g, k)	Require a complete stoppage of air
Fricatives	(f, v, th)	Require only a partial stoppage of air
Affricatives	(c, h, j)	Although involving only a partial stoppage of air, they require a rapid release of this air
Nasals	(m, n)	Require obstruction of the mouth with the nasal passages open
Laterals	(l)	Air forced to leave sides of mouth
Rolled	(r)	

Table 6.2 Classification of consonant sounds based upon place and manner of articulation

	Place of articulation													
Manner of articulation	Bilabial		Labiodental		Linguodentals				Linguopalatals					
	Dental		Alveolar						Alveolar		Palatal		Glottal	
Voicing	–	+	–	+	–	+	–	+	–	+	–	+	–	+
Plosives	p	b					t	D			k	g		
Fricatives			f	v	θ	ð	s	z	ʃ	3			h	
Affricatives							tʃ							
							tr	dr			j			
Nasals	m							n		ng				
Laterals								l						
Semivowels	w													

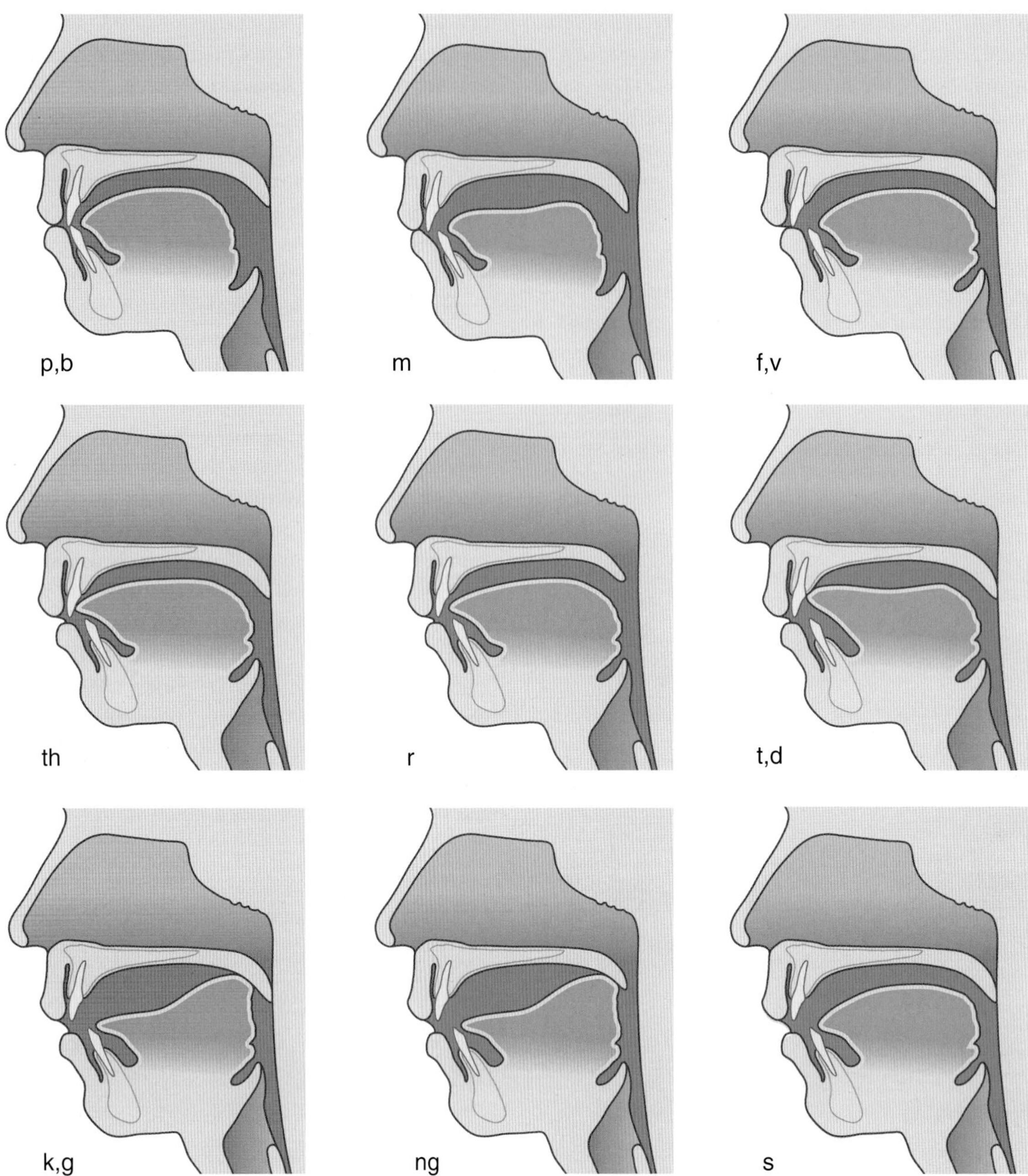

Fig. 6.15 Configuration of the oral structures during consonant articulations.

this area. Damage of Broca's area leads to the person being capable of deciding what he or she wants to say, but they cannot make the vocal system emit words instead of incoherent noises. This is called motor aphasia. Facial and laryngeal regions of the motor cortex activate the muscles involved in articulation, and the cerebellum, basal ganglia and sensory cortex all help to control the sequences and intensities of muscle contractions. Damage to any of these regions can cause either partial or total inability to speak distinctly.

That speech is probably the most complex movement in the body is indicated by the range of muscles involved, by the great number of nerves implicated and by the large areas of the cerebral hemispheres of the brain associated with speech (Fig. 6.17). The muscles involved include those in the chest that control breathing, the intrinsic muscles of the larynx that are concerned with phonation (i.e., those required to close the rima glottidis between the vocal cords, to put tension in the cords and to change the shape of the cords), the muscles in the pharynx and soft palate that help in resonance, and the muscles of the tongue, palate, jaws and facial musculature that produce meaningful speech. The nerves involved may include the intercostals and phrenic nerves; the recurrent laryngeal and superior (external) laryngeal branches of the vagus; nerves associated with the pharyngeal plexus; and the trigeminal, facial and hypoglossal cranial nerves.

The complexity of speech is further indicated by the fact that, although meaningful speech results from the bringing together of very simple sounds so that phonemes become syllables become words become whole sentences and concepts, the brain has to work in the opposite manner, so that whole concepts and ideas, if not entirely coherent sentences, have to be established before the physiological process of phonation and articulation. In addition, speech occurs alongside other means of communication – facial expression, hand movements, body posture – and requires feedback from the person(s) to whom one is speaking so that visual and auditory signals must be coordinated with speech.

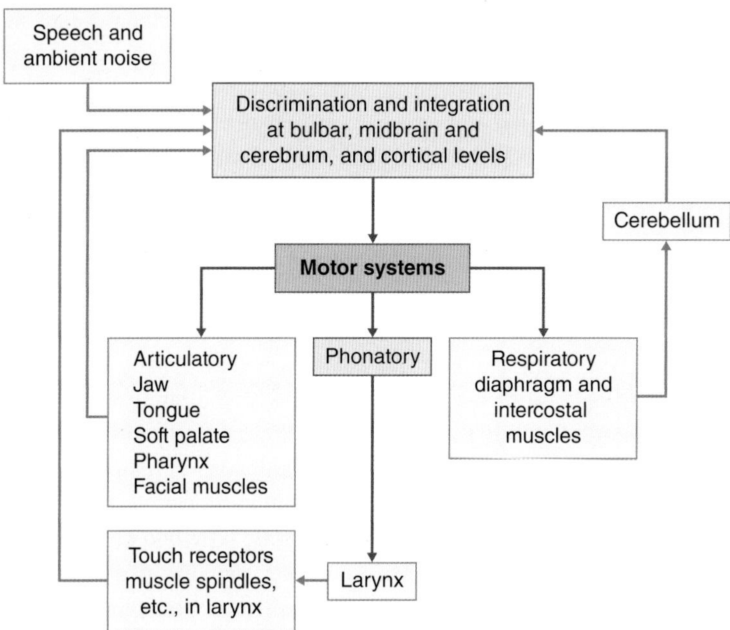

Fig. 6.16 The principal sensory and motor mechanisms in speech.

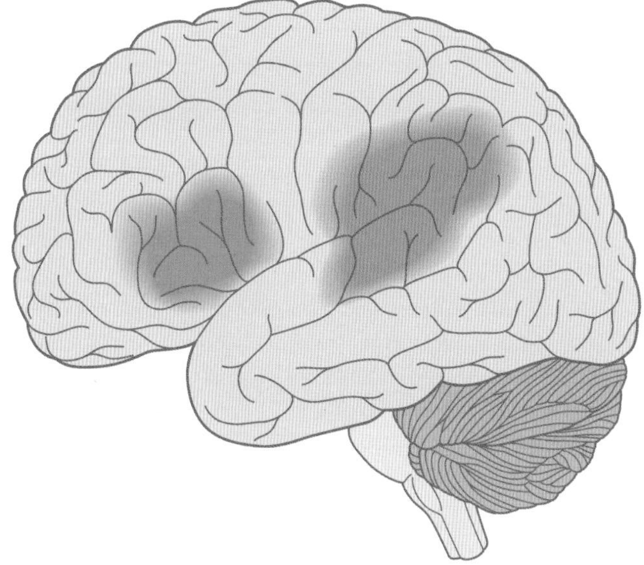

Fig. 6.17 Speech areas of the brain are located in the dominant cerebral hemisphere (i.e., left hemisphere for right-handed persons). The main areas are Broca's area (red), which is concerned with speech production, and Wernicke's area (blue), which is concerned with ensuring that spoken language is comprehensible. A third area (not illustrated), around the angular gyrus and posterior to Wernicke's area, is concerned with 'meaning'. In addition, the insula of the brain coordinates the activities of the speech areas. Note the large amount of the cerebral hemisphere given to speech.

The role of the tongue in the perception of taste and in thermoreception

The tongue is a muscular organ that, in addition to moving the food bolus around the mouth during mastication and into the pharynx during swallowing, is involved in the selection of food for ingestion (via taste) and with speech. In this section the role of the tongue in ingestion, in the sensation of flavours (including olfaction, as well as taste) and in thermosensation in the oral cavity is covered.

When we eat and drink, we experience a sensation that is commonly called taste, yet eating is a multisensory experience involving not only the chemical senses of taste (gustation) and smell (olfaction) but also the senses of texture and touch (mechanoreception), temperature (thermoreception), light (vision), pain (nociception) and even sound (audition). For example, when drinking champagne, we experience a combination of experiences – touch, fizziness, coolness, acidity, colour and exquisite smells, as well as the sound of the popping of the cork. Those who like spices in their food derive pleasure from the stimulation of receptors in the sensation of pain (nociceptors). These are stimulated by chemicals found in the common spices, such as chilli peppers, and the resulting sensation is referred to as the common chemical sense.

Taste (gustation) refers to the sensation experienced when chemicals come into contact with the gustatory end organs, the taste buds. Taste buds are embedded in the stratified epithelium of the tongue, soft palate, pharynx, larynx and epiglottis and are unevenly distributed around these regions. They are innervated by cranial nerves VII, IX and X. The lingual taste buds are associated with three of the four types of papillae (fungiform, foliate and circumvallate), whilst those associated with the other regions of the mouth are found on the smooth epithelial surfaces.

In humans the number of taste buds varies from person to person with on average between 2,000 and 5,000, but it can be as low as 500 and as high as 20,000 with no significant age or gender differences. The papillae in the different regions of the tongue have distinctive shapes and characteristic numbers of taste buds associated with them, as well as distinctive innervations related to their position on the tongue. Scattered over the main body of the tongue are approximately 200 small, mushroom-shaped fungiform papillae that have on average three taste buds each. The larger foliate papillae are found at the back and sides of the tongue. They comprise up to nine folds of epithelium and have as many as 600 taste buds each. Eight to 12 larger mushroom-shaped circumvallate papillae, each surrounded by a circular trough, lie at the back of the tongue in a V-shaped formation. The circumvallate papillae have on average 250 taste buds each.

Each taste bud is connected, at its base, by terminals of sensory nerve fibres. The nerve supply for most of the taste buds on the soft palate and on the anterior two-thirds of the tongue comes from a division of cranial nerve VII (the facial nerve), called the chorda tympani, because its route to the brainstem passes close to the tympanic membrane in the ear. Cranial nerve IX (the glossopharyngeal nerve) innervates the taste buds on the posterior third of the tongue and at the back of the mouth, whilst cranial nerve X (the vagus nerve) innervates taste buds in the pharynx and epiglottis.

Each taste bud is composed of 50–150 neuroepithelial cells arranged like the segments of an orange in a compact, pear-shaped structure (intragemmal cells). The taste bud complex is about 70 μm high and 40 μm in diameter and has a small 2- to 10-μm opening at the epithelial surface, called the taste pore, which allows direct contact between the chemicals dissolved in the saliva and the small tips of some of the neuroepithelial receptor cells within the taste bud. The exposed parts of the receptor cells are made up of many long corrugated folds in the membrane called microvilli and provide a large surface area for contact with the chemicals dissolved in the saliva. Saliva is essential for normal taste because it acts as the solvent for the chemicals, as well as a transport medium for the chemicals to reach the receptors. There is a layer of saliva that extends into the taste pore and that constantly bathes the receptor tips. The dissolved chemicals diffuse through this thin layer to reach the microvilli.

There is general agreement that there are four types of intragemmal cell: basal cells (stem cells) that give rise to the receptor cells, type I (dark) cells, intermediate cells and type II (light) cells. It has been suggested that these different types represent the separate stages in the life cycle of the taste receptor cell.

The taste bud complex is an extremely dynamic system in which there is a rapid turnover of receptor cells. The life span of an individual receptor cell is approximately 10 days, with cells being continually born through the division of epithelial stem cells (basal cells) within the bud, maturing, performing their gustatory function and then eventually dying.

The receptor cells do not in themselves have an axon or nerve fibre, but the base of each cell has specialised regions that look like terminals of nerve fibres. The cytoplasm at the base of the cell is packed with small vesicles filled with a chemical transmitter substance (possibly serotonin or vasoactive intestinal peptide), which is released when the potential inside becomes more positive (becomes depolarised). In most cases the depolarisation leads to an action potential followed by an increase in intracellular Ca^{2+} within the cell and the subsequent release of the neurotransmitter. In close association with these regions are the endings of the sensory nerve fibres (intragemmal nerve fibres) which make a synaptic-like connection with the receptor cells. The released neurotransmitter elicits generator potentials and action potentials in this primary afferent neurone, thereby transmitting impulses into the central nervous system. Each taste bud is innervated by more than one nerve fibre, and each single nerve fibre can innervate several receptor cells, taste buds and even papillae. This means that there is a high degree of convergence of inputs from taste buds onto the sensory nerve fibres. Because there is a rapid turnover of receptor cells, there are also constantly changing connections between the cells and the nerve fibres. The nerves are continually sprouting new processes, forming new synapses with young cells and retracting synaptic connections with dying cells. It has been calculated that, at any one time, less than one-third of the cells in a single taste bud are fully innervated. It has been shown that an intact nerve supply is necessary for the normal survival and function of taste buds. If the nerve supply is cut or damaged, the taste buds degenerate and slough off. After nerve regeneration, the taste buds reappear and can return to normal function.

Since Aristotle (384–322 BCE), there have been attempts to categorise taste into primary or basic qualities of taste. Although many hundreds of different chemicals can stimulate activity in taste receptor cells, the four basic qualities of taste (salt, sour, sweet and bitter) have stood the test of time. A fifth basic quality of taste has been recently described by Japanese researchers, that of umami (delicious taste), which is associated with the amino acid glutamate and some nucleotides.

Gustatory receptor cells have a dual role, that of detecting both nutrients and toxins. Because of this they have to be able to respond, both individually and collectively, to a wide variety of chemicals. These chemicals can be simple ions such as sodium ions (salt) and hydrogen ions (sour) or the more complex compounds that give the sensations of sweet (glucose), bitter (quinine) and umami (monosodium glutamate). The transduction mechanisms that convert the chemical stimuli into electrical events in the receptor cell are numerous, varied and sometimes complex. There does not appear to be a unique mechanism for each of the basic tastes: each seems to use several different mechanisms. There may even be similarities of mechanisms for different basic tastes. The way in which we perceive many subtle tastes and distinguish different compounds of the same basic taste category could be explained by the specificity and multiplicity of these mechanisms. However, we do know that simple Na^+ salts depolarise taste cells by Na^+ influx through channels in the apical and lateral cell membranes. Similar channels may be involved in the detection of H^+ ions, although the transduction mechanism for this ion shows a marked species variability. Transduction of more complex molecules such as sugars and bitter substances frequently involves membrane receptors linked to G proteins and second messengers, such as cyclic adenosine monophosphate (cAMP) and inositol trisphosphate/diacylglycerol that gate ion channels and cause depolarisation and action potentials to be initiated. Some artificial sweeteners are known to cause depolarisation by modulating ligand-gated ion channels directly. The response to glutamate (umami) is thought to involve *N*-methyl-D-aspartic acid and metabotropic glutamate receptors, similar to those found in the brain. In most cases the resultant depolarisation leads to an action potential in the receptor cell that in turn is followed by an increase in intracellular Ca^{2+} and the release of the neurotransmitter from the base of the cell associated with the intragemmal nerve ending. Recordings, using tiny electrodes, from individual nerve fibres innervating the taste buds, in anaesthetised animals, reveal that one does not get a burst of impulses only when a solution of just one of the basic taste substances is dripped onto the appropriate taste bud or buds. Such selectivity of response is rare. Most nerves respond to two or more of the basic taste stimuli, with the magnitude of the response varying from one taste substance to another (the so-called taste profile). This means that the activity of a single gustatory fibre does not provide unambiguous information to the brain about the quality and intensity of the stimulus. At some point the brain must perform a comparison between the activities in several different nerve fibres to determine what the taste actually is.

The primary afferent gustatory neurones have their first synaptic connection within the nucleus of the tractus solitarius, and it is here that approximately 82% of the neurones respond to three or four basic taste stimuli. There is also convergence here between gustatory and thermoreceptor inputs, with many neurones responding to cooling of the tongue, as well as to chemical stimuli. The second-order neurones in the nucleus of the tractus solitarius then project to the most medial part of the ventroposterior medial nucleus of the thalamus. There is a further projection to the brainstem reticular formation, the parabrachial nuclei and the cranial nerve nuclei involved in the reflexes associated with gestation. The thalamic neurones project to the primary gustatory cortex, which includes an area just anterior to the somatosensory area for the tongue, as well as to the nearby frontal operculum and anterior insular secondary cortex. There is evidence for a secondary gustatory area in the orbitofrontal cortex; studies suggest that neurones at these higher levels of the gustatory pathway respond more selectively, with 25% of the neurones in the primary cortex and 74% of the neurones in the secondary cortex responding to a single basic gustatory stimulus. Neurones in the orbitofrontal cortex that respond to gustatory stimuli are seen to be modulated by hunger and reduced when appetite is satiated. The orbitofrontal cortex receives inputs not only from the gustatory neurones but also from the olfactory, visual and somatosensory pathways, and neurones have been shown to respond to two or more modalities (touch, vision, smell, taste etc.). This area is thought to be involved in the learning of associations between stimuli, for instance, the association of the taste, smell, texture and sight of food substances, all of which are important in the appreciation of what is termed 'flavour'.

Several reviews on taste have, in the past, suggested that different areas of the tongue are more sensitive to the different basic tastes. These so-called tongue maps are now thought to be incorrect; their origin owes itself to a mistranslation of the early 20th century work of Hänig. His work referred to thresholds to the basic tastes and not to the exclusive nature of the loci. Subsequent misinterpretations have led to the impression that the tip of the tongue detects sweet, the sides sour and salt and the back bitter. This is clearly not true.

The *common chemical sense* is the sensation caused by stimulation of epithelial or mucosal free nerve endings by potentially harmful chemicals. The evidence suggests that free nerve endings are polymodal nociceptors that respond to a variety of different modalities of stimuli, such as mechanical, thermal and noxious stimuli. The major nerve that contributes to this sense in the mouth is cranial nerve V (the trigeminal nerve). The trigeminal nerve innervates almost all regions of the mouth, including the tongue, the hard and soft palate, and the mucosa of the lips and cheek. Free nerve endings are found throughout the oral cavity and amongst the chemicals that are known to stimulate these receptors, besides noxious, damaging chemicals, are alcohol, menthol, peppermint, capsaicin and piperine, which are found in chilli peppers and black pepper respectively.

Concerning *olfaction*, the human olfactory organ (namely, the olfactory epithelium or mucosa) comprises a sheet of cells 100–200 μm thick. It is situated high at the back of the nasal cavity and on a thin, bony partition called the central septum of the septum of the nose. This system responds to volatile, airborne molecules that make contact with the olfactory epithelium because of the in-out airflow during normal nasal breathing. There is a turbulent air flow in this region because of the nasal conchae on the lateral walls of the nose, and this leads to the odour molecules being distributed over the receptor sheet in an irregular pattern.

The olfactory epithelium contains olfactory receptors which are specialised, elongated cells. These cells have very fine, unmyelinated (0.1- to 0.4-μm-diameter) axons that run, in bundles, upwards through perforations in the skull (the cribriform plate of the ethmoid) that lies at the roof of the nasal cavity and below the frontal lobes of the brain. The olfactory nerve is short and ends in the olfactory bulbs, a pair of small swellings underneath the frontal lobes. The peripheral end of the olfactory receptors points down into the nasal cavity and is extended into a long process ending in small knobs that carry hair-like non-motile processes called cilia, which are 20–200 μm in length. These cilia are bathed in a 35-μm-thick layer of mucus, which has been secreted by specialised cells in the epithelium and in which the molecules of the odorous substances dissolve. The molecules diffuse through the surface layers of the mucus and interact with olfactory receptor proteins in the cilia membranes. This initiates a cascade reaction inside the cell that leads to a change of frequency of action potentials that pass along the olfactory nerve fibres. Hydrophilic (water soluble) molecules dissolve readily in the mucus, but the diffusion of less soluble molecules is assisted by odour-binding proteins in the mucus. These proteins are also thought to assist in removing the odour molecules from the receptor cell after stimulation. The mucous layer has been shown to move across the surface of the olfactory mucosa towards the nasopharynx at approximately 10–60 $mm\,min^{-1}$. The flow of mucus is increased and becomes more watery in conditions of infection of the nasal cavity. It is also thought to assist in the removal of odour molecules from the vicinity of the cilia after stimulation.

Contrasting with the limited number of taste sensations, human beings can detect 10,000 or more different odours. There have been attempts to classify these into a smaller number of basic or primary odours, but there is no universally accepted scheme. Unfortunately, there is no simple relationship between chemical structures and odours. Threshold concentrations of odours can be extremely low with many substances being detected at picomolar (10^{-12} mol L^{-1}) concentrations.

There are thought to be hundreds of different odorant membrane receptors located on the cilia of the olfactory cells. A large family of putative odorant receptor genes (perhaps as large as 1,000) has been cloned using oligonucleotide probes targeted to G protein–binding motifs. Binding of the odorant to the receptor leads to an increased conductance to Na^+ and to a depolarising generator potential, via a GTP-binding protein (G_{olf}) and cAMP. Although cAMP appears to be the major second messenger in olfactory transduction, there is increasing evidence for the involvement of phosphoinositide-derived second messengers as well.

Each olfactory receptor neurone spontaneously generates action potentials with between 3 and 60 impulses per second. When stimulated with a particular odour, they increase their firing frequency. Each receptor cell responds, but not equally, to many different types of odour. Single neurones appear to contain the gene for only one odorant receptor and are therefore selective for a particular set of odorants, which combines with that receptor. It has been shown that neurones containing the same receptor are dispersed within zones in the epithelium, and therefore different regions of the olfactory sheet (consisting of hundreds, if not thousands, of receptor cells) are maximally responsive to particular odours. The overall pattern of activity in the olfactory epithelium can be mapped using electro-olfactograms. Each distinctive odour produces its own fingerprint of activity across the epithelium. This so-called mapping reflects the patterns of activation (expression) of genes that make up the receptor proteins in the receptor cell membranes.

As in the gustatory system, the successive nerve cells in the pathway become more selective, each responding to fewer odours. The special coding of odour quality is transmitted to the first relay of the olfactory pathway, the olfactory bulb. There appears to be a loose topographical projection from the receptor sheet to the bulb. The primary olfactory neurones terminate in the spherical glomeruli (approximately 100–200 μm in diameter), where they synapse with the dendrites of neurones called mitral and tufted cells. Each olfactory neurone projects to only one glomerulus; however, each glomerulus can receive inputs from several thousand olfactory neurones widely dispersed throughout the olfactory epithelium. There is some evidence that each glomerulus may receive inputs from neurones expressing the same receptor, thus making the glomeruli functioning units, responding to a particular group of odorants. The olfactory bulb contains a complex network of nerve cells and is responsible for a considerable amount of sensory processing.

Neurones in the olfactory bulb respond with one distinctive temporal pattern of impulses to one odour and a completely different pattern of impulses to another. Besides the mitral and tufted neurones, the bulb also contains many interneurones (e.g., periglomerular and granule cells). It also receives descending projections from several higher brain regions, which, together with the interneurones, contribute to the processing of the sensory input. There is evidence of lateral inhibition between neighbouring glomeruli that sharpens olfactory acuity very similarly to the process of surround inhibition in other parts of the CNS. The mitral and tufted cells send their fibres into the olfactory tract to the thalamus, which in turn sends fibres to the primary olfactory cortex. The primary olfactory cortex includes the anterior olfactory nucleus, the olfactory tubercle and the piriform, periamygdaloid and entorhinal cortices. In addition, there are projections via the anterior commissures to the contralateral olfactory bulb. From the cortex there are projections to the orbitofrontal cortex. There is evidence that the piriform and the orbitofrontal cortices are involved in odour discrimination and combine with other stimuli to give the perception of flavour. Olfactory pathways also provide inputs to various regions of the limbic system around the region of the hypothalamus. Because the limbic system is thought to be responsible for regulating emotions, this may explain the observation that smells can evoke strong feelings of enjoyment or aversion (the hedonistic component of sensation).

The olfactory system occupies a smaller fraction of the brain in human beings than in many other species, and this is part of the evidence for the commonly held belief that humans are generally inferior in their sense of smell. Studies in other animals, from insects to monkeys, have revealed the importance of olfaction for many basic aspects of behaviour, especially reproduction. But, even in human beings, there is growing evidence that olfaction (mainly unconscious) is important in such functions as sexual preferences and recognition of other people.

The detection of change of temperature is the modality of *thermoreception*. Receptors within the mouth respond to the temperature of food and drink and are subjected to a wide range from less than 0°C to much greater than the threshold of pain at 46°C. However, thermal sensation is not a continuous variable but is divided into the sensations of warm and cold. The body surface and oral cavity are not uniformly sensitive to changes in temperature, but scattered all over the surface tissues and oral mucosa are small areas (about 1 mm^2) of heightened thermal sensitivity that respond either to warming or cooling of that area. Between these areas are areas of skin or mucosa that are totally insensitive to thermal stimulation. There appear to be about 10 times more cold-sensitive areas than warm-sensitive areas. The highest density of both cold and warm areas is found on the face, in particular the lips, with up to 19 cold areas per square centimetre. The tongue and lips have the highest sensitivity to both cooling and warming within the oral cavity, but overall the oral mucosa appears to be less sensitive to warming than other areas of the face. The sensitivity of different areas relates to the density of the thermoreceptors within the tissues but can also be attributed to the thickness and composition of the tissues in which they lie, as well as the depth of the receptors within that tissue.

Recordings from thermoreceptors in both skin and oral mucosa have confirmed the two separate types of thermoreceptor, namely, cold and warm receptors. Both receptor types are thought to be free nerve endings, unencapsulated except for a surrounding Schwann cell membrane. The cold receptors are thought to be derived from both small myelinated Aδ and unmyelinated C fibres and lie about 0.18 mm below the surface, whereas the warm receptors are thought to be derived from only unmyelinated C fibres and lie slightly deeper at about 0.22 mm below the surface. Both types of receptor are spontaneously active, firing impulses at a steady state to the ambient temperature. Cold receptors respond with an increase in discharge frequency on sudden cooling followed by an adaptation of discharge to a new set frequency as long as the stimulus is applied. On warming, the cold receptor responds with a transient inhibition of activity. In contrast, warm receptors respond with an increase in discharge frequency on a sudden warming followed by an adaptation of discharge to a new set frequency as long as the stimulus is applied. On cooling, the warm receptors respond with a transient inhibition of activity. These increases and decreases of discharge occur irrespective of the initial temperature of the tissues surrounding the free nerve endings. Receptors in the skin are important not only in detecting these dynamic and static changes in temperature but also in the maintenance of body temperature and initiating reflexes of sweating and shivering. In the mouth, they are particularly sensitive to sudden changes of temperature, such as when very hot coffee or an iced drink is imbibed.

Cold receptors are active over a wide range of surface temperatures (−5°C to 43°C), with the maximum static discharge frequency varying from receptor to receptor. Not all cold receptors respond maximally to the same temperature. For a large proportion of cold receptors, the temperature that gives rise to the maximum static discharge frequency of between 5 and 10 impulses per second is variable, ranging from −5°C to 40°C, giving a broad span of temperature ranges within the receptor population. The dynamic response of cold receptors when subjected to transient decreases of temperature results in a higher frequency of discharge, usually firing in bursts of activity separated by intervals of inactivity.

Warm receptors also have a static spontaneous discharge at ambient temperatures of the tissues in which they lie. The static discharge range begins at about 30°C and reaches a peak frequency when temperatures increase to 46°C. The maximum discharge is higher than that seen in cold receptor fibres at between 10 and 35 impulses per second. The dynamic response of warm receptors when subjected to transient increases of temperature can reach discharge frequencies of 200 impulses per second.

Thermoreceptive afferent neurones from the face and oral cavity form a synapse with second-order neurones in the trigeminal nucleus; these are located in the subnucleus interpolaris and marginal layer (lamina 1) of the medullary dorsal horn. The receptive fields of cold and warm neurones are on the ipsilateral side and cover a larger area than the first-order neurones of between 10 and 100 mm^2, suggesting a degree of convergence at the second-order level. The discharge patterns and static responses of the second-order neurones are similar to those of the first-order neurones, suggesting little, if any, processing except for a loss of bursting discharge in the second-order cold neurones. The trigeminal thermal neurones ascend farther in the trigemino-thalamic tract that terminates in the ventrobasal complex of the thalamus. Here, some of the neurones respond specifically to cooling, but others are multimodal and respond to touch and taste as well. Again, the response characteristics of the cold and warm receptors are preserved at this level. This specificity of peripheral thermal receptors is maintained even within the somatosensory cortex. There are single cortical cells in the oral region of the cortex that respond only to cold stimuli and nothing else. However, there is some evidence for central processing in that the neurones within the central nervous system appear to have a wider range of activity than the individual primary, first-order receptor neurones.

Further readings for Chapters 1 to 6 can be found in the accompanying eBook. Explore online Self-assessment quiz to test and reinforce your understanding of the material in your free ebook. Follow instructions in the Inside Front Cover to unlock your access.

Mastication (the act of chewing)

Mastication involves the coordination of teeth, jaw elevator and depressor muscles, temporomandibular joint, tongue, lips, palate and salivary glands (the so-called masticatory apparatus).

See Mind Map 2.1 for the jaws and Mind Map 3.2 for the muscles of mastication. Mind Maps 3.1 and 15.1 are concerned with the temporomandibular joint.

Control of mastication

Primarily a voluntary process, involving the cerebral cortex and motor neurones in the trigeminal motor nucleus.

Controlled by a central pattern generator and modulated by inputs from sensory feedback from the mouth and reflexes of mastication.

Mastication is a characteristic of mammals that show heterodonty. Humankind has a dentition reflecting an omnivorous diet.

Although it is thought that the primary function of mastication is to increase digestive efficiency, this depends on the type and consistency of the food ingested.

Tooth cusps may not be important for chewing but for guiding teeth during eruption and growth

Mastication does not usually involve both sides of the jaws – working and non-working sides. The pathway followed by the mandible during chewing is called the 'envelope of motion'.

Teeth are the main organ of mastication and adapted for the main functional requirement of the diet.

Masticatory forces:

- Maximum forces: 500–700 N between the molar teeth.
- During mastication, forces between 70 and150 N are achieved.

Involves both vertical and lateral movements of the jaws in human beings in so-called chewing cycle.

Chewing cycle involves:

- Opening phase
- Closing phase
- Occlusal or intercuspal phase

Puncture crushing and shearing stroke

Jaw reflexes

Jaw-jerk

Jaw-opening reflexes

Jaw uploading reflex

Mind Map 6.1 Mastication (the act of chewing).

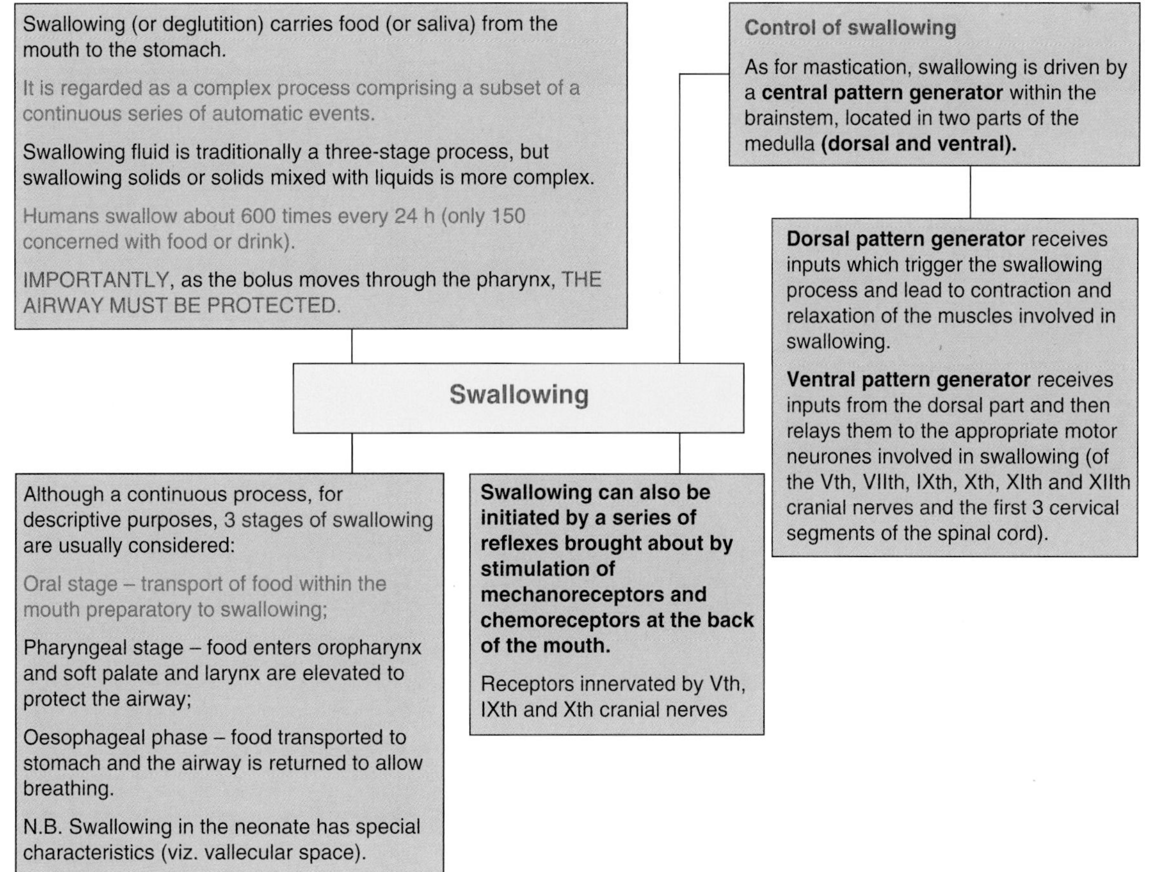

Swallowing (or deglutition) carries food (or saliva) from the mouth to the stomach.
It is regarded as a complex process comprising a subset of a continuous series of automatic events.
Swallowing fluid is traditionally a three-stage process, but swallowing solids or solids mixed with liquids is more complex.
Humans swallow about 600 times every 24 h (only 150 concerned with food or drink).
IMPORTANTLY, as the bolus moves through the pharynx, THE AIRWAY MUST BE PROTECTED.
Control of swallowing
As for mastication, swallowing is driven by a central pattern generator within the brainstem, located in two parts of the medulla (dorsal and ventral).
Dorsal pattern generator receives inputs which trigger the swallowing process and lead to contraction and relaxation of the muscles involved in swallowing.
Ventral pattern generator receives inputs from the dorsal part and then relays them to the appropriate motor neurones involved in swallowing (of the Vth, VIIth, IXth, Xth, XIth and XIIth cranial nerves and the first 3 cervical segments of the spinal cord).
Swallowing
Although a continuous process, for descriptive purposes, 3 stages of swallowing are usually considered:
Oral stage – transport of food within the mouth preparatory to swallowing;
Pharyngeal stage – food enters oropharynx and soft palate and larynx are elevated to protect the airway;
Oesophageal phase – food transported to stomach and the airway is returned to allow breathing.
N.B. Swallowing in the neonate has special characteristics (viz. vallecular space).
Swallowing can also be initiated by a series of reflexes brought about by stimulation of mechanoreceptors and chemoreceptors at the back of the mouth.
Receptors innervated by Vth, IXth and Xth cranial nerves

Mind Map 6.2 Swallowing.

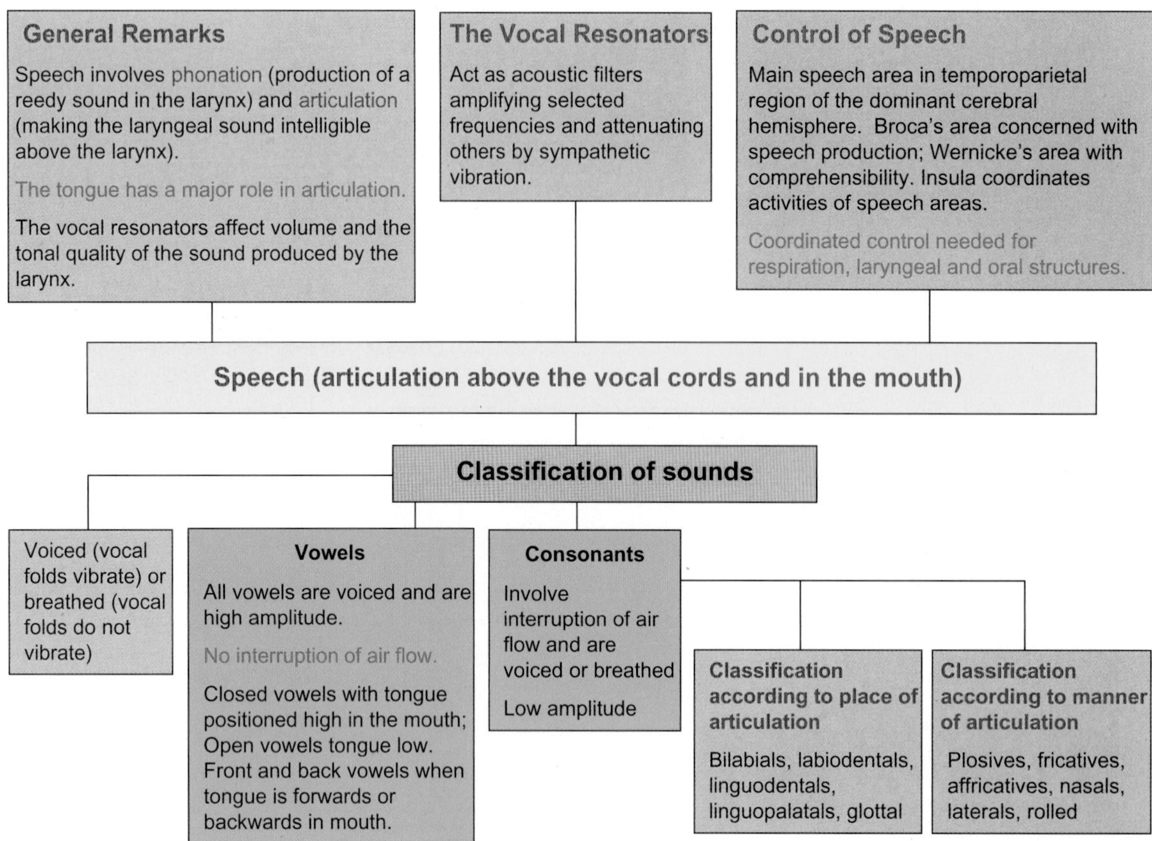

General Remarks
Speech involves phonation (production of a reedy sound in the larynx) and articulation (making the laryngeal sound intelligible above the larynx).
The tongue has a major role in articulation.
The vocal resonators affect volume and the tonal quality of the sound produced by the larynx.
The Vocal Resonators
Act as acoustic filters amplifying selected frequencies and attenuating others by sympathetic vibration.
Control of Speech
Main speech area in temporoparietal region of the dominant cerebral hemisphere. Broca's area concerned with speech production; Wernicke's area with comprehensibility. Insula coordinates activities of speech areas.
Coordinated control needed for respiration, laryngeal and oral structures.
Speech (articulation above the vocal cords and in the mouth)
Classification of sounds
Voiced (vocal folds vibrate) or breathed (vocal folds do not vibrate)
Vowels
All vowels are voiced and are high amplitude.
No interruption of air flow.
Closed vowels with tongue positioned high in the mouth; Open vowels tongue low. Front and back vowels when tongue is forwards or backwards in mouth.
Consonants
Involve interruption of air flow and are voiced or breathed
Low amplitude
Classification according to place of articulation
Bilabials, labiodentals, linguodentals, linguopalatals, glottal
Classification according to manner of articulation
Plosives, fricatives, affricatives, nasals, laterals, rolled

Mind Map 6.3 Speech (articulation above the vocal cords and in the mouth).

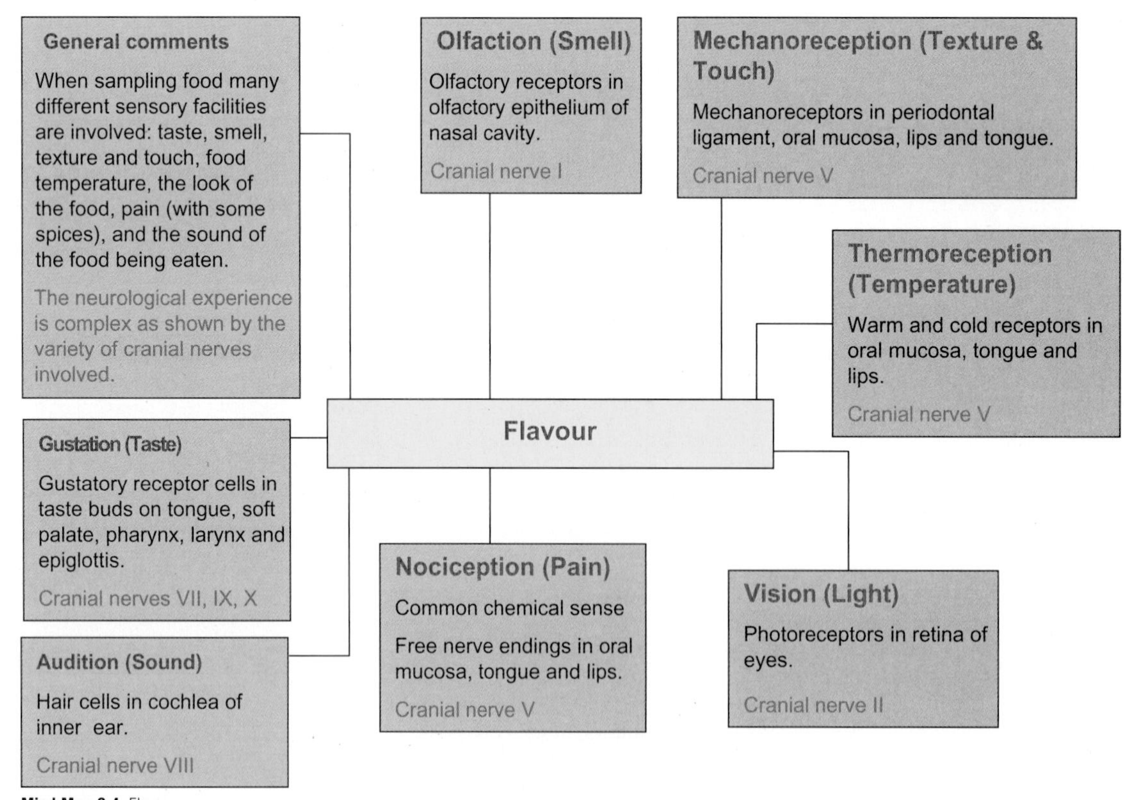

General comments
When sampling food many different sensory facilities are involved: taste, smell, texture and touch, food temperature, the look of the food, pain (with some spices), and the sound of the food being eaten.
The neurological experience is complex as shown by the variety of cranial nerves involved.
Olfaction (Smell)
Olfactory receptors in olfactory epithelium of nasal cavity.
Cranial nerve I
Mechanoreception (Texture & Touch)
Mechanoreceptors in periodontal ligament, oral mucosa, lips and tongue.
Cranial nerve V
Thermoreception (Temperature)
Warm and cold receptors in oral mucosa, tongue and lips.
Cranial nerve V
Flavour
Gustation (Taste)
Gustatory receptor cells in taste buds on tongue, soft palate, pharynx, larynx and epiglottis.
Cranial nerves VII, IX, X
Nociception (Pain)
Common chemical sense
Free nerve endings in oral mucosa, tongue and lips.
Cranial nerve V
Vision (Light)
Photoreceptors in retina of eyes.
Cranial nerve II
Audition (Sound)
Hair cells in cochlea of inner ear.
Cranial nerve VIII

Mind Map 6.4 Flavour.

Enamel

7

General introduction to the dental tissues

Before describing enamel, a few introductory remarks are required concerning the arrangement of the dental and supporting tissues. The teeth are composed of three mineralised tissues (enamel, dentine and cementum) surrounding an inner core of loose connective tissue, the dental pulp. Enamel is of ectodermal origin; dentine, cementum and the dental pulp are of ectomesenchymal origin. Enamel and dentine meet at the enamel–dentine (amelodentinal) junction: cementum and enamel meet at the cementum–enamel junction; cementum and dentine meet at the cementum–dentine junction.

The appearance of the tissues depends upon the method of specimen preparation: in ground sections the hard mineralised tissues remain intact, but the soft connective tissues and epithelia are lost; in demineralised sections the soft connective tissues and the organic matrices of the mineralised tissues remain. Because enamel is almost entirely mineral, it is lost completely after most demineralisation procedures and its structural features are mainly described as seen in ground sections (Fig. 7.1).

Dentine forms the bulk of the tooth and is covered in the crown with enamel and in the root with cementum (Figs. 7.1, 7.2). The dental pulp derives from the dental papilla and is responsible for the production of dentine, which continues throughout life. It also acts as a sensory organ detecting, when attacked by dental caries, significant physical stimuli and toxins. The dental pulp can respond to external stimuli by inducing an immune inflammatory response and by increasing the dentine thickness. If the dental caries infection persists, the pulp will be killed and become necrotic.

The tissues that support the teeth, known collectively as the periodontium (Figs. 7.1, 7.2), include the alveolar bone forming the tooth sockets, the periodontal ligament (a connective tissue that attaches the tooth to the alveolar bone) and the gingivae (the component of the oral mucosa that forms a collar around the tooth).

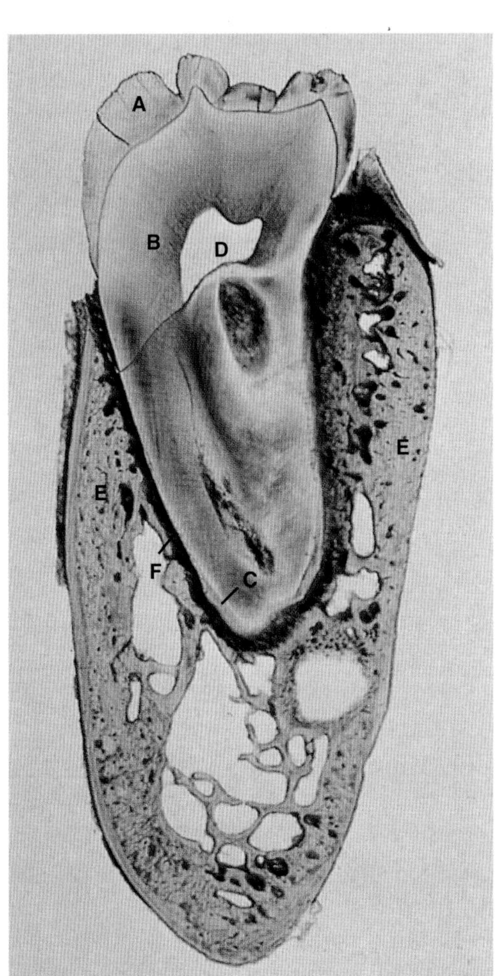

Fig. 7.1 Ground section of a tooth *in situ* showing the distribution of the dental tissues. A = enamel; B = dentine; C = cementum; D = dental pulp chamber; E = alveolar bone. As the section was embedded in plastic, part of the periodontal ligament (F) has been fortuitously retained (×4).

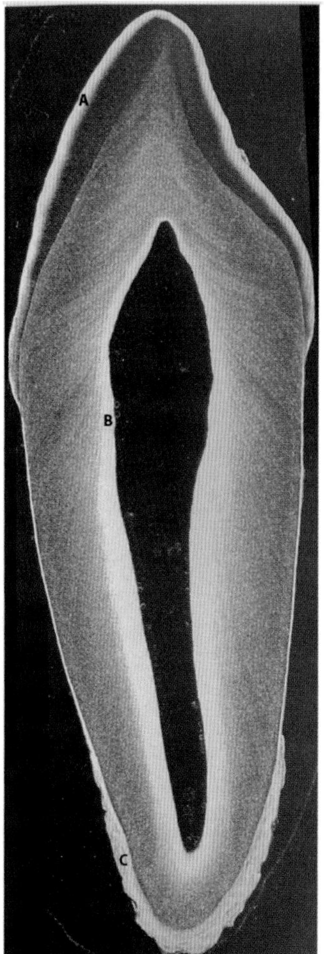

Fig. 7.2 Demineralised section of a tooth *in situ*. A = enamel–dentine junction; B = dentine; C = cementum; D = dental pulp; E = alveolar bone; F = periodontal ligament; G = gingiva. Compared with Fig. 7.1, the enamel has been lost (×6). Courtesy Dr D A Lunt.

Introduction to enamel

Enamel is a unique tissue. It differs from all other calcified tissues in the body by lacking cells within it or on its surfaces. It is the most highly mineralised tissue, containing only minute quantities of organic material, as compared with dentine and cementum (Fig. 7.3).

It develops from the internal enamel epithelium of the tooth germ (see pages 350–354) by a complex process of reciprocal epithelial/mesenchymal interactions.

Physical properties

Enamel covers the crown of the tooth (Fig. 7.4). It is thickest over cusps and incisal edges and thinnest at the cervical margin. Over the cusps of unworn permanent teeth, it is about 2.5 mm thick (over the cusps of deciduous teeth, 1.3 mm) and on lateral surfaces it is up to 1.3 mm thick (Fig. 7.5). The thickness declines gradually to become a very thin layer at the cervical margin. Enamel thickness varies between individuals and between teeth (Fig. 7.5), increasing from first to third molar. Although thickest in parts of the tooth that will suffer most attrition, it is also relatively thick in some protected areas, where it will add to the overall strength of the cusp and reduce the likelihood of fracture.

Research into the structure of enamel has been hampered by the difficulty of handling such a hard and fragile tissue. Sectioning techniques used on intact enamel result in disturbance of the architecture of the tissue. Although it is an inert tissue, enamel can be exposed to challenges and can change over a lifetime. In ancient times, and even now in some remote areas, diets contain a proportion of hard material that can lead to considerable abrasion on both occlusal and interproximal surfaces. Lengthy exposure to acidic elements of the diet (e.g., citrus juices and fizzy soft drinks) can lead to the dissolution of mineral that may not be remineralised. The most common cause of enamel loss in modern society is dental caries, and it is the ravages of this disease that many dentists spend time repairing.

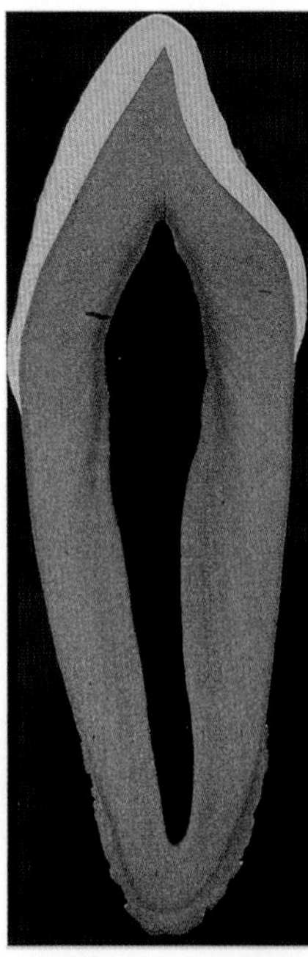

Fig. 7.3 Synchrotron X-ray fluorescence maps of calcium in a permanent canine tooth showing that calcium concentration is greater (appearing whiter) in enamel than in dentine and cementum. Courtesy Drs C Dean, F Elamin, A Le Cabec, and J Garrevoet and the DESY synchrotron facility, Hamburg, Germany.

Enamel is the hardest biological tissue and, although highly mineralised, withstands both shearing and impact forces well. Its abrasion resistance is high, allowing it to wear down only slowly, an important property because enamel can undergo neither repair nor replacement. Although enamel has a low tensile strength and is brittle, it has a high modulus of elasticity and this, together with the flexible support of the underlying dentine, minimises the possibility of fracture. Enamel has a high specific gravity (≈3). Enamel is a complex, bioceramic composite in which the hydroxyapatite crystal vastly predominates. Enamel is porous, and this relates to the presence of water-filled micropores between the crystals. This porosity can be visualized by the gradual buildup of water droplets on the dried surface of enamel.

The properties of enamel vary at different regions within the tissue. Surface enamel is harder, denser and less porous than subsurface enamel. Hardness and density also decrease from the surface towards the interior and from the cuspal/incisal tip towards the cervical margin.

Enamel is a birefringent crystalline material, with the crystals refracting light differently in different directions. Young enamel is white because, although light enters it readily, it is almost entirely internally reflected with no wavelengths differentially absorbed. This results in low translucency and the white colour. The translucency of enamel increases with age, and some of the colour of the underlying dentine is then transmitted, resulting in a more yellow appearance. The tissue has an average refractive index of 1.62. These optical properties considerably influence the histological appearance of enamel (e.g., explaining why there are differences with various mounting media). Some of the physical properties of enamel (and, for comparison, dentine) are listed in Table 7.1. Although softer than the geological materials, enamel resists fracture three times as well (Table 7.2) because of the arrangement of the crystals into prisms and the incorporation of an organic matrix.

Chemical properties

Hydroxyapatite crystals

The principal mineral component of enamel is calcium hydroxyapatite [$Ca_{10}(PO_4)_6(OH)_2$] in crystalline form. The crystals contain impurities in

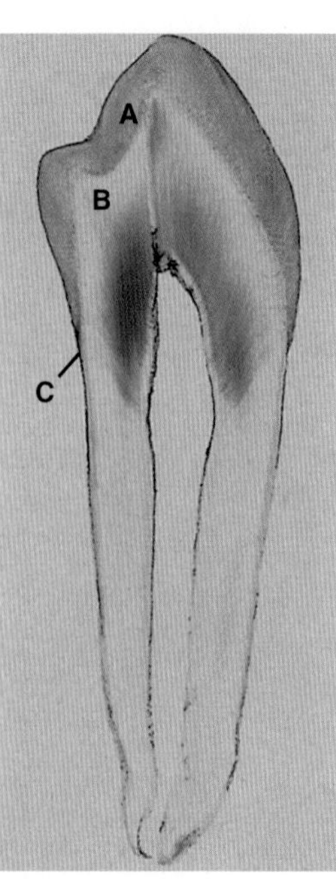

Fig. 7.4 The distribution of enamel. A = enamel; B = dentine; C = cementum–enamel junction (×3).

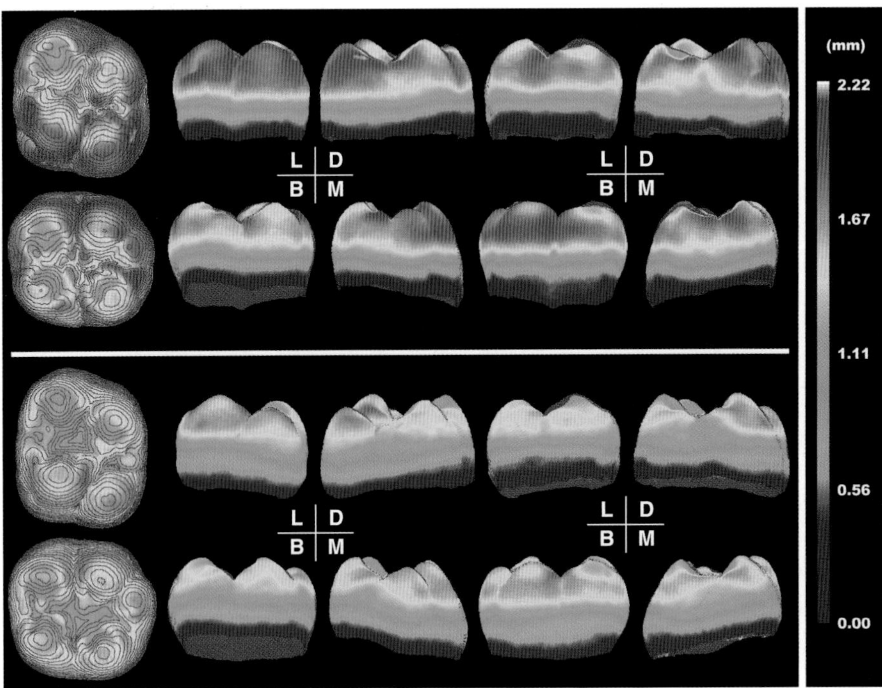

Fig. 7.5 Enamel thickness patterns of lateral and occlusal molar crown surfaces shown by colour grading. The colour scale to the right is common to all images. These images are obtained by taking an impression of each crown both before and after the enamel is removed by acid. Casts are made from these impressions and laser scanned. The inner and outer surface of the enamel of each crown is reassembled using three-dimensional reconstruction software, and the thickness of the enamel is measured and colour coded. The images show the lateral crown surfaces of two individuals. Each individual is shown in either the top or bottom rows, with the maxillary and mandibular molars in the left and the right quadrants respectively (L = lingual; D = distal; B = buccal; M = mesial). The variation in thickness within each tooth is clearly seen and follows a similar pattern in each tooth. The numerical values for thickness vary substantially between individuals and to a lesser extent between teeth from the same individual. From Kono et al., 2000. A three-dimensional analysis of enamel distribution patterns in human permanent first molars. *Archives of Oral Biology* 47: 867–875, with permission.

Table 7.1 A comparison of the physical properties of enamel and dentine (typical values)

	Enamel	Dentine
Specific gravity	2.9	2.14
Hardness (Knoop no.)	296	64
Stiffness (Young's modulus)	131 GN/m^2	12 GN/m^2
Compressive strength	76 MN/m^2	262 MN/m^2
Tensile strength	46 MN/m^2	33 MN/m^2

GN = giganewtons (N x 10^9); MN = meganewtons (N x 10^6).

Table 7.2 Mechanical properties of enamel, hydroxyapatite and fluorapatite

	Fracture toughness (MPa m$^{1/2}$)	Vickers microhardness (GPa)
Enamel along prisms	0.90	–
Enamel across prisms	1.30	–
Enamel	–	3.0
Geological hydroxyapatite	0.37	5.4
Geological fluorapatite	0.39	5.1

tiny amounts, such as carbonate substituting for phosphate in the crystal lattice.

Hydroxyapatite comprises about 88–90% of the tissue by volume, corresponding to about 95–96% by weight. The crystals approximately are 30 nm thick and 70 nm wide (Fig. 7.6). Field emission scanning electron microscopy (SEM) operated at high voltage (20–30 keV) produces

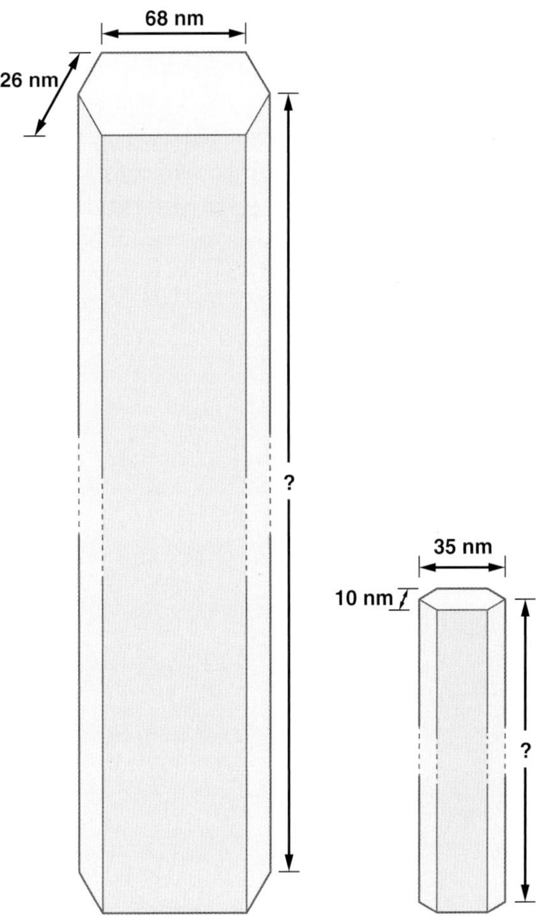

Fig. 7.6 The dimensions of an enamel crystallite (left) and a dentine crystallite (right). Both are impure hydroxyapatite.

topographic images of up to ×1,000,000 with good resolution. These show the crystals to be mainly in the form of long flat ribbons rhomboidal in cross-section, although some are distorted by crowding during development. The cores of the crystallites differ slightly in composition from the periphery, being richer in magnesium and carbonate. The core of the crystallite is more soluble than the periphery. Owing to technical problems associated with fracture, their length is not known for certain, but they may extend across the full width of the tissue (Figs. 7.6, 7.7). The mineral content increases from the enamel–dentine junction to the surface. Most crystallites are regularly hexagonal in cross-section (Figs. 7.8, 7.9), although some are distorted by crowding during development. The tooth shade is affected by crystal size and carbonation.

The molecular arrangement within each unit cell of the crystallite consists of a hydroxyl group surrounded by three uniformly spaced calcium ions, which in turn are surrounded by three similarly spaced phosphate ions. Six calcium ions in a uniform hexagon enclose the phosphate ions. The crystal consists of this arrangement of planes of ions repeated side by side and in stacked layers. Although the basic molecular arrangement of the crystal is highly organised, it is subject to variation. 'Normal' ions may be replaced by different ionic species. Carbonate may occur at a phosphate or hydroxyl site (about 90% being found at the phosphate position). Magnesium may occur in the place of a calcium ion or elsewhere in the lattice. Fluoride, being negatively charged, may substitute for hydroxyl ions, conferring greater stability and resistance to acidic dissolution. Fluoride levels (unlike magnesium and carbonate) decline from the outer surface towards the dentine, perhaps because the fluoride is acquired during enamel maturation. Chloride, lead, zinc, sodium, strontium and aluminium ions may also substitute into the apatite lattice. Trace levels of zinc are relatively enriched in outer enamel, secondary dentine and cementum (Fig. 7.10).

Another change in the molecular arrangement occurs if one plane of ions 'slips' from the usual uniform arrangement with its neighbour.

The concentration of trace elements varies throughout the enamel (see also page 148). Exchange of ions with saliva at the surface is important clinically, particularly relating to fluoride. Fluoride concentration increases again close to the enamel–dentine junction.

Enamel crystals increase in width from the enamel–dentine junction to the surface zone. The crystals are tightly packed with gaps (pores) of <5 nm between them which would be occupied by organic matrix and/or water.

A comparison of some of the characteristics of enamel with geological hydroxyapatite and fluorapatite is shown in Table 7.2.

Water

Water constitutes about 2% by weight of enamel, corresponding to 5–10% by volume. The presence of water is related to the porosity of the tissue. Some of the water may lie between crystals and surround the organic

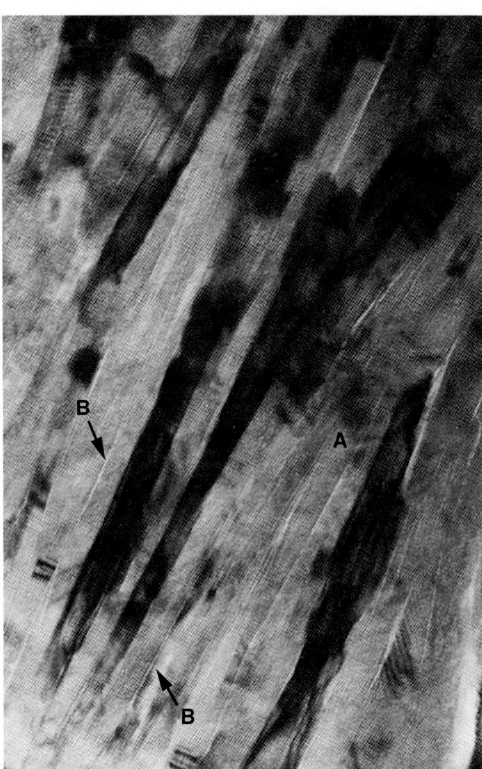

Fig. 7.7 Enamel crystallites in longitudinal section prepared by ion-beam thinning. For this technique a beam of ionised argon is directed obliquely onto the section so that it is etched. In such specimens, crystallites (A) up to 100 μm long are seen, and it is possible that some crystallites cross the full thickness of the enamel. B = pores between crystallites (TEM; ×100,000). Courtesy Dr H J Orams, Dr P P Phakey, Dr W Rachinger, and the editor of *Advances in Dental Research.*

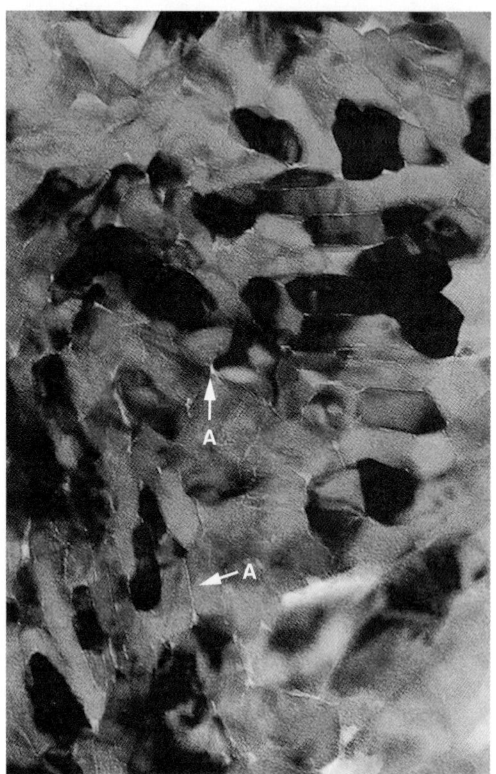

Fig. 7.8 TEM showing enamel crystallites in cross-section prepared by ion-beam thinning, showing the hexagonal pattern of the enamel crystallites (×120,000). Small gaps or pores (A), which may contain water and organic material, occur between crystallites. Courtesy Dr H J Orams, Dr P P Phakey, Dr W Rachinger, and the editor of *Advances in Dental Research.*

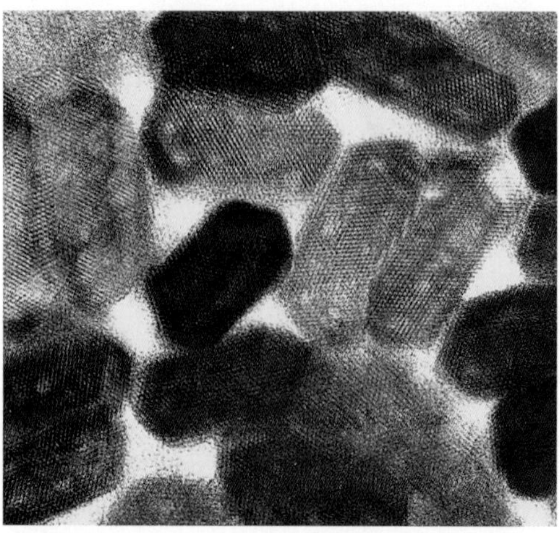

Fig. 7.9 TEM of isolated hexagonal enamel crystallites containing many hydroxyapatite molecules organised in a repeating pattern or lattice (×800,000). Courtesy Prof. H Warshawsky.

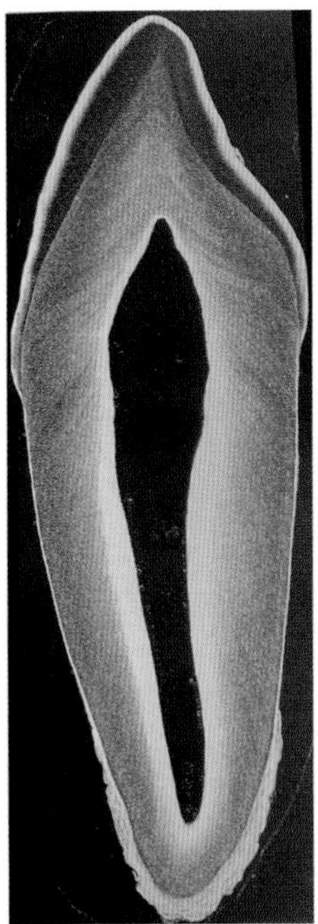

Fig. 7.10 Synchrotron X-ray fluorescence maps of zinc in a permanent canine tooth showing that zinc concentration is greater (appearing whiter) and is relatively enriched in outer enamel (A), secondary dentine (B) and cementum (C) compared with other parts of the tooth. Courtesy Drs C Dean, F Elamin, A Le Cabec, and J Garrevoet and the DESY synchrotron facility, Hamburg, Germany.

material, some may be trapped within defects of the crystalline structure and the remainder forms a hydration layer coating the crystals. The water component and its distribution are of clinical importance because ions such as fluoride travel through it.

Organic matrix

Mature enamel contains only 1–2% by weight of organic matrix. It may contribute to some of the mechanical properties of enamel, such as fracture toughness. The organic component of regions where the crystallite arrangement is straight and regular may be as low as 0.05% w/w; where the prisms and crystallites are more irregular it may be as high as 3%. The organic matrix is made up mainly of unique peptide groups termed amelogenins and non-amelogenins (amelogenins, ameloblastin, enamelin and other minor components). In the adult matrix, <10% is composed of amelogenins, whereas in developing enamel, 90% is composed of amelogenins. Thus the amelogenins are selectively reabsorbed during enamel maturation, allowing the enamel crystallites to grow to their large size, compared with the much smaller crystallites of dentine, cementum and bone, whose collagenous organic matrix remains throughout development. Although originally thought to be unique to enamel, enamel matrix components are also found in relation to the development of cementum (see page 443).

Amelogenin is encoded for by both chromosomes X and Y, with slight differences in their amino acid sequences. This means that protein analysis of the organic matrix of enamel removed by acid etching should enable the sex of an individual to be established. Not only is this true for modern individuals, but the stability of the organic matrix in fossils has allowed sex to be determined in material thousands, if not hundreds of thousands, of years ago (see Chapter 27).

Proteins are important indicators of physiological or pathological states. The use of mass spectrometry has allowed the identification of all proteins in enamel, even those present in minute quantities and which had remained unidentified in previous studies. Such proteomic analyses have revealed the presence of literally hundreds of proteins present in mature enamel matrix. Such proteins may have performed various roles in the complex process of enamel maturation, although their precise roles in amelogenesis have yet to be unraveled.

Enamel matrix is considered in more detail in reference to enamel formation on pages 409–412.

Although little studied, the lipid content of enamel appears to be a little less than that of protein. It too may represent the remnants of cell membranes remaining from development. Lipid material has been identified in the cross-striations, enamel striae (of Retzius), Hunter–Schreger bands and in the prism sheaths and prism cores of mature human enamel.

Enamel prisms

The basic structural unit of enamel is the enamel prism or rod (Fig. 7.11), consisting of several million crystallites, approximately 70 nm wide by 30 nm thick and of indeterminate length, packed into a long thin enamel rod (prism) 5–6 µm in diameter and up to 2.5 mm in length. Although the units are not strictly prismatic in outline, this term for the enamel unit has become accepted by widespread usage. Prisms run from the enamel–dentine junction to the surface. The boundaries of the prisms reflect sudden changes in crystallite orientation that give an optical effect different from that of the prism core or body: at the boundaries the crystallites deviate by 40–60 degrees from those inside the prism. Because of the resultant increased microporosity at the prism boundary, slightly more organic material can be accommodated.

Atomic force microscopy and nanoindentation techniques have been used to measure hardness and elastic modulus within single enamel prisms and the surrounding prism boundaries. The nanohardness and elastic modulus of the prism boundaries were approximately 75% and 50% lower than those within the prism cores.

In cross-section the shape of an enamel prism approximates to one of three main patterns (Fig. 7.12). Pattern I prisms have complete boundaries, and there is a clear distinction between prisms and interprismatic enamel. In patterns II and III the prism boundary is incomplete and in the cervical region there is a gradual change in orientation between the intraprismatic and interprismatic crystals. Different mammalian orders show a marked predisposition to the frequency at which these different prism packing patterns occur. The patterns also relate to the cross-sectional area of the cells: very roughly 20 µm^2 for pattern 2, 30 µm^2 for pattern 1 and 40 µm^2 for pattern 3.

All three patterns are present in humans, but pattern III (Figs. 7.11A, 7.13), the keyhole pattern, predominates. In pattern I enamel the prisms appear circular. The enamel between the prisms has been termed 'interprismatic'. Its composition is similar to that inside the prisms, but it has a different optical effect because the crystals deviate by 40–60 degrees from those in the prism. Pattern 1 (Fig. 7.14) is found near the enamel–dentine junction and near the surface, possibly because the enamel in these regions is formed slowly.

The keyhole pattern III of enamel shows clear 'head' and 'tail' regions, the tail of one prism lying between the heads of the adjacent prisms and pointing cervically. There is an abrupt change in crystal orientation (Figs. 7.15–7.17), which is responsible for the refraction of light and the appearance of the prism boundary. Because polarised light identifies changes in crystallite orientation, it is useful in highlighting features in enamel such as prisms (Fig. 7.18).

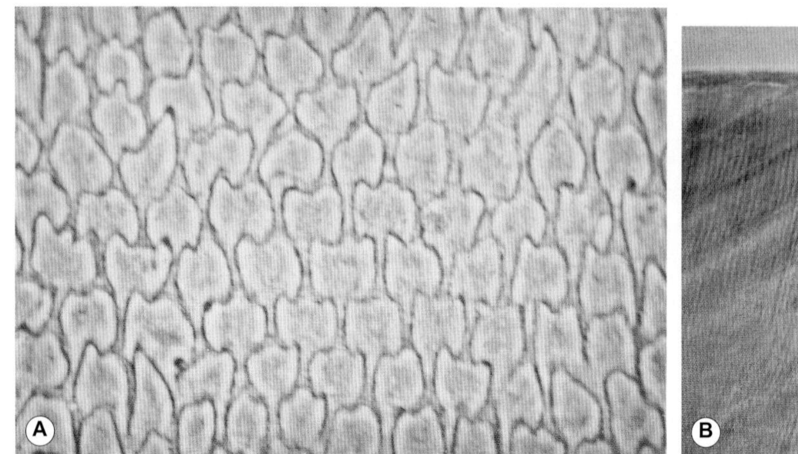

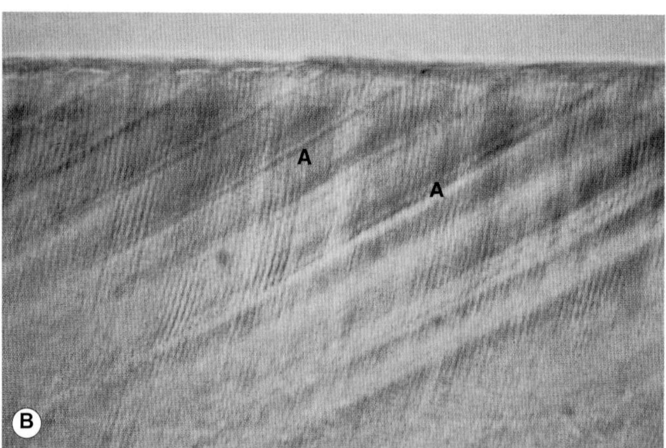

Fig. 7.11 (A) Enamel prisms in transverse section demonstrating the keyhole pattern seen in most regions of human enamel (phase contrast ×14,500). (B) Enamel prisms cut longitudinally and running perpendicularly towards the surface. The lines running obliquely (A) are enamel striae (×250). Courtesy Dr D F G Poole.

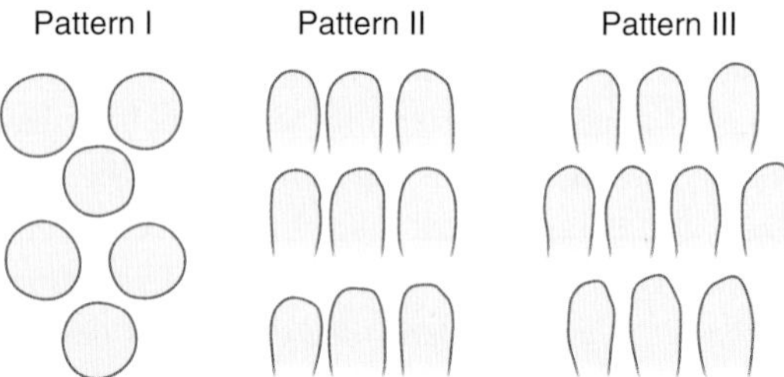

Fig. 7.12 The three prism patterns seen in human enamel. In pattern I enamel the prisms are circular. In pattern II enamel the prisms are aligned in parallel rows. In pattern III enamel the prisms are arranged in staggered rows such that the tail of a prism lies between two heads in the next row, giving a keyhole appearance.

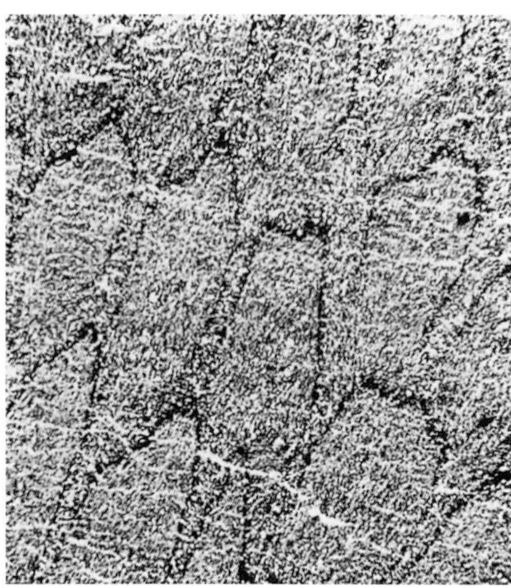

Fig. 7.13 Transverse section of prisms showing type III keyhole pattern (TEM with silver staining ×2,000). Courtesy Dr D F G Poole.

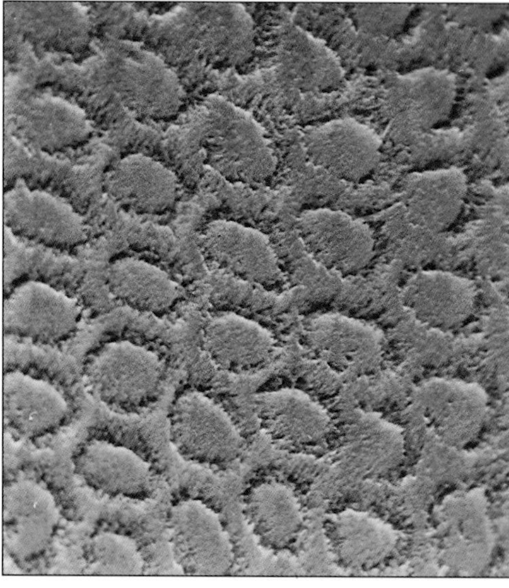

Fig. 7.14 Circular pattern I prisms (SEM ×4,300). Courtesy Prof. A Boyde.

In the head of the prism the crystals run parallel to the long axis of the prism. In the tail the crystals gradually diverge from this to become angled 65–70 degrees to the long axis (Fig. 7.15, face A). The change within a single prism is gradual such that there is no clear division between head and tail of the same prism; however, the crystals in the tail of one prism show a sudden divergence from the crystals in the head of an adjacent prism (Figs. 7.15, 7.16). In preparing histological material the enamel will be sectioned with varying degrees of obliquity, producing a wide variety of prism appearances. Although some areas may be termed interprismatic, what appears 'interprismatic' is often the tail of a prism from an adjacent row, and prismatic and interprismatic enamel are really continuous. In fractured enamel observed by SEM, peripheral crystallites (arrow in Fig. 7.19A) deviate from the long axes of the prism to form a continuum with interprismatic enamel (arrow in Fig. 7.19B). Interprismatic crystallites cross prisms at an angle of approximately 60 degrees.

When viewed in enamel fractured or sectioned parallel to the long axis of the tooth (see Fig. 7.23), most prisms appear to travel in a sinusoidal line from the enamel–dentine junction to the surface (however, see the following Hunter–Schreger bands section). The prisms meet the surface at varying angles depending on the relative shape of the enamel–dentine junction and the outer surface. Just above the cervical margin, prisms meet the surface at right angles, whereas more occlusally they meet the surface at an angle of about 60 degrees (Fig. 7.20). Within fissures, prisms make surface angles as acute as 20 degrees (Fig. 7.21).

Hunter–Schreger bands

Between 10 and 13 layers of prisms follow the same direction, but blocks above and below follow paths in different directions (Figs. 7.22–7.24). These periodic changes in prism direction give rise to a banding pattern termed the Hunter–Schreger bands (Fig. 7.25). These bands are approximately 50 µm wide and are visible because the different bands of prisms reflect or transmit light in different directions. In sections of enamel cut parallel to the long axis of the tooth, the individual crystallites will be oriented differently in the groups of prisms cut more transversely or more

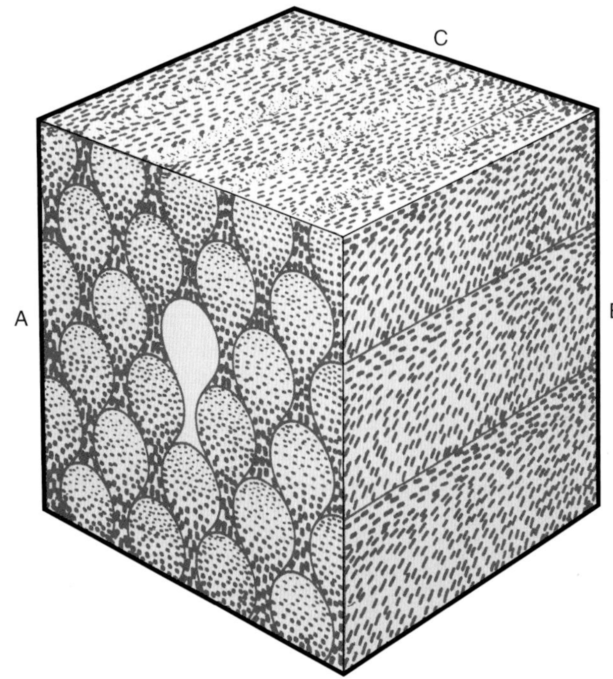

Fig. 7.15 Crystallite orientation and prism structure in a diagrammatic representation of a block of enamel. A = cross-sectional view; B = lateral surface; C = top surface. The cross-sectional view reveals the characteristic keyhole arrangement of enamel prisms with the tails pointing cervically and the heads occlusally. In the head of the prism the crystallites run parallel to the long axis of the prism. In the tail the crystallites gradually diverge from this to become angled 65–70 degrees to the long axis. The change within a single prism is gradual such that no clear division between head and tail of the same prism is seen. However, the crystallites in the tail of one prism show a sudden divergence from the crystallites in the head of an adjacent prism. The sudden change in crystallite orientation at the prism boundary can be seen most clearly in the lateral surface of the block (B). On this surface, where the prisms have been cut exactly centrally through the head–tail axis, there are rows of equal but wide prisms. On the top surface (C), where the plane of section has passed through adjacent heads and tails, there is the appearance of broad prisms separated by narrower bands of 'interprismatic' enamel. It must be noted that in preparing histological material the enamel will be sectioned with varying degrees of obliquity, producing a wide variety of prism appearances and crystallite orientations. Courtesy Dr A H Meckel, Dr W J Griebstein, Dr R N Neal and John Wright, Publishers.

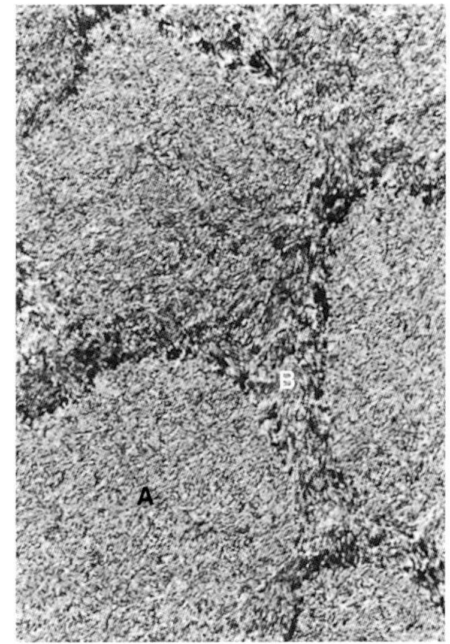

Fig. 7.16 TEM showing enamel prisms cut transversely showing variations in crystal orientation between head (A) and tail (B) regions (×7,000). Courtesy Dr D F G Poole.

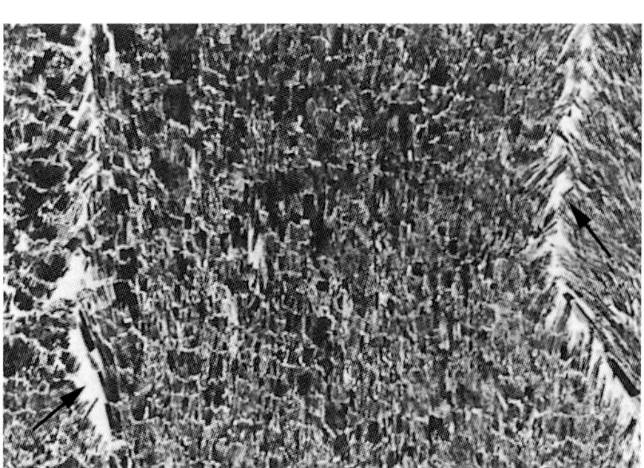

Fig. 7.17 TEM showing enamel prisms cut longitudinally showing sudden change in orientation (arrows) at the prism boundary. The apparent space at the prism boundary represents a preparation artefact (×13,500). Courtesy Dr D F G Poole.

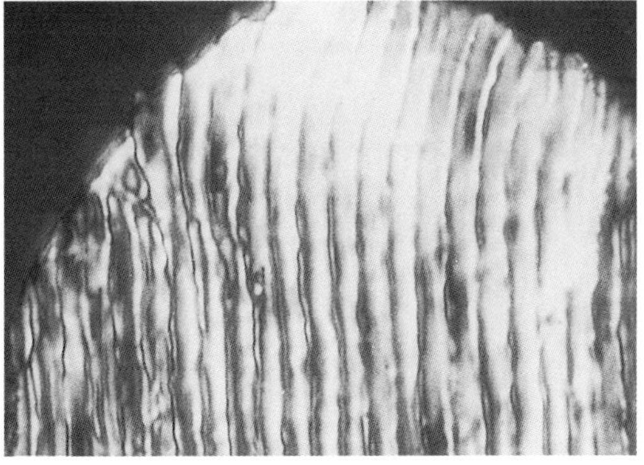

Fig. 7.18 In polarised light, enamel cut longitudinal to the prisms shows a series of light and dark lines that distinguish the prism cores from the prism boundaries. This appearance is owing to the abrupt change in orientation of the crystals at the prism boundary (and not to differential degrees of mineralisation). Indeed, the presence of the enamel prism as a subunit of enamel is entirely owing to these changes in crystal orientation (×600). Courtesy Dr D F G Poole.

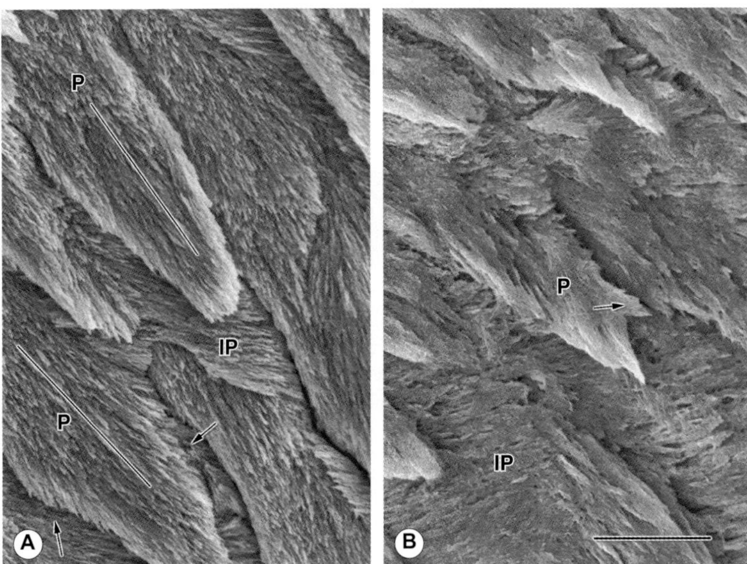

Fig. 7.19 SEMs of prismatic (P) and interprismatic (IP) enamel in sagittal section (scale bar = 5 μm). Peripheral crystallites (arrow in A) deviate from the long axes of the prisms to form a continuum with interprismatic enamel (arrow in B). Interprismatic crystallites cross prisms at an angle of approximately 60 degrees. Courtesy Dr S White and the *Journal of Dental Research*.

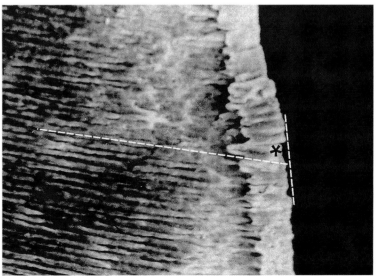

Fig. 7.20 SEM of lightly etched enamel showing enamel prisms reaching the surface at 60 degrees (*) (×320). Courtesy Dr R C Shore and the CRC Press.

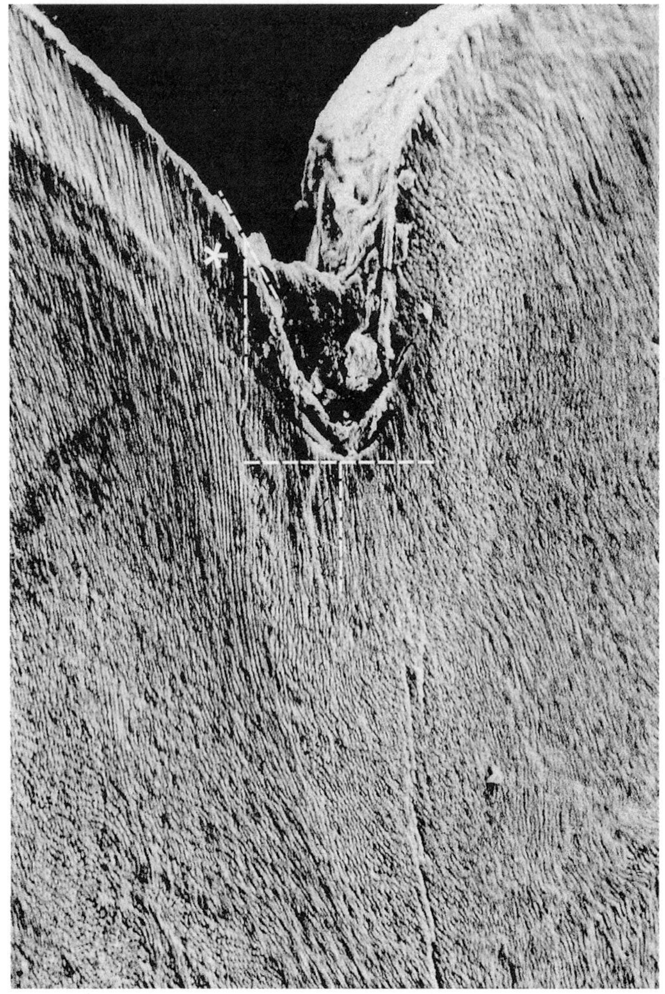

Fig. 7.21 SEM showing the orientation of enamel prisms within an occlusal fissure. Note the acute angle (*) at which the prisms reach the surface in this region (×100). Courtesy Dr R C Shore and the CRC Press.

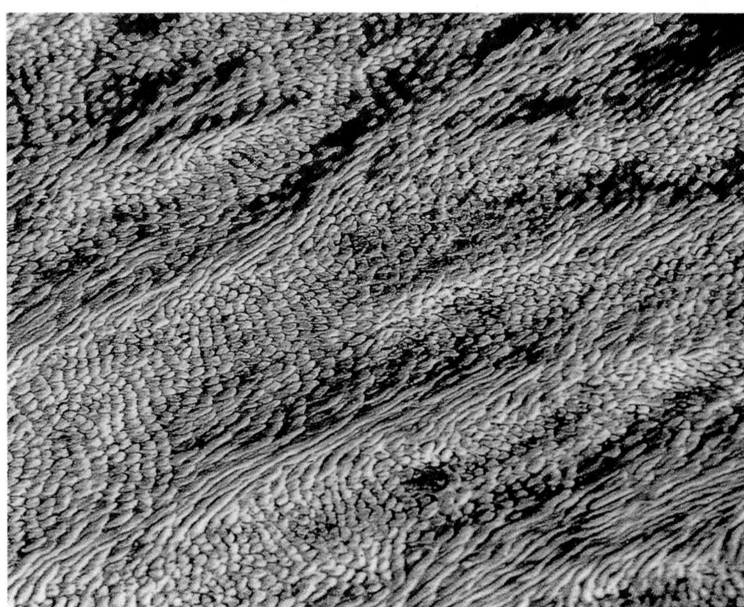

Fig. 7.22 SEM of longitudinally sectioned enamel lightly etched to show alternating bands of transversely sectioned (diazones) and longitudinally sectioned (parazones) prisms (×160). Courtesy Dr R C Shore and the CRC Press.

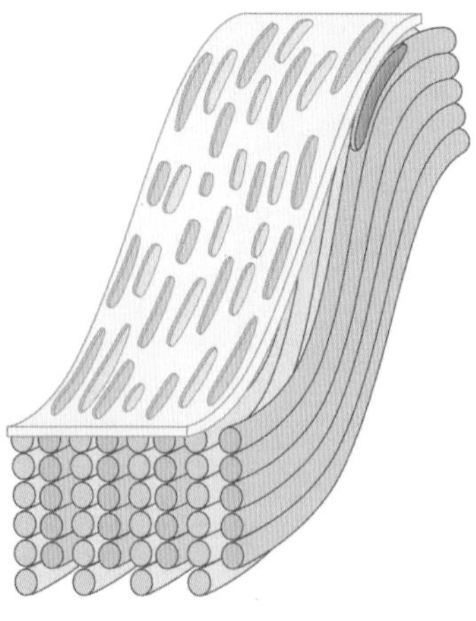

Fig. 7.23 The sinusoidal direction of the enamel prisms in alternating sheets results in alternately reflecting bands on the cut surface. Different sheets exhibit different crystal orientations and thus different degrees of polarisation.

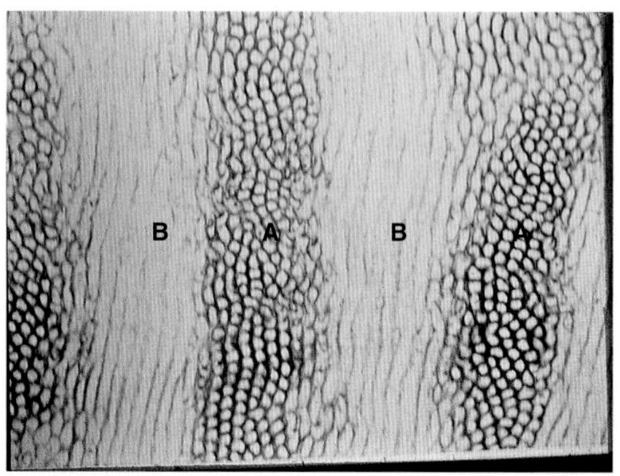

Fig. 7.24 Longitudinal section of enamel showing alternating regions with groups of prism sectioned more transversely (A) or more longitudinally (B) that give rise to the appearance of Hunter–Schreger bands (×300). Courtesy Dr B A W Brown.

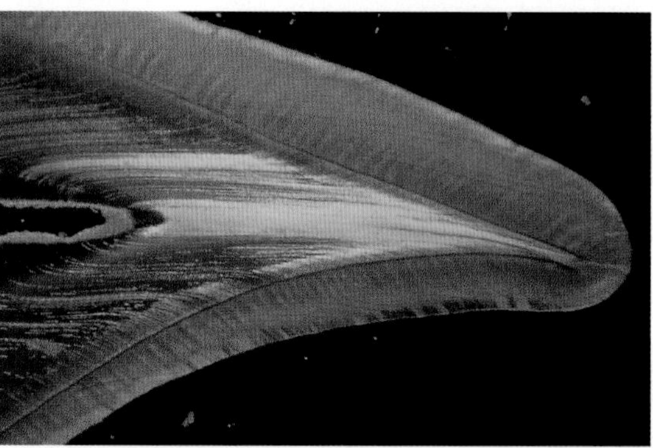

Fig. 7.25 Longitudinal section of enamel showing Hunter–Schreger bands in reflected light (×12).

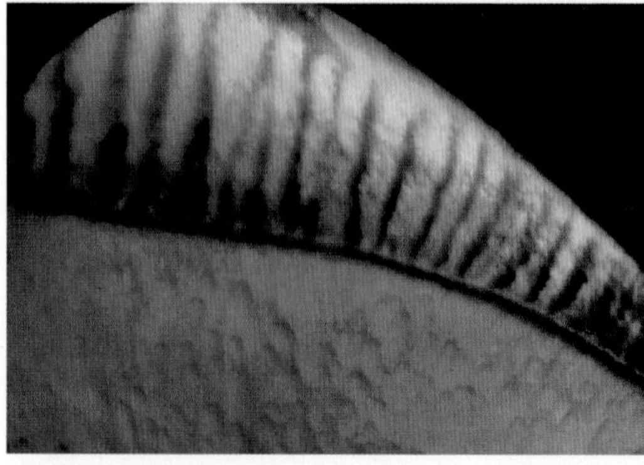

Fig. 7.26 Longitudinal section of enamel showing Hunter–Schreger bands in polarised light. Note that the bands do not completely reach the outermost surface of the enamel (×25).

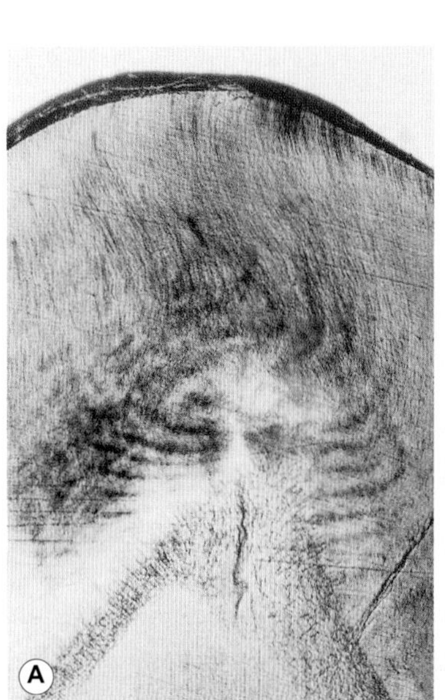

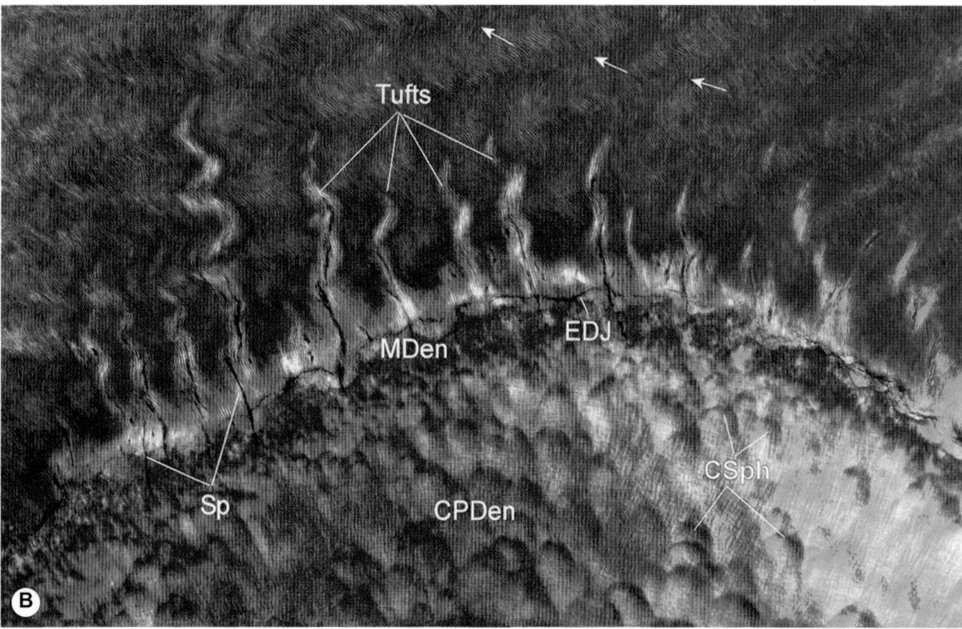

Fig. 7.27 (A) Longitudinal ground section of a cusp showing irregular spiralling of prisms over the tip of a cusp (gnarled enamel) (×25). (B) Ground section of tooth cusp, showing both enamel and dentine. The enamel over the cusp has a 'gnarled' structure: the prisms follow undulating paths, which are synchronised and give rise to numerous bands, which appear alternately red (see arrows) and blue in polarised light because of the change in prism direction. Enamel tufts, which consist of hypomineralised prism segments, radiate from the enamel–dentine junction (EDJ) and follow the same undulating paths as the normally mineralised prisms, so they appear wavy. The calcospheritic pattern of dentine formation (CSph) is evident (×75). CPDen = circumpulpal dentine; MDen = mantle dentine; Sp = enamel spindle. Courtesy Prof. T Bromage.

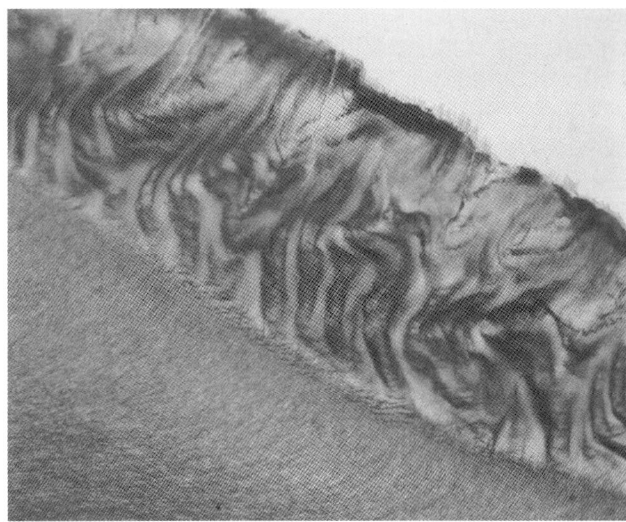

Fig. 7.28 Ground longitudinal section of molar of hyena showing complex appearance of Hunter–Schreger bands in the enamel. Copyright Royal College of Surgeons of England.

longitudinally. The bands of prisms that are cut longitudinally are known as parazones and those cut transversely as diazones. The angle between parazones and diazones is about 40 degrees. This complex pattern of prisms makes enamel resistant to fracture and, when exposed on the surface, leads to a microridged grinding surface. In approximately the outer quarter of enamel the prisms all run in the same direction, and no Hunter–Schreger bands are present (Fig. 7.26).

Because prisms are arranged in a spiral pattern, in some areas beneath the cusps and incisal edges the changes in direction of the prisms appear more marked and irregular. Groups of prisms seem to spiral around others, giving the appearance of 'gnarled' enamel (Fig. 7.27).

Hunter–Schreger bands are most conspicuous in the teeth of mammals whose diet contains hard material such as bone, as seen in the enamel of the hyena (Fig. 7.28).

Nonprismatic (aprismatic/prismless) enamel

The outer 20–100 µm of enamel of newly erupted deciduous teeth and the outer 20–70 µm of newly erupted permanent teeth are nonprismatic. Here the enamel crystallites are all aligned at right angles to the surface and parallel to each other. This surface layer is more highly mineralised than the rest of the enamel because of the absence of prism boundaries, where more organic material is located. Its thickness is variable (Fig. 7.29). A very thin layer of nonprismatic enamel, just a few microns wide, has also been reported to be present in the first enamel formed at the enamel–dentine junction. Nonprismatic enamel occurs as a result of the absence of Tomes processes from the ameloblasts in the first and final stages of enamel deposition (see Chapter 22).

Incremental lines

During changes in secretory rhythm during enamel development, chemical composition and/or the position of the developing enamel front are recorded as incremental features. There are two main types of incremental line: short period (cross-striations) and long period (enamel striae, also known as the striae of Retzius) (Box 7.1).

Cross-striations

Cross-striations are lines that cross enamel prisms at right angles to their long axes (Fig. 7.30) with a common interval of about 3–6 µm, being closer together near the enamel–dentine junction (see Fig. 7.31). Cross-striations are formed parallel to the secretory face of the ameloblast every 24 h, as evidenced by injections of labelling dyes administered at known time intervals. To provide further evidence that the circadian clock modulates enamel development, it has been demonstrated that the key genetic regulators of the circadian clock, Per2 and Bmal, are expressed in cultured ameloblasts.

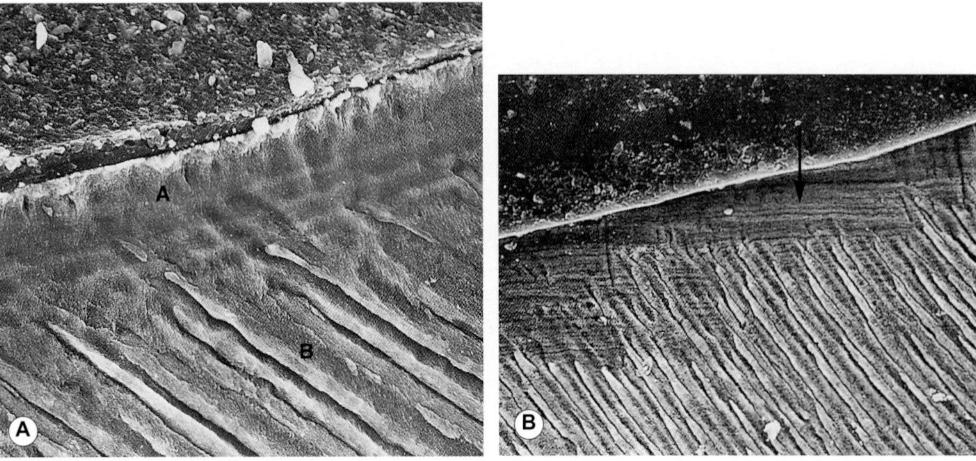

Fig. 7.29 (A) SEM showing a layer of aprismatic enamel (A) of even thickness overlying a layer of prismatic enamel (B) (×63). (B) SEM showing a layer of aprismatic enamel (arrow) of uneven thickness overlying prismatic enamel. Courtesy Dr D K Whittaker.

Box 7.1 Lines in enamel

Cross-striations	Enamel stria	Neonatal line
Short period incremental lines	Long period incremental lines	Reflects metabolic changes at birth
Transverse to prisms	Oblique to prisms	Oblique to prisms
Throughout enamel	Throughout enamel	A single line
3–6 μm apart	25–40 μm apart	About 20–40 μm thick
Represent daily increments	Represent weekly increments	Represents a few days after birth
Prism varies in width	Reach surface at perikymata	Prisms vary in width and direction

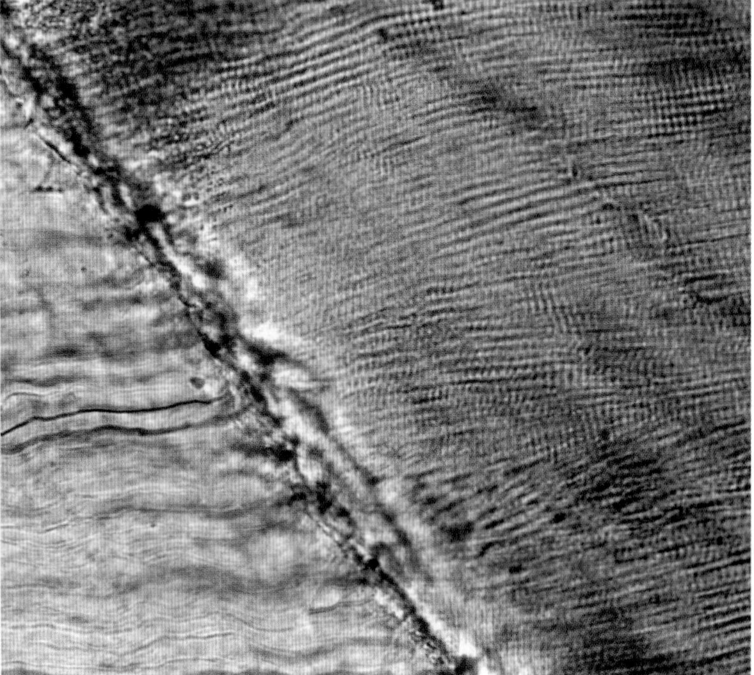

Fig. 7.31 The junction between dentine on the left and enamel on the right runs obliquely across this image. Thin brown enamel prisms (approximately 5 μm in diameter) pass from the enamel–dentine junction (EDJ) towards the enamel surface, and along their lengths small daily cross-striations that seem to divide the prisms into alternating varicosities and constrictions are easily visible in this image. Rarely in practice are they as good as this. Adjacent cross-striations are approximately 2.3 μm apart right up against the EDJ in this image but closer to 2.7 μm apart farther away from the EDJ (×300). From Dean, M.C., 2012. A histological method that can be used to estimate the time taken to form the crown of a permanent tooth. *Methods in Molecular Biology* 915: 89–100.

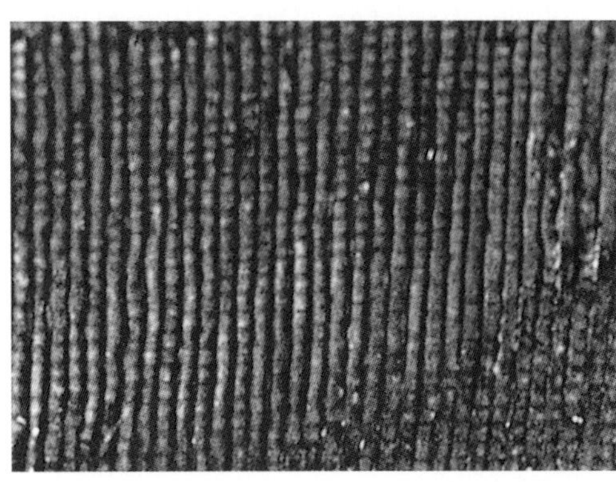

Fig. 7.30 Phase-contrast microscopy of longitudinal section of enamel showing cross-striations (horizontal lines) along the enamel prisms (×400). Courtesy Dr D F G Poole.

Furthermore, the expression of amelogenin in secretory ameloblasts oscillated with an approximate 24 hour period, with a twofold decrease in expression during the dark (night) period compared with the light (day) period.

The appearance of cross-striations may relate to regular variations in prism width (Figs. 7.32, 7.33). It has also been suggested that the appearance of cross-striations is the result of subtle changes in the nature of the organic matrix and/or crystallite orientation.

Enamel striae

In sections of enamel cut along the longitudinal axis of the crown the enamel striae (or striae of Retzius) are seen as prominent lines that run obliquely across the enamel prisms to the surface (Fig. 7.34). In horizontal sections they form concentric rings (Fig. 7.35). They represent the successive positions of the enamel-forming front. The periodic nature of this feature, which may be assessed by the number of cross-striations between successive enamel lines, has been one of the more contentious topics in the study of enamel microstructure. One unusual feature is that the spacing of the striae is species specific.

Although following routine demineralisation all enamel structure is lost because of the low content of the organic matrix, leaving an enamel space (Fig. 7.2), controlled (and probably incomplete) demineralisation will allow retention of some organic material for subsequent staining. Many of the structural features seen in ground sections will be retained. The keyhole pattern of the prisms can be clearly seen (Fig. 7.36A). Although it is known that the prism lacks an organic sheath, the level of organic material

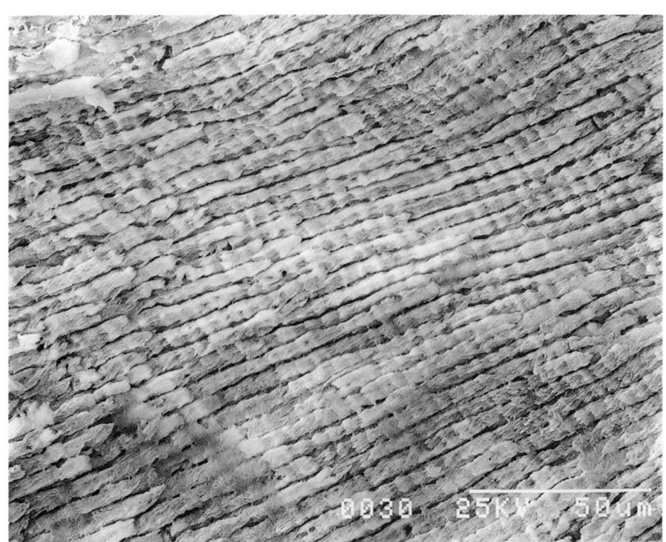

Fig. 7.32 SEM of fractured enamel surface showing cross-striations along the length of prisms seemingly corresponding to sites of narrowing of the prism width (×600). Courtesy Prof. M C Dean.

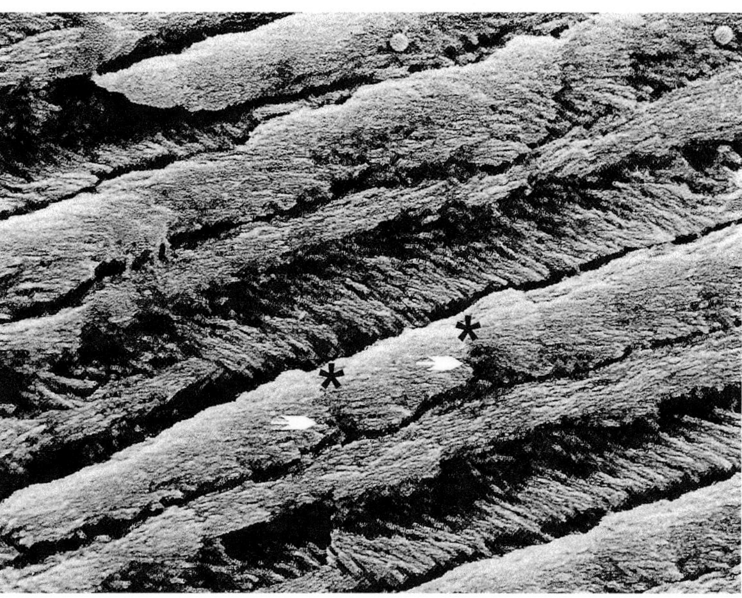

Fig. 7.33 SEM of lightly etched enamel showing individual enamel crystallites (arrows) terminating at constrictions of prisms (*) (×1,600). Courtesy Dr R C Shore and the CRC Press.

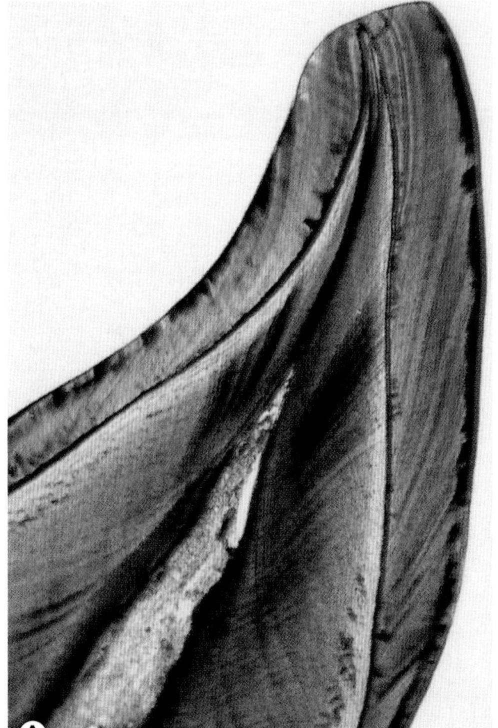

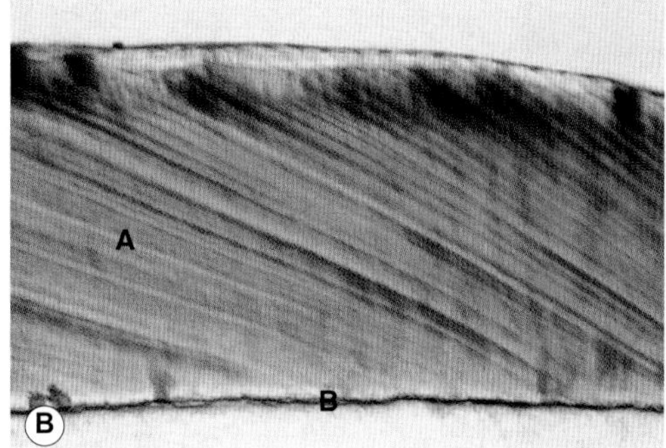

Fig. 7.34 (A) Longitudinal section of enamel showing enamel striae running obliquely across the tissue. Wear at the tip of the cusp has exposed some of the striae on the surface at this site. Along the slopes of the tooth the striae naturally reach the surface (×15). (B) Higher-power view (×40) of enamel striae in enamel (A) along the side of the tooth running from the enamel–dentine junction (B) to the surface.

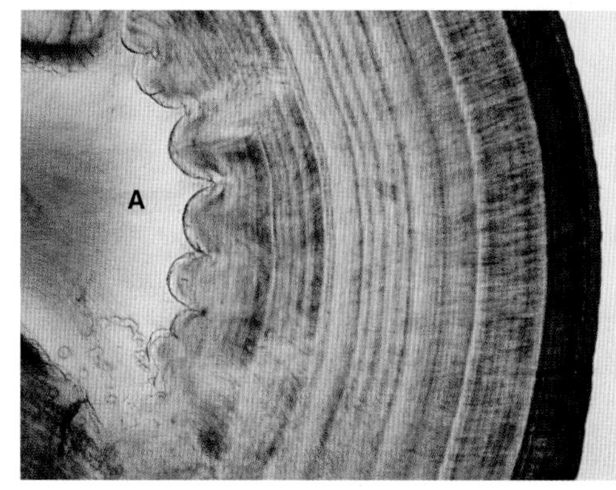

Fig. 7.35 Transverse section of enamel showing enamel striae running circumferentially. A = dentine (×120). Courtesy Dr M E Atkinson.

and water is likely to be higher at the prism boundary because of the larger pores produced by the abutment of hydroxyapatite crystallites at this junction. This, and the apparently lower solubility of the organic matrix at the prism boundary, can explain the deeper staining at these sites. Enamel striae are also observed in demineralised sections (Fig. 7.36B).

Owing to the manner in which enamel is deposited (see pages 415–416), the striae overlying the cusps and incisal edges do not reach the surface (Fig. 7.37) unless there has been enamel loss (Fig. 7.34A). In the case of unworn incisors the first 25–30 striae do not reach the surface.

In human teeth there are generally 7–9 cross-striations between adjacent striae in any one individual (Fig. 7.38), although this number can vary between 6 and 12 (Fig. 7.39). The striae are therefore formed at about weekly intervals. Because the average distance between two cross-striations is about 4 µm, enamel striae in the middle portion of enamel are about 25–35 µm apart. In cervical enamel, where enamel is formed more slowly and cross-striations may be only about 2 µm apart, the striae are closer together and may be separated by only 15–20 µm. Accentuated striae may be caused by metabolic disturbances occurring during the time of mineralisation.

Over the whole of the lateral enamel, enamel striae reach the surface in a series of fine grooves running circumferentially around the crown. These features are known as the perikymata grooves and are separated

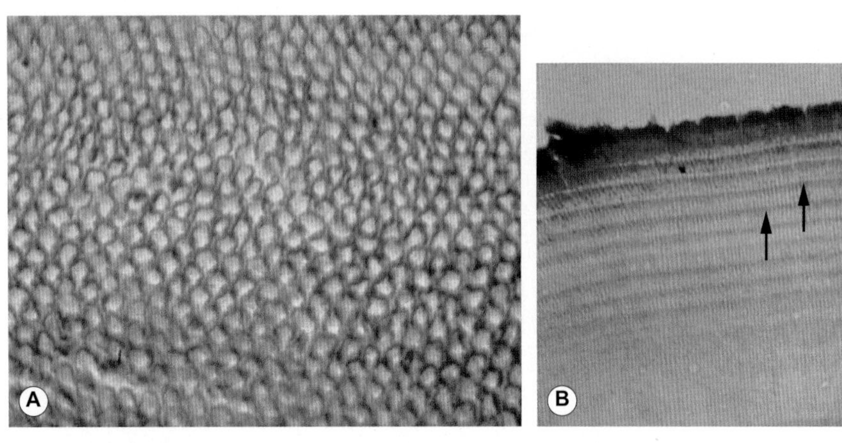

Fig. 7.36 (A) Demineralised section of enamel prisms cut transversely showing retained enamel matrix presenting a prismatic appearance (light blue stain; ×600). (B) Demineralised transverse section of enamel showing enamel striae patterns (arrows) in the retained enamel matrix (light blue stain; ×150).

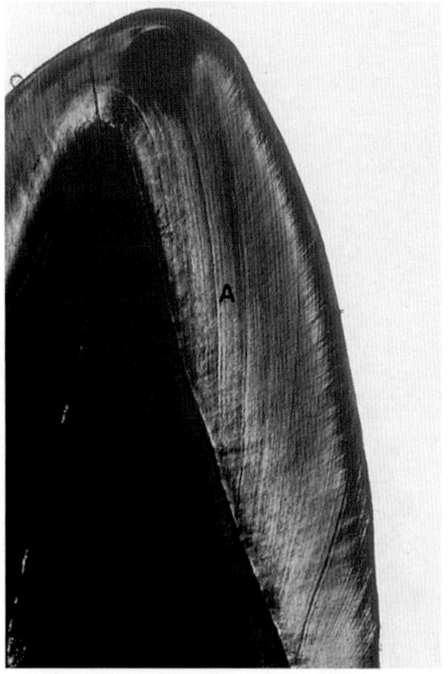

Fig. 7.37 Longitudinal section of unworn enamel (A) showing that striae passing over the cusp do not reach the outer tooth surface, but those more laterally do (×20). Courtesy Drs R J Hillier and G T Craig.

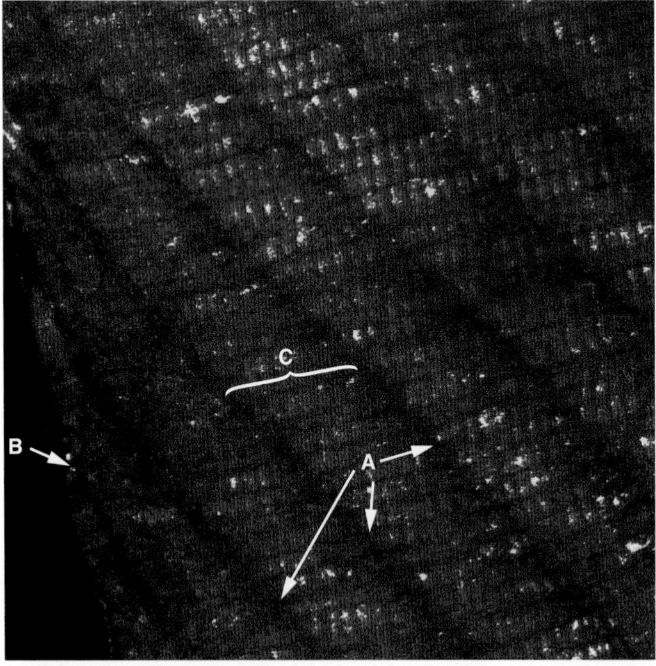

Fig. 7.38 Confocal image of a longitudinal section of enamel showing enamel striae (A) reaching the surface at perikymata grooves (B). Between adjacent striae, about seven cross-striations (C) are evident as vertical lines (×850). Courtesy Prof. M C Dean.

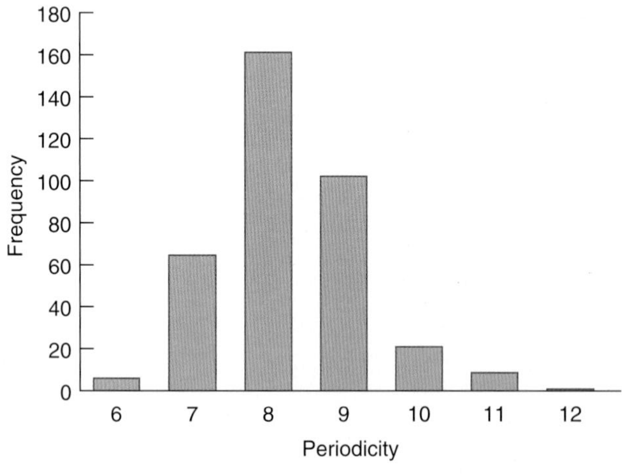

Fig. 7.39 Histogram showing number of cross-striations between enamel striae derived from measuring 365 modern human teeth. From Smith et al., 2007. New perspectives on chimpanzee and human molar crown development. In: Bailey, S. Hublin, J. (Eds.), *Dental perspectives on human evolution.* pp. 177–192 Springer.

by ridges, the perikymata ridges (Figs. 7.40–7.43). The distance between perikymata reflects the data already given for that of enamel striae: they are close together near the cervical margin (about 15–20 μm) but, as they reach the surface obliquely, may be up to 100 μm apart towards the cusp of the tooth. The process that results in the production of the enamel striae is unknown.

In deciduous teeth, enamel striae and perikymata are only ever clearly seen in the cervical enamel of deciduous second molars.

The exaggeration of striae in different teeth forming at the same time suggests a common systemic influence. One hypothesis is that there may be a rhythm with a 27-h cycle in addition to a diurnal daily rhythm. The two rhythms would coincide approximately every 7 or 8 days, producing a fault in the developing enamel. The underlying reason for the structural feature apparent as a stria in ground section is differential light-scattering effects at this fault line, possibly because of a slight change in prism direction/thickness, or slight differences in crystallite composition/orientation and/or differences in organic content. That the striae are seen in partially demineralised sections has been interpreted by some as being because of the site of striae having a higher carbonate content, which causes greater solubility of the crystals and greater porosity.

It is possible to use the incremental markings in enamel (cross-striations, enamel striae and perikymata) to assess the time taken to form the crown of the tooth and to help age material. Because impressions of the surface enamel can record the perikymata, rare teeth of fossil hominids have also been studied without the need to prepare destructive ground sections (Fig. 7.42). Assuming adjacent perikymata are separated by approximately 7-day intervals, the total number of perikymata on a crown indicates the time taken for the crown to form, if about 6–9 months are added to this total to account for the 25–30 striae over the top of the crown that do not reach the surface (Fig. 7.37). From such studies it has been found, for example, that the teeth of apes and many extinct hominids develop more quickly than those of modern humans, resulting in a shorter childhood period for learning (see also Chapter 27). If incremental markings from root development are also considered, age of death may be ascertained.

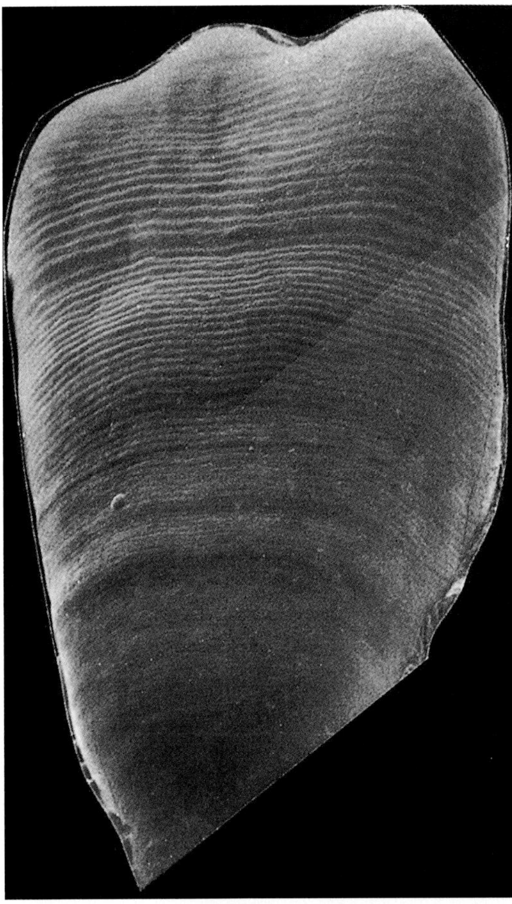

Fig. 7.40 SEM of enamel surface of a human lower incisor showing numerous transversely running perikymata grooves and ridges (×10). Courtesy Prof. M C Dean and the *Journal of Human Evolution*.

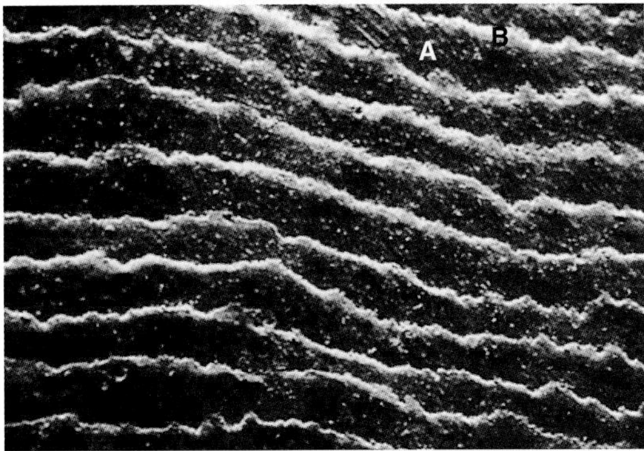

Fig. 7.41 Higher-power view of surface enamel with perikymata ridges (A) separated by perikymata grooves (B) (SEM ×400). Courtesy Dr D F G Poole.

For important fossil material, it is not often possible to section material to determine the periodicity of perikymata at the surface, which may vary from 6 to 12 days. For accurate determination of crown formation time, the number of cross-striations between adjacent striae is necessary. New non-destructive techniques have recently been developed whereby the whole thickness of enamel can be visualised and in which the enamel striae and cross-striations can be clearly seen (Fig. 7.44). This technique involves scanning a tooth using propagation-phase contrast X-ray synchrotron microtomography. The European Synchrotron Radiation Facility conducts such work in Grenoble, France. Using such a technique has provided more accurate data concerning crown formation times and age at death for many important australopithecines and some early fossil hominins, and confirms they fall below or at the low end of extant human values.

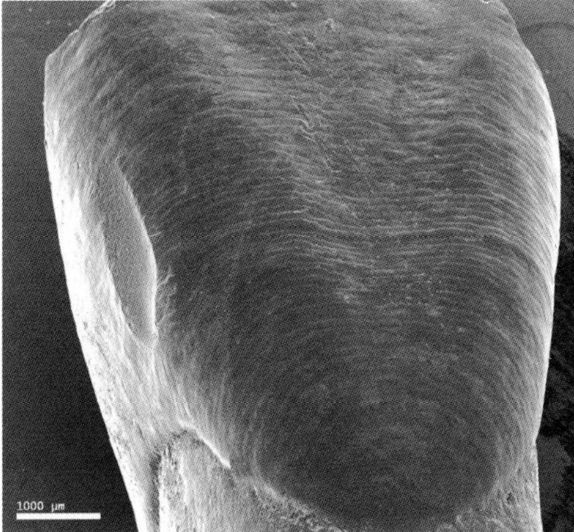

Fig. 7.42 SEM showing perikymata on the surface of a mandibular incisor from *Paranthropus robustus*. Scale bar = 1 mm. Courtesy Prof. M C Dean.

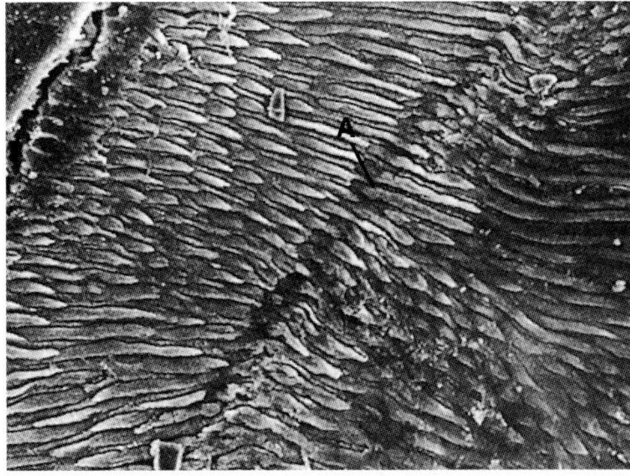

Fig. 7.43 SEM of an etched longitudinal section of deciduous enamel showing enamel prisms changing in both thickness and direction at the neonatal line (A) (×400). Courtesy Dr D K Whittaker.

Although it was once thought that striae periodicity was similar for all teeth of an individual, research has shown that there is often a decrease in this periodicity along the tooth row, such that the periodicity of anterior teeth may be 2 days higher than that of the molars. Such information must be borne in mind when using such features in ageing an individual. Similarly, recent research has also suggested that stria periodicity in deciduous molars is smaller than that of permanent molars.

It is thought that the deposition of the striation may reflect increases in both bone growth and body mass. There is some evidence in primates that the number of cross-striations between two adjacent striae reflects body size: in monkeys, there are only four to five cross-striations between striae.

Enamel striae are less pronounced or absent from enamel formed before birth. A particularly marked stria is formed at birth – this is the **neonatal line** (Fig. 7.45) and reflects the metabolic changes at birth. It is present in all deciduous teeth and is associated with the mesiobuccal cusp of first permanent molars. It is generally about 20–40 μm thick. Prisms appear to change both direction and thickness at the time of this event (Fig. 7.43). The neonatal line, as well as the enamel dentine junction and surface enamel, are all zinc rich. Thus identifying the distribution of the element zinc within teeth can help identify the presence of the neonatal line (Fig. 7.46). Within the neonatal line zinc may be associated with increased crystallinity.

The presence of a neonatal line represents enamel formed during the first few days of birth. It therefore has important forensic significance because its presence in a dead neonate indicates an infant lived for a few days, whereas its absence would indicate a stillbirth.

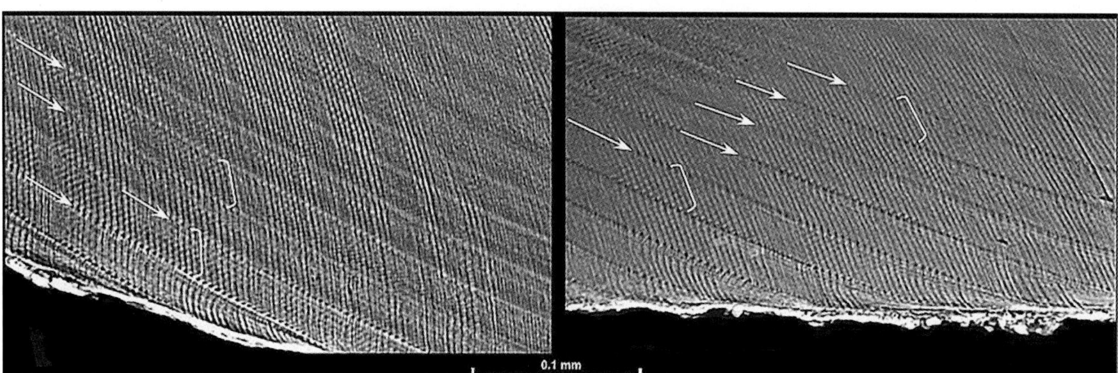

Fig. 7.44 Images showing enamel from the right lower first permanent molar (left image) and left upper first molar (right image) of juvenile fossil *Homo*. Using noninvasive multiscale synchrotron imaging, sections can be revealed showing enamel striae (arrows) and the presence of eight cross-striations between adjacent striae (brackets). From Smith, T.M. et al., 2015. Dental ontogeny in Pliocene and early Pleistocene hominins. *PLoS One* 10(2): e0118118.

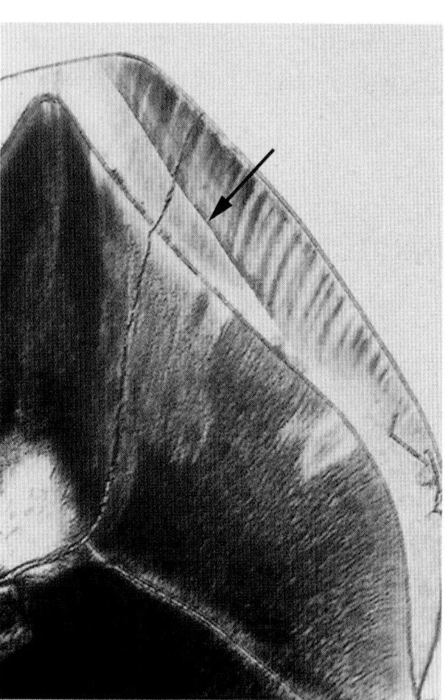

Fig. 7.45 Longitudinal section of a deciduous tooth showing a neonatal line (arrow) (×6). Courtesy Dr R J Hillier and Dr G T Craig.

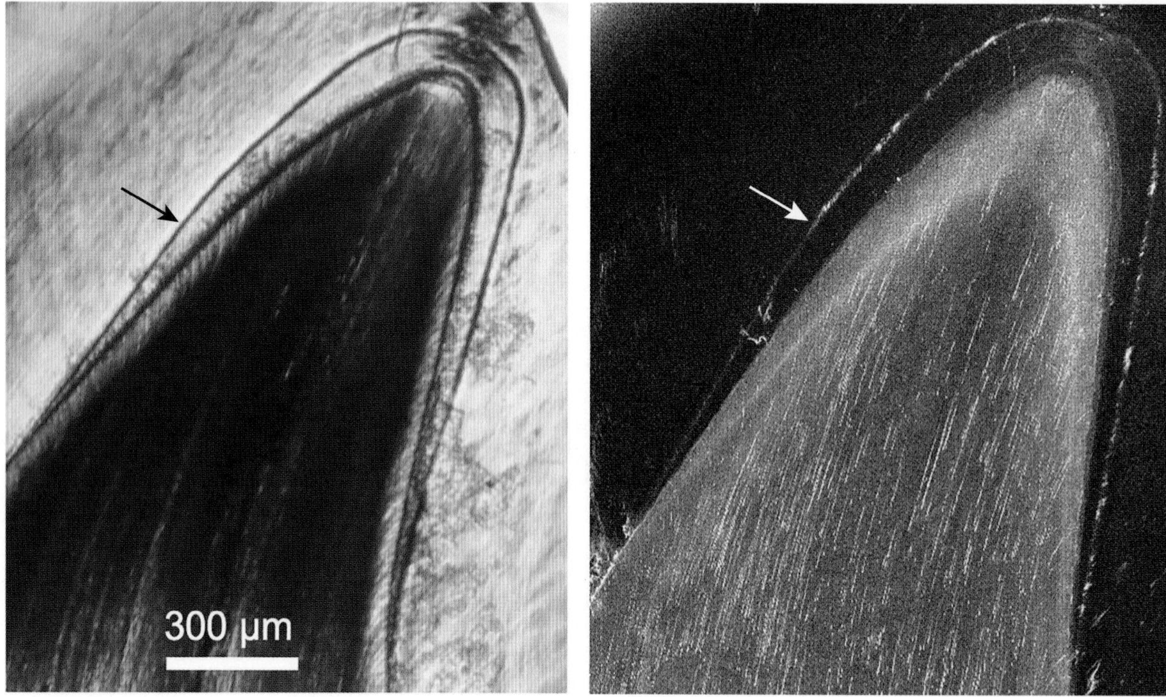

Fig. 7.46 Left image is a transmitted light micrograph (TLM) of the neonatal line (arrow) in the distobuccal cusp of an upper deciduous second molar. Right image is same section showing distribution of zinc highlighted in neonatal line (arrow) using synchrotron X-ray fluorescence to map elemental distributions. From Dean, M.C. et al., 2019. Synchrotron X-ray fluorescence mapping of Ca, Sr and Zn at the neonatal line in human deciduous teeth reflects changing perinatal physiology. *Archives of Oral Biology* 104: 90–102.

Physiological stress, such as malnutrition or illness, can disrupt normal enamel growth resulting in linear enamel hypoplasia that runs parallel with the striae.

Surface enamel

The surface of the enamel is perhaps its most clinically significant region. It is here that the tooth comes into contact with food, dental caries is initiated, restorations are attached or abutted, orthodontic brackets are cemented, and toothpaste, bleaches and fluoride/remineralisation preparations are applied.

Both physically and chemically, surface enamel differs markedly from subsurface enamel. Surface enamel is harder, less porous, less soluble and more radio-opaque than subsurface enamel. It is richer in some trace elements (especially fluoride) but contains less carbonate. The enamel surface presents a variable appearance, exhibiting features such as aprismatic enamel, perikymata, prism-end markings, cracks, pits and elevations.

The surface enamel, if unabraded, is in most areas aprismatic and thus more highly mineralised and resistant to caries (Fig. 7.29). This may help explain why acid etching, unless sufficient to penetrate to the prismatic enamel, may not always enhance adhesion. Although the surface enamel is aprismatic, the incremental striae of Retzius reach the surface and appear as perikymata grooves, wave-like concentric surface rings parallel to the cementum–enamel junction. The perikymata grooves are separated from each other by the wave-like perikymata ridges (Fig. 7.47, see also Figs. 7.40–7.42). Attrition and abrasion remove these features after eruption, but they may persist in protected cervical areas. In some areas, particularly cervically where the reduced enamel epithelium persists for some time after eruption, small pits are seen within the perikymata. These are the impressions of the ends of the ameloblasts and are 1–1.5 µm in depth (Fig. 7.48).

Small cracks are frequently found in surface enamel (Fig. 7.49), although it is difficult to know whether many of these were present *in vivo* or were induced by the procedures necessary to examine the tissue. They represent potential areas of weakness. The orientation of the enamel prisms as they reach the surface may determine whether small cracks extend easily. In areas where the prisms make an acute angle with the surface, such as in the intercuspal region, enamel will resist fracture best. Small elevations 10–15 µm across (enamel caps, Fig. 7.50) or depressions (focal holes, Fig. 7.51) are also found, particularly on lateral surfaces. The caps are thought to result from enamel deposition on top of small deposits of nonmineralisable debris late in development. The focal holes result from loss of the cap and underlying material by abrasion or attrition.

Larger surface elevations, enamel broches, 30–50 µm in diameter, also occur occasionally and consist of radiating groups of crystals (Fig. 7.52). They seem to be more common in premolars but are of unknown origin.

The loss of tooth structure can occur by four different mechanisms: attrition, abrasion, erosion and abfraction.

Attrition is tooth loss involving tooth-to-tooth contact. Attrition occurs both occlusally and interproximally. In molars, occlusal attrition is most commonly seen on the palatal surfaces of maxillary molars and the buccal surface of mandibular molars. The potential space to be expected during interproximal wear is generally closed up by mesial drift (see page 472). Thus, although initial tooth contact areas are small, these become broader with age. In people who habitually clench their teeth (bruxists) attrition may be severe and the occlusal plane flat (Fig. 7.53). There may also be exposure of sensitive dentine.

The progressive tooth substance loss caused by attrition is considered by some to be a normal ageing process as when teeth first erupt they are

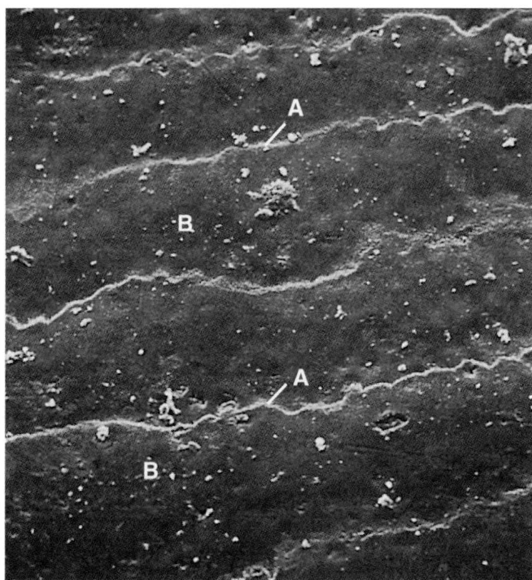

Fig. 7.47 SEM of enamel surface showing perikymata grooves (A) separated from each other by perikymata ridges (B) (×500). Courtesy Prof. H N Newman.

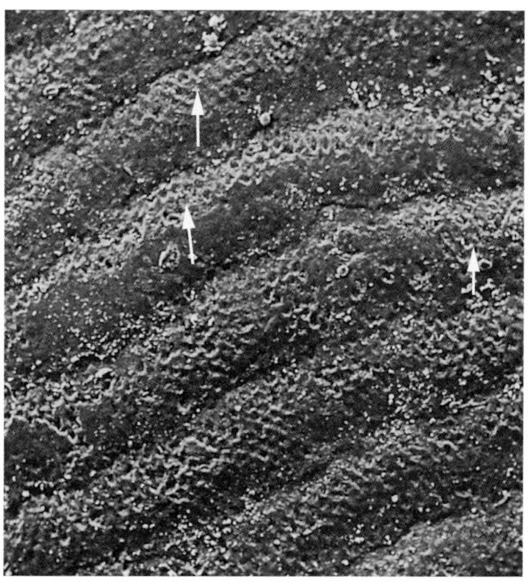

Fig. 7.48 SEM showing prism-end markings (arrows) on surface of enamel. Compare with Fig. 7.47, which lacks this feature (×300). Courtesy Prof. H N Newman.

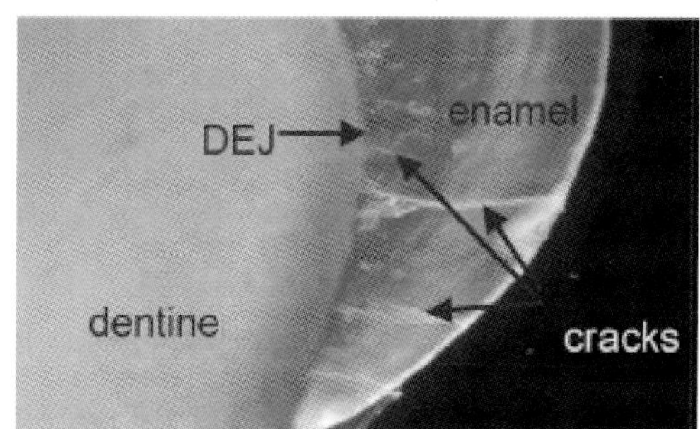

Fig. 7.49 Optical micrograph of a cross-section through a tooth, showing cracks that have propagated through the enamel but stop at the enamel–dentine junction (DEJ), without penetrating into the dentine. From Marshall, S.J. et al., 2003. The dentin–enamel junction—a natural, multilevel interface. *Journal of the European Ceramic Society* 23: 2897–2904, with permission.

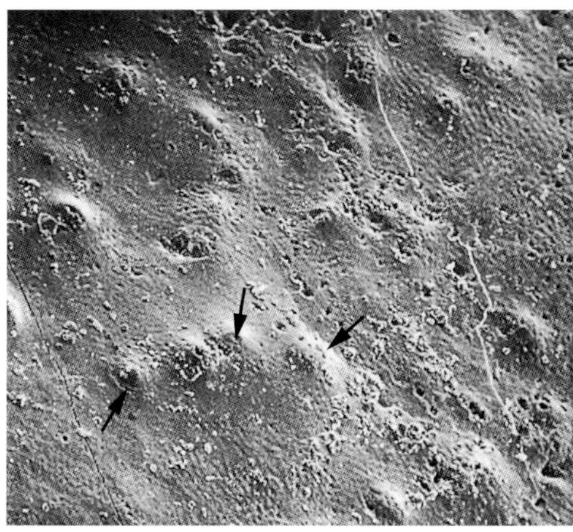

Fig. 7.50 SEM of enamel surface showing enamel caps (arrows) (×150). Courtesy Prof. H N Newman.

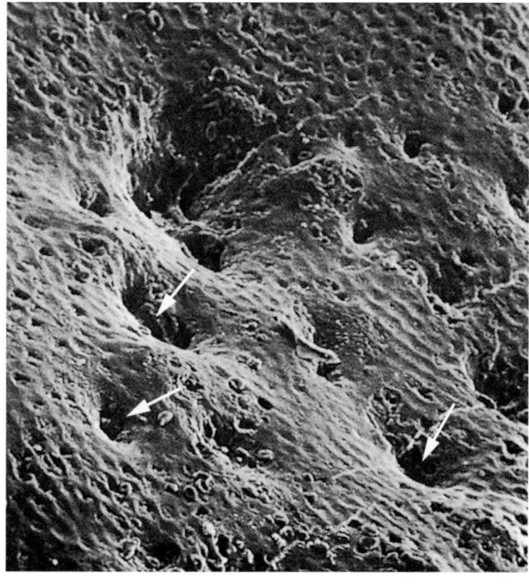

Fig. 7.51 SEM of enamel surface showing focal holes (arrows) (×400). Courtesy Prof. H N Newman.

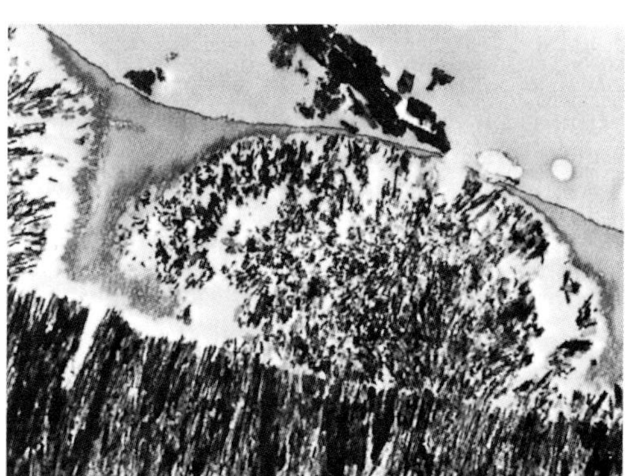

Fig. 7.52 TEM showing an enamel broch (×10,000). Courtesy Prof. H N Newman.

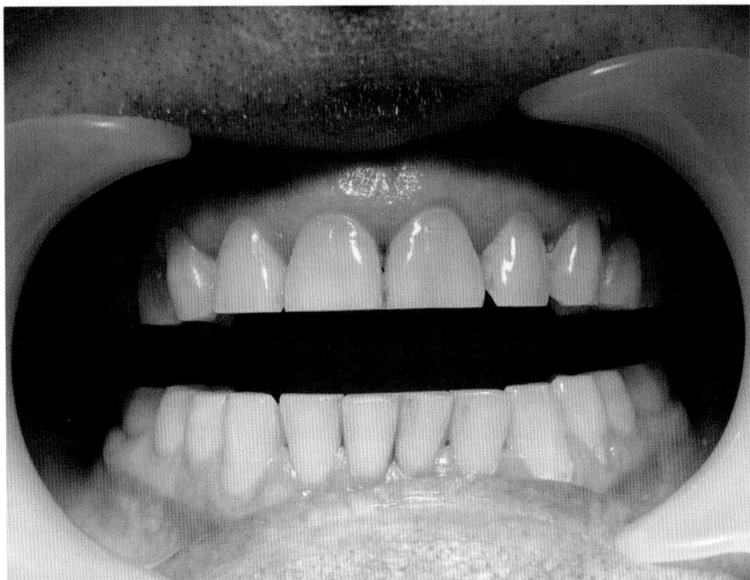

Fig. 7.53 Attrition in patient suffering from bruxism (tooth grinding). Note the flattened occlusal plane. Courtesy Prof. T J Watson.

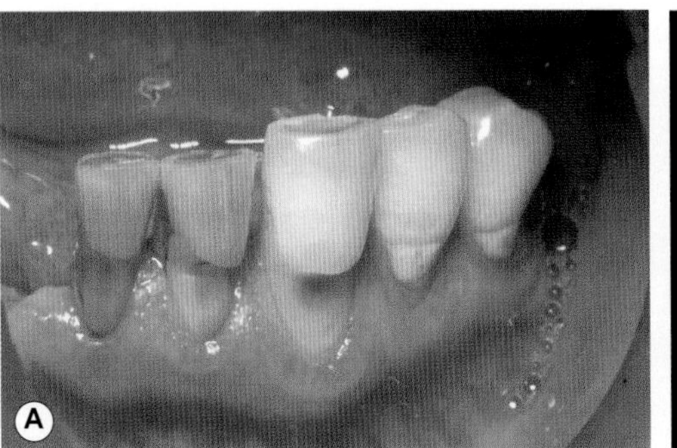

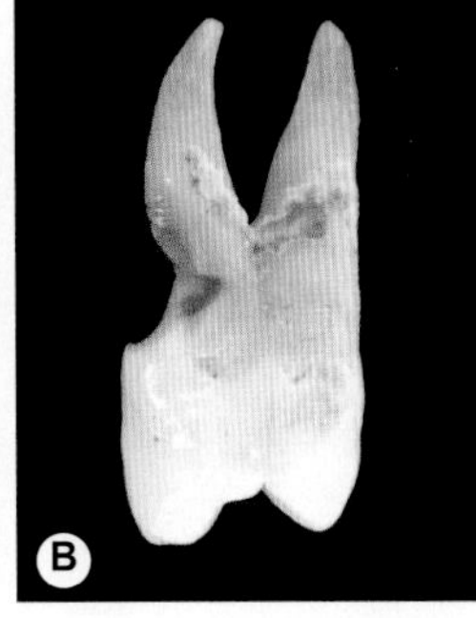

Fig. 7.54 (A) Toothbrush abrasion in the cervical region of the labial surfaces of the anterior teeth. (B) Side view of abrasion. Although this appearance is usually attributed to frictional contact with an outside material such as dental floss or a toothbrush, other factors such as occlusal stress or corrosion from bacterial plaque may also be involved. The term 'abfraction' is used to describe this kind of lesion with a multifactorial basis. (A) Courtesy Prof. T J Watson. (B) Courtesy Dr J Grippo.

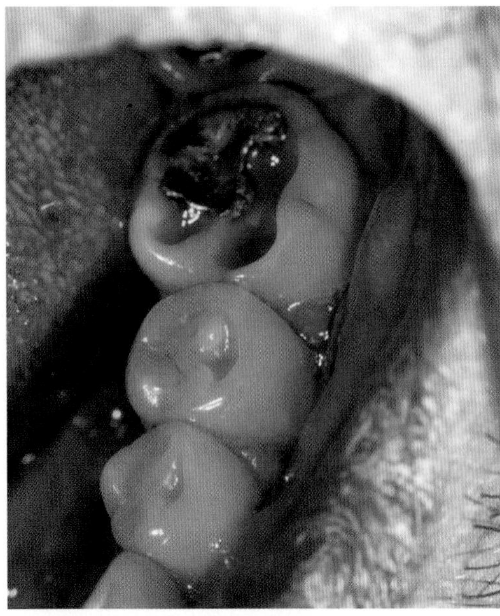

Fig. 7.55 Erosion of the teeth associated with the consumption of grapefruit producing irregular concavities on the occlusal surfaces. Courtesy Prof. T J Watson.

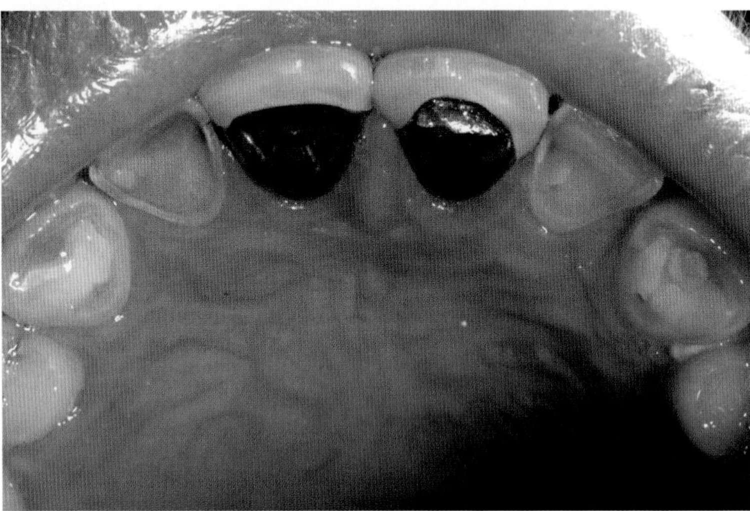

Fig. 7.56 Erosion of the upper anterior teeth in a patient suffering from bulimia. The central incisors have already been restored. Courtesy Prof. T J Watson.

not best suited to function and require a period of "wearing in" to achieve a more suitable morphology. Thus when restoring a tooth in someone showing attrition, it may be more appropriate not to return to the initial occlusal height.

Abrasion is tooth loss involving friction between the tooth and outside material. Maximum wear resistance will occur when the prisms are arranged perpendicular to the shearing force causing wear. Some types of dental abrasion may be related to habit or occupation, such as notching of incisal edges related to pipe smoking, nut cracking and nail biting. A common cause of abrasion is overvigorous tooth brushing or use of an abrasive dentifrice. The exposed dentine is shiny and smooth. Abrasion is typically seen on the labial and buccal surfaces (Fig. 7.54). As with attrition, the deposition of reactionary dentine protects the dental pulp (see page 181).

Erosion is tooth loss involving contact with acidic agents that may be extrinsic (e.g., soft drinks, citrus fruit [Fig. 7.55]) or intrinsic (gastric acids following chronic regurgitation). In cases of bulimia the erosion characteristically affects the palatal surfaces of the upper anterior teeth (Fig. 7.56). Some consider that an interval of 1 hour should be considered before toothbrushing after an acid attack, to allow a period of remineraliation from saliva necessary for improving the resistance of eroded enamel against brushing abrasion.

Although noncarious loss of cervical enamel is usually attributed to toothbrush abrasion and/or erosion, it has been suggested that such loss may also be the result of occlusal loading leading to cyclic, eccentric, occlusal forces in vulnerable cervical regions of teeth. Such loss has been termed **abfraction**. Its aetiology is controversial. Attrition, corrosion, abrasion and stress-corrosion might act alone or in combination to initiate and perpetuate lesions. If true, this may have to be taken into account when restoring noncarious cervical lesions, in that any evidence of excessive loading should also be treated.

Surface enamel may be damaged during orthodontic treatment by demineralisation beneath cemented brackets. This can be minimised by proper treatment of the surface, choice of adhesive and post-treatment remineralisation procedures.

Tooth loss by any of the four methods listed earlier may make a tooth hypersensitive (see page 187).

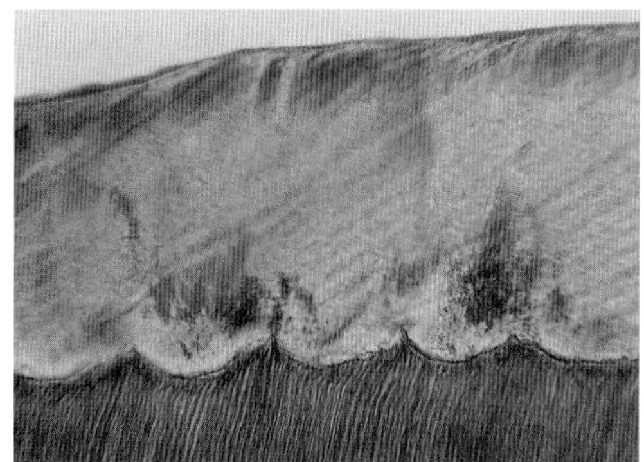

Fig. 7.57 Scalloped appearance of the enamel–dentine junction beneath the cusp of a tooth (×60).

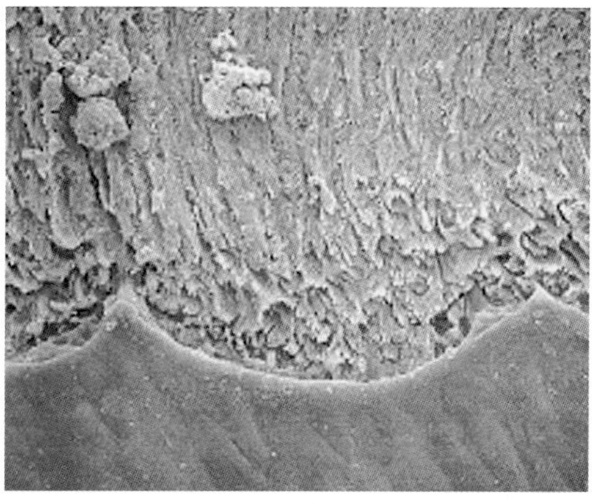

Fig. 7.58 SEM showing scallop structure in the enamel–dentine junction, with enamel on the top and dentine on the bottom (×700). From Marshall, S.J. et al., 2003. The dentin–enamel junction—a natural, multilevel interface. *Journal of the European Ceramic Society* 23: 2897–2904, with permission.

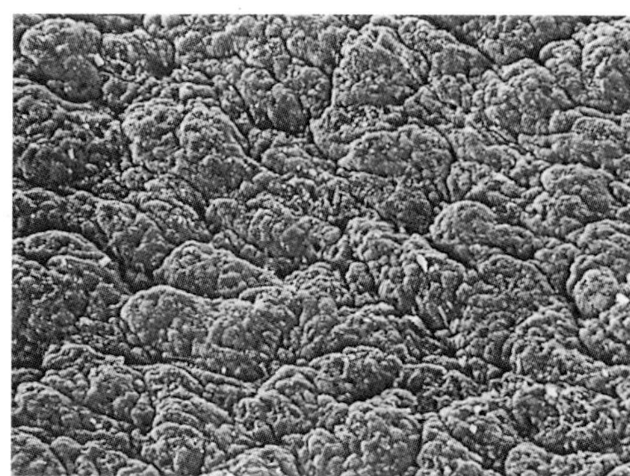

Fig. 7.59 SEM of the enamel surface that lies in contact with the dentine, with separation having been achieved after dehydration and fracture. The enamel surface is convex at this site (×250). Courtesy Dr D K Whittaker.

Enamel–dentine junction

In permitting the strong union of two dissimilar mineralised tissues, the enamel–dentine junction (alternatively termed the amelodentinal junction) exhibits some unique features, particularly those associated with retardation of crack propagation (Fig. 7.49). Structurally, there are three levels of features. The most obvious is the pattern of scallops 25 to 100 μm wide, that is particularly evident beneath cusps and incisal edges (Figs. 7.57, 7.58), areas where shearing forces would be high; the enamel–dentine junction is smoother on the lateral surfaces of the crown. The convexities of the scallops are on the enamel surface (Fig. 7.59), with the concavities on the dentinal surface (Fig. 7.60). With increased magnification, a second order of structure is the presence of smaller microscallops 2–5 μm in size. A third, nanostructural level of organisation yet to be fully determined also exists, with the ends of fine collagen fibrils from the dentine mingling with the initial crystals of enamel. Dentine crystals are much smaller than those of enamel, and the transition from one to the other at the junction of the two tissues is generally clear (Fig. 7.61). The enamel–dentine junction is less mineralised than either the enamel or dentine.

The shape of the junction is thought to determine the shape of the crown because the junction is the vestige of the internal enamel epithelium, although this can be modified by variations in the thickness of secreted enamel (Fig. 7.62). The junction between dentine and enamel appears to be crucial for limiting propagation of cracks through the tooth. Most cracks travelling inwards from the tooth surface terminate at this junction, and those which cross the junction seem to be arrested in the outer few micrometres of the dentine.

The enamel–dentine junction, together with the adjacent inner enamel layer (extending for 100–400 microns), has a higher organic content and a slightly lower mineral content. Using laser capture microdissection, proteomic analysis has revealed traces of 45 proteins in these two regions. The proteins identified have a variety of functions, including calcium ion binding, formation of extracellular matrix, formation of cytoskeleton, cytoskeletal protein binding, cell adhesion, and transport. Collagens were identified as the most dominant proteins (including collagen type XXII). Tissue-specific proteins, such as ameloblastin and amelogenin, were also detected. With such a complex array of proteins present, the reasons for the successful properties of the enamel-dentine junction await clarification.

Several other features can be seen at the enamel–dentine junction extending from the dentine surface into the enamel, including enamel spindles, enamel tufts and enamel lamellae (Fig. 7.63).

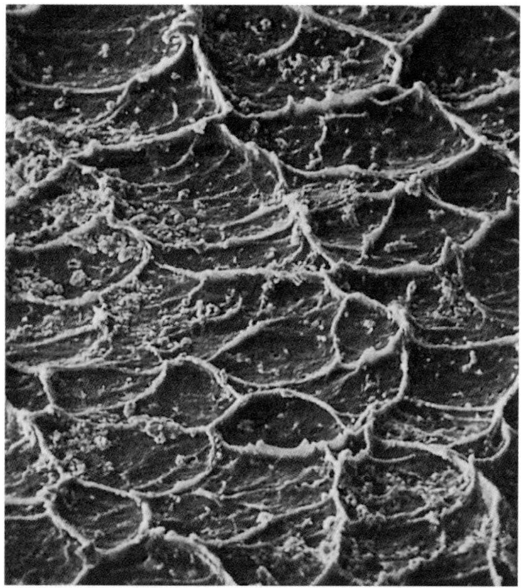

Fig. 7.60 SEM of dentine surface at the enamel–dentine junction, after removal of enamel by demineralisation. The dentine at this site shows a series of concavities (×400). Courtesy Dr B G H Levers.

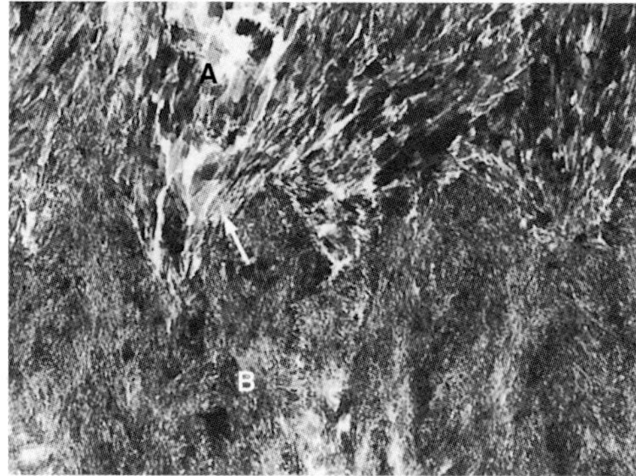

Fig. 7.61 TEM showing enamel (A) and dentine (B) crystallites at the enamel–dentine junction (arrow). Note the larger size of the enamel crystallites (×18,000). Courtesy Prof. H N Newman.

Enamel spindles

Narrow (up to 8 μm in diameter), round, sometimes club-shaped tubules – the enamel spindles – extend up to 25 μm into the enamel (Fig. 7.64). They are not aligned with the prisms and are thought to be the result of some odontoblast processes that, during the early stages of enamel development, insinuate themselves between the ameloblasts. The size of some would exceed the usual dimension of dentinal tubules. It has also been suggested that they may be dentinal collagen or the remnants of odontoblasts or ameloblasts (Fig. 7.65). Enamel spindles are most common beneath cusps where most crowding of odontoblasts would have occurred. In the erupted tooth these tubules do not contain cell processes. Because of their alignment they are best seen in longitudinal sections of enamel.

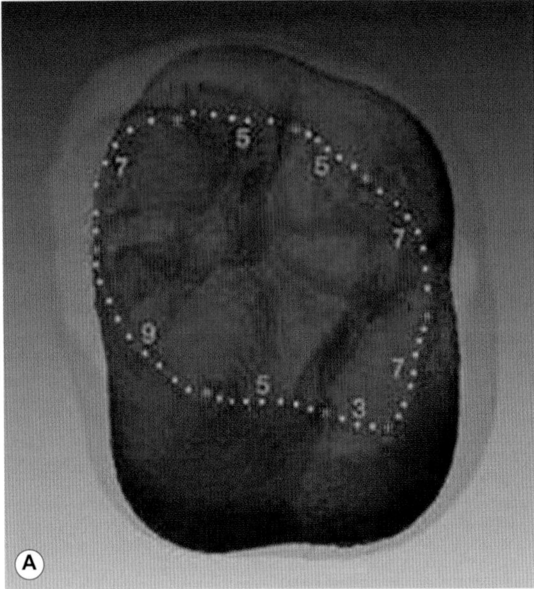

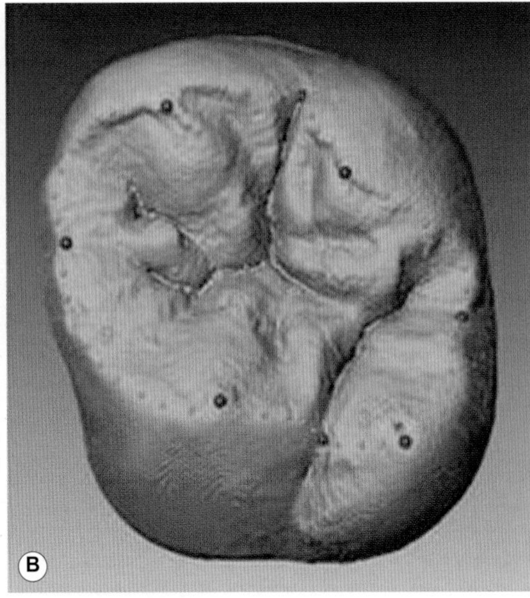

Fig. 7.62 Digital image of permanent maxillary first molar crown (occlusal view), (A) Enamel-dentine ridge curve digitised on the surface of the enamel-dentine junction. (B) The ridge curve of the outer enamel surface digitised on the outer enamel surface. Red circles are landmarks and yellow circles are semilandmarks. The images relate to how tooth crown patterning is governed by the growth and folding of the inner enamel epithelium and how overall dental crown shape is determined by processes that configurate shape at the enamel -dentine junction. From Morita et al., 2014. The boundary of the enamel–dentine junction as determined by morphometric analysis superimposed on the outer enamel surface. *Journal of Anatomy* 224: 669–680.

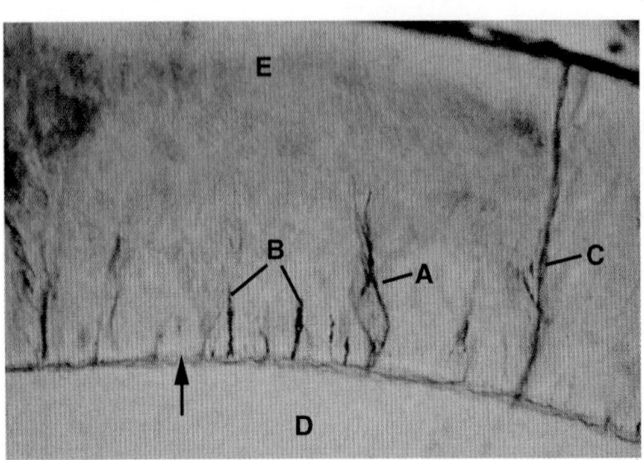

Fig. 7.63 Transverse section showing the enamel–dentine junction. A = enamel tuft; B = enamel spindle; C = enamel lamella; D = dentine; E = enamel (×60). Courtesy Dr R Sprinz.

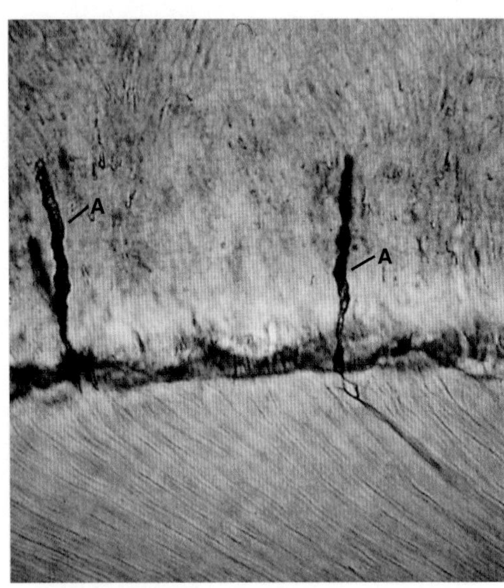

Fig. 7.64 Longitudinal section of enamel showing enamel spindles (A) (×250). Courtesy Dr R Sprinz.

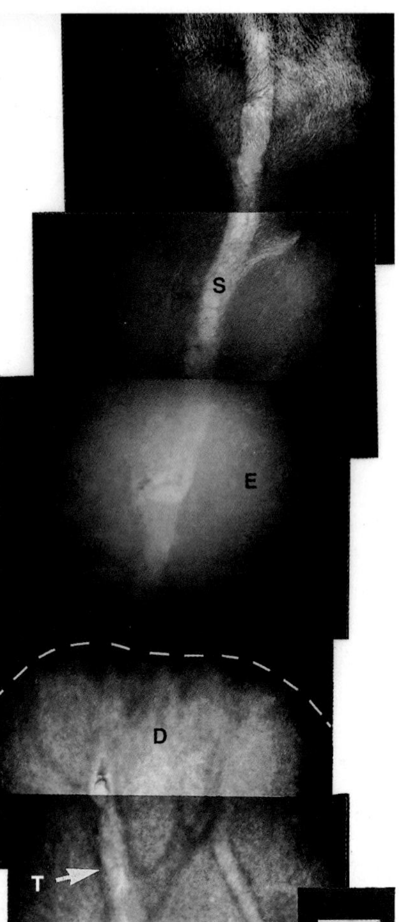

Fig. 7.65 TEM showing an enamel spindle (S) appearing as the continuation of a dentinal tubule (T) from dentine (D) into enamel (E) (×6500). Courtesy J Palamara, P P Phakey, W A Rachinger, H J Orams and the editor of *Advances in Dental Science*.

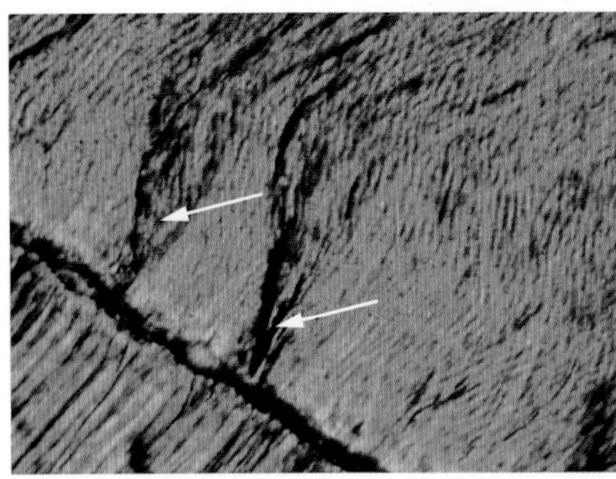

Fig. 7.66 Transverse section of enamel showing enamel tufts (arrows) (×200).

Enamel tufts

Enamel tuft is the term given to junctional structures in the inner third of the enamel that, in ground sections, resemble tufts of grass (Fig. 7.66). They appear to travel in the same direction as the prisms and, in thick sections, undulate with sheets of prisms. They are hypomineralised and recur at approximately 100-µm intervals along the junction. Each tuft is several prisms wide. It has been suggested that this appearance results from protein, presumed to be residual organic enamel matrix, at the boundaries of hypomineralised prisms (Fig. 7.67). Owing to their alignment, tufts are best visualised in transverse sections of enamel. Tufts contain 'tuftelin', a member of the nonamelogenin group of proteins.

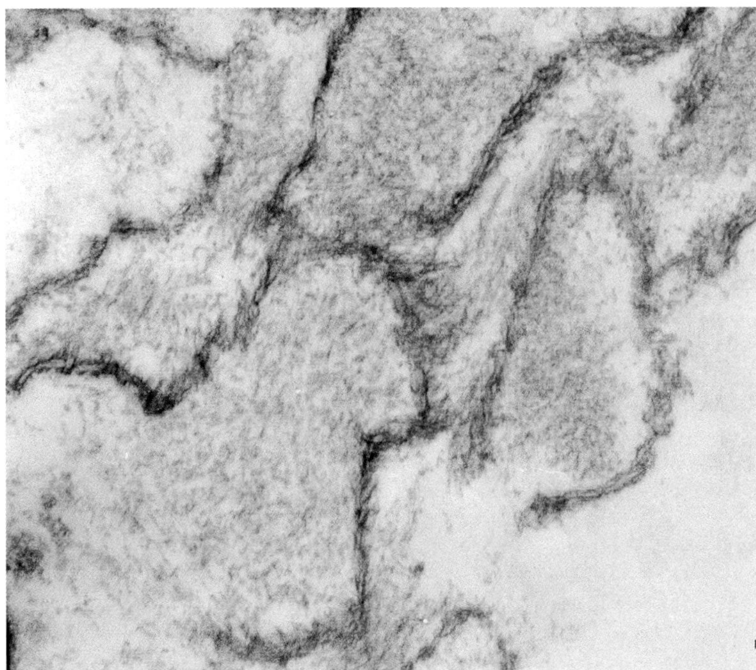

Fig. 7.67 TEM of an enamel tuft separated from the dentine surface after demineralisation of the enamel. The dense staining areas are presumptive prism boundaries representing organic matrix (×11,000). Courtesy Dr R C Shore and the CRC Press.

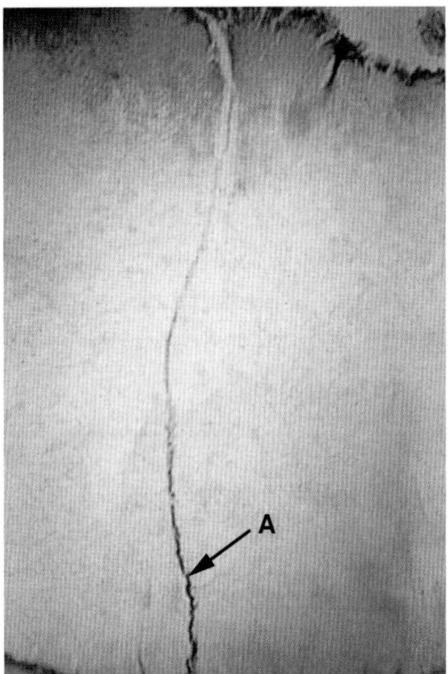

Fig. 7.68 Demineralised section of enamel sectioned transversely to show an enamel lamella (A) (light blue stain; ×150).

The protein content of enamel is highest in the region of the enamel tufts.

Enamel lamellae

Enamel lamellae are sheetlike, apparent structural faults that run through the entire thickness of the enamel (Fig. 7.68). They are hypomineralised and narrower, longer and less common than enamel tufts but, like tufts, are best visualised in transverse sections of enamel. In routine ground sections many lamella-like structures are simply cracks produced during section preparation. This can be confirmed by demineralising the section, when cracks (but not true lamellae) will disappear.

Lamellae may arise developmentally because of incomplete maturation of groups of prisms (in which case they would contain enamel proteins) or after eruption as cracks produced during loading of enamel and containing saliva and oral debris.

Microporosity of enamel

The enamel pores *in vivo* the pores in enamel are water-filled spaces between the crystallites. Based on thermogravimetric analysis, pore volume has been quoted as high as 10–12%. These values, however, may be inflated because of the release of water that is normally a structural part of the enamel crystallites. From studies based on water absorption techniques, enamel appears to have a porosity of about 3–5% by volume, but even this figure may not be a true reflection of the porosity because it may incorporate a factor related to water that is bound to the organic material. Within the prisms most pores exist as very narrow gaps between closely packed crystallites, but some, although they are still small, appear elongated and tube-like. Most of the pores are accessible only to small molecules such as water. Polarised light studies, internal surface area measurements and etching studies suggest that most, if not all, of the pores that are accessible to molecules larger than water are distributed in the prism boundaries, whereas those that are accessible only to small molecules are found throughout the rest of the enamel. The prism boundaries may thus be thought of as main highways through the enamel, whereas the rest of the porosity may be thought of as a fine network of footpaths connecting occasionally with the main highways so that access through them is slow and restricted. The pathways for diffusion and, to a lesser extent, electrochemical effects arising from the charge on the pore walls have an important influence on the formation of a carious lesion. Putative micropores are shown in Figs. 7.7 and 7.8.

Tooth whitening

Whether agents (food, drinks, tobacco, etc.) stain the enamel surface depends on the attraction of the materials to the tooth surface by such mechanisms as electrostatic charge, van der Waals forces and short-range interactions such as hydration and hydrogen bonds. These forces bring the chromogenic materials or their precursors to the tooth surface and determine whether adhesion will occur. The chromogens may then penetrate the enamel pores and bind to the organic matrix. Whitening agents such as hydrogen or carbamide peroxide produce reactive molecules (free radicals) that penetrate the enamel pores and act as both an oxygenator and an oxidant. This reduces the large chromogenic organic molecules in the enamel matrix to smaller, less noticeable molecules that may diffuse out from the enamel, or will absorb less light and hence give a whiter appearance. These agents are effective (Fig. 7.69). Their degree of effectiveness depends on the concentration of the whitening agent, the duration and number of applications, and the ability of the agent to reach the stain. They may, initially, cause a small reduction in the microhardness of enamel, but this soon returns to normal after the treatment.

Age changes in enamel

One of the unique properties of enamel is that, after the tooth has erupted, it loses its formative cells, the ameloblasts, and is therefore incapable of repair or regenerating. It does, however, undergo changes immediately after eruption as the surface enamel comes into equilibrium with its environment, the saliva. Both mineral and organic material may be absorbed into the surface enamel, resulting in posteruptive maturation. Enamel becomes less porous with age because of the infilling of micropores between the crystals and possible changes in the organic material. This results in surface hardening and the 'filling in' of prism boundaries such that the prismatic pattern is obscured. These are not age changes but related

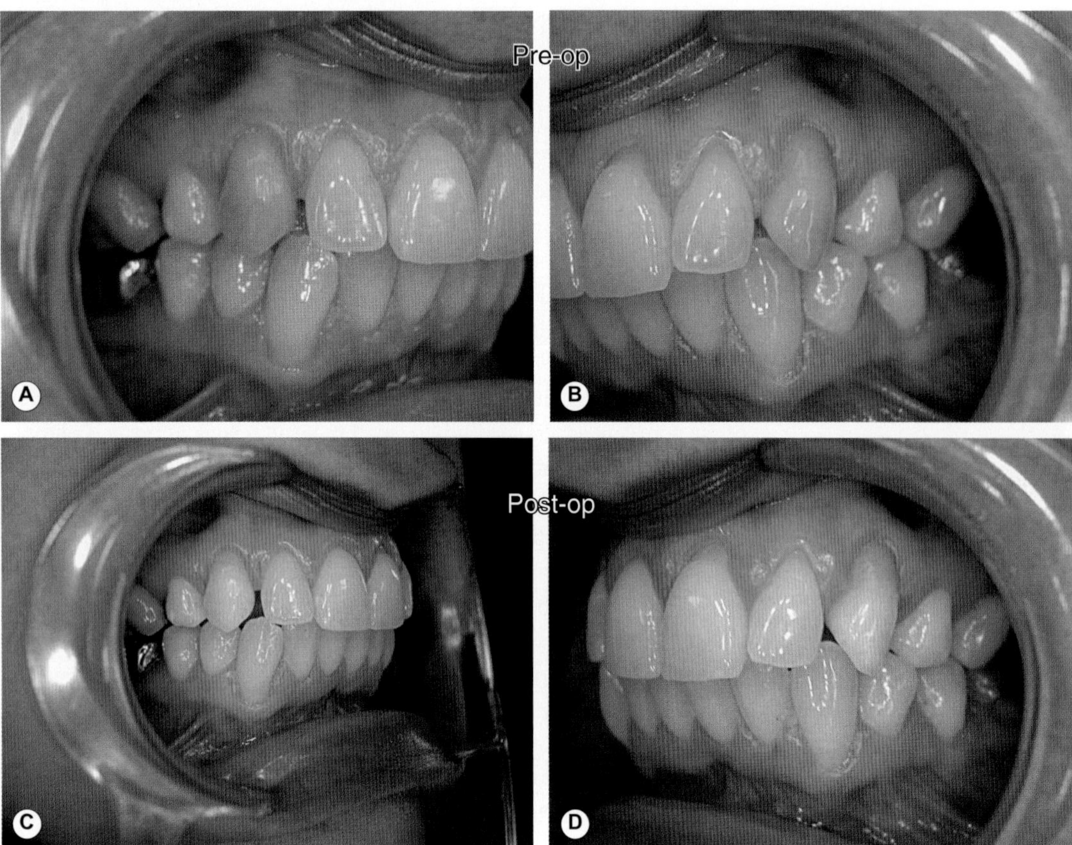

Fig. 7.69 Before (preoperative A, B) and after (postoperative C, D respectively) tooth-whitening procedures using 30% hydrogen peroxide. Courtesy Dr B Millar.

to the initial appearance of the crown in the mouth. Further exchanges occur with age that will largely be determined by the properties of the biofilm (plaque) that develops on the surface, particularly from the bacteria that inhabit it. Pigmented or stained organic material comes to be included in the surface enamel. These and other factors, such as the progressive thickening of the underlying dentine, reduce translucency and contribute to the darkening of teeth with age. This can be reversed temporarily, and to a limited extent, by the use of bleaches that oxidise the organic material. The exchange of ions between the saliva and enamel continues throughout life, depending on the composition (especially the pH of the saliva) and the activities of the plaque microorganisms. In general, surface enamel that is not affected by caries will become slightly more mineralised. Some ions will be exchanged, most significantly fluoride (from the saliva). This may explain, at least in part, why enamel in older individuals has a reduced vulnerability to caries. The presence of fluoride ions in saliva, whether from diet or toothpaste, will increase this effect. This movement of mineral elements into the enamel is applied in the remineralisation of early enamel lesions. One other clinical consideration with surface enamel is whether its adhesion to restorative materials changes over time. From the data currently available, the bonding of adhesive materials to enamel does not appear to change with age.

In health, the deeper portion of enamel is well protected from environmental changes. It has been shown that some materials can pass through the dentine and into the innermost layer of enamel. This has been shown in animal studies using blood-borne dyes, but its biological significance is unknown. The extent of this penetration is reduced with age, but this is more likely to be associated with changes in the thickness and composition of dentine than to changes in the enamel.

Enamel may be lost by attrition, erosion, abrasion and abfraction. Its thickness is reduced over time by both occlusal and interproximal attrition, although this will vary with both diet and occlusion. Toothbrush abrasion will lead to the loss of surface enamel. Thus perikymata will disappear, although some may be retained in protected areas such as interproximally. This loss of enamel may result in the tooth appearing darker as more of the underlying yellow dentine may be evident through the thinner translucent enamel

Cementum–enamel junction

The cementum–enamel junction is discussed with cementum on page 221.

Clinical considerations

Enamel structure and dental caries

In tooth decay (dental caries), acids produced by dental plaque dissolve enamel mineral. Because there is very little matrix, the histologically observable changes are due to demineralisation. The basic description of the structure of the carious lesion is based on the observation of ground sections in polarised light (Fig. 7.70), because this approach gives an appearance related to crystallite content. In early lesions, before cavitation occurs, the surface enamel shows relatively little change, but beneath it, in the 'body' of the lesion, 20–50% of the mineral is lost. When mineral is dissolved the loss begins at the periphery of the prism. The mineral is not necessarily lost permanently because remineralisation does occur (saliva is saturated with mineral). During carious attack a repeating cycle of demineralisation and remineralisation occurs: clearly, if demineralisation dominates, the caries progresses. That the possession of a relatively intact surface layer (despite considerable subsurface demineralisation) in the carious lesion does not reflect unique features of the surface enamel

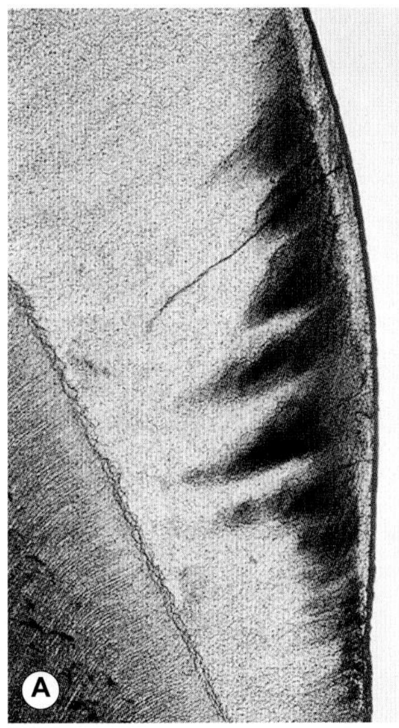

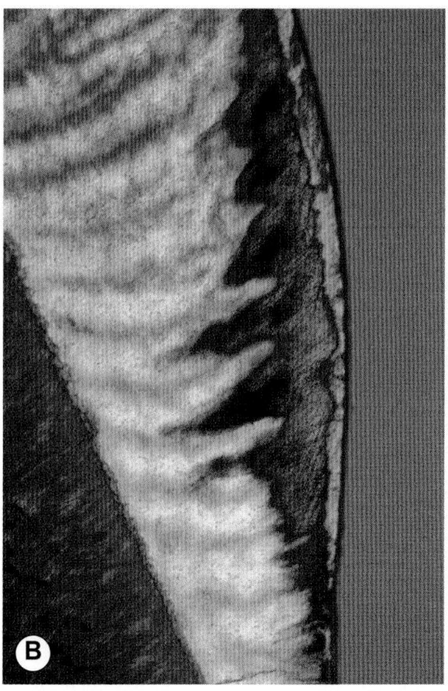

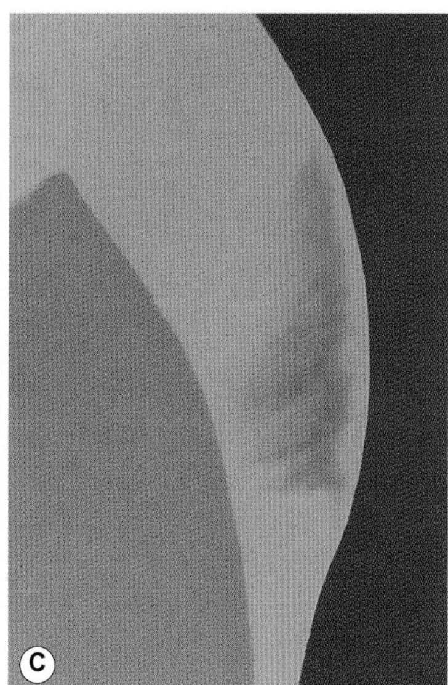

Fig. 7.70 An early carious lesion, which clinically would appear as a 'white spot' without cavitation. (A) A ground section showing an apparently intact surface zone but darker regions beneath it where mineral has been lost. (B) The same section seen in polarizing light. (C) The same section as a microradiograph with a darker (less radiodense) subsurface zone (×24). Courtesy Dr B H Clarkson.

(but more a process of reprecipitation of mineral) is evident from *in vitro* studies in which the surface layer of enamel was ground away to a considerable depth and carious-like lesions induced artificially. In such lesions an intact surface lesion still appeared as a characteristic feature of the carious process. In carious lesions, enamel striae, cross-striations and prism boundary markings become particularly prominent during the demineralisation and remineralisation processes.

Remineralisation of enamel

The important clinical topic of remineralisation of enamel is discussed in Chapter 28.

Enamel structure and restorative dentistry

Many of the structural features of enamel are important to restorative dentistry. The understanding of the initiation and progress of dental caries has been based on knowledge of enamel composition and morphology. This has led to a much more conservative approach by utilising the phenomenon of remineralisation and reducing the need for the removal of sound tissue. This reduced sacrifice of sound tooth structure has also been brought about by the development of adhesives that will bond to enamel, a process that is based on an understanding of the prismatic structure of enamel and the controllable effects of acids on it. Different acids at different concentrations can produce a variety of patterns of partial prism dissolution to provide a roughened surface suitable for adherence of restorative materials (acid conditioning). This reduces or eliminates the need for mechanical retention cutting into sound tissue. For agents mechanically binding to enamel, it is necessary to produce microporosities in the surface by acid-etch techniques (Fig. 7.71). Thus when bonding agents are applied to such a surface, microscopic tags can be seen invaginating into the roughened surface (Fig. 7.72).

When cavities are prepared, knowledge of the microanatomy of enamel, particularly in terms of prism orientation, is essential to conserve as much of the original strength of the tissue as possible. Cutting cavities into enamel with rotary instruments will inevitably lead to subsurface cracking. Fortunately, some of the adhesive materials are capable of reinforcing this weakened substrate (Fig. 7.73).

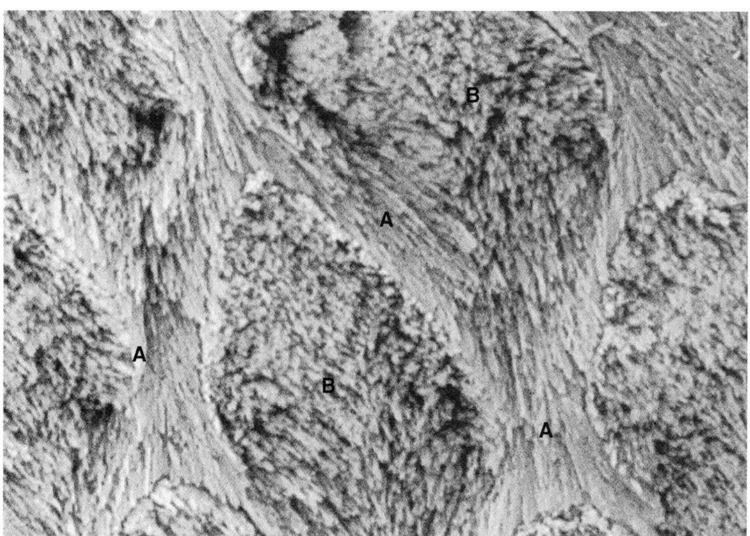

Fig. 7.71 SEM of enamel prisms etched end-on with an acid (maleic acid), showing a differential etch pattern between the prism boundary region (A) and the prism core region (B). This produces a microscopically rough surface suitable for the retention of a resin-based adhesive (×6,000). Courtesy Prof. B Van Meerbeek.

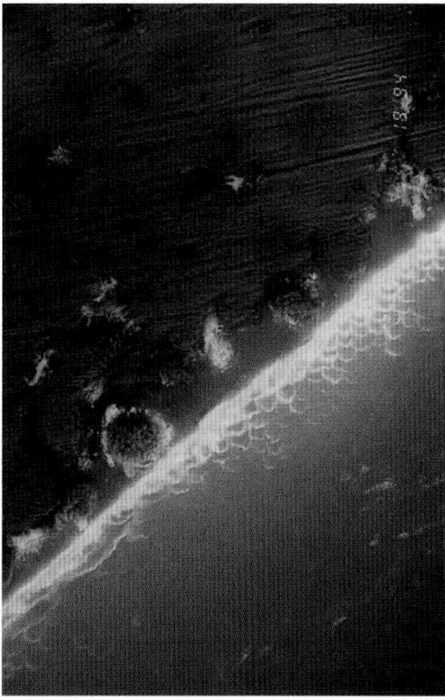

Fig. 7.72 Confocal microscope image showing the penetration of a (yellow) dye-labelled bonding agent into acid-etched enamel. Note tags of resin around the prism boundaries made porous by acid etching (×450). Courtesy Prof. T F Watson.

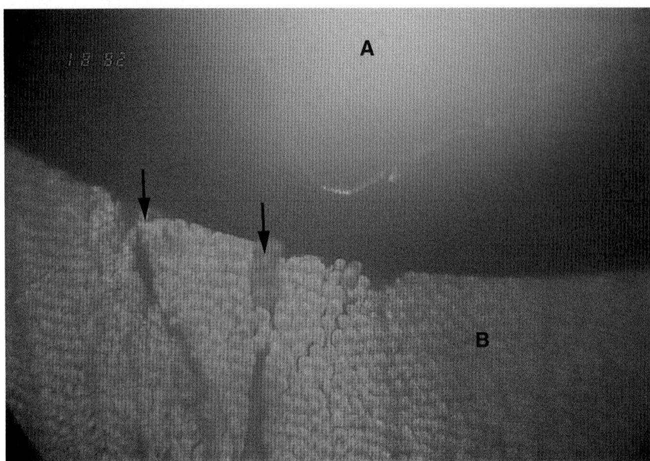

Fig. 7.73 Confocal microscope image of the interface between a dental bur (A) and the enamel wall (B) taken during the actual cutting of a cavity. Note the fracture lines (arrows), the prism boundaries, the enamel prisms being viewed in cross-section (×450). Courtesy Prof. T F Watson.

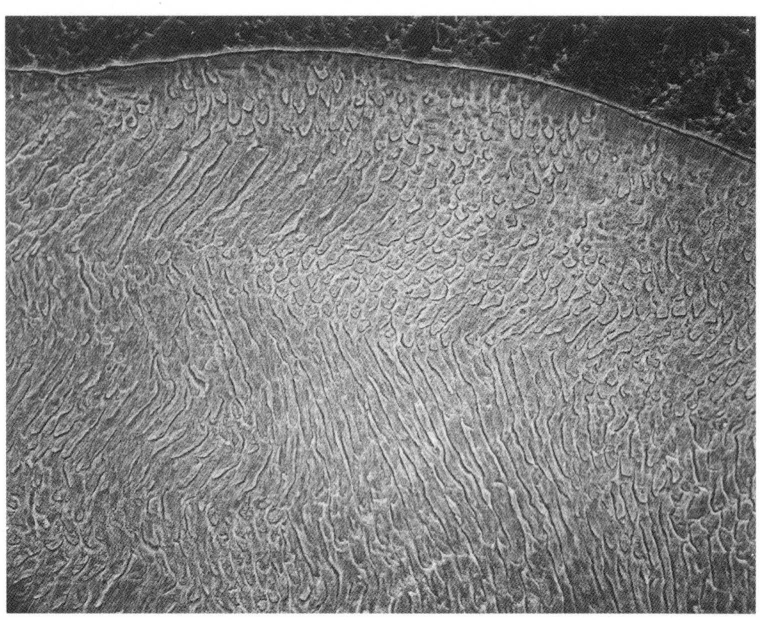

Fig. 7.75 Enamel from the central part of an enamel pearl showing the irregular course of prisms (×312). From Risnes, S. et al., 2000. Enamel pearls and cervical enamel projections on 2 maxillary molars with localized periodontal disease: case report and histologic study. *Oral Surgery Oral Medicine Oral Pathology Radiology & Endodontics* 89: 493–497.

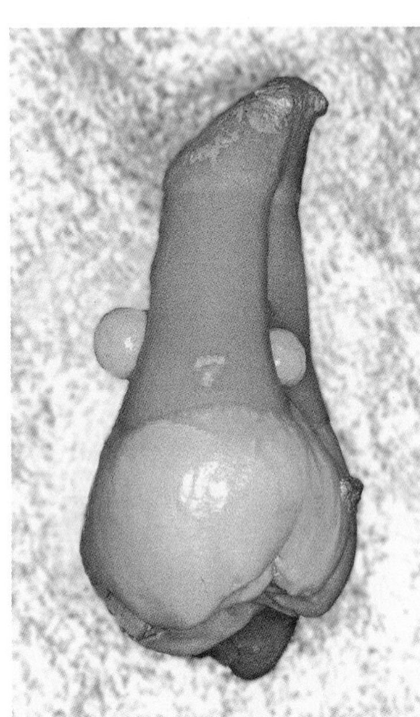

Fig. 7.74 Palatal view of a maxillary third molar with large enamel pearls on the mesial and distal surfaces. From Risnes, S. et al., 2000. Enamel pearls and cervical enamel projections on 2 maxillary molars with localized periodontal disease: case report and histologic study. *Oral Surgery Oral Medicine Oral Pathology Radiology & Endodontics* 89: 493–497.

Enamel pearls

Enamel pearls are small isolated spheres of enamel that occasionally are found on the root, generally towards the cervical margin (Fig. 7.74). The enamel is prismatic with the prisms following an irregular course (Fig. 7.75). They are particularly common in the root bifurcation region.

Because there will be a deficiency in the attachment apparatus at this site, gingival recession and dental plaque accretion may result in the onset of periodontal disease.

Developmental defects in enamel

Defects are considered with the development of enamel in Chapter 22.

Further readings for this chapter can be found in the accompanying eBook. Explore online Self-assessment quiz to test and reinforce your understanding of the material in your free ebook. Follow instructions in the Inside Front Cover to unlock your access.

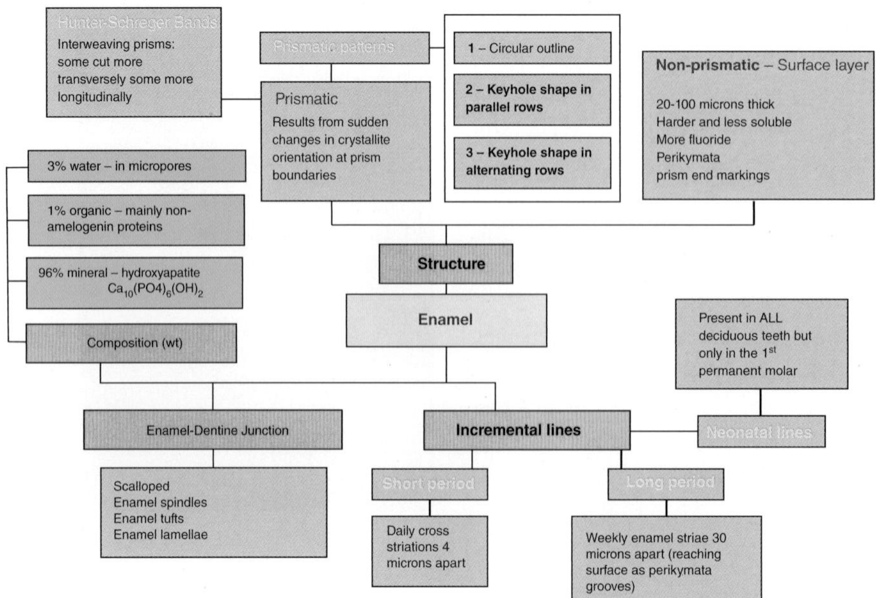

Mind Map 7.1 Enamel.

Investing organic layers on enamel surfaces

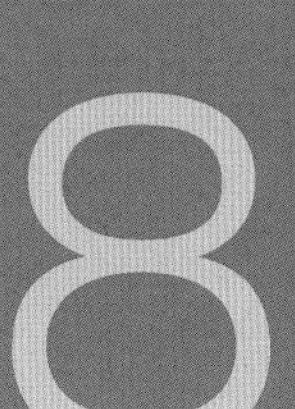

Introduction

Throughout its life, the crown of a tooth is covered by an organic layer or integument. Before the tooth erupts into the oral cavity, the crown is covered by the overlying oral mucosa, the coronal part of the dental follicle and the vestiges of the enamel organ (plus its associated primary enamel cuticle). For information concerning the origins of the enamel organ and the dental follicle during early tooth development, see Chapter 21. After emerging into the mouth, parts of the integument of enamel organ origin are lost by degeneration of its epithelial component and by attrition or abrasion of the underlying cuticular component. In the region of the gingival crevice or sulcus the primary (or pre-eruptive) enamel cuticle acquires additional matter from the lining epithelium and, coronal to the gingival margin, from saliva. The salivary layer is known as the acquired pellicle. Oral bacteria adhere initially to the enamel cuticle, and later to the acquired pellicle, to form dental plaque.

Investing layers associated with the crowns of unerupted teeth

The soft tissues covering an erupting tooth comprise the oral mucosa and the subjacent connective tissue of the dental follicle. Between the dental follicle and the enamel is an epithelial layer that is the remains of the enamel organ – the reduced enamel epithelium (Fig. 8.1). The appearance of this epithelium varies from a thin, flattened layer of cells to a more organised layer of recognisable cuboidal or columnar reduced ameloblasts, deep to which may be additional cell layers (Fig. 8.2). Although it is not evident at the light microscope level, a basal lamina (primary enamel cuticle) is interposed between the enamel surface and the reduced enamel epithelium. The reduced enamel epithelium and the basal lamina comprise Nasmyth's membrane. The enamel organ associated with an occlusal fissure appears to be the last to change to a reduced enamel epithelium, and the cells adjacent to the enamel in this region may retain a columnar appearance for some considerable time (Fig. 8.3). The reduced enamel epithelium covering the crown of unerupted teeth can be demonstrated with special staining (Fig. 8.4).

Investing layers associated with the crowns of erupted teeth

The organic layers covering the erupted healthy tooth can be revealed by special stains (Fig. 8.5). That part of the crown well exposed in the mouth is covered by loosely adherent reduced enamel epithelium. This is soon lost, leaving the primary enamel cuticle that immediately acquires an organic element of salivary origin, the acquired pellicle. Passing towards the gingiva but above the gingival margin, the tooth is likely to be covered by plaque. In the region of the gingival crevice the tooth will be covered only by the primary enamel cuticle. Below this layer the tooth will be covered by the junctional epithelium, its extent being related to the stage of tooth development. Using careful demineralising techniques, it is possible to lift off the organic integument; consequently the plaque, primary enamel cuticle and junctional epithelium appear as a single continuous entity (Figs. 8.6, 8.7). The surface of this organic film adjacent to the enamel may even show prism-end markings in the region of the gingival crevice, where it is formed only by the primary enamel cuticle, indicating its intimate association with the enamel surface (Fig. 8.8).

The three distinct zones forming the enamel integument as seen in Figs. 8.5 and 8.6 are clearly distinguishable at the ultrastructural level. Beneath the gingival crevice in the region of the junctional epithelium, the enamel integument covering the enamel surface consists of the junctional epithelial cells and the primary enamel cuticle (Fig. 8.9). The junctional epithelium is described further on pages 302–305. Immediately coronal to this, in the region of the gingival crevice, the enamel surface is covered only by the primary enamel cuticle, the junctional epithelium having been lost (Fig. 8.10).

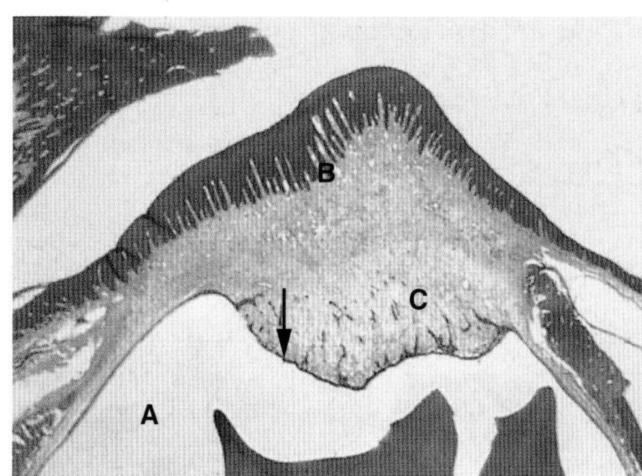

Fig. 8.1 Demineralised, longitudinal section of an erupting tooth. A = enamel space; B = oral epithelium, immediately beneath which is its associated lamina propria and submucosa; C = dental follicle associated with the underlying erupting tooth. Reduced enamel epithelium (arrow) (H & E; ×10.)

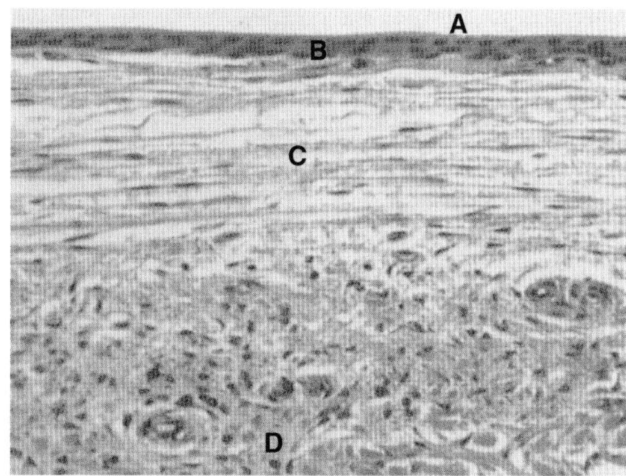

Fig. 8.2 Immediately adjacent to the enamel space (A) is the reduced enamel epithelium (B). In this section the reduced enamel epithelium appears flattened. Superficial to the reduced enamel epithelium is the fibrous connective tissue of the dental follicle (C), and superficial to this is the oral submucosa (D). (Demineralised section, H & E; ×160.)

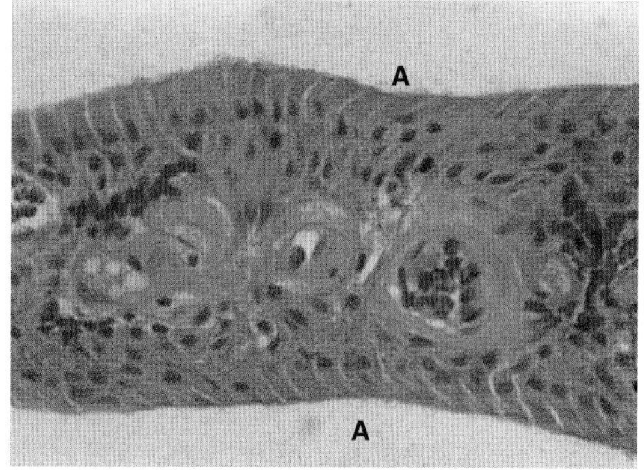

Fig. 8.3 The reduced enamel epithelium from within an occlusal fissure. Although the reduced enamel epithelium covering the rest of the crown comprises cells with a flattened morphology, the cells immediately adjacent to the enamel space (A) still retain a columnar appearance. Note the vascularity of the tissue in this region. (Demineralised section, Mallory's trichrome; ×80.) *Courtesy Prof. H N Newman.*

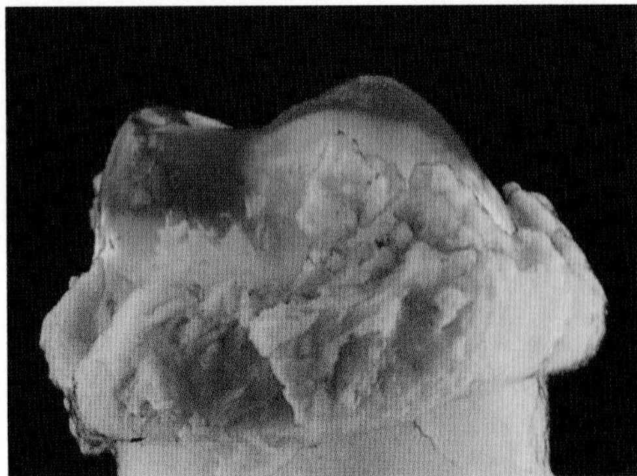

Fig. 8.4 This unerupted permanent third molar has been stained to show the remains of the dental follicle (yellow) and the vestigial enamel organ (blue). Note that part of the follicle has been lost during the surgical removal of the tooth, and that the underlying vestigial enamel organ covers the entire crown (Alcian blue after fixation in Bouin's solution; ×4). *Courtesy Prof. H N Newman.*

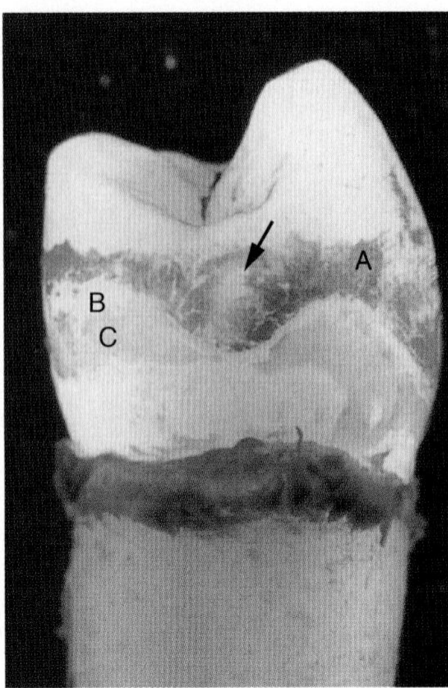

Fig. 8.5 Approximal view of a partially erupted premolar, showing the zones of its organic integument. Two zones are stained. The dark blue layer (A) is the plaque. The light blue layer (C) is the attachment or junctional epithelium, which in life links the tooth to the gingiva coronal to the periodontal ligament. The unstained zone between them (B) comprises the primary (or pre-eruptive) enamel cuticle. Note that the plaque corresponds to a position above the crest of the gingival margin and around the contact point (arrowed) where adjacent teeth meet. Also note that the cuticle lies in the region of the gingival crevice. Apical to the junctional epithelium, the enamel was covered *in vivo* by loosely adherent reduced enamel epithelial cells, which were lost during extraction. Coronal to the plaque the crown is covered by the primary enamel cuticle together with an organic element of salivary origin (the acquired pellicle) (Alcian blue–aldehyde fuchsin; ×4). *Courtesy Prof. H N Newman.*

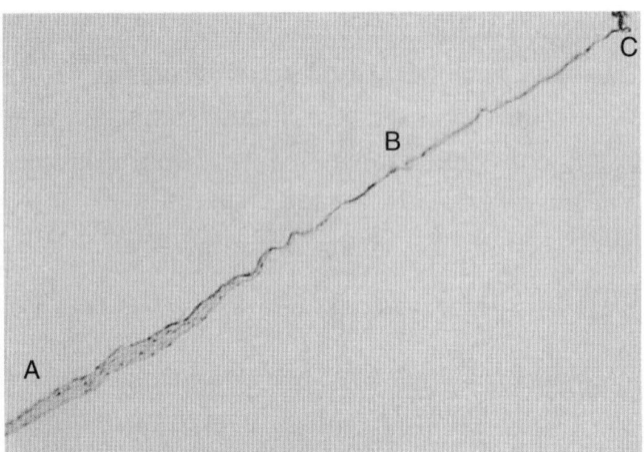

Fig. 8.6 The organic integument removed from the enamel surface of an erupted tooth after careful demineralization. A = epithelium; B = primary enamel cuticle; C = plaque. (Ollett's modification of Twort; ×100.) *Courtesy Prof. H N Newman.*

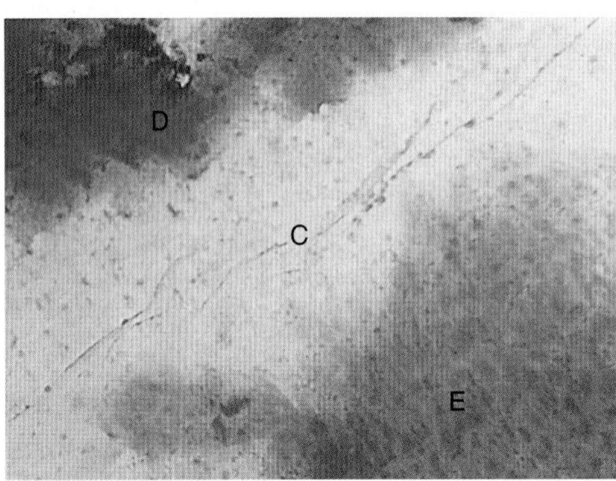

Fig. 8.7 High-power view of the external surface of part of the organic integument removed from enamel by careful demineralization. C = primary (pre-eruptive) enamel cuticle; D = dental plaque; E = junctional epithelium (toluidine blue and erythrosin; ×20). *Courtesy Prof. H N Newman.*

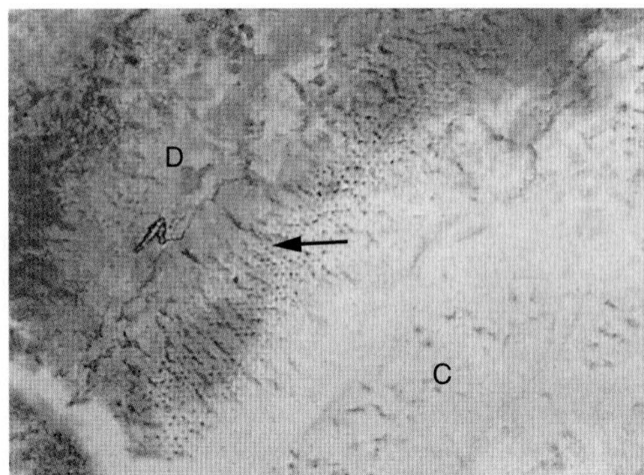

Fig. 8.8 Deep enamel-related surface of organic integument removed from enamel by careful demineralization, revealing a zone of prism-end markings (arrowed) in the primary enamel cuticle (C) just beneath the dental plaque (D) (Alcian blue and erythrosin; ×20). *Courtesy Prof. H N Newman.*

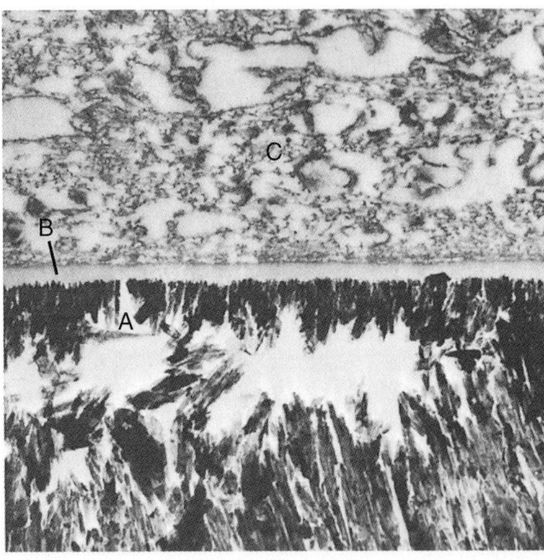

Fig. 8.9 The enamel integument at the level of the junctional epithelium. This micrograph is taken from a region at the coronal limit of the gingival crevice. The enamel surface (A) is covered by the primary enamel cuticle (B) and the remaining vestige of an attachment or junctional epithelial cell (C) (TEM; ×13,000). *Courtesy Prof. H N Newman.*

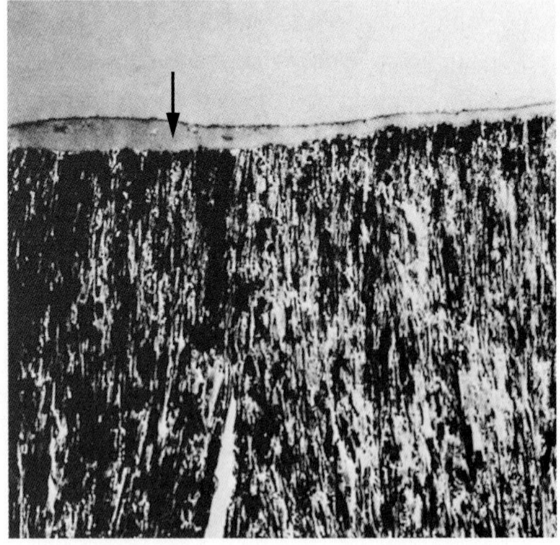

Fig. 8.10 The enamel integument immediately coronal to the junctional epithelium showing the primary enamel cuticle (arrowed) on the enamel surface. This section is in the region of the gingival crevice coronal to that illustrated in Fig. 8.9 and therefore lacks a junctional epithelial cell. Note that the cuticle usually has an electron-dense outer border (TEM; ×10,000). *Courtesy Prof. H N Newman.*

Primary enamel cuticle

Above the gingival crest, the primary enamel cuticle exposed in the mouth will become coated with an acquired pellicle derived from saliva, and this will become colonised by bacteria to form dental plaque (Fig. 8.11). The firm apposition of the gingiva to the tooth limits the plaque to the gingival margin (Fig. 8.12). Excessive plaque accumulation is associated with both dental caries and chronic inflammatory periodontal disease.

The primary enamel cuticle is in intimate contact with the underlying organic enamel matrix. Generally approximately 30 nm thick, the cuticle acquires accretions in the region of the gingival crevice, which derive from crevicular epithelium and plasma and may increase the cuticle to about 5 µm thick (Fig. 8.13). Localised thickening of the primary enamel cuticle may also occur on its deep aspect, where enamel maturation is incomplete, because of the presence at this site of enamel striae reaching the surface (Fig. 8.14). The primary enamel cuticle is thought to be composed of

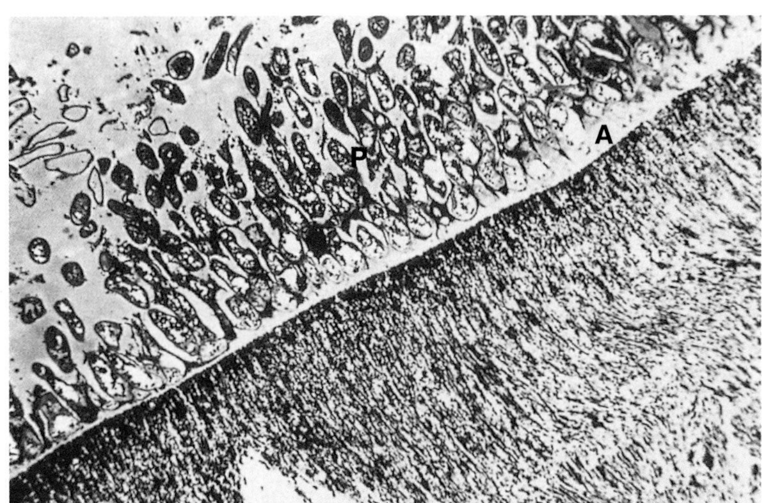

Fig. 8.11 The enamel integument above the gingival crest showing bacterial colonisation forming dental plaque. This micrograph shows early approximal surface plaque on a clear layer (A), which is probably combined primary enamel cuticle and pellicle, above which is a layer of plaque (P) (TEM; ×1,250). *Courtesy Prof. H N Newman.*

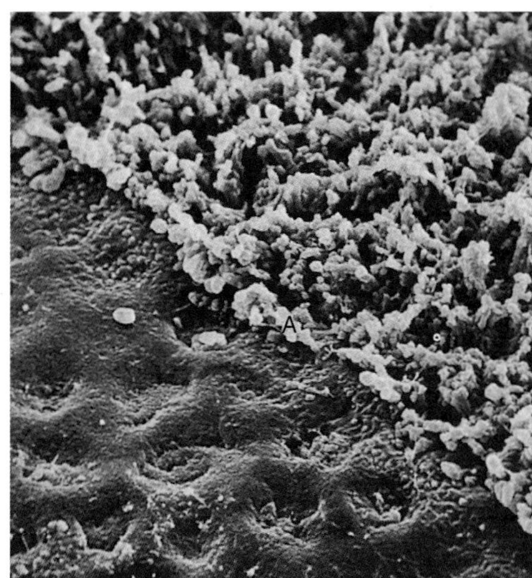

Fig. 8.12 In health the firm apposition of the gingiva to the tooth limits the dental plaque to the gingival margin. There is a sharp boundary to the dental plaque (A), below which lies the plaque-free surface of enamel in the region of the gingival sulcus (SEM; ×1,500). *Courtesy Prof. H N Newman.*

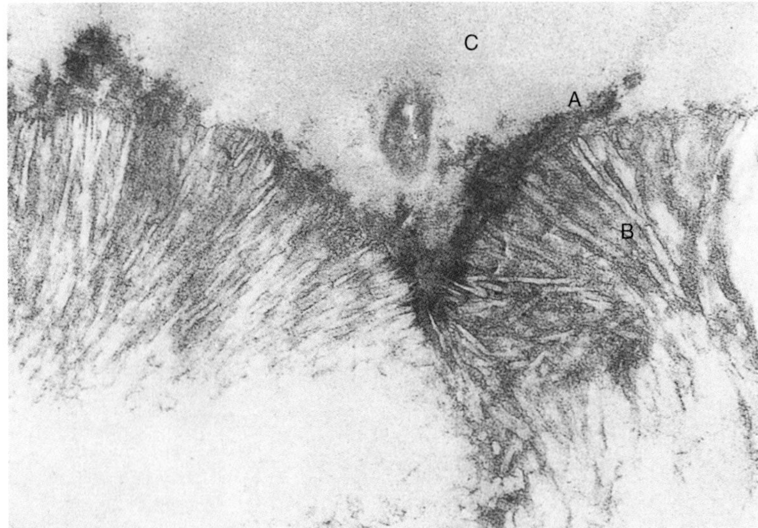

Fig. 8.13 The thin primary enamel cuticle (A) is in intimate contact with the underlying organic enamel matrix (B). Note the lathe-like spaces occupied *in vivo* by enamel crystals. In the region of the gingival crevice the cuticle acquires accretions (C) and appears thicker (demineralised section, TEM ×30,000.) *Courtesy Prof. H N Newman.*

protein. Its accretions are mainly proteoglycan and glycoprotein elements from the contiguous soft tissues. Plasma contributions include immunoglobulins, which form part of the host defence system against plaque (Fig. 8.15).

Where the enamel surface is exposed to wear, either by attrition or abrasion, the vestigial enamel organ is worn away, but the enamel rapidly gains a layer of acquired pellicle. Indeed, this pellicle always forms a protective coat following any wear. This acellular layer is derived mainly from salivary proteins but includes elements from crevicular fluid and bacteria.

Acquired pellicle

Above the gingival crest the primary enamel cuticle exposed in the mouth will become coated with an acquired pellicle. The acquired (enamel) pellicle is a bacteria-free, organic film formed on the tooth surface as the result of selective adsorption of salivary proteins and glycoproteins. Other macromolecules are also present, such as lipids. The pellicle can protect the tooth surface from acid attack. Caries-susceptible individuals appear to have a higher number of peptide fragments in their saliva, suggesting higher

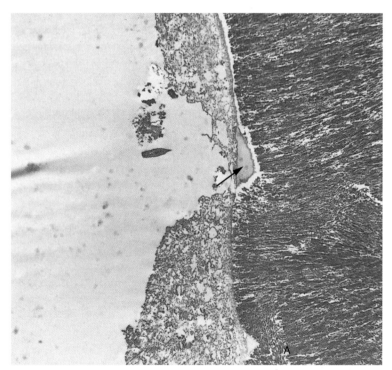

Fig. 8.14 Localised thickening of the primary enamel cuticle at the enamel surface in relation to an enamel stria reaching the surface (arrow) (TEM micrograph; ×5,100). *Courtesy Prof. H N Newman.*

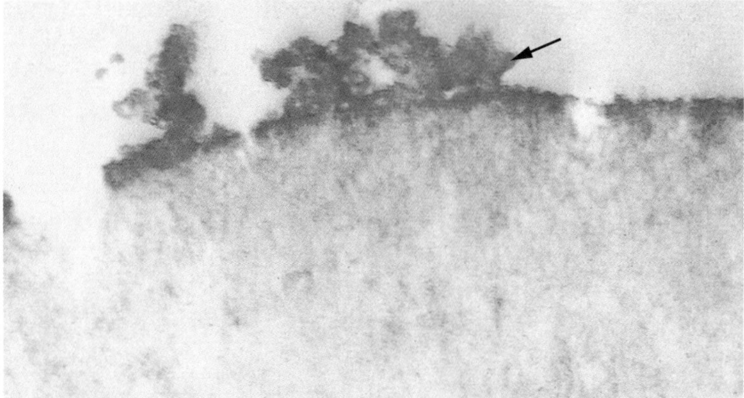

Fig. 8.15 The primary enamel cuticle at the enamel surface showing positive staining for the immunoglobulin G (IgG; arrow). This forms part of the host defence system against dental plaque (TEM with antibody to human IgG; peroxidase method for localization of IgG; ×34,500). *Courtesy Prof. H N Newman and S J Challacombe.*

proteolytic activity. In addition, they have reduced amounts of proline-rich proteins (PRPs), histatins and statherins than caries-free volunteers, suggesting a potential role of these proteins to maintain tooth integrity.

Proteomic analysis has been undertaken on the acquired pellicle to evaluate which proteins are present within the acquired pellicle and which remain after acidic challenges that mimic erosive and cariogenic conditions. A total of 72 proteins were identified, the precise function of many being unknown. The proteins that are increased after exposure to the acids were PRPs, histatins and statherins. Cystatins are a group of proteins present in saliva that have antimicrobial properties and were identified only in the pellicle of caries-free volunteers. Cystatin B was also the protein with the highest increase in the pellicle after acidic exposure, suggesting a high affinity of this protein to hydroxyapatite, even under acidic conditions. Thus this protein is a potential candidate to be used in new preventive protocols against caries and erosion.

Dental plaque

The main stages of dental plaque formation are indicated in Box 8.1.

Dental plaque is the combination of bacteria embedded in a matrix of salivary proteins and bacterial products superimposed on the acquired pellicle (Fig. 8.11). Dental plaque is an example of a biofilm, a term used to describe communities of microbes attached to surfaces. Early plaque is composed of mainly Gram-positive, facultative, anaerobic cocci and filaments (Fig. 8.16). With time, the deposit will thicken, although in nonpathological, supragingival situations its microfloral composition is unlikely to vary greatly (Fig. 8.12). Dental plaque accumulates in areas that lack self-cleansing, such as pits, fissures and the gingival third of smooth surfaces.

Box 8.1 Stages in the formation of dental plaque

1) Initial transport of bacteria to tooth surface
2) Reversible adsorption of the bacteria onto the pellicle surface
3) Less reversible attachment of bacteria to tooth surface
4) Buildup of new bacterial layers
5) Growth of the attached organisms to produce a biofilm
6) Organisms within plaque synthesise extracellular polymers

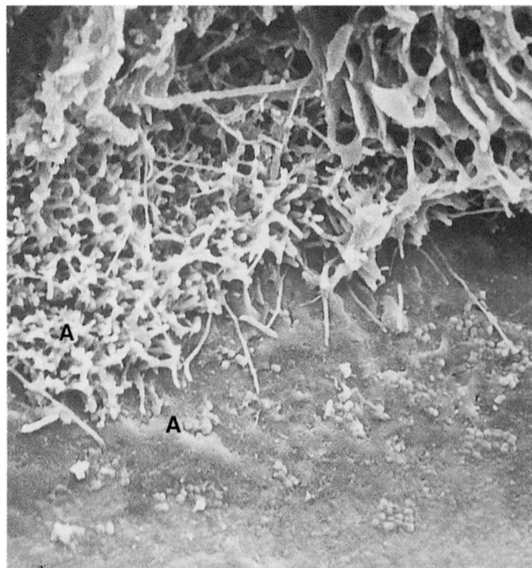

Fig. 8.16 SEM showing apical border of early plaque composed mainly of cocci (A) and filaments (×1,300). *Courtesy Prof. H N Newman and the editors of British Dental Journal.*

Where the plaque is associated with chronic inflammatory periodontal disease and becomes subgingival, a more complex flora develops with anaerobic Gram-negative organisms predominating, to include cocci, rods, filaments and many motile forms (particularly spirochaetes) (Figs. 8.17, 8.18). The microbial composition of dental plaque will vary, not only with the stages of maturity of the deposit but also from individual to individual, from tooth to tooth, from site to site and from surface to surface. Dental plaque can be seen on all tooth surfaces that are not subject to constant abrasion, especially in areas that are difficult to clean (such as occlusal pits and fissures, interproximal regions and at the

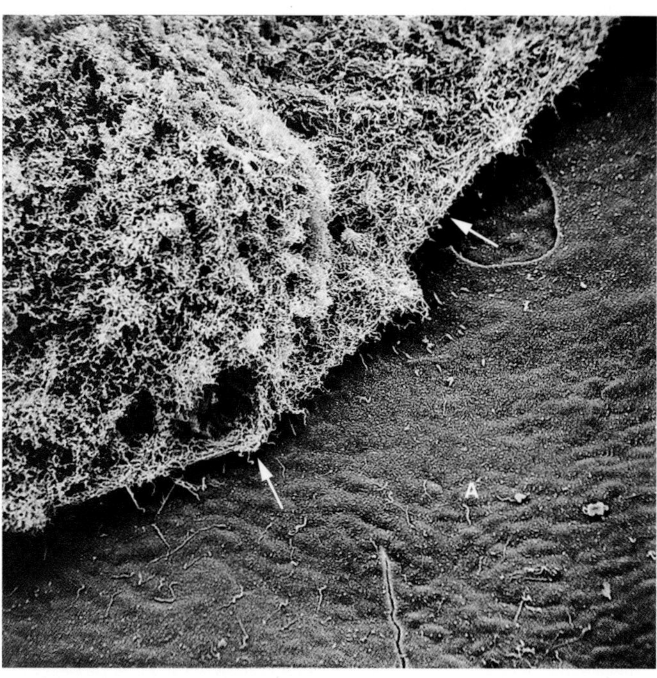

Fig. 8.17 SEM showing apical border of subgingival plaque (arrows) associated with advanced chronic inflammatory periodontal disease. The predominant organisms are spirochaetes. The details of cementum (A) are obscured by a dental cuticle on which isolated spirochaetes can be seen (×430). *From Newman, H.N., 1977. Ultrastructure of the apical border of dental plaque. In Lehner, T. (Ed.), Borderland Between Caries and Periodontal Disease, Vol. 1. Academic Press, London, pp. 73–103.*

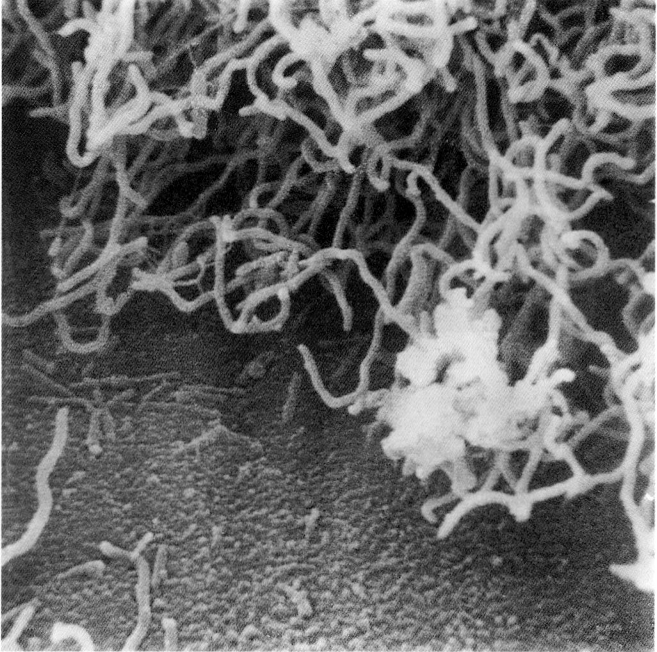

Fig. 8.18 SEM showing high power of the apical border shown in Fig. 8.17. The subgingival plaque is composed mainly of spirochaetes (×4,000). Newman, H.N. 1977. Ultrastructure of the apical border of dental plaque. In Lehner, T. (Ed.), *The Borderland Between Caries and Periodontal Disease*, Vol. 1, Academic Press, London, pp. 73–103.

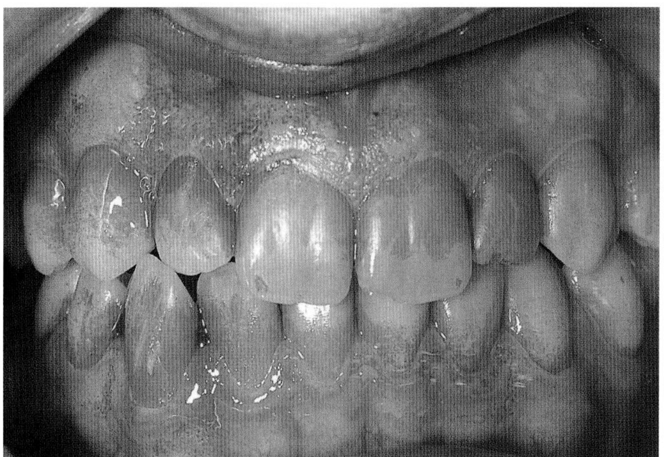

Fig. 8.19 Dental plaque stained red and exposed by the use of a disclosing solution. *Courtesy Prof. R Palmer.*

gingival margin). Its presence may be more readily visualised clinically by the use of disclosing solutions (Fig. 8.19). Many dental plaque bacteria metabolise dietary carbohydrates, often producing polysaccharides, which may be stored intracellularly on the cell surface and extracellularly in the matrix.

The transport of microorganisms to the pellicle-coated tooth is via passive means, and local variations in the chemical composition of the pellicle can influence the pattern of microbial deposition.

Attachment of bacteria

Initial reversible attachment of bacteria to the tooth surface involves the formation of long-range, physicochemical interactions between microorganisms and pellicle proteins. Such interactions include electrostatic interactions (ionic and hydrogen bonds), Van der Waals forces (induced dipole formation) and hydrophobic bonds. Because microorganisms are generally negatively charged due to the nature of the cell-surface molecules, and acidic proteins are present in acquired pellicle, these interactions usually involve the formation of calcium bridging between the pellicle proteins and bacterial membranes for successful interaction. Less reversible attachment of bacteria to the tooth surface involves short-range interactions between adhesins on the microbial surface and receptors in the acquired pellicle. These are usually specific and irreversible.

Plaque matrix and extracellular polysaccharides

Plaque matrix and extracellular polysaccharides are as important in the functions of dental plaque as the microorganisms. The plaque matrix is the intercellular material between bacteria. It can be directly related to the diet consumed and be a key source of carbohydrates for acid production during caries. The matrix consists of carbohydrates from foodstuffs, as well as polysaccharides produced by bacterial metabolism. It also contains salivary proteins and glycoproteins that have precipitated out of solution. The dental plaque matrix is directly related to the diet, and indeed both its consistency and composition may vary with the diet. In the absence of a diet taken orally (e.g., stomach tube feeding), the dental plaque matrix is thin and porous and composed mainly of precipitated salivary glycoproteins. These are incorporated onto the tooth surface and into the dental plaque because they have a strong negative charge due to terminal sialic acid sugars on side chains and thus low pH. In more mature dental plaque, acid production by bacteria may cause some precipitation of salivary glycoproteins and incorporation into the matrix. High levels of calcium in dentalplaque may also help precipitation.

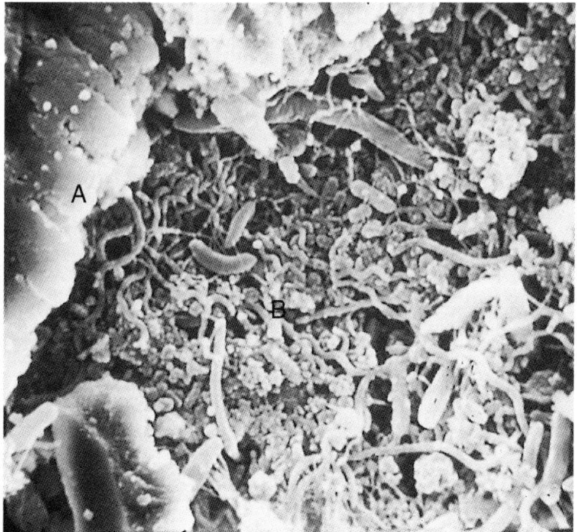

Fig. 8.20 SEM of dental calculus showing mineralised (A) and unmineralised areas of dental plaque composed of a mixed flora (B) (×3,000). Newman, H.N., 1977. Ultrastructure of the apical border of dental plaque. In Lehner, T. (Ed.), *The Borderland Between Caries and Periodontal Disease*, Vol. 1. Academic Press, London, pp 73–103.

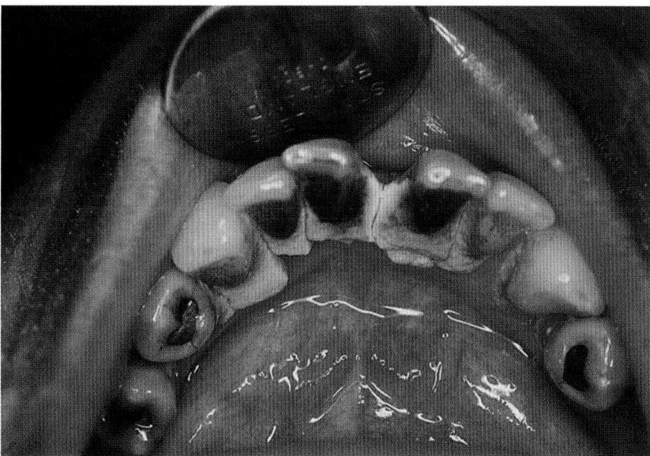

Fig. 8.21 View of mouth showing the presence of supragingival dental calculus associated with the lingual surfaces of heavily stained anterior mandibular teeth. *Courtesy Dr M Ide.*

Dental calculus

Dental calculus is mineralised dental plaque and may become attached to the enamel of the crown or the cementum (or dentine) of the root (Figs. 8.20, 8.21). Approximately 20% dry weight of dental calculus is organic and includes a range of proteins, carbohydrates and lipids, most associated with the dental plaque matrix. The remaining 80% dry weight is inorganic mineral, of which only 50% is hydroxyapatite.

Saliva is supersaturated with minerals (such as calcium and phosphate) that have the potential to mature newly erupted enamel, protect exposed tooth surfaces from acid action and remineralise areas in the early stages of demineralisation. Salivary inhibitors prevent precipitation and crystallisation of minerals in saliva, but bacterial enzymes can degrade these inhibitors. Thus, under suitable conditions (e.g., with high concentrations of minerals derived from saliva), precipitation and crystallisation may occur within dental plaque. Whereas the mineral in enamel consists of carbonated hydroxyapatite, that in dental plaque consists of a number of different mineral forms because of the variety of local factors associated with its formation. There is thus regional variation in the Ca:P ratio of dental calculus. Early calculus formation involves deposition in the matrix of poorly crystalline calcium phosphate types, including dicalcium phosphate dehydrate (brushite) and octacalcium phosphate, together with dying bacterial cells. With time, more structured crystalline elements, dental including carbonated hydroxyapatite and whitlockite, are formed. In supragingival calculus, hydroxyapatite and octacalcium phosphate are most abundant, whereas in subgingival dental calculus, whitlockite is most abundant, with little brushite being present. Supragingival dental plaque is less mineralised than subgingival dental plaque (approximately 40% versus 60%).

The organic component of dental calculus, originating from dental plaque, will therefore be derived from saliva, gingival crevicular fluid, desquamated epithelial cells, blood cells, food debris, bacteria and their products.

Dental calculus can be classified into supragingival (above the free gingival margin and attached to enamel) and subgingival (below the free gingival margin and therefore attached to cementum). Supragingival dental calculus is cream coloured and found adjacent to the opening of the major salivary glands. Thus it is seen predominantly on the lingual surfaces of the anterior mandibular teeth, near the opening of the submandibular and sublingual glands (Fig. 8.21), as well as on the buccal surfaces of the maxillary molars (near the openings of the parotid glands). Subgingival dental calculus is darker in colour and can occur throughout the dentition from minerals in the inflammatory exudate associated with periodontal disease.

The different distribution of supragingival and subgingival calculus deposits relates to the causes of mineralisation: supragingivally, an increase in salivary pH, due to evaporation of dissolved CO_2 on entering the mouth (together with the greater viscosity and higher Ca:P ratio of the saliva coming out from the submandibular duct), promotes dental calculus formation, whereas subgingival calculus formation, promoted by formation of alkaline bacterial waste products within periodontal pockets, may occur anywhere in the mouth.

Large deposits of subgingival dental calculus are sometimes identified on interproximal surfaces in dental radiographs (Fig. 8.22). Subgingival dental calculus may also be exposed when the gingiva recedes from the teeth after chronic inflammatory periodontal disease (Fig. 8.23). Dental calculus is always covered with a biofilm of living organisms (Fig. 8.20).

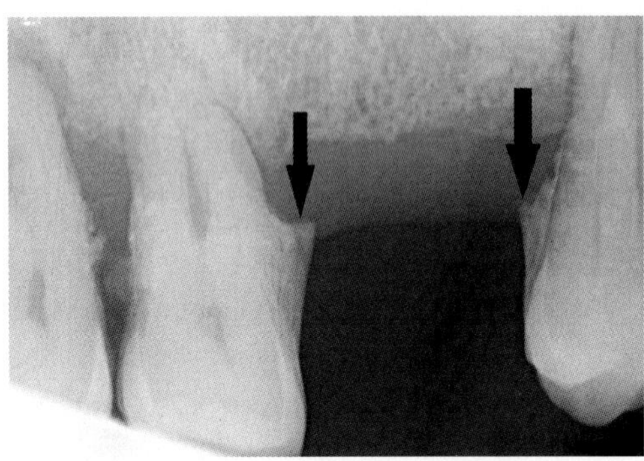

Fig. 8.22 Dental calculus (arrowed) evident in a periapical radiograph. *Courtesy Dr J Makdissi.*

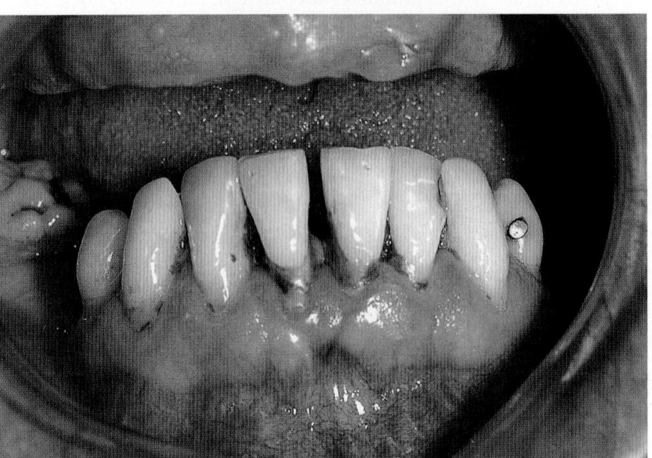

Fig. 8.23 Subgingival dental calculus exposed after gingival recession associated with chronic inflammatory periodontal disease. *Courtesy Prof. R Palmer.*

Clinical considerations

Dental plaque and caries

The presence of dental plaque predisposes to the onset of the two main dental pathologies: dental caries and periodontal disease. However, different microorganisms are involved in the two diseases.

Dental caries is associated with the metabolism of dietary sugar to acid by predominantly Gram-positive organisms (e.g., *Streptococcus mutans*) in supragingival dental plaque. Numerous studies have been undertaken to determine which bacteria in the dental plaque are associated with the onset and progression of dental caries. The solution is complicated by the fact that there are very large numbers of different types of bacteria present in dental plaque at different concentrations. Earlier studies depended on identifying bacteria by culture methods in Petri dishes, with many proving difficult to culture and therefore identify. However, present methods of identifying bacteria employ DNA analysis to provide a microbiome. The number of bacteria present, together with variation between patients and between tooth sites, means that it is usually only viable to survey a limited number of patients. However, some information has been obtained comparing the microbiome (the combined genetic material of microorganisms in dental plaque) between caries-free and caries-active individuals. More than 1,300 different types of bacteria were identified. Approximately half of the bacteria identified were common to both caries-free and caries-active patients and present at similar abundance. However, the analysis identified 87 phylotypes that are represented in either the caries-free or caries-active subjects (Fig. 8.24). New techniques associated with proteomics allow information of the oral microbiome to be determined from samples of saliva (salivaomics; see pages 352–353). A Human Oral Microbiome Database has now been established online (https://www.ehomd.org) to provide the scientific community with comprehensive curated information on the bacterial species present in the human oral cavity. The database lists 2,109 genomes representing 539 taxa.

Among the bacterial pathogens associated with dental caries are *Streptococcus mutans* and *S. sobrinus*, *Lactobacillus acidophilus* and *Actinomyces viscosus*. Attempts are being made to develop a safe and workable vaccine against these cariogenic bacteria or other strategies to limit their presence and growth in dental plaque.

The nature of the dental plaque matrix reflects the diet, and its cariogenic potential is determined by the type of carbohydrate consumed. Frequent intake of sugar induces a cariogenic dental plaque in which organisms capable of surviving at low pH are favoured. If the carbohydrate source is primarily glucose, the dental plaque is thin, whereas if the carbohydrate is sucrose, the plaque is much thicker and gelatinous with 'sticky' properties. This thick and sticky matrix is far more cariogenic due to extracellular polysaccharides produced by the plaque bacteria. Extracellular polysaccharides increase the bulk of dental plaque and may play a role in caries by aiding bacteria to stick/agglutinate within the matrix. They may also act as a source of carbohydrate for bacterial acid production. These extracellular polysaccharides improve the structural integrity of dental plaque and are formed by bacterial glucosyltransferases or fructosyltransferases that are found in the bacterial cell wall and are cell wall enzymes. Action of these enzymes on sucrose gives rise to dextrans/glucans, which are polymers of glucose or levans/fructans (polymers of fructose).

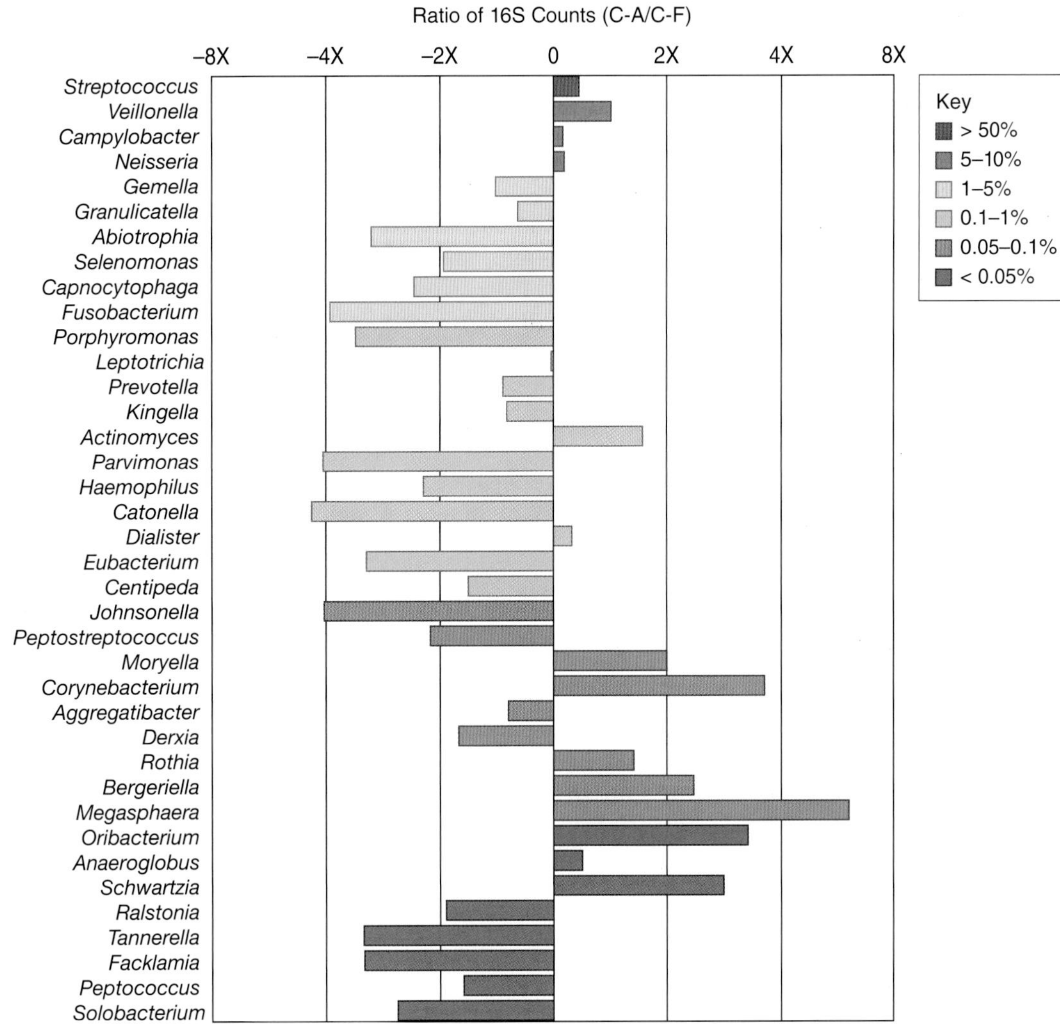

Fig. 8.24 Differential representation of genera of bacteria in the caries-free (C-F) and caries-active (C-A) microbiomes. Bars to the left correspond to over-representation of genera in the C-F subject pool. Bars to the right correspond to over-representation in the C-A pool. Bar colour key references percentage. *From Peterson, S.N. et al., 2013. The dental plaque microbiome in health and disease. PLoS One 8: e58487.*

Dental plaque and periodontal disease

Periodontal disease is associated with the persistent presence of mature dental plaque at the gingival margin and exacerbated by an increase in Gram-negative organisms and obligate anaerobes, which are favoured by the environment of periodontal pockets. Gingival inflammation and periodontal destruction are the result of direct action of bacterial products (such as proteases) and indirect promotion of potentially damaging immune responses.

Because of the intricate bacteriology, the associated inflammation and the immune factors of the host response, periodontal disease is complex and multifactorial, and the combination of factors leading to disease is likely to differ among patients, making comparisons of treatment regimens difficult.

Control of Plaque control

The challenge of dental plaque can be limited by reducing dietary sugar intake, employing mechanical removal of the plaque, and modifying the pathogenic potential. Toothbrushing, flossing or professional scaling and root planing may achieve mechanical removal. However, because of the intimate contact of its crystals with those of the tooth surface, dental calculus may be difficult to remove completely. In this context, plaque-control agents should encourage the formation of calcium phosphates that are most easily removed, being either more soluble or less strongly attached to the tooth surface. Pathogenic potential may be modified by the use of personal oral hygiene products, such as toothpastes, mouth rinses and gels containing antimicrobials, or the delivery of antibiotics as local or systemic treatments by the dental practitioner.

Further readings for this chapter can be found in the accompanying eBook. Explore online Self-assessment quiz to test and reinforce your understanding of the material in your free ebook. Follow instructions in the Inside Front Cover to unlock your access.

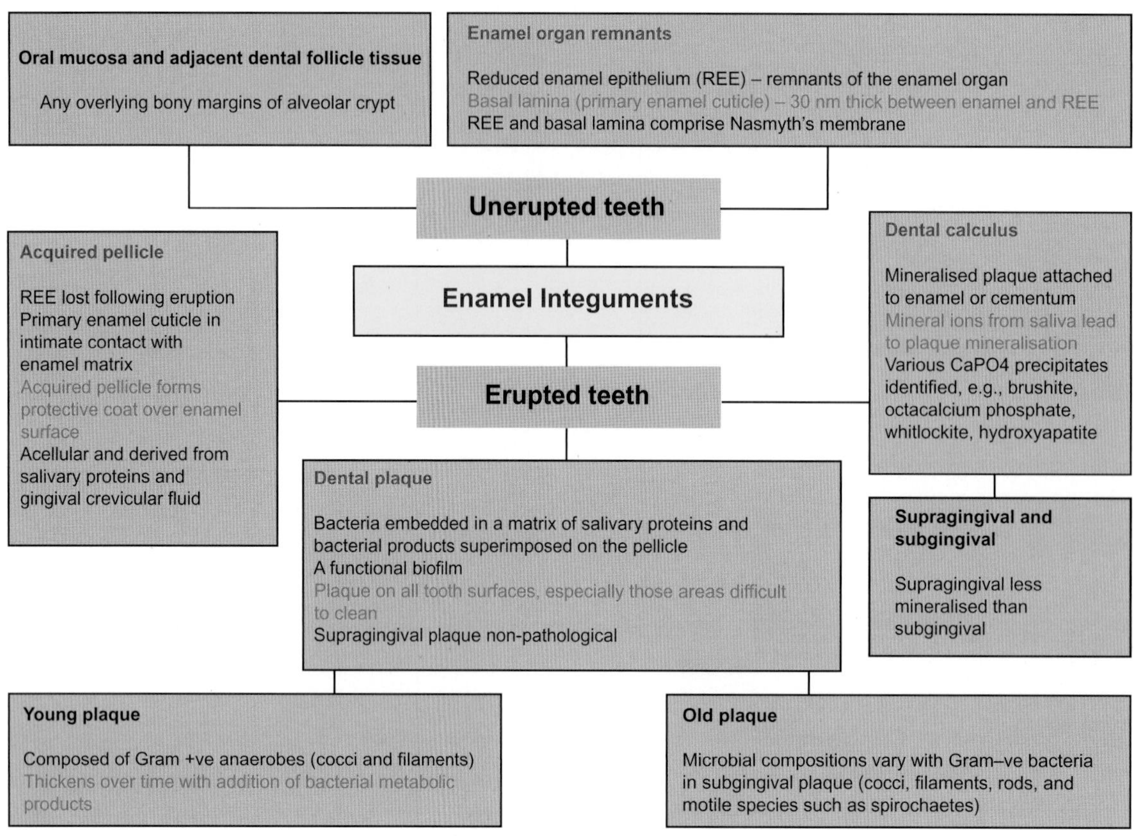
Oral mucosa and adjacent dental follicle tissue
Any overlying bony margins of alveolar crypt
Enamel organ remnants
Reduced enamel epithelium (REE) – remnants of the enamel organ
Basal lamina (primary enamel cuticle) – 30 nm thick between enamel and REE
REE and basal lamina comprise Nasmyth's membrane
Unerupted teeth
Enamel Integuments
Erupted teeth
Acquired pellicle
REE lost following eruption
Primary enamel cuticle in intimate contact with enamel matrix
Acquired pellicle forms protective coat over enamel surface
Acellular and derived from salivary proteins and gingival crevicular fluid
Dental calculus
Mineralised plaque attached to enamel or cementum
Mineral ions from saliva lead to plaque mineralisation
Various CaPO4 precipitates identified, e.g., brushite, octacalcium phosphate, whitlockite, hydroxyapatite
Dental plaque
Bacteria embedded in a matrix of salivary proteins and bacterial products superimposed on the pellicle
A functional biofilm
Plaque on all tooth surfaces, especially those areas difficult to clean
Supragingival plaque non-pathological
Supragingival and subgingival
Supragingival less mineralised than subgingival
Young plaque
Composed of Gram +ve anaerobes (cocci and filaments)
Thickens over time with addition of bacterial metabolic products
Old plaque
Microbial compositions vary with Gram–ve bacteria in subgingival plaque (cocci, filaments, rods, and motile species such as spirochaetes)

Mind Map 8.1 Enamel integuments.

Dentine

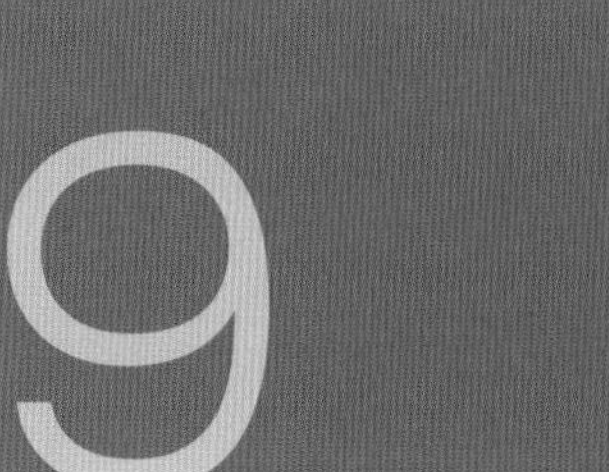

Introduction

Dentine is the mineralised tissue that forms the bulk of the tooth. In the crown it is covered by enamel, in the root by cementum (Fig. 9.1). It is a rigid but elastic tissue consisting of large numbers of small, parallel tubules in a mineralised collagen matrix. The tubules contain the long processes of the cells responsible for forming the tissue, the odontoblasts, as well as a small volume of extracellular (dentinal) fluid. The cell bodies of the odontoblasts line the deep surface of the dentine, defining the outer border of the dental pulp. The combination of enamel and dentine provides a rigid, hard structure suitable for tearing and chewing that resists both abrasion and fracture. The cementum covering the dentine of the root anchors the tooth to the bone of the socket via the periodontal ligament. The junctions of the dentine with these two other hard tissues are biologically unique, as is the tissue itself. Two major properties distinguish dentine from enamel. Firstly, dentine is sensitive. Secondly, dentine is formed throughout life, increasing in thickness at the expense of the dental pulp. This is reflected in the presence of an unmineralised layer of dentine matrix at the pulpal surface known as predentine. The physical properties of enamel and dentine are complementary. Thus, although enamel is extremely hard it is unyielding and may fracture during mastication if the underlying dentine did not provide a degree of deformability.

For convenience, dentine and pulp are considered as separate tissues. However, they are so closely interlinked as to be considered one functional unit, the dentine–pulp complex. Thus:

1) Developmentally, they both originate from the dental papilla (see Chapter 21).
2) Structurally, although the cell body of the odontoblast lies at the periphery of the dental pulp, the odontoblast process continues along the dentinal tubule. Other structures passing from the dental pulp into the dentinal tubule are nerve fibres and the dendritic processes of antigen-presenting cells.
3) Nutritionally, the tissue fluid that passes along the dentinal tubules is derived from the vasculature of the dental pulp.
4) Responsiveness of dentine to external stimuli resulting in the formation of tertiary dentine is mediated by the recruitment of stem cells within the dental pulp.

Physical properties

Fresh dentine is pale yellow in colour and contributes to the appearance of the tooth through the translucent enamel. Dentine is harder than bone and cementum but softer than enamel. Dentine is much more resistant to propagation of cracks than enamel (higher fracture toughness) because of the intimate association of small apatite crystals with strong protein fibres. Dentine's organic matrix and tubular architecture provide it with greater compressive, tensile and flexural strength than enamel. Dentine can sustain large stresses owing to its crystals having smaller unit cells near pulp compared with crystals near enamel. Dentine is permeable, with the permeability depending on the size and patency of the tubules, which will decline with age. Cracking occurs in dentine when it has been weakened by dental caries or cavity preparation and can result in an unrestorable tooth. The development of cracks is more likely in older teeth and in teeth in which the dentine has become dehydrated by root canal therapy. Stresses parallel to the direction of the dentinal tubules are more likely to result in fracture than those at right angles to them. Some of the physical properties of dentine (compared with those of enamel) are listed in Table 7.1, page 137.

Chemical properties

Dentine, like cementum and bone, is a composite material, consisting of apatite crystals on an organic scaffold predominantly composed of collagen. The gross composition of dentine approximates to 70% inorganic, 20% organic and 10% water by weight and 50% inorganic, 30% organic and 20% water by volume.

The inorganic mineral component is in the form of calcium hydroxyapatite crystals. The percentage dry weight of some of the important elements is shown in Table 9.1. The crystallites are calcium-poor and carbonate-rich in comparison to pure hydroxyapatite and, although similar in shape, are very much smaller (approximately 35 nm × 10 nm or less and of indeterminate length) than those in enamel (see Fig. 7.6). The crystallites contain other trace elements, including fluoride. The hydroxyapatite crystallites in the mineralised dentine are found on and between the collagen fibrils.

Organic matrix

The organic matrix of dentine in which the crystallites are embedded has a composition similar to that of bone. The organic matrix consists of fibrils embedded in an amorphous ground substance. The fibrils are collagen and comprise over 90% of the organic matrix.

The collagen molecule consists of three polypeptide chains that are coiled around each other to form a right-handed helix. Although over 90% of collagen in the body is type I collagen, there are 28 types of human collagen. They can be divided into two main groups according to whether the collagen is fibrillar or non-fibrillar, with further subdivisions indicating the diverse functionality of the collagen as follows:

- Fibrillar collagens (type I, II, III, V, XI)
- Non-fibrillar collagens
- FACIT (fibril-associated collagens with interrupted triple helices) (type IX, XII, XIV, XIX, XXI)
- Short chain (type VIII, X)
- Basement membrane (type IV)
- Multiplexin (multiple triple helix domains with interruptions) (type XV, XVIII)
- MACIT (membrane-associated collagens with interrupted triple helices) (type XIII, XVII)
- Microfibril forming (type VI)
- Anchoring fibrils (type VII)

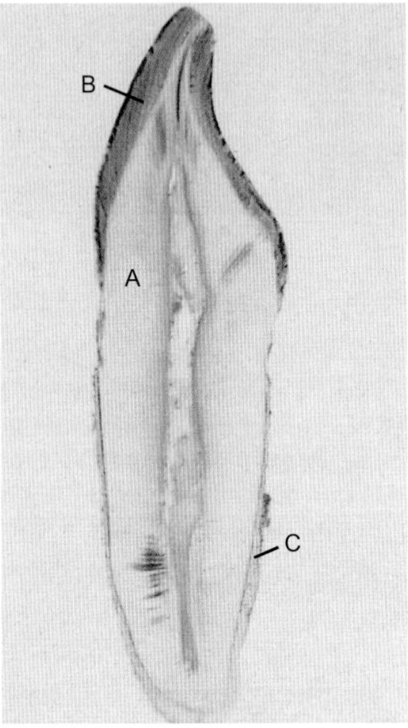

Fig. 9.1 Ground longitudinal section of a tooth showing dentine (A) forming the bulk of the tooth, covered in the crown by enamel (B) and in the root by cementum (C). The dental pulp has been lost during preparation, and the pulp chamber and root canal are empty (×4).

Table 9.1 The major inorganic components of dentine

Constituent	% of dry weight
Calcium	26.9
Phosphorus	13.2
Carbonate	4.6
Sodium	0.6
Magnesium	0.8

The three polypeptide chains of collagen may be identical (homotrimers), as in collagens II, III, VII, VIII, X and others, or different (heterotrimers), as in collagen types I, IV, V, VI, IX and XI. Each of these chains shows a repetitive sequence of amino acids with glycine at every third position (Gly-X-Y), and X and Y are mostly proline and hydroxyproline. The collagen molecule has a stagger of 65 nm between adjacent rows. The length of the stagger is a quarter of the length of the molecule, and this quarter stagger arrangement gives the 65-nm banding characteristic under the electron microscope (see Fig. 12.9). The larger collagen molecule is cleaved extracellularly by proteinases and stabilised through the cross-linking by oxidation of the lysine and hydroxylysine residues by lysyl oxidase.

The principal collagen fibril in the dental hard and soft tissues (including periodontal ligament, oral mucosa and temporomandibular disc) is the ubiquitous type I collagen. However, dentine collagen has more hydroxylysine than the equivalent in soft tissue collagen. Traces of type III and type V collagen, which are present in sizeable amounts in the pulp, have also been detected. Most of the collagen fibrils in dentine run parallel to the pulpal surface (Fig. 9.2). In mineralised dentine the collagen fibrils are of larger diameter (100 nm) and are more closely packed than in predentine. Collagen fibrils in dentine are not assembled into bundles as they are in many non-mineralised connective tissues such as tendons or the periodontal ligament.

Non-collagenous proteins

Though comprising only a relatively small percentage of the organic matrix compared with collagen (8%), the non-collagenous proteins of

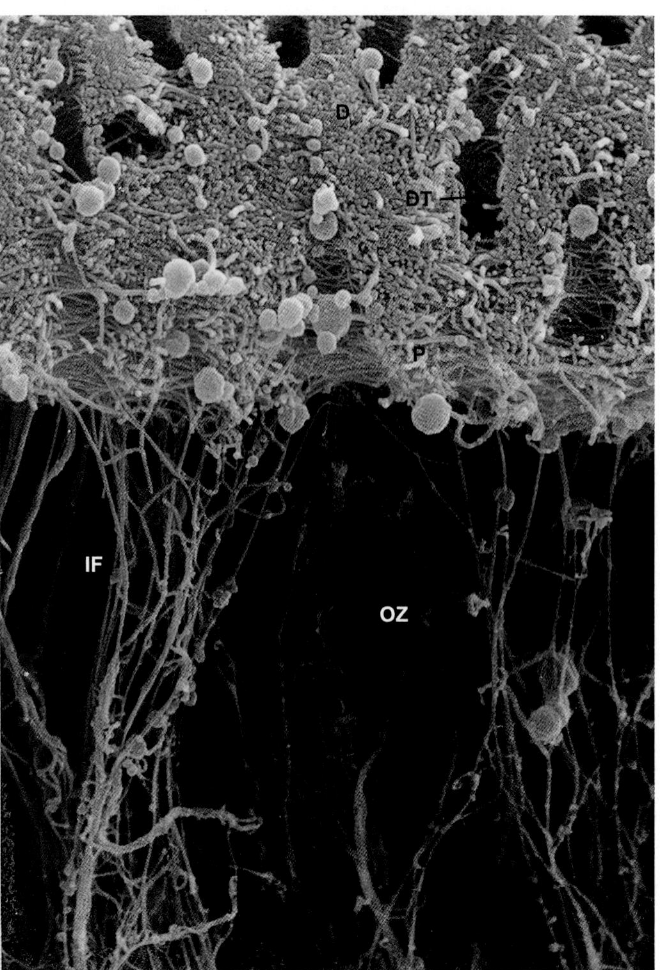

Fig. 9.2 SEM of predentine (P) with mineral and odontoblast cells removed revealing the pattern of collagen fibrils. In predentine, most of the dentinal collagen fibrils run parallel to the pulpal surface. Collagen fibrils in the odontoblast layer parallel the long axis of the cell bodies; D = dentine; DT = dentinal tubule; IF = intercellular fibrils; OZ = odontoblast zone (×3,500). Courtesy B Sogaard-Pedersen, H Boye, M Matthiessen and the editor of the *Scandinavian Journal of Dental Research*.

dentine have important, yet poorly understood, biological functions. They include dentine phosphoproteins, proteoglycans, Gla-proteins, other acid proteins and growth factors. Although many are involved in mineralisation, they may have other functions. Some act as both inhibitors and promotors of mineralisation, depending on concentration and posttranslational modification. Amino acids undergo changes with age, in which they convert from one racemic form to another. This can be measured very accurately by gas chromatography. Measuring these changes in aspartate in dentine is an accurate way of determining the age of human remains (see page 482).

Dentine phosphoproteins

These represent the main non-collagenous protein. There are several types, but the term *dentine phosphoprotein* (phosphophoryn or PP-H) relates to the highly phosphorylated protein species. Owing to its very high phosphate content, it represents the most acidic protein known. Indeed, about 80% of the amino acid residues carry negatively charged phosphate or carboxyl groups. Its high calcium ion–binding properties have implicated PP-H in the process of mineralisation. The dentine sialophosphoprotein gene synthesises both dentine phosphoprotein and dentine sialoprotein.

Dentine matrix protein 1 (DMP-1), present in dentine and bone, is thought to play a pivotal role in mineralisation as it can initiate apatite nucleation. It has an Arg–Gly–Asp (RGD) cell attachment sequence and may act as a morphogen for odontoblast differentiation and intertubular dentine formation for both primary and tertiary dentine. It is present in only small amounts in predentine and intertubular dentine but is strongly represented in peritubular dentine. DMP-1–null mice show abnormalities in mineralisation and structural organisation of dentine. It may also play a role in fracture healing in bone.

As DMP-1 and dentine phosphophoryn are found at different sites, they are likely to have different actions during mineralisation.

Proteoglycans

These also form a significant component of the non-collagenous proteins. In dentine they are represented by the smaller-molecular-weight types known as *biglycan* and *decorin*, also known as the small leucine-rich proteoglycans (SLRPs). The glycosaminoglycans are primarily chondroitin-4-sulphate and chondroitin-6-sulphate. Among the important functions of proteoglycans in general are their roles in collagen fibril assembly and their cell-mediated effects such as cell adhesion, migration, proliferation and differentiation. As significant biochemical changes occur at the mineralising front, it can be assumed that proteoglycans have an important but, as yet, incompletely understood role in mineralisation. They appear to bind calcium nonspecifically. They may be inhibitors of calcifications that need to undergo some degree of degradation before mineralisation will occur.

Glycoproteins/sialoproteins

Dentine also contains other acidic proteins such as osteonectin, osteopontin and dentine sialoprotein. Osteonectin, a protein containing high levels of glutamic and aspartic acid, is found in dentine at levels of about 5% of total protein. Osteopontin, a phosphorylated glycoprotein, has been identified in predentine and contains the receptor-binding sequence RGD. The precise roles of osteonectin and osteopontin in dentine (as in bone) are unknown.

Gamma-carboxyglutamate-containing proteins (Gla-proteins)

Little is known about the function of these small proteins, present in low amounts in dentine. They bind strongly, but reversibly, to hydroxyapatite crystallites and may play some role in mineralisation.

SIBLING family

Several of the non-collagenous proteins have been regrouped together as the SIBLING (small integrin-binding ligand N-linked glycoproteins) family, including osteopontin, bone sialoprotein, DMP-1, matrix extracellular phosphoglycoprotein and dentine sialophosphoprotein. The genes for these proteins are located on human chromosome 4q21-23. The proteins contain the RGD motif, because of the presence of an Arg-Gly-Asp tripeptide, which interacts with cell-surface integrins mediating cell adhesion and signalling. This family of proteins is known to regulate hydroxyapatite crystal formation and act as nucleating factors for mineralisation

The group members contain a large fraction of aspartic and glutamic acids and numerous serines that are 90% phosphorylated. They are therefore extremely acidic. They adopt an open and random configuration in solution, providing freedom for interaction with other molecules. Accumulating evidence has implicated the SIBLING proteins in matrix mineralisation of dentine and bone. Clinically, they may play a role in cancer progression through malignant transformation, invasion and metastasis.

Growth factors and cytokines

Several growth factors can be isolated from the dentine matrix, as they can from bone matrix, and are presumably absorbed from circulating tissue fluid. These include insulin growth factor (IGF)-II, bone morphogenetic protein (BMP)-2 and transforming growth factor (TGF)-beta. During dentine development, these growth factors are involved in important processes such as cell proliferation and differentiations, chemotaxis neuronal growth and angiogenesis. Once entombed in fully formed dentine, as dentine does not turn over like bone, it is unlikely that these factors play an everyday role in the tissue's metabolism, but they could be released during the progress of dental caries and induce the production of reactionary or reparative dentine. They appear to be very stable, having been found in teeth from Neolithic times.

Cytokines are also present in dentine. These pro- and anti-inflammatory cytokines, including interleukins and tumour necrosis factor alpha (TNF-α), lie sequestered within the dentine matrix and can be released by various dental materials and bacterial acids.

Metalloproteinases

The organic matrix of dentine contains small amounts of the enzymes collagenase (MMP-1) and enamelysin (MMP-20). Trace amounts of tissue inhibitors of matrix metalloproteinases (TIMPs) can also be found.

Serum-derived proteins

Dentine matrix will also contain some serum-derived proteins, such as albumin.

Lipids

These comprise about 2% of the organic content of dentine and, as they are conspicuous at the mineralising front, are thought to play a role in mineralisation. They are in the form of phospholipids and cholesterol. Phospholipids have been detected in both predentine and mineralised dentine. They occupy the spaces between collagen fibrils along with the proteoglycans. In the predentine, they are most heavily concentrated near the mineralising front. In dentine, phospholipids are needle-like 'crystal ghosts' and may be involved in the formation and growth of crystals. They seem to be absent from the centres of calcospherites but present in interglobular dentine.

Proteomics

As with enamel (see page 412), new and advanced technologies in proteomic analysis have allowed the detection of proteins present in the smallest quantities to be determined in dentine matrix. A recent analysis detected a total of 813 proteins, with large numbers being detected for the first time. With so many proteins present, it would be necessary to determine which are exogenous and which are endogenous. Although the functions of many proteins can be related to cell growth, maintenance of odontoblasts, cell communication, signal transduction, protein metabolism, immune response, transport and nucleic acid metabolism, the function of other proteins remains unknown. Fig. 9.3 denotes the protein classes detected in human dentine with respect to function, while the numbers in parentheses indicate the number of proteins in each family.

Dentinal tubules

Dentine is permeated by the dentinal tubules that run from the pulpal surface to the enamel–dentine and cementum–dentine junctions (Fig. 9.4).

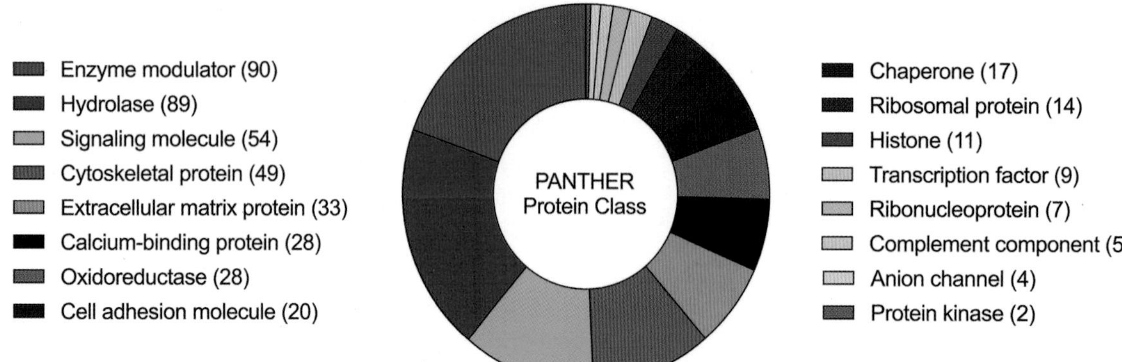

Fig. 9.3 Protein classes detected in dentine at the most general level and, in parentheses, the number of proteins in each family. From Widbiller, M., Schweik, H., Bruckmann. A., et al. 2019. Shotgun proteomics of human dentin with different prefractionation methods. *Nature Scientific Reports 9, 4457.*

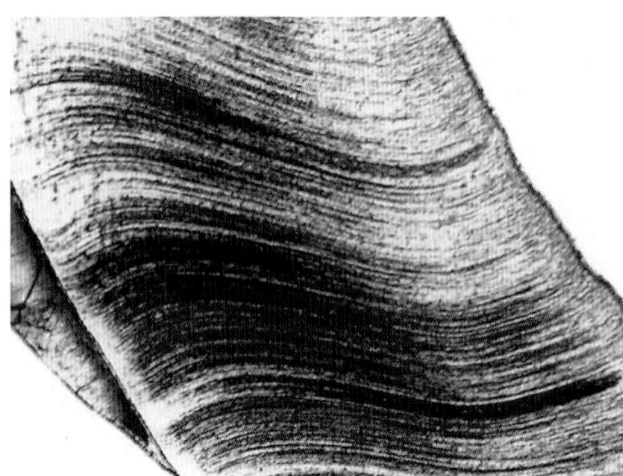

Fig. 9.4 Ground section showing dentinal tubules cut longitudinally and demonstrating the sinusoidal primary curvatures (×25).

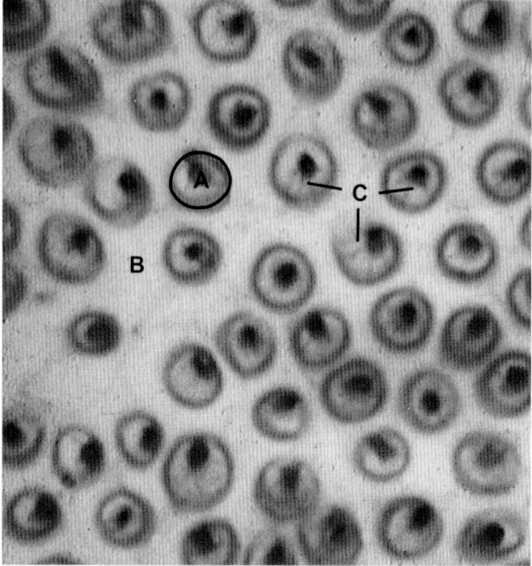

Fig. 9.5 Ground, partially demineralised section of dentinal tubules cut transversely. A = perimeter of a tubule as initially laid down; B = intertubular dentine; C = peritubular/intratubular dentine. (Eosin stain; ×1,500.) Courtesy Dr. R Sprinz.

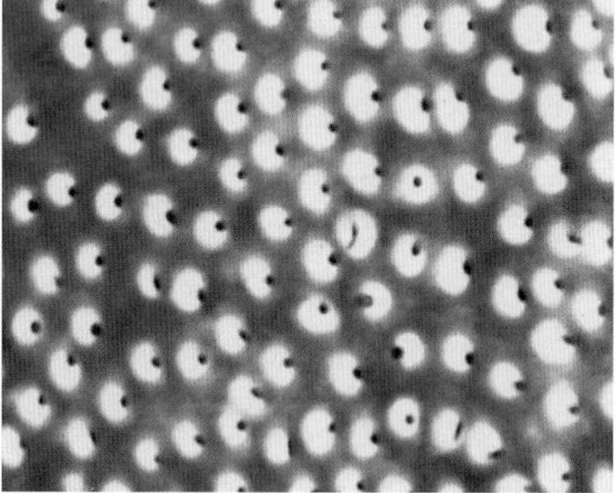

Fig. 9.6 A demineralised section of dentinal tubules cut transversely. This treatment results in the loss of the peritubular/intratubular dentine, which has little organic matrix. The dark-staining odontoblast processes occupy only a small proportion of the resulting lumen. (Haematoxylin; ×1,000.) Courtesy Prof. E W Bradford.

The dentinal tubules follow a curved, sigmoid course – the primary curvatures. The convexity of the primary curvatures nearest the pulp chamber faces rootward. In the root and beneath the cusps, the primary curvatures are less pronounced, with the tubules running a straighter course. In transverse section the tubules are approximately circular, although their appearance is obviously dependent on the plane in which the tissue is sectioned (Figs 9.5, 9.6). The dentine between the tubules is termed *intertubular dentine*.

The tubules taper from approximately 2.5 µm in diameter at their pulpal ends to 1 µm or less peripherally. During the formation of dentinal tubules by the odontoblasts, the cells migrate inwards and occupy a smaller surface area. Hence, the tubules are more widely separated at their peripheries. Approximately 22% of the cross-sectional area of the dentine near the pulp is composed of tubules, while near the enamel–dentine junction, the tubules comprise only about 2.5%. Estimates of the number of tubules vary somewhat between reports because of differences in tooth age and type and the thickness of the dentine. A reasonable rounding of the numbers in the crown suggests 20,000/mm^2 in outer dentine, 50,000/mm^2 in inner dentine and 40,000/mm^2 in the middle. The number in root dentine is lower, being about 8,000 mm^2, and lowest in the apical region.

The tubules also show changes in direction of a much smaller (a few micrometres) amplitude. These are known as the *secondary curvatures* (Fig. 9.7). In some regions the secondary curvatures may coincide in adjacent tubules. At low magnification, this gives the appearance of a line crossing the dentine, a contour line (of Owen) (Fig. 9.7). These are not commonly seen in most of the dentine, but one such line is usually evident at the junction of primary and secondary dentine where, during deposition, all the odontoblasts seem to take a simultaneous and similar change in direction (see Figs 9.51, 9.52, 9.64).

Dentinal tubules branch. The most profuse branching is in the periphery near the enamel–dentine junction (Fig. 9.8), presumably a reflection of the numerous processes the early odontoblast has. Many small side branches appear to end blindly, but some may unite with branches of other tubules. In the root, the terminal part of the tubule branches and the branches loop. This looping is thought by some to be responsible for the appearance of the granular layer (of Tomes) seen in this region in ground section (see page 177). Branching is not obvious in much of the dentine beneath the periphery but becomes notable in the uncalcified predentine near the pulp. Presumably during mineralisation many of the odontoblastic branches retract or atrophy and the small canals they occupied fill in.

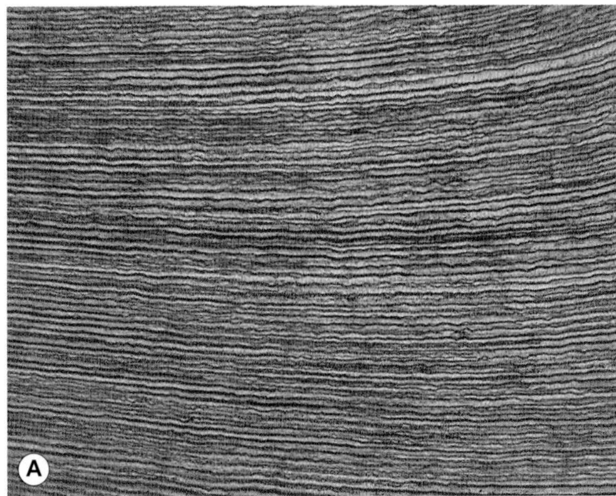

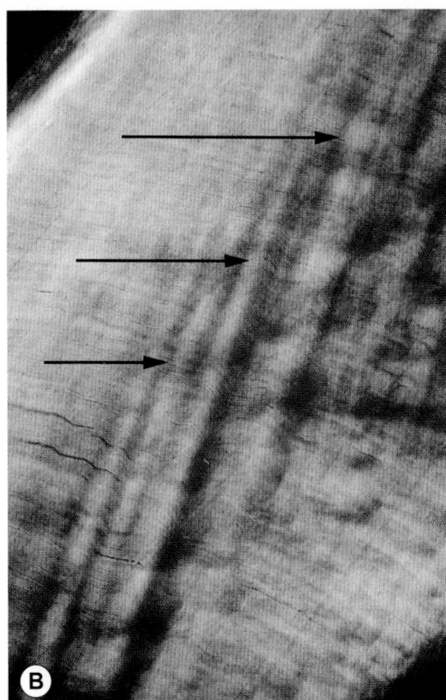

Fig. 9.7 (A) Decalcified section showing dentinal tubules cut longitudinally. The lumens of the tubules have been stained with picrothionin and demonstrate secondary curvatures (×200). (B) Ground section showing dentinal tubules cut longitudinally and exhibiting contour lines *(arrows)* due to coincidence of secondary curvatures (×150). (A) Courtesy Prof. M M Smith. (B) Courtesy Dr. R P Shellis.

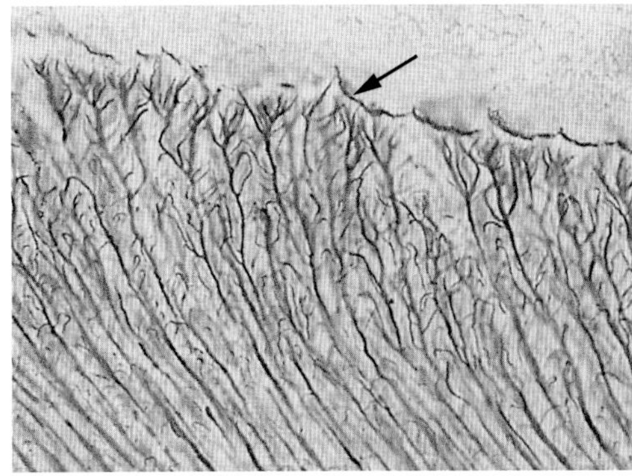

Fig. 9.8 Ground section of dentine near the enamel–dentine junction *(arrow)* showing branching of dentinal tubules (×320).

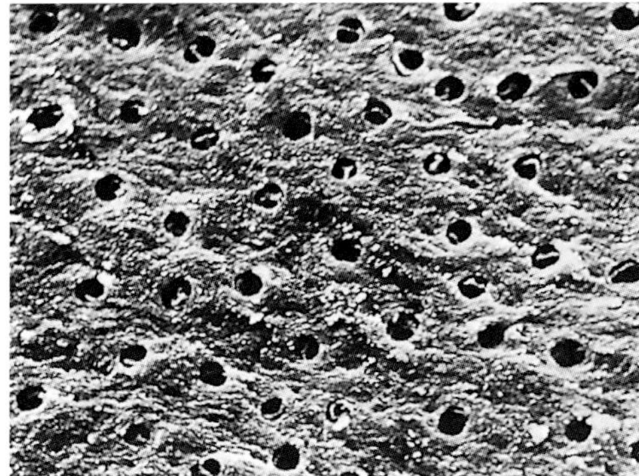

Fig. 9.9 SEM of transversely sectioned dentinal tubules close to the pulp and lacking peritubular dentine (×540). Courtesy Prof. B R R N Mendis.

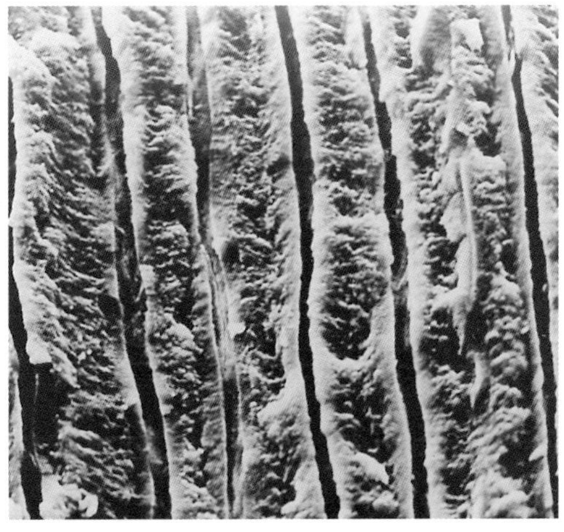

Fig. 9.10 SEM of longitudinally sectioned dentinal tubules close to the pulp showing little evidence of peritubular dentine (×540). Courtesy Prof. B R R N Mendis.

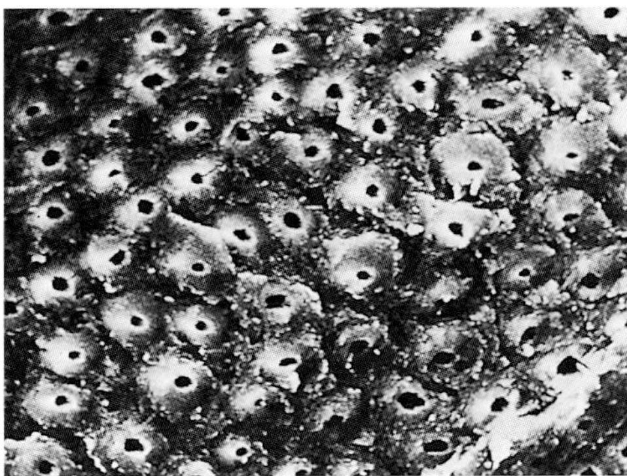

Fig. 9.11 SEM of dentinal tubules cut in cross-section in the middle of the dentine. They reveal a distinctive zone of peritubular dentine, narrowing the original tubule (×1,200). Courtesy Prof. B R R N Mendis.

Peritubular dentine

The walls of the dentinal tubules in recently formed intertubular dentine at the pulp surface are composed of mineralised type I collagen. With maturation, another type of dentine is deposited on the walls of the dentinal tubule, narrowing the lumen (Figs 9.9–9.12). This type of dentine is known as *peritubular dentine* (also known as intratubular dentine), and its formation gradually leads to obliteration of the tubule (Fig. 9.13).

Peritubular dentine differs from intertubular dentine in lacking a collagenous fibrous matrix. This also relates to the finding that it exhibits no piezoelectricity. Its matrix is rich in glutamic acid and serine. It lacks dentine phosphophoryn but is rich in DMP-1. Together with its lipid content, its composition has been classified as a proteolipid–phospholipid complex.

Peritubular dentine can be distinguished from intertubular dentine as a zone of increased radiographic (Fig. 9.14) and electron (Fig. 9.15) density lining the internal surface of the dentinal tubule. It can be clearly distinguished in sections that have been specially prepared by ion beam milling and have thus not undergone destructive chemical processing (Figs 9.16, 9.17). Peritubular dentine is about 5–12% more mineralised than intertubular dentine and has a higher elastic modulus (29–45 versus 12–25 GPa).

When dentine is routinely demineralised, the peritubular dentine will be lost, as it lacks the stabilising feature of collagen. The dimensions of the dentinal tubules will thus be increased to their initial dimensions (compare Figs 9.5 and 9.6). Peritubular dentine is found in unerupted teeth. This, with its predominant distribution in apical dentine, indicates that it is an age change rather than a response tissue.

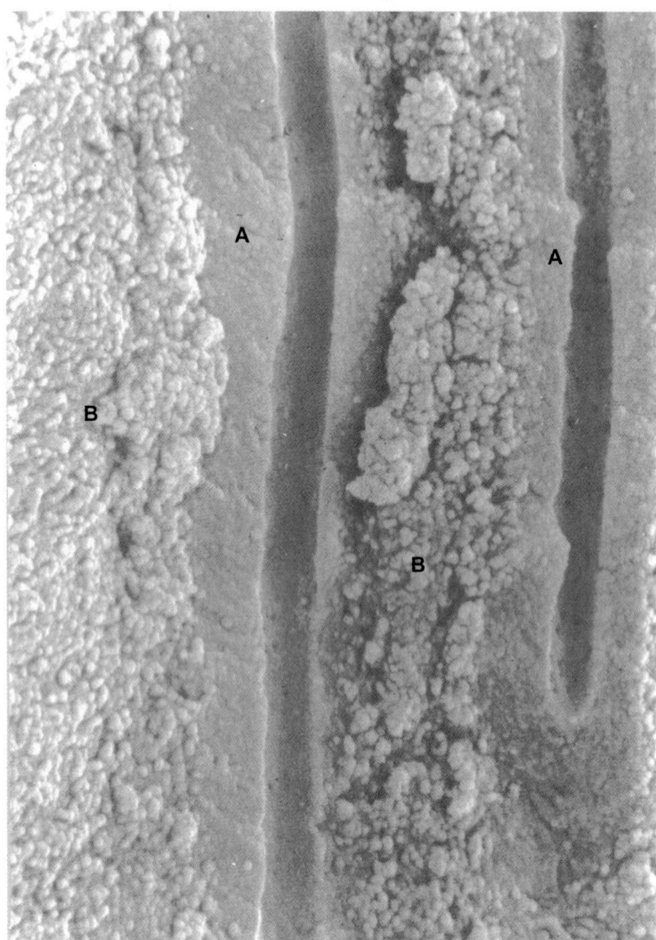

Fig. 9.12 SEM of dentinal tubules cut longitudinally and showing peritubular dentine (A) deposited on the tubule wall. B = intertubular dentine (×7,000). Courtesy Prof. M M Smith.

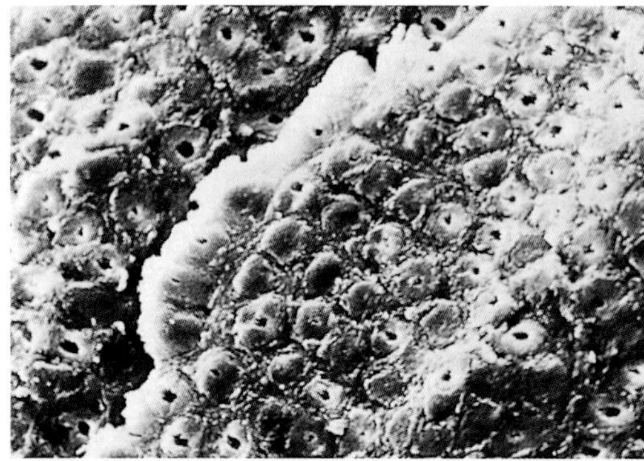

Fig. 9.13 Dentinal tubules sectioned transversely close to the enamel–dentine junction showing peritubular dentine formation obliterating the lumen (×1,200). Courtesy Prof. B R R N Mendis.

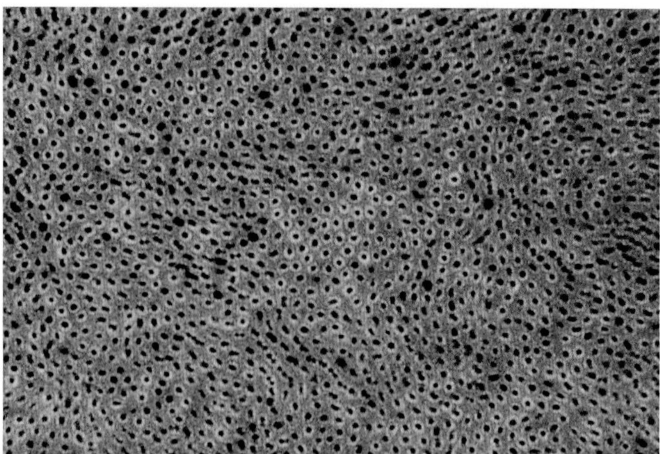

Fig. 9.14 Microradiograph of transversely sectioned dentinal tubules surrounded by a more radio-opaque (and therefore denser) zone of peritubular dentine (×650). Courtesy Dr. G McKay.

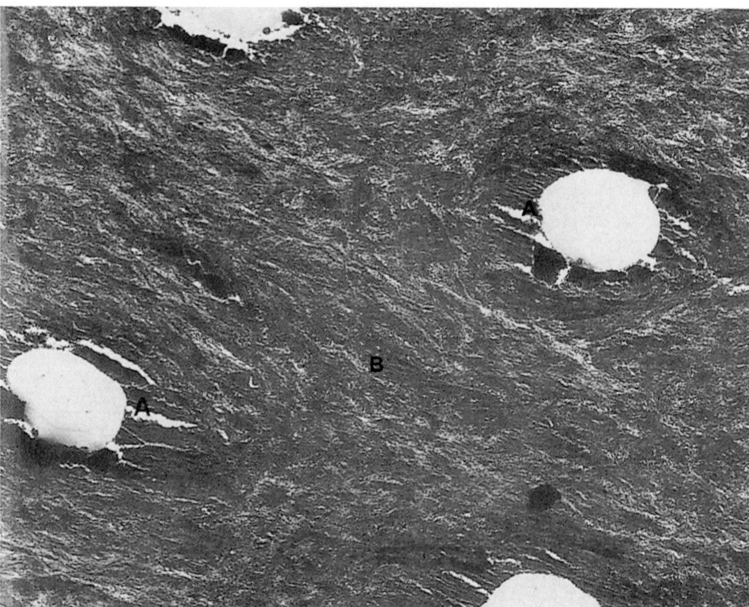

Fig. 9.15 TEM of peritubular dentine (A) seen in an ultrathin undecalcified section. The peritubular dentine appears nonfibrillar and more electron opaque. It is more fragile than intertubular dentine (B) and shatters during sectioning (×6,000). Courtesy Prof. N W Johnson.

In demineralised sections at the electron microscope level, the matrix appears as an amorphous material. The mineral component of peritubular dentine is mainly carbonated apatite, but its crystalline form is distinct from that of intertubular dentine. Some crystallites have an hexagonal shape and appear as compact platelets slightly smaller than (but similar to) those of intertubular dentine. Other crystalline species may also be present. In tubules exposed by attrition, some occluding components may be derived from saliva. Although the bulk of peritubular dentine is hypercalcified relative to the intertubular dentine, hypocalcified areas bound its inner and outer surfaces. Peritubular dentine is formed at about the same time as (or soon after) intertubular dentine. By the time primary dentine formation is complete, all peripheral tubules have a lining of peritubular dentine that extends from the enamel–dentine junction to within 50–100 μm of the predentine. In outer dentine (Fig. 9.13), peritubular dentine occupies two-thirds of the cross-sectional area of the tissue; near to the predentine, it occupies only approximately 3% (Fig. 9.9).

Associated with physiological ageing, especially in root dentine, the dentinal tubules become completely occluded by peritubular dentine formation. The contents of the tubule acquire the same refractive index as the intertubular dentine. When a ground section of a root is placed in water (which has a refractive index different from that of dentine), regions blocked by peritubular dentine will appear translucent ('translucent dentine'), while regions with patent tubules will fill with water and appear opaque (Fig. 9.18). Dentinal tubules become infilled at the root apex adjacent to the cementum and extend cervically and towards the root canal with age. In cross-section, translucent zones have a butterfly shape owing to the convergence of the tubules pulpally, being wider at the mesial and distal margins (Fig. 9.19). The amount of translucent dentine increases linearly with age and is not affected by function or external irritation. This feature is used in forensic dentistry to age teeth. Translucent dentine is also referred to on page 183; sclerotic dentine, which has features similar to translucent dentine, is discussed on pages 183–184.

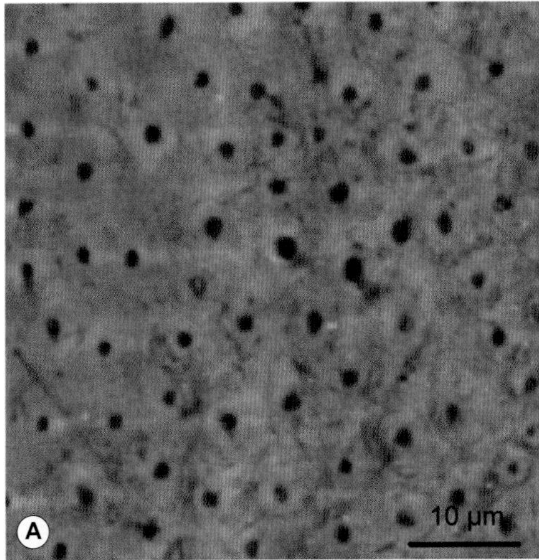

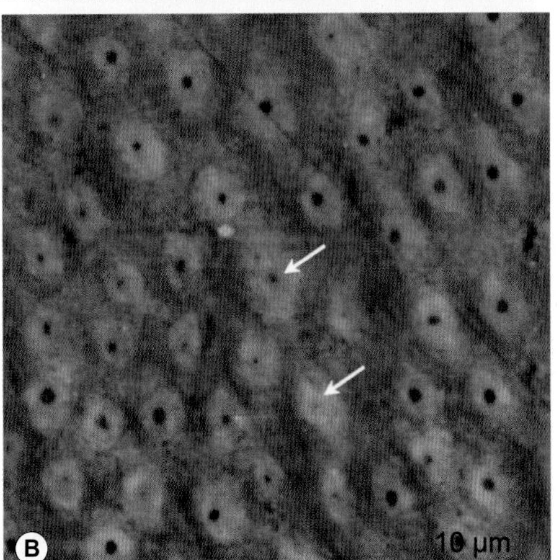

Fig. 9.16 Atomic force microscopic images of (A) normal (donor age 25 years) and (B) translucent (donor age 67 years) dentine. The dark contrast indicates the tubule sites, and the *white arrows* in (B) show representative tubule lumens occluded with peritubular mineral. Atomic force microscopy is a technique that scans a sample and builds up an image of resolution much higher than that achieved by scanning electron microscopy. From Porter, A.E. 2006. Nanoscale characterization of the interface between bone and hydroxyapatite implants and the effect of silicon on bone apposition. *Micron* 37, 681–688, with permission.

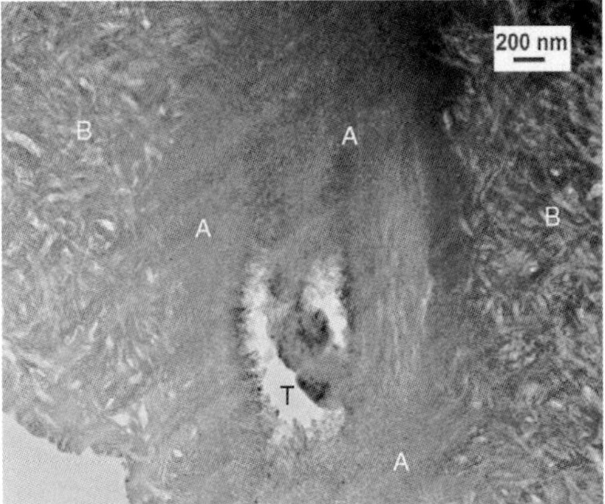

Fig. 9.17 A partially filled dentinal tubule in a section thinned by less damaging ion beam milling. The very different structure of the peritubular dentine can be clearly seen. A = peritubular dentine; B = intertubular dentine; T = tubule. From Porter, A.E. 2006. Nanoscale characterization of the interface between bone and hydroxyapatite implants and the effect of silicon on bone apposition. *Micron* 37, 681–688, with permission.

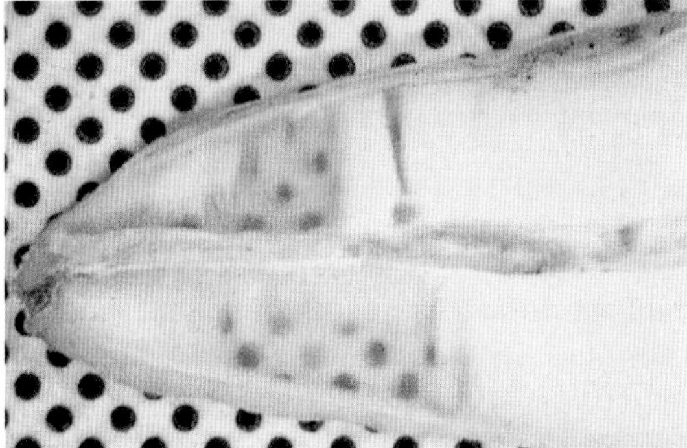

Fig. 9.18 Old tooth root sectioned longitudinally and placed in water. The presence of peritubular dentine completely occluding the tubules in much of the apical tissue on the left side of this image results in this part appearing translucent as water is excluded. Towards the cervical margin (right side), patent tubules become filled with water, which has a refractive index that differs from that of the intertubular dentine. This results in the tissue appearing opaque (×5). Courtesy Prof. A G S Lumsden.

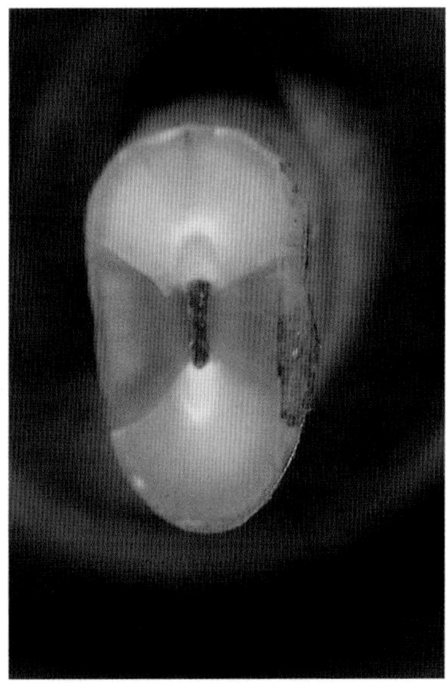

Fig. 9.19 Transverse section of mandibular premolar showing butterfly-shaped outline of translucent dentine. Courtesy Dr. R O'Sullivan.

Contents of the dentinal tubules

The dentinal tubules contain the processes of the odontoblasts that are responsible for their formation. In some parts of the tissue they also contain afferent nerve terminals (Fig. 9.20). It is also possible that processes from antigen-presenting cells in the peripheral pulp may extend for a short distance into the tubules. Technical limitations prevent a definitive figure being given for what proportion of the tubule is occupied by cell processes and how far along the tubule the processes extend. It seems likely, however, that there is a periodontoblastic space, and possibly a postodontoblastic space, from which the process has receded. These spaces are thought to be filled with extracellular 'dentinal' fluid, the precise composition of which is unknown. Some studies have suggested a composition that differs from extracellular fluids elsewhere in having a relatively higher concentration of potassium ions and a relatively lower concentration of sodium ions. Such a balance could affect the membrane properties of the nerve endings and odontoblast processes in the tubules. If dentine is fractured, fluid exudes from the tubules and forms droplets on the surface of the dentine. This suggests that there is a positive force, presumably pulpal tissue pressure, that is exerted outwards (page 204). This could help limit the progress of chemicals or toxins on, or in, dentine towards the dental pulp.

The cell body of the odontoblast is described in detail in the section on the dental pulp (pages 195–198). The process of the odontoblast that extends into the dentine varies in structure at different levels in the tissue, with organelles being most numerous in the predentine (Fig. 9.21), whereas in mineralised dentine, few are present.

Two technical problems limit the interpretation of available histological data on the contents of the dentinal tubules. One is the difficulty of fixing small amounts of tissue deep in mineralised tissue. Fixation tends to shrink tissue, and even when this can be minimised, the slowness with which most fixatives penetrate means that postmortem changes will often occur. The second problem is that in extracting a tooth, it is often compressed by forceps. Releasing the compression often draws tissue up into the tubules (e.g., 'aspiration' of odontoblast nuclei) that is not normally there. Thus, the interpretation of images of tubule contents should be approached with caution. More indirect approaches, such as labelling the tissue *in vivo* with, for example, a radioactive tag or using immunohistochemical techniques that mark the presence of cell components, can add considerably to our understanding.

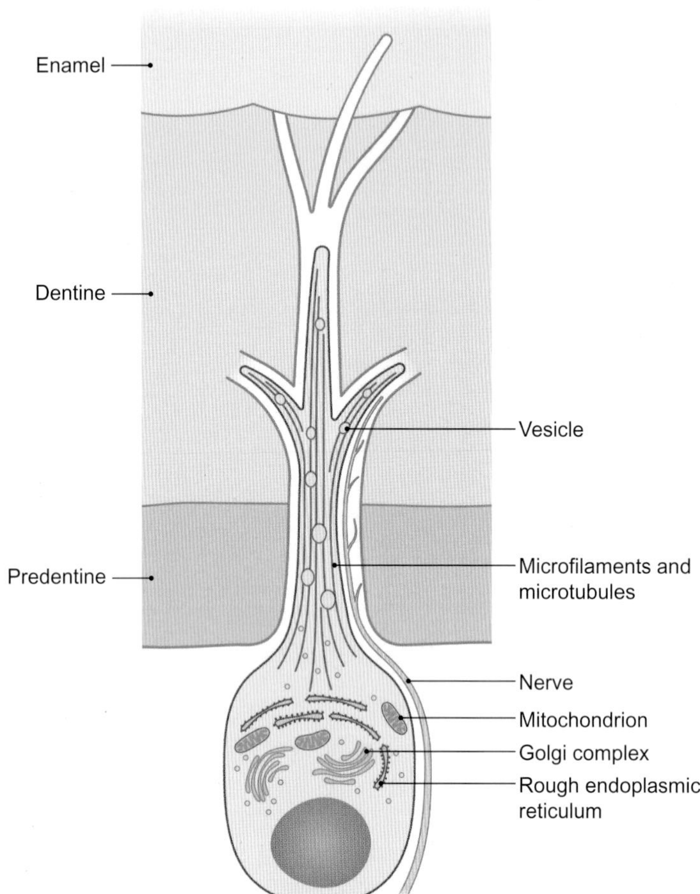

Fig. 9.20 Diagram of an odontoblast and its main process extending into the dentine. The true extent of the process is controversial, as is the existence of the periodontoblastic space.

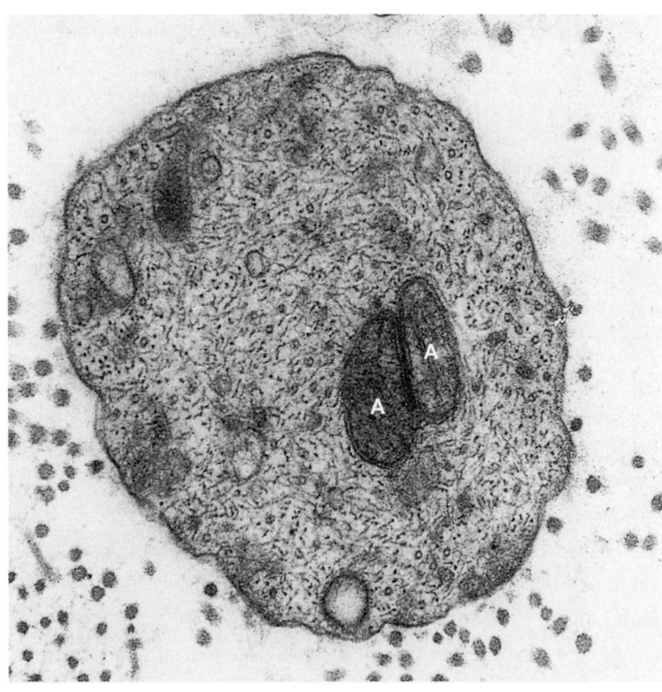

Fig. 9.21 TEM of an odontoblast process from the predentine in cross-section. A = mitochondrion (×80,000).

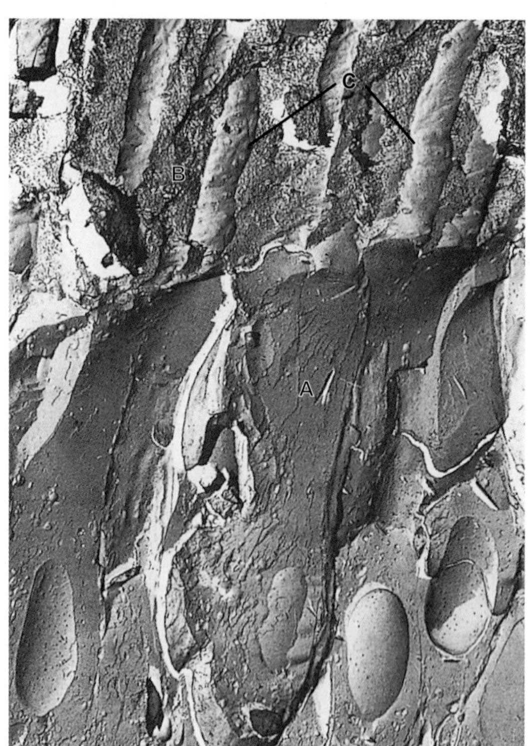

Fig. 9.22 TEM of a surface replica of the pulp–predentine junction. The odontoblasts (A) form a continuous layer on the surface of the predentine (B), and their processes (C) completely fill the dentinal tubules with no evidence of a periodontoblastic space. The technique involves fracturing the frozen tissue, coating the surface with vaporised metal and then separating the ultrathin coating for examination in the microscope. This complex technique is thought to cause minimal, if any, shrinkage (×2,000). Courtesy Dr. A Riske-Anderson, Dr. A Koling and the editors of *Acta Scandinavica Odontologica*.

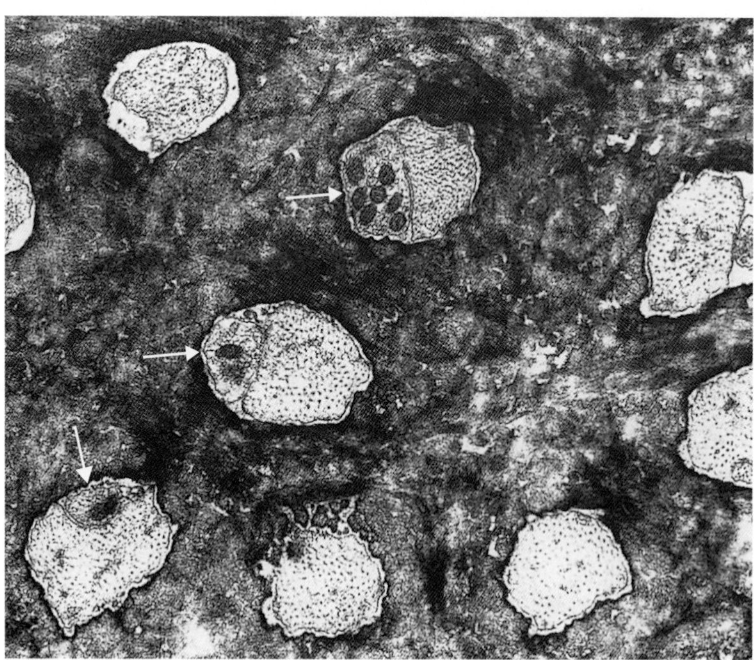

Fig. 9.23 TEM of dentinal tubules in inner calcified dentine in cross-section. Three of the tubules contain naked nerve endings (arrows) as well as odontoblast processes. The periodontoblastic space is either small or absent (×10,000).

Microtubules and intermediate filaments run longitudinally throughout the odontoblast process. Mitochondria are sometimes present in the process in the predentine; strands of rough endoplasmic reticulum are also occasionally seen. Vesicles of a variety of sizes are present, being denser near the cell membrane. Their incidence declines in the more distal parts of the process.

In the predentine and very innermost mineralised circumpulpal dentine, the odontoblast process seems to occupy the full width of the dentinal tubule with no discernible periodontoblast space (Figs 9.22, 9.23). At these levels afferent nerve axons are also seen within the tubule and in close apposition to the odontoblast process. The axons contain several mitochondria and an occasional vesicle. They do not contain large accumulations of vesicles, as are found in synapses, although proteins associated

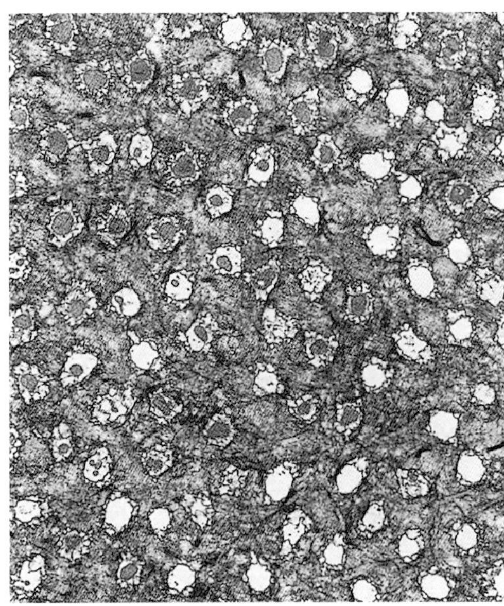

Fig. 9.24 TEM of dentinal tubules from the middle region of coronal circumpulpal dentine. Some tubules appear to contain cell processes, some contain noncellular material and some are empty (×3,000).

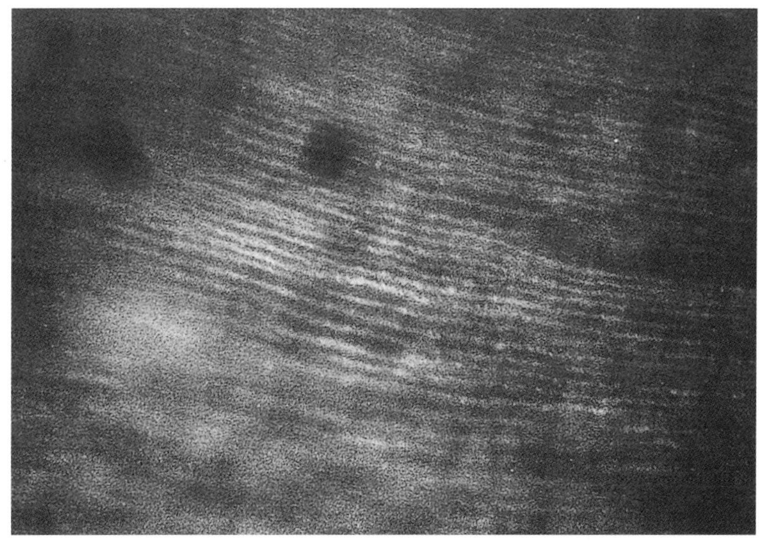

Fig. 9.26 Components of the cytoskeleton in peripheral dentine. A fluorescent label *(white)* marks the presence of tubulin, a component of intracellular microtubules (×4,200). Courtesy Dr. M Sigal, Dr. S Pitaru, Dr. J Aubin, Dr. A R Ten Cate and the editor of the *Anatomical Record*.

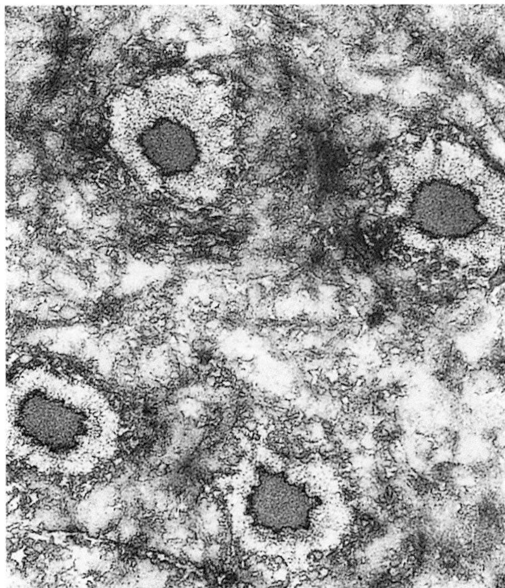

Fig. 9.25 TEM of dentinal tubules in peripheral dentine. The tubules contain amorphous, noncellular material (×8,000).

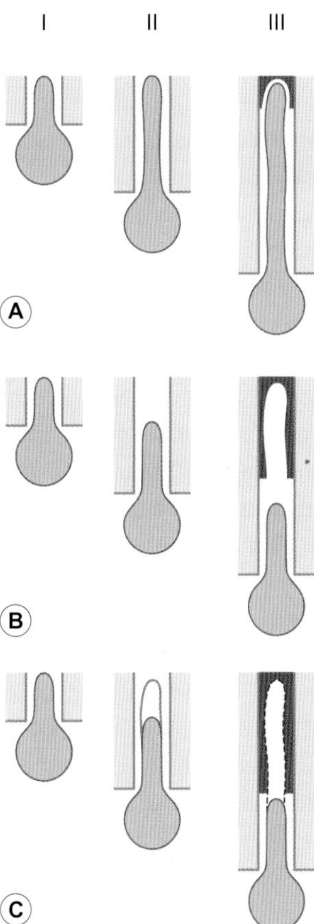

Fig. 9.27 Three hypotheses describing the pulpward migration of the odontoblast as dentine is deposited (see text for details).

elsewhere with synaptic vesicle exocytosis have been demonstrated in dentinal tubules. It is not possible by electron microscopy to recognise cell processes in the dentinal tubules of peripheral dentine (Figs 9.24, 9.25).

Although the structural characteristics of cells may be lost because of poor fixation, remnants characteristic of cells may still be found (e.g., tubulin – Fig. 9.26). The microtubule and intermediate filament systems are characteristic of cell processes and are made up of proteins such as actin, tubulin and vimentin. Some of these proteins can be demonstrated in peripheral dentinal tubules even though no structurally recognisable process can be seen. One possible interpretation for this finding might be that the odontoblast process has degenerated, leaving remnants containing tubulin or microfilamentous material behind. Some studies using this approach suggest that the process extends farthest in the dentine below the cusps.

Clearly, the odontoblast process must occupy the entire dentinal tubule it forms in the early stages of development when the dentine is thin. There are three hypotheses for what might happen later, and these are illustrated in Fig. 9.27. In Fig. 9.27A, the process grows in length as dentine is deposited, and its peripheral termination remains at the outer end of the tubule. This would result in a metabolically unsupported cell process several millimetres long, an arrangement unknown elsewhere in the body where axons (except at their terminations) are supported by Schwann cells. In Fig. 9.27B, the process reaches a predetermined length and then moves pulpally as dentine is formed, leaving behind an empty tubule in which peritubular dentine forms. Perhaps peritubular dentine differs from intertubular dentine in being formed by a process that does not directly involve the odontoblast. In Fig. 9.27C, the peripheral end of the processes degrades sequentially, and its remains form part of the matrix for the peritubular dentine.

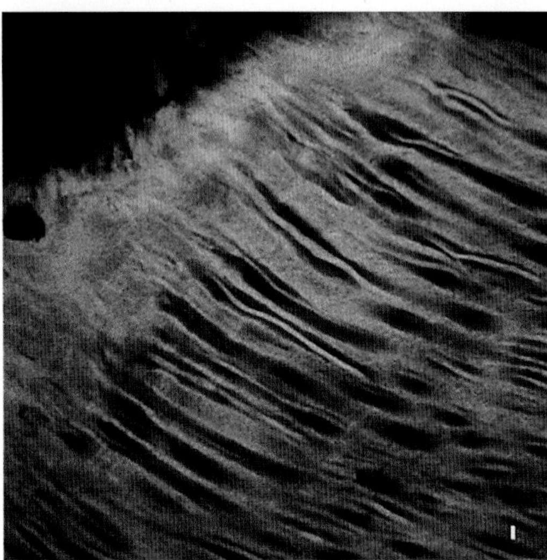

Fig. 9.28 Dentinal tubules in a region of tertiary dentine showing the presence of tubular structures in an area from which the odontoblasts have been lost and which probably represent the lamina limitans (confocal microscopy of a demineralised section ×1,700). Courtesy Dr. G Goracci, Dr. G Mori, Dr. F Marci, Dr. M Baldi and the editor of *Minerva Stomatologica*.

The possible existence of an odontoblast process in outer dentine is also complicated by the presence of a very thin, apparently proteinaceous, membrane termed the *lamina limitans* that lines the wall of the dentinal tubule. In certain preparations, it may give rise to the erroneous impression of an odontoblast process (Figs 9.28, 9.29). The lamina limitans is composed primarily of proteoglycans, unlike the organic matrix of peritubular dentine that is composed mainly of glycosaminoglycans.

In some parts of the dentine, most commonly beneath cusps, the tubules in inner dentine can contain additional small processes (Fig. 9.30). Some of these could be smaller odontoblastic processes that are lost during later deposition; others will be the processes of the immunocompetent antigen-presenting cells that are found in several areas of the pulp, particularly in the periphery within and beneath the odontoblast layer (see pages 199–201). These, and their extensions into the dentinal tubules, are found in small numbers even in unerupted teeth, with intratubular processes limited to the predentine in the coronal pulp. In intact erupted teeth, these processes are present over a much wider area, although still limited to predentine. In dentine beneath dental caries, the processes of the immunocompetent cells extend much deeper into the tubules of the circumpulpal dentine. However, in all tubules there is one large odontoblast process.

Sensory terminals have been firmly identified within the dentinal tubule, but special techniques are needed to distinguish them from smaller branches of the odontoblast process. As for odontoblast process, their extent into dentine is not known for certain. Nerve terminals are limited mainly to the dentine of the crown beneath the cusps, where they may be found in over 40% of the tubules. In the cervical part of the crown, nerves are found in 4% to 8% of tubules, while in the root dentine only 0.02% to 0.2% of dentinal tubules contain nerves. The axon in an innervated tubule is narrower than the odontoblast process and contains microtubules, a few microfilaments and often mitochondria. Vesicles are rare in nerve terminals (or in the odontoblast process adjacent to them), and structurally specialised contacts between the nerve terminal and the odontoblast process seem to be absent (Fig. 9.30).

The sensory nature of intratubular axons can be demonstrated by tracer techniques. Radioactive amino acids (e.g., tritium-labelled proline) injected into the trigeminal ganglion are converted into proteins and transported down the axons to the peripheral terminations (Fig. 9.31).

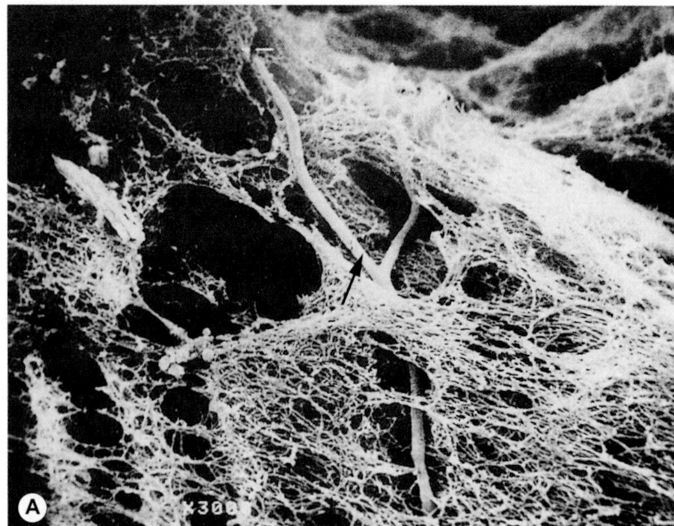

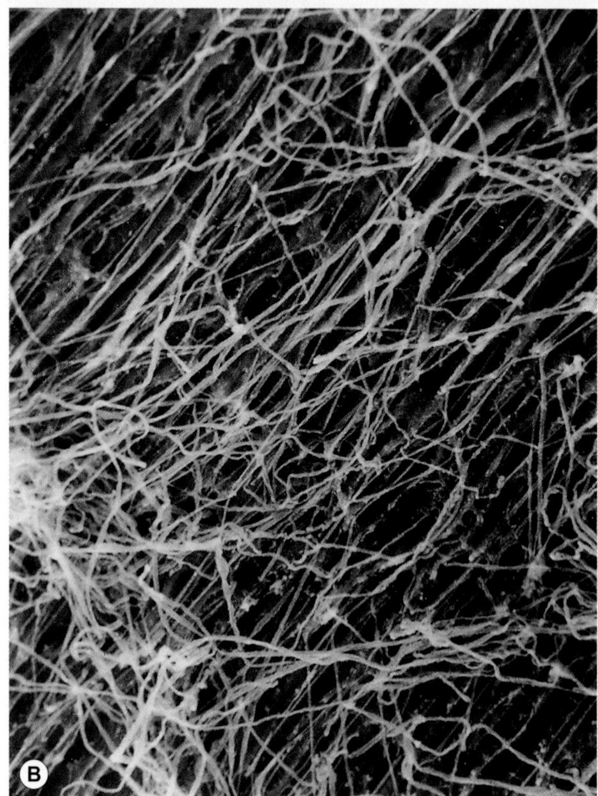

Fig. 9.29 (A) SEM of a tubular branching structure in peripheral dentine *(arrowed)* following collagenase treatment. It is difficult to establish whether this is a true odontoblast process or the lamina limitans (×3,000). (B) SEM of demineralised dentine also treated with collagenase to remove the bulk of the organic matrix. The remaining tubular structures seen in this micrograph are thought to represent the lamina limitans, as complementary TEM studies show them to possess no cellular characteristics (×1,000). (A) Courtesy Dr. M Sigal, Dr. S Pitaru, Dr. J Aubin, Dr. A R Ten Cate and the editor of the *Anatomical Record*. (B) Courtesy Dr. H F Thomas.

Regional variations in dentine structure and composition

The properties and composition of mineralised dentine vary with distance from the predentine to the enamel–dentine junction, allowing for the division of dentine into different zones (Table 9.2). The mineral content of dentine decreases and the thickness of mineral crystals increases towards the enamel–dentine junction. Hardness and elastic moduli both decrease towards the junction. Several different regions can be recognised in dentine (Fig. 9.32). The most peripheral region beneath the enamel and cementum has special characteristics bestowed on it by being the earliest

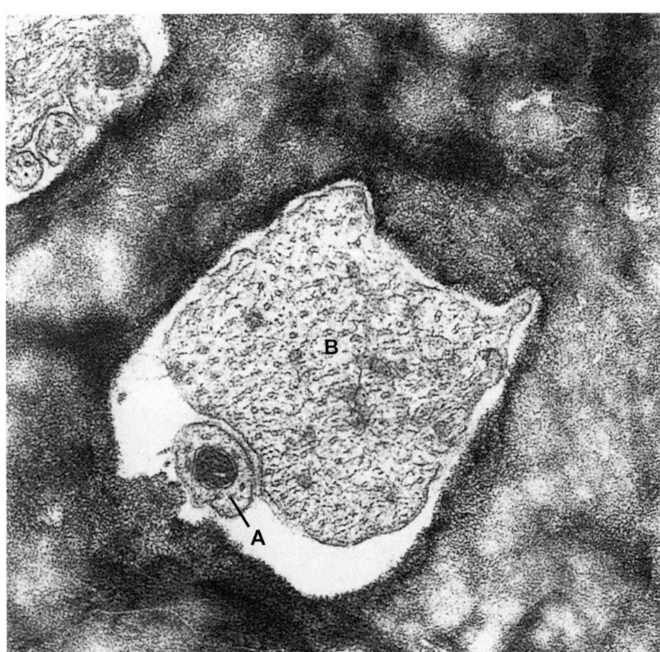

Fig. 9.30 TEM showing two processes within a single dentinal tubule. The larger process (B) is the odontoblast process; the smaller one (A) a presumptive nerve terminal (×65,000).

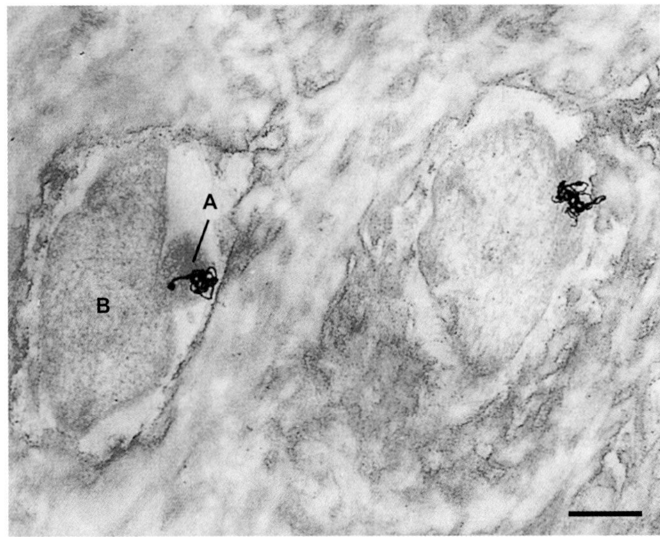

Fig. 9.31 TEM showing autoradiographically labelled nerve (A) adjacent to an odontoblast process (B). The labelled amino acid was originally injected into the trigeminal ganglion (×20,000). Courtesy Dr. M R Byers.

Table 9.2 Regional variations in dentine

Zone	Position in tooth
Mantle dentine (Fig. 9.33)	Periphery of dentine in crown
Interglobular dentine (Fig. 9.35)	Typically in outer part of crown
Granular layer in dentine (Fig. 9.37)	In outer part of root dentine beneath hyaline layer
Hyaline layer in dentine (Fig. 9.37)	Outermost part of root dentine
Circumpulpal dentine (Fig. 9.63)	Bulk of dentine in crown and root
Predentine (Fig. 9.40)	Unmineralised innermost dentine in crown and root
Secondary dentine (Fig. 9.63)	Innermost layer of dentine between circumpulpal dentine and predentine
Tertiary dentine (Fig. 9.56)	Inner layer of dentine formed mainly in crown response to serious insult (e.g., severe attrition, fracture and dental caries)

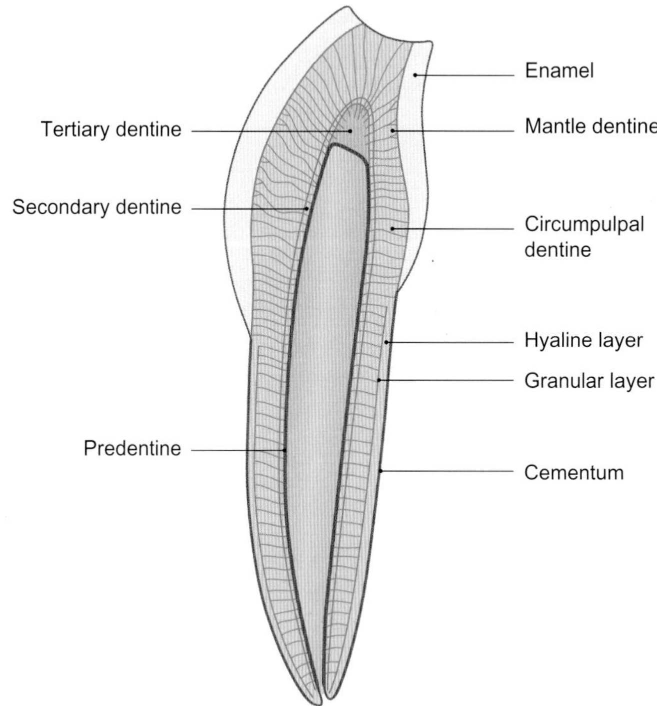

Fig. 9.32 The regions of varying dentine structure.

formed part of the tissue. In the crown this first-formed layer is known as *mantle dentine*. In the root there are two morphologically recognisable outer zones: the *hyaline layer* and the *granular layer* (of Tomes). There is some controversy (discussed later) as to whether the hyaline layer is properly a component of dentine or cementum or is a mingling of components of both tissues. Predentine is the innermost unmineralised layer, where new dentine is being deposited throughout life. Just peripheral to the predentine is a zone of mineralisation, which is recognisable even in decalcified tissue samples because, simultaneously with mineral deposition, the matrix undergoes considerable modification that results in different staining properties. This region has sometimes been called *intermediate dentine*. The bulk of the dentine between the mantle layer and the zone of mineralisation is the *circumpulpal dentine*. The outer part of the circumpulpal dentine beneath the mantle layer is often incompletely mineralised and has a characteristic appearance when seen in ground sections, referred to as '*interglobular dentine*'. A peripheral region in root dentine, the granular layer (of Tomes) is also hypomineralised but to a lesser extent than the interglobular dentine. In older teeth the inner, pulpal part of the circumpulpal dentine differs somewhat in structure from the bulk of the tissue. This *secondary dentine* is laid down as an age-related change in the rate of dentine formation once a (presumably) genetically predetermined thickness of primary circumpulpal dentine has been deposited and root development (at least in terms of length) is complete. The rate and amount of secondary dentine laid down vary with tooth type, between the crown and root (higher) and, of course, with age. Very approximately in the tooth of an older individual, the dentine thickness might be 2.5 mm of which 0.5 mm would be secondary dentine. In teeth that have been subject to severe external stimuli (such as attrition, dental caries and cavity preparation), another layer of dentine is found pulpal to the circumpulpal (and in older teeth secondary) dentine and restricted to the region beneath the irritation. When of the reparative type (see pages 181–183), this tertiary dentine is not formed by the original odontoblasts but by odontoblast-like cells that have differentiated from the dental pulp. It is much more irregular than circumpulpal dentine and has been given a variety of names such as reactionary dentine, reparative dentine, response dentine and irregular secondary dentine. There has been acceptance of the term *tertiary dentine* in preference to other terms (see page 183).

Mantle dentine

The outer layer of dentine in the crown differs from the bulk of the circumpulpal dentine in four features:

- It is slightly (approximately 5%) less mineralised.
- The collagen fibrils are largely oriented perpendicular to the enamel–dentine junction (see also page 422). For this reason, it can be distinguished from the circumpulpal dentine beneath using polarised light (Fig. 9.33).
- The dentinal tubules branch profusely in this region (Fig. 9.34).
- It undergoes mineralisation in the presence of matrix vesicles (see pages 424–426).

The mantle layer varies in width from 20 μm to 150 μm. The special properties of mantle dentine prevent small cracks developing in the enamel near the junction from spreading into the dentine. The three-dimensional scalloped architecture of the enamel–dentine junction and the extension of some dentinal tubules into the enamel as enamel spindles have been described in Chapter 7.

Interglobular dentine

Much of the mineral in dentine is deposited as globules or calcospherites (see Figs 23.14, 23.15 and pages 177, 427). These can be identified at the mineralising front on the pulp predentine border when the organic matrix is removed by hypochlorite. Six patterns at the mineralisation front have been described:

1) Partially fused calcospherites
2) Almost or completely fused calcospherites
3) Network-like mineralised appearance
4) Ridge-like mineralised appearance
5) Spherically mineralised appearance
6) Structureless mineralised appearance.

In most areas, calcospherites fuse to form a uniformly calcified tissue. However, in some areas, usually beneath the mantle layer in the crown and beneath the granular layer in the root, the fusion may be incomplete. When ground sections are viewed in transmitted light, internal reflection of the light makes the uncalcified, interglobular areas appear dark (Fig. 9.35). Dentinal tubules pass without deviation through interglobular areas (Fig. 9.36). As interglobular areas remain uncalcified, peritubular dentine is also absent from the tubules as they pass through interglobular dentine.

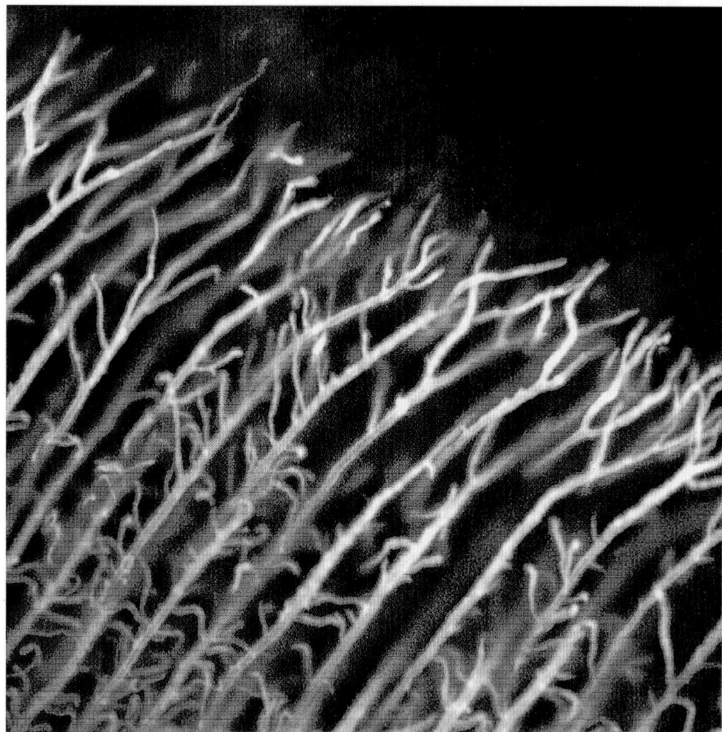

Fig. 9.34 Confocal image of dentinal tubules branching in the region of the mantle dentine (alizarin red; ×1,200). Courtesy Dr. M Kagayama, Dr. Y Sasao, Dr. S Kamakura, Dr. K Motegi, Dr. I Mizoguchi and the editor of *Anatomy and Embryology*.

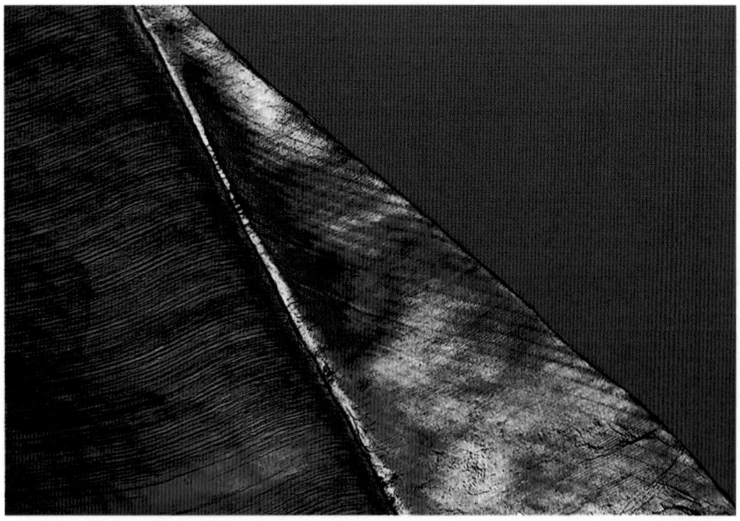

Fig. 9.33 Ground longitudinal section of the crown of a tooth viewed in polarised light (with a quartz filter). Owing to the different orientation of the collagen, the mantle layer immediately beneath the enamel–dentine junction appears red, in contrast to the blue appearance of the rest of the circumpulpal dentine (×50).

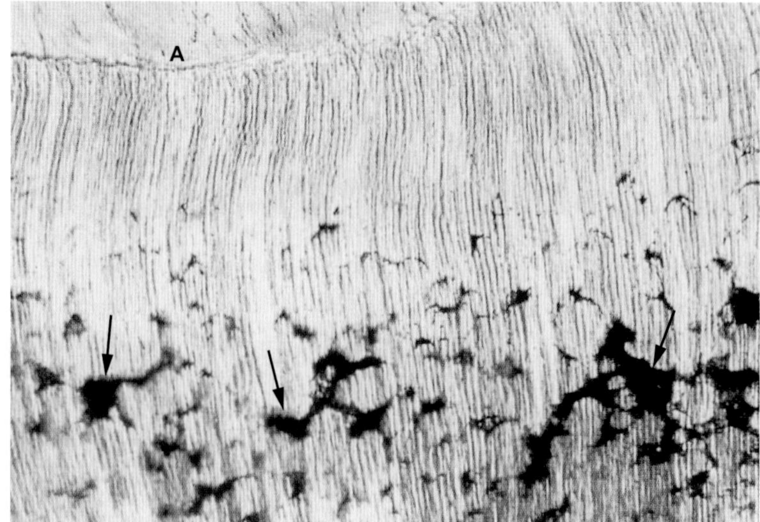

Fig. 9.35 Ground section of outer dentine showing areas of interglobular dentine *(arrowed)*. A = Enamel (×300). Courtesy R V Hawkins.

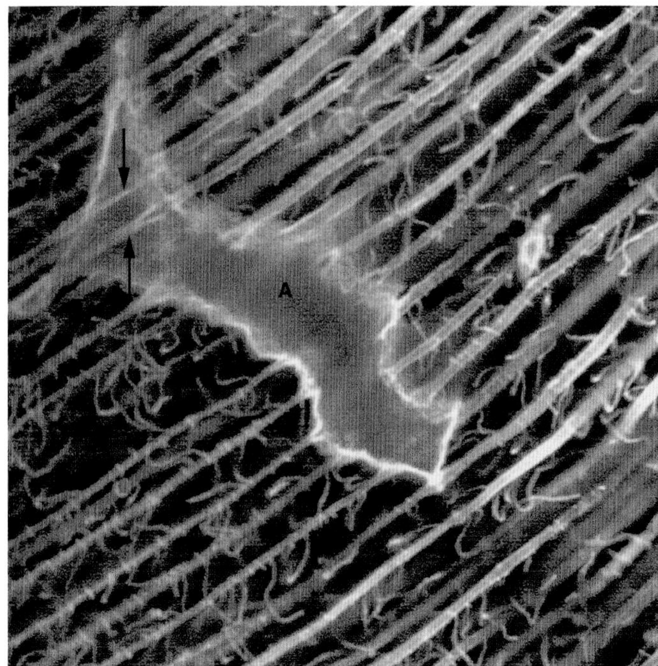

Fig. 9.36 Confocal image of dentinal tubules *(arrows)* passing through an area of interglobular dentine (A) (alizarin red; ×1,200). Courtesy Dr. S M Kagayama, Dr. Y Sasao, Dr. S Kamakura, Dr. K Motegi, Dr. I Mizoguchi and the editor of *Anatomy and Embryology.*

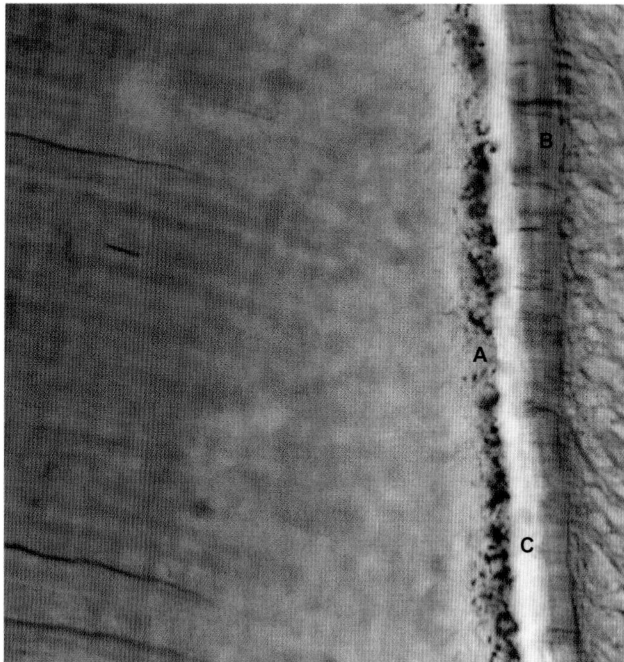

Fig. 9.37 Ground longitudinal section of a root showing the granular (A) and hyaline (C) layers beneath a layer of acellular cementum (B) (×160).

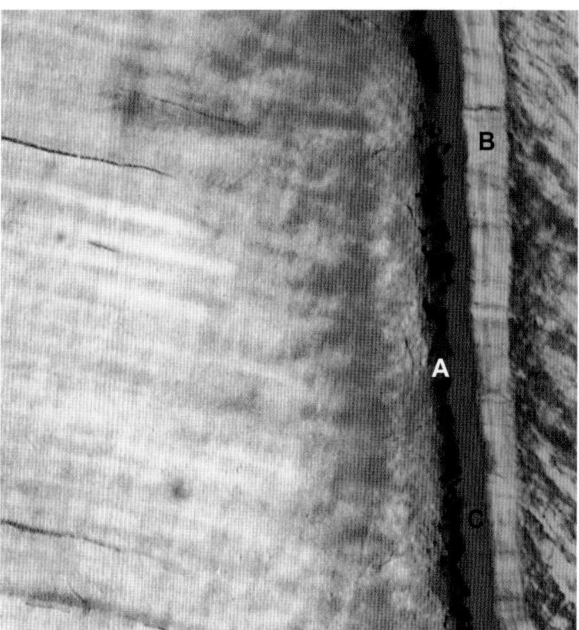

Fig. 9.38 The same section as in Fig. 9.37 viewed in polarised light with a quartz tint. The hyaline layer can be distinguished from the rest of the underlying dentine and the cementum, suggesting a difference in the orientation of its collagen fibres. A = granular layer; B = acellular cementum; C = hyaline layer (×160).

Granular layer

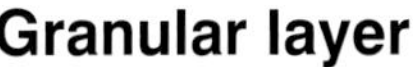

In ground sections the periphery of the dentine in the root is marked by the presence of a dark granular zone: the granular layer (Figs 9.37, 9.38). Various explanations for this appearance have been suggested. The most currently accepted is that the dentinal tubules in this area branch more profusely and loop back on themselves, creating air spaces in ground sections that result in internal reflection of transmitted light. Differences in the rate of formation of coronal and radicular dentine could explain why this appearance is seen in the root but not the crown. Stain-filled tubules viewed in thick sections have a 'tree-top' appearance somewhat supporting this idea (Fig. 9.39). The granular layer is hypomineralised in comparison to circumpulpal dentine, but this may be the result of the presence of more tubular branches. An alternative explanation for the granular appearance is that it results from the incomplete fusion of calcospherites.

Hyaline layer

Outside the granular layer is a clear hyaline layer. This is usually considered to be a component of the dentine but whose origin is obscure. The hyaline layer is narrow (up to 20 µm wide) and appears to be non-tubular and relatively structureless (Figs 9.37, 9.38). The hyaline layer may serve to bond cementum to dentine and may be of considerable clinical significance when considering periodontal regeneration. It is discussed further on page 443.

Circumpulpal dentine

The basic structure of dentine as described throughout this chapter is that of circumpulpal dentine. It forms the bulk of the dentine and is uniform in structure except at its edges where, peripherally, interglobular dentine marks incomplete initial mineralisation and, centrally, the mineralising front represents ongoing mineralisation. In older teeth its tubular pattern is modified on the pulpal surface owing to the age-related deposition of secondary dentine.

Dentine at root apex

Because of its importance in the root canal therapy, researchers have investigated the nature of the dentine in this region compared with that more cervically has been investigated. At the root apex, accessory root canals are common. Apical dentine often deviates from the long access of the tooth (dilacerations – see pages 63, 65). There may be localised areas of dentine resorption and repair. The dentinal tubules themselves

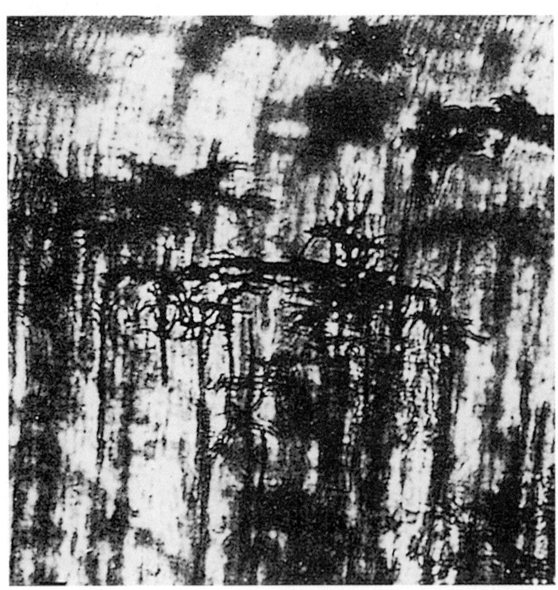

Fig. 9.39 Ground thick section of root impregnated with silver stain in the region of the granular layer showing peripheral terminations of tubules exhibiting profuse branching in three dimensions (×490).

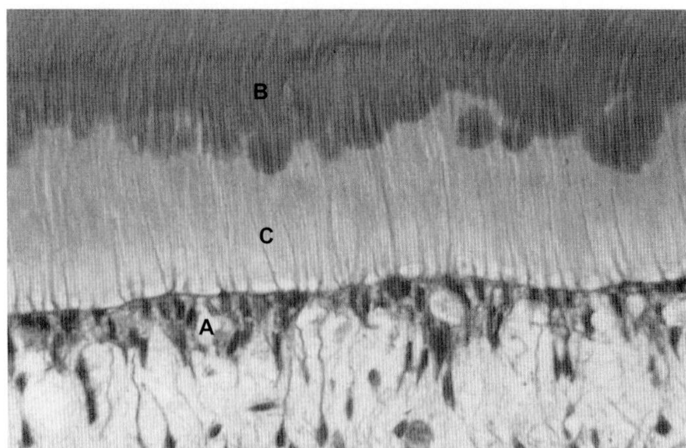

Fig. 9.40 Decalcified section of the pulpodentinal region showing the odontoblast layer (A) and predentine (C). Note the different staining reaction of the predentine to that of the mineralised dentine matrix (B). The mineralising front at B is globular (H & E; ×500).

may show irregularities in direction and density. Indeed, some areas may be devoid of tubules. Cementum at the root apex may be reflected to line the innermost surface of the pulp for a short distance. This produces a narrowing known as the *apical constriction*, which is a landmark used during root canal therapy (see page 34).

Predentine

In demineralised sections stained with haematoxylin and eosin, the innermost layer of dentine, the predentine, has a distinct pale-staining appearance (Fig. 9.40). This reflects a difference in the composition of its matrix from that of the matrix of the mineralised circumpulpal dentine. The mineralising front may show a globular (Fig. 9.40) or a linear outline, reflecting the mineralisation process (see page 427). The predentine is the initially laid down dentine matrix before its mineralisation. During mineralisation the matrix undergoes considerable modification. The principal role of the odontoblast process in predentine is the secretion of matrix components. In mineralising dentine the role of the odontoblast process is to participate in the modification of that matrix and perhaps also in its mineralisation (see pages 424–426). The width of the predentine can vary from 10 μm to 40 μm, depending on the rate at which dentine is being deposited: it is, for example, thicker in young teeth.

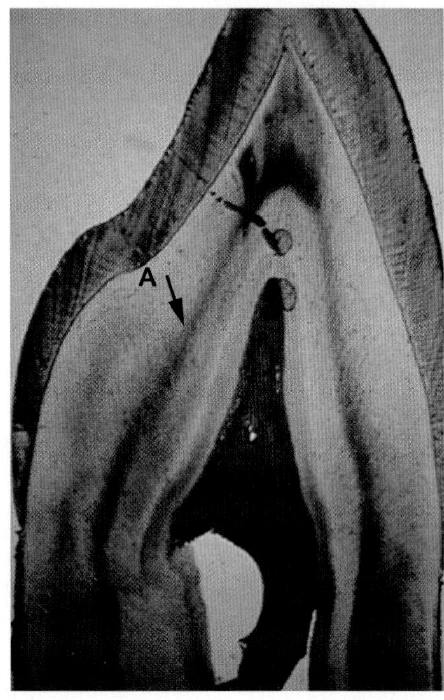

Fig. 9.41 Ground longitudinal section of a crown showing a broad Schreger line (A), coincident with the apex of one of the primary curvatures of the dentinal tubules. Only one is visible, although hypothetically, two are possible (×5).

Structural lines in dentine

In sections of dentine viewed by different techniques, a variety of lines approximately perpendicular to the dentinal tubules can be seen. The descriptions and explanations of these lines vary considerably. Some have had the name of the individual who first described them attached to them, causing confusion when later investigators use those names to include somewhat different structures. The description given here will rely on the functional origin of the lines as best understood but will include the eponym to retain the historical flavour these lines have acquired.

There are two related groups of lines: those originating from curvatures in the dentinal tubules and those arising from the incremental deposition of dentine and its subsequent mineralisation.

Lines associated with the primary curvatures of the dentinal tubules

In some longitudinal sections, the peaks of the sigmoid primary curvatures coincide to form broad bands in the dentine. These are not apparent in many sections, and rarely can two be seen. They are more difficult to see in horizontal sections, where they would be seen as broad concentric bands in the circumpulpal dentine. These lines are known as *Schreger lines* (Fig. 9.41).

Lines associated with the secondary curvatures of the dentinal tubules

When the secondary curvatures coincide, they also give rise to an optical effect, resulting in the appearance of lines, the contour lines of Owen (Fig. 9.42). They are unusual in primary dentine but are sometimes seen. An exaggerated line is found at the border of primary and secondary dentine (see page 181) and between dentine formed before and that formed after birth. This latter neonatal line may include compositional variations in the matrix and mineralisation.

Incremental lines associated with matrix deposition and mineralisation

Dentine has regular, incremental, short-period and long-period markings. The lines may be seen in normal ground sections (Fig. 9.43), demineralised sections, under polarised light (Fig. 9.44) and in microradiographs. They can be attributed to circadian fluctuations in acid–base balance that affect both the mineral content and the refractive index of forming hard tissues. The long-period lines, at least, are greatly enhanced when viewed in polarised light (Fig. 9.44), suggesting that they are associated with changes in collagen fibril orientation.

Short-period markings may be seen as alternating dark and light bands, with each pair reflecting the diurnal rhythm of dentine formation (Fig. 9.45). Similar to enamel (see page 143), this suggests the involvement of a circadian clock mechanism during dentinogenesis. This is supported by evidence showing that odontoblasts express clock proteins. These fine lines are sometimes referred to as *von Ebner lines*. In cuspal dentine, where deposition is most rapid, the amount of dentine formed each day and the distance between adjacent dark bands are approximately 4 μm (Fig. 9.46). In the root peripherally near the granular layer where the dentine has a calcospheritic pattern, the distance between lines is nearer to 2 μm (Fig. 9.47). In demineralised sections the values are smaller, presumably because of shrinkage caused by processing of the tissue.

The coarser, long-period lines (Andresen lines) are approximately 16–20 μm apart (Figs 9.43, 9.44, 9.48). Between each long-period line there are 6–10 pairs of short-period lines (Fig. 9.48). The cause for the 6- to 10-day periodicity is unknown. The same periodicity exists between the long-period striae of Retzius in enamel and the long-period Andresen lines in dentine, making it likely that a common mechanism exists.

As with enamel, an exaggerated line, the neonatal line (Fig. 9.49), can be seen in teeth mineralising at birth. The neonatal line is rich in zinc.

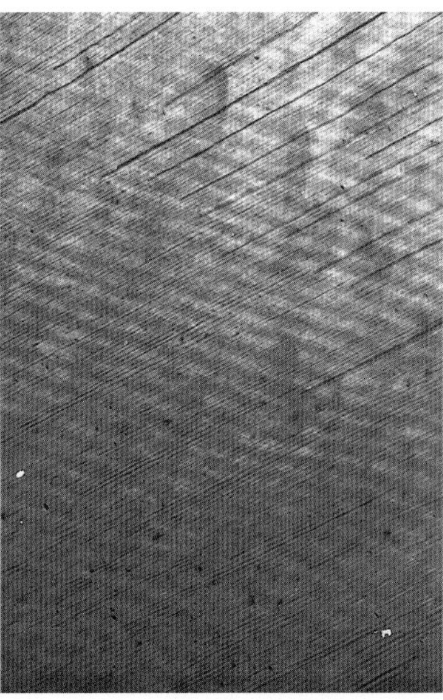

Fig. 9.44 Ground longitudinal section of dentine viewed in polarised light showing alternate light and dark bands representing long-period incremental lines. The bands are approximately orientated at right angles to the direction of the dentinal tubules (×250).

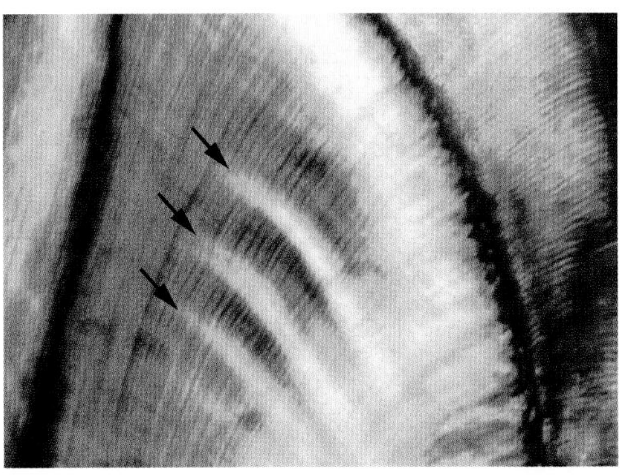

Fig. 9.42 Ground longitudinal section viewed in polarised light of a crown showing contour lines associated with the coincidence of secondary curvatures *(arrows)* of the dentinal tubules (×120).

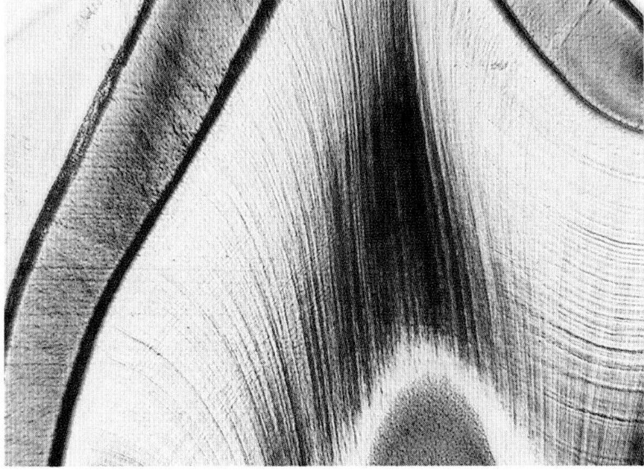

Fig. 9.43 Ground longitudinal section of a crown showing, on the right side, horizontally running, long-period incremental lines (×12). Courtesy Dr. B A W Brown.

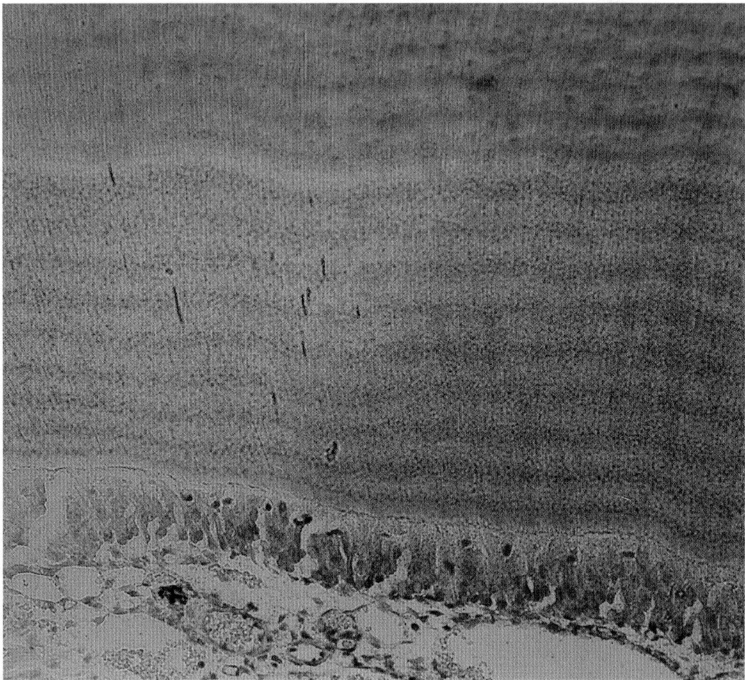

Fig. 9.45 This decalcified section is taken from a rat injected with tritiated proline. The amino acid is incorporated rhythmically into the collagen of the dentine matrix, as shown by the periodic presence of silver grains developed by the radioactivity from the photographic emulsion layered onto the section. The section is also lightly stained to show incremental lines and how these coincide with the incorporation of proline (H & E; ×350). Courtesy Dr. M Ohtsuka, Dr. S Saeki, Dr. K Igarashi, Dr. H Shinoda and the editor of the *Journal of Dental Research*.

Age-related and posteruptive changes

Once the tooth is erupted and fully formed, dentine can undergo changes that are either related to age or occur as a response to a stimulus applied to the tooth, such as caries or attrition. With regard to physiological age changes, secondary dentine and translucent dentine will be considered. Concerning the response of dentine to stimuli, tertiary dentine, sclerotic dentine and dead tracts will be discussed.

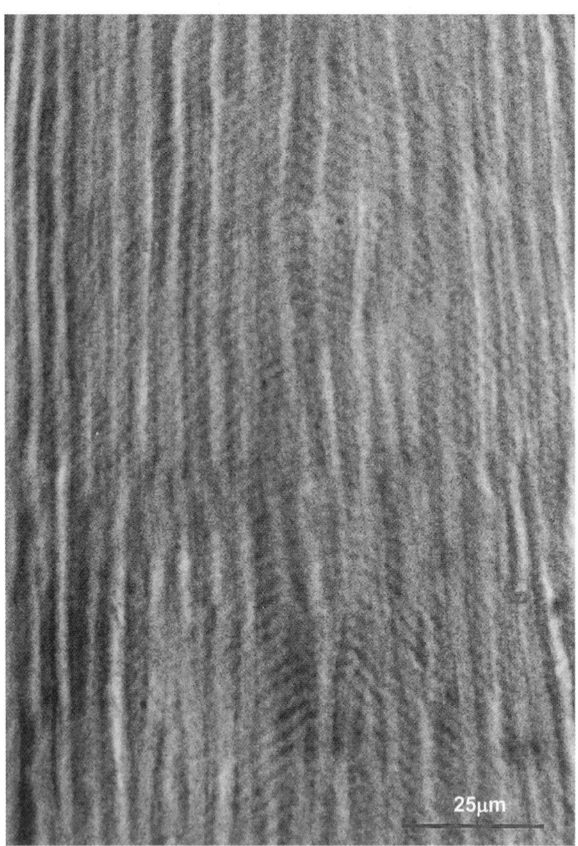

Fig. 9.46 Anorganic ground section of dentine high over the cuspal region of a premolar showing short-period incremental lines running across the field approximately 4 μm apart (×720). Courtesy Prof. M C Dean and the editor of the *Archives of Oral Biology*.

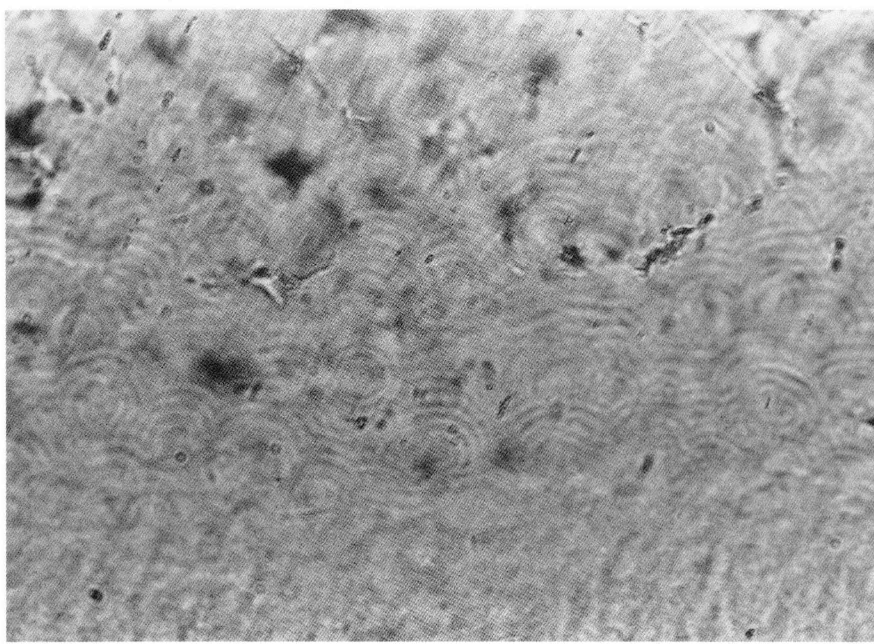

Fig. 9.47 Anorganic preparation of root dentine near the granular layer (at the lower part of the field) showing short-period incremental lines about 2 μm apart and having a calcospheritic outline (×800). Courtesy Prof. M C Dean and the editor of the *Archives of Oral Biology*.

Secondary dentine

The most conspicuous age-associated change in dentine is the formation of secondary dentine. Its structure is very similar to that of primary dentine, and it may be difficult to distinguish between the two. However, primary and secondary dentine are often delineated as a result of a change in direction of the dentinal tubules with coincidence of secondary curvatures. This produces a particularly pronounced contour line (of Owen) (Figs 9.50–9.53). The same odontoblasts continue to lay down similar dentine, and the tubules of primary and secondary dentine are continuous. The increased crowding of odontoblasts as secondary dentine formation continues throughout life, and the slower rate of deposition makes the tubular pattern of secondary dentine a little less regular than that of primary dentine and the incremental markings somewhat closer together. Secondary dentine formation begins at the completion of root formation as the tooth comes into occlusion. The main coincidence would seem to be

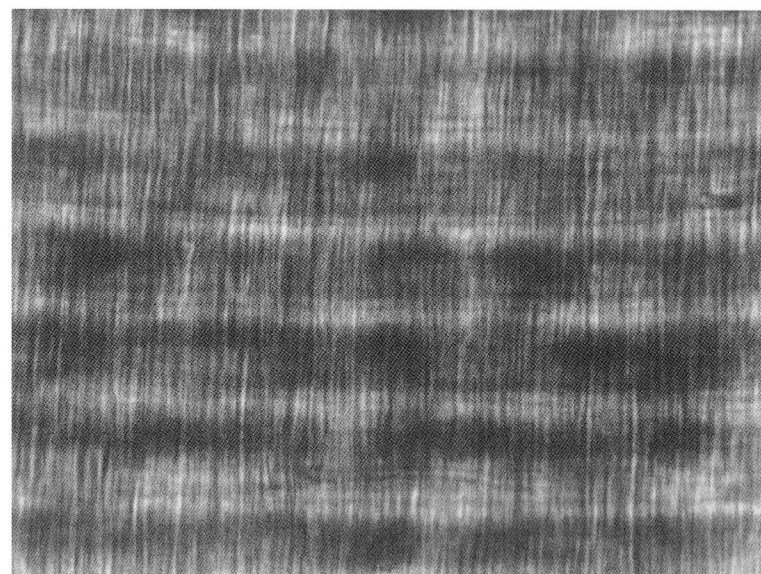

Fig. 9.48 Ground section of dentine viewed in polarised light. The long-period (horizontal) lines are about 20 μm apart and between them are seven or eight short-period incremental lines (×900). Courtesy Prof. M C Dean and the editor of the *Archives of Oral Biology*.

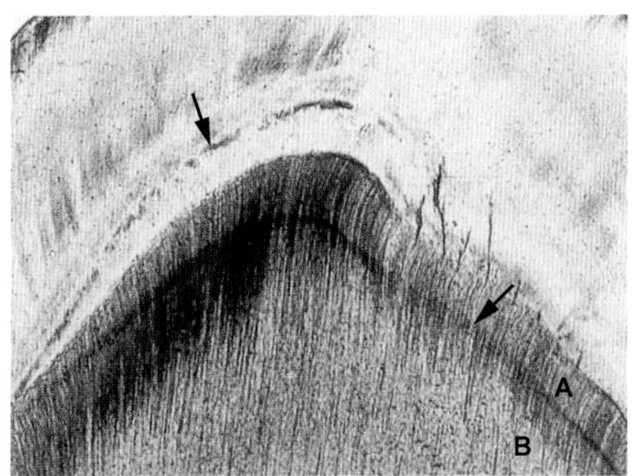

Fig. 9.49 Ground longitudinal section of a deciduous tooth showing neonatal lines *(arrows)* in enamel and dentine. These are exaggerated in this example, as the tooth came from a patient who suffered from *icterus neonatorum* (newborn jaundice) (×25). A = dentine formed prenatally; B = dentine formed postnatally.

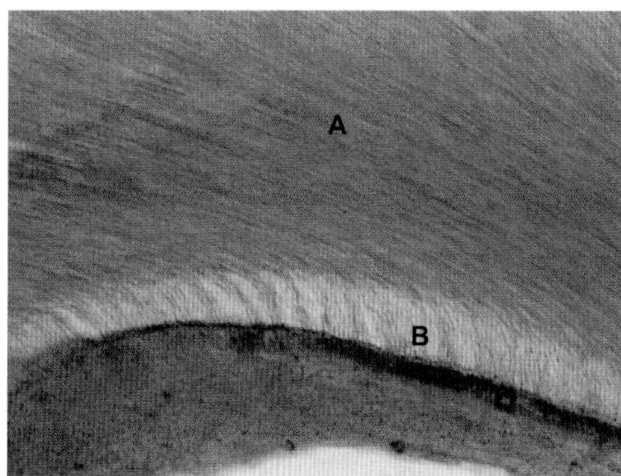

Fig. 9.52 Ground longitudinal section showing primary (A) and secondary (B) dentine (×80).

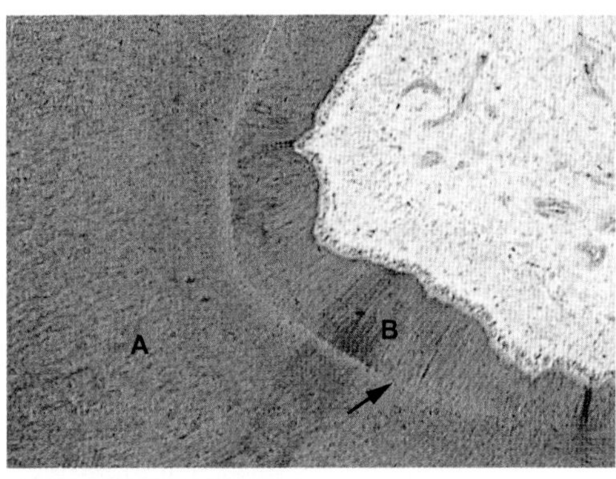

Fig. 9.50 A decalcified cross-section of dentine showing a pronounced contour line *(arrow)* separating primary dentine (A) from secondary dentine (B) (silver staining; ×32).

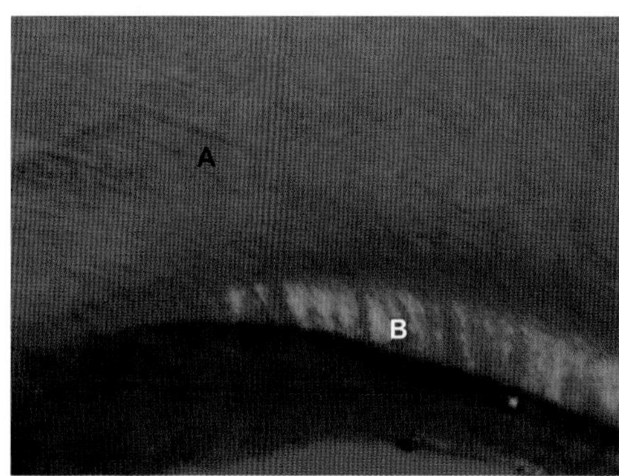

Fig. 9.53 Same section as Fig. 9.52, but viewed in polarised light with a quartz tint. The difference in colour between primary (A) and secondary (B) dentine is presumably owing to the difference in orientation of collagen and/or crystals (×80).

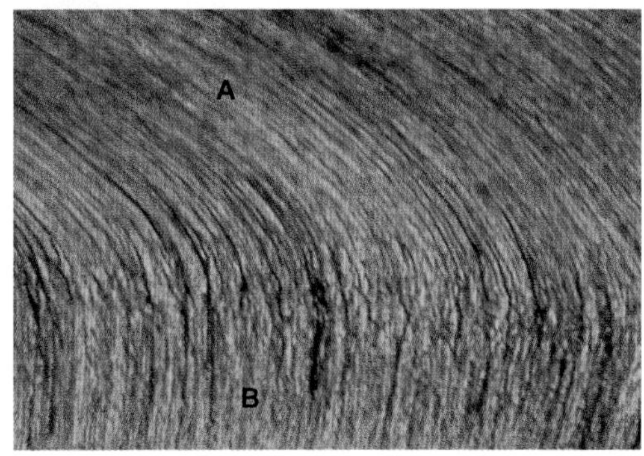

Fig. 9.51 Ground longitudinal section of dentine illustrating the change in direction of dentinal tubules as they pass from primary (A) to secondary (B) dentine (×125).

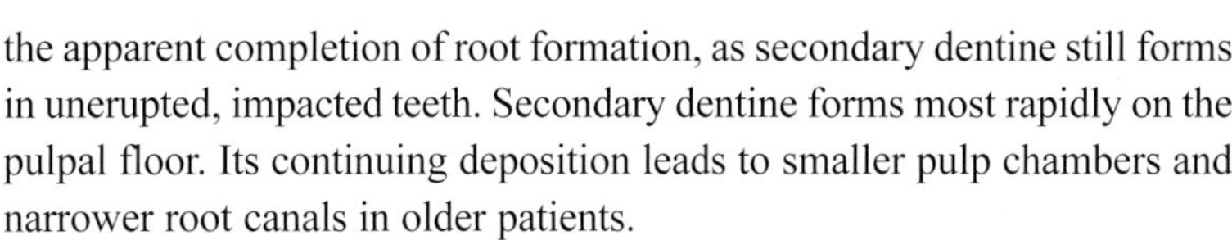
the apparent completion of root formation, as secondary dentine still forms in unerupted, impacted teeth. Secondary dentine forms most rapidly on the pulpal floor. Its continuing deposition leads to smaller pulp chambers and narrower root canals in older patients.

In physiological ageing, especially in root dentine, the tubules can become completely occluded with peritubular dentine to form translucent dentine. With age, translucent dentine is particularly pronounced at the root apex and increases linearly with age (Figs 9.54, 9.55). For this reason it is used in forensic dentistry to help determine the age of a person from the teeth. Translucent dentine is discussed further on pages 170, 183–184, 479.

Tertiary dentine

The dental pulp may be induced to produce calcified material in addition to its 'usual' primary and secondary dentine by a variety of outside stimuli, including dental caries, attrition, cavity preparation, microleakage around restorations and trauma. Stimuli of different types and extent may be applied to teeth at different stages of development or ageing, resulting in a response tissue that may vary considerably in appearance and composition: it may resemble secondary dentine in having a regular tubular structure, it may have few and/or irregularly arranged tubules or it may

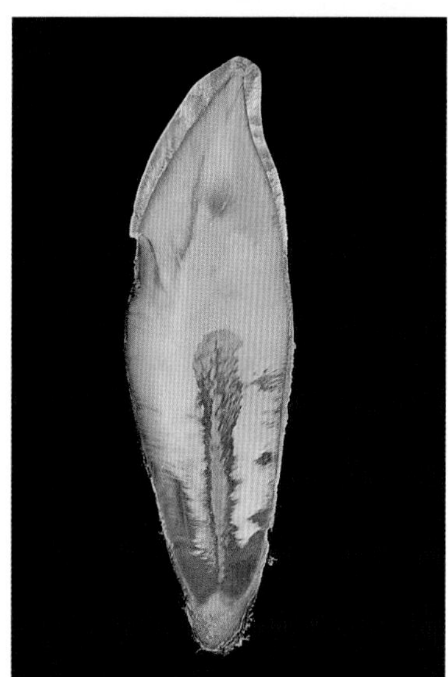

Fig. 9.54 A section of a whole tooth showing the translucent dentine predominantly in the apical part of the root (ground section). Courtesy Dr. A M Sengupta, Dr. D K Whittaker, Dr. P R Shellis and the editor of the *Archives of Oral Biology*.

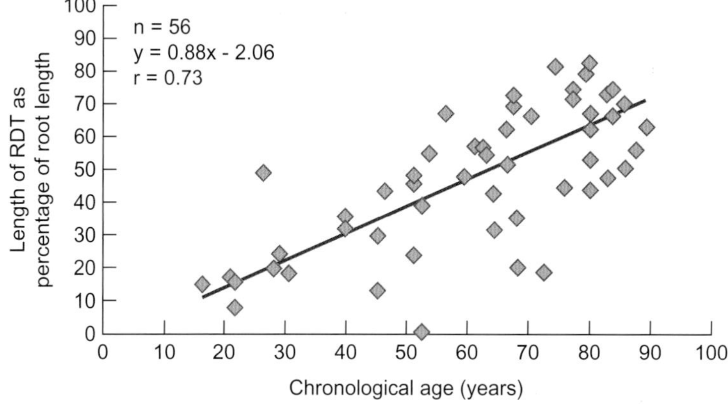

Fig. 9.55 The relationship between age and the area of translucent dentine (RDT). Courtesy Dr. A M Sengupta, Dr. D K Whittaker, Dr. P R Shellis and the editor of the *Archives of Oral Biology*.

be relatively atubular (Figs 9.56–9.58). Continuity of dentinal tubules between normal dentine and tertiary dentine will therefore be lost in many instances (Fig. 9.59).

Because of this wide range of presentations, this response tissue has been given a variety of names, including irregular secondary dentine, reparative dentine, reactionary dentine, response dentine and osteodentine. It seems sensible to rationalise this nomenclature and use the term 'tertiary dentine' for all hard tissue deposited on the pulpal surface in response to an external stimulus.

The pulp does not seem to respond to stimuli by increasing the rate of deposition of secondary dentine, but by inducing previously quiescent odontoblast-like cells to produce mineralised tissue. The different appearances of tertiary dentine are thus probably owing to its production by newly differentiated mesenchymal cells rather than by the odontoblasts that have produced primary and secondary dentine (although studies suggest that, at least on some occasions, primary odontoblasts may be involved in the initial stages of tertiary dentine formation). The newly differentiated cells responsible for tertiary dentine formation are similar to odontoblasts in that they produce type I collagen and dentine sialoprotein, a dentine-specific protein.

The term *reactionary dentine* refers to the dentine forming in response to an insult in which, although some damage has been sustained and some odontoblasts die, the existing odontoblasts recover and continue to form dentine. There will be some irregularity in dentine structure depending on the strength of the stimulus, and the dentine will have an irregular appearance with fewer tubules.

The term *reparative dentine* relates to dentine forming after a stimulus in which the original odontoblasts in the associated region have been destroyed and new calcified tissue (reparative dentine) has been formed by newly differentiated cells referred to here as 'odontoblast-like' cells. In considering the origin of odontoblasts during normal tooth formation (see pages 420–421), reciprocal epithelial/mesenchymal interactions are an essential feature. However, it is clear that odontoblast-like cells arising from the adult pulp after a suitable stimulus do so in the absence of epithelial cells. There are two possible explanations for this. It might be that during initial dentine formation epithelial/mesenchymal interactions guide some cells on the path to becoming odontoblasts but that these cells remain dormant in the pulp, awaiting a later stimulus for them to complete their life cycle and form reparative dentine. A more likely explanation, however, is that odontoblast-like cells are differentiated from a stem cell population in the absence of any epithelial contribution. It is envisaged that the appropriate bioactive molecules necessary for such differentiation (e.g., cytokines, growth factors) are locally synthesised and released during the inflammatory process accompanying the stimulus (such as dental caries). To this effect, several factors have been shown to induce the formation of repair dentine in the pulps of experimental animals, such

Fig. 9.56 Demineralised section showing tertiary dentine (A) having an irregular appearance in a pulp horn (H & E; ×50).

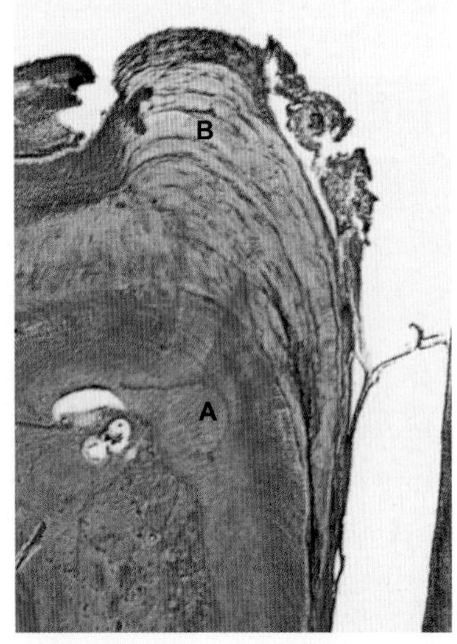

Fig. 9.57 Tertiary dentine (B) overlying primary dentine (A) on the floor of a pulp chamber extending around the orifice of a root canal (demineralised section stained with Weigert and van Gieson; ×20).

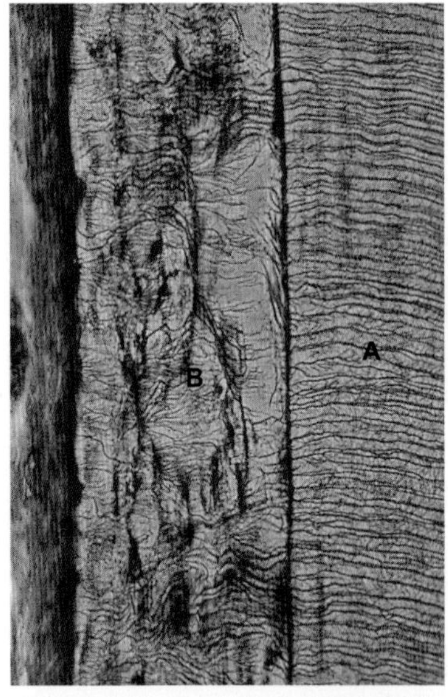

Fig. 9.59 Demineralised section showing loss of continuity of many dentinal tubules between normal dentine (A) and tertiary dentine (B) (picrothionin stain; ×100). Courtesy Prof. M M Smith.

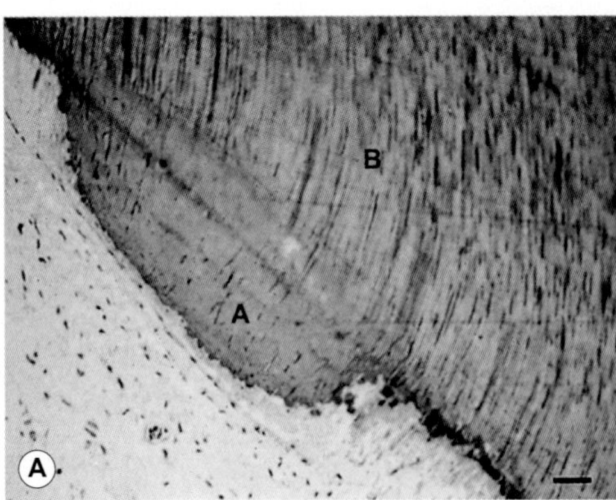

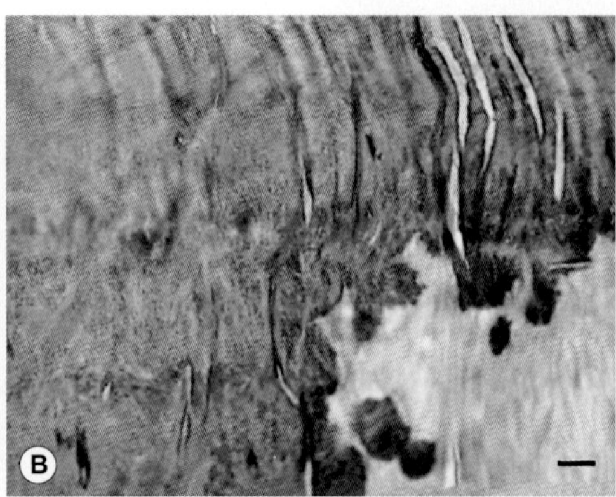

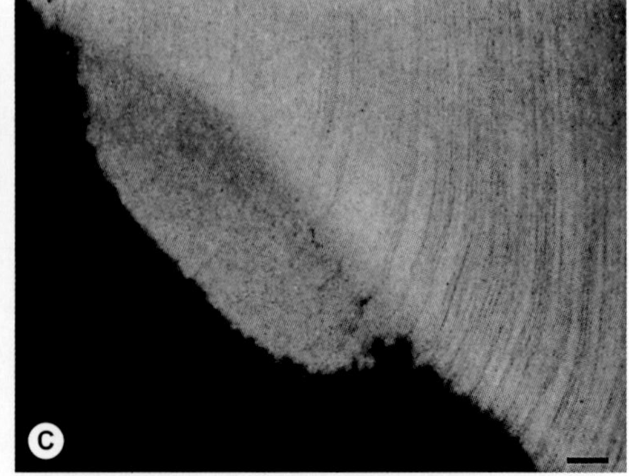

Fig. 9.58 Tertiary dentine formation in response to deep caries. Fig. 9.59A. Zone of tertiary dentine (label A) at the dentine–pulp interface projecting from normal dentine (label B) (H & E; ×300). Fig. 9.59B. Higher-power view, showing calcospherites in tertiary dentine (H & E; ×1500). Fig. 9.59C. Microradiograph of undemineralised lesion similar to that seen in (A), revealing a difference in mineralisation levels between normal and tertiary dentine, there being less mineral in tertiary dentine (×300). Courtesy Dr. L Bjorndal, Dr. T Darvann and the editor of *Caries Research*.

as pieces of native dentine, pieces of demineralised dentine, crude extracts of dentine matrix, fibronectin products and bone morphogenetic protein. It might be envisaged that the addition of suitable activating substances to the region of pulp exposures might aid and speed up clinically the formation of repair dentine over pulp exposures. However, also research suggests that healing can occur naturally providing that the cavity is completely sealed at its margins.

Sclerotic dentine

In addition to infilling with peritubular dentine as a physiological response to ageing (eventually forming translucent dentine – see page 170), dentinal tubules commonly fill in as a response to an external stimulus such as under slowly advancing caries or beneath areas of severe attrition (Figs 9.60, 9.61). This type of dentine is termed *sclerotic dentine* and, like translucent dentine, will present as areas that lack structure and appear transparent (Fig. 9.62). Little is known about the precipitated material, but it appears to differ from peritubular dentine and is thus thought not to be formed by the odontoblast. The mineral is crystalline and possibly an apatite, although plate-like crystals of octocalcium phosphate have also been reported. The mineral concentration, as measured by X-ray computed microtomography, is significantly higher in sclerotic than in young dentine, consistent with the closure of the tubule lumens. Crystallite size, as

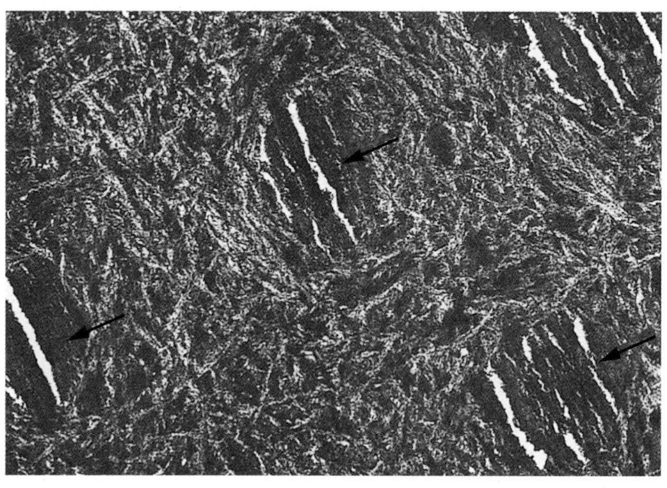

Fig. 9.60 TEM of a zone of sclerotic dentine adjacent to a carious cavity showing transversely sectioned tubules completely occluded *(arrows)*, forming a zone of sclerotic dentine (×7,000). Courtesy Prof. N W Johnson.

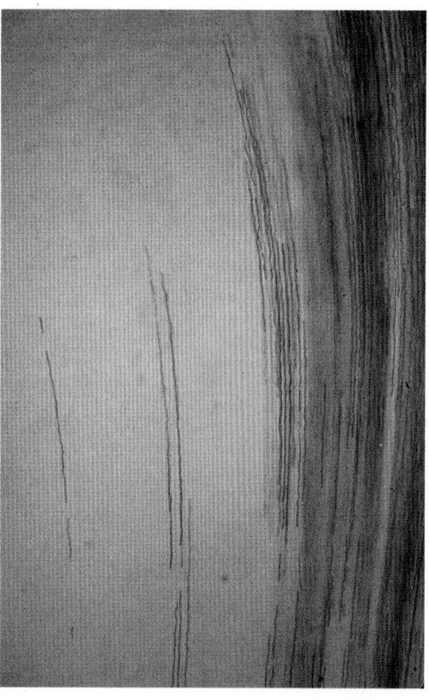

Fig. 9.62 A longitudinal ground section (mounted in water) of sclerotic dentine on the left of the micrograph showing a loss of tubular structure and appearing transparent, as the dentinal tubules have been completely occluded by mineral. The unaffected right edge of the micrograph shows a more normal tubular morphology (×20).

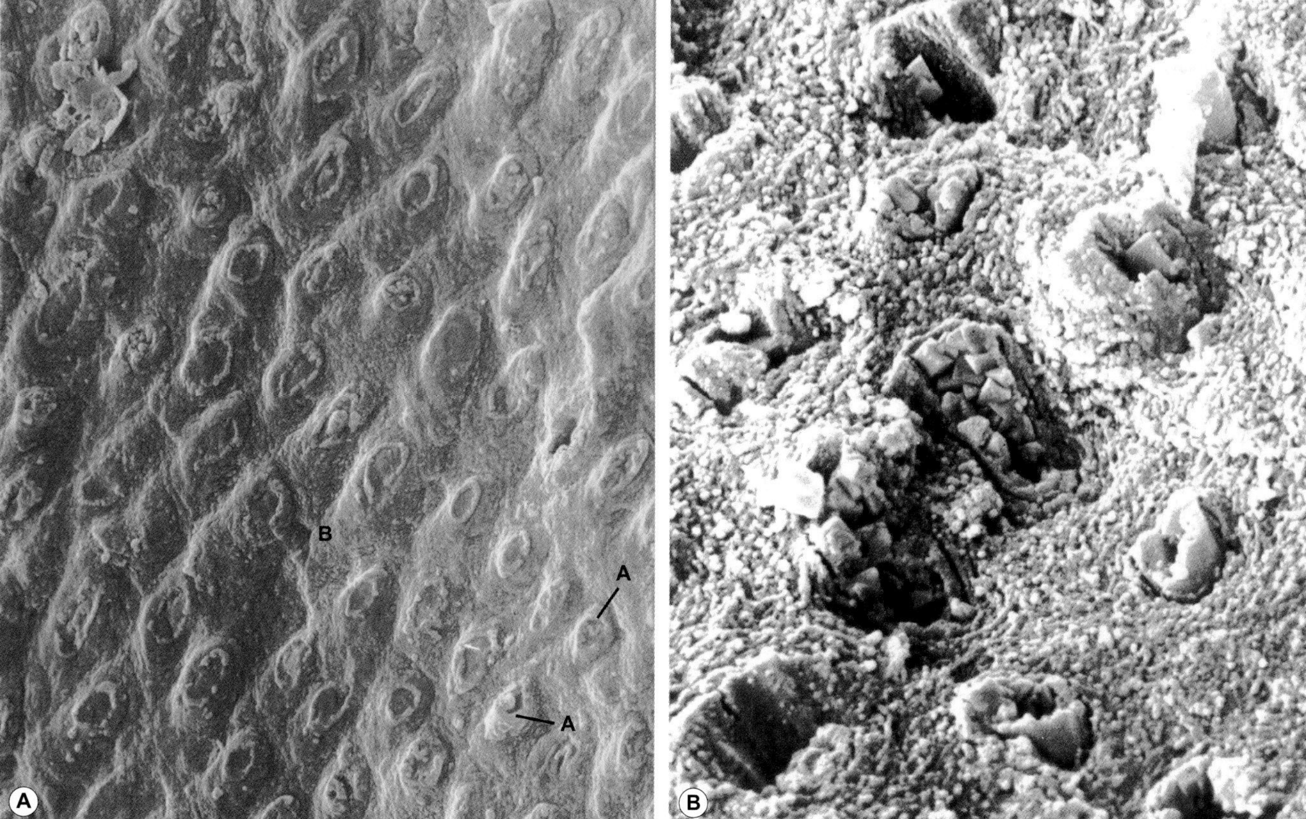

Fig. 9.61 (A) SEM of the fractured surface through a region of sclerotic dentine. In the lower part of the micrograph, within an initial layer of peritubular dentine (Label A), an additional central plug of mineral has been deposited to occlude the tubule. Label B = Intertubular dentine. In the upper part of the micrograph, the dentinal tubules remain patent (×1,500). (B) High-power view of sclerotic dentine from (A), showing central plug of dentinal tubules containing large rhombohedral crystals (probably whitlockite) (×5,000). Courtesy Prof. M M Smith.

measured by small-angle X-ray scattering, is slightly smaller in sclerotic dentine. The elastic properties of dentine are unchanged by transparency; however, sclerotic dentine, unlike normal dentine, exhibits almost no yielding before failure. In addition, the fracture toughness is lowered by roughly 20%. In tubules exposed by attrition or caries, some occluding components may be derived from saliva.

Dead tracts

If the primary odontoblasts are killed by an external stimulus or retract before peritubular dentine occludes the tubules, empty tubules will be left. They may be sealed at their pulpal end by tertiary dentine. When ground sections are prepared and mounted, the mounting medium will not enter these sealed-off tubules and they will remain air-filled. Under the microscope, transmitted light will be totally internally reflected, and these tubules will appear dark (Figs 9.63, 9.64). This appearance, which is due partly to the pulpal response and partly to the preparatory procedure, has been termed a 'dead tract'.

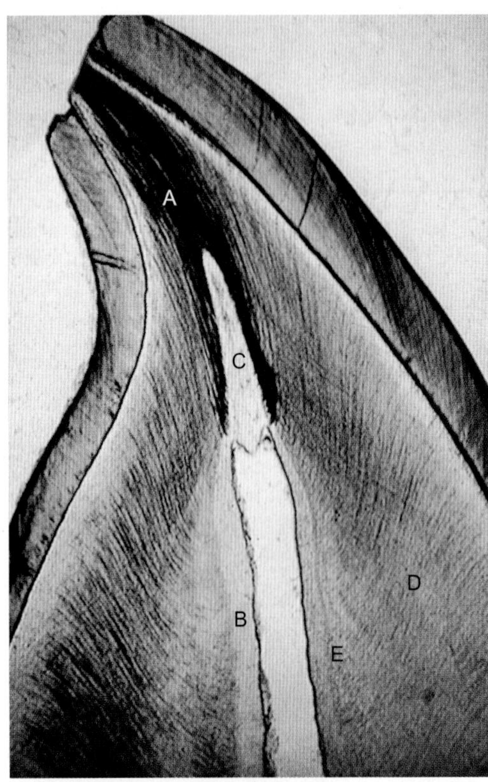

Fig. 9.63 Ground longitudinal section of a crown showing a dead tract (A) beneath a region of attrition that is sealed pulpally by tertiary dentine (C). Secondary dentine (B) lines the rest of the pulp chamber. D = circumpulpal dentine. E = Owen line (×15).

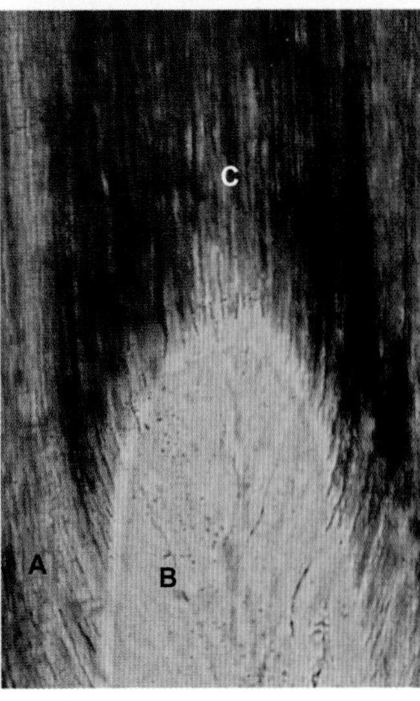

Fig. 9.64 Ground longitudinal section of coronal dentine showing secondary dentine (A) and tertiary dentine (B) beneath a dead tract (C) (×50).

Age changes in dentine

Unlike enamel, dentine is a living tissue and has a layer of cells; the odontoblasts on its inner surface continue to be active throughout life, while stem cells in the pulp can generate new odontoblast-like cells. Two major changes in dentine are closely related to age. One is the formation of secondary dentine, which is tubular and whose tubules are continuous with those of the primary dentine. The demarcation of secondary from primary dentine is often visible as a line of Owen (see page 168), where there is a coincidence of a change in secondary curvatures. This coincides in time with the completion of root formation. Secondary dentine continues to be laid down throughout life, and its thickness can be used to determine approximately the age of a tooth. The number of tubules in secondary dentine is reduced over time as the number of odontoblasts declines. As the surface area of the inner dentine is much less than the outer, the number of tubules per unit area is increased towards the pulp. The deposition of secondary dentine is of considerable clinical significance, as it will, perhaps in concert with the formation of any tertiary dentine, reduce the size of the pulp chamber and root canals. Often the pulp chamber becomes completely occluded and the root canals reduced to a size only visible through a microscope. These changes make the endodontic treatment of older teeth a considerable challenge.

The second major change related to age is the infilling of the tubules by peritubular (more correctly termed intratubular) dentine. The difference in appearance and composition of peritubular dentine has been discussed elsewhere (see pages 169–171). As the infilling of the tubules continues, dentine can become as translucent as glass (sclerotic or translucent dentine – see page 170). That peritubular dentine is an age change rather than a response to external irritation or injury and is supported by two simple observations:

1) Translucent dentine is found most abundantly in roots.
2) Peritubular dentine is found in (older) unerupted teeth.

The mechanism by which peritubular dentine is formed is a mystery. Whether it is the last product of a retreating odontoblast process or is produced by some form of precipitation only after the process has retracted is unclear. The first hypothesis is supported to some extent by the occasional observation of odontoblast processes in tubules lined by peritubular dentine. The difficulty of preserving cellular structure in this tissue obscures a clear answer to this question. As for secondary dentine, the extent of translucent dentine is related to chronological age. The production of both secondary dentine and peritubular dentine may result in the aged tooth being less sensitive.

While calcospherites are small, discrete and quantifiable at the mineralising front of predentine in young teeth up to 30 years of age, above this the calcospherites fuse and enlarge so that above 50 years of age, they are not quantifiable.

The presence and concentration of a large number of trace elements (grouped as potentially toxic or essential) and their relationship with age have been studied in human dentine. They show an increase in the concentration of toxic (Pb, Li and Sn) and essential (B, Ba, K, Sr, S and Mg) elements in coronal dentin related to the age of the teeth, regardless of sex. The concentrations of Pb and K in the dentine of molars and premolars are the elements that best related their variations with age and could be considered in age dating studies in different forensic situations.

Tertiary dentine, whether reparative or regenerative, is not an age change but a response to injury.

Clinical considerations

Permeability of dentine

The tubular structure of dentine allows for the possibility of substances applied to its outer surface being able to reach and affect the dental pulp. This depends on several factors:

- That the dentine surface is exposed by dental caries, attrition, abrasion or trauma.
- That the tubules are patent. Tubules may be occluded physiologically by peritubular (intratubular) dentine or by exogenous material precipitated in them peripherally. They may also be sealed off from the pulp by tertiary dentine.
- That the outward movement of interstitial 'dentinal' fluid does not wash them out of the tubule.
- That they are able to pass through the odontoblast layer, which presents a barrier to molecules of higher molecular weight.

Given that these factors are overcome, the most significant materials to travel down the tubules are the bacteria of dental caries and, more importantly, the toxins they produce. It is possible, but unproven, that molecules capable of exciting sensory nerves in the pulp may follow this route and induce pain. Components of dental materials, or etchants used to prepare for their placement, may pass through the dentine and kill or damage the dental pulp. This does not appear, however, to be as great a concern as it may seem. The weak pulpal response to some restorative materials is more likely to be owing to the poor marginal seal the material provides, allowing microleakage and the presence of bacteria on the surface of the dentine, whose toxins affect the pulp. Although *in vitro* some components of dental materials pass through dentine, *in vivo* the outward flow of dentinal fluid opposes this.

Response to external stimuli (eg. dental caries)

The response to outside stimuli comes from the dental pulp but is manifest in the structure of the dentine it produces. The deposition of tertiary dentine provides a barrier to the progress of dental caries and toxins. The presence of secondary dentine and its continuing deposition throughout life, although not a response to external stimuli, contributes to the barrier function of the dentine.

Cavity preparation

An overall understanding of the structure of the dentine–pulp complex is essential when undertaking cavity preparation to ensure the best patient outcome. Any drilling through dentine will potentially open a pathway towards the pulp. The greater the distance between the floor of the cavity and the surface of the pulp, the less the dental pulp will be affected. The deeper the cavity, the greater the surface area of exposed dentinal tubules and potentially the greater harm done to the dental pulp. Age can significantly affect the outcome, as the younger the patient, the thinner the layer of dentine and the lesser amount of peritubular dentine. As heat is generated during drilling, the thinner the intervening dentine, the greater the dental pulp may be affected. The term 'residual dental thickness' refers to the amount of dentine separating the floor of the dental cavity from the periphery of the dental pulp. A residual dentine thickness of about 0.5 mm is thought to be a reasonable estimate to ensure the dental pulp is unlikely to be compromised. When the residual dental thickness is less than 0.5 mm, care must be taken in treating any residual dental caries.

Adhesion of dental materials to dentine

Many of the advances in restorative dentistry are a result of the development of materials that will adhere to enamel and dentine. This allows more conservative cavity preparations, less pulpal injury and improved aesthetic results. Adhesion to dentine is more complex than that to enamel because of the high organic and water content of the tissue, its tubular architecture, its heterogeneity, its age changes and its reactions to dental caries. In addition, when dentine is cut with a dental bur, a smear layer (Fig. 9.65) forms on its surface, consisting of dentine that has been melted and reset; it may also contain embedded in it bacteria from dental caries being removed. Smearing has an advantage in that it occludes the dentinal tubules but a disadvantage in that it may harbour bacteria and provides a difficult surface for adherence. Removing the smear layer is therefore a prerequisite before applying bonding agents. Like enamel, dentine is first etched with strong acids to remove the smear layer.

This acid treatment also exposes collagen fibrils and provides a porous surface that can be infiltrated by the bonding agent (Fig. 9.66). This thin resin impregnation creates a transitional 'hybrid' layer (Fig. 9.67) that locks the two dissimilar substances together at a molecular level, sealing the surface against leakage and imparting a high degree of acid resistance. The final quality of dental restoration depends greatly on the properties of the hybrid layer. The bonding material will also penetrate the etched intertubular dentine up to a depth of about 7 microns, further enhancing the retention of the restoration as well as having significantly longer resin tags within the dentinal tubules (Figs 9.67, 9.68).

The exposed collagen forming the hybrid layer contains small amounts of various collagenases (MMP-2, MMP-3, MMP-8, MMP-9, MMP-20) and cathepsins (B and K) normally present in dentine that, with release over time, may weaken the bond between the restoration and dentine. For this reason, the exposed dentine may be treated with enzyme inhibitors, such as chlorhexidine and dimethyl sulphoxide, to avoid subsequent weakening of the bond. Laboratory studies show promising results with these and other MMP inhibitors, but the potential clinical advantages are, as yet, unproven.

Endodontics

The continuing deposition of secondary dentine throughout life and the development of tertiary dentine in response to dental caries and restorative procedures can lead to a reduction in size – even obliteration of the pulp chamber and root canals (Fig. 9.69). Root canal therapy (endodontics) consists of cleaning, shaping and filling the root canal system. Care must

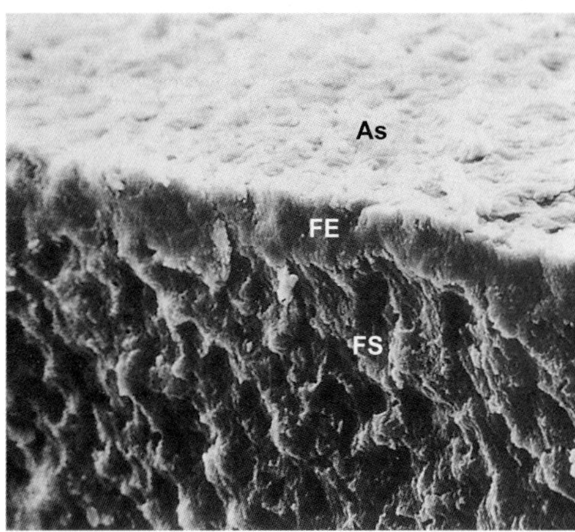

Fig. 9.65 SEM showing a smear layer on the surface of dentine cut with a high-speed bur. As = abraded surface; FE = smear layer on fractured edge; FS = fractured surface (×35). Courtesy Dr. J Dennison.

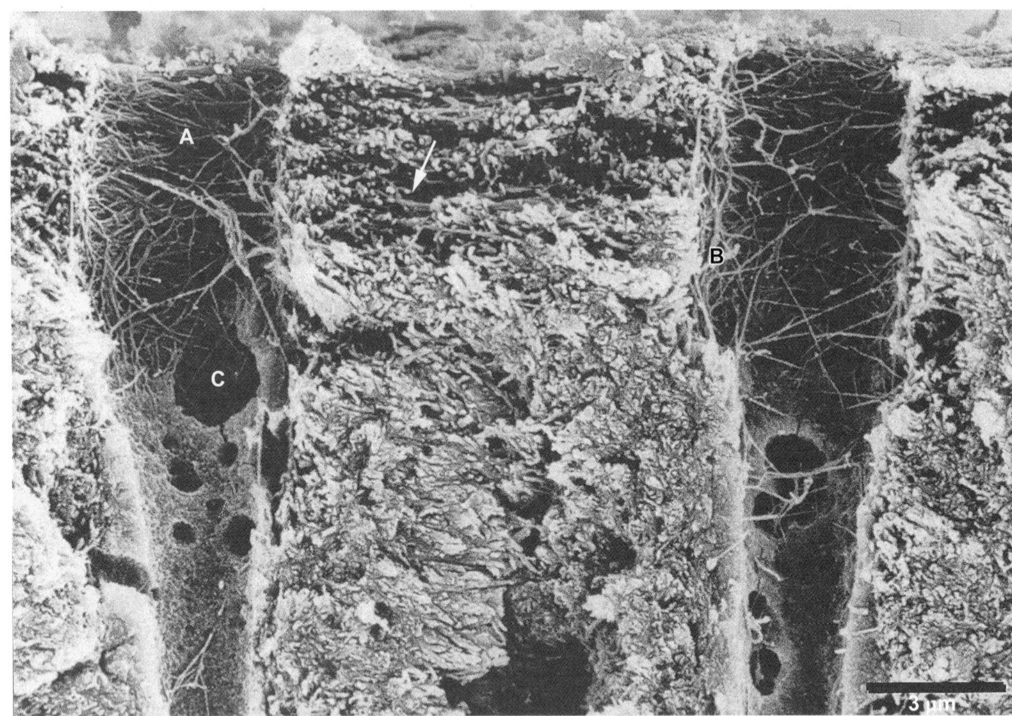

Fig. 9.66 SEM of a fractured surface of dentine after etching with 37% phosphoric acid. Notice the exposed collagen fibrils in the superficial layers (A) and loss of peritubular dentine (seen in deeper layers) (B). Open lateral tubules (C) are visible. Mineralised collagen fibrils *(arrow)* are evident in the intertubular dentine (×6,500). Courtesy Prof. B Van Meerbeek.

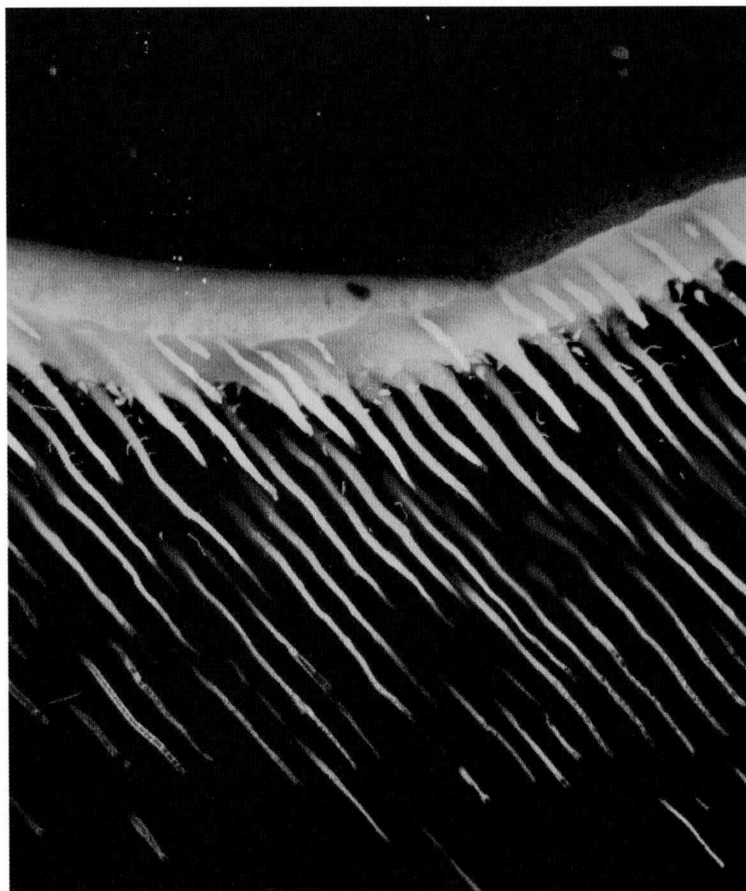

Fig. 9.67 Confocal image of acid-etched dentine infiltrated with a multiple dye-labelled bonding agent. Notice the penetration of the bonding agent into the tubules and the intertubular region at the surface forming a 'hybrid zone' (×1,000). Courtesy Prof. T F Watson.

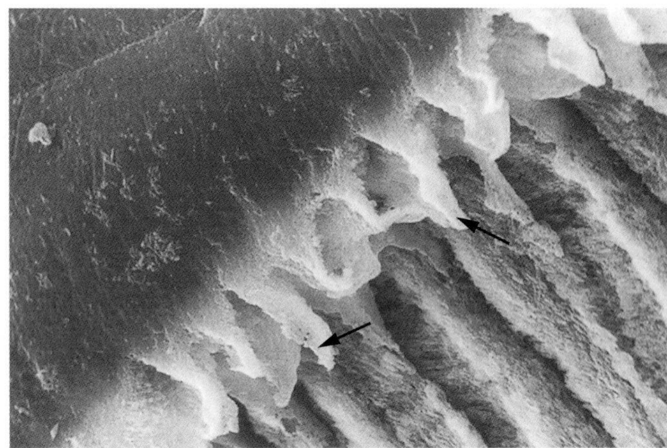

Fig. 9.68 SEM showing tags of resin in a restorative material *(arrows)* conforming to the dentinal tubules in etched dentine and enhancing retention of the restoration (×35). Courtesy Dr. J Dennison.

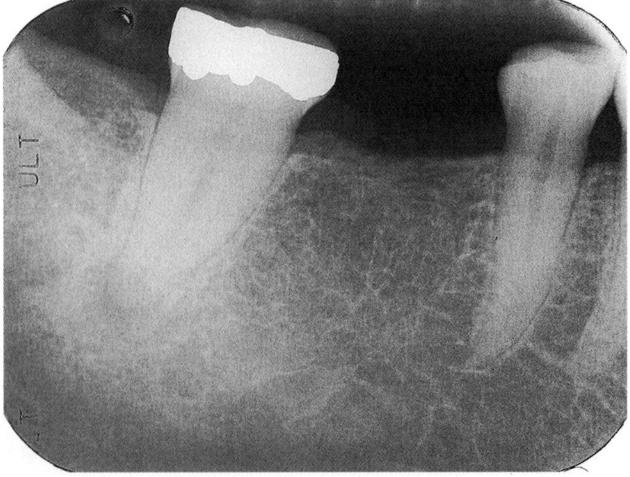

Fig. 9.69 Clinical radiograph of a molar tooth in which the root canals have almost been obliterated by mineralisation.

be taken since smaller, lateral canals (Fig. 9.70) may exist that enter the main canal and that may not be cleaned during treatment. As the repair and regeneration of dentine are properties of odontoblasts in the dental pulp, this topic is considered in detail on pages 492–493.

Sensitivity

Exposed dentine is often (but not always) sensitive. Three main hypotheses have been put forward to account for its sensitivity, implicating:

1. Nerves in dentine
2. The odontoblast processes
3. Fluid movements in the dentinal tubules (Fig. 9.71)

Arguments against the view that pain results from direct stimulation of nerves in the dentine relate to their relative scarcity and to the fact that they appear to be absent in the outer parts of dentine. In addition, the application of local anaesthetics to the surface of dentine does not abolish the sensitivity.

With regard to the second hypothesis, there is no physiological evidence to date that indicates that the odontoblast process is analogous to a nerve fibre and can similarly conduct impulses pulpwards. Furthermore, the process may not extend to the enamel–dentine junction, nor is the application of substances designed to prevent transmission of such impulses effective. Odontoblasts have not been shown to be synaptically connected to nerve fibres.

The most plausible hypothesis to explain the transmission of sensory stimuli suggests that all effective stimuli applied to dentine cause fluid movement through the dentinal tubules and that this movement is sufficient to depolarise nerve endings in the inner parts of tubules, at the pulp–predentine junction and in the subodontoblastic neural plexus. Some stimuli, such as cold, osmotic pressure and drying, would tend to cause fluid movement outwards, while others, such as heat, would cause movement inwards (Fig. 9.71). Movement in either direction would mechanically distort the terminals. These stimuli have been shown to cause such fluid movement *in vitro*. Chemicals (in strong solution) and thermal stimuli induce a response much more quickly than can be explained by conduction or diffusion. This also is consistent with the hydrodynamic hypothesis. In animal experiments, however, the response of intradental nerves to chemical stimuli is often slow and may be more readily explained by diffusion. It may be that both 'direct' and 'hydrodynamic' mechanisms operate, but that the hydrodynamic force predominates whenever there is pulpal inflammation and a lowering in the threshold of intrapulpal nerves to the small mechanical forces generated by fluid flow.

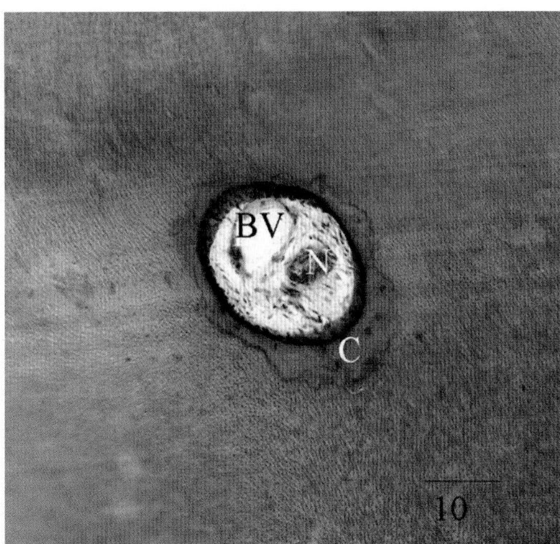

Fig. 9.70 A small (lateral) canal of the root canal system containing a blood vessel (BV) and nerve bundle (N) and lined by cementum (C).

Hypersensitivity

Hypersensitivity is defined as a short, sharp pain arising from exposed dentine in response to a stimulus such as thermal (especially cold), tactile, osmotic and chemical that cannot be ascribed to any other form of dental defect or pathology, such as dental caries or lateral pulp canals. Its reported incidence in the population varies considerably but averages between 10% and 20% and is most commonly associated with the buccal surfaces of canines and premolars, especially in teeth that show gingival recession. Such dentine has tubules that are patent (Fig. 9.72A). Exposed dentine in which the tubules are not patent is not sensitive (Fig. 9.72B).

Eliminating or reducing the sensitivity of exposed dentine requires the patent tubules to become infilled and occluded with calcium phosphate material. Desensitising toothpastes can be used and/or special mouthwashes and/or topical application of solutions containing, amongst other substances, fluoride and calcium phosphate ions, such as diamine silver fluoride or a mixture of 8% arginine, calcium carbonate and fluoride. The use of bioactive glass has recently been suggested to treat dentine hypersensitivity (Fig. 9.73). Bioglass is composed of silicon, sodium, calcium and phosphorus oxides and

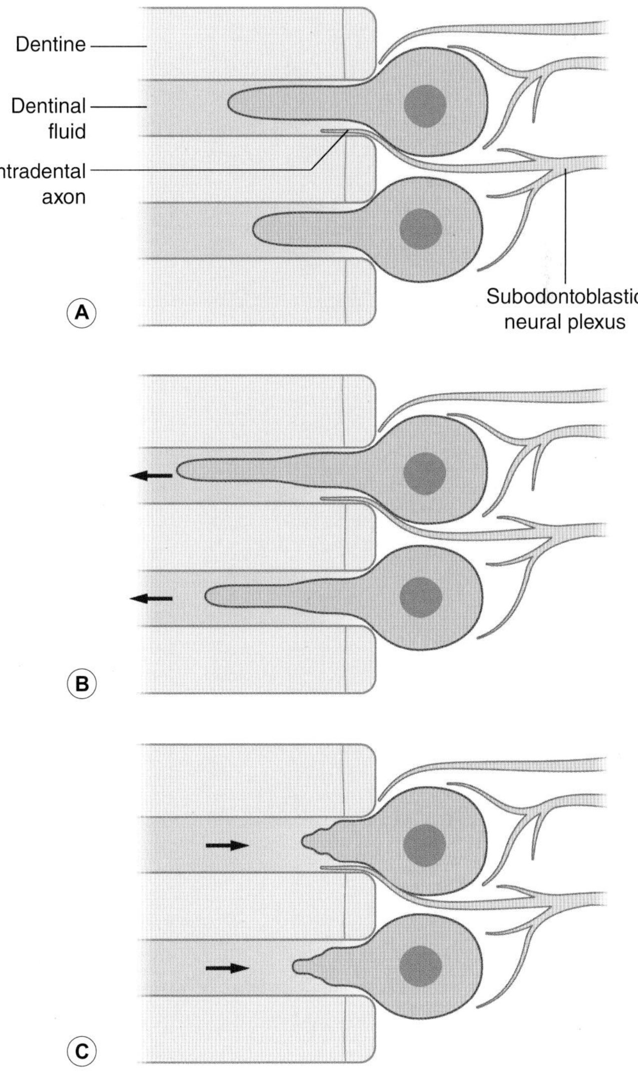

Fig. 9.71 The effects of outward (B) and inward (C) fluid movement in the dentinal tubules.

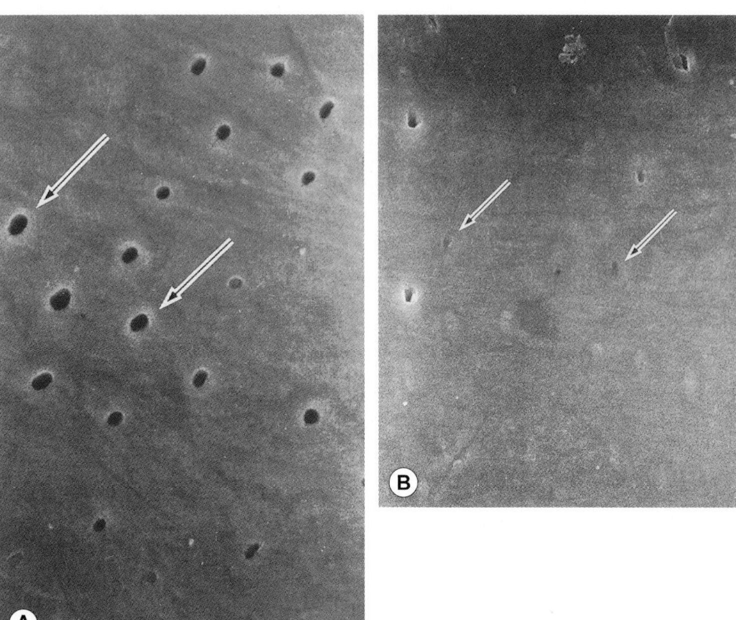

Fig. 9.72 (A) SEM of an exposed dentine surface of a hypersensitive area. A large proportion of dentinal tubules *(arrows)* are seen to be open. (B) SEM of exposed dentine from a nonsensitive area. The tubules are occluded *(arrows)* (×2,400). Courtesy Dr. M Yoshiyama and the editor of the *Journal of Dental Research*.

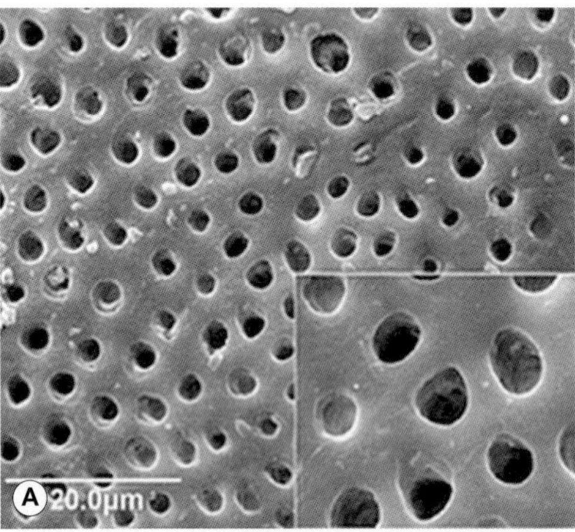

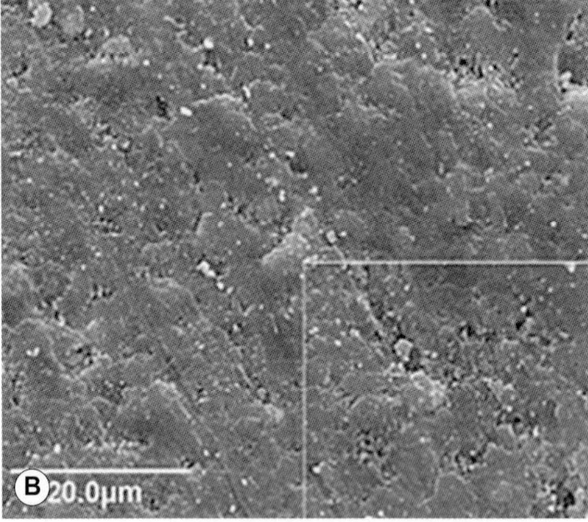

Fig. 9.73 Scanning electron microscope images of partially demineralised dentine showing the effects of immersion for 7 days in artificial saliva alone (A) or artificial saliva containing bioglass (B). Note the remineralisation with bioactive glass that has resulted in blockage of the dentinal tubules in B compared with artificial saliva alone (A). From Wang, Z., Jiang, T., Sauro, S., et al. 2011. Dentine remineralization induced by two bioactive glasses developed for air abrasion purposes. *Journal of Dentistry* 39, 746–756.

fluoride. New glasses (e.g., Biomin F) contain polymers that bond them to the calcium while the calcium phosphate and fluoride are released. The glass particles are extremely small, allowing them to enter and block off the dentinal tubules, preventing fluid flow through them. Bioglass has the ability to release dentine matrix components that are bioactive, such as growth factors and enzymes.

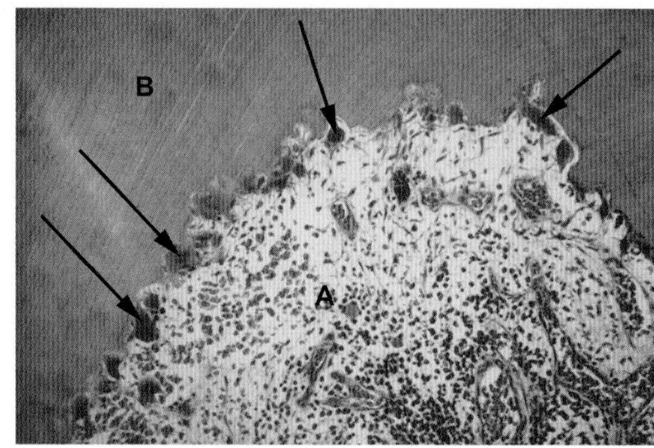

Fig. 9.74 Section of tooth undergoing internal dentine resorption. The pulp (A) has lost its peripheral odontoblast layer and is replaced by a vascular granulation tissue. The dentine (B) is undergoing resorption by large, multinucleated, odontoclast-like cells *(arrows)* (H & E stain; ×200). Courtesy Dr. H Trowbridge.

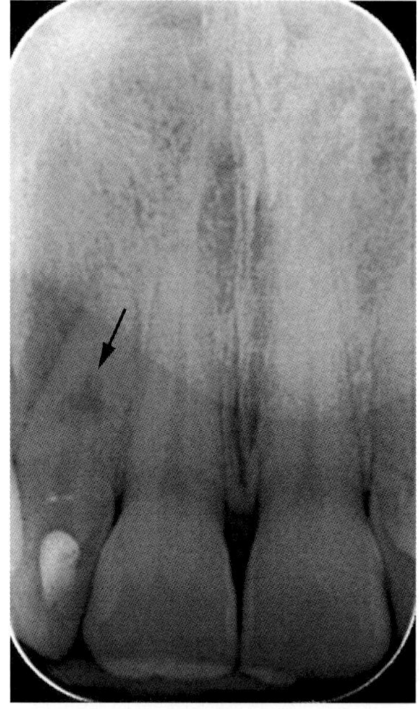

Fig. 9.75 Radiograph showing a central radiolucent area *(arrow)* in the root of a maxillary lateral incisor continuous with the outline of the central pulp canal, indicating internal dentine resorption. Courtesy Dr. J Makdissi.

Dentine resorption

Apart from the dentine that is resorbed during the shedding of deciduous teeth, dentine in permanent teeth is normally stable throughout adult life. However, it can be resorbed in permanent teeth. This resorption is usually associated with inflammation. However, when the cause is unknown, this condition is termed *idiopathic resorption*. Dentine resorption may be initiated from two sites: from the pulpal surface, when it is known as *internal dentine resorption*, or from the root surface, when it is known as *external dentine resorption*.

Internal dentine resorption

In the case of internal resorption, the pulp at the pulp–dentine surface contains multinucleated cells known as odontoclasts that are responsible for resorbing the dentine (Fig. 9.74). This will be evident radiologically as an enlarged radiolucency in the pulp continuous with the outline of the pulp canal (Fig. 9.75).

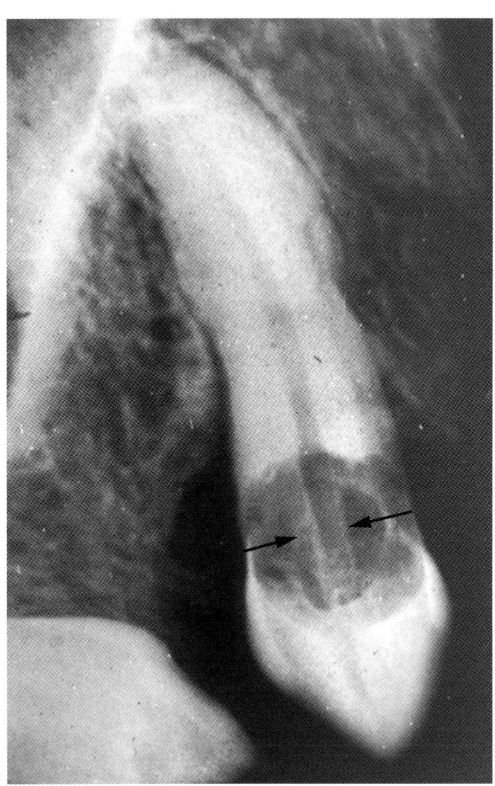

Fig. 9.76 Radiograph of tooth showing external dentine resorption. The presence of a radiopaque layer of dentine internally *(arrows)* helps distinguish this case from one of internal dentine resorption (compare with Fig. 9.75). Courtesy Dr. J D Harrison.

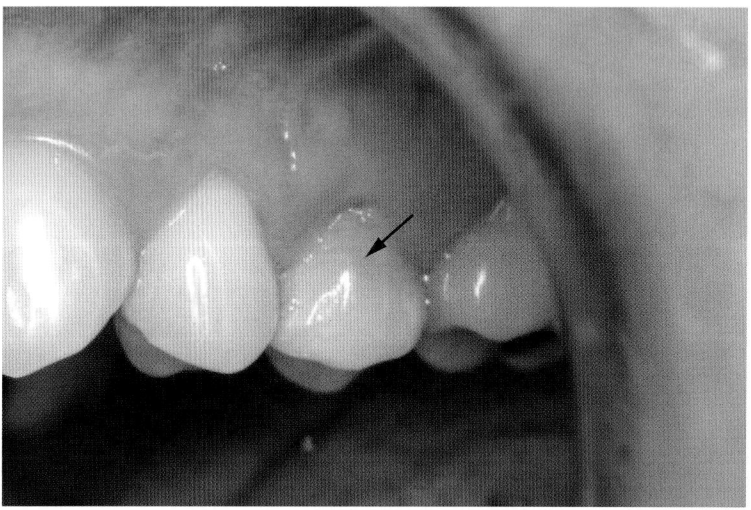

Fig. 9.77 Patient with underlying dentine resorption involving a second maxillary premolar *(arrow)*. The crown shows a pinkish colouration compared with the normal adjacent teeth. The cause may be either internal or external resorption. Courtesy Dr. N McDonald.

External dentine resorption

External resorption of the dentine begins on the external surface of the root and penetrates through the cementum into dentine. It does not normally penetrate the pulp and, radiologically, is difficult to distinguish from internal resorption. However, a thin shell of dentine may be visible on a radiograph, and the area of resorption is not continuous with the pulp outline (Fig. 9.76). If resorption proceeds far enough, the crown may have a pinkish coloration as the vascular granulation tissue is seen beneath the translucent enamel (Fig. 9.77).

Root resorption may be seen following periapical inflammation, orthodontic treatment (see Fig. 13.51) and tooth implantation.

Further readings for this chapter can be found in the accompanying eBook. Explore online Self-assessment quiz to test and reinforce your understanding of the material in your free ebook. Follow instructions in the Inside Front Cover to unlock your access.

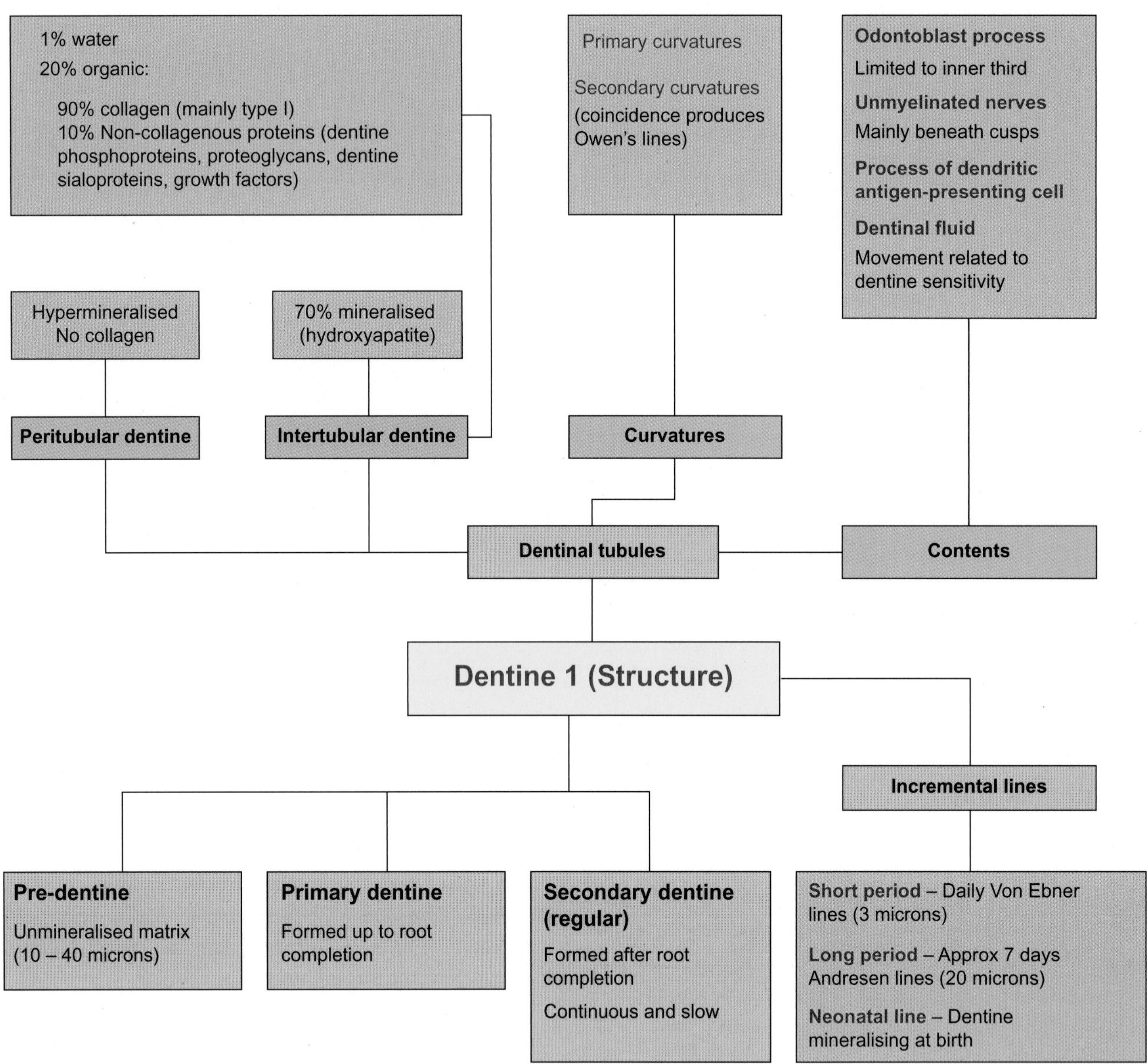
1% water
20% organic:
90% collagen (mainly type I)
10% Non-collagenous proteins (dentine phosphoproteins, proteoglycans, dentine sialoproteins, growth factors)
Primary curvatures
Secondary curvatures
(coincidence produces Owen's lines)
Odontoblast process
Limited to inner third
Unmyelinated nerves
Mainly beneath cusps
Process of dendritic antigen-presenting cell
Dentinal fluid
Movement related to dentine sensitivity
Hypermineralised
No collagen
70% mineralised (hydroxyapatite)
Peritubular dentine
Intertubular dentine
Curvatures
Dentinal tubules
Contents
Dentine 1 (Structure)
Incremental lines
Pre-dentine
Unmineralised matrix (10 – 40 microns)
Primary dentine
Formed up to root completion
Secondary dentine (regular)
Formed after root completion
Continuous and slow
Short period – Daily Von Ebner lines (3 microns)
Long period – Approx 7 days Andresen lines (20 microns)
Neonatal line – Dentine mineralising at birth

Mind Map 9.1 Dentine 1 (Structure).

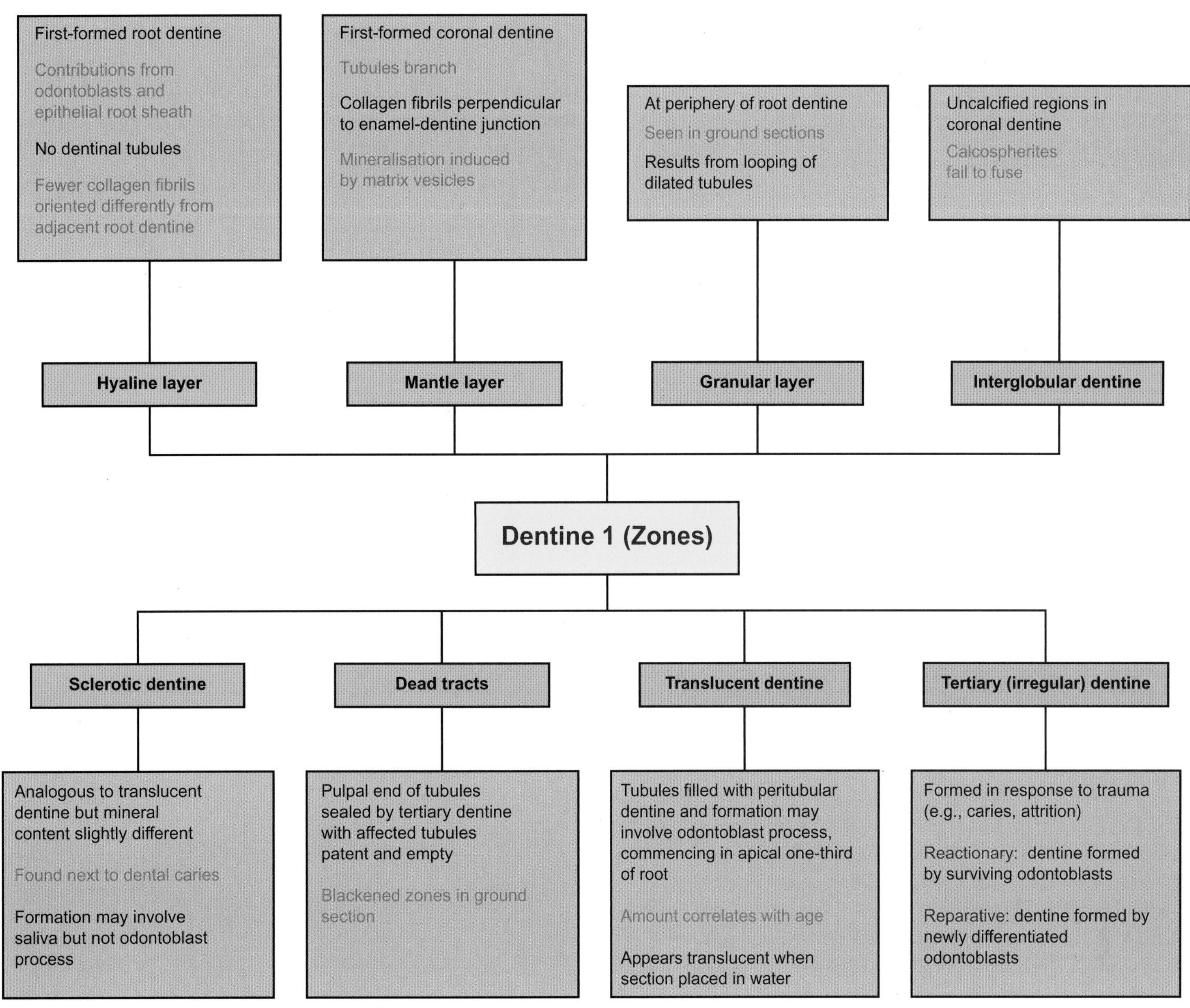

Mind Map 9.2 Dentine 1 (Zones).

10 Dental pulp

Introduction

The dental pulp is the tissue derived from the dental papilla and is responsible for the formation of dentine. It is contained within the pulp chamber and root canals of the tooth (see pages 33–34) and, because of its unyielding walls, is a system of low compliance. At the apical constriction of the root canal, it becomes continuous with the periodontal ligament (see Fig. 2.59). Although the pulp is most obviously active during development and eruption of the tooth, it remains productive throughout life, forming secondary dentine slowly but regularly. It is able to respond (within certain important limits) to stimuli such as caries, trauma, tooth movement and restorative procedures by producing tertiary dentine (see pages 181–183). Different cell types within the dentine–pulp complex are able to detect invading bacteria, and at early disease stages, odontoblasts will respond to bacterial components. As the disease progresses, other pulpal cells, including fibroblasts, endothelial cells, immune cells and stem cells, will become involved. The close association of the dental pulp and dentine gives rise to the concept of a dentine-pulp complex (see page 165).

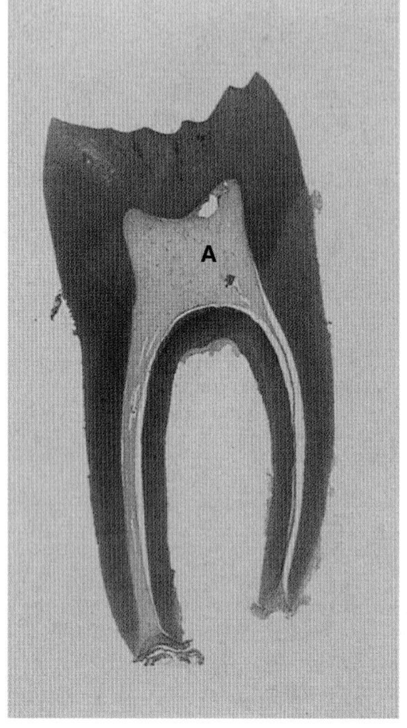

Fig. 10.1 Decalcified section of a whole tooth showing the general disposition of the dental pulp (A) (H & E; ×3).

Organisation

The dental pulp is a specialised connective tissue with a unique anatomical arrangement determined by its position inside a rigid chamber and by its role in forming hard tissue on the walls of that chamber (Fig. 10.1). The cells responsible for dentine deposition, the odontoblasts, lie at the periphery of the tissue. Also at the periphery are two elements capable of detecting external stimuli and initiating a response initiating a response. These are the nerve terminals of trigeminal afferents and specialised dendritic antigen-presenting cells. The odontoblasts themselves may also be able to detect the presence of foreign antigens. The rest of the dental pulp acts as a support system for these three components. Blood vessels and nerves enter and leave the root canals through an apical foramen at the root apex. Each root has at least one main canal and apical foramen; many have two. Smaller accessory canals branch from the main canal and have their own foramina. They are most commonly found in the apical third of the root (Fig. 10.2). In multirooted teeth some small vascular canals enter the pulp chamber from the bone between the roots.

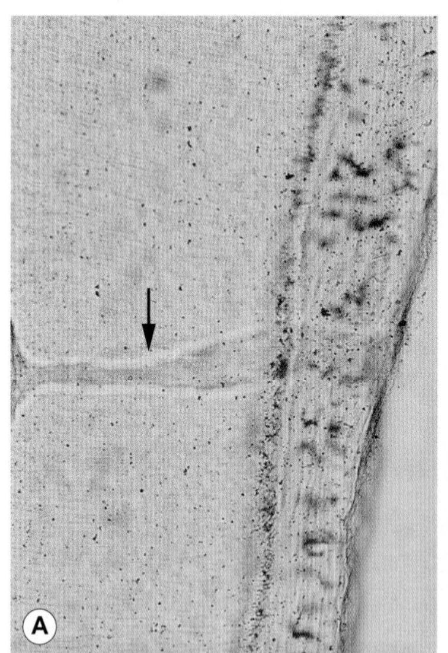

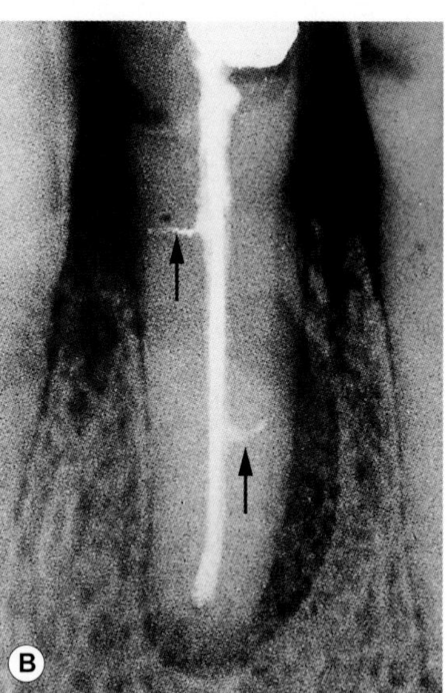

Fig. 10.2 (A) Ground section of root showing a lateral branch from the main root canal (arrow) (×12). (B) Radiograph of a root-filled tooth showing accessory canals (arrows). (A) *Courtesy Dr M E Atkinson. (B) Courtesy Dr J Souyave.*

Composition

The composition of any connective tissue varies during development and with ageing. It changes when the tissue is injured or challenged with a bacterial toxin. Different cells may be activated, migrate to the tissue or develop from stem cells. It is impossible to study all the elements of a tissue at the same time. Each cell type may contribute different products to the extracellular matrix at different times. Often cells are observed in culture separated from all other components. In this situation they may produce extracellular materials that they do not create in the intact tissue. Larger molecules are built up from smaller components and, conversely, some smaller molecules may be breakdown products from larger molecules. The end result is that the composition is dynamic and will vary depending on when and how it is studied. What follows is a static description, some of which may be correct all the time, but some of which will be correct only some of the time!

The dental pulp is a loose connective tissue and is made up of a combination of cells embedded in an extracellular matrix of fibres in a semifluid gel. It contains 75% water and 25% organic material by weight. As with most connective tissues, the matrix is more plentiful than the cells. The extracellular matrix is made up of a versatile group of polysaccharides and proteins secreted by the cells of the tissue and assembled into a complex framework closely associated with the cells. The extracellular matrix forms a scaffold that stabilises the structure of the tissue, but it is far from inert: indeed, in the dental pulp, where there is a rigid supporting and protecting hard shell, the skeletal function is minimal. The matrix plays a very active role in controlling the activity of the cells within it. It affects their development, migration, division, shape and function. Collagen is the predominant extracellular matrix component, comprising 25–32% of the dry weight. The composition of the dental papilla and dental pulp changes during development and can vary between tooth types. Much of the data that are available derive from animal tissues, which may differ somewhat from human. In addition, much of the published work is on the products of isolated cell types maintained *in vitro*. Their output may differ in the intact tissue.

Fibres

The principal fibrous component of the dental pulp is a combination of collagen types I (60%) and III (40%) (Figs. 10.3, 10.4; see Fig. 10.8B) present as fibrils 50 nm in diameter grouped into fibres thinly and irregularly scattered throughout the tissue. The arrangement becomes more organised at the periphery, with the fibres aligned parallel to the forming predentine surface. Type III collagen has a similar 67 nm banding pattern to type I but differs from it by having only α1 chains rather than α1 and α2 chains. The functional significance of the high levels of type III collagen is not known. In other sites it has been associated with rapid remodelling. Overall, collagen forms 3–5% of the wet weight of the pulp, a low proportion in comparison with other loose connective tissues. Small amounts of type V and type VI collagen are also present as a meshwork of fine microfibrils. Type IV collagen is nonfibrous and present in the basement membranes of blood vessels.

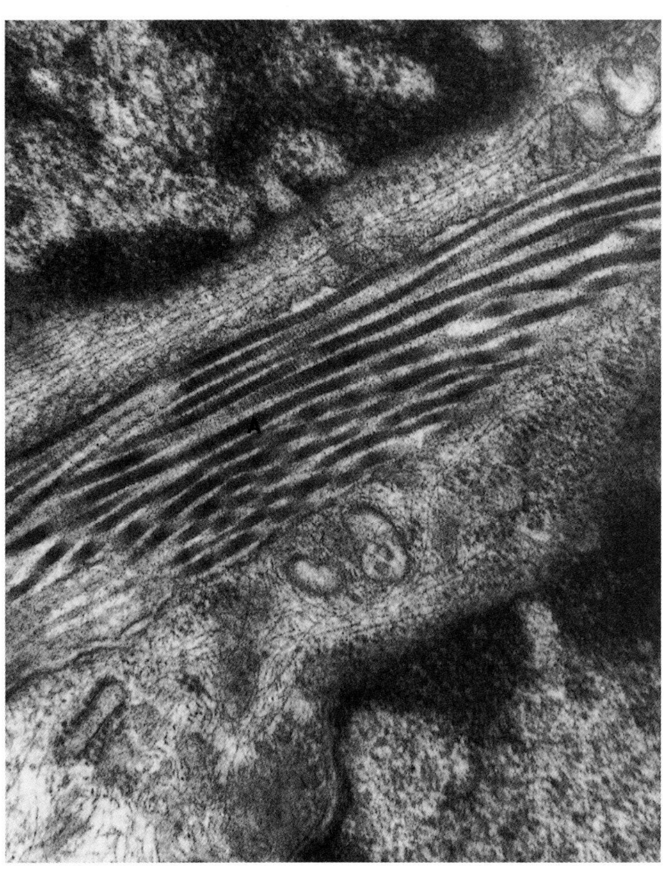
Fig. 10.3 TEM showing collagen fibrils (A) within the pulp (×134,000).

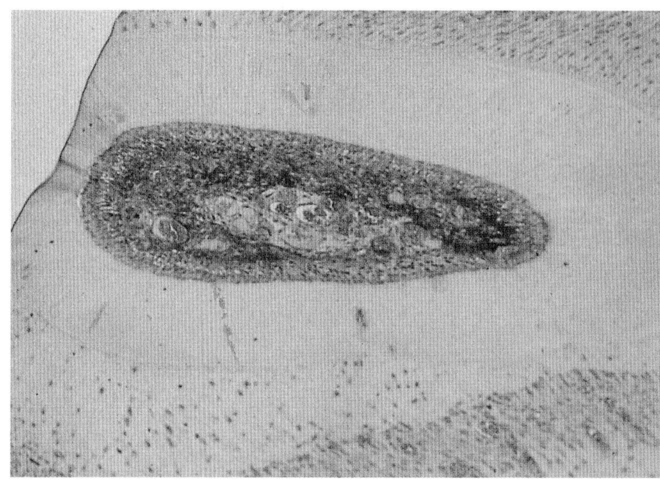
Fig. 10.4 Section of developing mouse molar root showing type III collagen stained brown by immunohistochemical methods (×30). *Courtesy Dr Y Ohsaki and the editor of Anatomical Record.*

Fibronectin is a glycoprotein found in several forms, one of which is fibrous and distributed throughout the pulp. It anchors cells and may be important in determining their shape.

Noncollagenous beaded microfibrils 10–14 nm in diameter are also present. These are formed from fibrillin, a large glycoprotein that, in other tissues, is associated with elastic fibres. There has been no convincing demonstration of elastic fibres in the pulp.

Nonfibrous matrix

The macromolecules that make up the bulk of the nonfibrous component of the extracellular matrix are proteoglycans, glycoproteins and unbound glycosaminoglycans (GAGs).

Glycosaminoglycans

GAGs are unbranched polysaccharide chains composed of repeating disaccharide units. There are four GAGs: chondroitin sulphate, dermatan sulphate, heparan sulphate and hyaluronan. All are present in the dental pulp. Most of the GAGs are covalently bound to a protein core to form proteoglycans. These are bulky hydrophilic molecules that swell when hydrated and form gels that fill most of the extracellular space. They readily allow the movement of water and ions and probably act as a reservoir for holding growth factors and other bioactive molecules. Hyaluronan is the only GAG found unbound to protein in any quantity. As well as having a mechanical function, it is thought to facilitate cell migration, particularly during development.

In the mature pulp, 60% of the GAG content is hyaluronic acid, 20% dermatan sulphate, 12% chondroitin sulphate (Fig. 10.5) and the remainder heparin sulphate. In the developing pulp, chondroitin sulphate is the major GAG, with hyaluronic acid only a minor component.

Proteoglycans

Proteoglycans (GAGs attached to a protein core) are functionally diverse molecules. Some, such as versican (Fig. 10.6), contribute to the bulk of the matrix; others may bind to fibres, to other nonfibrous components of the tissue, or contribute (e.g., syndecan) to the basement membranes of epithelially derived cells, such as Schwann cells and endothelial cells.

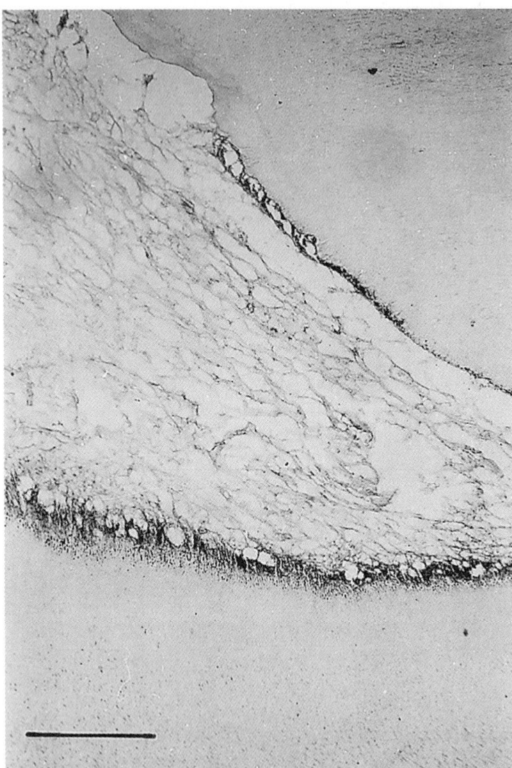

Fig. 10.5 Adult human dental pulp stained by immunohistochemical methods for chondroitin sulphate (staining black at the pulp–dentine junction), showing widespread presence but a greater concentration peripherally in the odontoblast layer, suggesting (circumstantially) a role for this molecule in the development of dentine (×40). *Courtesy Dr P M Bartold, Dr U Schlagenhauf and the editor of International Endodontic Journal.*

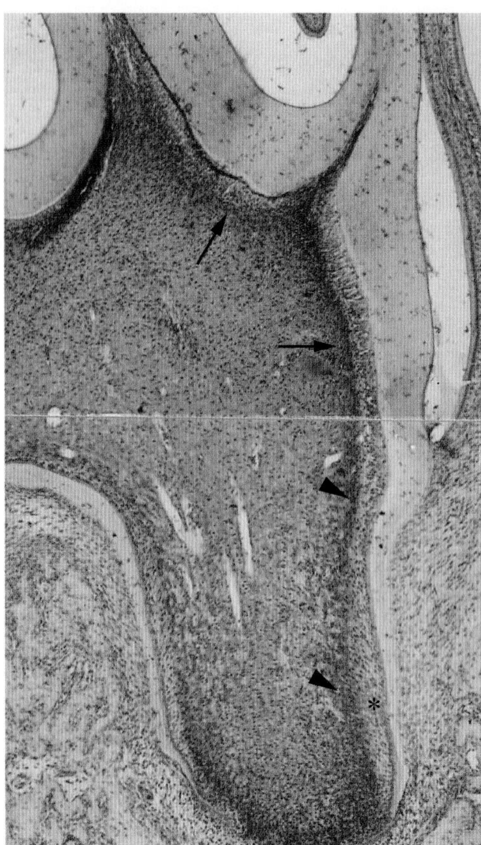

Fig. 10.6 A section of rat pulp stained immunohistochemically for the proteoglycan versican (dark stain). Staining is most intense in the subodontoblastic zone of the coronal pulp (arrows). The staining moves centrally in the cervical region (arrowheads) and is weak in the subodontoblastic zone of the root (*) (×1,000). *Courtesy Dr S Shibata and the editor of International Journal of Endodontics.*

They cement the various components of the tissue together and are largely responsible for limiting its permeability. Table 10.1 summarises the proteoglycans present in the pulp and their possible functions.

Table 10.1 Proteoglycans of the dental pulp

Versican and Syndecan	Form large hydrated aggregates creating a gel
Decorin	Binds to type I collagen
Biglycan	May help regulate collagen fibrillogenesis
Integrins	Cell surface adhesion receptors
Fibronectin	Concentrated near the odontoblast layer. Binds cells to extracellular matrix.
Tenascin	Associated with cell movement. Concentrated near the odontoblast layer.
Osteoadherin	Associated with mineralisation

Glycoprotein

Collagen is a glycoprotein (saccharides attached to a protein core). Two other glycoproteins, fibronectin (Figs. 10.7, 10.8C) (which also occurs in fibrous form; see earlier) and tenascin (Fig. 10.8D), have been described in the pulp and are at their highest concentration near the odontoblast layer. This has led to the suggestion that they may be involved in the deposition of dentine.

An important group of molecules described by function as cell adhesion molecules are predominantly glycoproteins. Four groups of cell adhesion molecules are generally recognised: the immunoglobulin superfamily, the selectins, the cadherins and the integrins (Fig. 10.9). They are responsible (along with structurally specialised cell junctions) for cell-to-cell adhesion. The selectins have a very special role in guiding the diapedesis of leukocytes during inflammation. The large family of integrins anchors cells to the matrix.

The basement membranes of the epithelial cells in the pulp, the Schwann cells and the endothelial cells, consist of a meshwork created from collagen type IV in which many adhesion and bioactive molecules are embedded.

Molecules more intimately associated with dentine, dentine sialoprotein and dentine phosphoprotein, are produced by the odontoblasts and can be detected at the periphery of the pulp.

Proteomics of dental pulp

As for other dental tissues the new technique of proteomics has allowed the total quantification of proteins present within the dental pulp. One study has identified 342 different proteins within the dental pulp. Of these, the majority of the proteins identified are involved in metabolism and energy pathways (23.7%) and cell growth and/or maintenance (20.5%). The next most significant functions are protein metabolism (14.0%), cell communication and signal transduction (12.3%), and immune response (7.9%). Some proteins have unknown functions (5.3%). The proteomics of the dental pulp with that of dentine in which they identified 289 proteins. Of these latter proteins, 140 are shared with the dental pulp, 95 proteins are specific to dentine, while 137 proteins are specific to the dental pulp.

Initial studies have been undertaken using proteomics analysis to compare the normal with the diseased pulp. The most prevalent protein functions in the normal pulp group are metabolic and energetic pathways; the most prevalent protein functions in the inflamed pulp group are cellular communication and signal transduction, and regulation and repair of DNA/RNA; whereas in the necrotic pulp the most prevalent group of proteins is associated with the immune response. The most expressed proteins in the inflamed pulp group in relation to the normal pulp group are hemoglobin, peroxiredoxins and immunoglobulins, whereas the less expressed are the tubulins.

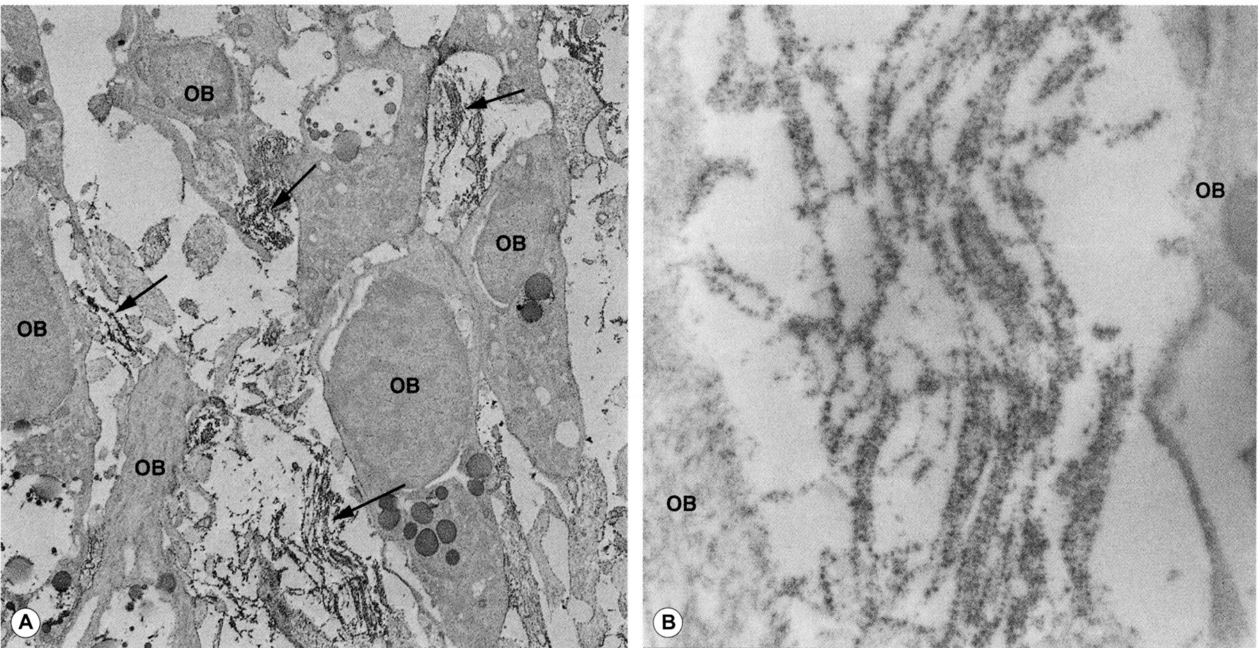

Fig. 10.7 (A) Electron micrograph showing immunolabelling for fibronectin (dark staining, arrows) on surface of collagen fibres of the odontoblast (OB) layer. There is little staining in the predentine (×170). (B) Immunoelectron micrograph showing presence of fibronectin as dark staining fibrillar fascicles between odontoblasts (OB) (×3,600). *Courtesy Dr N Yoshiba et al. and the editor of Archives of Oral Biology.*

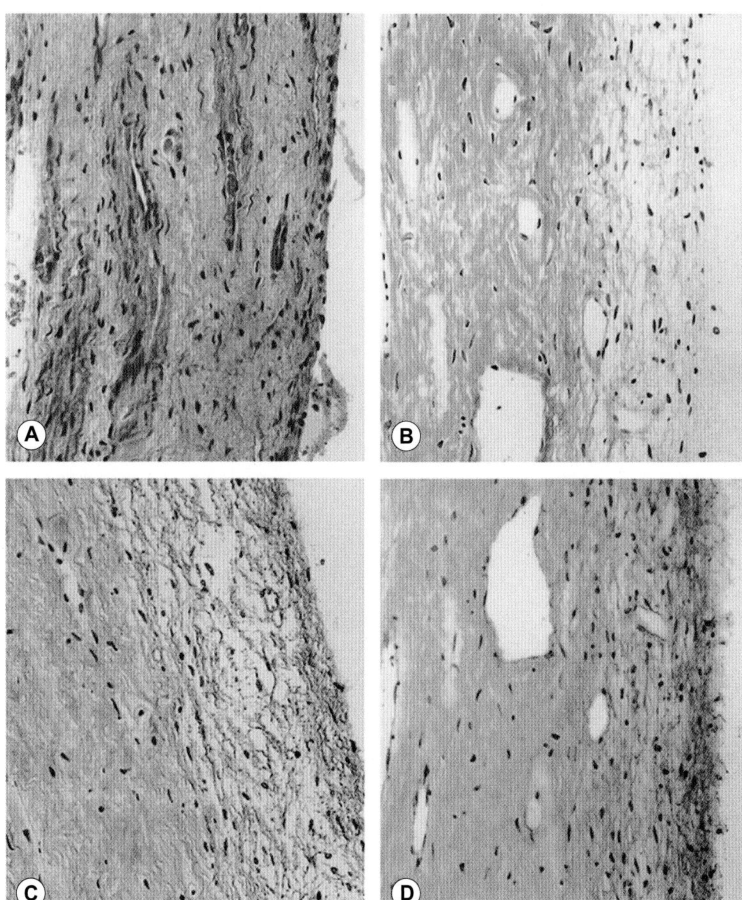

Fig. 10.8 (A) H & E staining. (B) Immunolabelling (brown) for collagen type III. The periphery of the pulp is unstained. (C) Immunolabelling for fibronectin. There is strong labelling in the cell-free zone. (D) Immunolabelling for tenascin. The peripheral tissue is negative (×250). *Courtesy Dr E F Martinez and the editor of Journal of Endodontics.*

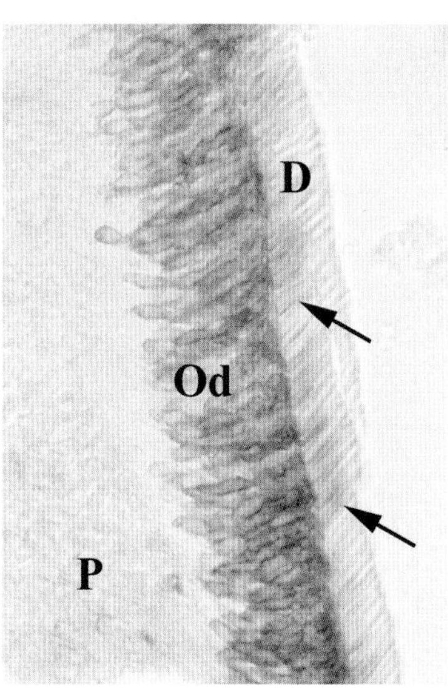

Fig. 10.9 Immunolocalisation of an integrin in human dental pulp. An intense membrane labelling (brown) with an anti-integrin antibody in mature odontoblasts (Od) of the pulp horn, including processes in dentine tubules (arrows). D = dentine (×1,000); P = pulp. *Courtesy Dr J C Farges and the editor of Journal of Dental Research.*

Cells

Odontoblasts

The odontoblast (Figs. 10.10–10.13) is responsible for the formation of dentine and secretes type I collagen. The origin and differentiation of these cells are described on pages 420–422. In the fully developed tooth the odontoblasts continue to lay down secondary dentine throughout life and survive for as long as the tooth remains vital. If the tooth is subjected to a mild insult, such as dental caries, the odontoblast is able to respond by laying down tertiary reactionary dentine, which is essentially an accelerated deposition of secondary dentine. The odontoblast is a postmitotic cell and cannot divide: more severe injury will result in the death of odontoblasts.

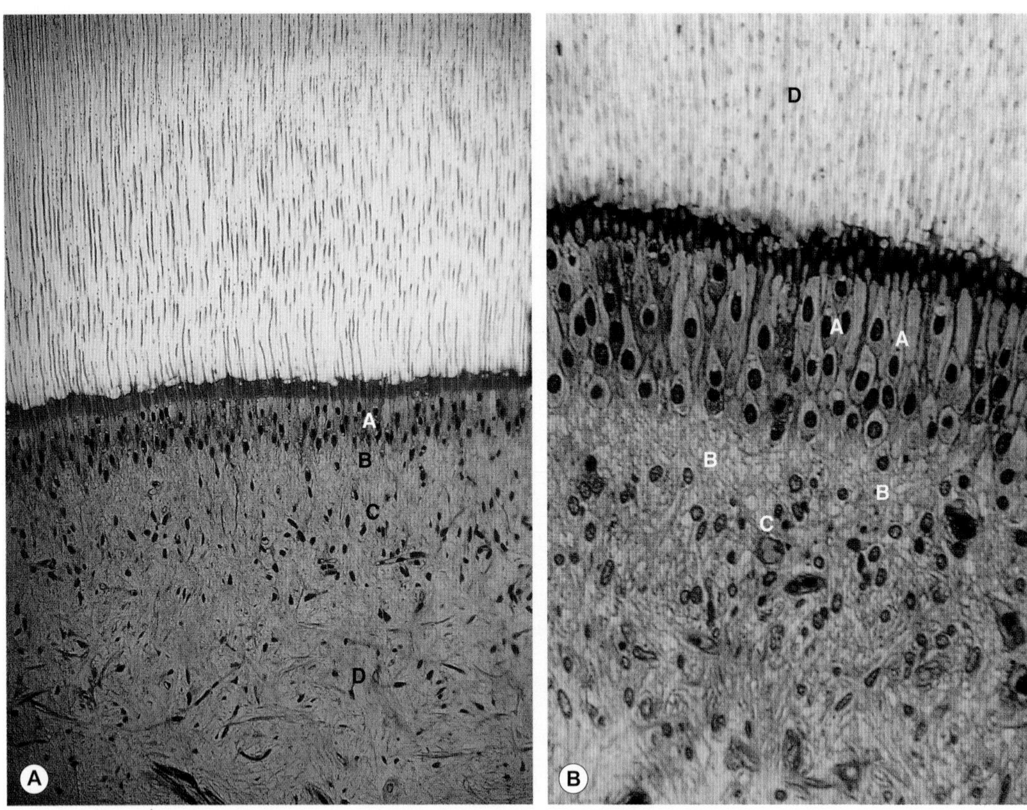

Fig. 10.10 (A) Low-power micrograph showing some cell types and their distribution in the pulp. A = odontoblast layer adjacent to dentine; B = cell-free zone; C = cell-rich zone; D = central pulp showing principally fibroblasts (toluidine blue; ×200). (B) Higher-power view showing pseudostratified odontoblast layer (A). B = cell-free zone; C = cell-rich zone; D = dentine (toluidine blue; ×650).

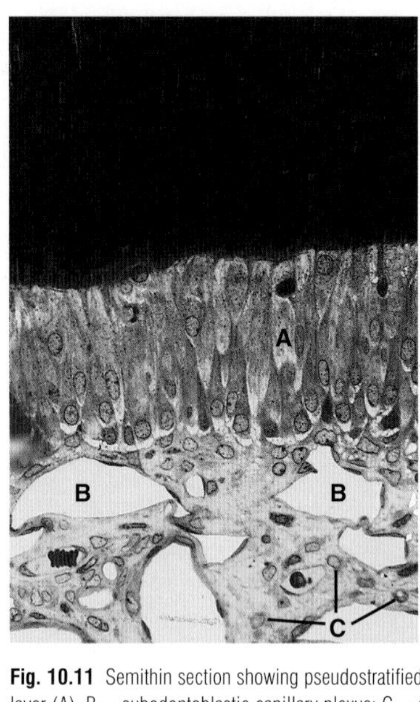

Fig. 10.11 Semithin section showing pseudostratified odontoblast layer (A). B = subodontoblastic capillary plexus; C = pulp fibroblasts; D = dentine (toluidine blue; ×450).

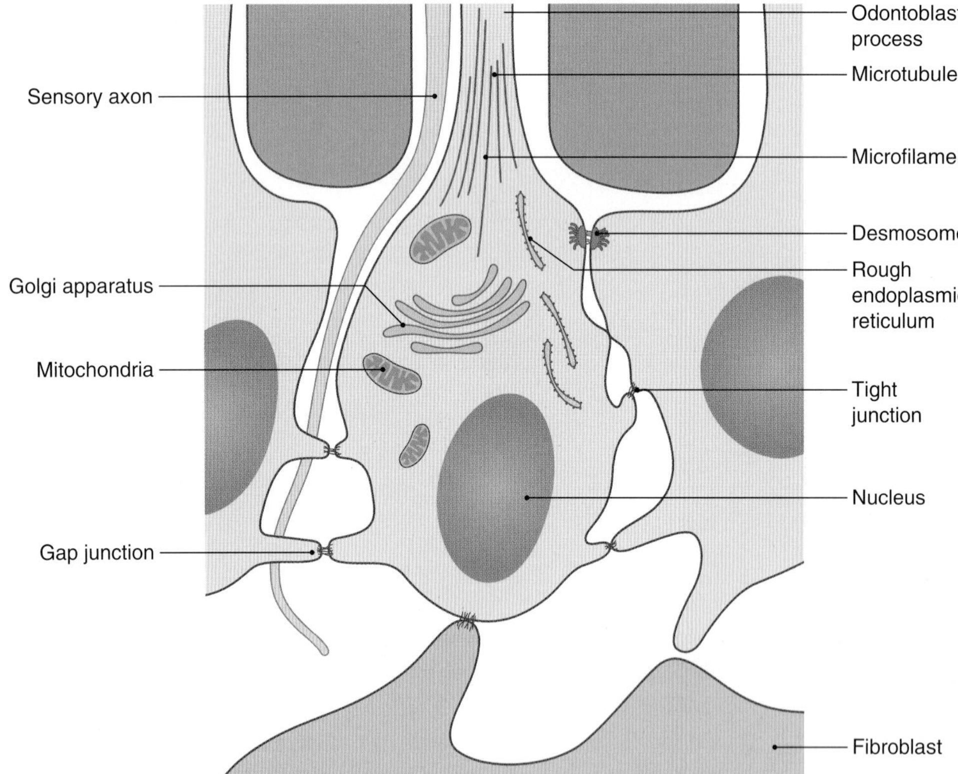

Fig. 10.12 The ultrastructure of the odontoblast in a mature tooth is typical of a polarised protein-synthesising cell of low activity containing all the organelles associated with this process (mitochondria, rough endoplasmic reticulum, Golgi apparatus) in the supranuclear region. One large process enters a dentinal tubule, but many smaller ones link the odontoblast to its neighbouring odontoblasts and fibroblasts.

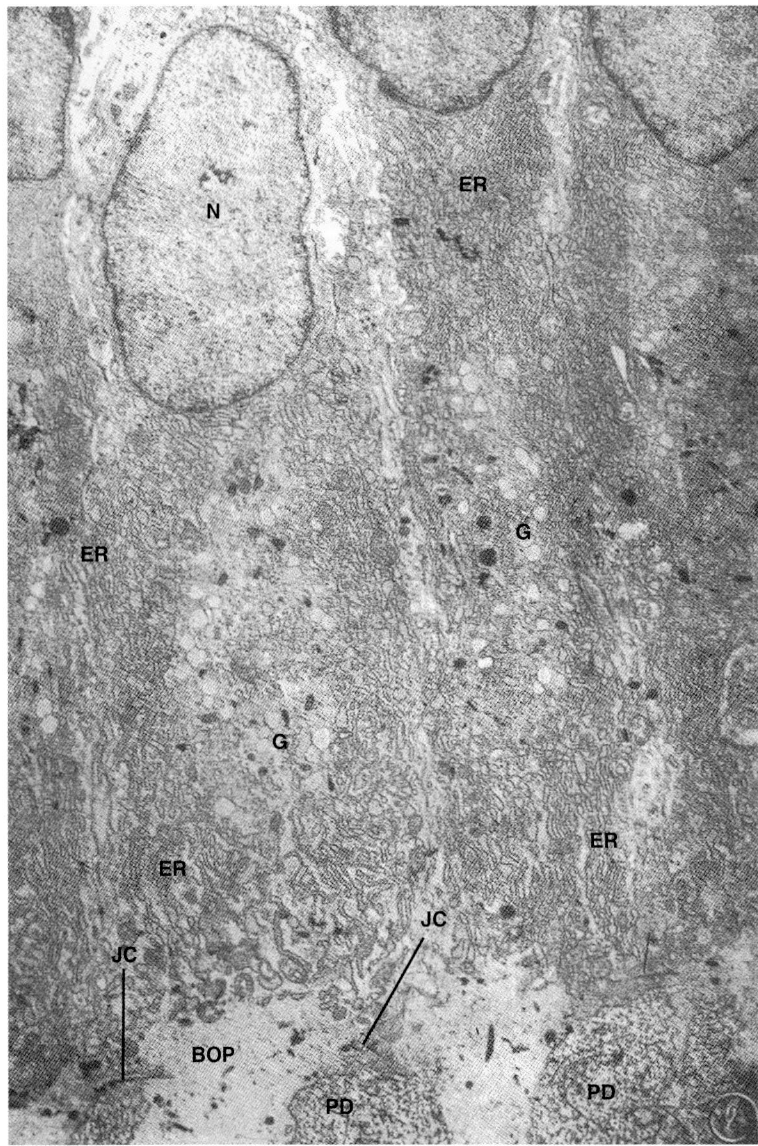

Fig. 10.13 TEM of an odontoblast. BOP = base of odontoblast process; ER = rough endoplasmic reticulum; G = Golgi apparatus; JC = junctional complex; N = nucleus; PD = predentine (×12,000). *Courtesy Prof. M M Smith.*

However, subodontoblastic stem cells can, in these circumstances, divide and differentiate and lay down a protective barrier of reparative tertiary dentine. Growth factors, especially members of the transforming growth factor (TGF)-β family, play an important role in controlling the synthetic activity of odontoblasts during development. They may also be significant in initiating the production of tertiary dentine in response to dental caries because they seem to be sequestered within mature dentine and may be released during carious breakdown. Odontoblasts in both healthy and diseased teeth express membrane receptors for the TGF-β family well above the level of other cells in the pulp.

The fully differentiated odontoblast is a polarised columnar cell with a long cell process that extends into the predentine and dentine within a dentinal tubule. It also has numerous smaller processes that link it to adjacent odontoblasts and other pulp cells.

The cell body is approximately 50 μm long and 5–10 μm in width. The nucleus sits in the basal (pulpal) half of the cell with the other organelles involved in dentine synthesis, the rough endoplasmic reticulum, Golgi complex and mitochondria, above it. These organelles are much more pronounced in an actively secreting cell (Fig. 10.13).

In the mature tooth the odontoblasts form a single layer of cells attached to the predentine surface. Coronal odontoblasts are columnar in outline; in the root they are commonly more cuboidal. The nuclei of adjacent cells in the layer lie at different levels, and when the layer is sectioned obliquely this gives the false appearance of multiple layers ('pseudostratification'; Figs. 10.10 and 10.11).

Dentine is formed almost exclusively by the odontoblasts, except possibly during the initial dentine formation that results in the mantle layer when some products from other cells are included (see page 176). The odontoblast continues to lay down secondary dentine at a slow rate throughout life. As it does so the pulp chamber becomes smaller and root canals narrower. The odontoblast layer becomes a flatter layer of cells, and the number of cells declines by apoptosis. It has been estimated that half the odontoblasts in a premolar will die in the 4 years after the completion of root formation. Although the odontoblast layer's prime role is dentinogenesis, it has other significant properties that help preserve the well-being of the pulp. It acts as a selective barrier reducing the speed with which toxins can reach the pulp while at the same time allowing tissue fluid from the pulp to enter and perhaps circulate within the dentinal tubules. There is a potential outward pressure of this 'dentinal fluid' that, should the dentine lose its enamel or cementum covering, would lead to an outward fluid flow that would dilute and wash away toxins diffusing along the tubules from the surface. The dentinal fluid differs in composition from the tissue fluid within the pulp, suggesting that the odontoblasts have a role in controlling its composition.

Because odontoblasts are located in the outermost layer of dental pulp, they are the first to recognise caries-related pathogens and sense external irritations. They possess a specialised innate immune system to fight oral pathogens invading into dentine. Generally, the rapid initial sensing of microbial pathogens, especially pathogen-associated molecular patterns shared by microorganisms, is mediated by pattern recognition receptors, such as Toll-like receptor and the nucleotide-binding oligomerisation domain. In response to bacterial toxins from dental caries, such as lipopolysaccharides, odontoblasts synthesise proinflammatory mediators, producing a range of cytokines (such as IL-1β, IL-6, IL-8, IL-12 and TNF-α) and chemokines (such as CCL1, CCL3-5, CCL8, CXCL1, CXCL3 and CXCL5). Cytokines and chemokines mediate the cross-talk between odontoblasts and cells of the innate immune system, such as neutrophils, monocytes/macrophages, dendritic cells, and natural killer cells. These proteins are secreted by both odontoblasts and immune cells in response to bacterial stimuli to attract additional immune cells, as well as initiate and modulate inflammatory responses.

It has been suggested that the odontoblast could act as a sensory receptor passing on information from the outer dentine to nerve fibres in the peripheral pulp. Odontoblast cell membranes contain numerous potassium channels in their apical end. These channels may have a role not only in mineralisation but also in the transduction of mechanical displacement into an electrical signal. Odontoblasts also express several classes of ion channels involved in nociception and signal propagation. However, it is not clear whether/how they can transduce the noxious signal to adjacent nerve fibre. Furthermore, there is no convincing evidence of synaptic junctions between odontoblasts and nerves, but because at least in the crown axons and odontoblast processes occupy the same narrow dentinal tubule, it is possible that the odontoblast could affect the excitability of the axon by modifying the ionic environment.

Cell junctions on odontoblasts

The odontoblast layer provides a controlled barrier between the pulp and the dentine. The integrity of the odontoblast layer and its limited permeability are maintained by numerous cell-to-cell junctions (Fig. 10.14). These are of three types:

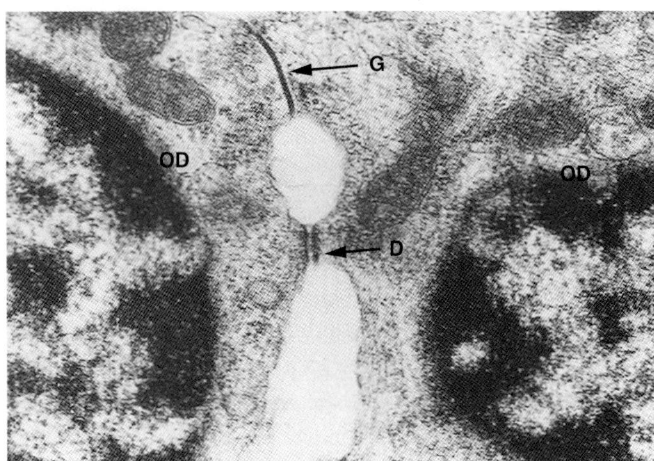

Fig. 10.14 TEM illustrating cell junctions between two odontoblast cell bodies (OD). D = desmosome; G = gap junction (×45,000).

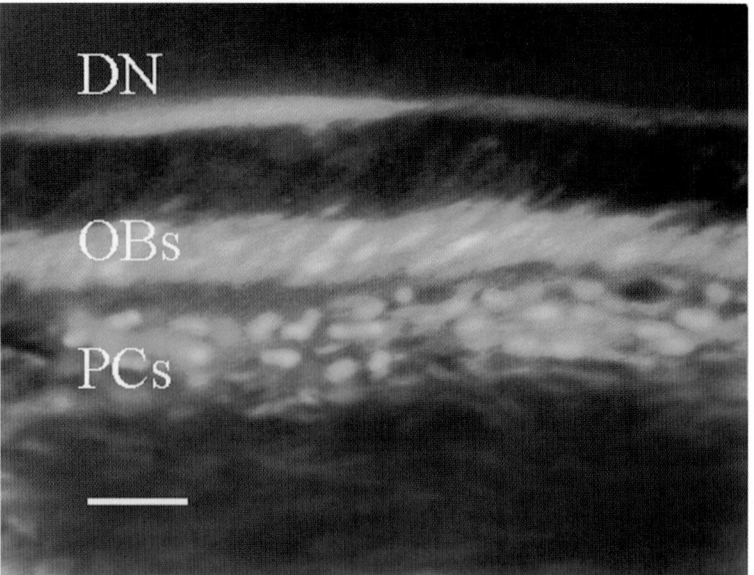

Fig. 10.15 A fluorescent dye, Lucifer yellow, has been applied to enamel. It is taken up by underlying odontoblasts (OBs) and passed on to other odontoblasts and other pulpal cells (PCs). DN = dentine (×50). *From Ikeda, H. et al. 1995. Three groups of afferent pulpal feline nerve fibres show different electrophysiological response properties. Archives of Oral Biology 40: 895–904, with permission.*

- The macula adherens junctions **(desmosomes)** have a clear intercellular component, as well as an intracellular system of anchoring fibrils, and they are largely responsible for mechanical union. Junctions that completely encircle the cells (zonula type) are not present.
- **Tight junctions** appear as a near fusion of apposing cell membranes and limit the permeability of the cell layer. The more tight junctions there are and the closer they are together, the lower is the permeability. These junctions do not completely encircle the odontoblasts and so limit rather than eliminate permeability. The tight junctions also add to the mechanical integrity of the layer. An arrangement like the 'terminal bar' apparatus found in epithelia (in which a regular pattern of both tight and adherens type junctions is arranged uniformly at the outer margin of the cell layer) is not found in the odontoblast layer. The odontoblast layer is not an epithelium.
- The third type of junction seen between odontoblasts is the **gap junction**. This allows the movement of small molecules directly between adjacent cells. It is important in cell-to-cell communication and would presumably have a role in synchronising the activity of all the odontoblasts in the layer.

As well as forming junctions with themselves, odontoblasts are also linked to other pulpal cells. In histological sections it is difficult to recognise the origin of most of the cell processes. Small processes from an odontoblast, fibroblast, stem cell and possibly even a defence cell or an unsheathed axon have a superficially similar appearance. Odontoblasts do have a close relationship with dendritic antigen-presenting cells (see pages 199–201), although the functional nature of this relationship has not been demonstrated. Fig. 10.15 shows that the odontoblast layer and the underlying pulpal cells form a kind of syncytium. A low-molecular-weight fluorescent dye, Lucifer yellow, was placed on the enamel surface of a tooth for 30 minutes. The tooth was then sectioned and examined under ultraviolet light. The dye fluoresces with a green colour. This is present within the cells of the odontoblast layer and the underlying pulpal cells, demonstrating that they are linked by junctions permitting the passage of small molecules.

During tooth development the activity of the odontoblasts is affected by many signalling and growth factors. In mature odontoblasts the genes for several growth factors, including TGF-β and bone morphogenetic protein (BMP), are expressed, suggesting perhaps that these cells are primed to activate other cells. Odontoblasts do not produce nerve growth factor (NGF) but may have it transferred to them because the odontoblast cell membrane contains NGF receptors. Injured odontoblasts produce heat shock proteins, metalloproteinases and the enzymes responsible for nitric oxide production.

Odontoblasts contain specialised pattern recognition receptors. These can initiate an immune response by secreting chemokines that recruit immature dendritic cells and beta defensins that kill bacteria.

Although the odontoblast cell itself is not thought to be directly associated with the transduction of sensory impulses (see page 187), the cell expresses several classes of ion channels involved in other sites with nociception and signal propagation. The functional significance of these in the odontoblast awaits further explanation.

The odontoblast process found in the dentinal tubule is described on pages 171–174.

Fibroblasts

The fibroblast is the ubiquitous cell of nonmineralised connective tissues. In the dental pulp, fibroblasts form a loose network throughout the tissue linked by adherens-type junctions and gap junctions. Pulpal fibroblasts secrete the collagen of the pulp, which is mainly types I and III. Their morphology is highly variable but is most aptly described as stellate, with the arms of the stars linking fibroblast to fibroblast or fibroblast to odontoblast (Fig. 10.16). Their most obvious role in the development of the tissue is the production of extracellular fibres and ground substance for the dental pulp. Because this production (and presumably turnover) is relatively slow, pulpal fibroblasts show only moderate amounts of associated intracellular organelles, such as endoplasmic reticulum, Golgi complex or mitochondria. They make little or no contribution to the production of dentine. Like fibroblasts in other sites, pulpal fibroblasts release growth factors and signalling agents, such as vascular endothelial growth factor (VEGF), fibroblast growth factor (FGF)-2, platelet-derived growth factor, BMP, TGF, and NGF.

Much of what is known about pulpal fibroblasts has been obtained from experiments in which they have been maintained in cell culture. These studies show that the pulpal fibroblast, as well as being able to secrete the components that form the extracellular matrix, can participate in their degradation. It thus seems likely that, in the mature tooth, the

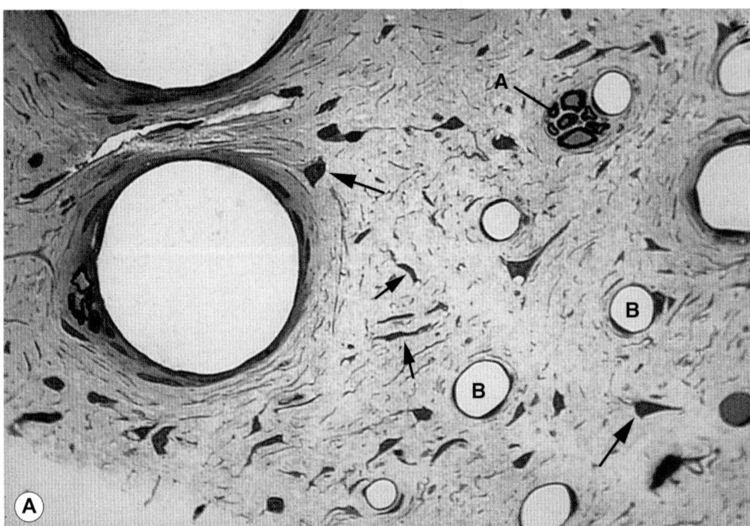

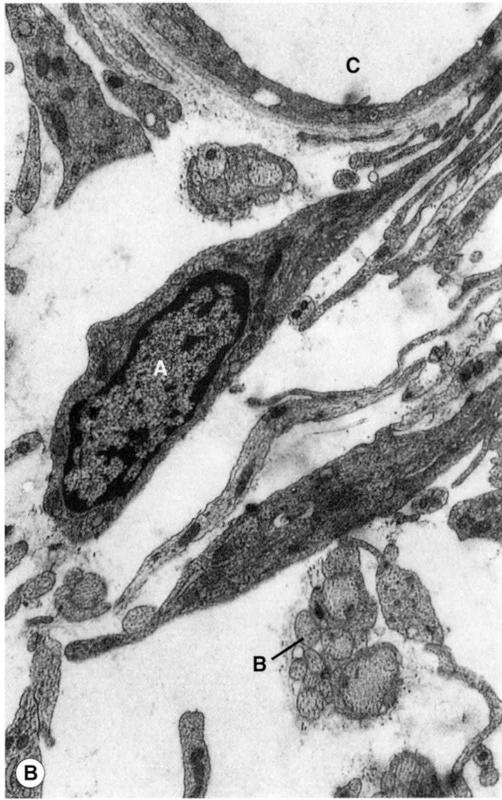

Fig. 10.16 (A) Semithin section of the central portion of the pulp showing the appearance of pulpal fibroblasts, which may vary from spindle-shaped (small arrows) to a more rounded and stellate shape (large arrow). A = myelinated fibres; B = capillary (toluidine blue; ×450). (B) TEM illustrating spindle-shaped pulpal fibroblasts (A). B = unmyelinated nerve axons; C = capillary. Note the absence of collagen fibrils in the extracellular matrix (×20,000).

fibroblasts slowly turn over the matrix. Cultured pulpal fibroblasts do undergo cell division, although mitotic figures are rarely encountered in the normal, uninjured dental pulp. Apoptosis (programmed cell death) has been demonstrated in the continuously growing incisor of the rat. It seems reasonable to expect cell turnover in the pulps of mature teeth of limited eruption.

Stem cells

In routinely stained sections the connective tissue cells in the pulp below the odontoblast layer all have a similar morphology. There are, in fact, significant functional differences in that subsets of this population are stem cells (Fig. 10.17). Many of the cell types in the dental pulp, including the odontoblasts, defence cells and possibly many fibroblasts, are terminally

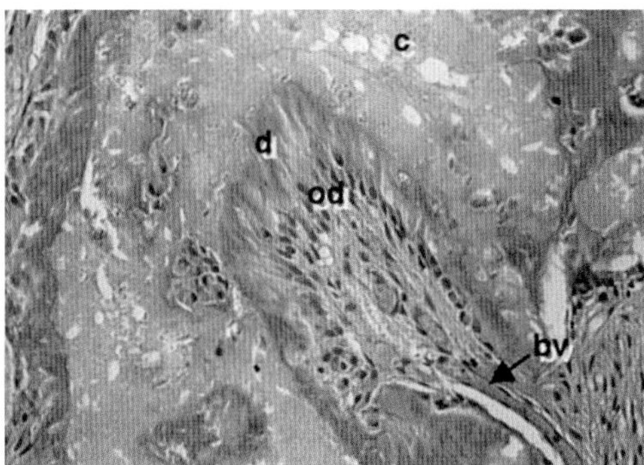

Fig. 10.17 Stem cells that were isolated from the dental pulp and then grown in culture were placed subcutaneously in mice in contact with a ceramic powder. The stem cells (od) lay down a dentine-like tissue (d) in contact with the ceramic (c). bv = blood vessel. (Polarised image.) *Courtesy Dr S Gronthos et al. and the editor of Proceedings of the National Academy of Sciences of the USA.*

differentiated and, although able to respond to stimuli in a predetermined manner, are unable to differentiate into another cell type. It has long been known that there is a population of precursor cells in the dental pulp that can, in response to a severe challenge, produce tertiary dentine. Under the influence of signaling molecules released in response to injury and cell death, these precursor cells migrate to the site of injury and differentiate into odontoblasts. Key signaling molecules in this process are members of the BMP family and TGF-β. These cells, in the past, have been given a variety of names, including 'pluripotential mesenchymal' and 'ectomesenchymal' cells, but they are now recognised as stem cells (See Chapter 28). They are defined by a similarity in gene expression to odontoblasts and by their ability to differentiate and form dentine under appropriate stimulation.

Dental pulp stem cells (DPSCs) may be found in two regions of the dental pulp: peripherally beneath the odontoblast layer and more centrally around blood vessels. Whether these represent a single population of stem cells awaits clarification. DPSCs are multipotent and can differentiate into cells of the adipogenic, osteogenic and chondrogenic lineage. They can also be made to differentiate into both neural and vascular endothelial cells. Thus, dental pulp cells have been cultured and used to replace nerve defects. Mesoblast, a leading global stem cell therapy development company, has taken out exclusive rights to patents covering DPSCs with the hope of treating conditions such as Parkinson's disease and stroke. It has been found that hydrogen sulphide increases hepatic differentiation in DPSCs so that they may provide a future form of treatment for kidney disease. Unusually, DPSCs show more developed and metabolically active cells than human bone marrow–derived cells.

The significance of DPSCs is considerable, because they may be harnessed in treatment using known signalling molecules to initiate or enhance the regenerative process. Stem cells are considered further in Chapter 28.

Defence cells

T lymphocytes are present in small numbers in the normal dental pulp (Fig. 10.18). Their numbers increase enormously when the pulp is injured or subjected to toxins.

Macrophages (Fig. 10.19) are a substantial presence. In their resting form (sometimes termed histiocytes or pericytes) they can appear in a variety of morphological forms and are difficult to distinguish from fibroblasts in routine histological preparations. Immunohistochemical techniques, however, show that they are widely distributed in considerable numbers.

Dendritic antigen-presenting cells (Figs. 10.20–10.23) are also an important component of the normal dental pulp. They are at least 50 μm long and have three or more main dendritic processes that branch. Like the macrophages, they are distributed throughout the pulp but most densely in the periphery and around nerves and blood vessels (Figs. 10.20, 10.21). Some dendritic cells extend processes into the dentinal tubules (Figs. 10.21, 10.22).

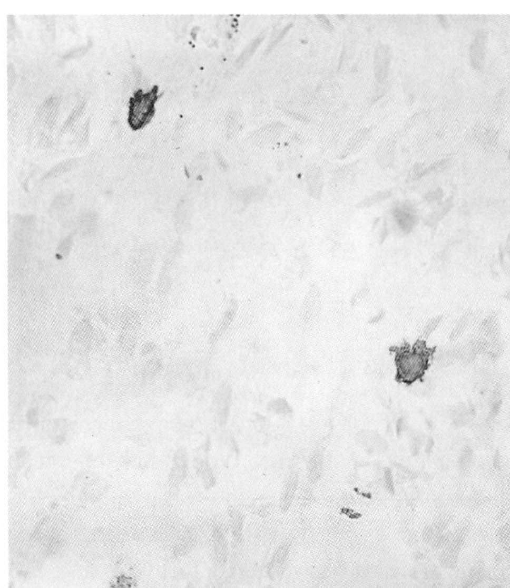

Fig. 10.18 Antibody staining (black) to identify T lymphocytes in the dental pulp (×500). *Courtesy Dr T Okiji and the editor of Journal of Dental Research.*

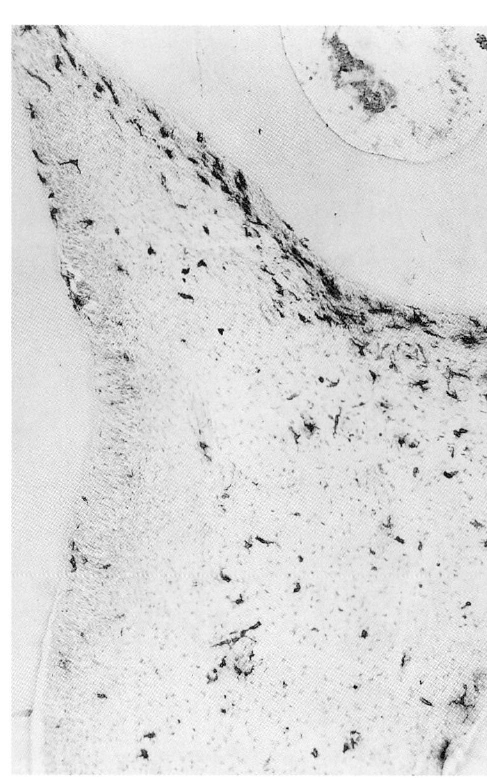

Fig. 10.20 Immunohistochemical stain (black) identifying antigen-presenting cells particularly prominent at the periphery of rat molar pulp (×70). *Courtesy Dr T Okiji and the editor of Journal of Dental Research.*

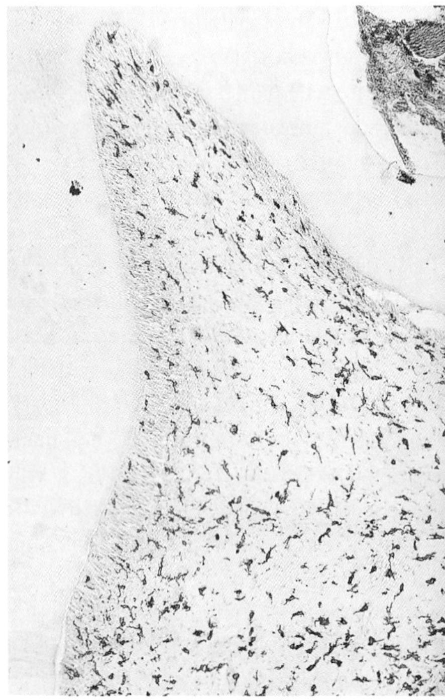

Fig. 10.19 Antibody staining (black) to demonstrate the wide distribution of macrophages in healthy rat dental pulp (×50). *Courtesy Dr T Okiji and the editor of Journal of Dental Research.*

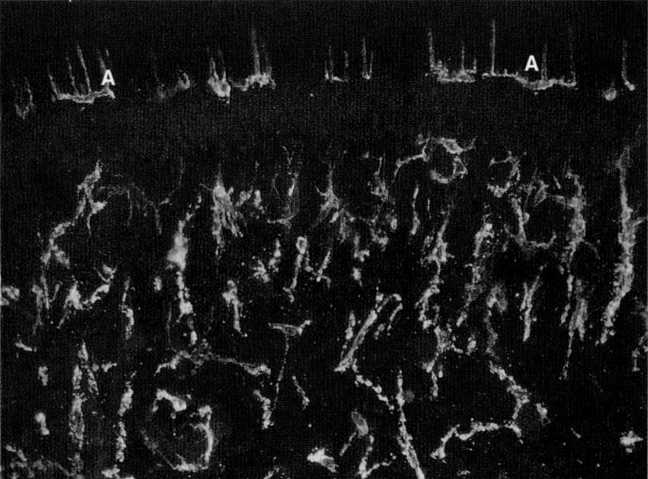

Fig. 10.21 Immunohistochemical stain (white) viewed under fluorescent light showing the distribution of antigen-presenting cells. Note the cells (A) at the periphery of the odontoblast layer have processes extending into the dentine (×200). *Courtesy Dr N Yoshiba and the editor of Journal of Dental Research.*

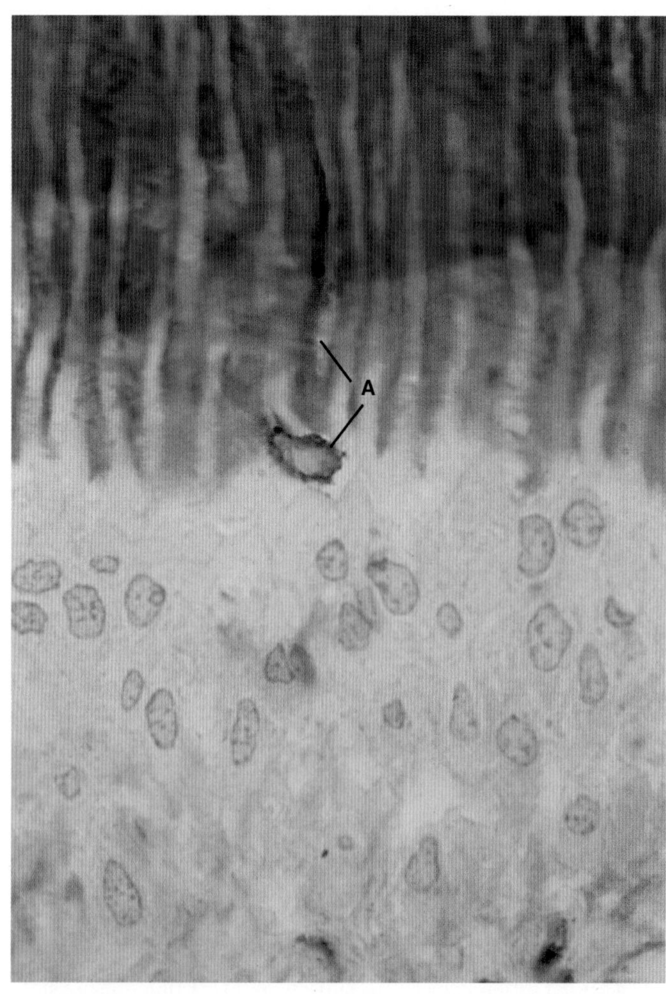

Fig. 10.22 Immunohistochemical stain (brown) identifying an antigen-presenting cell (A) in the outer odontoblast layer and extending a process into the inner dentine (methylene blue; ×500). *Courtesy Dr N Yoshiba and the editor of Journal of Dental Research.*

The dendritic cells act, at least primarily, as antigen-presenting cells stimulating the division and activity of naive T lymphocytes. Mature dendritic cells initiate the primary immune response and can migrate, with trapped antigen, to regional lymph nodes within 16 hours and induce T lymphocyte division and differentiation there. Following exposure to cariogenic bacteria, dental pulp dendritic cells migrate to regional lymph nodes in 16 hours. The cells that migrate represent mature cells expressing the highest levels of CD273 and CD86 costimulators and MHC class II.

Mast cells are difficult to demonstrate in the dental pulp because they are fragile and destroyed during processing for histology.

There is an intimate relationship between the immune and neural systems. After pulp injury, nerves release neuropeptides and other molecules that participate in the immune response. In animal experiments, removing the sympathetic innervation to the pulp increases the number of lymphocytes present even in the uninjured tissue. Many of the signalling molecules released by cells of the immune system have an effect on nerves, either increasing their excitability or in some cases reducing it. There is a close structural relationship between nerve fibres and immunocompetent cells (Fig. 10.23).

Blood vessels of the dental pulp

The pulp has a rich blood supply occupying about 40% of the total volume. The architectural arrangement of the blood vessels of the dental pulp closely parallels that of the nerves. The arrangement is clearly seen in pulps perfused with Indian Ink and cleared (Figs. 10.24, 10.25). Arterioles and venules enter the dental pulp via the apical foramina (Fig. 10.25B) and lateral canals as components of neurovascular bundles. The size of the blood vessels varies according to author and the techniques used; one stating that the largest vessels were approximately 150 microns in diameter, whereas another said diameters varied from 2 to 30 microns. Such variation may relate to different techniques of fixation and preparation. The blood vessels run longitudinally through the root canals (Fig. 10.24). Within the root canals, they send off side branches to the periphery (Figs. 10.24, 10.25). The vessels divide and narrow to some degree in the root canal but branch profusely once they are within the coronal pulp. Capillary loops extend towards the dentine. This looping is most easily demonstrated in animal preparations because plastic resins can be perfused through the vascular system and casts prepared (Figs. 10.26, 10.27).

A network of vessels beneath the odontoblasts (the subodontoblastic capillary plexus) is more evident in sectioned histological material than it is in three-dimensional casts. These capillaries are 6–8 μm in diameter. Capillaries are present both within (Fig. 10.28) and below the odontoblast layer (Fig. 10.29) and between the odontoblasts and the predentine. Capillaries do not enter the dentinal tubules. The fluid that is present in the dentine is probably an ultrafiltrate of the pulpal interstitial fluid. The arrangement of the blood vessels supplies oxygen and nutrients where they are most needed during dentinogenesis. The capillary network beneath the odontoblasts is dense enough to be known as the subodontoblastic

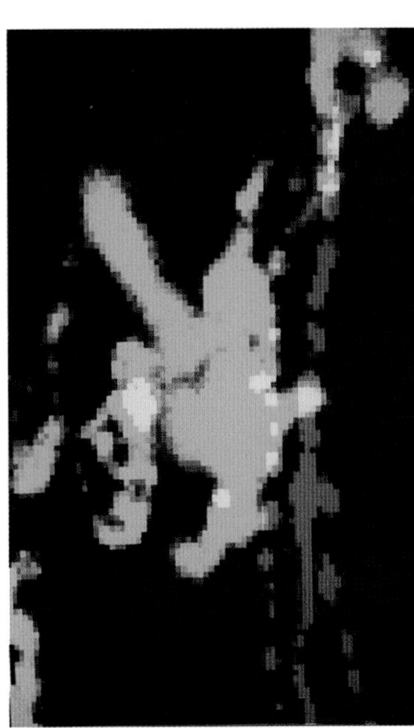

Fig. 10.23 Confocal laser scanning micrograph of a section of dental pulp from the pulp horn of a rat. It is double stained with two fluorescent dyes staining macrophages (green) and substance P–containing nerve fibres (red). This technique allows great depth of focus and, in this case, shows areas (in yellow) where the nerve and macrophage are in close contact (×1,000). *Courtesy Dr T Okiji and the editor of Journal of Dental Research.*

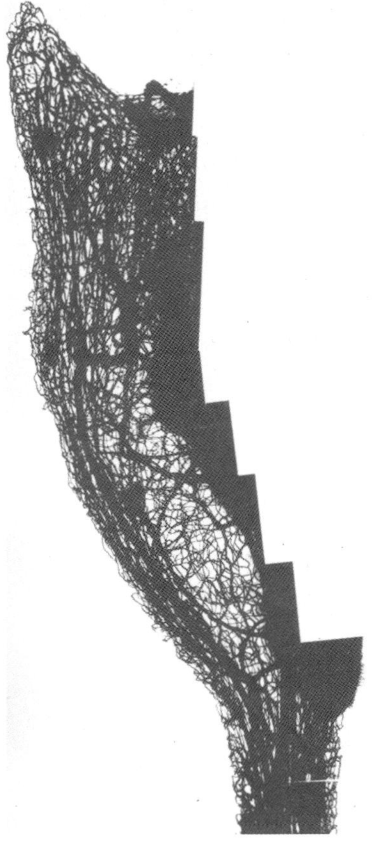

Fig. 10.24 India ink has been drawn into the vessels of the pulp in a human premolar, which has subsequently been cleared. This image is a montage of several micrographs. A large vessel, an arteriole, is seen running through much of the pulp with a network of branches arising from it. *Ikeda, H. et al. 1995. Three groups of afferent pulpal feline nerve fibres show different electrophysiological response properties. Archives of Oral Biology* 40: 895–904, with permission.

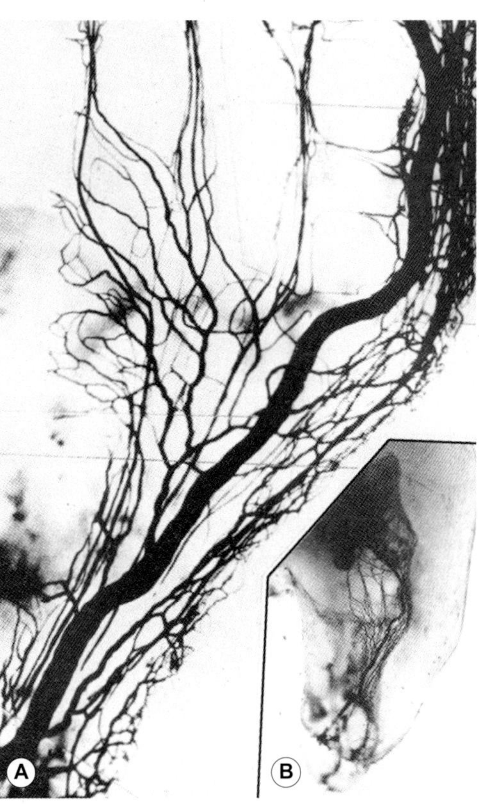

Fig. 10.25 (A) A molar root prepared as for Fig. 10.24. Note that the apex has two tips with one apical foramen in one and two in the other. (B) An enlargement of part of (A) showing a large central vessel and to the right a capillary plexus that would be below the odontoblast layer. *Ikeda, H. et al. 1995. Three groups of afferent pulpal feline nerve fibres show different electrophysiological response properties. Archives of Oral Biology 40: 895–904, with permission.*

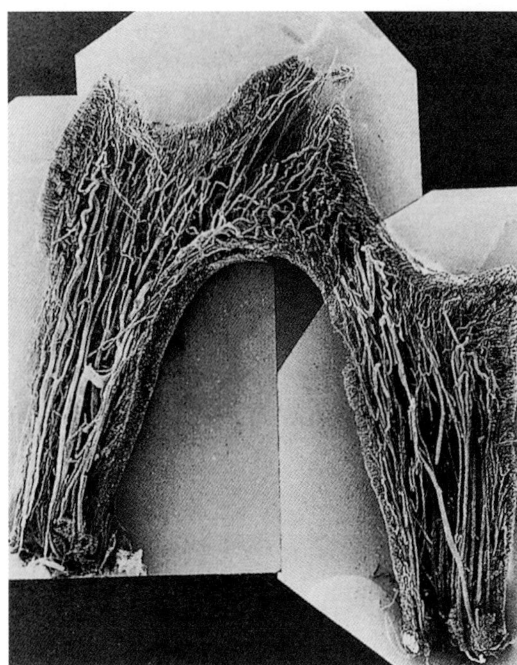

Fig. 10.26 SEM of a vascular cast of a dog mandibular molar. Arterioles run coronally along the sides of the root canal; venules drain in the centre. Larger vessels follow relatively straight pathways. Side branches subdivide to form a capillary network beneath the dentine (×8). *Courtesy Dr Y Kishi, Dr K Takahashi, Dr K. Kanagawa and the editor of Journal of Dental Research.*

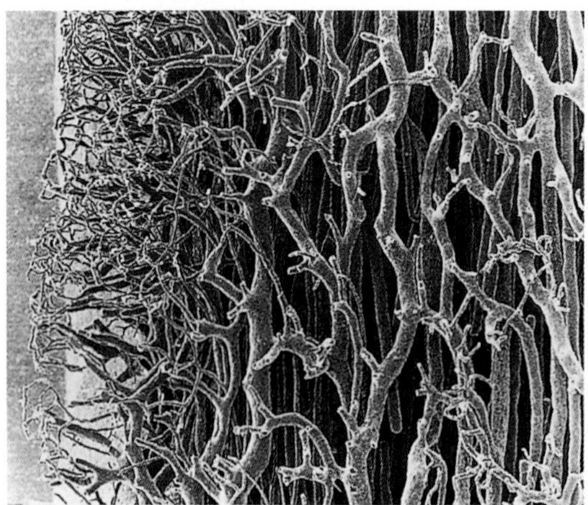

Fig. 10.27 SEM of a vascular cast of terminal capillary network in pulp. There are three layers of the terminal supply to the odontoblast layers: most superficially the flat-ended capillary loops, beneath these the capillary network and under these the venular network. Deep to all these layers are straight arterioles (×11). *Courtesy Dr K Takahashi, Dr Y Kishi, Dr S Kim and the editor of Journal of Endodontics.*

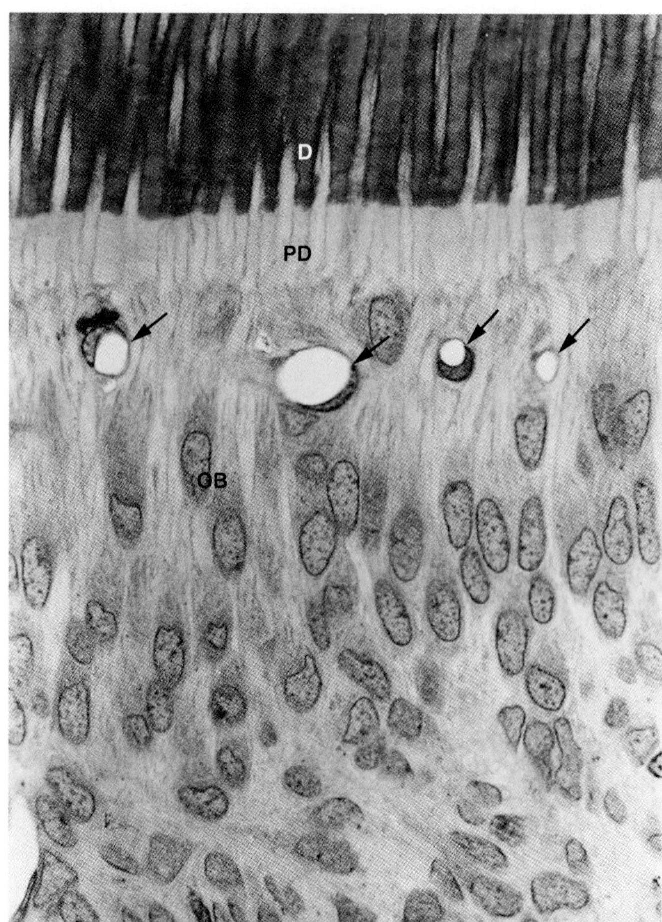

Fig. 10.28 TEM showing capillaries (arrows) in the odontoblast layer (OB). D = Dentine; PD = predentine (×1,200). *Courtesy Dr S Yoshida, Dr H Oshima and the editor of Anatomical Record.*

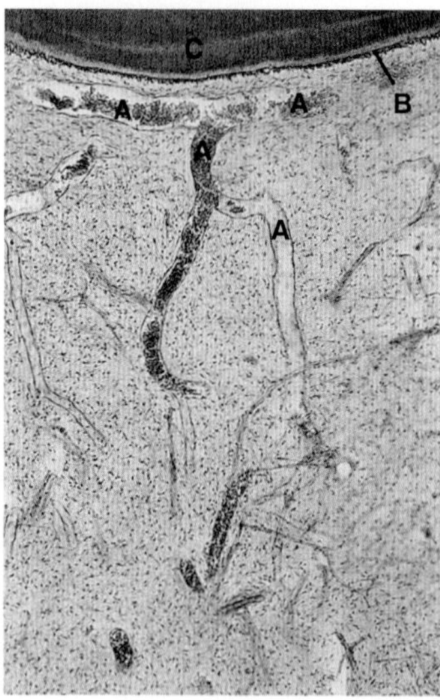

Fig. 10.29 Section of the dental pulp showing branching capillaries (A) below the odontoblast layer (B). C = dentine (H & E; ×100). *Courtesy Prof. L Fonzi.*

capillary plexus. Approximately 4–5% of the capillaries in the subodontoblastic zone are fenestrated (Fig. 10.30). Fenestrations are 60–80 nm in diameter. Only a basement membrane is present at the fenestrations, presumably allowing rapid diffusion of materials out of the capillary.

Numerous arteriovenous and venous–venous anastomoses (Fig. 10.31) are found between peripheral pulpal vessels, presumably to allow rapid changes in blood perfusion. The blood supply of the pulp is regulated largely by the sympathetic innervation associated with precapillary sphincters.

Lymphatic vessels in the pulp are small, blind-ended, thin-walled vessels. There are discontinuities in their walls, and this porosity permits the passage of interstitial tissue fluid and lymphocytes (Fig. 10.32). Lymphatics exit as one or two larger vessels through the apical foramen. The lymphatics assist in the removal of inflammatory exudates.

The presence of lymphatics in the dental pulp has also been confirmed using antibody stains that can distinguish lymphatics from blood vessels (Figs. 10.33, 10.34).

The presence of lymphatics in the pulp has been established by tracing particulate material from the pulp to regional lymph nodes. Retrograde lymphography deposits material into pulpal vessels.

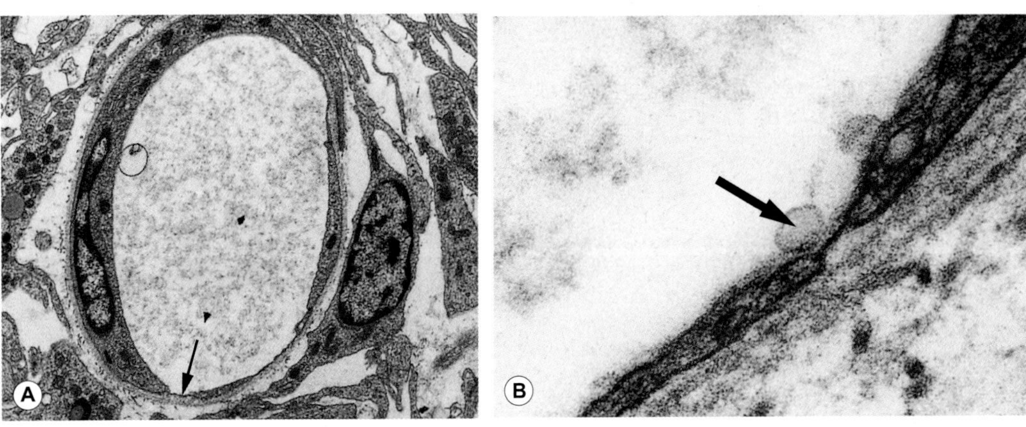

Fig. 10.30 (A) TEM of a subodontoblastic capillary with fenestration (arrowed) (×12,600). (B) TEM showing a fenestration (arrow) in a capillary wall (×31,500).

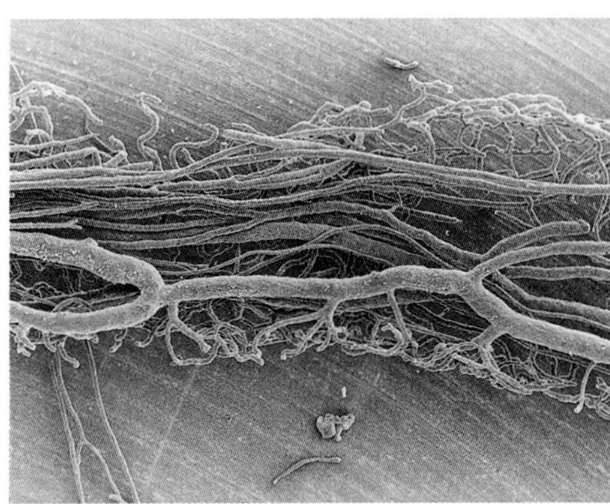

Fig. 10.31 SEM of a vascular cast showing a venous–venous anastomosis (×160). *Courtesy Drs Y Kishi and K Takahashi.*

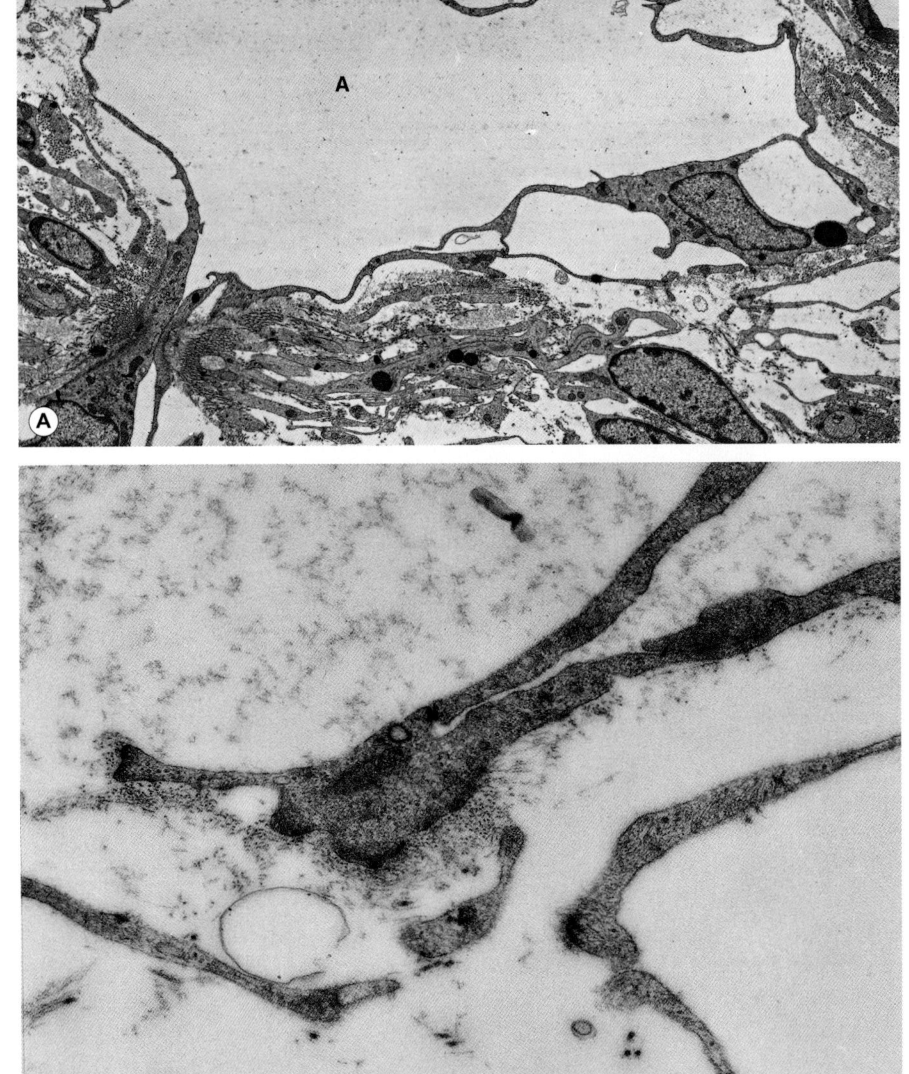

Fig. 10.32 (A) TEM of a lymphatic vessel (A) in the central dental pulp (×400). (B) Higher-power TEM of part of the wall of the lymphatic vessel, showing incomplete junctions between the cells and absence of a basement membrane (×3,000). *Courtesy Dr M Bishop.*

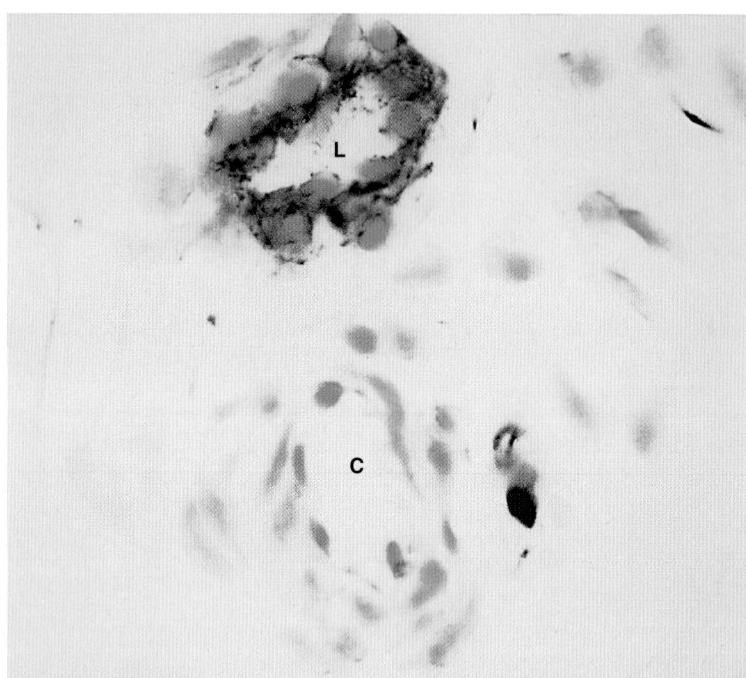

Fig. 10.33 A lymphatic vessel (L) from human dental pulp stained with an antibody against human thoracic duct. The dark-blue stain attaches to the endothelium. Another vessel, presumably a blood capillary (C), remains unstained (×1,000). *Courtesy Dr Y Sawa, Dr S Yoshida, Dr Y Ashikaga, Dr T Kim, Dr Y Yanaoka, Dr M Suzuki and the editor of Tissue and Cell.*

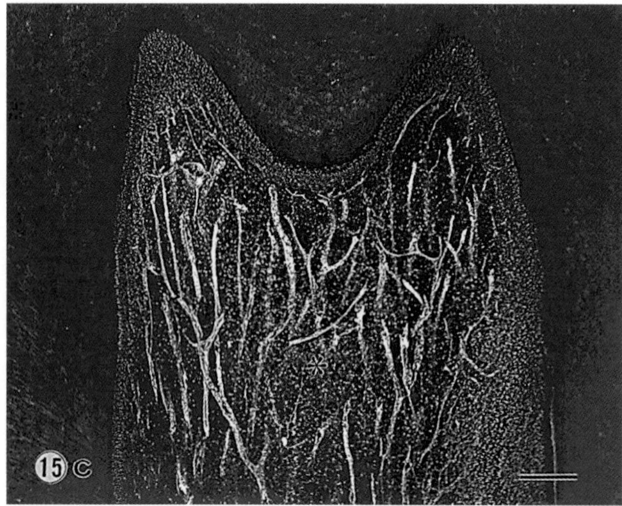

Fig. 10.34 SEM of secondary and backscattered electron imaging of the residual tissue block of a decalcified tooth after cryosectioning. Using 5′-nucleotidase alkaline phosphatase (ALPase) double staining allows the lymphatic vessels to appear white and be differentiated from blood vessels. Scale bar = 200 mm. From Matsumto, Y., Zhang, B., Kato, S. 2002. Lymphatic networks in the periodontal tissue and dental pulp as revealed by histochemical study. *Microscopy Research and Technique* 56: 50–59.

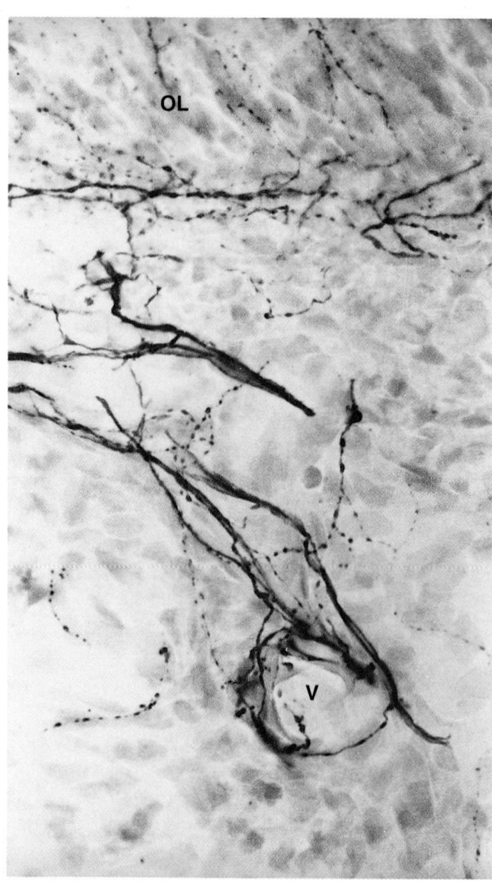

Fig. 10.35 Immunohistochemical method demonstrating varicose calcitonin gene–related peptide (CGRP)-immunoreactive nerve fibres (black) around a blood vessel (V) and in the odontoblast layer (OL) (×1,600). *Courtesy Dr J-Q Zhang, Dr K Nagata, Dr T Iijima and the editor of Anatomical Record.*

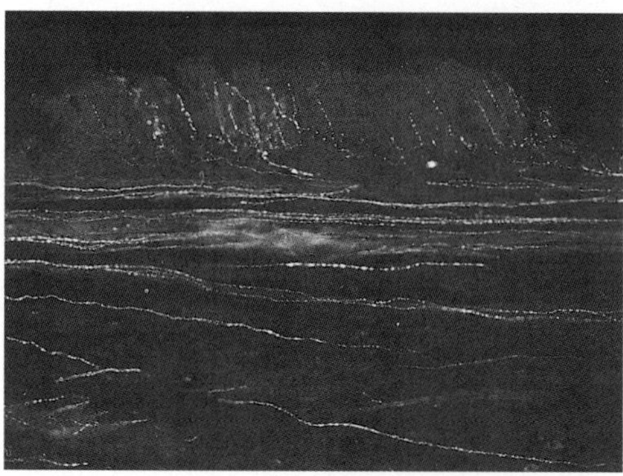

Fig. 10.36 Immunohistochemical staining demonstrating substance P–containing nerve fibres (white) in the odontoblast layer (top) and in the subodontoblastic plexus (dark field illumination; ×300).

In the healthy pulp, blood flow is under nervous control. The smooth muscle of the arterioles (present in the central radicular pulp) is innervated by terminals of sympathetic nerves, which maintain a vasoconstrictor tone as they do in most other sites. The neurotransmitters are noradrenaline (norepinephrine) and neuropeptide Y. There is little evidence for parasympathetic innervation of the pulp. Vasoconstrictor tone probably accounts for most of the vascular control, but afferent (sensory) nerves also have effects not only on vessel dilatation but also on capillary permeability. The vasoactive contribution of the afferent nerves is largely in the peripheral pulp and becomes significant when there is inflammation. The most prominent neuropeptides in these nerves are calcitonin gene–related peptide (CGRP) (Fig. 10.35) and substance P (Fig. 10.36), both of which induce vasodilatation and increased capillary permeability. Nitric oxide also acts as a vasodilator. It is too volatile to demonstrate directly, but the presence of the enzyme responsible for forming it, nitric oxide synthetase, has been found in nerve fibres in the coronal pulp (Fig. 10.37). Neuropeptide Y has also been demonstrated in peripheral axons (Fig. 10.38), including some within the odontoblast layer. Their role in this position is unknown.

Pulpal blood flow has been estimated to be 20–60 mL/min per 100 g of tissue. The pulp has a high, pulsatile interstitial tissue fluid pressure. This pressure would allow dentinal fluid to move outwards whenever the dentinal tubules were patent peripherally. It may also slow the inward movement of toxins during the progression of dental caries.

Nerves of the dental pulp

The dental pulp is richly innervated. For example, approximately 2,500 axons enter the apical foramen of a mature premolar; 25% of these are

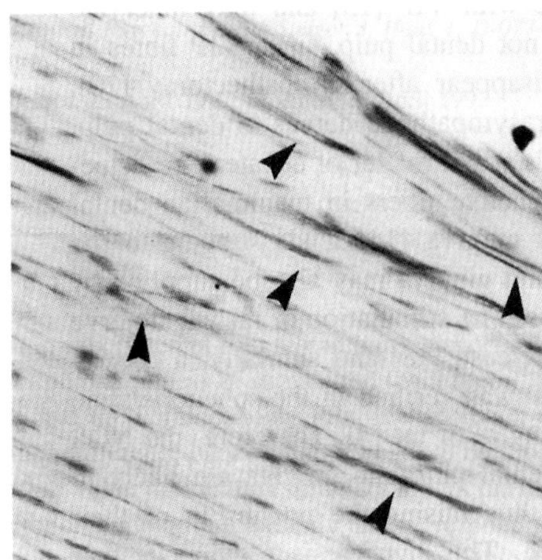

Fig. 10.37 Immunohistochemical staining to show nerve fibres (arrowed) staining for nitric oxide synthetase in dog coronal pulp (×140). *Courtesy Dr Z Lohinai et al and the editor of Neuroscience Letters.*

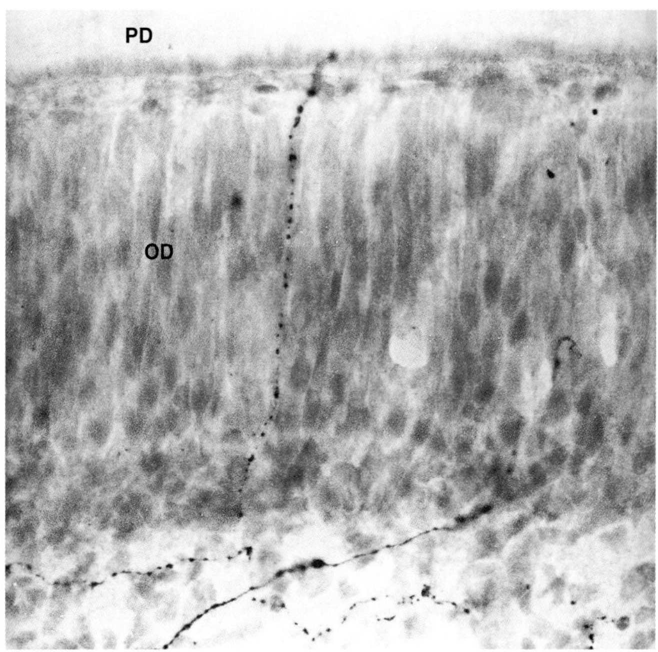

Fig. 10.38 Immunohistochemical labelling (black) showing neuropeptide Y–containing nerve fibres in and below the odontoblast layer (OD). PD = predentine (×1,600). *Courtesy Dr J-Q Zhang, Dr K Nagata, Dr T Iijima and the editor of Anatomical Record.*

myelinated afferents whose cell bodies lie in the trigeminal ganglion. Of these 90% are narrow Aδ fibres (1–6 μm in diameter), with the rest belonging to the wider Aβ group (6–12 μm in diameter). The unmyelinated C fibres are either afferent or autonomic. Although the nerve fibres enter the dental pulp in bundles, there is only a scant perineurium or epineurium.

The apical neural bundles have an average diameter of 25 microns (range 2–35 microns) and collectively occupy near 40% of the dental pulp volume. The average diameter of the nerve bundles in the mid-root and coronal areas is 12 and 7 microns, respectively.

The nerve bundles run centrally in the pulp of the root in close association with the blood vessels. A few fibres leave the central bundles in the root and travel to the periphery. Most continue to the coronal pulp where they spread apart and branch profusely (Fig. 10.39). Most of the branches end in the odontoblastic or subodontoblastic region (Fig. 10.40). In the crown, there is a pronounced plexus of nerves beneath the odontoblasts known as the plexus of Raschkow. This plexus is not evident until after the tooth has erupted. Branches from the plexus pass into the odontoblast layer and form the marginal plexus between the odontoblast layer and the predentine; others continue into the dentine to accompany odontoblast processes in the dentinal tubules. This subodontoblastic plexus may be one of the sites of sensory activation in the pulp. Many of the axons are devoid of a Schwann cell covering, either completely or partially, rendering them susceptible to changes in the extracellular environment (Fig. 10.41). The axons branch profusely, providing a broad surface area for activation. Within the Schwann cell, there are often many axons in a single pocket, and the spread of signals from axon to axon is possible.

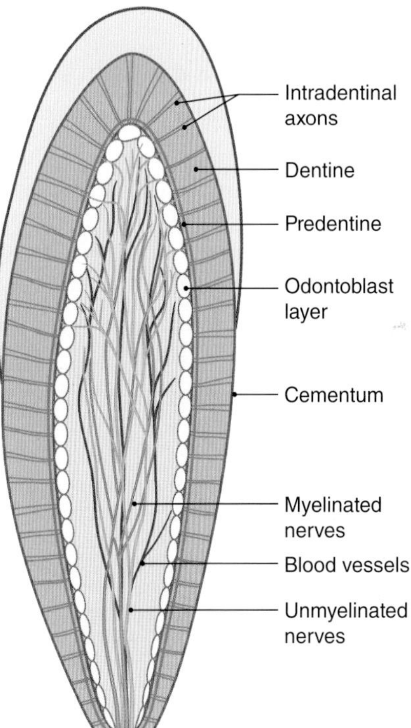

Fig. 10.39 General distribution of myelinated nerves (green), nonmyelinated nerves (yellow) and blood vessels (red) in the pulp.

Nerve fibre types

Afferent nociceptors

The myelinated nerves in the dental pulp (Fig. 10.16A) are trigeminal afferents. They are all thought to be nociceptive and carry sensations of sharp pain centrally. The larger-diameter Aβ afferents in some regions carry other nonnoxious sensations, but there is no clear evidence that any sensation other than pain can be experienced from the pulp with physiological stimuli. Pain and nociception are not synonymous. Pain is a subjective sensation and is defined as 'an unpleasant sensory and emotional experience associated with actual or potential tissue damage, or described in terms of such damage'. Nociception, in contrast, describes a series of objective neuronal processes and is defined as the reception, conduction and central processing of noxious signals. Nociceptors are essentially receptors that respond to harmful or potentially harmful (noxious) stimuli. Pain clearly can be a result of stimulation of nociceptors, but so are some reflexes and changes in arousal state without the organism sensing pain.

Nociceptors are thought to be free nerve endings and appear to respond specifically to noxious heat, intense pressure, or irritant chemicals, but not by innocuous stimuli such as warming, cooling or light touch. Fibres innervating the region of the head arise from cell bodies in the trigeminal ganglion.

There are considered to be three major classes of nociceptors: thermal, mechanical and polymodal.

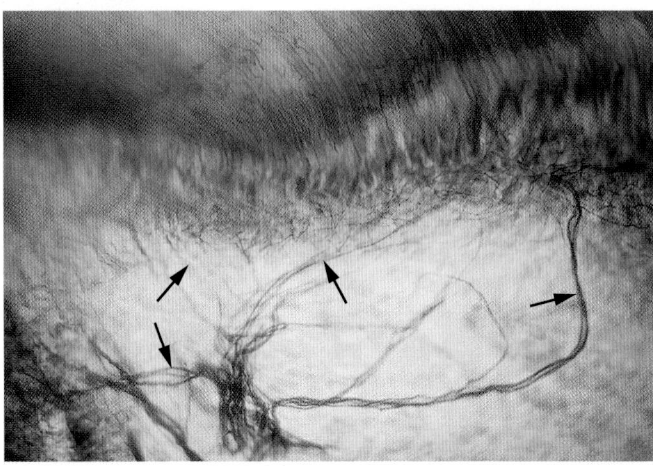

Fig. 10.40 Terminal branching of sensory fibres (arrows) in the dental pulp. This very thick section allows the axons at several levels to be seen, including the subodontoblastic nerve plexus of Raschkow (silver stain; ×140).

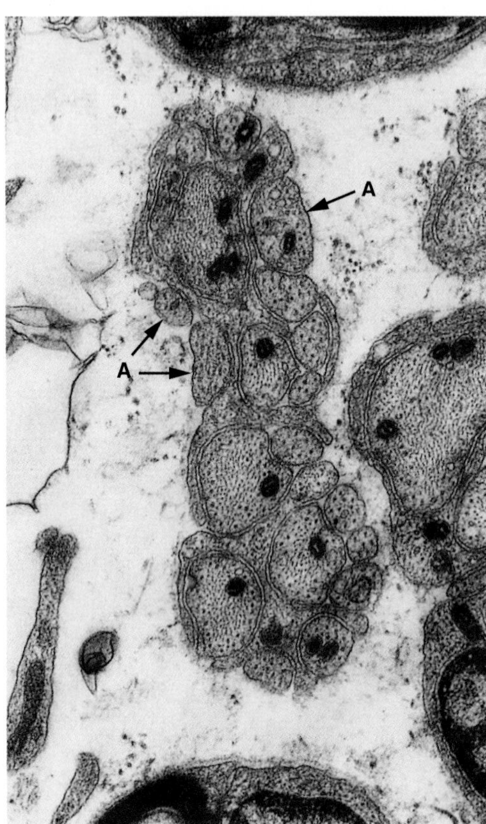

Fig. 10.41 TEM showing nerve fibres in the subodontoblastic plexus. Many of the axons are incompletely sheathed by Schwann cells (A), perhaps making them more susceptible to changes in the local environment (×40,000).

- Thermal nociceptors, which are activated by extreme temperatures >45°C or <5°C, are innervated by small myelinated Aδ fibres that conduct impulses at about 5–30 m/s.
- Mechanical nociceptors are activated by intense pressure applied to the tissues in which they lie and are also innervated by small myelinated Aδ fibres.
- Polymodal nociceptors are activated by high-intensity mechanical, chemical or thermal (both hot and cold) stimuli and are innervated by either Aδ fibres or unmyelinated C fibres with conduction velocities of less than 0.5–2 m/s.

The cell bodies of nociceptor neurones in the oral and facial regions are to be found in the trigeminal ganglion, and the central axons project via the trigeminal sensory root to synapse in the trigeminal spinal nucleus and, in particular, the subnucleus caudalis. Nociceptive neurones in the nucleus caudalis fall into two distinct types: those that receive inputs specifically from nociceptors, the so-called nociceptive-specific cells, and a second group of cells that receive inputs from a wide range of receptors such as nociceptors, mechanoreceptors and thermoreceptors, the so-called nociceptive-nonspecific cells. It is thought that the nociceptive-specific neurones signal the presence and location of the noxious stimulus, whilst the nociceptive-nonspecific neurones may grade the overall severity of the stimulus. There is evidence of primary afferent divergence and convergence within the nucleus caudalis onto second-order neurones, with each primary afferent branching and synapsing with several second-order neurones and each second-order neurone receiving inputs from a number of primary afferent fibres. These phenomena may explain why pain appears to radiate and come from a larger area than that injured or inflamed. Convergence of primary afferent neurones can also explain the phenomenon of referred pain, where pain appears to come from structures other than the injured or inflamed tissue.

Most of the nonmyelinated C fibres (Fig. 10.16B) are also afferent and involved in the conduction of noxious information centrally. At least as important as the sensory functions of both these afferent nerve groups is their role in axon reflexes. In these reflexes, action potentials generated in one terminal branch travel centrally and then pass anterogradely (central to peripheral) down other branches, resulting in the release of neuropeptides important in the local control of blood flow (but perhaps with other functions as well). It has been suggested that some pulpal nerves may have direct trophic effects, perhaps controlling, in part, the activity of odontoblasts. There is, however, no convincing evidence of an effect other than one that might be mediated by blood flow changes.

Autonomic fibres

Some of the C fibres are sympathetic efferents and supply arteriolar smooth muscle. Because there are only a few arterioles within the dental pulp, sympathetic fibres are scarce (Fig. 10.42). They seem to mediate their vasoconstrictive effect by the release of noradrenaline (norepinephrine)

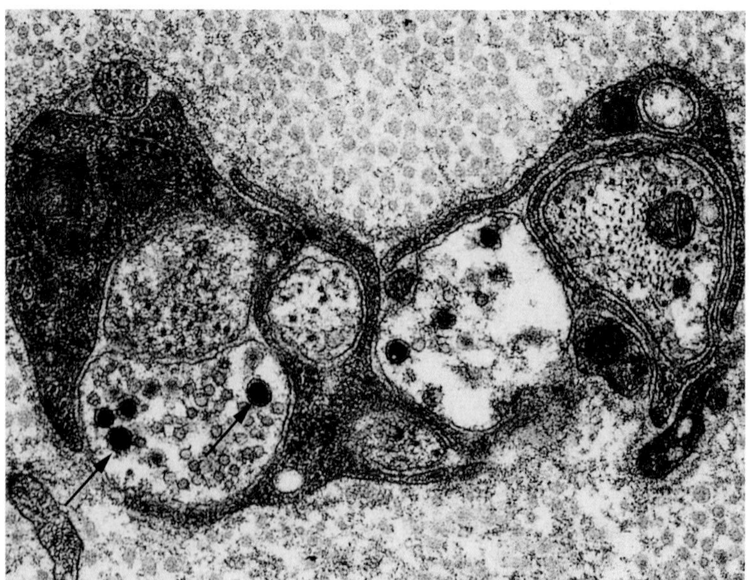

Fig. 10.42 TEM demonstrating sympathetic axons from an animal injected with a false neurotransmitter, 6-hydroxydopamine, which is taken up, but not released, by noradrenergic axons. The false neurotransmitter accumulates as dense-cored vesicles (arrowed) identifying the sympathetic axons. In this nerve fibre the sympathetic axons are contained in the same Schwann cell pocket as unlabelled, presumably sensory, axons. Simultaneous activation of sympathetic axons amplifies the activity in sensory nerves. The close approximation of sensory and sympathetic axons may explain this interaction (×31,000).

and neuropeptide Y. Evidence for parasympathetic innervation of the dental pulp is weak. Acetylcholine, the principal mediator for the parasympathetic system, is rarely detected in the dental pulp. Vasodilatation seems to be affected by axon reflexes involving afferent nerves, as well as (presumably as in other tissues) by the buildup of metabolites locally. Nitric oxide produced after hypoxia and tissue injury in the dental pulp is the signalling molecule most likely to induce vasodilatation under these conditions.

Nerve endings

It is difficult to determine where all nerve fibres end. Autonomic nerves end on the smooth muscle of the arterioles, and special neuromuscular junctions are present. Some of the afferent fibres (probably a proportion of the Aδ fibres) enter the tubules largely in the coronal dentine and predentine. Others may end at the pulp–predentine junction in what is sometimes known as the marginal plexus (Fig. 10.43). Both of these groups would be in an ideal position to detect stimuli applied to the outside of the dentine.

Many axons end in close proximity to odontoblasts. It has been suggested that there are specialised junctions between odontoblasts and nerves, but confirmatory evidence is lacking, although recent studies describe the proteins synapsin and synaptotagmin, characteristic of neural junctions, in the dentinal tubules. Although odontoblasts participate in many gap junctions (which elsewhere can act as electrical synapses), the cell processes involved in these junctions seem to come from other odontoblasts or from fibroblasts. The nerve–odontoblast relationship may be functionally, if not structurally, significant because the odontoblast or its process would dominate the local environment in which naked axons were present, especially in the dentinal tubules.

The nerves in the dentinal tubules, at the pulp–predentine border and among the odontoblast cell body, have all lost their ensheathing Schwann cells, and their axolemmas are exposed directly to the extracellular environment (Fig. 10.43). Changes in the composition of, or movement within, the extracellular fluid could readily affect the membrane properties of these terminals. Most activity in these terminals probably does not reach the level of sensation but presumably results locally in the release of neuropeptides by axon reflexes. The variety of neuropeptides found in the dental pulp is considerable. The most widely distributed, and possibly the most significant functionally, is CGRP (Fig. 10.44A), whose name derives from its first discovery and does not represent the widespread role it is now known to have.

CGRP is a potent vasodilator and quite possibly the principal agent controlling blood flow locally in the periphery of the dental pulp. CGRP is synthesised in the cell bodies of the nerves in the trigeminal ganglion and moved peripherally by axonal transport. Clearly a message, presumably a signalling molecule such as NGF, is carried from the periphery of the dental pulp to the ganglion cell body to modulate the production of CGRP. As well as having a role in pulpal blood flow, CGRP may participate in initiating or controlling hard-tissue production. Dental pulp cells, when maintained *in vitro*, respond to the application of CGRP with increased production of BMP-2, a signalling molecule known to be involved in dentine formation. NGF and NGF receptors have been detected in the peripheral dental pulp. Both NGF and receptors for it are found on odontoblasts, as well as pulpal nerves. NGF appears not to be produced by odontoblasts but donated by neighbouring fibroblasts. The expression of both NGF and its receptors increases in the injured pulp. Apart from a direct neural role, NGF may be a chemoattractant for leukocytes in the damaged pulp.

Although something of a paradigm shift from the original division of sensory and motor functions between different components of the nervous system, it seems reasonable to suggest that the major role of the trigeminal afferents in the dental pulp is in controlling the local environment rather than in carrying sensory information centrally. Some neuropeptides may function to control the flow of sensory activity centrally. The experience of toothache makes one realise that the balance of activities is flexible.

Several other neuropeptides and transmitters have been found in the normal dental pulp, and it is possible, based on their known activities in other sites, to speculate on their role in the pulp (Table 10.2). We are a long way from understanding what such a large number of agents contributes to the intact pulp and how they interact. In the injured pulp the number of biologically active molecules present increases substantially, and many of those detectable in normal pulps increase in quantity and distribution. It is likely that the continuous release of such peptides plays a role in the homeostasis of the dental pulp (Fig. 10.44).

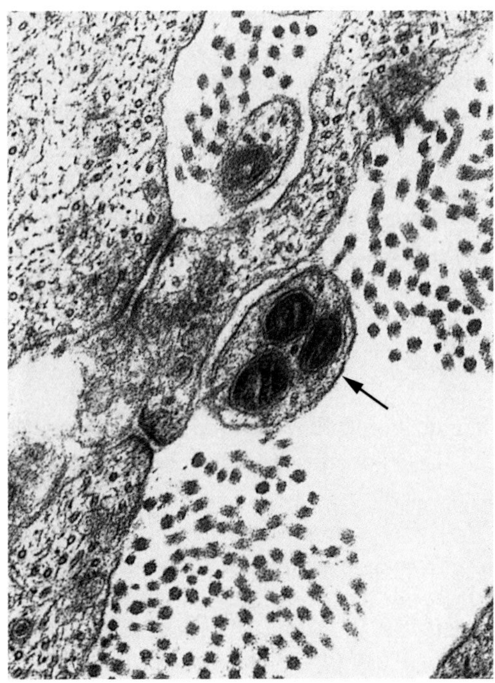

Fig. 10.43 Unsheathed, unmyelinated axon (arrowed) at the pulp (left) predentine border. Such axons may be activated by stimuli applied to dentine that cause fluid movement through the dentinal tubules (TEM; ×85,000).

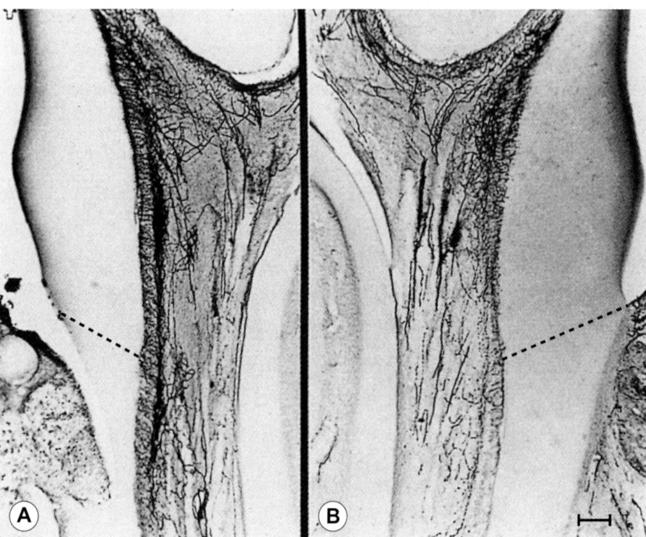

Fig. 10.44 Pulpal nerves stained immunohistochemically (black) for calcitonin gene–related peptide (CGRP). (A) A tooth in which a cervical cavity was cut 12 days earlier; (B) a normal control tooth. The broken line approximates the boundary between coronal and radicular dentine. There are many more CGRP-staining nerves after cavity preparation. Marker bar = 0.1 mm. *Courtesy Dr R Taylor, Dr M Byers and the editor of Brain Research.*

Table 10.2 Neuropeptides and neurotransmitters identified in the dental pulp with possible roles (largely interpolated from actions in other tissues)

Neuropeptide/small molecule transmitter	Possible role
Calcitonin-gene-related peptide	Vasodilatation, stimulates cell division in pulpal fibroblasts
Substance P	Vasodilatation, ?nociceptive transmitter, stimulates cell division in pulpal fibroblasts
Neuropeptide Y	Sympathetic vasoconstrictor
Noradrenaline (norepinephrine)	Sympathetic vasoconstrictor
Enkephalin	Silencer of nociceptors
Somatostatin	Silencer of nociceptors
Endorphin	Silencer of nociceptors
Dopamine	Vasoactive or a precursor of adrenaline (epinephrine)
Adrenaline (epinephrine)	Vasoconstrictive via smooth muscle in arterioles
Cholecystokinin	Unknown
Vasoactive intestinal polypeptide	?Parasympathetic
Secretoneurin	Axon reflexes
Neurokinin A	Vasodilatation, ?nociceptive transmitter, stimulates cell division in pulpal fibroblasts
Peptide histidine isoleucine amide	?Parasympathetic
?Acetylcholine	?Parasympathetic

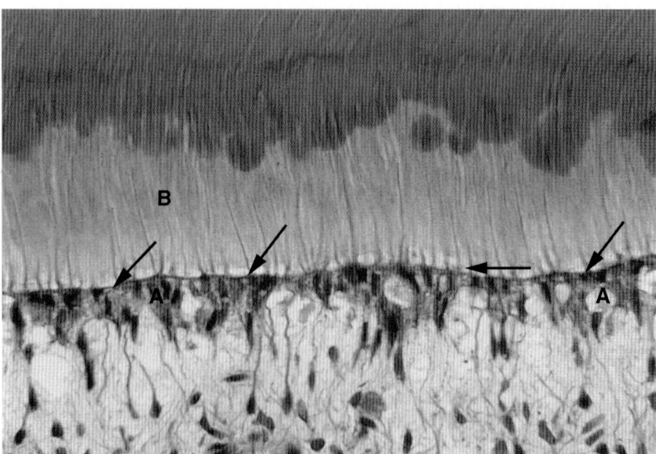

Fig. 10.45 Micrograph of the pulp–dentine boundary exhibiting slight shrinkage and showing continuity of odontoblast processes (arrows) with odontoblast cell bodies (A). B = predentine. Note the globular (calcospheritic) nature of the mineralising front (H & E; ×400).

Regions

The structure of the dental pulp can be described on a regional basis (Fig. 10.11). Beginning from the outside, the potential space between the odontoblast layer and the predentine could be described as the supraodontoblast region. In most histological preparations there is shrinkage of the soft pulp away from the dentine, creating a space in this region that is not present in the vital tissue. However, such preparations are useful in demonstrating the presence of odontoblast processes (Fig. 10.45). Two important structures are located in this region:

- Unsheathed axons, found almost exclusively in the crown. These have been described as the predentinal plexus (of Bradlaw). They are not a true plexus (network) but an area where axons congregate. It is not clear whether many axons end in this plexus. Most, presumably, continue to enter and end within dentinal tubules. These axons are in an ideal position to sense changes in fluid movement through the dentinal tubules, as well as changes in the extracellular fluid composition, which, because of the barrier properties of the odontoblast layer, will be delayed in reaching the core of the pulp.
- Dendritic antigen-presenting cells (described earlier).

This region thus deserves some special recognition because (after the odontoblast process) it is the first level at which external stimuli can be detected in the pulp.

The odontoblast layer (Figs. 10.11, 10.12) is, self-evidently, the effector system of the pulp. All other elements of the pulp are supportive or protective of the cells forming dentine or those programmed to replace them should they be lost.

The subodontoblastic zone (Fig. 10.11) has several terms associated with it. Immediately beneath the odontoblast layer a cell-free zone (of Weil) is commonly described in which, in standard paraffin-embedded sections, no cells are apparent. Many routine stains (such as haematoxylin and eosin) mainly stain nuclei, and consequently areas that lack nuclei appear empty: this is the case with the area immediately beneath the odontoblasts. Electron microscopy reveals that many cell processes of fibroblasts, odontoblasts, axons and capillaries cross this region. More correctly, this area could be described as anuclear. The cell-free zone is usually absent from the radicular pulp and generally appears in the coronal pulp once the tooth has erupted. There is no apparent reason for this feature, and it has been suggested that it is an artefact of histological processing produced by differential shrinkage of the odontoblast and the deeper pulp.

Immediately deep to the 'cell-free' zone is another region in which there are, apparently, many cells – the so-called cell-rich zone (Fig. 10.13). This too may be an artefact induced by contrast with the cell-free zone. In this region there is a high concentration of both capillaries (the subodontoblastic capillary plexus) and axons (the subodontoblastic neural plexus). The Schwann cells, endothelial cells, etc. associated with these 'plexi' could result in the 'cell-rich' appearance.

Central to the subodontoblastic region is the bulk of the dental pulp, which, devoid of its peripheral structures and its central neurovascular core, would be similar to loose connective tissue in many other sites, although having a richer nerve and blood supply. The central core itself is most evident in the root canal. Once it enters the crown, repeated branching of both nerves and blood vessels renders the neurovascular bundle less obvious.

Role of the dental pulp

Once differentiated from the dental papilla, the dental pulp is a single industry organ dedicated to the production of dentine: rapidly during development, slowly during adult life or suddenly in response to insult. The presence of a soft-tissue core in a tooth affects its physical properties. A young tooth with a large vital pulp is more elastic than a tooth in which most of the pulp has been replaced with secondary dentine or all of the pulp with a filling material (as occurs during root canal therapy).

Age-related changes in the dental pulp

The most obvious change in the dental pulp related to age is a progressive decrease in its size as secondary dentine is laid down. As an example, Table 10.3 shows the changes with age in length and width of mandibular central incisors. The number of odontoblasts declines in line with this by apoptosis such that, between the ages of 20 and 70 years, approximately 50% of the number of original odontoblasts is lost. Because the pulp is prone to artefactual changes, phenomena, such as wheatsheafing of the odontoblasts or reticulation, have been described that are not biological in origin. The rest of the pulp tissue undergoes a similar decline in cellularity of about 50%. Ageing also affects the DPSCs, which exhibit typical senescence features such as enlarged cell shape, decreased proliferation and decreased differentiation potential.

As for other connective tissues, both the vascularity and the innervation of the pulp decline with age. Whether this is related to the constriction at the root apex because of continued deposition of secondary dentine and cementum is not known. Ultrastructurally, the endothelial cell cytoplasm of older pulpal vessels shows more numerous pinocytotic vesicles, microvesicles and microfilaments. In addition, lipid-like vacuoles and extensive Golgi complexes with dilated cisterns are also present in older endothelial cells. Pulpal blood flow and the ability to respond to injury is reduced with age.

The teeth become less sensitive with age. It is not clear whether this is the result of a reduced number of nerves and/or the result of an increase in the thickness of dentine (secondary dentine) and the presence of peritubular dentine.

The pulp becomes more fibrous with age. Collagen in the coronal pulp of human third molars has been analysed for age changes, when it was found that there was a decrease in the reducible cross-link dihydroxylsino-norleucine (DHLNL). Based on the premise that collagen synthesis is characterized by the presence of reducible crosslinks, the study implied that coronal pulp collagen synthesis decreases with age; this was also accompanied by a decrease in collagen concentration in terms of dry weight and total protein.

Many older human teeth show some degree of mineralisation, which can occur as numerous tiny spicules of mineralised tissue throughout the pulp ('snow storm' calcification) or as discrete pulp stones either singly or in small groups. Pulp stones may occasionally resemble dentine in being, at least partially, tubular ('true' denticles) but usually lack tubules or resemble bone by having cells embedded within them ('false' denticles; Fig. 10.46). In some (lamellated pulp stones), accretion by layers is evident. Some larger pulp stones may be attached to the dentine. The incidence of pulpal calcifications increases with age, and they are generally regarded as an age-related change rather than being pathological. Pulp stones can usually be detected on radiographs (Fig. 10.47). If detected in the absence of symptoms or pathological change, pulp stones are not an indication for root canal therapy. The presence of pulp stones can complicate root canal therapy when it is indicated for other reasons. The factors determining why some individuals and not others produce pulp stones are not known – nor why, when present, one form or another occurs. If an individual has pulp stones in one tooth, it is likely that they have pulp stones in other teeth. Widespread mineralisation of the pulp may be associated with genetically determined dentine dysplasias.

Table 10.3 Changes in the length and width of the dental pulp with age in the mandibular central incisors with age

Age (years)	Pulp length (mm)	Pulp width (mm)
11–20	18.75	1.82
21–30	18.30	1.74
31–40	17.47	1.34
41–50	16.41	0.98
51–60	14.30	0.88

Each age group contains measurements from 20 teeth.
Data modified from Gupta, S., Gupta, G., Gupta, N. 2018. Age changes in dentin and dental pulp: a radiographic study. *Journal of Mahatma Gandhi University of Medical Sciences & Technology* 3: 82–87.

Clinical considerations

Pulpal responses to disease

Genetic, congenital, nutritional and traumatic factors that affect dentinogenesis exert that effect via the dental pulp. In the mature tooth the pulp is the sense organ that mandates the use of anaesthesia during cavity preparation. It is the tissue that defends (or at least tries to defend) the integrity of the tooth in response to dental caries, attrition and trauma. After pulp exposures and restorations it will, under the right conditions, form tertiary dentine and maintain tooth vitality. When dental caries begins, the pulp responds at a very early stage. Pulpal inflammation can often be detected when caries is limited to the enamel. On some occasions pulpal inflammation (pulpitis) is painful and induces a memorable experience for the patient, and sometimes a therapeutic challenge for the dentist. Pain from the dental pulp is difficult to localise and is commonly referred to other sites, either teeth or elsewhere. Sometimes pain in other sites is referred to the dental pulp (even angina). On many occasions pulpitis is painless and the dental pulp necroses. Necrotic pulp tissue can induce inflammation and sepsis in the supporting tissues around the tooth with possibly serious sequelae. It is not known why pulpal inflammation on some occasions results in severe pain and on other occasions is silent.

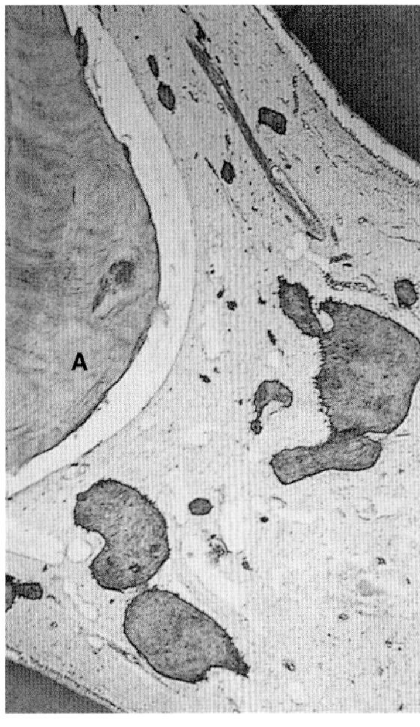

Fig. 10.46 Multiple free pulp stones present in the dental pulp and lacking dentine structure (false denticles). A = dentine (H & E; ×40).

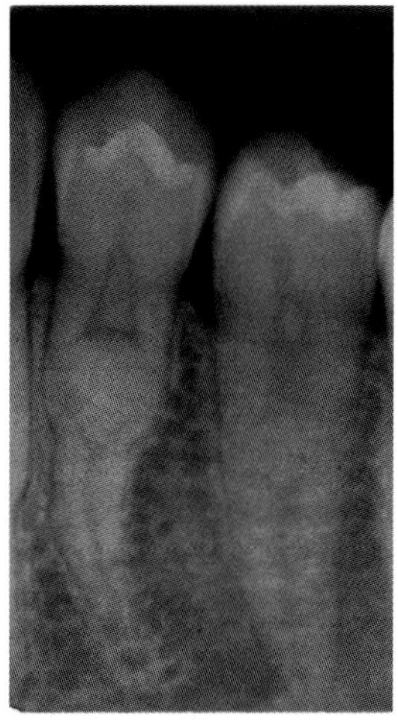

Fig. 10.47 Radiograph showing large calcifications in the pulp chambers of lower premolars in a young individual. *Courtesy Dr S Parekh and the editor of Oral Surgery, Oral Medicine, Oral Pathology, Oral Radiology, and Endodontics.*

The lack of sensitivity associated with older teeth, whether because of the increased thickness of dentine or the reduced innervation of the pulp, may allow, on some occasions, for the restorative treatment of teeth without anaesthesia.

Where the effects of pulpal inflammation result in death of the pulp and a non-vital tooth, over time a symptomless periapical granuloma may develop involving the periodontal ligament (apical periodontitis). Subsequently, epithelial cell rests at the apex may be stimulated to divide and a radicular cyst may develop. These cells release prostaglandins which cavitate the bone (Fig. 10.48). Dendritic cells are potent regulators of the immune system, and their presence in periapical lesions could be an indication of the severity of the lesion, with a constant presence of antigen in the periradicular region. The failure to successfully treat periapical lesions may be because of the continued presence of an infectious biofilm.

Lateral root canals

Gingival recession may expose the opening of a lateral root canal, especially in the furcation area of cheek teeth, causing pain and the possible spread of infection into the pulp (Fig. 10.2). Infection associated with periodontal disease may also affect the pulp and vice versa. The successful treatment of these endodontic–periodontic lesions is dependent on determining in which of the tissues the disease process originated.

Regeneration after dental pulp exposures

If an uninfected pulp is exposed during cavity preparation in a tooth, it can, if treated appropriately, repair and form a bridge of dentine over the exposure. New odontoblast-like cells differentiate and lay down tertiary (reparative) dentine.

Some materials, such as calcium hydroxide, seem to facilitate dentine bridge formation. This effect may be more by their ability to protect the pulp and their biocompatibility rather than any direct stimulation of dentine-producing cells. MTA, a modified preparation of Portland cement, has also been employed to induce reparative dentinogenesis. Compared with calcium hydroxide, it may be more efficient in the natural wound healing process of exposed pulps and may stimulate hard-tissue-forming cells to induce matrix formation and mineralisation. It can interact with phosphate-containing fluids to form apatite precipitates.

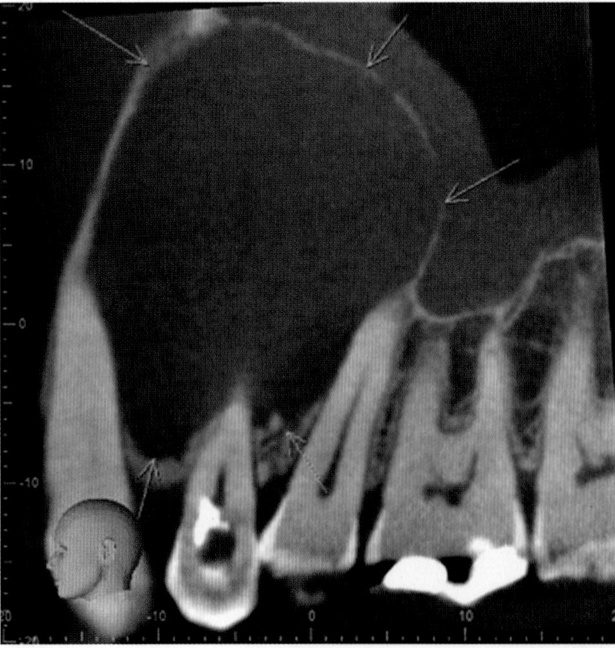

Fig. 10.48 Radiograph of a large, radicular cyst arising from a non-vital maxillary first premolar. *From Sengupta, A. Coulthard, P., Theaker, E.D. et al. 2022. Master Dentistry: Oral and Maxillofacial Surgery, Radiology, Pathology and Oral Medicine, 4th ed. Elsevier, London.*

Other, more biologically active molecules, such as BMP, TGF-β and some other components of the dentine matrix, seem to have a direct and positive effect on the differentiation and activation of hard-tissue-forming cells. During the demineralisation of dentine with caries and during clinical procedures such as acid etching, these bioactive molecules sequestered in dentine may be released to play a role in dentine bridge formation. These bioactive molecules have not, as yet, been widely applied clinically.

If the exposed pulp is infected or contaminated, the likelihood of successful bridge formation is much reduced, and removal of the dental pulp may be necessary, followed by its replacement with a suitable root canal filling material. However, research is being undertaken with the hope of eventually replacing a root canal filling with a new dental pulp using the principles of tissue engineering (see Chapter 28). Two strategies are under investigation. Having removed the original dead pulp and prepared the root canal space in the best way to retain the positive features of the dentine surface to encourage pulp regeneration, one may attempt filling it with transplanted stem cells (preferably derived from the patient) in a suitable scaffold and with morphogenetic signalling agents, such as BMPs and FGFs. An alternative and less complex strategy is to just fill the root canal with a suitable scaffold and morphogenetic signalling agents that may chemotactically encourage stem cells from the environment of the root apex to populate the scaffold. Because developing a blood supply is crucial to the success of both strategies, the addition of proangiogenic factors such as FGF-2 and VEGF may be considered.

It may, in the future, be possible to control infection and inflammation in the pulp. It might also be possible to replace or regenerate all or part of a diseased pulp that has been removed using biological matrices carrying growth factors and/or cultures of pulpal cells. Currently, the definitive treatment of the irreversibly diseased or necrotic pulp is to remove it and replace it with an inert root canal filling material (see page 64).

Apexification

In addition to dealing with pulp exposures, as described earlier, it may also be desirable to seal off the apex of the root and any deficiency associated with the presence of internal resorption or root fractures. This can be achieved by using bioactive materials such as MTA. As with other bioactive materials (see Chapter 28), their success relates to the ability to deposit calcium phosphates after an increase in pH and to upregulate genes associated with biological mineralisation.

Regeneration after dental pulp exposures in young teeth with incompletely formed roots

A common clinical situation that has proven difficult to successfully treat concerns pulpal necrosis occurring in permanent but immature teeth. A typical case history is of a young patient who presents with an anterior tooth which has been knocked out in an accident and in which the root has not completed its development. Although it may be possible to successfully reimplant the tooth, the pulp often undergoes necrosis and, even if it can be root-filled, the long-term prognosis is not always good, and no existing method of treatment is likely to result in the completion of root development. However, application of stem cell treatment has recently suggested a possible way of successfully treating the condition and resulting in a tooth with a completed and vital root apex. In such reimplanted teeth, the incompletely formed root apex may still harbour apical stem cells. The aim is to irrigate and remove the necrotic pulp tissue and fill the root canal with antibiotic paste, but seal off and cover any vital tissue at the growing root apex with calcium hydroxide. This apical region should contain stem cells of the apical papilla (SCAPs). After a period of healing, the apical region is accessed again, and apical bleeding intentionally induced to form a blood clot immediately below and around the root apex. The apical region is again sealed off, and the root canal is finally sealed above it. It is anticipated that the formation of the blood clot at the root apex will bring in large numbers of stem cells and, in addition to the SCAPs already present, will eventually lead to a completed and vital root apex (see also Chapter 28).

If the dental pulp undergoes death and necrosis, degradative products may pass along the dentinal tubules, giving the crown a darker appearance (Fig. 10.49).

Tests for pulp vitality

In many clinical situations it is important to know whether the tooth is vital and reactive or is nonvital and may be considered for endodontic treatment. Because the dental pulp cannot be directly inspected, indirect methods need to be applied. There are three main methods. Two use either temperature or electrical stimulation to test for the presence of nerves, whereas a third tests for the presence of blood flow through the tissue. The thermal test usually involves application of an ice refrigerant spray (tetrafluoroethane) on a cotton pellet applied to the middle of the crown to stimulate any vital nerves present in the pulp. Although heat in the form of hot water or heated gutta-percha has also been used to test vitality, cold is a more reliable test than heat. The electrical test employs a suitable electrical pulp tester to pass a current to stimulate any vital nerves in the pulp. A pulp oximeter is an electrical device that tests for the existence of blood flow through the tooth by directly measuring blood oxygen saturation levels.

Comparisons have been made between the three types of test and, although the temperature and electrical methods are very useful, the most reliable is the pulp oximeter. Recently traumatised teeth may temporarily lose their nerve supply and give a false negative result to temperature and electrical testing, even though the blood system is intact. Conversely, a dental pulp that is partly necrotic with no blood supply may give a false positive response to temperature and electrical testing if there are some surviving nerves.

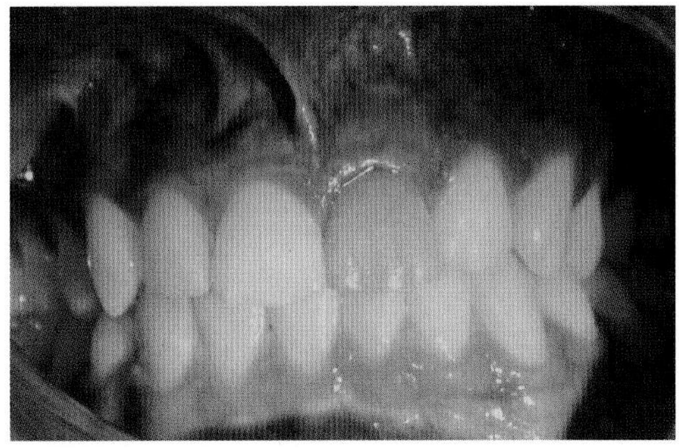

Fig. 10.49 Patient with a maxillary left permanent central incisor, the dental pulp of which necrosed after trauma. It is darker than the adjacent tooth.

Gerodontology

Gerodontology is a specialised area of dentistry which deals with the diagnosis, management and treatment of dental conditions relating to older adults. In various chapters of this book, we have described the age changes that occur. For many dental tissues, the decline in stem cells with age means that healing of any dental lesions may well be slower and incomplete. Thus, the regeneration of dental tissues must take this into account (see Chapter 28). Because of the age changes in dentine and dental pulp, the tooth is less sensitive and may not even require a local anaesthetic during treatment. Similarly, much of the crown can be removed without fear of exposing the dental pulp. In contrast, root canal treatment in the elderly is more difficult because the pulp cavity may be very small and irregular.

Pulp testing is a more difficult procedure in the teeth of older patients because of the associated age changes in pulp. The pulp may, to all intents and purposes, be dead and practically unresponsive, but it may contain one or two viable nerves that can respond to temperature and electrical stimulation and give a false positive test.

Further readings for this chapter can be found in the accompanying eBook. Explore online Self-assessment quiz to test and reinforce your understanding of the material in your free ebook. Follow instructions in the Inside Front Cover to unlock your access.

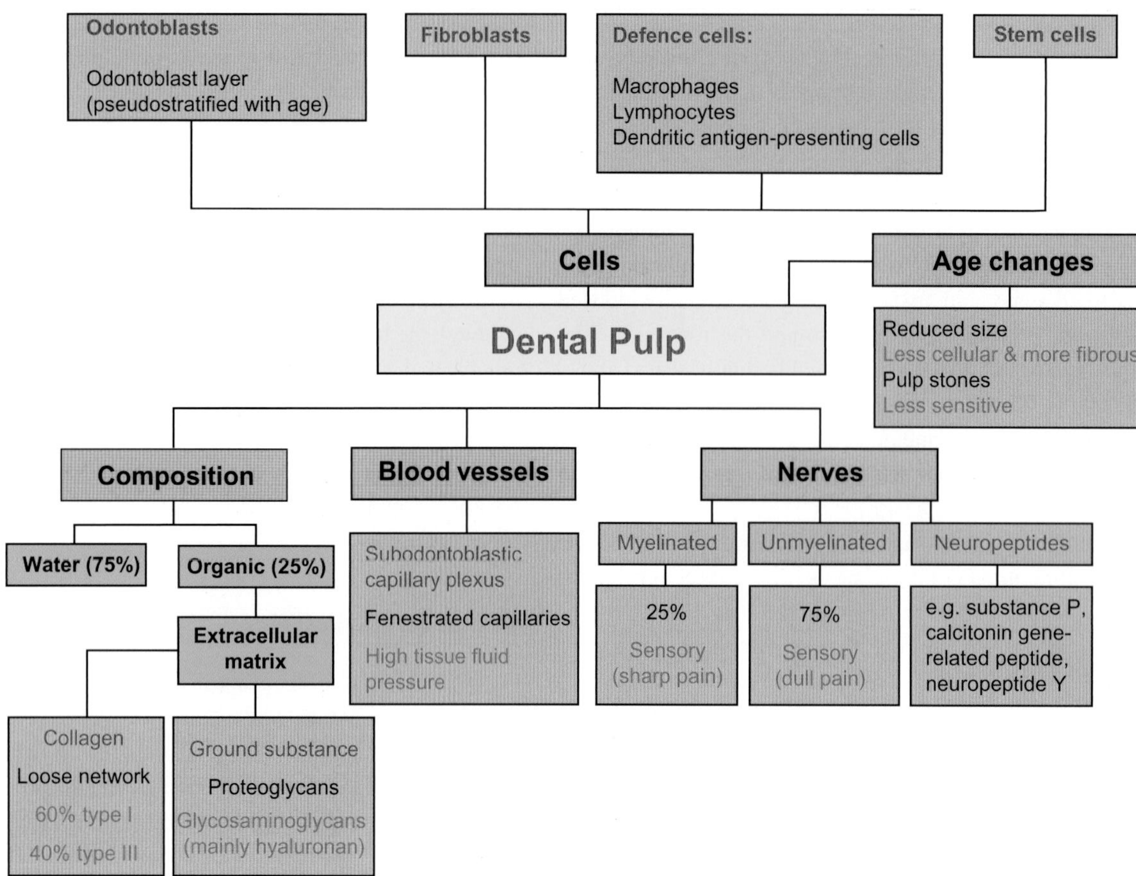

Mind Map 10.1 Dental pulp.

Cementum

11

Introduction

Cementum is the thin layer of calcified tissue covering the dentine of the root (Fig. 11.1). It is one of the four tissues that support the tooth in the jaw (the periodontium), the others being the alveolar bone, the periodontal ligament and the gingiva. Although many of these periodontal tissues have been extensively studied, cementum remains the least known. Indeed, it is the least known of all the mineralised tissues in the body. For example, very little is known about the origin, differentiation and cell dynamics of the cementum-forming cell (the cementoblast), and it has been questioned whether these cells are a subpopulation of osteoblasts or have a unique phenotype. It is known that both cementoblasts and osteoblasts have receptors for parathormone (PTH) and parathormone receptor protein (PTHrP). Furthermore, they respond similarly to many of the factors that regulate cell activity. This, however, does not mean that the cells are of the same lineage.

Although restricted to the root in humans, cementum is present on the crowns of some mammals as an adaptation to an herbivorous diet. Cementum varies in thickness at different levels of the root. It is thickest at the root apex and in the interradicular areas of multirooted teeth and thinnest cervically. The thickness cervically is 10–15 μm and apically 50–200 μm (although it may exceed 600 μm).

Cementum is contiguous with the periodontal ligament on its outer surface and is firmly adherent to dentine on its deep surface. Its prime function is to give attachment to collagen fibres of the periodontal ligament. It therefore is a highly responsive mineralised tissue, maintaining the integrity of the root, helping to maintain the tooth in its functional position in the mouth and being involved in tooth repair and regeneration.

Cementum is slowly formed throughout life, and this allows for continual reattachment of the periodontal ligament fibres – some regard cementum as a calcified component of the ligament. Developmentally, cementum is said to be derived from the investing layer of the dental follicle. Like dentine, there is always a thin layer (3–5 μm) of uncalcified matrix on the surface of the cellular variety of cementum (see page 447). This layer of uncalcified matrix is called *precementum* or *cementoid* (Figs 11.2, 11.25). Similar in chemical composition and physical properties to bone, cementum is, however, avascular and has no innervation. It also shows little ability to remodel and is also less readily resorbed, a feature that is important for permitting orthodontic tooth movements. The reason for this feature is unknown but it may be related to:

- Differences in physicochemical or biological properties between bone and cementum
- The properties of the precementum
- The increased density of Sharpey fibres (particularly in acellular cementum)
- The proximity of epithelial cell rests to the root surface

Unlike bone cells, cementoblasts do not have the required receptors for remodelling mediators.

Unlike bone, cementum does not have a lamellar appearance and has no marrow spaces.

The arrangement of tissues at the cementum–enamel junction is shown in Figs 11.3–11.5. In any single section of a tooth, three arrangements of the junction between cementum and enamel may be seen. Pattern 1, where the cementum overlaps the enamel for a short distance, is the predominant arrangement in 60% of sections. Pattern 2, where the cementum and enamel meet at a butt joint, occurs in 30% of sections. Pattern 3, where the cementum and enamel fail to meet and the dentine between them is exposed, occurs in 10% of sections. Although one of these patterns may predominate in any individual tooth, all three patterns can be present.

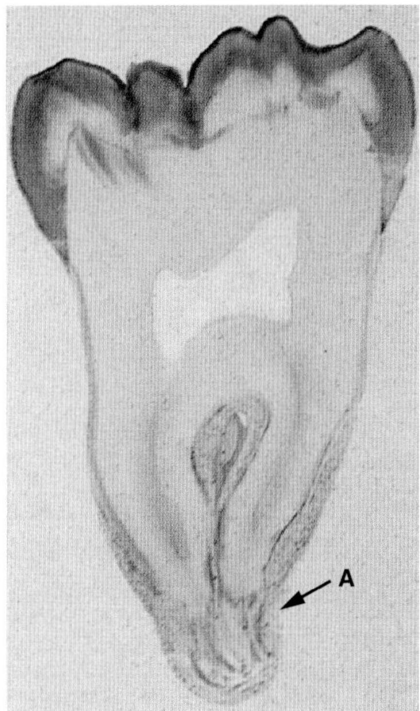

Fig. 11.1 The distribution of cementum (A) along the root of a tooth (ground longitudinal section of a tooth; ×4).

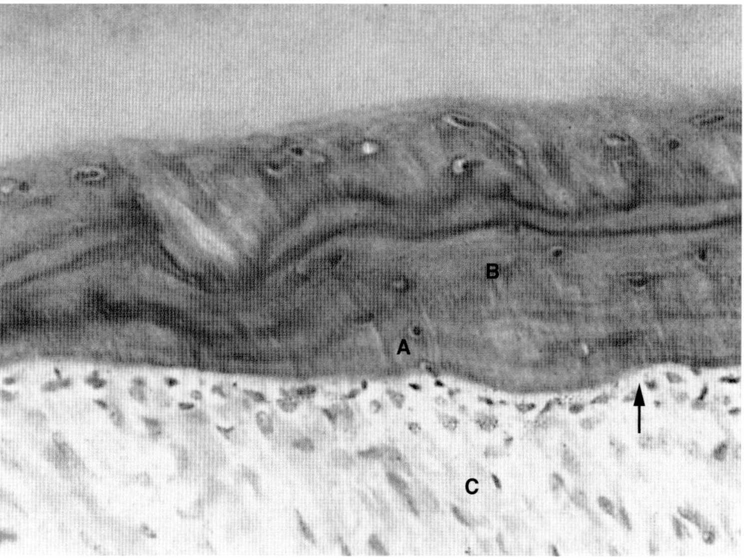

Fig. 11.2 The relationship between cementum (B), precementum *(arrow)*, a layer of cementoblasts (A) and the periodontal ligament (C) (decalcified section; H & E; ×200).

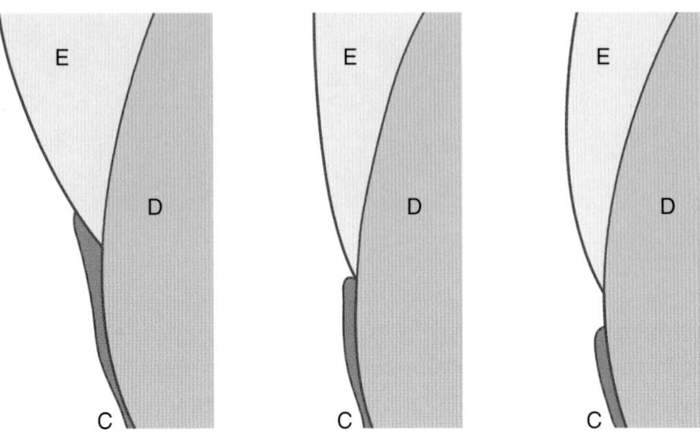

Fig. 11.3 Three patterns for the arrangement of the cementum–enamel junction. C = cementum; D = dentine; E = enamel. See text for further details.

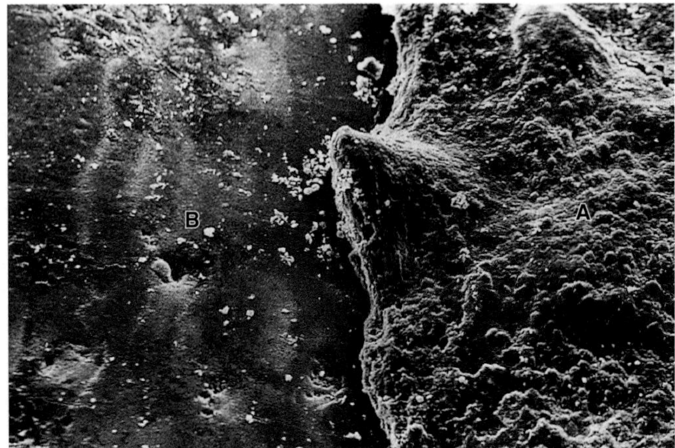

Fig. 11.4 Scanning electron micrograph of the cementum–enamel junction where the cementum overlaps the enamel. A = cementum; B = enamel (SEM; ×250).

Physical properties

Cementum is pale yellow with a dull surface. It is softer than dentine. Permeability varies with age and the type of cementum, with the cellular variety being more permeable. In general, cementum is more permeable than dentine. As for the other dental tissues, permeability decreases with age. The relative softness of cementum, combined with its thinness cervically, means that it is readily removed by abrasion when gingival recession exposes the root surface to the oral environment. Loss of cementum in such cases will expose dentine.

Chemical properties

Cementum contains on a wet-weight basis 65% inorganic material, 23% organic material and 12% water. By volume, the inorganic material comprises approximately 45%, organic material 33% and water 22%. The degree of mineralisation varies in different parts of the tissue; some acellular zones may be more highly calcified than dentine. The principal inorganic component is hydroxyapatite, although other forms of calcium are present at higher levels than in enamel and dentine. The hydroxyapatite crystals are thin, platelike and similar to those in bone. They are on average 55 nm wide and 8 nm thick. Their length varies, but values derived from sections cut with a diamond knife are underestimated owing to

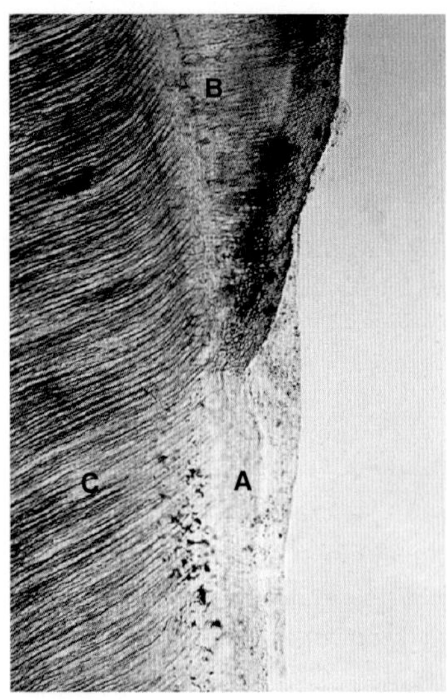

Fig. 11.5 Ground longitudinal section through a tooth to show cementum (A) overlapping enamel (B). C = dentine (ground section; ×80). Courtesy Prof. A G S Lumsden.

shattering of the crystals along their length. The crystallinity of the apatite in cementum is lower than the other dental tissues and is demineralised more easily. As with enamel, the concentration of trace elements, such as zinc, tends to be higher at the external surface. Indeed, fluoride levels in cementum are higher than any of the other mineralised tissues. Fluoride levels are higher in acellular than in cellular cementum.

The organic matrix is primarily collagen. The collagen is virtually all type I (although types III, V, VI and XII have been found in small quantities). In addition, the non-collagenous elements are assumed to be similar to those found in bone (see pages 262–263). However, because of the difficulties in obtaining sufficient material for analysis, less information is available. Nevertheless, among the important molecules known to be present are bone sialoprotein, dentine sialoprotein, fibronectin, tenascin, osteopontin and possibly other cementum-specific elements that are conjectured to be involved in periodontal reattachment and/or remineralisation. Such molecules contain the well-recognised adhesion domain arginine–glycine–aspartic acid that targets specific integrin receptors on cells. Sialoproteins are located in the cementum matrix and osteopontin in the incremental lines.

Cementum-derived attachment protein (CAP) is a 56-kDa or 65-kDa collagenous protein in cementum that promotes the attachment of mesenchymal cells to the extracellular matrix. It is located in the matrix of mature cementum and in cementoblasts (but not in bone). Although initially thought to be a marker to differentiate bone and cementum, CAP is also expressed in periodontal ligament cells and alveolar bone cells and shares homology with some collagen domains.

Cementum is rich in glycosaminoglycans, predominantly chondroitin sulphate. This glycosaminoglycan is primarily located around the lacunae of cementum. In addition, dermatan sulphate and hyaluronan can be found. Among the proteoglycans found in cementum are lumican, versican, decorin, biglycan and fibromodulin. These are also found in bone and, for both tissues, are located especially at the peripheries of lacunae and canaliculi. It appears that fibromodulin and lumican are more abundant in cementum.

As for bone, cementum also contains many growth factors. Unlike bone, these are normally locked up and remain inactive because of the low turnover rate. However, they may be activated where cementum is locally resorbed.

Recent proteomic analysis has revealed much more detail about the protein composition of cementum matrix, highlighting differences between cementum from deciduous and permanent teeth. A total of 510 proteins have been identified: 259 (50.8%) commonly expressed in the cementum of both deciduous and permanent teeth, 123 (24.1%) exclusive to deciduous teeth and 128 (25.1%) exclusive to permanent teeth. Of the 259 commonly expressed proteins, 60 (11.8%) have been found to be differentially expressed. One of these important proteins, osteocalcin, is increased in the cementum of permanent teeth, with the highest concentration in the cellular-perilacunar regions around cementocytes. Among many proteoglycans present in cementum, asporin and biglycan are more detectable in the cementum of deciduous teeth, whilst decorin is present in greater amounts in the cementum of permanent teeth. By analysing the proteins of both deciduous and permanent teeth, it may eventually indicate why deciduous teeth resorb while permanent teeth do not.

Classification of cementum

The various types of cementum encountered may be classified in three different ways: the presence or absence of cells, the nature and origin of the organic matrix and a combination of both.

Classification based on the presence or absence of cells: cellular and acellular cementum

The cells forming both acellular and cellular cementum lie on the surface and are known as *cementoblasts* (Fig. 11.2). When they become incorporated into cellular cementum, the cells are known as *cementocytes* (see Fig. 11.12). These cells are discussed in detail in Chapter 25.

Cellular cementum, as its name indicates, contains cells (cementocytes); acellular cementum does not. In the most common arrangement, acellular cementum covers the root adjacent to the dentine, whereas cellular cementum is found mainly in the apical area and overlying the acellular cementum (Fig. 11.6). Deviations from this arrangement are common, and sometimes several layers of each variant alternate. The mechanism responsible for the shift from acellular to cellular cementum is not known, but it may involve occlusal forces transmitted to the tooth.

Being formed first, the acellular cementum is sometimes termed *primary cementum* and the subsequently formed cellular variety *secondary cementum*. Cellular cementum is especially common in interradicular areas.

Acellular cementum appears relatively structureless (Fig. 11.7). In the outer region of the radicular dentine, the granular layer (of Tomes) can be seen, and outside this, the hyaline layer (of Hopewell-Smith). These layers are also described on page 177. A dark line may be discerned between the hyaline layer and the acellular cementum; this may be related to the afibrillar cementum that is patchily present at this position. The usual arrangement at the apical region of the root is of a layer of cellular cementum overlying acellular cementum (Fig. 11.8). Many of the structural differences between cellular and acellular cementum are thought to be related to the faster rate of matrix formation for cellular cementum. Indeed, a major difference is that as cellular cementum develops, the formative cells (the cementoblasts) become embedded in the tissue as cementocytes. The different rates of cementum formation are also reflected in the presence of a precementum layer and in the more widely spaced incremental lines in cellular cementum.

Although the usual relationship between acellular and cellular cementum is for the cellular variety to overlie the acellular, the reverse may occur (Fig. 11.9). Furthermore, it is also common for the two variants of cementum to alternate (Fig. 11.10), probably representing variations in the rate of deposition.

The spaces that the cementocytes occupy in cellular cementum are called lacunae and the channels that their processes extend along are the canaliculi (Fig. 11.11, 11.12). Adjacent canaliculi are often connected, and the processes within them exhibit gap junctions. In ground sections (Fig. 11.11), the cellular contents are lost, with air and debris filling the

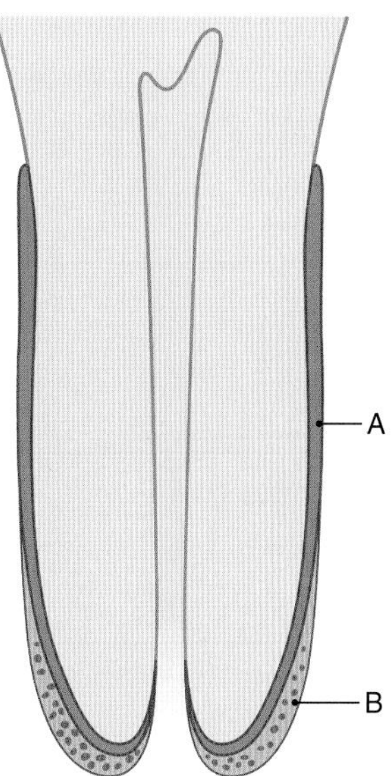

Fig. 11.6 The distribution of acellular (A) and cellular (B) cementum.

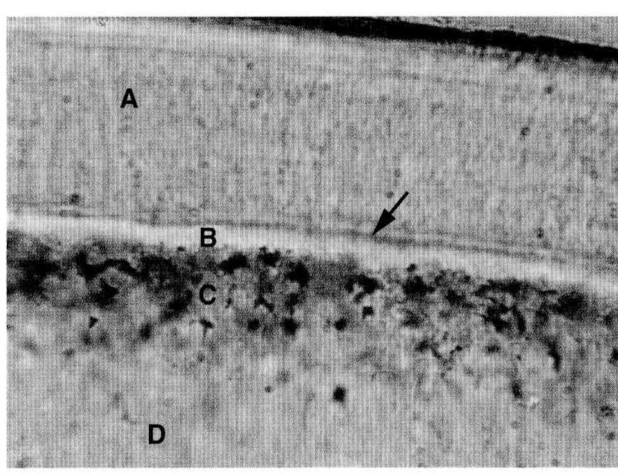

Fig. 11.7 The appearance of acellular cementum (A). B = hyaline layer (of Hopewell-Smith); C = granular layer (of Tomes); D = root dentine. Note that the dark layer arrowed between the hyaline layer and the acellular cementum may be related to the afibrillar cementum patchily present at this position (ground section; ×200).

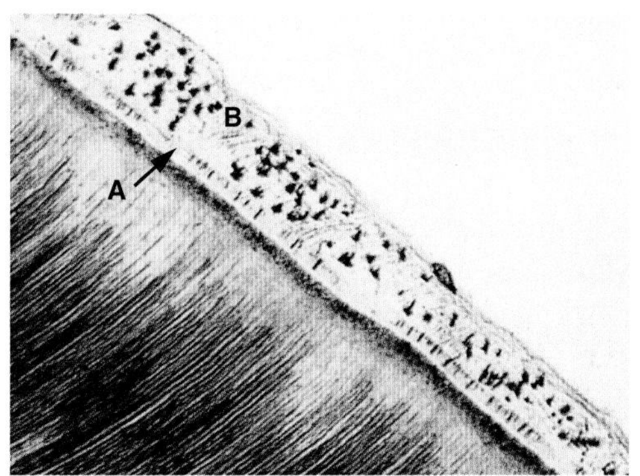

Fig. 11.8 Cellular cementum (B) overlying acellular cementum (A). Note the greater thickness of the cellular layer (ground section; ×50).

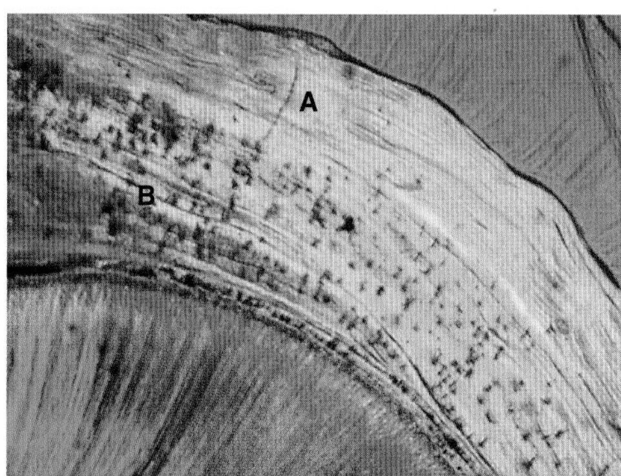

Fig. 11.9 Acellular cementum (A) overlying cellular cementum (B) (ground section of the root; ×50).

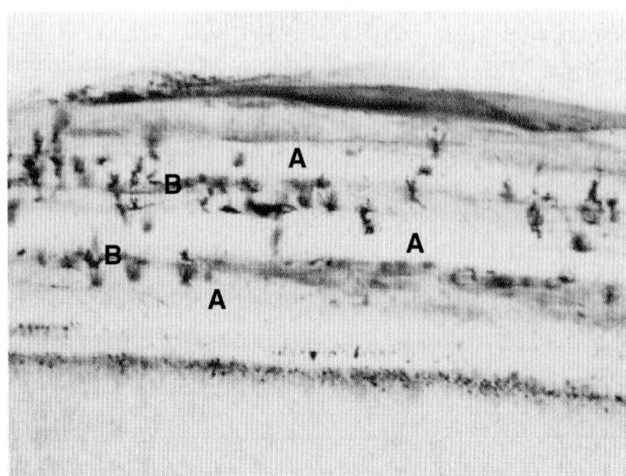

Fig. 11.10 Alternating acellular (A) and cellular cementum (B). Note the presence of incremental lines (ground section; ×60).

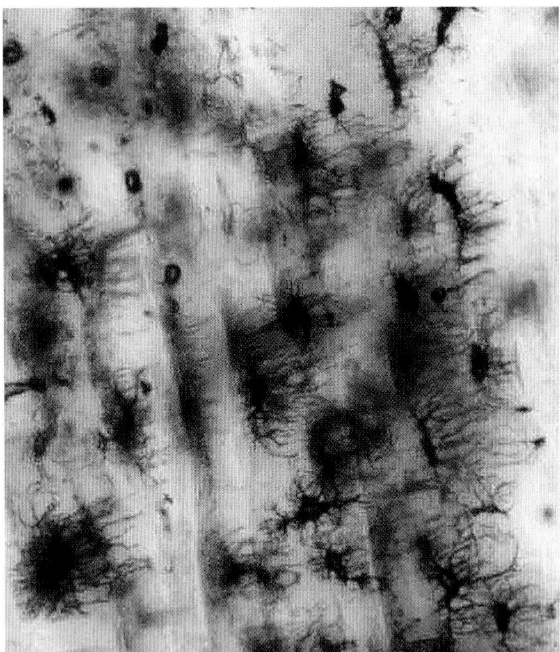

Fig.11.11 Lacunae and canaliculi in cellular cementum. In this section, the preferential orientation of the lacunae indicates that the external surface is to the right (ground section). Courtesy Dr. A. Leblanc.

voids to give the dark appearance. In thicker layers of cellular cementum, it is highly probable that many of the lacunae do not contain vital cells. This contrasts with the situation in bone. Furthermore, compared with osteocytes in bone, cementocytes are more widely dispersed and more randomly arranged. In addition, their canaliculi are preferentially oriented towards the periodontal ligament, their chief source of nutrition (Fig. 11.11). Unlike bone, the cementocytes are not arranged circumferentially around blood vessels in the form of osteons (Haversian systems). In decalcified sections (Fig. 11.2), the cellular contents of the lacunae are retained, albeit in a shrunken condition.

Fig. 11.12 illustrates the ultrastructural appearance of a cementocyte within a lacuna. Although derived from active cementoblasts, once they become embedded within the cementum matrix, cementocytes become relatively inactive. This is reflected in their ultrastructural appearance. Their cytoplasmic/nuclear ratio is low, and they have sparse, if any, representation of the organelles responsible for energy production and for synthesis. Some unmineralised matrix may be seen in the perilacunar space. The cementocyte processes can extend for distances several times longer than the diameter of the cell body. There is presently no evidence that cementocytes have a function in tissue homeostasis.

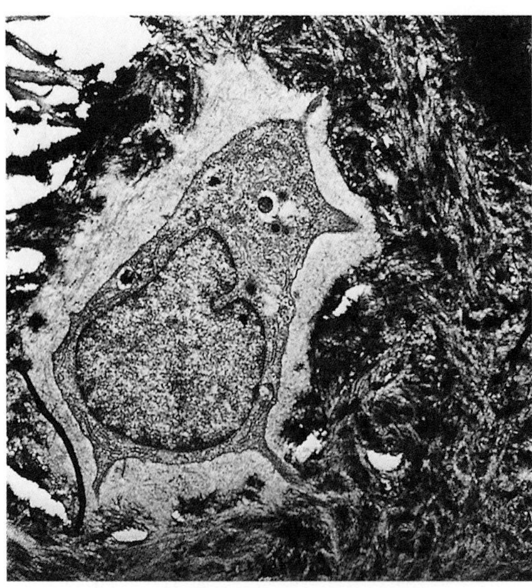

Fig. 11.12 TEM of a cementocyte within a lacuna. Note that the cementocyte processes here appear short only because they extend out of the plane of section (×4,500).

Age changes and cementum annulations

As cementum is deposited slowly throughout life, its thickness increases about threefold between the ages of 16 and 70, although whether this proceeds in a linear manner is not known. Cementum may be formed at the root apex in much greater amounts as a result of compensatory tooth eruption in response to attrition (wear) at the occlusal surface. Such hypercementosis may cause problems during tooth extraction. Most roots of permanent teeth show small, localised areas of resorption, and these are said to increase with age. The cause of this is not known.

Cementum is deposited rhythmically throughout life, producing a series of incremental lines seen in both ground (Fig. 11.10, Fig. 11.13) and demineralised sections (Fig. 11.14). In acellular cementum, incremental lines tend to be close together, thin and even. In the more rapidly formed cellular cementum, the lines are farther apart, thicker and more irregular.

In many mammals, these incremental lines (often also produced in dentine) reflect annual periods of growth, allowing many species to be aged and hence are also termed *cementum annulations*. Each annual growth consists of two lines/bands: a darker band and a lighter band.

Dark bands have been attributed to hypermineralisation linked to a slowing down of cementoblast activity during late autumn, winter and early spring. The lighter and wider bands are thought to result from a less well-organised collagen network combined with hypomineralisation that occurs during rapid tissue growth in spring and summer. Together, each dark and light pair is thought to represent one calendar year.

The existence of incremental lines relates to a transient disruption of hard tissue formation. In temperate or polar regions, the lines form during winter, when food is short. However, annual lines also occur in teeth of tropical animals and seem to be correlated with dry seasons. Seasonal fluctuations in availability of foods, especially of fruits, are experienced in the tropics, even if less severe than in more seasonal temperate regions.

The phenomena underlying the formation of annual and sub-annual lines in cementum have not been fully elucidated and may be multifactorial. There is evidence for variations in mineral concentration, although these are reflected only in calcium concentration but not phosphorus concentration. It has also been suggested that the incremental lines in cementum result from variations in orientation of Sharpey fibres, which are correlated

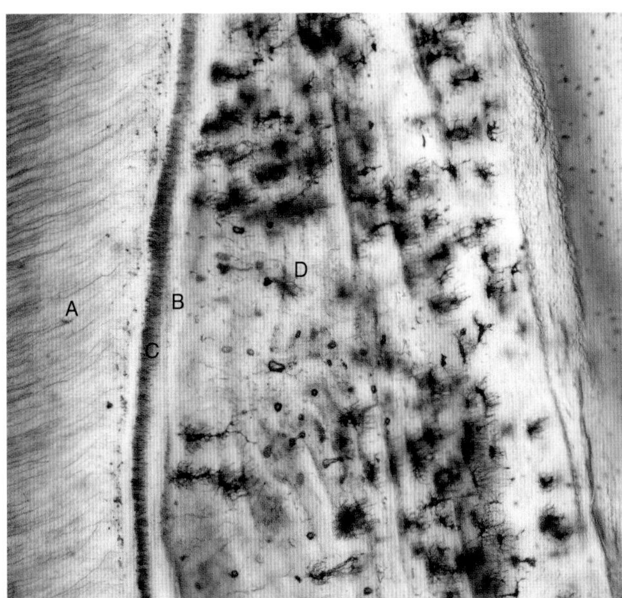

Fig. 11.13 Ground longitudinal section of tooth showing incremental lines in cementum. A = dentine, B = hyaline layer, C = granular layer, D = cellular cementum with incremental lines ×100. Courtesy Dr. A. Leblanc.

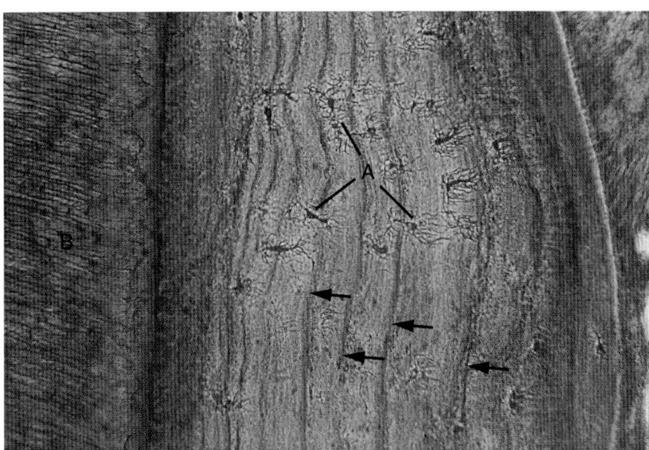

Fig. 11.14 Incremental lines (of Salter) in cementum *(arrows)*. A = cementocytes; B = dentine (decalcified section; picrothionin; ×75). Courtesy Prof. M M Smith.

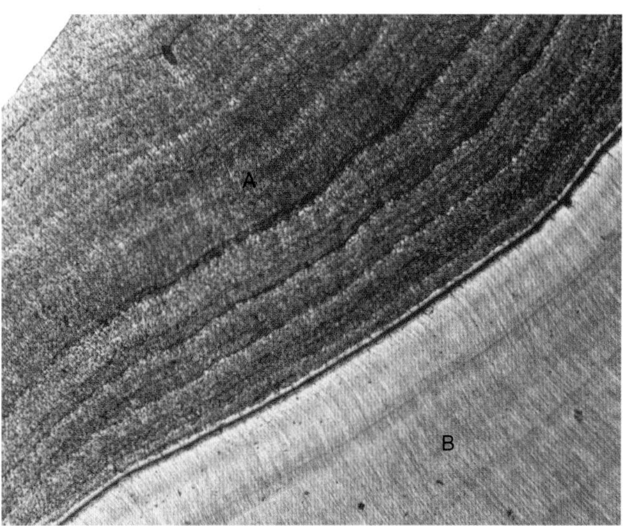

Fig. 11.15 Sperm whale *(Physeter microcephalus)*. Ground transverse section of tooth showing incremental layers in dentine *(lower right, A)* and cementum *(upper left, B)*. Image width = 4.3 mm. Copyright the Royal College of Surgeons Tomes slide collection RCSOMA/ 795. From Berkovitz, B., Shellis, P., 2018. *The teeth of mammalian vertebrates*. Elsevier, San Diego.

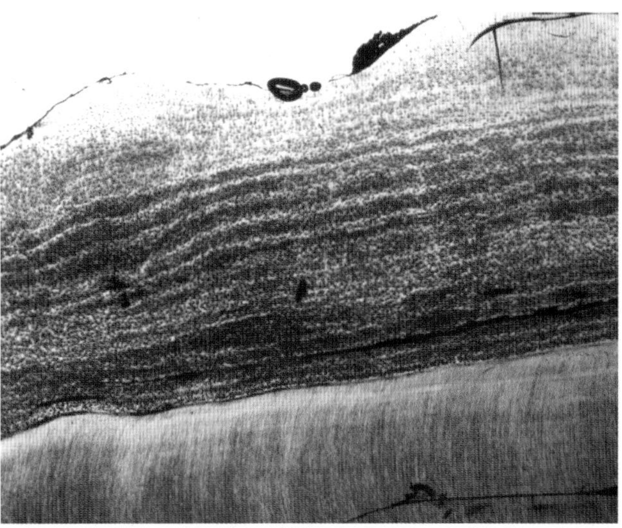

Fig. 11.16 Brown bear *(Ursus arctos)*. Ground longitudinal section of tooth, showing the presence of numerous growth rings in the cementum. Image width = 4.3 mm. Copyright the Royal College of Surgeons Tomes slide collection RCSOMA/ 1271. From Berkovitz, B., Shellis, P., 2018. *The teeth of mammalian vertebrates*. Elsevier.

with varying mechanical demands on the tooth. Fluctuations in the trace metal zinc are also associated with incremental lines, which may be rich in osteopontin to aid the cohesion of the matrix molecules at these sites.

Ageing mammals may be straightforward when the annual layers consist of a pair of bands: a thin band marking the period of slow growth and a wide band marking the period of normal growth. This is the case with age determination in mammals such as many species of seal, sperm whales (Fig. 11.15) and brown bears (Fig. 11.16). However, the presence of numerous or less regular lines of unknown origin between the principal lines tends to increase the difficulty of counting and may make counting impossible. In orca whales, numerous accessory growth layers in dentine frequently obscure any annual pattern of growth layers (Fig. 11.17).

Concerning the possibility of ageing human teeth, there is evidence both for and against this possibility. Thus, there are references that state that human annulation counts in an age group up to 55 years appeared to be very close to the actual ages, though annulations for individuals who were above 55 years of age showed an increased tendency to be inaccurate – maybe because of a decreased apposition of cementum. As destructive techniques may not be applicable to much important archaeological material, nondestructive visualisation of cementum annulations has successfully been

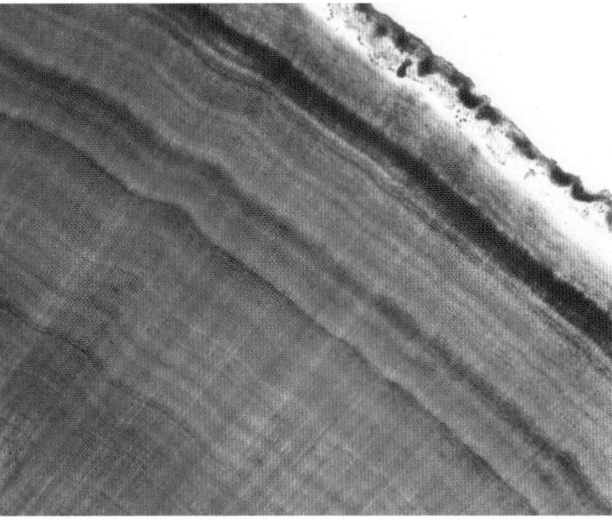

Fig. 11.17 Orca *(Orcinus orca)*. Ground cross-section of tooth. The presence of many accessory growth lines in the dentine and the lack of regularity between successive layers make ageing difficult. Image width = 2.1 mm. Courtesy Royal College of Surgeons Tomes slide collection RCSOMA/ 784. Copyright the Royal College of Surgeons Tomes slide collection RCSOMA/ 1271. From Berkovitz, B., Shellis, P., 2018. *The teeth of mammalian vertebrates*. Elsevier.

Table 11.1 Summary of differences between acellular and cellular cementum

Acellular cementum	Cellular cementum
No cells	Lacunae and canaliculi containing cementocytes and their processes
Border with dentine not clearly demarcated	Border with dentine clearly demarcated
Rate of development relatively slow	Rate of development relatively fast
Incremental lines relatively close together	Incremental lines relatively wide apart
Precementum layer virtually absent	Precementum layer present

undertaken using synchrotron X-ray microtomography However, the results give a significant underestimate of actual age, especially for the old age group.

Table 11.1 summarises the differences between acellular and cellular cementum.

Classification based on the nature and origin of the organic matrix

Cementum derives its organic matrix from two sources: the inserting Sharpey fibres of the periodontal ligament and the cementoblasts. It is therefore possible to classify cementum according to the nature and origin of the fibrous matrix. When derived from the periodontal ligament, the fibres are referred to as the *extrinsic fibres*. These Sharpey fibres continue into the cementum in the same direction as the principal fibres of the ligament (i.e., perpendicular or oblique to the root surface; see page 232). When derived from the cementoblasts, the fibres are referred to as *intrinsic fibres*. These run parallel to the root surface and approximately at right angles to the extrinsic fibres. Where both extrinsic and intrinsic fibres are present, the tissue may be termed *mixed fibre cementum*.

Classification based on the presence or absence of cells and on the nature and origin of the organic matrix

AEFC grows throughout the life of a tooth, with a rate of between 0.005 μm and 0.01 μm per day. During its formation, CIFC grows about 50 times as fast. In comparison, bone grows by 1 μm to 2 μm per day (faster for woven bone).

This classification, which is becoming more widely used, contains several types of cementum. For human teeth, two main varieties of cementum are found – acellular extrinsic fibre cementum (AEFC) and cellular intrinsic fibre cementum (CIFC). AEFC is located mainly over the cervical half of the root and constitutes the bulk of cementum in some teeth (e.g., in premolars). AEFC is the first formed cementum (see pages 442–447), and layers attain a thickness of approximately 15 μm.

Acellular extrinsic fibre cementum (Fig. 11.18)

For this type of cementum, all the collagen is derived as Sharpey fibres from the periodontal ligament (the ground substance itself may be produced by the cementoblasts). This type of cementum corresponds with primary acellular cementum and therefore covers the cervical two-thirds of the root (Fig. 11.7). It is formed slowly, and the root surface is smooth (Fig. 11.4). The fibres are generally well mineralised. As shown in Fig. 11.19, however, the extrinsic fibres seen in ground sections may have unmineralised cores. These may be lost during preparation of a ground section and replaced with air or debris. This results in the total internal reflection of transmitted light, giving the appearance of thin black lines.

Cellular intrinsic fibre cementum (Figs 11.20, 11.21)

This type of cementum is composed only of intrinsic fibres running parallel to the root surface. The absence of Sharpey fibres means that intrinsic fibre cementum has no role in tooth attachment. It may be found in patches in the apical region. It may be a temporary phase, with extrinsic fibres subsequently

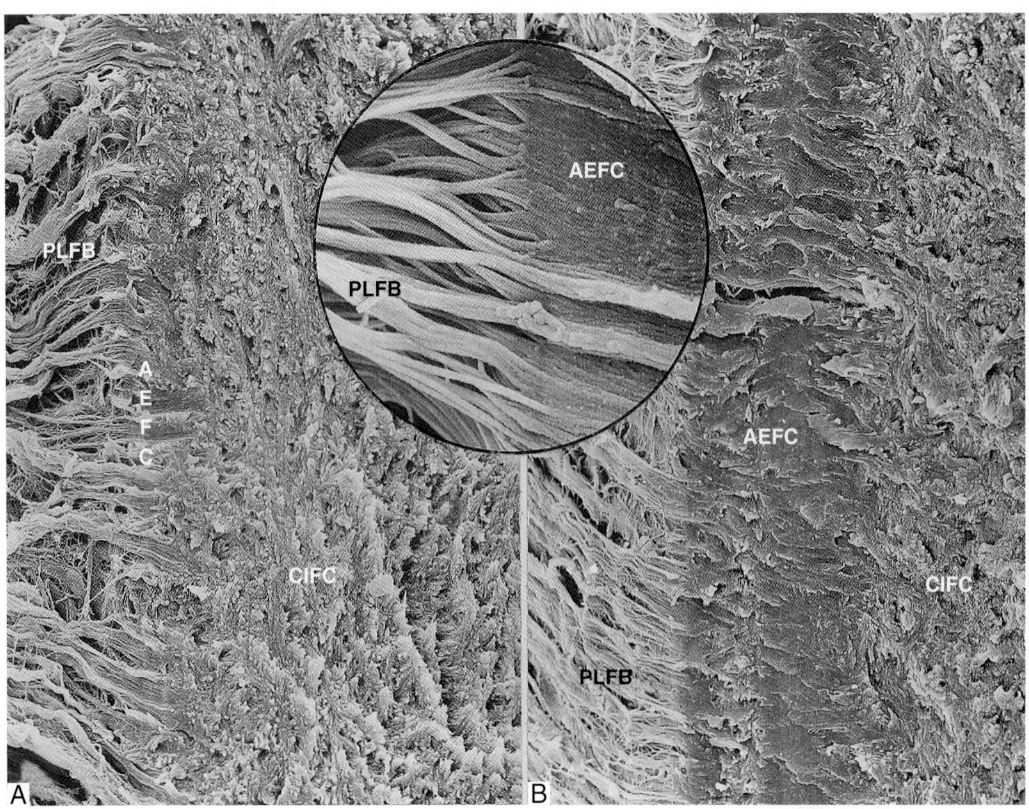

Fig. 11.18 SEMs of fractured surface of root illustrating acellular extrinsic fibre cementum (AEFC). PLFB = inserting periodontal ligament fibre bundles; CIFC = underlying cellular intrinsic fibre cementum (A, B, ×630; inset, ×1,650). From Schroeder, H.E., 1993. Human cellular mixed stratified cementum: a tissue with alternating layers of acellular extrinsic and cellular intrinsic fiber cementum. *Schweizer Monatsschrift fur Zahnmedizin* 103, 550–560.

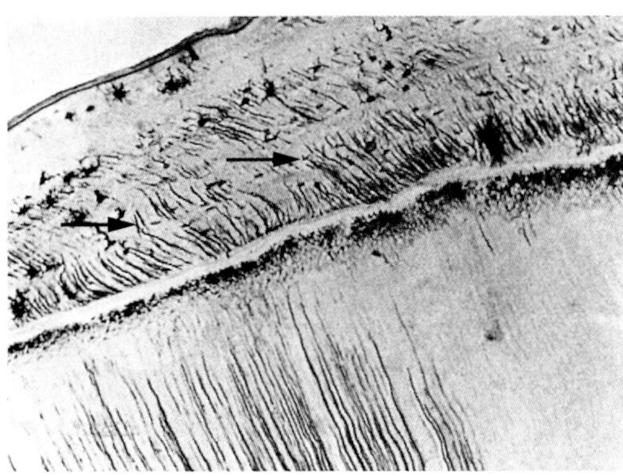

Fig. 11.19 Extrinsic fibres in ground sections. The *arrows* indicate that the core of the extrinsic fibre bundle has been lost during preparation of the ground section and replaced with air or debris (ground section; ×100). Courtesy Dr. P D A Owens.

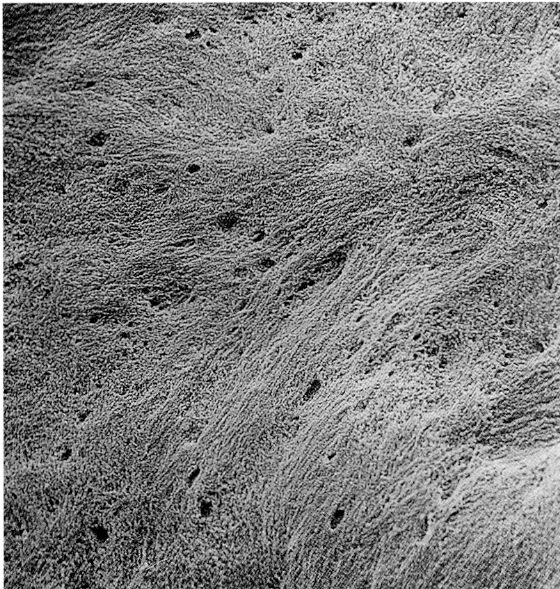

Fig. 11.20 SEM showing the appearance of intrinsic fibre cementum at the surface of the root apex. Note the absence of Sharpey fibres and the parallel distribution of the bundles of mineralised intrinsic fibres (anorganic preparation; ×150). Courtesy Prof. S J Jones.

gaining a reattachment, or may represent a permanent region without attaching fibres. It generally corresponds to secondary cellular cementum and is found in the apical third of the root and in the interradicular areas. Although intrinsic fibre cementum is generally cellular because of the rapid speed of formation, sometimes intrinsic fibre cementum is formed more slowly and cells are not incorporated (acellular intrinsic fibre cementum). CIFC is less cellular than bone and has a cementoid seam on its outer surface (Fig. 11.2). This cementoid seam is similar to the osteoid seam seen in bone. Note that a cementoid seam is not present on the surface of AEFC.

Towards the root apex and in the furcation areas of multirooted teeth, the AEFC and the CIFC are commonly present in alternating layers known as *cellular mixed stratified cementum* (Fig. 11.22).

Mixed fibre cementum (Fig. 11.23)

For this third variety of cementum, the collagen fibres of the organic matrix are derived from both extrinsic fibres (from the periodontal ligament) and intrinsic fibres (from cementoblasts). The extrinsic and intrinsic fibres can be readily distinguished. First, the intrinsic fibres run between the extrinsic fibres with a different orientation. Indeed, the fewer the number of intrinsic fibres in mixed fibre cementum, the closer the extrinsic fibre bundles. Second, the fibre bundles are of different sizes: the extrinsic fibres are ovoid or round bundles about 5–7 µm in diameter; the intrinsic fibres are 1–2 µm in diameter.

If the formation rate is slow, the cementum may be termed *acellular mixed-fibre cementum* and is generally well mineralised. If the formation rate is fast, the cementum may be called *cellular mixed-fibre cementum* and the fibres are less well mineralised (especially their cores).

Fig. 11.24 shows the fibre orientation in acellular and cellular cementum as seen in polarised light, with the different colours reflecting different orientations of the collagen fibres. The acellular cementum contains primarily extrinsic fibres arranged perpendicular to the root surface. The overlying cellular cementum contains mainly intrinsic fibres running parallel to the root surface. Thus, there is a colour difference between the two layers.

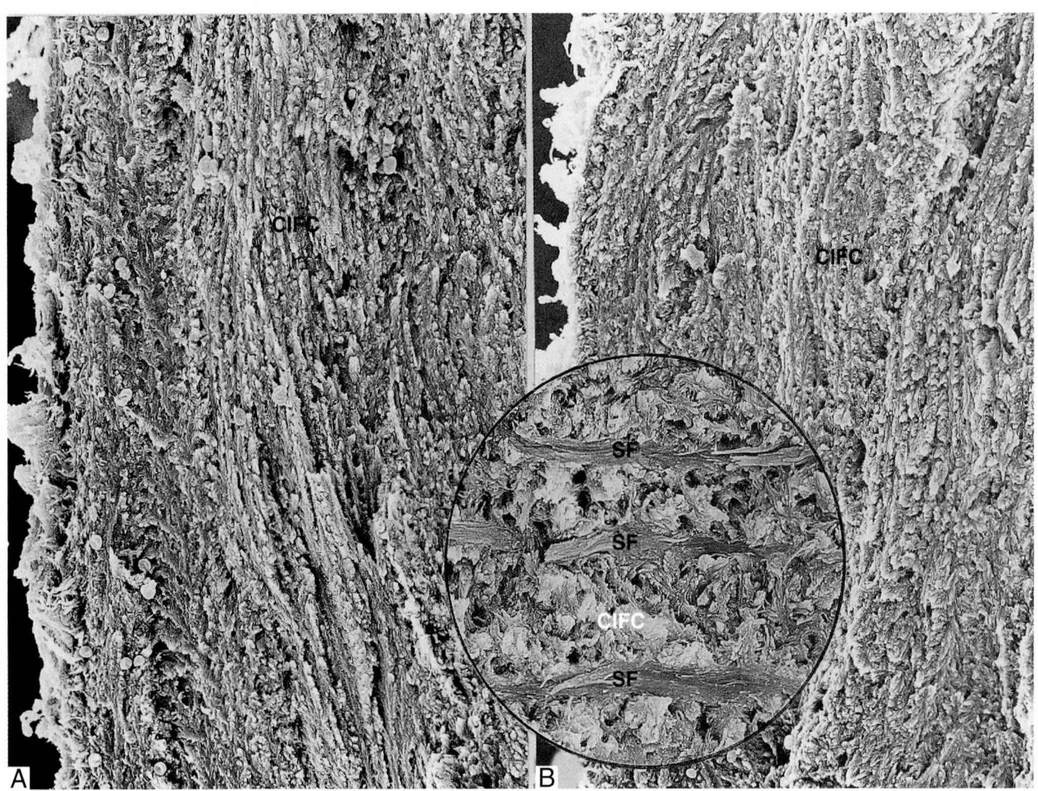

Fig. 11.21 SEMs of fractured surface of root showing the appearance of cellular intrinsic fibre cementum (CIFC). Note the absence of Sharpey fibres and the parallel distribution of the bundles of mineralised intrinsic fibres (A, B, ×470; inset shows that Sharpey fibres [SF] can occasionally be seen inserting into CIFC ×1,650). From Schroeder, H.E., 1993. Human cellular mixed stratified cementum: a tissue with alternating layers of acellular extrinsic and cellular intrinsic fiber cementum. *Schweizer Monatsschrift fur Zahnmedizin* 103, 550–560.

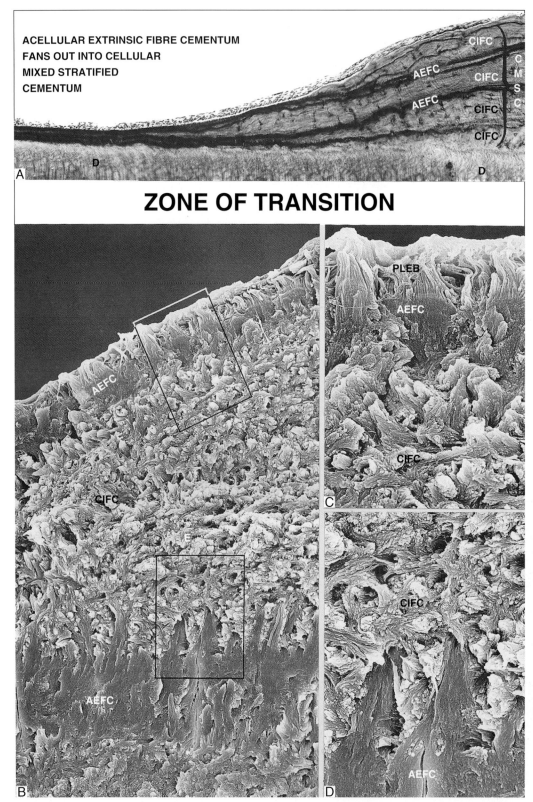

Fig. 11.22 (A) The appearance of mixed fibre cementum. A light micrograph to show the alternating distribution of acellular extrinsic fibre cementum (AEFC) and cellular intrinsic fibre cementum (CIFC), forming cellular mixed stratified cementum (CMSC) (ground section; ×80). (B–D) SEMs illustrating mixed fibre cementum; (C) and (D) are highlighted areas provided by the boxes in (B) (SEM; B, ×900; C, D, ×2,450). From Schroeder, H.E., 1993. Human cellular mixed stratified cementum: a tissue with alternating layers of acellular extrinsic and cellular intrinsic fiber cementum. *Schweizer Monatsschrift fur Zahnmedizin* 103, 550–560.

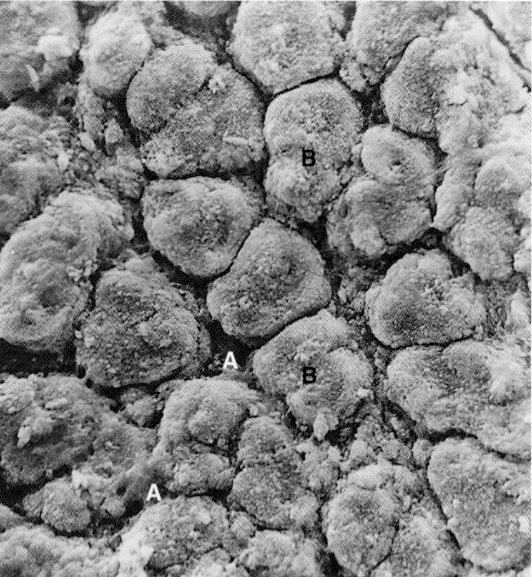

Fig. 11.23 SEM of the surface of a root showing the appearance of mixed fibre cementum. A = mineralised intrinsic fibres (present here in small amounts); B = mineralised extrinsic fibres. Note the smaller dimensions of the intrinsic fibre bundles (anorganic preparation; ×3,000). Courtesy Prof. S J Jones.

Finally, a variety of acellular intrinsic fibre cementum has been characterised, and this, like CIFC, displays a cementoid seam.

Chemical differences exist between the different forms of cementum. Dentine sialoprotein, fibronectin and tenascin are not present in AEFC but are found in CIFC. Furthermore, AEFC is deficient in lumican, versican, decorin, biglycan and fibromodulin. These differences probably reflect differences in the secretory activities of the cells involved in the development of these two varieties of cementum. It has also been reported that enamel matrix components, possibly secreted by epithelial root sheath cells and their derivatives, can result in cells synthesising AEFC.

Afibrillar cementum

The extrinsic, intrinsic and mixed fibre cementum types all contain collagen fibres. However, there is a further type of cementum that contains no collagen fibres. This afibrillar cementum is sparsely distributed and consists of a well-mineralised ground substance that may be of epithelial origin. Afibrillar cementum is a thin, acellular layer (difficult to identify at the light microscope level), which covers cervical enamel or intervenes between fibrillar cementum and dentine. Afibrillar cementum is thought to be formed at this site following the loss of the reduced enamel epithelium (see page 447).

Attachment of the periodontal ligament fibres to cementum

The fibres of the periodontal ligament run into the organic matrix of precementum that is secreted by cementoblasts. Subsequent mineralisation of precementum will incorporate the extrinsic fibres as Sharpey fibres into cementum (Figs 11.25, 11.26). It has been estimated that for AEFC there are approximately 30,000 principal fibres of the periodontal ligament attached into the cemental tissue per square millimetre.

Cementum–dentine junction

The nature of the cementum–dentine junction is of particular importance, being of interest biologically because it forms an interface (a 'fit') between two very different mineralised tissues that are developing contemporaneously. It is also of clinical importance because of the processes involved in maintaining tooth function while repairing a diseased root surface. The cementum–dentine junction appears to have a lower mineral content and is a composite of inorganic and organic components (including dermatan sulphate and collagen fibrils).

It is often reported that an 'intermediate layer' (Fig. 11.27) exists between cementum and dentine and that this layer is involved in 'anchoring' the periodontal fibres to the dentine. A variety of names has been given to the 'intermediate layer' (including 'innermost cementum layer', 'superficial layer of root dentine' and 'intermediate cementum'). Indeed, it appears that the term has even been used to describe the hyaline layer of dentine (see page 177).

The intermediate layer is said to be characterised by wide, irregular, branching spaces (Fig. 11.28) and is most commonly found in the apical region of cheek teeth. The spaces may interconnect with dentinal tubules. The nature and origin of the spaces are controversial; they may be related to entrapped epithelial cells (cell remnants containing filaments characteristic of epithelial cells have been described in this region). Alternatively, they may be enlarged terminals of dentinal tubules.

There are marked species differences with respect to the intermediate layer. In rat molars, a distinct intermediate layer exists that is rich in sialoprotein and osteopontin (both these glycoproteins being normally bone related), although the role of these glycoproteins remains unclear. The origin of this layer in rat molars is also unclear, with some suggesting that it is derived from the epithelial root sheath that lines the developing root (see pages 436–439) and others claiming that it is cementoblast-derived. Indeed, there are reports suggesting that, in humans, the region between the cementum and the root dentine contains enamel matrix protein and is a product of the epithelial root sheath. However, it seems that for many human teeth, the collagen within the AEFC layer intermingles with the dentine matrix. Furthermore, there is no sialoprotein and osteopontin, and there is no obvious zone between dentine and cementum.

Where an intermediate layer exists, it has been suggested that this functions as a permeability barrier, that it may be a precursor for cementogenesis

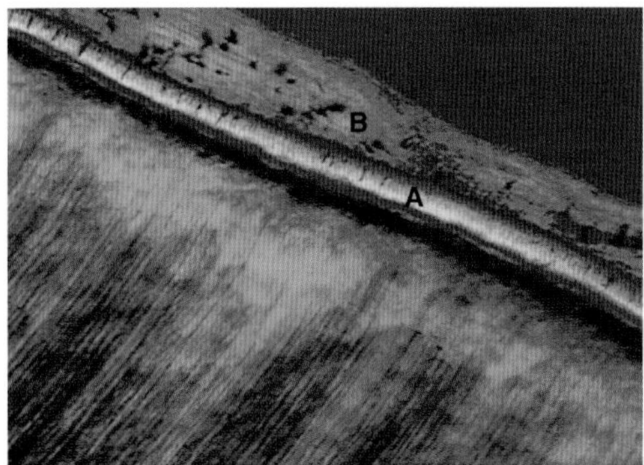

Fig. 11.24 Fibre orientation in acellular and cellular cementum. The root surface is seen in polarised light, with the different colours reflecting different orientations of the collagen fibres. A = acellular cementum; B = cellular cementum (ground longitudinal section; ×50).

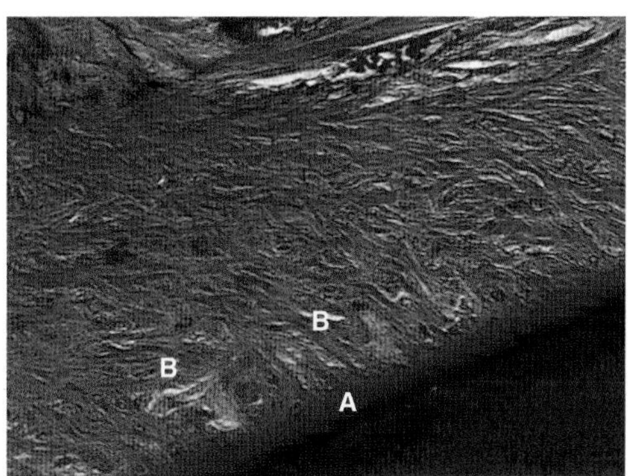

Fig. 11.25 Attachment of the periodontal ligament fibres to cementum. The fibres of the periodontal ligament (B) are seen to run into the organic matrix of precementum (A) (decalcified section; Masson blue trichrome; ×200).

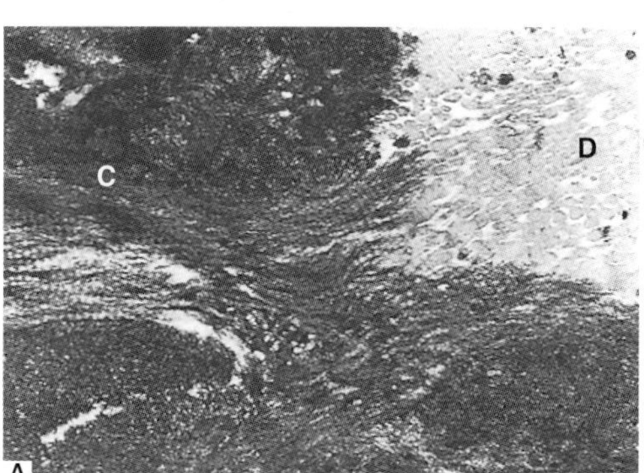

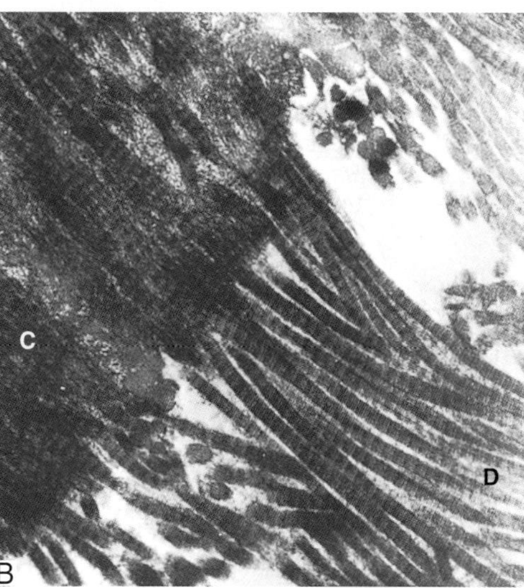

Fig. 11.26 Electron microscopic appearance of the insertion of Sharpey fibres into cementum. (A) Ground section showing that the inserting collagen fibres darken as they enter the cementum because of their partial mineralisation. (B) Decalcified section showing the grouping of collagen into a bundle and collagen cross-banding. C = cementum; D = periodontal ligament (TEM; A, ×8,000; B, ×15,000). Courtesy Dr. D K Whittaker.

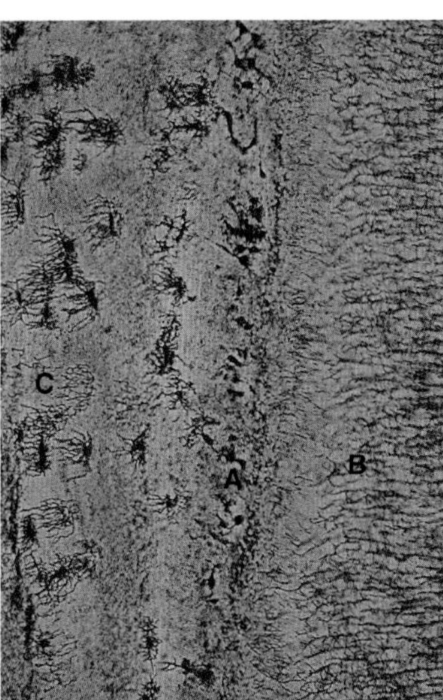

Fig. 11.27 Intermediate cementum (A). B = root dentine; C = cellular cementum (demineralised section; picrothionin; ×75). Courtesy Prof. M M Smith.

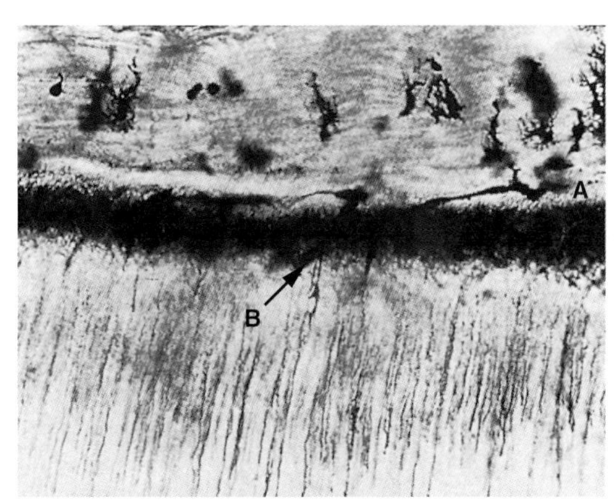

Fig. 11.28 Intermediate cementum (A) near the cementum–dentine junction. B = granular layer (ground section; ×250). Courtesy Dr. P D A Owens.

and that it is a precursor for cementogenesis in wound healing. These potential functions remain speculative. If, however, there is doubt about the very presence of an intermediate zone in human teeth, then either human teeth do not require such functions (which is highly unlikely) or too much is being conjectured with too little experimental evidence.

The clinical significance of the interface between cementum and dentine relates to regeneration of the periodontium following periodontal surgery. Although a layer of cementum may regenerate, subsequent histological examination may show a 'space' between regenerated cementum and surface dentine, perhaps indicating an absence of a true union.

Ultrastructural appearance of cementum

This varies with the level of the tissue examined. Near the periodontal surface (Fig. 11.29), cementum is not homogeneous because of ongoing calcification and the presence of Sharpey fibres. The calcification of precementum is probably initiated in the early phases by the presence of the underlying root dentine mineral and continues on and around the collagen fibres (both those formed by the cementoblasts and those included as attachment fibres from the periodontal ligament). The outer part of the cementum, where Sharpey fibres predominate, may be considered calcified periodontal ligament. Unlike dentine, no calcospherites are present within precementum. At deeper levels (Fig. 11.30), closer to the cementum–dentine junction, acellular cementum resembles peripheral dentine, and a demarcation is often difficult to see. The small channels seen at this level may be canaliculi derived from more superficial cementocytes, but some may be the terminals of dentinal tubules that traverse the border between the two tissues.

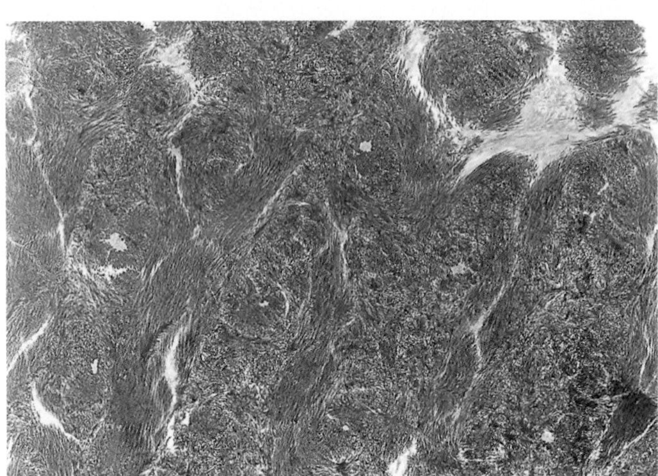

Fig. 11.29 Appearance of cementum near the periodontal surface (TEM; ×2,000).

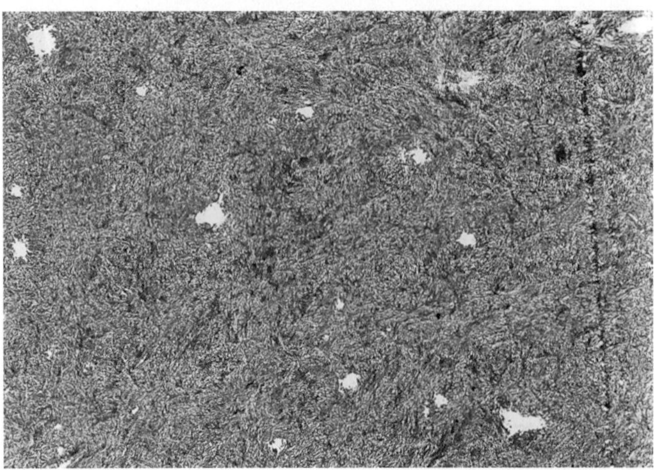

Fig. 11.30 Appearance of cementum near the cementum–dentine junction (TEM; ×2,000).

Resorption and repair of cementum

Although cementum is less susceptible to resorption than bone under the same pressures (e.g., with orthodontic loading), most roots of permanent teeth still show small, localised areas of resorption (Figs 11.31–11.33). The cause of this is not known but may be associated with microtrauma. The resorption is carried out by multinucleated odontoclasts (see pages 188–189) and may continue into the root dentine. It has been suggested that the different levels of fluoride in cementum and bone (higher in cementum) may explain why cementum is less susceptible to resorption. Alternatively, the greater resistance to resorption might relate to the fact that the surface of the cementum is covered by a layer of tightly packed collagen, and therefore the mineralised surface is relatively inaccessible.

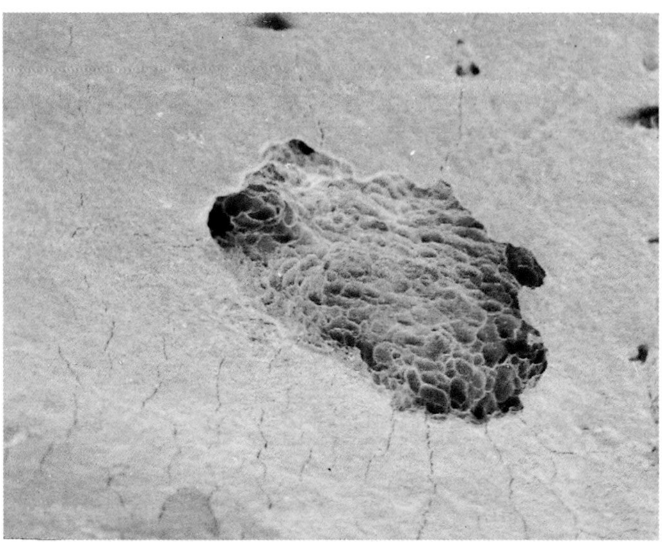

Fig. 11.31 The surface of a root showing localised area of resorption of cementum (SEM; ×250). Courtesy Prof. S J Jones.

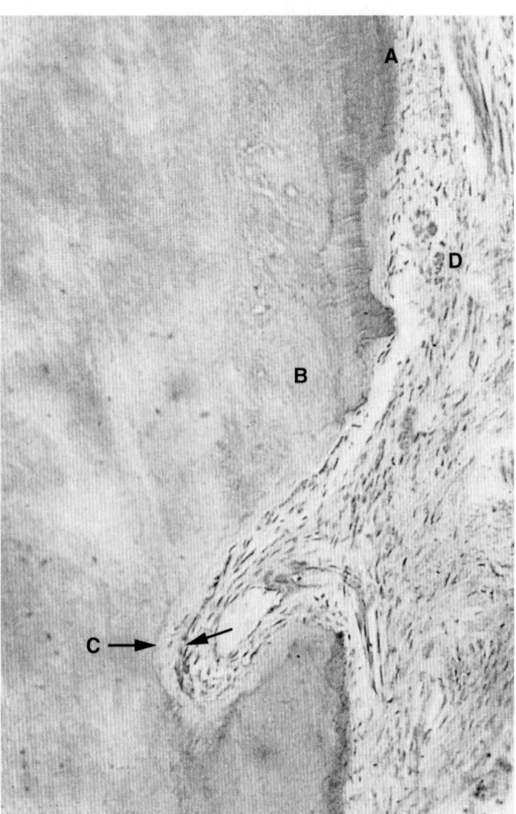

Fig. 11.32 Repair of cementum following a localised region of root resorption. A = acellular cementum; B = root dentine; C = reversal line separating repair tissue from underlying dental tissues; D = periodontal ligament; *arrows* indicate cementoblasts depositing layer of precementum in resorption deficiency (decalcified section of a root; H & E; ×90).

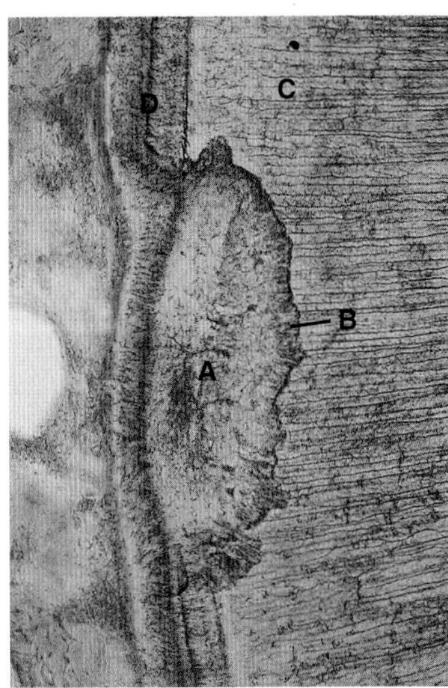

Fig. 11.33 Demineralised section of root showing infilled area of repair cementum (A). B = reversal line; C = dentine; D = cementum (picrothionin; ×75). Courtesy Prof. M M Smith.

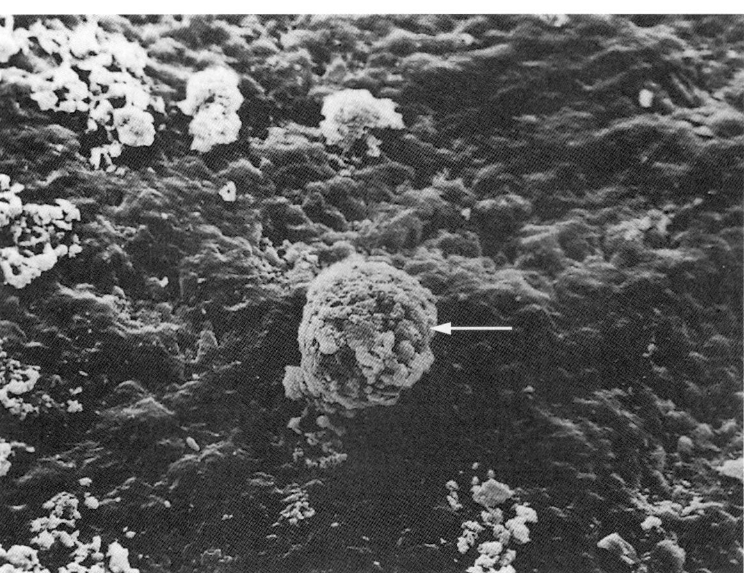

Fig. 11.34 SEM appearance of a cementicle *(arrowed)*. This cementicle is attached to the root surface (×1,000).

The unmineralised surface layer of collagen thus protects against the action of odontoclasts. It has also been suggested that cementoblasts lining the root surface do not retract from this surface in response to PTH and that therefore the surface is not exposed to odontoclasts.

Resorption deficiencies may be filled by deposition of mineralised tissue. Indeed, a line known as a *reversal line* may be seen separating the repair tissue from the normal underlying dental tissues. The repair of cementum following a localised region of root resorption is illustrated in Fig. 11.32. In this section, odontoclasts have resorbed through the thin layer of acellular cementum and penetrated into the root dentine. Repair is occurring, and a layer of formative cells (cementoblasts) have deposited a thin layer of matrix (precementum) in the deficiency. An irregular and dark-staining reversal line separates the repair tissue from the underlying dental tissues. Fig. 11.33 shows an infilled area where dentine has been resorbed.

The repair tissue resembles cellular cementum. The formative cells have a similar ultrastructure to cementoblasts. Lines resembling incremental lines may be seen, and there is a zone of uncalcified repair tissue homologous to precementum. However, differences can be noted between the repair tissue and cementum: the width of the uncalcified zone of reparative cementum (15 μm) is greater than that for precementum (5–10 μm); its degree of mineralisation is less (as judged by electron density); its crystals are smaller; and calcific globules are present, suggesting that mineralisation is not proceeding evenly.

These differences may be related to the speed of formation of the repair tissue. Where this is very slow, the repair tissue cannot be distinguished histologically, or in its mineralisation pattern, from primary cementum. However, where the repair tissue is formed rapidly (as in resorbing deciduous teeth), it closely resembles woven bone.

Clinical considerations

Exposed root dentine

Developmentally, cementum may not completely cover dentine around the entire circumference of the cervical margin (see page 213). Furthermore, it may easily be abraded. These conditions lead to the exposure of dentinal tubules to the oral environment and, if the tubules are patent, may give rise to the painful symptoms of hypersensitivity (see page 187).

Root fractures and cementicles

The most common cause of root fractures is physical trauma resulting from sporting events, falls or fights. It is most commonly seen in patients between 10 and 20 years and most often involves the anterior teeth. The plane of the fracture may be horizontal or vertical and may lead to mobility in the fractured part of the tooth. The dental pulp often retains its vitality, although initially it may be unresponsive to some forms of pulp testing. In other instances, the pulp may become necrotic. Root fractures may, on some occasions, repair by the formation of a cemental callus. Unlike the callus that forms around fractured bone, the cemental callus does not usually remodel to the original dimensions of the tooth.

Cementicles (Fig. 11.34) are small, globular masses of cementum found in approximately 35% of human roots. They are not always attached to the cementum surface but may be located free in the periodontal ligament. Cementicles may result from microtrauma, when extra stress on the Sharpey fibres causes a tear in the cementum. They are more common in the apical and middle third of the root and in root furcation areas.

Hypercementosis and cementoblastomas

Cementum continues to be deposited slowly throughout life, with its thickness increasing about threefold between the ages of 16 and 70, although whether this proceeds in a linear manner is not known. Undue thickening of cementum is referred to as *hypercementosis* and is found particularly at the root apex and also at the interradicular region of molar teeth. Cementum may be formed at the root apex in much greater amounts as a result of compensatory tooth eruption in response to attrition (wear) at the occlusal surface. It may also be found in impacted teeth and teeth without antagonists (where the increased thickness may be associated with overeruption). Where there has been a history of chronic periapical inflammation, cementum formation may be substantial, giving rise to local hypercementosis (Fig. 11.35; see also Fig 2.179A). This may cause problems during tooth extraction. If interdental bone is lost, continued cementum formation may result in fusion of the roots of adjacent teeth. Such a condition is known as *concrescence* (see Fig. 2.179B) and will lead to difficulties during tooth extraction. Hypercementosis affecting all the teeth may be associated with Paget disease.

Cementoblastomas, now more correctly categorised as fibro-osseous lesions, are benign neoplasms forming a mass of cementum-like tissue attached to the root apex of a tooth, usually a mandibular permanent first molar. The patients are often young adults. The lesion may be rounded or more irregular (Figs 11.35, 11.36). Resorption of related roots is common.

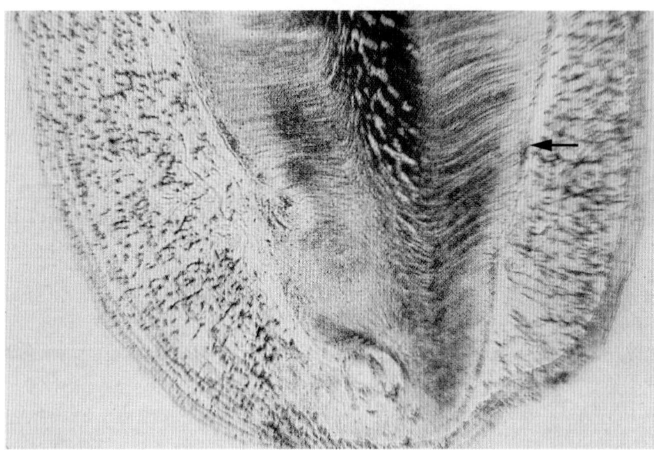

Fig. 11.35 Ground section near the root apex showing hypercementosis. *Arrow* shows cementum–dentine junction (×25).

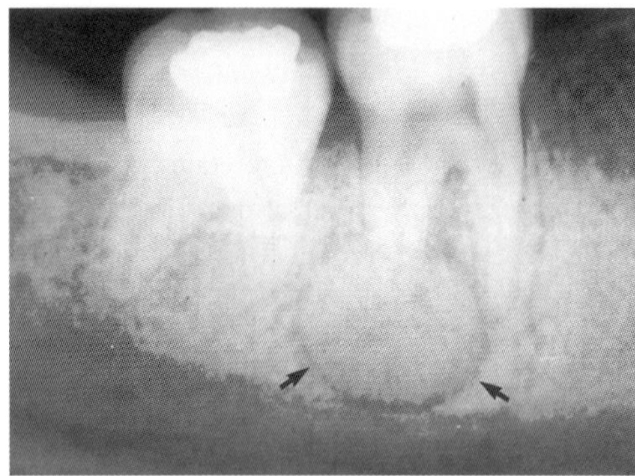

Fig. 11.36 Periapical radiograph showing the typical appearance of a cementoblastoma *(arrows)*, being a radio-paque mass with a radiolucent rim attached to the root apex. Courtesy Dr. E Whaites. From *Cawson's essentials of oral pathology and oral medicine,* eighth ed., Elsevier, London 2008.

Hypophosphatasia

Hypophosphatasia is a rare condition in which there is a reduction in the activity of tissue-nonspecific alkaline phosphatase. The gene for this enzyme is located on chromosome 1. The condition is characterised by a significant reduction in the amount of cementum formed and affects both acellular and cellular cementum (Fig. 11.37). As a result, the attachment of the principal fibres of the periodontal ligament is compromised, with premature loss of the deciduous teeth. Permanent teeth are similarly affected.

Caries of cementum

Dental plaque adhering to the cervical region of teeth, particularly in association with exposure of dental cementum following periodontal disease, may result in root caries. The lesion is similar to that seen in enamel, with a radiolucent area being evident below a well-mineralised layer of AEFC. Treatment of this condition may require conservation and the use of bonding materials. Although much research on bonding of materials to the tooth has understandably concerned enamel and dentine, bonding to cementum, which differs significantly in both structure and composition, may require different clinical procedures to gain the maximum clinical outcome and is a source for future research. For example, prior to any adhesive treatment, it may be necessary to remove any organic layers from the surface.

Apical constriction

Where the root canal exits at the apex of the tooth, cementum is deposited not only over the apex but also for a short distance (usually 0.5–1.5 mm) from the anatomical apex. This results in a narrowing of the canal at this point – the apical constriction (see Fig. 2.59 and Fig. 2.69). This represents the junction of the pulp and periodontal tissue (although there is no visible demarcation in the soft tissue). In clinical procedures of root canal therapy that call for the removal of a diseased or decayed pulp, this is the point to which the cleansing should be extended.

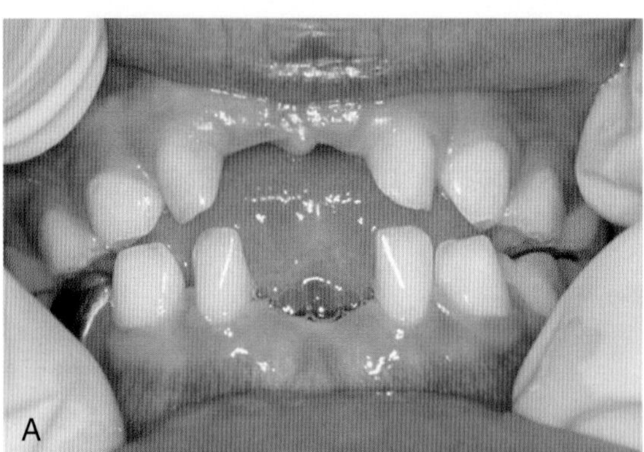

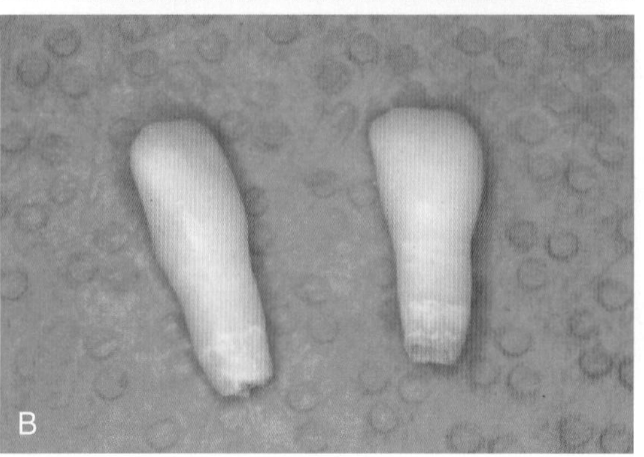

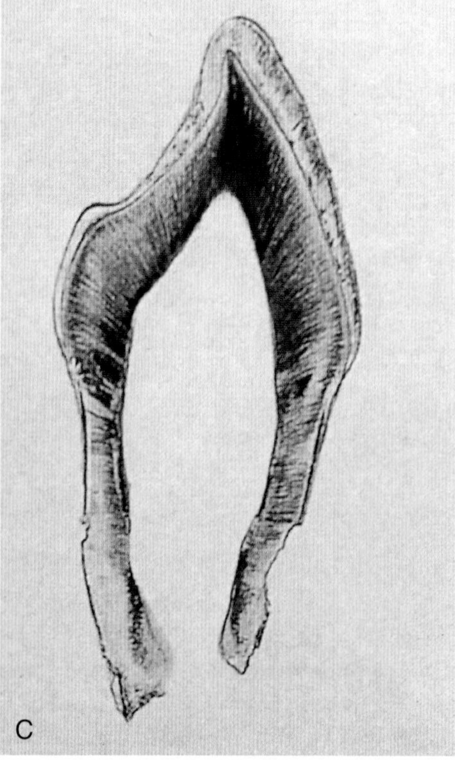

Fig. 11.37 (A) The dentition of a 4-year-old child with early loss of upper and lower central incisors due to hypophosphatasia. (B) The lower incisors, exfoliated at 13 months of age. Note the incomplete root development at the time the teeth were exfoliated. From Nowak, A.J., Christensen, J.R., Mabry, T.R., et al., 2019. *Pediatric dentistry: infancy through adolescence,* sixth ed. Elsevier. C. Ground longitudinal section of a tooth with hypophosphatasia. Note the absence of cementum. From Odell, E.W. 2017. *Cawson's essentials of oral pathology and medicine*, 9th ed. Elsevier, London.

Regeneration of cementum

Because of the widespread occurrence of chronic periodontal disease, much research has focussed on treatment of this condition in terms of tissue engineering a new periodontal ligament. The accumulation of dental plaque and subgingival calculus are aetiological factors associated with the onset of the disease and will require cleansing. In the removal of subgingival calculus, care must be taken to limit removal of cementum.

Modern-day treatment aims not only at limiting further loss of affected periodontal tissue but also at trying to regenerate new attachment tissues. This involves generating, in addition to the periodontal ligament itself, the attachment tissues comprising cementum and alveolar bone. In the case of cementum, not only must it be engineered on the surface of the tooth, but it must also become securely attached to the adjacent root surface formed by the hyaline layer. Hence, the need for understanding how the hyaline layer develops during normal ontogeny (see pages 442–445).

The stem cells associated with the formation of cementum reside in the periodontal ligament. However, as yet it is not known whether cementum has its own unique stem cells or whether there is a common stem cell for cementoblasts, osteoblasts and periodontal fibroblasts (see page 247). Furthermore, the surface of the root in periodontally affected teeth is considered to undergo changes deleterious to successful periodontal repair, including cementum resorption, and there is a considerable literature related to improving this surface by various clinical procedures during root conditioning. Cementum regeneration is considered further in Chapter 28.

Further readings for this chapter can be found in the accompanying eBook. Explore online Self-assessment quiz to test and reinforce your understanding of the material in your free ebook. Follow instructions in the Inside Front Cover to unlock your access.

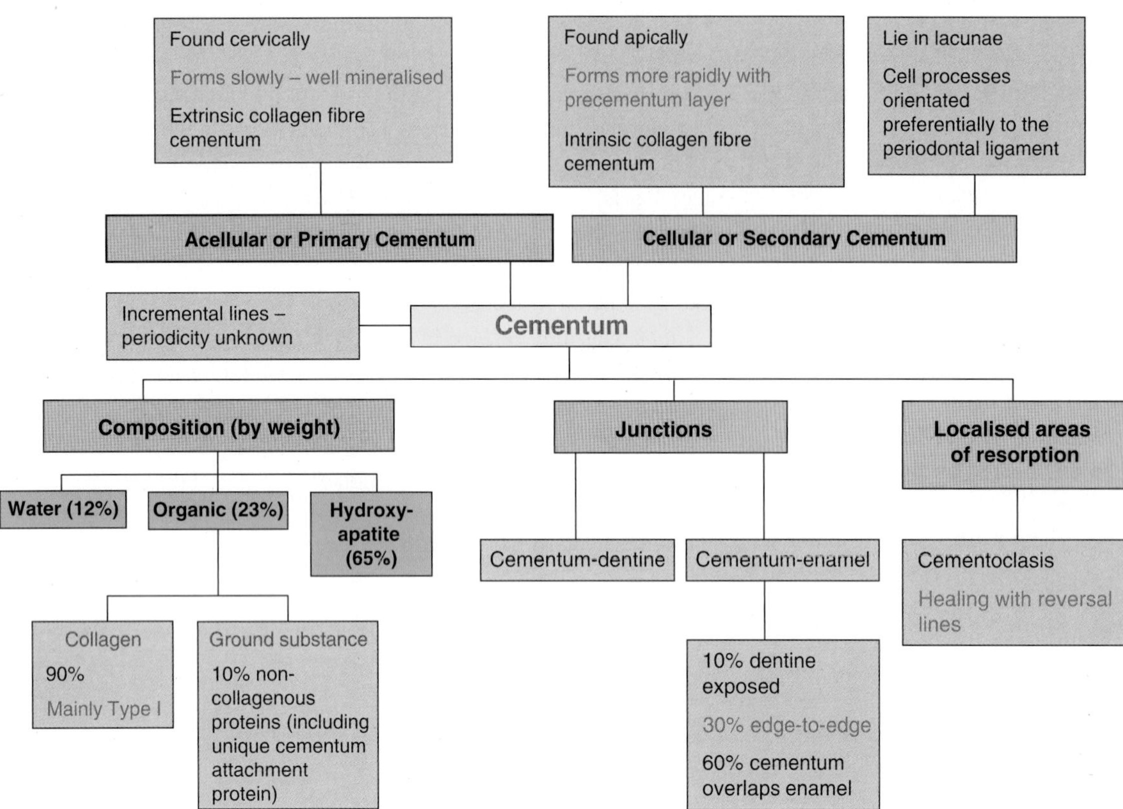

Mind Map 11.1 Cementum.

Periodontal ligament

12

Introduction

The periodontal ligament is the dense fibrous connective tissue that occupies the periodontal space between the root of the tooth and the alveolus (Fig. 12.1). It is derived from the dental follicle (see page 383). Above the alveolar crest, the periodontal ligament is continuous with the connective tissues of the gingiva; at the apical foramen, it is continuous with the dental pulp. The continuity with the gingiva is important when considering the progression of periodontitis from gingivitis. The continuity with the pulp explains why inflammation from this dental tissue (often related to dental caries) spreads to involve the periodontal ligament and the other apical supporting tissues.

Like other fibrous connective tissues, the periodontal ligament is composed of cells embedded in an extracellular matrix of collagen fibres and ground substance. The fibres are chiefly collagen.

There are several cell types, the most numerous representing fibroblasts. Unusually, there are also epithelial cells lying freely within the ligament. For a connective tissue the periodontal ligament has some unusual features including a very high rate of turnover and a very rich blood and nerve supply.

The average width of the periodontal space is said to be 0.25 mm, although there is considerable variation both between teeth and within an individual tooth. The width of the periodontal ligament in molars ranges from 0.15 to 0.38 mm. The space has been described as hourglass in shape, being narrowest in the mid-root region and near the fulcrum about which the tooth moves when an orthodontic load (tipping load) is applied to the crown. The width of the periodontal space also varies according to the functional state of the periodontal tissues. The space is reduced in nonfunctional and unerupted teeth and is increased in teeth subjected to heavy occlusal stress. With age, the periodontal space narrows slightly. The periodontal spaces of the permanent teeth are said to be narrower than those of the deciduous teeth.

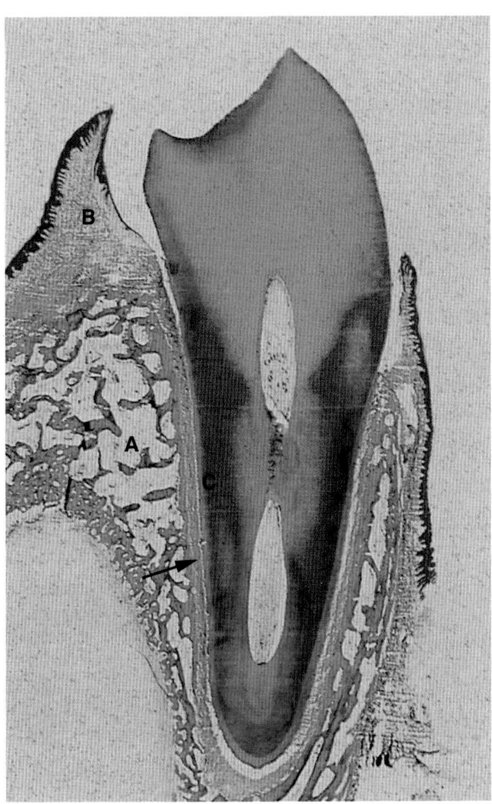

Fig. 12.1 The relationship of the periodontal ligament and the periodontal space (arrow) to the other tissues of the periodontium. A = alveolar bone; B = gingiva; C = root of tooth lined by cementum (decalcified, longitudinal section of a tooth *in situ*; H & E; ×4). Courtesy Dr. D A Lunt.

Although we are only now beginning to understand the extent of specialisation of the periodontal ligament (see pages 254–255), we still do not know why the ligament remains a soft connective tissue and does not calcify, even though it is enclosed by bone externally and cementum internally. Indeed, the width of the periodontal space essentially is preserved over time, and the alveolar bone rarely 'colonises' this space. It is evident that there must be some 'signalling systems' to accurately 'measure' and maintain the periodontal space. Failure of such a system is implicated in tooth ankylosis. That heat killing of periodontal cells induces ankylosis provides some crude evidence that periodontal fibroblasts may regulate periodontal ligament width. More convincingly, periodontal cells can inhibit the formation of mineralised bone nodules by bone stromal cells, and there is evidence to suggest that the block exerted by periodontal cells may be the result of prostaglandin production. Research also indicates that bradykinin and thrombin can stimulate prostanoid synthesis by periodontal ligament cells. Contrariwise, periodontal ligament cells are capable of producing bone-like tissue *in vitro*, can form mineralised nodules and can express alkaline phosphatase. Indeed, alkaline phosphatase, an enzyme expressed by mineralised tissue-forming cells, is expressed constitutively by periodontal ligament cells. Periodontal fibroblasts possess the capacity to differentiate into cementoblasts and osteoblasts, and this may be related to alkaline phosphatase activity.

That the ground substance can be implicated in preventing mineralisation may be deduced from *in vitro* experiments in which, after the administration of hyaluronidase, mineralisation can be produced in the remaining periodontal ligament connective tissue.

Much research has been conducted into the structure, function and composition of the periodontal ligament because the tissue is associated with important dental functions (in particular, the mechanisms of tooth support and tooth eruption; see pages 256–257 and 460–463, respectively) and for clinical reasons. The tissue is involved with inflammatory periodontal disease (a common cause of tooth loss), and there is considerable interest in tissue reattachment following such disease. Furthermore, with the application of orthodontic loads, the periodontal tissues must adjust to permit tooth relocation. Despite the amount of research undertaken, many of the important features of the periodontal ligament are not well understood, and consequently there is much controversy. The functions of the periodontal ligament are shown in Box 12.1.

The periodontal ligament has been likened to a fibrous joint (a gomphosis) and to periosteum. As will become apparent, however, such comparisons are not accurate either from a structural or a functional point of view.

Box 12.1 Functions of the periodontal ligament

1) It is responsible for resisting displacing forces (the tooth support mechanism) and for protecting the dental tissues from damage caused by excessive occlusal loads (especially at the root apex).
2) It is responsible for the mechanisms whereby a tooth attains, and then maintains, its functional position. This includes the mechanisms of tooth eruption, tooth support (particularly the recovery response after loading) and drift.
3) Its cells form, maintain and repair alveolar bone and cementum.
4) Its mechanoreceptors are involved in the neurological control of mastication (see page 122 for reflex jaw activities).

Box 12.2 The fibres in the periodontal ligament

1) Collagen
   i) Type I (about 70%)
   ii) Type III (about 20%)
   iii) Types V, VI, VII, XII (trace amounts)
2) Oxytalan, elastin and elaunin
3) Reticulin

In common with other dense fibrous connective tissues, the periodontal ligament consists of a stroma of fibres and ground substance containing cells, blood vessels and nerves.

There is some non-uniformity of structure within the periodontal ligament. For example, in furcation areas sustaining repeatedly high compression, there are fewer collagen fibres and large blood vessels that may leave more volume for non-collagenous components such as proteoglycans and glycosaminoglycans, which may better function as load dissipators.

Fibres

The connective tissue fibres are mainly collagenous (comprising over 90% of the periodontal ligament fibres), but there may also be small amounts of oxytalan, elaunin and reticulin fibres and, in some species, mature elastin fibres. Box 12.2 summaries information concerning the extracellular fibres in the periodontal ligament.

Collagen

Types

There are 29 genetically distinct types of collagen present in animal tissues. They can be broadly divided into fibrillar and nonfibrillar collagens. The most commonly found are the fibrillar collagens termed types I -III, V and XI.

The main types of collagen in the periodontal ligament are types I and III. Approximately 70% of the periodontal collagen is type I collagen. This variety of collagen is the major protein component of most connective tissues (including bone and skin) and contains two identical α_1 chains and a chemically different α_2 chain. It is low in hydroxylysine and glycosylated hydroxylysine. Unusually, however, the periodontal ligament is rich in type III collagen (about 20%). This variety consists of three identical α_1 III chains. It is high in hydroxyproline, low in hydroxylysine and contains cysteine. The function of type III collagen is not properly understood, although it is associated in other sites of the body with rapid turnover (e.g., granulation tissues and fetal connective tissue). Type III collagen is not localised to any specific region of the periodontal ligament but is covalently linked to type I collagen throughout the tissue. It is found in the periphery of Sharpey's fibre attachments into alveolar bone (page 277) and around nerves and blood vessels. *In vitro* studies have shown that there is clonal heterogeneity for expression of type I and type III collagens and for fibronectin in periodontal ligament cell populations.

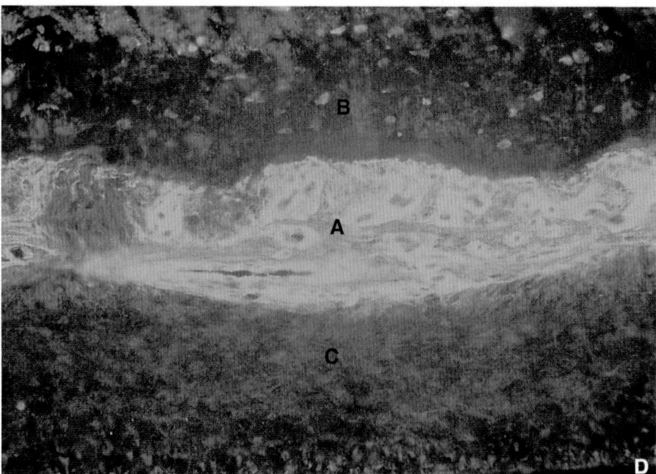

Fig. 12.2 Longitudinal cryosection of rat incisor periodontal ligament with immunofluorescent staining for type VI collagen showing strong positive yellow staining (A) towards the alveolar bone surface (B) with an absence of staining (C) in the ligament towards the tooth surface (D) (×80). From Sloan, P., Carter, D.H., 1995 Structural organisation of the fibres of the periodontal ligament. In: Berkovitz, B.K.B., Moxham, B.J., Newman, H. (Eds), The Periodontal Ligament in Health and Disease, second ed. Mosby–Wolfe, London, pp 35–53.

Small amounts of types VI (4%), V (2%) and XII (1%) collagens have been found in the periodontal ligament, as well as traces of basement membrane collagens (types IV and VII) associated with epithelial cell rests (see pages 243–245) and blood vessels. Type V collagen coats cell surfaces and other types of collagen. This collagen may increase in amount with inflammatory periodontal disease. Although located in all zones of the periodontal ligament in fully erupted teeth, type VI collagen is absent from the middle zone of erupting molars and from the tooth-related portion of the ligament of continuously growing incisors of rats (Fig. 12.2). This type of collagen forms part of the oxytalan fibre system and can promote proliferation of fibroblasts.

It has been proposed that periodontal cells regulate the periodontal ligament's connective tissue architecture through expression of type XII collagen (Fig. 12.3). Type XII collagen is a nonfibrous collagen (known as a fibril-associated collagen) with interrupted helices. It may function by linking together other collagens. There is evidence to suggest that type XII collagen occurs within the periodontal ligament only when the ligament is fully erupted and functional. Furthermore, it appears on the pressure side of the periodontal ligament after orthodontic loading and remodelling of the tissue. Transgenic mice with a mutation of collagen type XII show disruption of the normal architecture of the collagen fibre system within the periodontal ligament. Type XIV collagen can also be expressed in the periodontal ligament.

Size and arrangement

Much of the collagen is gathered together to form bundles approximately 5 µm in diameter. These bundles are termed the 'principal fibres'. They appear to be more numerous (but smaller) at their attachments to cementum than at the alveolar bone (Fig. 12.19). Fig. 12.4 shows principal collagen fibres passing across the periodontal space from the root to the alveolar bone. The close association between the principal fibres and the fibroblasts of the periodontal ligament is shown in Figs. 12.5 and 12.6. The fibroblasts are responsible for the synthesis and degradation of collagen. Cellular processes surround, or envelop, the fibre bundles; indeed, processes from adjacent cells are joined by intercellular contacts (see page 237) to form a cellular network. Many of the isolated islands of cytoplasm present in the section in Fig. 12.5 are cell processes from fibroblasts whose cell bodies are beyond the plane of section.

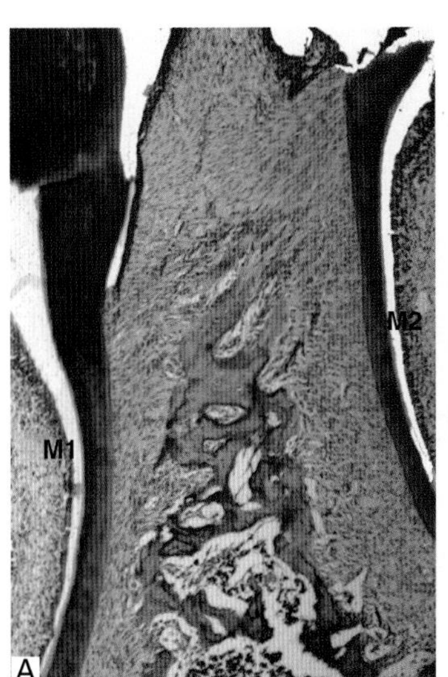

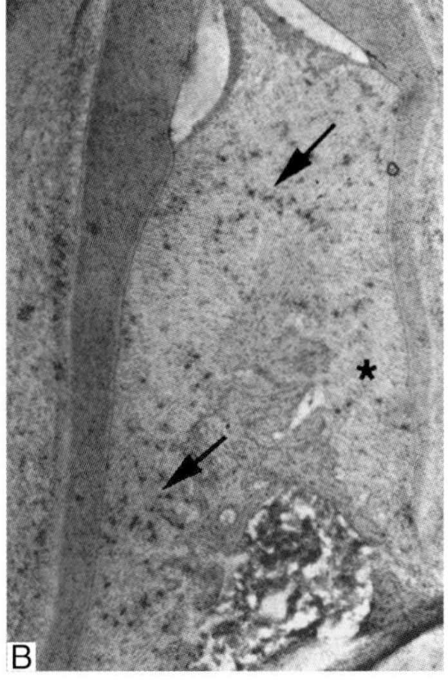

Fig. 12.3 The presence of type XII collagen within the periodontal ligament. (A) Developing periodontal ligament of maxillary first molar (MI) and second molar (M2) in a 25-day-old rat. In this specimen, the first molar has completed eruption and its periodontal ligament is more organised, whereas the second molar has not yet erupted. (B) *In situ* hybridisation of the S35-labelled type XII collagen cDNA probe. The type XII collagen probe hybridised to fibroblasts in the periodontal ligament of the first molar (arrows). Fibroblasts in the second molar periodontal ligament (*) were less active in type XII collagen synthesis. It has been postulated that type XII collagen may contribute to the organisation of the mature and functional ligament collagen fibre architecture, which serves to resist unidirectional force. Courtesy Dr. Ichiro Nishimura and the UCLA Weintraub Centre for Reconstructive Biotechnology.

Within each collagen bundle, subunits of structure called *collagen fibrils* can be seen. The individual collagen fibrils illustrated in Fig. 12.7A are sectioned longitudinally and show the classical banding characteristic of collagen. The collagen fibrils are formed by the packing together of individual tropocollagen molecules. The diameters of the collagen fibrils reflect the mechanical demands put upon the connective tissue. The collagen fibrils of the periodontal ligament are small and of uniform diameter (Fig. 12.7B). The histogram provided in Fig. 12.8 shows that for the rat periodontal ligament, there is a sharply unimodal distribution of collagen fibrils (range ≈20–70 nm) with a mode of approximately 42 nm. For humans, the mean is only slightly larger (50 nm). This confirms that the periodontal fibrils are small and of essentially uniform diameter. The pattern of distribution is reminiscent of collagen in connective tissues placed under compression and differs markedly from the bimodal distribution with large fibrils usually associated with tissues under tension (e.g., tendon). Research indicates that this distribution of periodontal collagen alters neither with changes in periodontal function nor with age. The lack of change with age differs from many other fibrous connective tissues.

The principal collagen fibres show different orientations in different regions of the periodontal ligament (Figs. 12.9–12.13). They comprise dentoalveolar crest fibres, horizontal fibres, oblique fibres, apical fibres and interradicular fibres. It has been usual to ascribe specific functions to each of the groups of principal fibres. For example, it has been suggested that the orientation of the oblique fibres shows that they form a suspensory ligament, which translates pressure on the tooth into tensional forces on the alveolar wall. However, no physiological evidence exists to support such a concept, and many of the structural features of the periodontal ligament (e.g., the collagen fibril diameters) suggest that the ligament acts in compression (see page 256).

Controversy exists concerning the extent of individual fibres across the width of the periodontal ligament. One view holds that there are distinct tooth-related and bone-related fibres and that these intercalate near the middle of the ligament at an intermediate plexus (Fig. 12.14). However, most evidence suggests that the fibres cross the entire width of the periodontal space but branch en route and join neighbouring fibres to form a complex three-dimensional network. While remodelling of fibres in the intermediate plexus provides a convenient model to explain how such

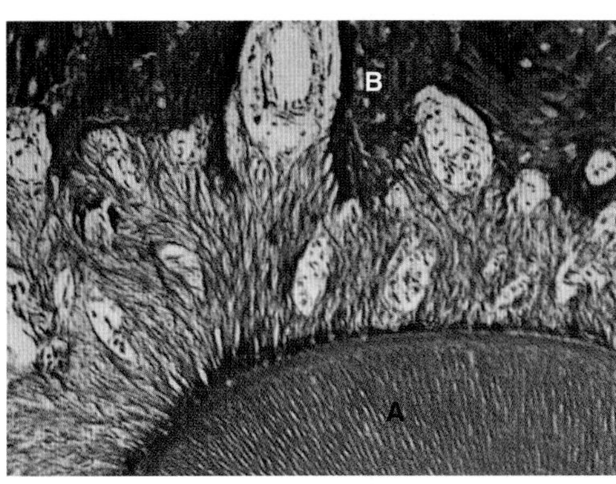

Fig. 12.4 Principal collagen fibres passing across the periodontal space from the root (A) to the alveolar bone (B). Note also the vascular nature of the periodontal ligament (decalcified, transverse section through the periodontal ligament; Gomori's silver stain; ×250).

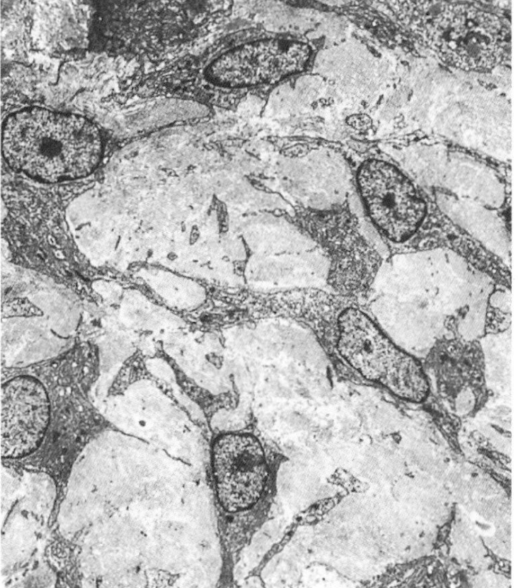

Fig. 12.5 TEM showing the close association between the principal fibres and the fibroblasts of the periodontal ligament (×3,000).

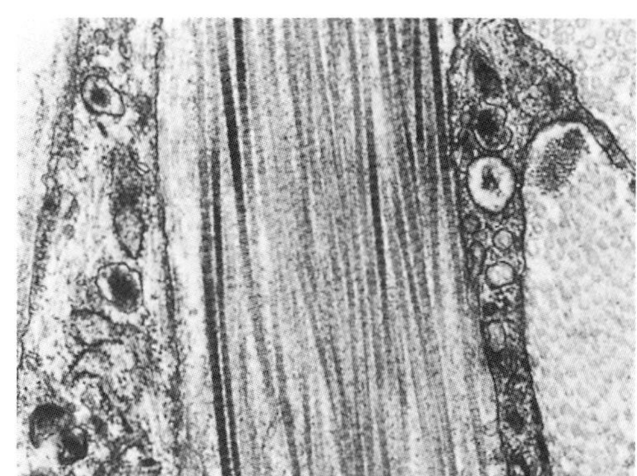

Fig. 12.6 High-power view of a fibroblast process enveloping a principal fibre. Note the individual collagen fibrils within the principal bundle sectioned longitudinally (TEM; ×10,000).

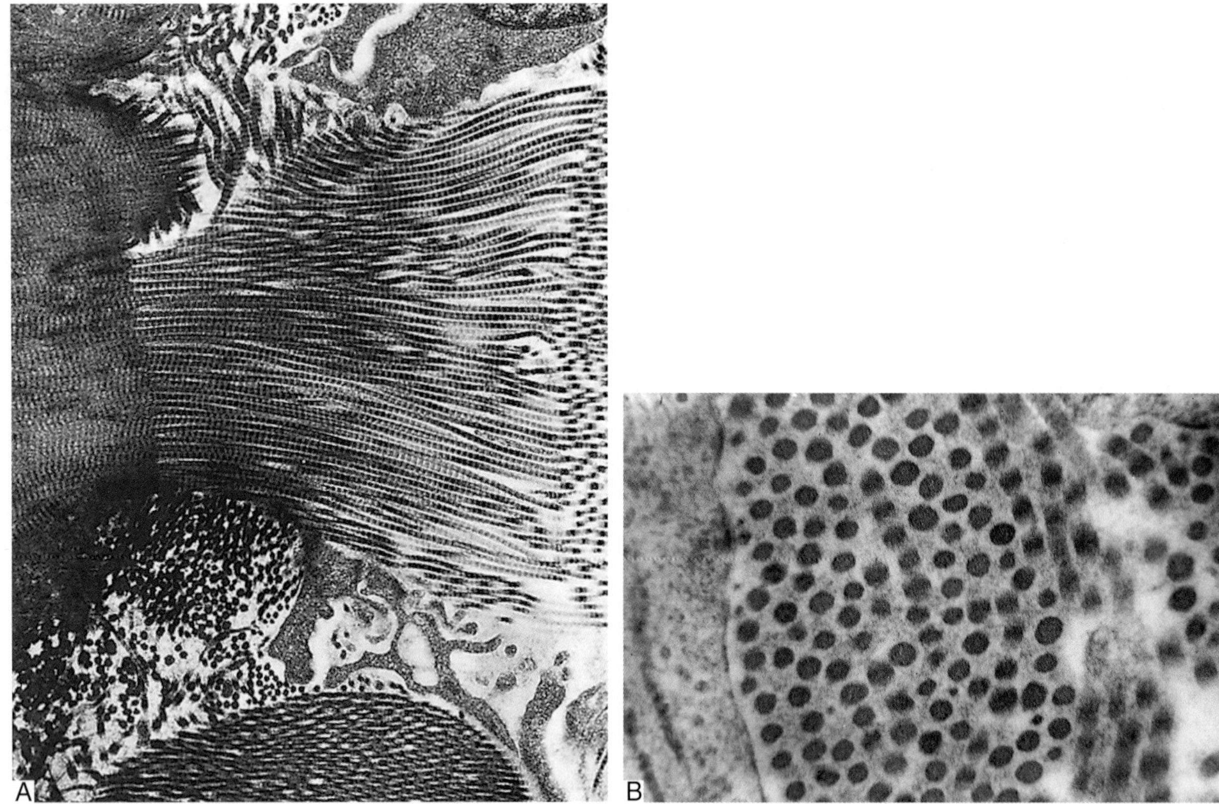

Fig. 12.7 High-power view of collagen fibrils within a principal fibre of the periodontal ligament. (A) Fibrils sectioned longitudinally. (B) Fibrils sectioned transversely. The fibrils in longitudinal section display the banding characteristic of collagen. The fibrils in transverse section appear to be small and of uniform diameter (TEM; A, ×16,000; B, ×100,000).

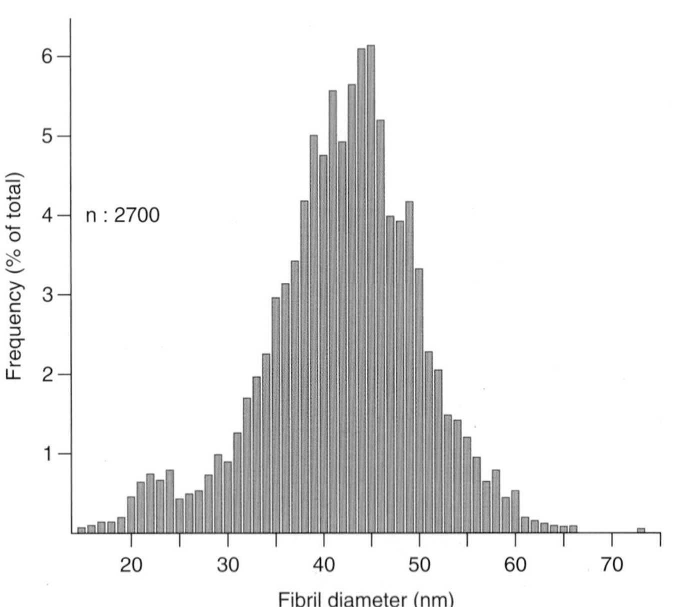

Fig. 12.8 Histogram showing the range of collagen fibril diameters in the periodontal ligament.

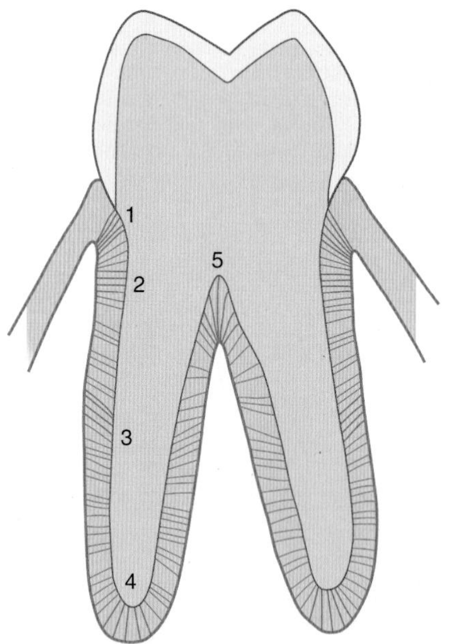

Fig. 12.9 The orientation of the principal fibres of the periodontal ligament seen in longitudinal section of a multirooted tooth: 1 = dentoalveolar crest fibres; 2 = horizontal fibres; 3 = oblique fibres; 4 = apical fibres; 5 = interradicular fibres.

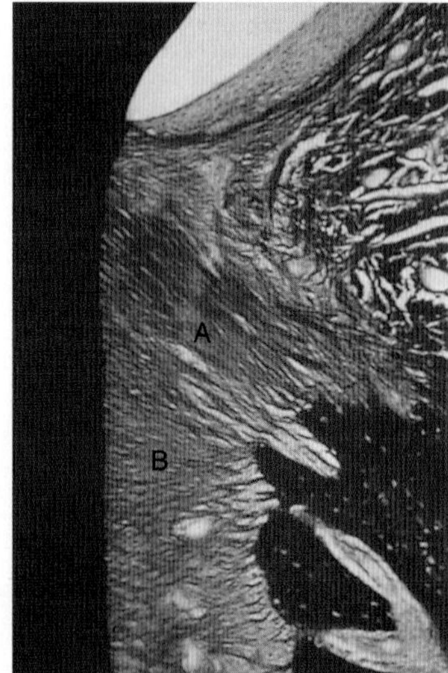

Fig. 12.10 The dentoalveolar crest fibres (A) and the horizontal fibres (B) of the periodontal ligament (decalcified, longitudinal section through the ligament in the region of the alveolar crest; aldehyde fuchsin and van Gieson; ×80).

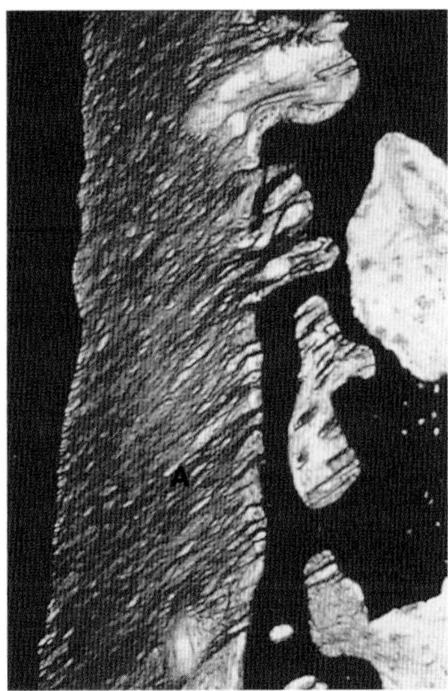

Fig. 12.11 The oblique fibres (A) of the periodontal ligament (decalcified, longitudinal section; aldehyde fuchsin and van Gieson; ×80).

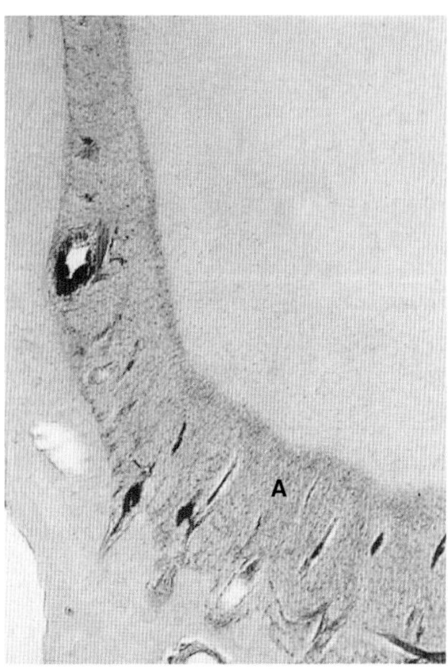

Fig. 12.12 The apical fibres (A) of the periodontal ligament (decalcified, longitudinal section through the ligament in the region of the root apex; aldehyde fuchsin and van Gieson; ×30).

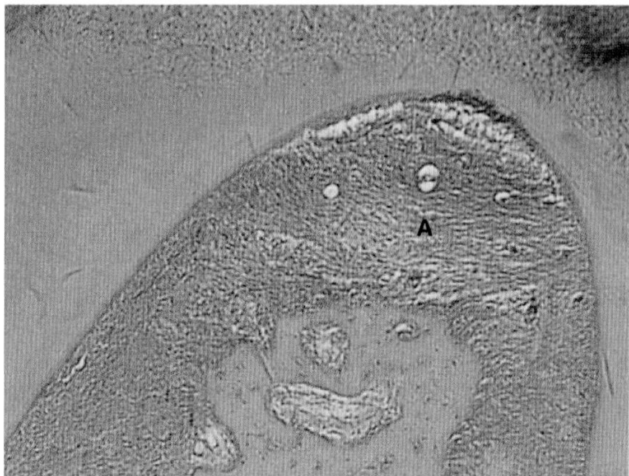

Fig. 12.13 Interradicular fibres (A) of the periodontal ligament (decalcified, longitudinal section of the ligament in the region of a root bifurcation; orange green and light green; ×40). Courtesy Dr. R O'Sullivan.

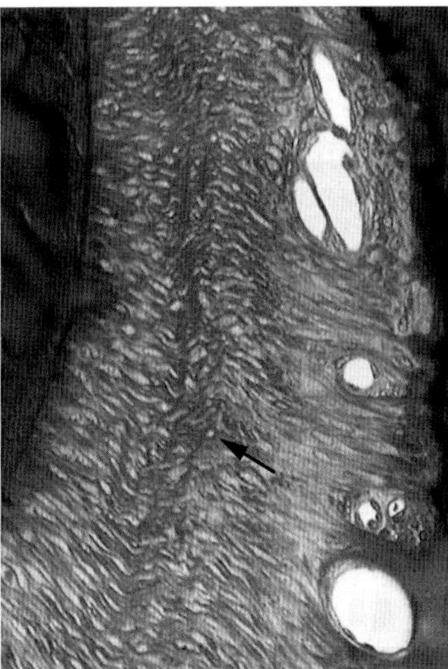

Fig. 12.14 Longitudinal section through the periodontal ligament producing an appearance of an intermediate plexus (arrowed) (decalcified, longitudinal section; Alcian blue; ×200).

axial tooth movements as eruption may be sustained, the plexus is usually seen only in longitudinal sections of continuously growing incisors (of rodents and lagomorphs): it is not seen in cross-sections. Thus, the plexus is an artefact, probably related to the fact that the collagen fibres in the periodontal ligaments of continuously growing incisors are arranged mainly in the form of sheets rather than bundles. The continuity of the principal fibres across the periodontal space in teeth of noncontinuous growth is displayed in Fig. 12.15. Here, no intermediate plexus can be seen, with the fibres branching and joining with each other.

Despite the lack of histological evidence for an intermediate fibre plexus, it has been proposed that there is a 'zone of shear' – a site of remodelling during eruption. However, the location of this zone is in dispute. Some believe that it lies near the centre of the periodontal ligament, the relatively avascular, tooth-related part of the ligament moving with the erupting tooth. Studies using tritium-labelled proline might suggest that there is increased uptake in a zone in the mid-region of the periodontal ligament. However, other studies have been unable to support this, demonstrating uniform uptake of various labels over the whole width of the ligament.

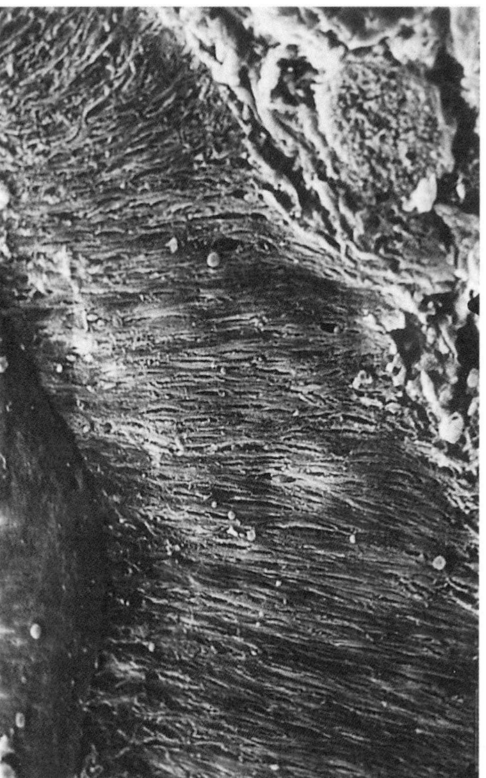

Fig. 12.15 Continuity of the principal fibres across the periodontal space seen in a periodontal ligament cut transversely (SEM; ×500). Courtesy Prof. P Sloan.

The physiological significance of a central location for the zone of shear is thrown into doubt by experiments on the resected rodent incisor, which indicate that the zone of shear is close to the root surface (Fig. 12.16). Root resection involves surgical removal of the growing base of the incisor. Because this tooth continues to erupt, it passes up the socket, leaving a space below its base. Accordingly, if the zone of shear occurs centrally within the periodontal ligament, the tooth-related part of the ligament should move with the tooth, leaving behind the bone-related tissue only. In fact, the whole width of the ligament is left behind the erupting tooth, indicating that the zone of shear is close to the tooth surface. That the zone

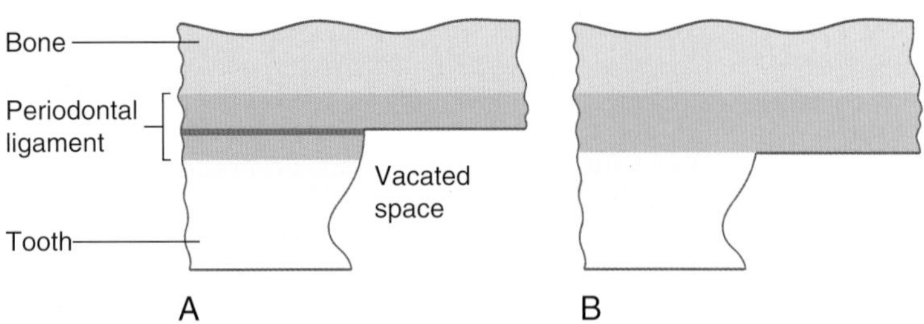

Fig. 12.16 The effects of root resection on the periodontal ligament and its significance to the 'zone of shear' and tissue remodelling. (A) The situation that would pertain if the zone of shear occurs centrally within the periodontal ligament – the tooth-related part of the ligament should move with the tooth, leaving behind the bone-related tissue only. (B) The whole width of the ligament is left behind the erupting tooth, indicating that the zone of shear is close to the tooth surface.

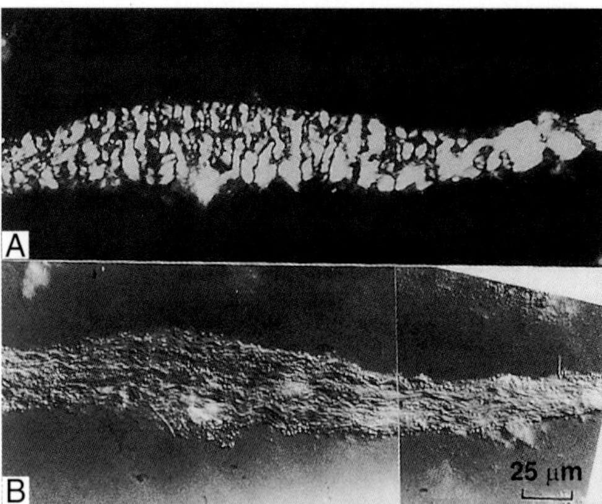

Fig. 12.18 Crimping displayed in a single teased-out collagen fibre from the periodontal ligament. (A) Polarising optical micrograph. (B) Nomarski differential interference contrast of same field as (A) (×200). Courtesy Dr. L J Gathercole.

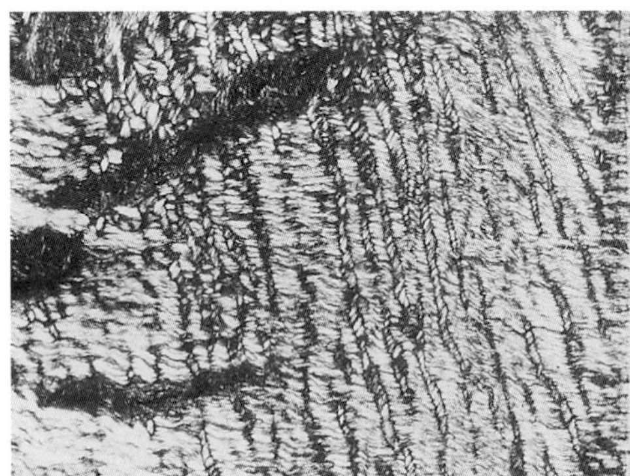

Fig. 12.17 Crimping of collagen in the periodontal ligament as viewed under polarised light. The fibres are seen to be banded between crossed polars, reflecting an underlying periodicity along the fibre (transverse section of the central region of the rabbit incisor periodontal ligament; polarising optical micrograph; ×200). Courtesy Prof. P Sloan.

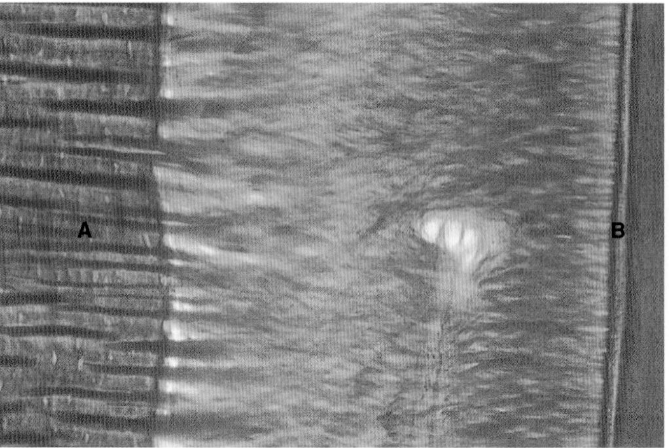

Fig. 12.19 The insertion of periodontal fibres into alveolar bone (A) and cementum (B). The horizontal lines in the bone and cementum represent the Sharpey's fibres (decalcified section; aldehyde fuchsin and van Gieson; ×250).

of shear is close to the tooth surface is further supported by experiments where lathyrogens – drugs that inhibit the formation of collagen cross-links – are administered in the rodent diet: the lathyritic rat periodontal ligament is characterised by a longitudinal cleft down the ligament adjacent to the tooth surface.

Crimping

The principal fibres of the periodontal ligament do not run a straight course as they pass from the region of the alveolar bone to the tooth. Indeed, they are said to be wavy, although it is not known whether the waviness is real or is an artefact of histological preparation. If real, it could have important implications for the biomechanical properties of the ligament and consequently the mechanism of tooth support (see pages 256–257). A specific type of waviness seen in collagenous tissues (including the periodontal ligament) is crimping. Collagen crimps are best seen under the polarising microscope (Fig. 12.17). The fibres are banded in polarised light, reflecting an underlying periodicity along the fibre. The period is about 16 μm, and the angular deflection from the fibre axis is in excess of 20 degrees. It is important to realise that the banding does not rely on seeing shapes (waves in particular); the alternating dark and bright bands are evident in otherwise straight and smooth cylindrical fibres. Indeed, crimping can be displayed in a single, teased-out collagen fibre from the periodontal ligament (Fig. 12.18), and the banding relates to the wavy course of the fibrils in the bundle. In functional terms, it has been proposed that the crimp is gradually pulled out when the ligament is subjected to the early phase of mechanical tension.

Sharpey's fibres

The principal fibres of the periodontal ligament that are embedded into cementum and the bone lining the tooth socket are termed *Sharpey's fibres* (Fig. 12.19). The principal fibres are more numerous, but smaller, at their attachments into cementum than at the alveolar bone. Under the electron microscope, the mineralised parts of the Sharpey's fibres in alveolar bone (Fig. 12.20) appear as projecting stubs covered with mineral clusters. The occurrence of mineralisation at approximately right angles to the long axes of the fibres may indicate that, in function, the fibres are subjected to tensional forces. The location and distribution of Sharpey's fibres from the periodontal collagen along the tooth socket is illustrated in Fig. 12.21. This diagram is conjectured from data obtained from a variety of species and suggests that the fibres near the alveolar crest show pronounced Sharpey's fibre insertions. Elsewhere, however, many of the principal fibres in the periodontal ligament do not insert into bone but appear to terminate around the blood vessels of the ligament.

Turnover

The rate of turnover of collagen within the periodontal ligament is faster than virtually all other connective tissues (half-life of collagen 3–23 days). The rate appears to vary in different parts of the same tooth, being highest towards the root apex. However, turnover seems to be relatively even across the width of the periodontal ligament, perhaps providing evidence against the existence of separate tooth-related and bone-related parts to the

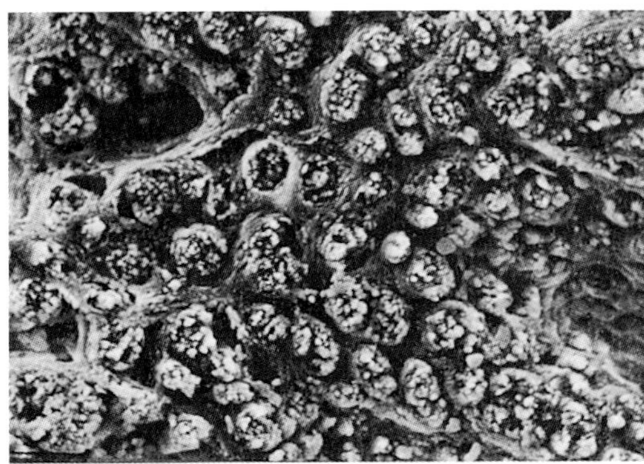

Fig. 12.20 SEM of Sharpey's fibres at the surface of alveolar bone showing 'stublike' appearance (×300). Courtesy Prof. P Sloan.

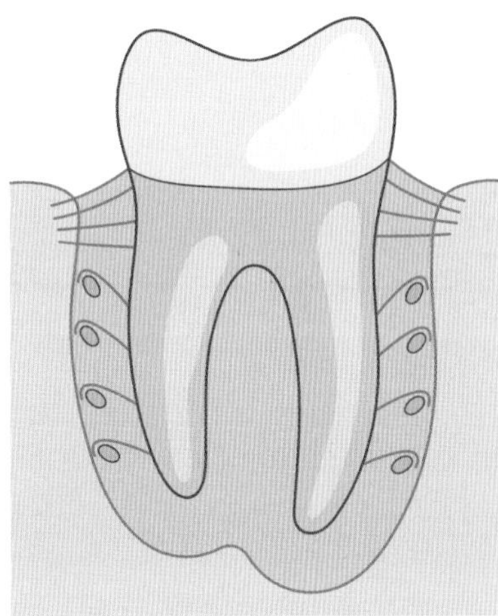

Fig. 12.21 The location and distribution of Sharpey's fibres from the periodontal collagen along the tooth socket.

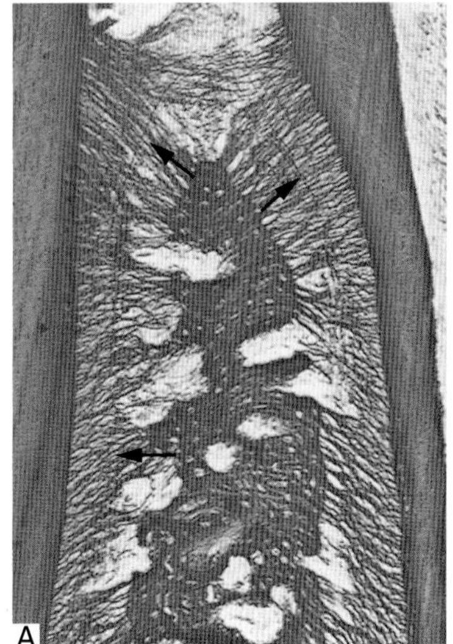

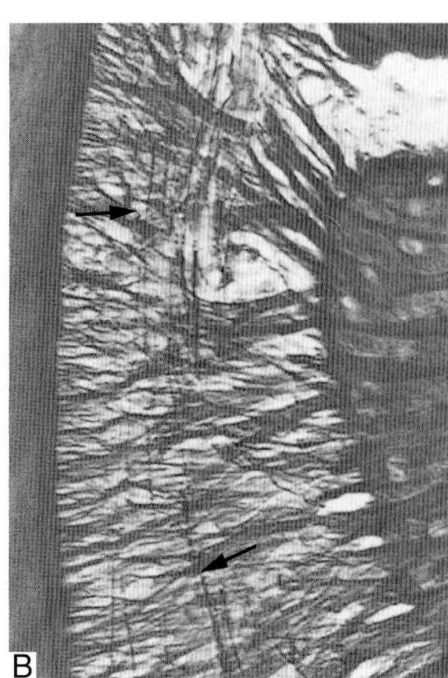

Fig. 12.22 The course of oxytalan fibres (arrowed) (decalcified, longitudinal section through the periodontal ligament; potassium monopersulphate, aldehyde fuchsin counterstained with van Gieson; (A) ×40; (B) ×120). Courtesy Dr. A D Beynon.

tissue (see pages 229–232). The explanation for the high rate of turnover is not known, but it is reasonable to suppose that the high rate may relate to the considerable functional demands placed upon the tooth in terms of remodelling as a reaction to occlusal stress and to tooth movements. However, the ligaments of teeth subjected to greatly reduced masticatory loads do not show different rates of turnover from teeth subjected to normal loads. Furthermore, the turnover rate in teeth erupting very rapidly is no different from that in the ligaments of fully erupted teeth.

Research indicates that measuring rates may not reflect total protein turnover and that there may be several protein pools having different turnover rates, each contributing to a different extent to overall protein turnover in the periodontal ligament. Indeed, control of matrix morphostasis may be more dependent on extracellular processing (e.g., fibrillogenesis, proteolysis) than upon the initial rate of protein secretion. For example, far more collagen may be synthesised than is eventually secreted, with the excess being degraded intracellularly without ever leaving the cell.

The high rate of turnover may also be reflected in the type of reducible cross-link found in the periodontal collagen (i.e., dehydrodihydroxy lysinonorleucine).

The possible role of the periodontal collagen in tooth support and tooth eruption is considered further on pages 256–257 and 460–463, respectively.

Oxytalan and elaunin

Elastic system fibres are composed of elastin, elaunin, and oxytalan fibres. Depending upon the species, the periodontal ligament contains either oxytalan fibres or elastin fibres. In humans, both oxytalan and elaunin fibres have been reported.

Oxytalan, whose name indicates its resistance to acid, is composed of fibrillin-rich microfibrils, chiefly microfibrils 1 and 2, and contains no elastin. Fibrillin, synthesised by fibroblasts, is a large, cysteine-rich glycoprotein that is composed of several extracellular protein domains such as epidermal growth factor (EGF). The mechanism by which extracellular fibrillin-1 assembles into microfibrils is not fully understood. Fibrillin-1 contains the Arg-Gly-Asp (RGD) motif, which may allow binding to RGD-recognising integrins on the surface of periodontal ligament fibroblasts. To test this hypothesis, periodontal ligament fibroblasts were treated with an alpha v beta3–specific antagonist to examine fibrillin-1 assembly. Such treatment abolished fibrillin-1 deposition. These results provide evidence that integrin alpha v beta3 regulates extracellular assembly of fibrillin-1, thereby modulating cell-mediated homeostasis of microfibrils.

In order to demonstrate periodontal oxytalan fibres at the light microscope level, it is necessary to oxidise tissue sections strongly before staining with certain elastin stains. Unlike collagen, oxytalan fibres are not susceptible to acid hydrolysis. Although little is known about their composition, their ultrastructural characteristics suggest that they are immature elastin fibres (pre-elastin), and they appear to have elastin and type VI collagen components.

Oxytalan fibres are attached into the cementum of the tooth and course out into the periodontal ligament in various directions (Fig. 12.22), rarely being incorporated into bone. In the cervical region, they follow the course of gingival and transseptal collagen fibres but within the periodontal ligament proper they tend to be more longitudinally oriented, crossing the oblique fibre bundles more or less perpendicularly. In the outer part of the ligament, they are said to often terminate around blood vessels and nerves. Oxytalan fibres vary from 0.5 µm to 2.5 µm in diameter (as assessed with the light microscope) and constitute no more than about 3% of the extracellular fibre composition. The oxytalan fibre can be recognised at the ultrastructural level (Fig. 12.23) as a collection of unbanded fibrils arranged parallel to the long axis of the fibre. Each fibril is approximately 15 nm in diameter, and an interfibrillar amorphous material is present in variable amounts. In cross-section, the oxytalan fibre is oval and its dimensions are smaller than reported using the light microscope. They are thought to resemble pre-elastin in that, unlike mature elastin, there is no central amorphous core.

The functions of oxytalan fibres remain unknown, and there is a paucity of experimental data. They are said to be thicker and more numerous

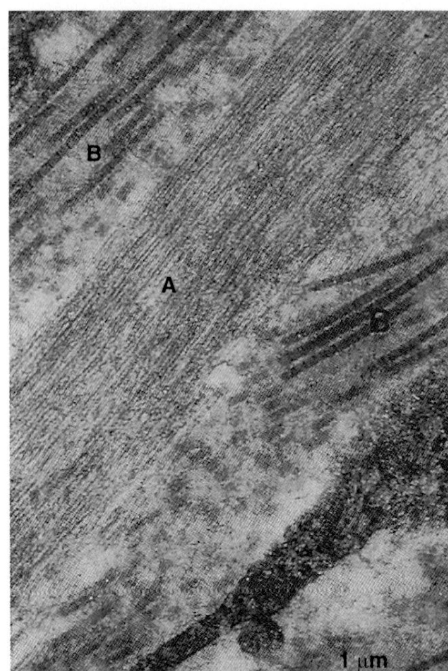

Fig. 12.23 TEM of an oxytalan fibre (A). B = collagen fibres (×25,000).

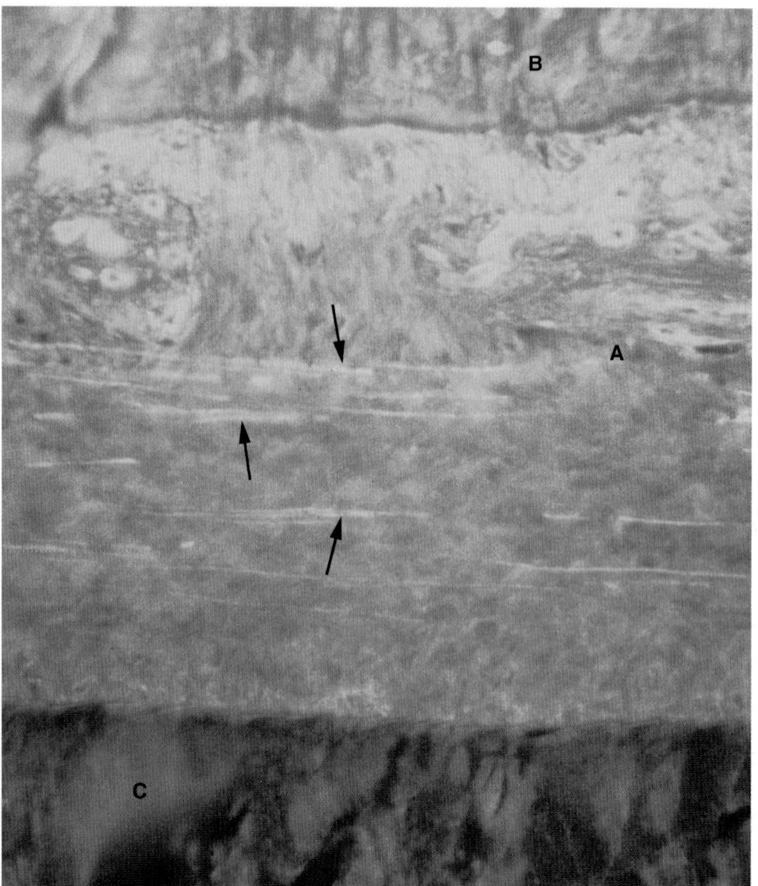

Fig. 12.24 Longitudinal cryosection of rat incisor periodontal ligament (A) with immunofluorescent labelling for fibronectin showing positive labelling (arrows) with the same longitudinal orientation as for oxytalan fibres. B = alveolar bone; C = tooth (×55). From Sloan, P., Carter, D.H., 1995. Structural organisation of the fibres of the periodontal ligament. In: Berkovitz, B.K.B., Moxham, B.J., Newman, H. (Eds.), The Periodontal Ligament in Health and Disease, second ed. Mosby–Wolfe, London, pp 35–53.

in teeth that carry abnormally high loads, including abutment teeth for bridges and teeth being moved for orthodontic reasons. Thus, it appears that oxytalan may have a role in tooth support (perhaps also indicated by the relationship with the periodontal vasculature). However, experimental evidence shows that oxytalan fibres do not change with age or reduction in masticatory loading. Oxytalan microfibrils have a similar ultrastructure to the fibrils of fibronectin. In addition, they are stained strongly by immunohistochemical stains for fibronectin (Fig. 12.24). As fibronectin is important in fibroblast adhesion and migration, this would support the suggestion that oxytalan fibres aid fibroblast migration in the periodontal ligament.

When cultured fibroblasts are subjected to tension, there is an increase in the levels of fibrillin-1 and fibrillin-2. This might suggest that tension functionally regulates microfibril assembly in periodontal ligament fibroblasts and thus may contribute to the homeostasis of oxytalan fibres.

Elastin fibres are restricted to the walls of the blood vessels, although in some animals (e.g., herbivores) they replace the oxytalan fibres. Elaunin is a component of elastic fibres found in the periodontal ligament and in the connective tissue of the dermis (particularly in association with sweat glands). Elastin-positive fibres (characteristic of elaunin) are found primarily around the blood vessels in the apical region of the periodontal ligament, but fibrillin-positive fibres (characteristic of oxytalan) are more widely distributed throughout the tissue. Thus, elaunin in the periodontal ligament might provide mechanical protection for the vascular system.

Reticulin

Reticulin is an argyrophilic fibre that is now known to be type III collagen. Within the periodontal ligament, reticular fibres cross-link and form a fine meshwork to aid tissue support. Reticulin fibres are also related to basement membranes within the periodontal ligament (i.e., associated with blood vessels and epithelial cell rests).

Ground substance

Because of its relative inaccessibility, small volume and complex biochemical nature, little detailed information exists concerning the functions of this important component of the periodontal ligament. Although we are used to thinking of the ligament as a collagen-rich tissue, in reality it is a tissue rich in ground substance. Indeed, even the collagen fibre bundles are composed of about 60% ground substance by volume (Fig. 12.25). Furthermore, 70% of the ground substance comprises bound water. The turnover rate of the components of the periodontal ligament ground substance is more rapid than that for the collagens. Components of the ground substance play an important role in all aspects of fibrillogenesis, including orientation, diameter of fibrils and turnover of collagen. They

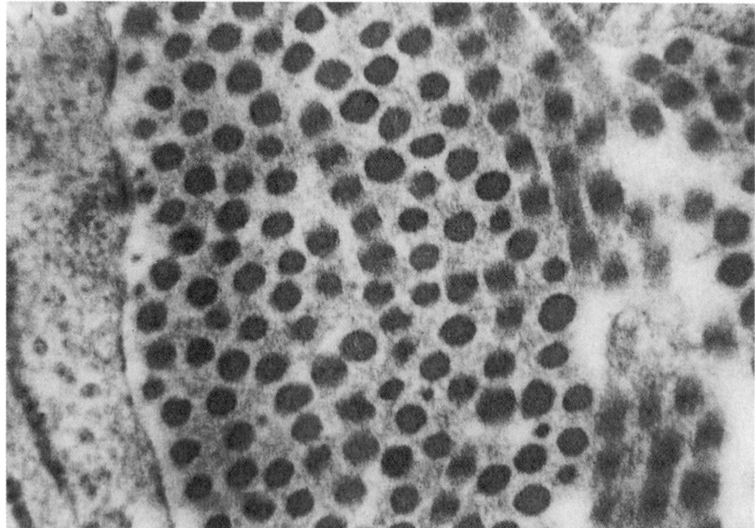

Fig. 12.25 Electron micrograph of a collagen fibre in the periodontal ligament showing that 60% by volume of the fibre is ground substance (TEM; ×100,000).

also control the movement, proliferation, differentiation and activity of the cells of the periodontal ligament (particularly fibroblasts) in addition to controlling the activity of bioactive molecules released into the extracellular milieux. The high tissue fluid pressures recorded within the periodontal ligament may be related to the ground substance and be responsible for tooth support (see page 256) and tooth eruption (see page 460). Ground substance molecules may also be responsible for maintaining an unmineralised periodontal ligament (see bottom of page).

The ground substance of the periodontal ligament consists of glycosaminoglycans, proteoglycans and glycoproteins. All components of the periodontal ligament ground substance are presumed to be secreted by fibroblasts.

Glycosaminoglycans

The main type of glycosaminoglycan is hyaluronan, although dermatan, chondroitin and heparin sulphates are also found. Much of the glycosaminoglycan is located near the surfaces of the collagen fibrils. Hyaluronan is a highly charged molecule, and this type of glycosaminoglycan occupies a large volume of the periodontal ligament. Consequently, it has a major influence on the permeability of the tissue. It can also influence cell motility.

Proteoglycans

Proteoglycans are proteins that are heavily glycosylated. The anionic polysaccharides (glycosaminoglycans) are covalently attached to a protein core. The chains are long, linear carbohydrate polymers that are negatively charged under physiological conditions. The ratio of main proteoglycans present in the periodontal ligament are asporin (ASPN) (30%), lumican (LUM) (26%), decorin (DCN) (15%) and osteomodulin (OMD) (11%).

Asporin is so named because of the unique aspartic acid repeat at the N terminus of the mature protein. Asporin binds to type I collagen and also binds calcium. This latter property may allow asporin to play a major role as a negative regulator for mineralisation. Lumican is a major keratan sulphate proteoglycan found in the periodontal ligament and most mesenchymal tissues throughout the body and is involved in collagen fibril organisation and circumferential growth. Decorin is a small cellular or pericellular matrix proteoglycan and is closely related in structure to biglycan protein. Decorin (and biglycan) is thought to bind to type I collagen fibrils, playing a role in matrix assembly.

Glycoproteins

Glycoproteins studied in the periodontal ligament include fibronectin, tenascin and vitronectin.

Fibronectin is thought to promote attachment of cells to the substratum, especially to collagen fibrils. Furthermore, as cells preferentially adhere to fibronectin, it may be involved in cell migration and orientation. Considering these functions together with the high rate of turnover in the periodontal ligament, it is not surprising that fibronectin may have considerable biological significance within the periodontal ligament. Immunofluorescent techniques at the light microscope level have revealed that fibronectin is uniformly distributed throughout the periodontal ligament in both erupting and fully erupted teeth. Ultrastructural studies have localised the glycoprotein over collagen fibres and at sites on the cell–collagen interface. As loss of fibronectin has been observed during the terminal maturation of many connective matrices, its continued presence within the periodontal ligament may be indicative of the ligament retaining immature, fetal-like characteristics (see page 254). Clinically, fibronectin has been employed therapeutically to 'condition' the roots of teeth in expectation of improving periodontal wound healing.

Like fibronectin, **tenascin** is more characteristic of a fetal-like connective tissue than a fully 'mature' connective tissue. Unlike fibronectin, tenascin is not uniformly localised throughout the ligament but is concentrated adjacent to the alveolar bone and the cementum.

Vitronectin is associated with elastin fibres. The role of these glycoproteins in the periodontal ligament still awaits clarification. However, they may play a role in tissue remodelling since there are important reactions between the matrix and fibroblast surface receptors that can change cell secretion of collagen to secretion of extracellular matrix degradative enzymes.

Other non-collagenous proteins

The two most highly expressed non-collagenous proteins (NCPs) present in the ground substance of the periodontal ligament were periostin (POSTN) and osteonectin (SPARC). In addition, small amounts of other NCPs include osteocalcin (OCN), osteopontin (OPN) and matrix Gla protein.

The term *matricellular proteins* (MCPs) has been recently introduced to describe the group of non-collagenous proteins that regulate cell–matrix interactions and cell function by interactions with cell-surface receptors, such as integrins, with other bioeffector molecules and with structural matrix proteins. In normal tissues, they are present in low concentrations. As they are not directly involved in tissue homeostasis, animal knock-out genetic deletions normally show no major phenotypic changes. MCPs in the periodontal ligament include Gla-containing proteins (such as periostin), osteonectin (SPARC), tenascin and SIBLINGS (see page 167)

Ground substance and mineralisation

The ground substance is thought to have many important functions (ion and water binding and exchange, control of collagen fibrillogenesis and fibre orientation, binding of growth factors). Tissue fluid pressure is high in the periodontal ligament, about 10 mm Hg above atmospheric pressure, and the tissue fluid has been implicated in the tooth support and eruptive mechanisms (see pages 256–257 and 460–463). Furthermore, the composition of the ground substance in the periodontal ligament varies according to the developmental state of the tissue (Fig. 12.26) and according to location (Fig. 12.27). The data suggest that there is a marked change in the amount of hyaluronan as development proceeds from the dental follicle to the initial periodontal ligament, a trend that occurs during embryonic development of other connective tissues. Furthermore, a significant increase in the amount of proteoglycans occurs during eruption.

The nature of the ground substance may also explain why the periodontal ligament rarely mineralises, as it may act as an inhibitor of this process. This is suggested by *in vitro* experiments whereby enzymes that degrade elements of the ground substance (hyaluronidase and chondroitinase) have been applied and, following the addition of mineralising solutions, mineral crystals appear within the periodontal ligament (but do not appear within the normal ligament). Calcium-binding proteins such as S100A4 in the extracellular matrix have also been implicated in inhibiting mineralisation in the periodontal ligament. In cases of ankylosis, the homeostasis controlling the width of the ligament is disrupted. Experimentally, ankylosis can be produced by the administration of a bisphosphonate, which may act by reducing cell numbers and by inducing the expression of osteogenic factors in the body of the periodontal ligament.

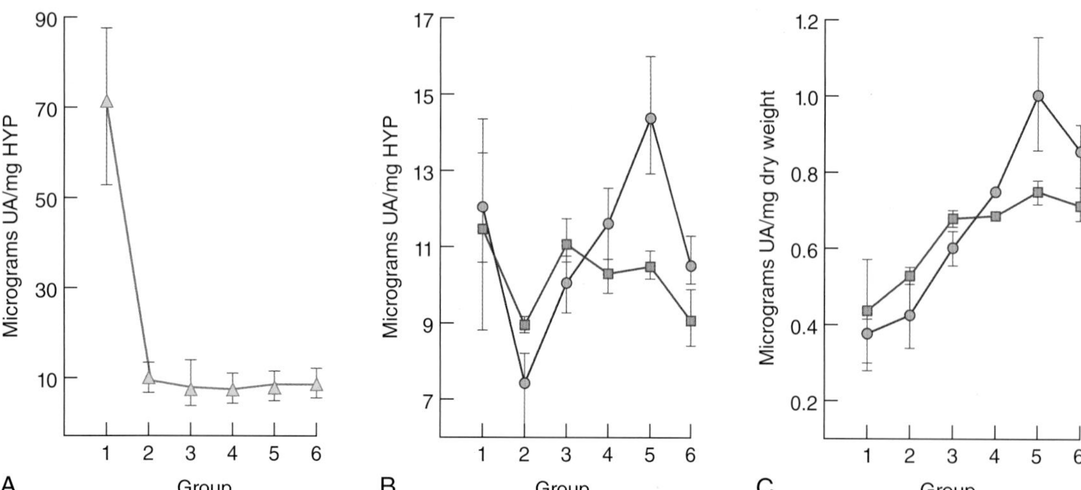

Fig. 12.26 Glycosaminoglycans in the periodontal ligament at different stages of development (from bovine incisors). Hyaluronate in green; proteodermatan sulphate in blue and PG1 proteoglycan in red. Group 1 specimens are of dental follicle. Group 2 is the initial stage of formation of the periodontal ligament. Sharpey's fibre attachments were discernible in group 3. Groups 4 and 5 were for erupting teeth (the typical orientation of collagen fibres being first observed in group 5). Group 6 specimens were from fully erupted teeth. HYP = hydroxyproline, enabling determinations of ground substance components relative to collagen content. From Pearson, C.H., 1982. The ground substance of the periodontal ligament. In: Berkovitz, B.K.B., Moxham, B.J., Newman, H.J. (Eds.), The Periodontal Ligament in Health and Disease. Pergamon Press, Oxford, pp 119–149.

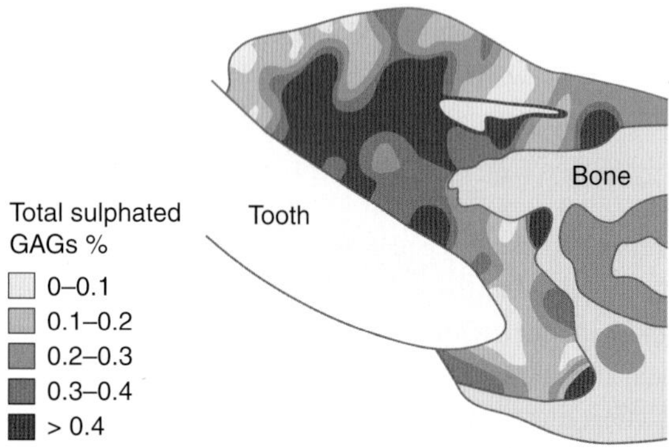

Fig. 12.27 Glycosaminoglycans (sulphated GAGs) at different sites in the periodontal connective tissues (from sheep incisors). From Kirkham, J., Robinson, C., Spence, J., 1989. Site-specific variations in the biochemical composition of healthy sheep periodontium. Archives of Oral Biology 34, 405–411.

Ground substance changes in disease

Analysis of the ground substance following the onset of periodontal disease indicates that there may be a decrease in the dermatan sulphate content and an increase in chondroitin sulphate. Occlusal hypofunction results in remodelling of the ligament with a significant decrease of chondroitin sulphate, decorin and heparin sulphate. That there are differences in the ground substance (and in the nature of collagen) between the periodontal ligament and adjacent alveolar bone may provide a clinical diagnostic tool when analysing gingival crevicular fluid to assess, and predict, patient susceptibility to further progress of the disease.

Cells

Although the predominant connective tissue cell within the periodontal ligament is the fibroblast, the tissue presents a heterogeneous population (Fig. 12.28). Formative cells covering the surface of both cementum and alveolar bone (i.e., cementoblasts and osteoblasts) are considered part of the ligament and have a similar mesenchymal origin. Resorbing cells on the surface of bone and cementum are osteoclasts and odontoclasts (also referred to as *cementoclasts*); these are derived from a monocyte/macrophage lineage from the blood. In addition, the periodontal ligament contains undifferentiated mesenchymal cells (stem cells and precursors such as preosteoblasts and precementoblasts), defence cells and epithelial cells (the rests of Malassez). The type and number of cells vary according to the functional state of the ligament.

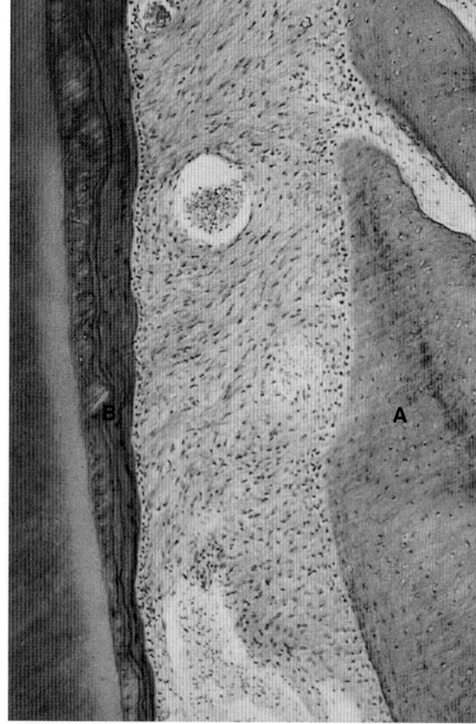

Fig. 12.28 The distribution of cells in the periodontal ligament. In addition to the numerous fibroblasts within the ligament, the surfaces of the alveolar bone (A) and cementum (B) are lined with osteoblasts and cementoblasts respectively, indicating active deposition of bone and cementum in this specimen (decalcified, longitudinal section through the periodontal ligament; H & E; ×80).

Fibroblasts

The fibroblast is the most common cell in the periodontal ligament and is responsible for the synthesis and secretion of the extracellular matrix and for its breakdown during remodelling. It is not yet known whether the fibroblasts are a more or less homogenous population or whether they represent subsets of cells with different properties. They are derived from a population of stem cells lying within the periodontal ligament

Microscopic appearance

The fibroblasts in the periodontal ligament are responsible for regeneration of the tooth support apparatus and have an essential role in the adaptive responses to mechanical loading of the tooth (including orthodontic loading). The periodontal ligament fibroblasts (Figs. 12.29, 12.30) seem to have a variety of shapes with many fine cytoplasmic processes, although they are usually described as being fusiform. However, the overall shape can only be determined by consideration of the cell outlines in different planes. When

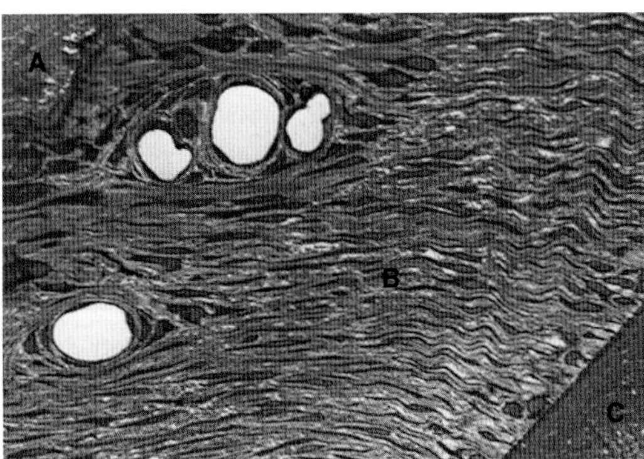

Fig. 12.29 Periodontal ligament (B) with comprising numerous fibroblasts. A = alveolar bone; C = cementum (decalcified, longitudinal section through the periodontal ligament; toluidine blue; ×300).

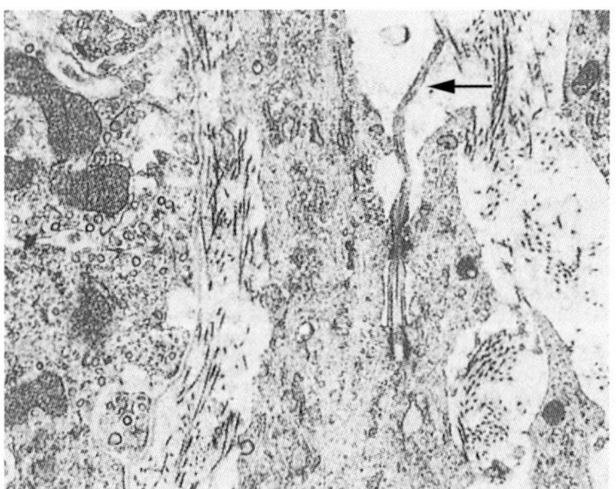

Fig. 12.31 A cilium (arrowed) lying within an invagination of the cell membrane of a periodontal ligament fibroblast (TEM; ×11,000).

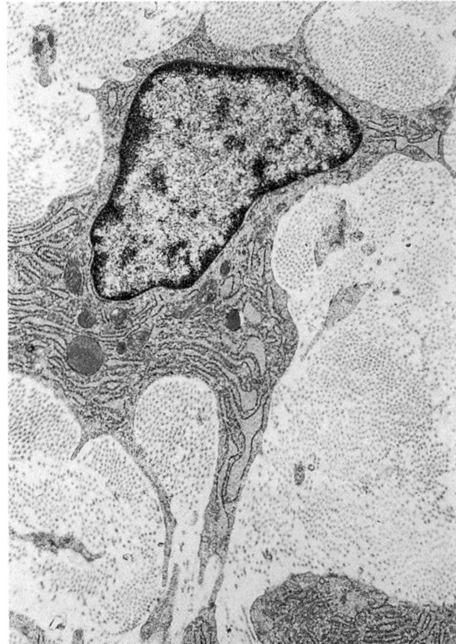

Fig. 12.30 Electron microscopic appearance of a periodontal fibroblast in vivo (TEM; ×4,000).

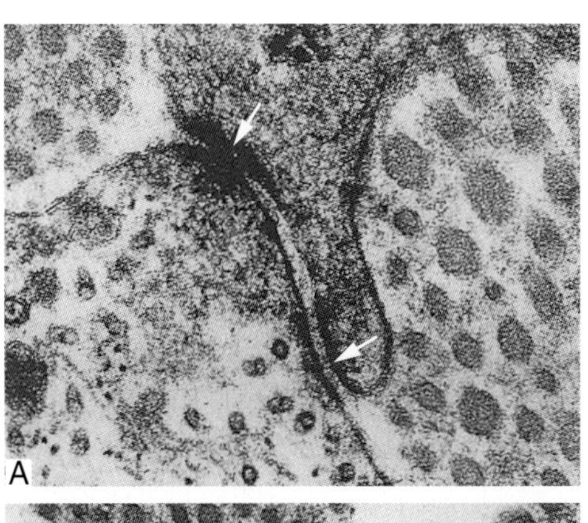

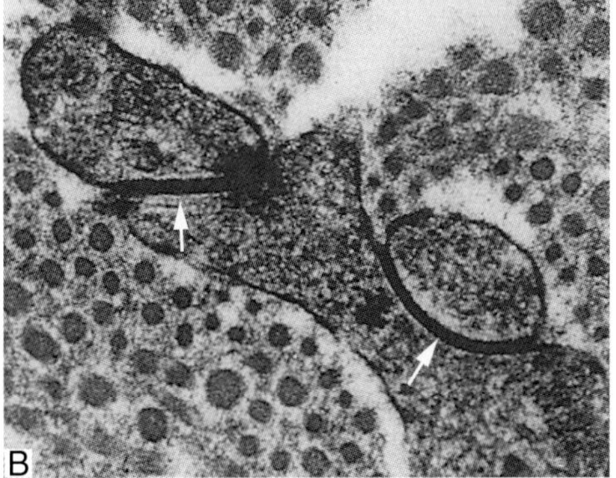

Fig. 12.32 Intercellular contacts (arrowed) between the fibroblasts of the periodontal ligament. A = shows simplified desmosome; B = shows gap junction. (TEM; ×80,000.)

this is done, the periodontal fibroblasts often appear as flattened, disc-shaped cells. *In vitro* studies (see later) have led to the suggestion that the periodontal ligament fibroblasts are polarised with respect to the site of secretion of collagen, which appears to take place preferentially at one end of the cell.

Periodontal fibroblasts, being very active cells metabolically, have low nuclear:cytoplasmic ratios, and each nucleus contains one or more prominent nucleoli. The typical periodontal fibroblast is rich in the intracytoplasmic organelles associated with the synthesis and export of proteins: rough endoplasmic reticulum, Golgi material and mitochondria (Fig. 12.30). Indeed, the high rate of protein synthesis in the periodontal ligament is shown by autoradiographic studies involving tritiated proline or glycine. The findings indicate that within 30 minutes of the injection of the tritiated amino acids, labelled collagen appears in the extracellular matrix of the periodontal ligament. Progenitor fibroblasts are said to be smaller than the mature fibroblasts in the periodontal ligament and have a less distinct Golgi apparatus and rough endoplasmic reticulum.

The fibroblasts of the periodontal ligament have cilia and many intercellular contacts, a feature that is not particularly common in the fibroblasts of other fibrous connective tissues (intercellular contacts are a feature of fibroblasts in fetal-like connective tissues). Fig. 12.31 shows a cilium lying within an invagination of the cell membrane of a periodontal ligament fibroblast. The cilium differs from those seen in other cell types in that it contains no more than nine tubule doublets (compared to the usual 'nine plus two' configuration). The significance of the cilia in periodontal fibroblasts is unknown, although they may be associated with control of the cell cycle or inhibition of centriolar activity. The intercellular contacts (simplified desmosomes and gap junctions) between the fibroblasts of the periodontal ligament are shown in Fig. 12.32. The simplified desmosome is the most frequently seen of the contacts. There is little information concerning the functional significance of these organelles in the periodontal fibroblast. In general terms, tissue differentiation and remodelling depend upon intercellular adhesion and communication. They are essential for the maintenance of tissues in addition to cell recognition and, during development, cell sorting. Gap junctions represent small, round areas where two opposing membranes lie close together but separated by a gap of about 3 nm. Tubules with lumina about 2 nm link the interiors of adjacent cells. Ions and small water molecules pass across the gap junction and are crucial for facilitating intercellular signalling in nonexcitable cells during development, growth and cell differentiation.

Comparison with gingival fibroblasts

Periodontal ligament fibroblasts differ in several respects from gingival fibroblasts. First, they are derived from different sources. Periodontal ligament fibroblasts are ectomesenchymal, being derived from the neural crest (see page 383), whereas gingival fibroblasts are mesodermal in origin. Second, the gingival fibroblasts are less proliferative. Third, the expression of alkaline phosphatase and cyclic adenosine monophosphate (cAMP) is greater in periodontal ligament fibroblasts. Other features distinguishing fibroblasts from the periodontal ligament and the gingiva are shown in Table 25.2 and page 452.

Motility and *in vitro* culture

Much has been made of the possibility that the periodontal fibroblasts are motile or contractile cells and that they are thereby capable of generating a force responsible for tooth eruption. Much of the evidence for migratory or contractile activities comes from research on the behaviour and appearance of periodontal fibroblasts *in vitro*. However, major changes take place upon transfer from tooth to cell culture environment, when periodontal cells undergo significant alterations in their morphology and biochemical behaviour. Considerable care must be taken before extrapolating from results obtained from *in vitro* experiments to the in vivo situation.

In vitro, periodontal fibroblasts can organise a fibrous network and can generate significant forces. However, their behaviour and appearance depend upon the method of culture. For example, cells cultured on plastic (Fig. 12.33) assume the properties of motile cells and are thin and highly polarised with respect to both shape and location of organelles. In particular, there are numerous microtubules and microfilaments (as stress fibres) that run along the length of the cell. Cells with these characteristics have not been seen in the periodontal ligament in vivo. Periodontal fibroblasts cultured on collagen gels (Fig. 12.34), during contraction of the gel, assume the appearance of myofibroblasts (see also pages 462–463), cells that have the properties of both fibroblasts and smooth muscle cells, and are found in contracting wounds. Myofibroblasts are characterised ultra-structurally by having a polarity of shape, crenulated (folded) nuclei and numerous microfilaments. Adjacent cells contact by means of gap junctions. While periodontal fibroblasts in vivo may show occasional gap junctions (Fig. 12.32B), they show no other features characteristic of myofibroblasts. Thus, although the evidence from *in vitro* studies suggests that the periodontal fibroblasts have the potential to be migratory or contractile cells, under normal functional conditions, the cells are primarily involved in protein synthesis and secretion.

There is sufficient evidence, however, to show that there may be some localised movement of cells in the periodontal ligament in vivo and that the migration may be directed along the collagen fibres in an apicocoronal direction. Such migration is likely to be dependent on appropriate chemotactic stimuli. Evidence suggests that extracts from both bone and cementum have a potent chemotactic influence upon periodontal fibroblasts. The dependence of migratory behaviours upon the cytoskeleton and upon surface integrins has also been suggested. New populations of periodontal fibroblasts, osteoblasts and cementoblasts appear to arise from stem cells in the vicinity of blood vessels and then migrate to other regions of the ligament. However, how much the change in position of periodontal cells is the result of active, rather than passive, movements (i.e., being carried with tooth movements) awaits clarification.

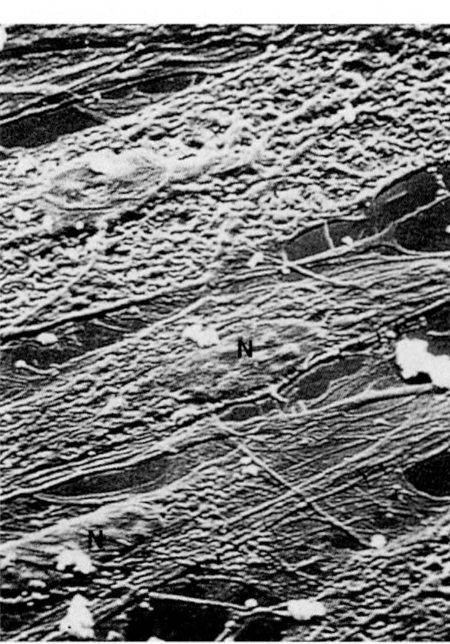

Fig. 12.33 The appearance of motile periodontal fibroblasts cultured on plastic. N = nucleus (SEM; ×1,200).

Intracellular collagen degradation

There is evidence that in addition to synthesising and secreting proteins, the periodontal fibroblasts are responsible for collagen degradation. This contrasts with earlier views that degradation was essentially an extracellular event involving the activity of proteolytic enzymes such as collagenases. The main evidence indicating that the periodontal fibroblasts are also 'fibroclastic' is the presence of organelles termed *intracellular collagen profiles* (Figs. 12.35, 12.36). These profiles show banded collagen fibrils

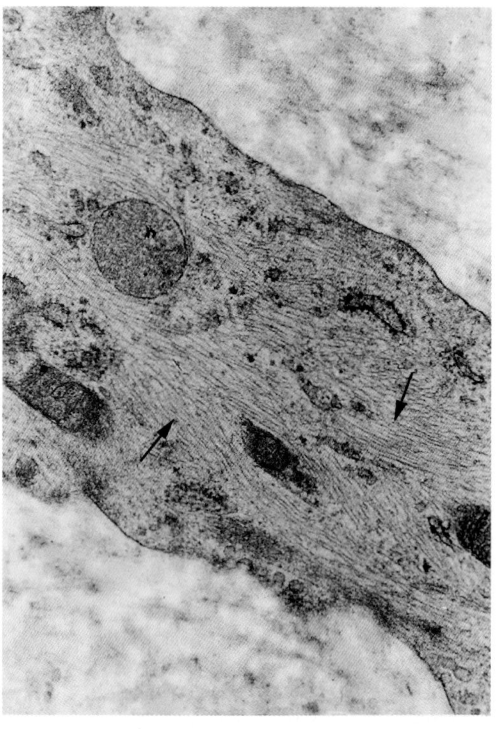

Fig. 12.34 The appearance of contractile periodontal fibroblasts cultured on collagen gels. Note the numerous microfilaments (arrows) (TEM; ×30,000). Courtesy Dr. C A Shuttleworth.

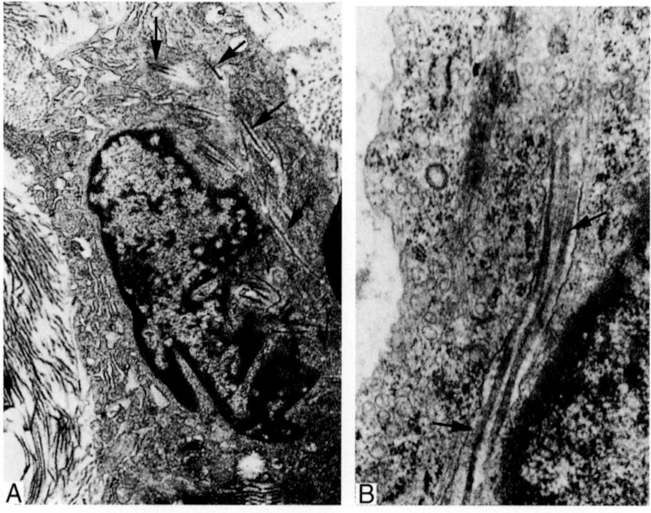

Fig. 12.35 (A) Periodontal fibroblast showing intracellular collagen profiles (arrowed) (TEM; ×5,000) (B) Banded collagen fibrils (arrowed) seen within an elongated membrane-bound vacuole (TEM; ×25,000). Courtesy Dr. J D Harrison.

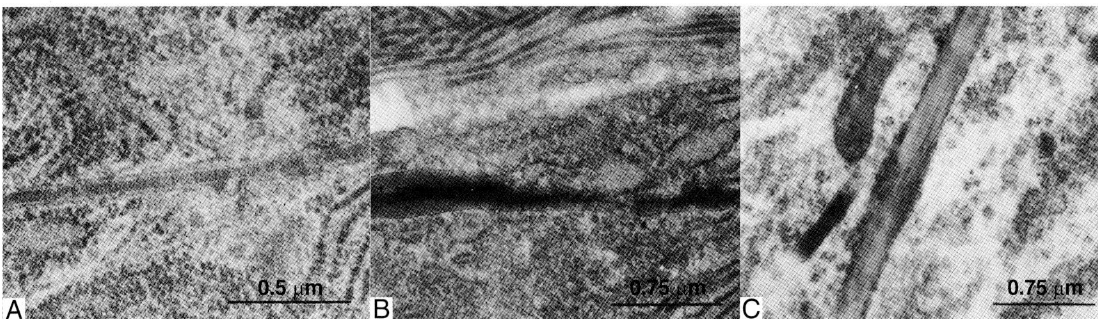

Fig. 12.36 The temporal sequence for intracellular digestion of collagen in the periodontal ligament. (A) Banded fibril surrounded by an electron-lucent zone. (B) Banded fibrils surrounded by an electron-dense zone. (C) Fibrils with indistinct banding surrounded by an electron-dense zone (TEM). From Berkovitz, B.K.B., Shore, R.C., 1995. Cells of the periodontal ligament. In: Berkovitz, B.K.B., Moxham, B.J., Newman, H.J. (Eds.), The Periodontal Ligament in Health and Disease, second ed. Mosby–Wolfe, London, pp 9–33.

within an elongated membrane-bound vacuole. It is thought that the intracellular collagen vacuoles are associated with the degradation of collagen that has been 'ingested' from the extracellular environment. The temporal sequence for intracellular digestion of collagen in the periodontal ligament is illustrated in Fig. 12.36. When a collagen fibril is first phagocytosed by the fibroblast, a banded fibril surrounded by an electron-lucent zone is seen. Subsequently, the banded fibril is surrounded by an electron-dense zone. At this stage, the phagosome fuses with primary lysosomes to form a phagolysosome in which there is a gradual increase in electron density of the matrix. At the terminal stage, the fibril shows indistinct banding and is surrounded by an electron-dense zone: enzymic degeneration of the fibril has proceeded to the point where the fibril loses its characteristic structure. The time taken to degrade collagen intracellularly is not known, although about 30 minutes has been suggested (a time similar to that required for synthesis). Evidence suggests that, biochemically, the internal degradation of collagen does not involve matrix metalloproteinase (MMP-1), but acid phosphatase and cathepsins. In addition, cell surface–located alkaline phosphatase and MMPs may be involved in the process of internalising a collagen fibril from the extracellular matrix. In support of the view that the intracellular collagen profiles lined by dense material do represent extracellular collagen that has been phagocytosed, blocking lysosomal enzymes in the periodontal ligament (e.g., with leupeptin) results in accumulation of intracellular vacuolar fibrils.

It has been argued that the collagen profiles within periodontal fibroblasts are not truly intracellular and that the collagen merely lies in surface invaginations. If this were so, the degradation would still be an extracellular phenomenon. It has also been suggested that, because the periodontal fibroblasts may be synthesising collagen in excess of requirements, the profiles contain collagen that is being degraded without ever having been secreted extracellularly. Overall, however, the evidence suggests that the collagen is ingested from the extracellular compartment of the periodontal ligament and that the profiles are intracellular. Nevertheless, it is not known whether all periodontal fibroblasts are capable of phagocytosis.

The degradation of collagen may be expected to include both extracellular and intracellular events. There is, however, little evidence for the presence of the enzyme collagenase within the normal periodontal ligament, and other experimental data suggest that collagenase is not essential for collagen remodelling. If this is correct, then other enzymes (e.g., cysteine proteinase) and other MMPs are involved in collagen remodelling in the normal physiological situation. Fibroblasts in the periodontal ligament secrete MMP-1, which degrades extracellular matrix collagen under physiological conditions. The fibroblasts can also secrete tissue inhibitors of metalloproteinases (TIMPs). TIMPs are found in high concentrations at healthy periodontal sites.

Collagenase production and phagocytosis can be upregulated after exposure to cytokines such as prostaglandin E_2, interleukin (IL)-1 or lectin concanavalin A. Furthermore, because fibroblasts are induced to secrete prostaglandin when mechanical loads are applied (e.g., with orthodontic loads), the periodontal fibroblasts may have 'intrinsic' mechanisms for remodelling the matrix. However, the precise role of collagenase in physiological remodelling awaits clarification, as inhibition of its activity *in vitro* does not prevent the ingestion of collagen by fibroblasts.

Some lysosomes within periodontal fibroblasts relate to the process of autophagy, which is the lysosomal protein degradation system in which the cell self-digests its protein components and organelles to maintain cellular homeostasis. This mechanism for the clearance of damaged organelles is the most important function of autophagy in mammalian cells. It may also allow for the clearance of misfolded or unfolded collagen. When autophagy is inhibited, there is an accumulation of intracellular collagen.

Despite the high turnover rate of collagen within the periodontal ligament, if one obtains periodontal ligament tissue from a normal healthy periodontal ligament and cultures it on collagen gels, no collagenolytic activity can be measured. However, if periodontal ligament is taken from the roots of resorbing deciduous teeth and cultured on collagen gels, collagenic activity can be observed to occur in the absence of any inflammatory infiltrate, suggesting the periodontal ligament is directly involved in the resorptive process.

Importantly, inflammation associated with periodontal disease may lead to an increased expression of MMPs and to aggressive loss of collagen in the periodontal ligament that results in tissue destruction. As the amount of collagen present within the periodontal ligament must represent a balance between the rate of synthesis and the rate of degradation, the loss of collagen during periodontal disease could result from either a more rapid rate of breakdown and/or a slower rate of synthesis and/or the loss of fibroblasts. Furthermore, the process of collagen loss during periodontal disease probably represents a different process, as in the diseased inflammatory state there is evidence of the activity of collagenase. The presence of TIMPs in the periodontal ligament, some produced by its fibroblasts, provides the rationale for the use of drugs that have a similar activity to combat periodontal disease, such as the designer tetracycline drug doxycycline.

Cytoskeleton

As expected for cells of mesenchymal origin, periodontal ligament fibroblasts label for vimentin intermediate cytoskeletal filaments at all stages of development (Fig. 12.37), and there is no labelling for cytokeratins, tubulin or F-actin in the 'mature' periodontal ligament. However, labelling for cytokeratin 19 (an intermediate filament usually associated with epithelial cells) occurs during the active stage of tooth eruption (Fig. 12.38).

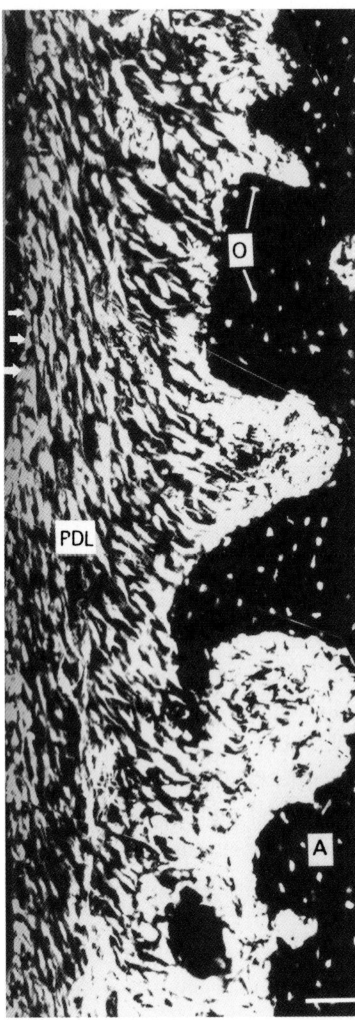

Fig. 12.37 Immunolabelling for vimentin intermediate cytoskeletal filaments in cells of the mature (non-aged) periodontal ligament. The labelling (white areas) is observed in all the fibroblasts of the periodontal ligament (PDL), osteocytes (O) within alveolar bone (A) and cementoblasts (arrows) lining the root surface. Bar = 100 μm.

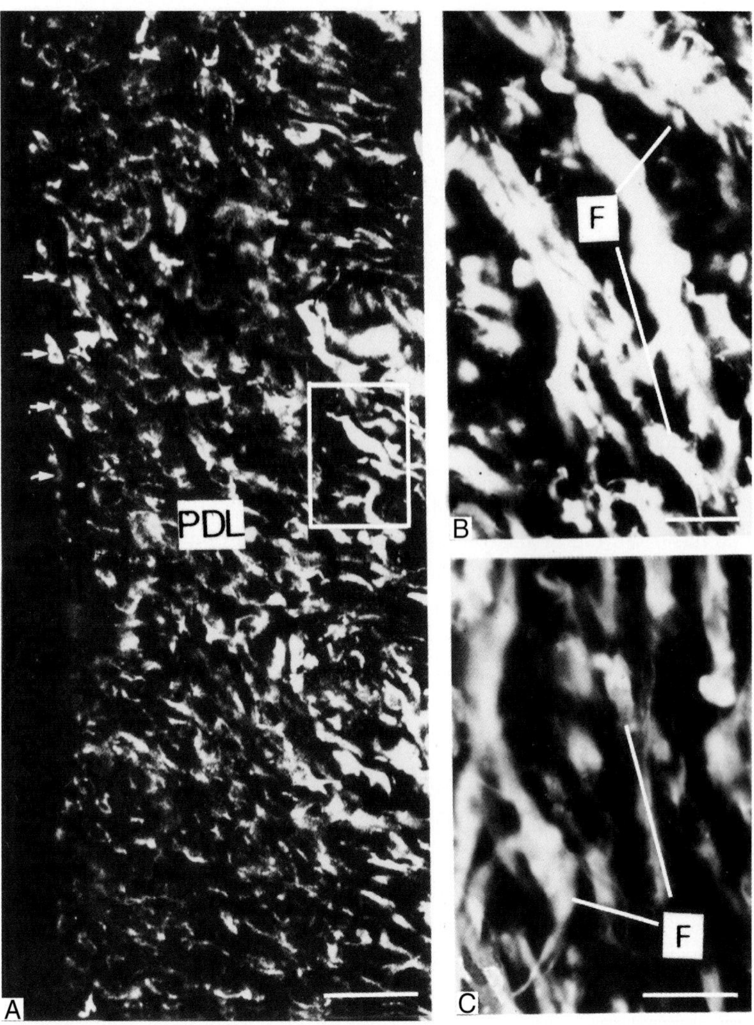

Fig. 12.39 Immunolabelling for intermediate filaments (white areas) in cells of the aged periodontal ligament. (A) Vimentin labelling in the periodontal ligament (PDL) and cementoblasts (arrows) was reduced in comparison with earlier stages (see Fig. 12.37). Bar = 100 μm. (B) Higher-power view of the region enclosed by the rectangle in (A) showing labelling for vimentin in fibroblasts (F) of the periodontal ligament. Bar = 10 μm. (C) Cytokeratin-19 labelling (white areas) in periodontal ligament fibroblasts (F). Bar = 15 μm.

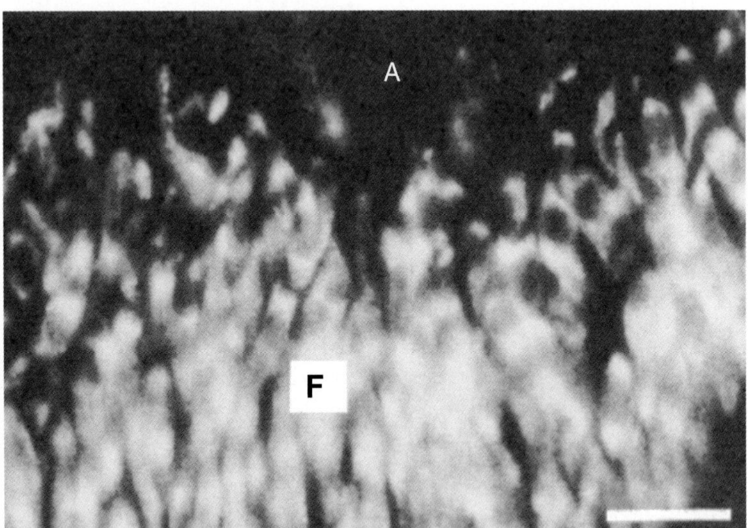

Fig. 12.38 Immunolabelling for cytokeratin-19 intermediate cytoskeletal filaments in periodontal ligament fibroblasts (F) (white areas) during an active stage of eruption. The dark area (A) beyond the periodontal ligament is alveolar bone. Bar = 25 μm.

Furthermore, transient expression for cytokeratin 19 can be observed in the aged periodontal ligament (Fig. 12.39). Some changes in labelling for vimentin are also detected in the aged tissues, with labelling being weaker in cementoblasts and fibroblasts contained in the cementum-related portion of the periodontal ligament. The coexpression of cytokeratins and vimentin is not unknown for mesenchymal cells, being reported for those of the eye, choroid plexus fibroblasts, chondrocytes and regenerating organs.

The functions of intermediate filaments are poorly understood but are presumed to be structural. There is some evidence to suggest that cells may increase their intermediate filament content in response to mechanical loading. Where coexpression of different intermediate filaments occurs, these cytoskeletal elements have been associated with the cell environment, cell shape or possible secretory activity of the cell. The specific distribution of different intermediate filaments indicates particular functions for these elements within tissues. For instance, the presence of cytokeratins could be related to the combined shear and compressive forces to which they are subjected. The accumulation of vimentin may also be related to mechanical loading.

That periodontal fibroblasts transiently express cytokeratin 19 during the active phase of tooth eruption could relate to the fact that the periodontal ligament must undergo major structural reorganisation of its extracellular matrix. It has been suggested that intermediate filaments could form part of a mechanotransduction system that enables the cells to respond to external forces and sense changes in the extracellular matrix. Thus, the expression of an additional type of filament could be related to the effects of periodontal ligament remodelling and the changing conditions during tooth eruption. In epithelia, cytokeratin 19 commonly occurs at sites of rapid cell proliferation. This may also be the case in the periodontal ligament at the time of eruption. However, this explanation for the expression of cytokeratin 19 in the aged periodontal tissue is difficult to sustain. To understand the processes involved, we need to know much more about the biomechanical properties and remodelling characteristics of the periodontal ligament with age. However, despite the obvious importance (both biologically and clinically) of investigating the effects of ageing on the oral fibrous connective tissues, our understanding of this subject is poor at present. There have been, for example, remarkably few studies concerned with the changing composition and functions of the periodontal ligament, and the effects of ageing upon the turnover rates of the extracellular matrices have yet to be assessed.

Integrins

Integrins are transmembrane receptors that facilitate cell–cell and cell–extracellular matrix adhesion. Thus, integrins function as links between the extracellular matrix and the cytoskeleton. Integrins are heterodimers assembled from 18 α and 8 β subunits in different combinations with specificity for various extracellular matrix molecules. Several are present on the surface of periodontal fibroblasts, including α1β1, α2β1, α11β1 and αVβ6.

For most of integrins, the linkage is to the actin cytoskeleton. Periodontal ligament fibroblasts interact with the extracellular matrix via integrin binding of different collagenous and non-collagenous substrates. Interaction of integrins with the extracellular matrix extracellularly and with cytoskeletal components intracellularly are considered to be force-transducing elements in fibroblasts. Integrins therefore play an important role in assembling and maintaining the complex pattern of collagen in the periodontal ligament. Integrins can act as mechanosensors and generate signals that affect cell physiology via complex intracellular signalling mechanisms, including autocrine and paracrine mechanisms. Mechanical tension can also increase integrin affinity. Integrins can act as regulators of MMPs and cathepsins

Growth factors and cytokines

The activities of periodontal ligament fibroblasts are modulated by numerous bioactive molecules. These molecules may be produced by the cells themselves, be produced by local inflammatory cells or be present within the extracellular matrix of the periodontal ligament or of bone and cementum. They include growth factors and cytokines. The cell membrane also contains a multitude of receptors to bioactive molecules. At the cell–matrix interface are found a group of adhesion molecules, the integrins that regulate many cellular activities, including those relating to cell spreading, cytoskeletal reorganisation and apoptosis. Through the activities of bioactive molecules and receptors, the fibroblast is involved in maintaining homeostasis. There may be rapid upregulation or downregulation of activities following, for example, the application of mechanical stress associated with orthodontic tooth movement or the onset of periodontal inflammation. Periodontal ligament fibroblasts produce numerous growth factors and cytokines, such as insulin-like growth factor (IGF)-I, bone morphogenetic proteins (BMPs), platelet-derived growth factor (PDGF) and IL-1. Transforming growth factor (TGF)-β, for example, stimulates the synthesis of collagen and inhibits the synthesis of MMPs such as collagenase. It is not surprising, therefore, that increased production of cytokines is related to the onset of tissue damage. Fibroblasts may release factors that inhibit osteoclastic differentiation and function (e.g., osteoprotegerin), while supporting it by expressing receptor activator nuclear factor kappa B ligand (RANKL) on its surface. The cells also release prostaglandins, which may influence bone cell activity. Periodontal ligament fibroblasts are rich in substances such as alkaline phosphatase (which might be related to the formation of acellular cementum), cellular retinoic acid–binding protein, and receptors to EGF (which may inhibit the fibroblast from differentiating into a cementoblast/osteoblast that lacks such receptors). Presumably, periodontal ligament fibroblasts have the genome to produce any of the proteins in the body, but most of these are inactivated. For example, whereas the cell does not normally produce elastin in vivo (or only in negligible amounts), *in vitro* tropoelastin messenger RNA (mRNA) is transcribed. This transcription is suppressed by basic fibroblast growth factor (FGF), suggesting one possible role for this growth factor. Bioactive molecules, such as TGF-β, IGF-I, PDGF, BMP-2, BMP-7 and FGF-2, that can regulate the proliferation and differentiation of fibroblasts, osteoblasts and cementoblasts, in addition to promoting angiogenesis, have been applied in animal models, alone and in combination. This is in the hope of inducing or improving periodontal regeneration, with varying degrees of success being reported. However, whether any of these growth factors will be found to be suitable for promoting periodontal regeneration in humans remains to be seen (see also pages 450–454 and 495–499).

Tissue culture experiments suggest that the ability of periodontal fibroblasts to produce cytokines may allow them to interact with local immune cells (e.g., dendritic cells and macrophages). This has been achieved under both noninflammatory and inflammatory conditions by enhancing their migration, by facilitating their phagocytic capacities and by affecting their phenotypic maturation both through cell–cell contact and released soluble mediators.

Cementoblasts

The connective tissue cells of the periodontal ligament also include cementoblasts, cementoclasts, osteoblasts and osteoclasts. Cementoblasts are the cement-forming cells lining the surface of cementum (Figs. 12.40, 12.41).

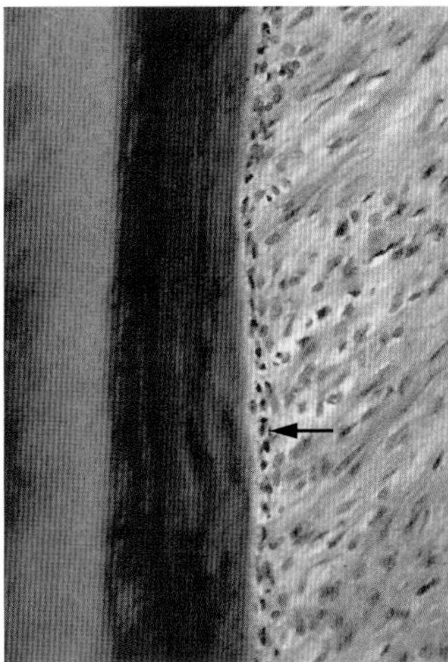

Fig. 12.40 A layer of cementoblasts (arrowed) lining the cementum (decalcified, longitudinal section of periodontal ligament; H & E; ×160).

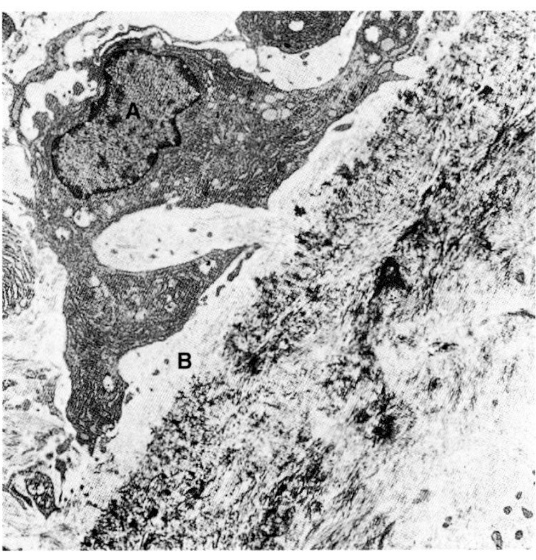

Fig. 12.41 A cementoblast (A) lining cementum. B = precementum (TEM; ×3,700).

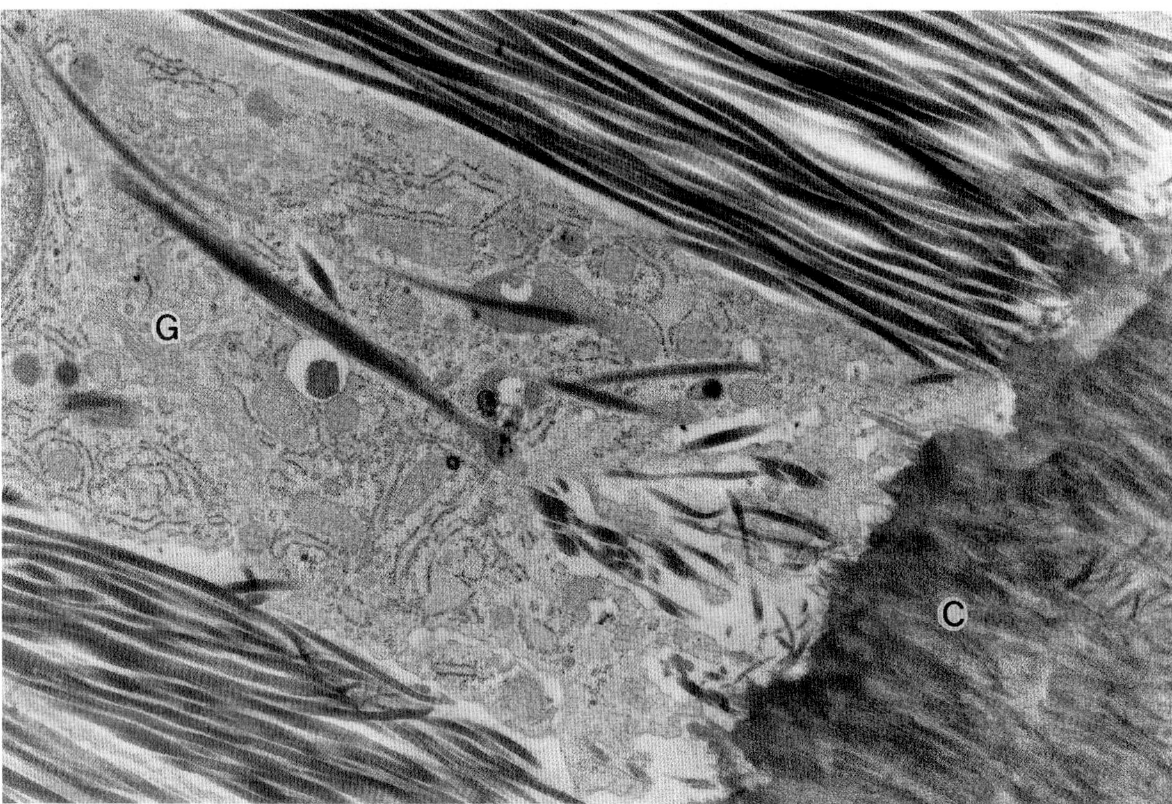

Fig. 12 42 Part of a cementoblast demonstrating the degradation of collagen fibrils. Note the presence of electron-dense phagolysosomes containing collagen fibrils. C = cementum, G = Golgi complex. (×15,000). From Yajima, T., Matsuo, A., Hwai, T., 1989. Collagen phagocytosis by cementoblasts at the periodontal ligament-cementum interface. Archives of Histology and Cytology 52, 521–528.

Cementoblasts are not as elongated as periodontal fibroblasts, being squat cuboidal cells. They are rich in cytoplasm and have large nuclei. Like fibroblasts, they contain all the intracytoplasmic organelles necessary for protein synthesis and secretion. The nucleus of a cementoblast is distinctly vesicular, with one or more nucleoli. The appearance of a cementoblast will depend upon its degree of activity. Cells actively depositing acellular cementum do not have prominent cytoplasmic processes. However, cells depositing cellular cementum exhibit abundant basophilic cytoplasm and cytoplasmic processes, and their nuclei tend to be folded and irregularly shaped (see also page 448, Fig. 25.33).

When present, actively secreting cementoblasts are producing protein to be incorporated in newly forming cementum and/or periodontal ligament. As with periodontal ligament fibroblasts, cementoblasts have also been shown to contain membrane-bound collagen fibrils surrounded by an electron-dense material and interpreted as representing phagolysosomes (Fig. 12.42). Such structures have been interpreted as representing collagen at various stages of degradation. To confirm this interpretation, acid phosphatase activity is present within the phagolysosomes. Therefore, in addition to synthesising connective tissue matrix, cementoblasts also participate in its degradation and turnover.

Osteoblasts

Osteoblasts are the bone-forming cells lining the tooth socket (Fig. 12.43), closely resembling cementoblasts. The layer of osteoblasts is prominent only when there is active bone formation. Each osteoblast appears cuboidal and exhibits a basophilic cytoplasm that is related to the extensive endoplasmic reticulum within the cell. The prominent, round nucleus tends to lie towards the basal end of the cell. A pale, juxtanuclear area indicates the site of the Golgi apparatus. When bone is not forming, its surface is occupied by flattened, inactive, bone-lining cells. Like the periodontal fibroblasts, active osteoblasts contain an extensive rough endoplasmic reticulum and numerous mitochondria and vesicles (Fig. 12.44), although their Golgi apparatus appears more localised and extensive. Microfilaments are prominent beneath the cell membrane at the secreting surface. The cells contact one another by means of desmosomes and tight junctions. The cell surface adjacent to bone has many fine cytoplasmic processes, some of which contact underlying osteocytes by tight junctions to form part of a transport system throughout the bone (see also pages 265–268).

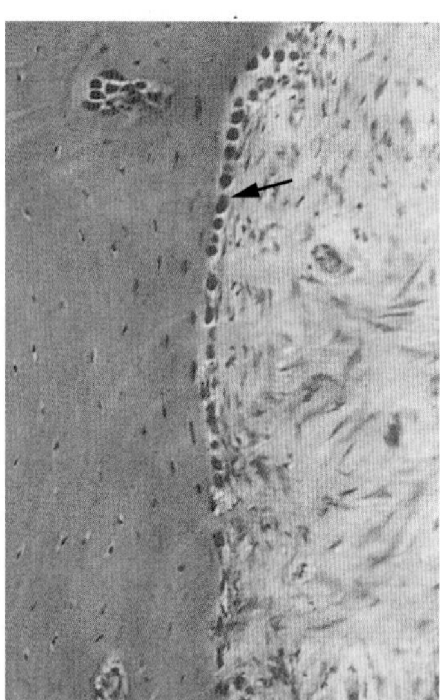

Fig. 12.43 A layer of osteoblasts (arrowed) lining the alveolar bone (decalcified, longitudinal section of periodontal ligament, H & E; ×230).

As for cementoblasts (see earlier), cells identified as osteoblasts lying on the surface of the alveolar bone have been seen possessing collagen-containing phagosomes. These intracellular collagen profiles

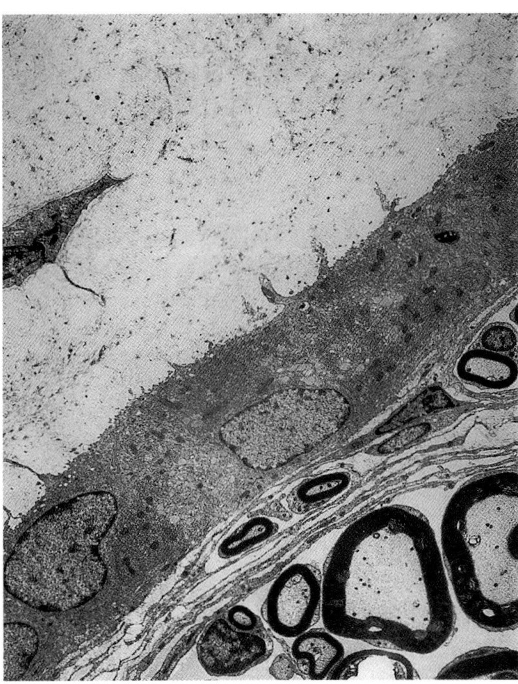

Fig. 12.44 Ultrastructural features of the osteoblast (A). B=osteocyte"(TEM; decalcified section. ×6,000).

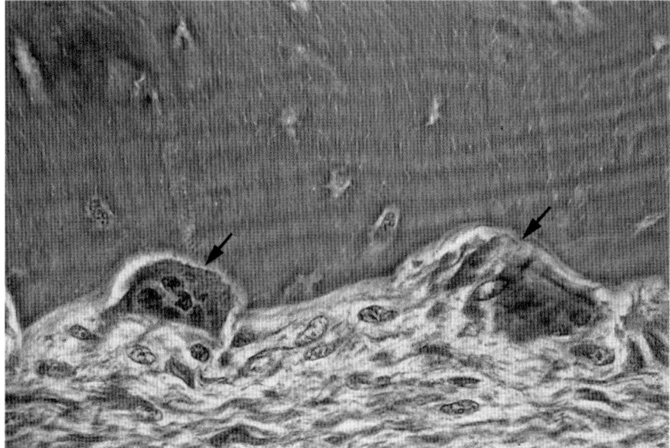

Fig. 12.45 Resorbing alveolar bone and the osteoclast. Resorption concavities termed Howship's lacunae in which lie osteoclasts are arrowed (decalcified, longitudinal section of the periodontal ligament; H & E; ×250). Courtesy Prof. M M Smith.

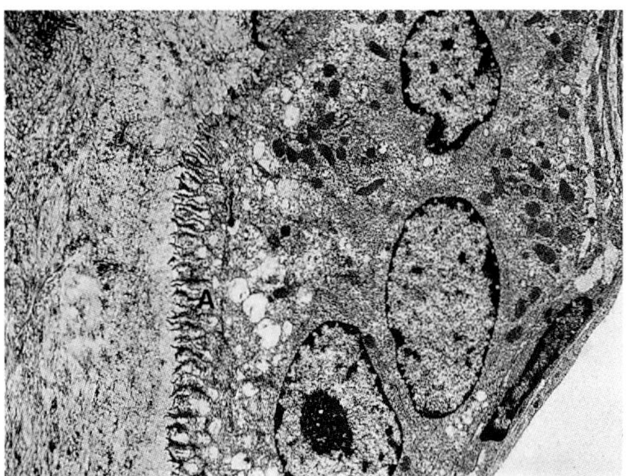

Fig. 12.46 Ultrastructural features of a multinucleated osteoclast. A = brush border (TEM; ×3,000). From Berkovitz, B.K.B., Shore, R.C., 1995. Cells of the periodontal ligament. In: Berkovitz, B.K.B., Moxham, B.J., Newman, H.J. (Eds.), The Periodontal Ligament in Health and Disease, second edn. Mosby-Wolfe, London, pp 9–33.

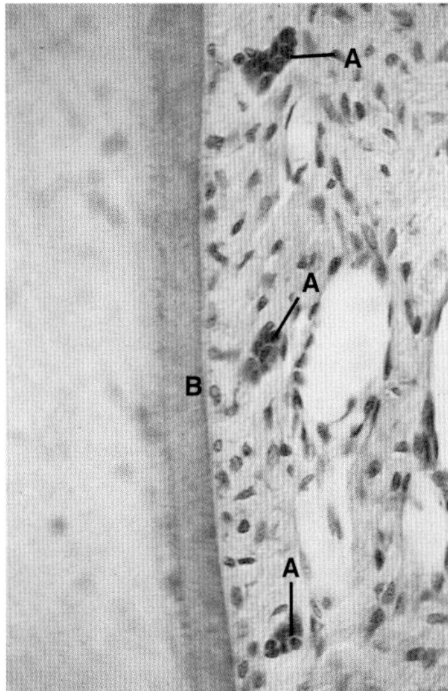

Fig. 12.47 The position of the epithelial rests (A) close to the cementum (B) (decalcified section through periodontal ligament; H & E; ×240).

are at various stages of degradation. Acid phosphatase and cathepsin B activity are associated with the phagosomes. This suggests that osteoblasts are capable of phagocytosis and intracellular degradation of collagen.

Osteoclasts and cementoclasts

Osteoclasts and cementoclasts (or odontoclasts) are found in areas where bone and cementum are being resorbed. These cells are actively involved in the resorption process. Osteoclasts and cementoclasts have the same cytoplasmic features. These cells are now known to arise from blood cells of the macrophage type. When osteoclasts resorb alveolar bone (Fig. 12.45), the surface of the alveolar bone shows resorption concavities termed Howship's lacunae, in which lie the osteoclasts. Osteoclasts show considerable variation in size and shape, ranging from small mononuclear cells to large multinuclear cells. The part of the cell that lies adjacent to bone often has a striated appearance, the so-called 'brush border' (Fig. 12.46). The brush border comprises many tightly packed microvilli, which may be coated with fine, bristle-like structures. At the circumference of the brush border the plasma membrane tends to become smooth and the cytoplasm beneath it denser. This modified annular zone may serve to limit the diffusion of hydrolytic enzymes, thereby creating a microenvironment in which resorption can take place. The osteoclast contains numerous mitochondria distributed throughout the cytoplasm, except for the region immediately beneath the brush border. The rough endoplasmic reticulum is less conspicuous than in osteoblasts, but Golgi material is prominent (especially in juxtanuclear areas). Most of the remaining cytoplasm contains large numbers of vesicles of different sizes and types; some contain acid phosphatase (Fig. 13.22).

Epithelial cells

Aggregations of epithelial cell rests, the rests of Malassez (Fig. 12.47), are a normal feature of the periodontal ligament. They are the remains of the developmental epithelial root sheath (of Hertwig) (see pages 436–437). Although the term 'rests' may imply that the epithelial cells are relatively inert and have little functional significance, research indicates that they may have important functions in the homeostasis of the periodontal ligament.

Structure

Epithelial cell rests are unusual in that they are completely surrounded by connective tissue of the periodontal ligament, whereas in other parts of the body, epithelial cells form a surface layer that covers mesenchymal tissues.

Epithelial rests can be distinguished from adjacent fibroblasts by the close packing of their cuboidal cells and their tendency to stain more deeply. The rests lie about 25 μm from the cementum surface. That the cell rests are epithelial in origin is indicated by using immunofluorescent techniques for the detection of cytokeratins (Fig. 12.48).

In cross-section, the epithelial cells appear cluster-like (Fig. 12.49), although tangential or serial sections show a fishnet arrangement of interconnecting strands parallel to the long axis of the root and extending along its complete length (Fig. 12.50).

The ultrastructural appearance of the epithelial cell rests is illustrated in Fig. 12.51. The cluster arrangement of the cells is reminiscent of a duct-like structure. The cells are separated from the surrounding connective tissue by a basal lamina. The nucleus of each cell is prominent and often shows invaginations. The scanty cytoplasm is characterised by the presence of tonofibrils, some of which insert into the desmosomes that are frequently found between adjacent cells and others into hemidesmosomes between the cells and the basal lamina. Tight junctions are also found between the cells. Mitochondria are distributed throughout the cytoplasm, while the rough endoplasmic reticulum and Golgi apparatus are poorly developed. A primary cilium is often present, although its function is not understood. *In vitro*, the cell rests are capable of phagocytosing collagen.

Following orthodontic movement, there is no regeneration of the epithelial rests, although there is regeneration of connective tissue on the compression side.

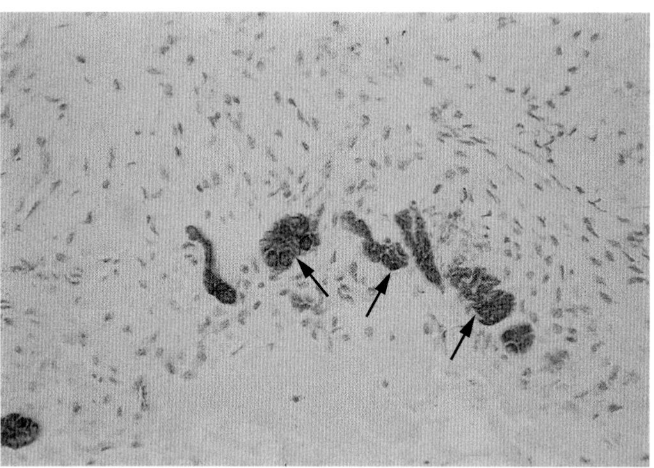

Fig. 12.48 Decalcified section of the periodontal ligament showing positive brown staining for simple cytokeratins in epithelial cell rests (arrowed) (immunohistochemistry; ×300). Courtesy Dr. A E Barrett.

Cell turnover

Differences have been observed in the distribution of epithelial cells according to site and age: during the first and second decades they are most prevalent in the apical zone; between the third and seventh decades the majority are located cervically in the gingiva above the alveolar crest. This might imply that they have a slow rate of turnover, which may be related to the presence of receptors for EGF. However, they can be readily cultured and can proliferate to form cysts or tumours if appropriately stimulated (e.g., by chronic inflammation). This would imply the presence of epithelial stem cells, and epithelial stem cell–related genes have been identified. Indeed, *in vitro* studies have shown that epithelial cell rests are pluripotent and can differentiate into mesenchymal cells such as cementocytes and osteocytes. Furthermore, there may be heterogeneity among stem cells, as epithelial cloned cell rests have been shown to have different properties.

Epithelial cell rests have been shown to strongly express clock genes that control circadian functions (such as the circadian transcription repressor, Period (PER)).

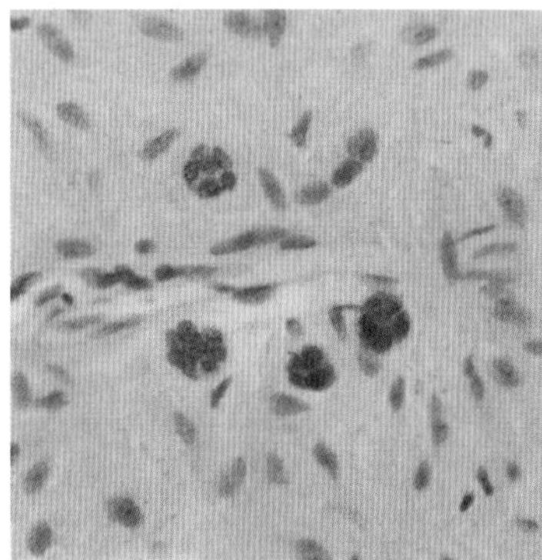

Fig. 12.49 Cluster-like appearance of epithelial rests (decalcified section through periodontal ligament; H & E; ×250).

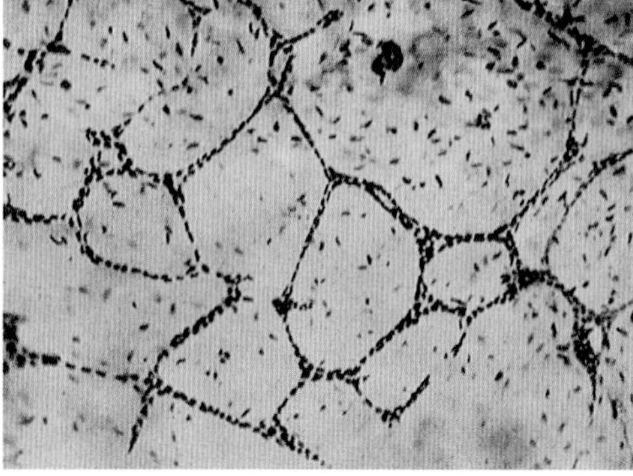

Fig. 12.50 Tangential section through the epithelial rests showing a network appearance (iron haematoxylin; ×60).

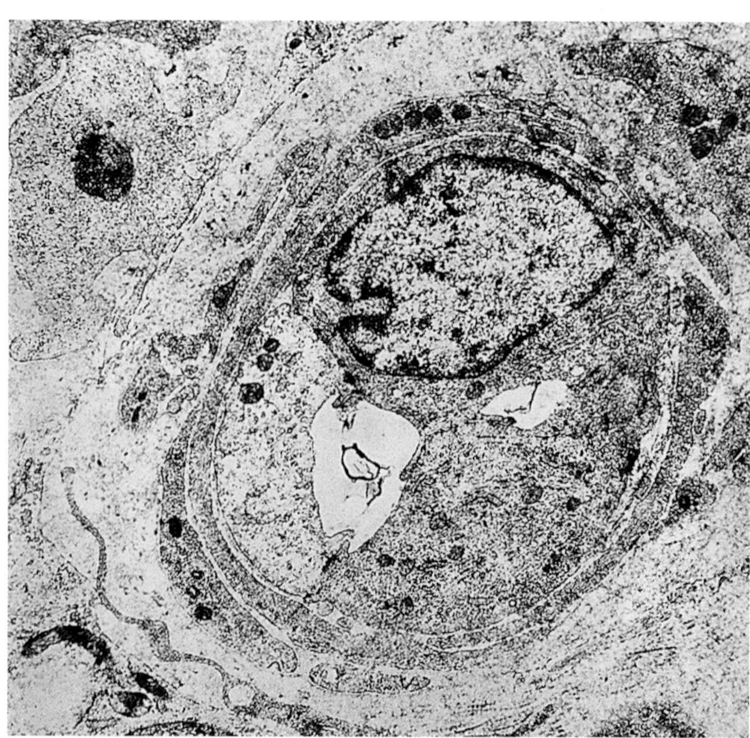

Fig. 12.51 Ultrastructural appearance of the epithelial cell rest (TEM; ×6,100).

Protein expression

Epithelial cell rests have been shown to produce matrix molecules (such as hyaluronan, fibronectin and laminin), proteins (such as osteopontin, bone sialoprotein and MMPs), growth factors (such as EGF and BMPs), cytokines (such as ILs and prostaglandins) and neuropeptides (such as substance P and calcitonin gene–related peptide). Other important proteins released from epithelial cell rests are enamel-related proteins such as amelogenin and amelin. These proteins are thought to play an important role in root formation (see Chapter 25) and have been implicated in the regeneration of the periodontal ligament (see pages 257–258 and Chapter 28).

Functions

It has been suggested that the network of epithelial cell rests plays an important role in homeostatic mechanisms within the periodontal ligament, and this is supported by the many important molecules that the cell rests have been shown capable of producing. Furthermore, when epithelial cell rests are co-cultured with periodontal ligament fibroblasts, protein expression of both cell types is different compared with the proteins expressed by each cell type cultured individually, suggesting the possibility of interaction in the in vivo ligament.

The cells play a critical role in root development, particularly in the initial development of cementum (see Chapter 25). Moreover, there is evidence that epithelial cell rests are capable of epithelial/mesenchymal transformation into cementoblasts and cementocytes. When transplanted in vivo, cell rest populations have the capacity to differentiate into a mesenchymal phenotype and thus represent a unique stem cell population within the periodontal ligament.

Of particular significance are the various molecules that the epithelial cells secrete such as EGF, ameloblastin, osteopontin, osteoprotegerin and osteonectin, which are all involved in regulating mineralisation and osteoclast function. In this context, the epithelial cell rests have been implicated in being responsible for maintaining the normal dimensions of the periodontal space and are active during orthodontic tooth movement. EGF released by the epithelial cell rests is directly implicated in osteoclastogenesis, and hence bone resorption, through the inhibition of osteoprotegerin (OPG), a well-established decoy receptor for RANKL.

In further support of this view is an experiment where the inferior alveolar nerve is sectioned, with a resultant decrease in the number of epithelial cell rests, a decrease in the width of the periodontal ligament and ankylosis of the tooth.

Owing to these varied possible functions, the epithelial cell rests have been given importance in the subject of periodontal ligament regeneration.

Clinically, the cell rests are also involved in the formation of dentigerous and periodontal cysts (see page 274) when inflammatory cytokines stimulate their proliferation.

Defence cells

Defence cells within the periodontal ligament include macrophages, mast cells and eosinophils. These are similar to defence cells in other connective tissues.

Monocytes/macrophages

These make up about 4% of the periodontal ligament cell population (Fig. 12.52), and they are preferentially located near the nerves and blood vessels and not in the dense connective tissue of the periodontal ligament. Indeed, monocytes are blood-borne cells that enter the periodontal ligament from the blood vessels. Monocytes are oval cells with a ruffled border produced by numerous microvilli. They have prominent Golgi apparatus and rough endoplasmic reticulum, and they contain many vesicles and lysosomes. There is some evidence that fibroblasts produce a chemoattractant protein that, as its name implies, attracts monocytes into the tissue and is synthesised in response to inflammation. Monocytes contain many enzymes that can degrade connective tissue extracellular matrix. Macrophages are derived from monocytes and are responsible for phagocytosing particulate matter and invading organisms and synthesising a range of molecules with important functions such as interferon (the antiviral factor), prostaglandins and factors that enhance the growth of fibroblasts and endothelial cells. Their structure depends upon their site of activity. The resting macrophage differs from the fibroblast in that there is a paucity of rough endoplasmic reticulum; there are thin, finger-like projections from the cell surface; and many lysosomes and other membrane-bound vesicles of varying density. When active, macrophages have many mitochondria and vesicles and may possess many branching processes. It has been speculated that the 'looser' arrangement of the periodontal connective tissues near the alveolar bone and the blood vessels relates to the presence of monocytes/macrophages.

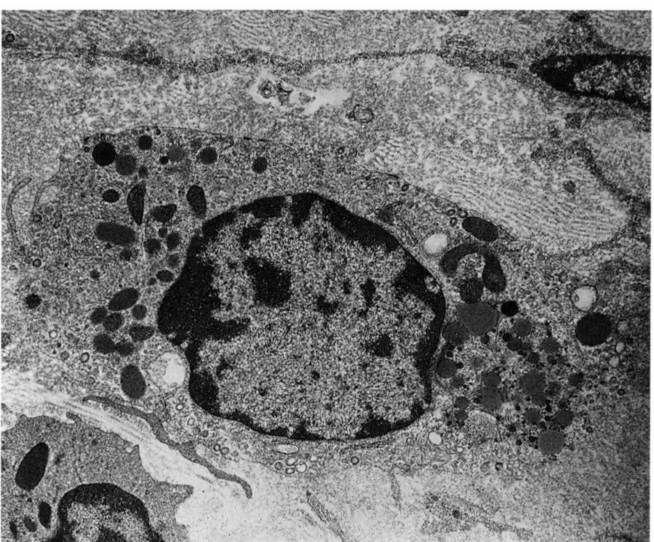

Fig. 12.52 Ultrastructural features of a macrophage (TEM; ×6,000).

Mast cells (Fig. 12.53)

These cells are often associated with blood vessels. They show a large number of intracytoplasmic granules (which explains the intense staining reaction with basic aniline dyes for light microscopy). The granules are dense, membrane-bound vesicles of varying sizes. Other cytoplasmic organelles are relatively sparse. When the cell is stimulated, it degranulates. Numerous functions have been ascribed to the mast cell, including the production of histamine, heparin and factors associated with anaphylaxis.

Eosinophils (Fig. 12.54)

These are only occasionally seen in the normal periodontal ligament. Characteristically, they possess granules (peroxisomes) that consist of one or more crystalloid structures. The cells are capable of phagocytosis.

Dendritic cells (Fig. 12.55)

As for the soft tissues of the dental pulp, gingiva and skin, the periodontal ligament possesses dendritic cells derived from the bone marrow. These

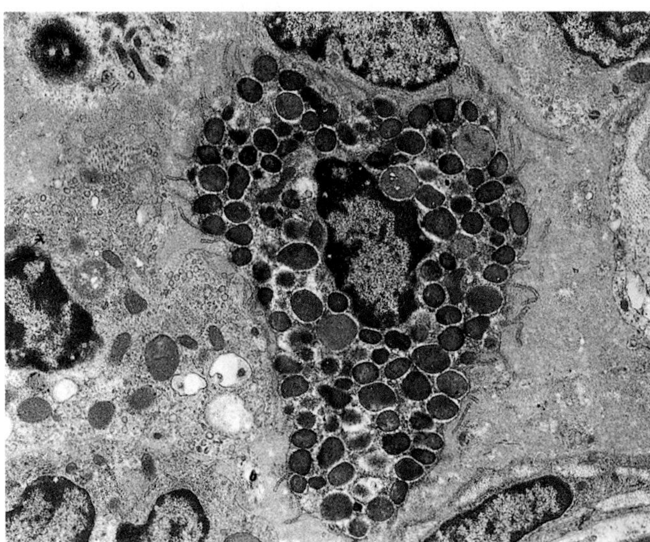

Fig. 12.53 The ultrastructural appearance of the mast cell. Note the numerous dense membrane-bound vesicles (TEM; ×5,000).

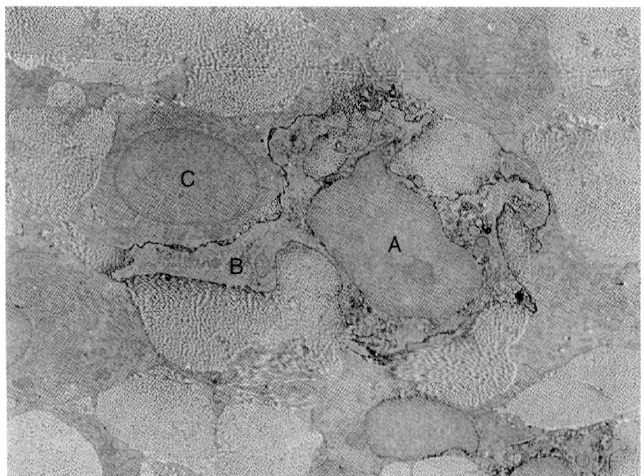

Fig. 12.55 Electron micrograph of a dendritic cell in the periodontal ligament. Specific immunoreaction products for antibodies for OX6 and ED1 localised as dark granules along cytoplasmic membrane and around cytoplasmic vesicles belonging to the phagolysosome apparatus. The dendritic antigen-presenting cells are distinguished from macrophages by the presence of several cytoplasmic processes of different lengths and thickness and possessing less well-developed ED1 positive phagolysosomal structures. A = nucleus of dendritic cell; B = dendritic processes: C = nucleus of unlabelled fibroblast. Note large bundles of collagen fibres cut in cross-section. Courtesy Dr. T Kaneko.

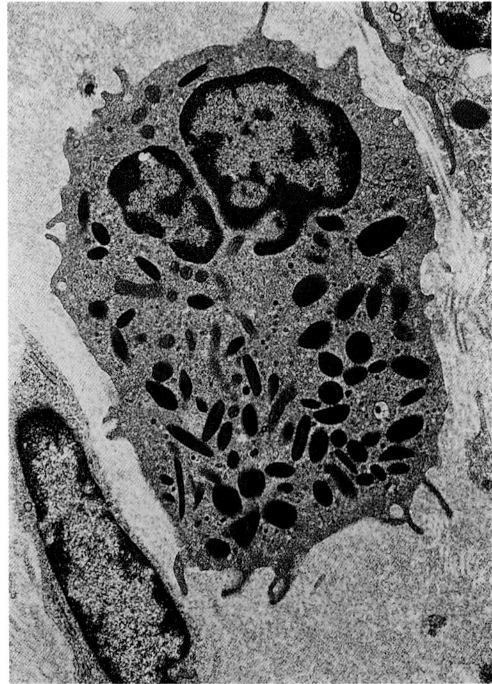

Fig. 12.54 The ultrastructural features of an eosinophil. Note the characteristic granules (peroxisomes) (TEM; ×2,500).

dendritic cells present antigens to naive T cells during primary and secondary immune responses. The few studies undertaken indicate that there are regional differences in their distribution and variation in their degree of maturation/activation that may reflect microenvironmental differences (e.g., the amount of external antigens).

The various defence cells of the periodontal ligament are capable of synthesising and releasing bioactive molecules such as cytokines, growth factors and cell adhesion molecules. These are important when considering the biology of the tissues. Many of these substances are upregulated during orthodontic tooth movement. Neutrophils and lymphocytes can also be seen within the periodontal ligament in response to inflammation.

Cell kinetics

Periodontal ligament fibroblasts need replenishing. Furthermore, as osteoblasts and cementoblasts of the periodontal ligament become incorporated into alveolar bone and cellular cementum, replacement cells must be provided within the ligament to permit osteogenesis and cementogenesis to continue. In contrast to periodontal ligament fibroblasts, gingival fibroblasts belong to two progenitor cell populations: one with limited proliferative capacity and the other having extensive self-renewal capacity. Periodontal ligament fibroblasts are larger than gingival fibroblasts, exhibit more filamentous actin and display smooth muscle myosin. Further differences between the two cell types are listed in Table 25.2.

The actual mechanisms that contribute to the development of cellular lineages in the periodontal ligament are largely unknown. During the development, the cells populating the dental follicle (see page 283) are probably ectomesenchymal (neural crest) in origin and migrate from the dental papilla (see page 283). In the mature periodontal ligament, progenitor cell populations of the periodontal ligament are located adjacent to the blood vessels near the surface of the alveolar bone and in the contiguous endosteal spaces. At the blood vessels, some of the cells exhibit the classical features of stem cells – small size, responsiveness to stimulating factors and slow cycle time.

Surprisingly, mesenchymal stem cells in the periodontal ligament have a higher growth potential than bone marrow–derived mesenchymal stem cells, Furthermore, they are highly multipotent stem cells, having the capacity to differentiate into osteoblasts, adipocytes, chondrocytes, fibroblasts (tenocytes), pancreatic islet cells, endothelial cells, retinal ganglion cells, neural cells, myocytes and cementoblasts (Fig. 12.56).

Grafting experiments suggest that the periodontal ligament near the tooth also contains cementoblast precursors (which have no paravascular association), while the ligament near the bone contains osteoblast precursors. Tritiated thymidine injections show that mitotic cells appear at paravascular sites and then migrate towards the bone surface. In addition, cells from the vascular channels within alveolar bone migrate towards the periodontal ligament. It has also been reported that there is a significant migration of periodontal cells to the surface of the alveolar bone with orthodontic tooth movement. In the normal periodontal ligament, the rate of cell generation (mitotic index) is modest (0.5–3%); the higher level has been found in the central part of the periodontal ligament where there is the least cell density. Such variation may be related to diurnal periodicity or to location within the ligament, in addition to individual variation. There is a reduction of the

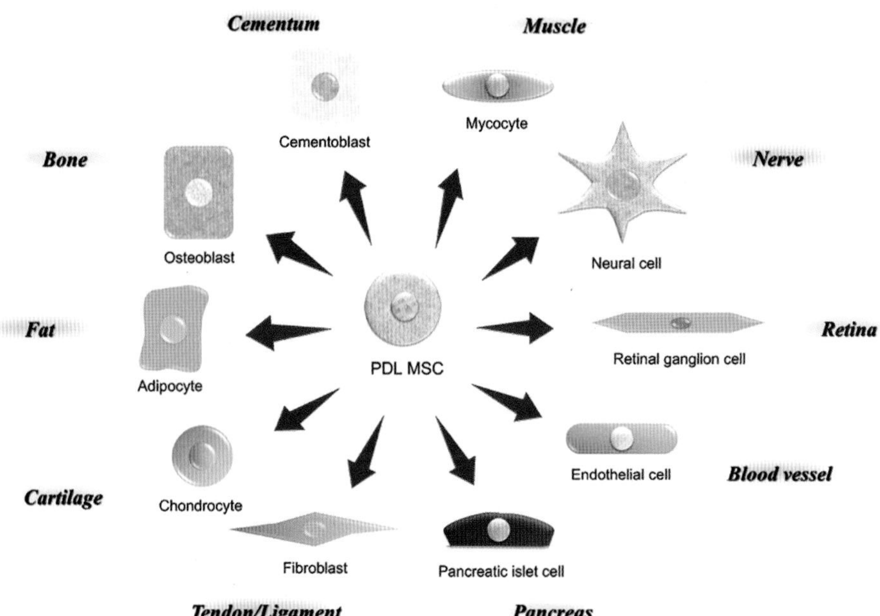

Fig. 12.56 Mesenchymal stem cells of the periodontal ligament (PDLMSC) are highly multipotent cells, having the capacity to differentiate into osteoblasts, adipocytes, chondrocytes, fibroblasts (tenocytes), pancreatic islet cells, endothelial cells, retinal ganglion cells, neural cells, myocytes and cementoblasts. From Tomokiyo, A., Yoshida, S., Hamano, S., et al., 2018. Detection, characterization, and clinical application of mesenchymal stem cells in periodontal ligament tissue. Stem Cells International 2018, 5450768.

mitotic index with age, although this rate is relatively rapid for a soft connective tissue. Cell mitosis and cell differentiation increase markedly with wounding or after the application of orthodontic loads, while different stimuli may recruit progenitors giving rise to different cell types (e.g., an osteoblastic rather than fibroblastic response following orthodontic loading).

For the fibroblasts, the cellular hierarchies in fibroblast populations of adult mammalian periodontal tissues are poorly understood, in part because of the lack of clear-cut phenotypic markers. Nevertheless, some reports suggest that there is significant morphological heterogeneity among periodontal cells. For example, there are said to be varying nuclear sizes (perhaps related to different capacities for undergoing cell division), a feature that has been claimed to provide a system for identifying the various cells in the osteoblast lineage. Other quantitative electron microscopy studies, however, indicate that the cells are remarkably homogeneous. Furthermore, morphological diversity is not itself indicative of functional heterogeneity. Periodontal fibroblasts comprise a renewal cell system in steady state, and the progenitors can generate multiple cell types of more differentiated, specialised cells. Renewal systems are characterised by a balance between newly generated cells and cells lost by apoptosis and migration out of the tissue.

For cementoblasts and osteoblasts, a major question concerns whether periodontal fibroblasts, cementoblasts and osteoblasts all arise from a common precursor or whether each cell type has its own specific precursor cell. Although progenitor cells can be identified by their ability to incorporate tritium-labelled thymidine, little is known about their origin and life cycle. One of the problems with answering this question is the lack of specific markers to distinguish fibroblasts, osteoblasts and cementoblasts (and their precursors). However, progress is being made, and the combined use of markers such as types I and III collagens (present in periodontal fibroblasts), bone sialoprotein and osteocalcin (present in cementoblasts and osteoblasts) and receptors for EGF (present in periodontal fibroblasts and possibly osteoblasts) may help to alleviate the problem. Table 12.1 summarises some of the features that help to distinguish fibroblasts, cementoblasts and osteoblasts in the periodontal ligament.

The presence of binding sites for EGF on periodontal fibroblasts is said to have an important role in their differentiation, and it has been shown that numerous receptors for EGF (EGFRs) are expressed on the cells of the periodontal ligament (particularly for fibroblasts, paravascular cells and preosteoblasts). However, they are not expressed on fully differentiated cementoblasts and osteoblasts. Such observations have led to the hypothesis that the fibroblast phenotype in the periodontal ligament requires the continued expression of EGFRs and that they inhibit their differentiation into mineralised tissue-forming cells. When exposed to EGF, periodontal fibroblasts show slightly increased mitogenic and chemotactic responses but decreased collagen synthesis. It has also been reported that PDGF-AB, PDGF-BB and IGF-I have potent mitogenic and chemotactic effects on the cells of the periodontal ligament. Furthermore, PDGF stimulates collagen synthesis. In contrast, TGF-β has only slight chemotactic effects and inhibis mitogenic responses.

Table 12.1 Groups of markers helping to distinguish cementoblasts, fibroblasts and osteoblasts within the periodontal ligament

	Cementoblasts	Periodontal ligament fibroblasts	Osteoblasts
Bone sialoprotein	+	–	+
Osteopontin	+	–	+
Osteocalcin	+	–	+
Osteonectin	?	+	+
Epithelial growth factor receptors	–	+	±
Parathyroid hormone receptors	+	–	+
Vitamin D responsive	+	?	+
Alkaline phosphatase	±	+	+
Collagens:			
Type I	+	+	+
Type III	–	+	–
Type V	–	+	–

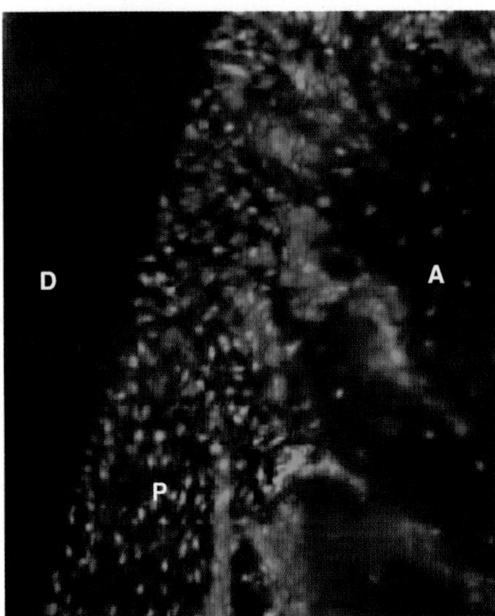

Fig. 12.57 Labelling for apoptosis within the periodontal ligament using the TUNEL technique. D = root dentine of a rat second molar in an aged animal; P = periodontal ligament showing many positively labelled green apoptotic cells (such cells are absent in the nonaged tissue); A = alveolar bone (TUNEL fluorescent micrograph; ×120).

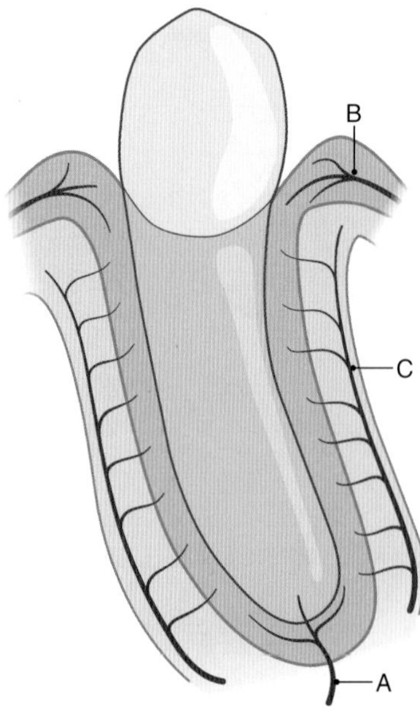

Fig. 12.58 The blood supply to the periodontal ligament. A = arteries from dental pulp; B = arteries from gingiva; C = arteries from alveolar bone.

Further information regarding stem cells within the periodontal ligament is provided on pages 255 and 496 in relation to the notion that the ligament retains fetal-like characteristics.

Apoptosis

Apoptosis (programmed cell death) is not a common feature in the mature connective tissues of the periodontal ligament. In the aged animal, however, many of the cells are apoptotic (Fig. 12.57), and this is supported by immunocytochemical studies, which show a reduced level of focal adhesions in the cells of the aged tissues. Upregulation of the enzyme focal adhesion kinase within the periodontal ligament is seen during a phase of maximum eruption of the tooth (particularly at the root apex), and this feature is associated with upregulation of proliferating cell-nuclear antigen.

Regeneration of the periodontal ligament

Knowledge of the basic cell biology of the periodontal ligament is important for clinical practice in enabling a detailed understanding of the principles involved in obtaining periodontal regeneration (as opposed to repair) and in developing successful clinical strategies towards this end. During regeneration, cells such as fibroblasts, cementoblasts and osteoblasts must be induced in appropriate numbers, at the right time and in the right place, and then synthesise their appropriate extracellular matrices. New Sharpey's fibres must gain a functional attachment into new bone and cementum. In addition, epithelial downgrowths must be excluded from the cementum surface. Unfortunately, *in vitro* studies to advance the development of these clinical strategies are often scientifically suspect. For example, when papers describe studies obtained by culturing cells scraped from the roots of extracted teeth (and often calling them periodontal ligament fibroblasts), it is difficult to know precisely what cell types are involved and how homogeneous the population is. Furthermore, as different culture techniques (with different passage numbers and different culture media) are used, it is not surprising that different authors report different results. A clinical procedure said to be important in the attainment of periodontal regeneration is that of tissue-guided regeneration. This is discussed on page 497.

Blood vessels and nerves

Blood vessels

Arteries

The rich blood supply to the periodontal ligament is derived from the appropriate superior and inferior alveolar arteries, although arteries from the gingiva (such as the lingual and palatine arteries) may also be involved (Fig. 12.58). The arteries supplying the periodontal ligament are primarily derived not from those entering the pulp at the apex of the tooth, but from a series of perforating arteries passing through the alveolar bone. This source of blood supply allows the periodontal ligament to function following removal of the root apex as a result of various endodontic treatments. The coronal part of the periodontal ligament is supplied by vessels from the gingival tissues.

The volume of the periodontal ligament occupied by blood vessels varies between about 10% and more than 30% according to species, tooth type, whether the tooth is erupting or is fully erupted and site within the periodontal ligament.

The vessels found near the root surface are said to form a capillary plexus. Vessels nearer the bone surface form a postcapillary plexus from which venules pass into the alveolar bone. Many of the vessels of the periodontal ligament lie between the principal fibre bundles and closer to the alveolus than the tooth (Fig. 12.59 and Fig. 12.64A). They have an average diameter of about 20 µm. The vessels branch and anastomose to form a capillary plexus around the teeth. Semithin sections of periodontal ligament show that the blood vessels are seen as large spaces (Fig. 12.60). Indeed, the volume of the periodontal space occupied by blood vessels and by blood may be so great that we should perhaps think of the periodontal ligament as a 'blood space' as much as a 'connective tissue'!

Special features

Specialised features of the vasculature of the periodontal ligament are a crevicular plexus of capillary loops and the presence of large numbers of fenestrations in the capillaries. A crevicular plexus of capillary loops (Fig. 12.61) completely encircles the tooth within the connective tissue beneath the region of the gingival crevice. Each loop consists of one or

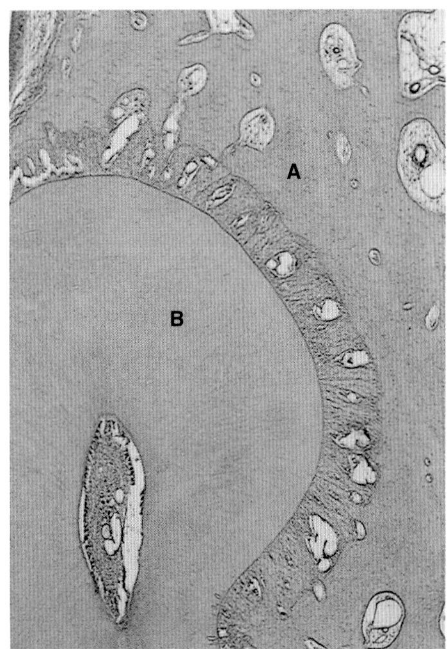

Fig. 12.59 Transverse section through a periodontal ligament to show blood vessels lying close to alveolar bone. A = alveolar bone; B = dentine (van Gieson; ×30).

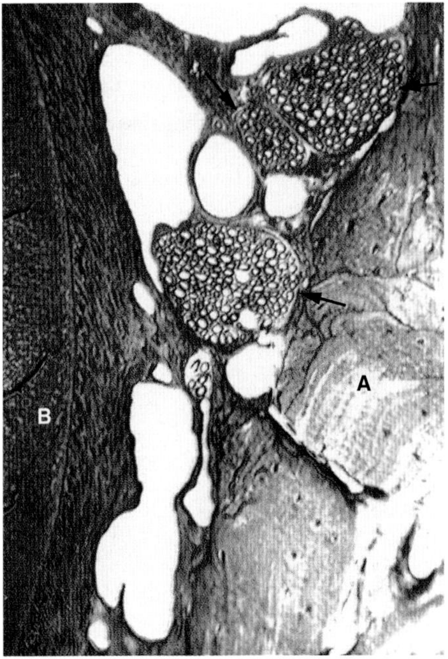

Fig. 12.60 Semi-thin section of periodontal ligament showing large blood volume in the periodontal space. Nerve bundles are arrowed. A = alveolar bone; B = dentine (toluidine blue; ×100).

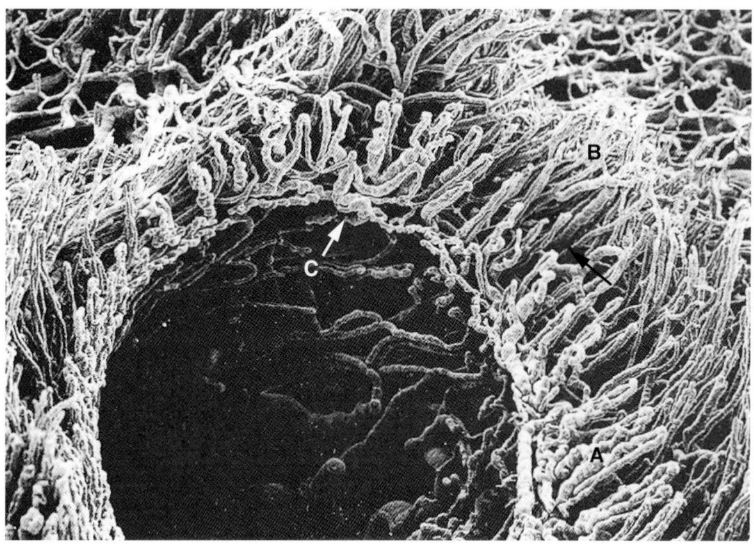

Fig. 12.61 A crevicular plexus of capillary loops (A). B = capillary loops in the gingival surface; C = circular plexus; arrow indicates a gap between crevicular and circular plexuses (SEM of vascular cast; ×80). Courtesy Prof. M R Sims.

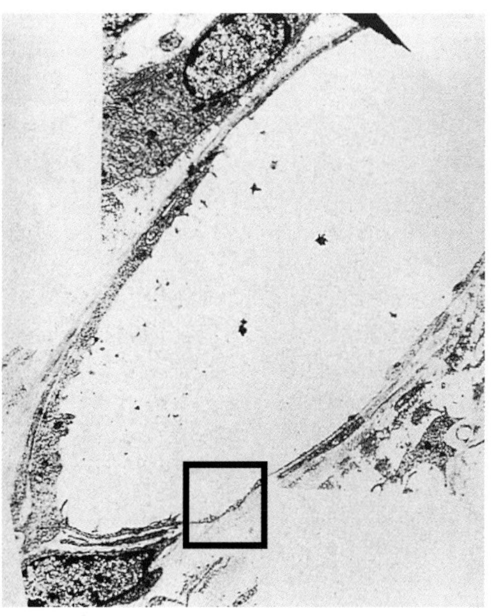

Fig. 12.62 Fenestrated capillaries within the periodontal ligament. Note the thinning of the endothelium in the boxed area where fenestrations are present (TEM; ×10,000).

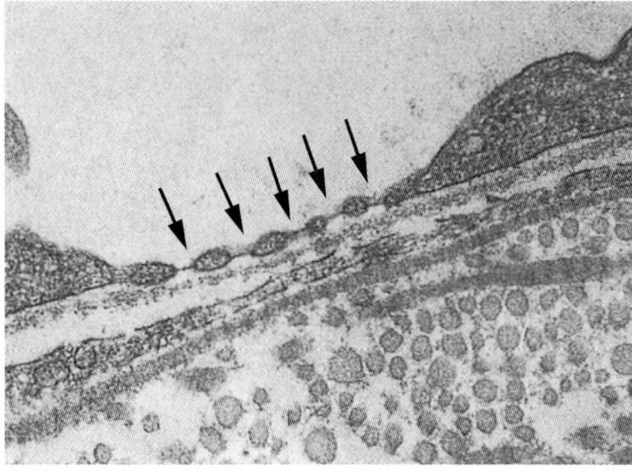

Fig. 12.63 Fenestrated capillaries within the periodontal ligament. This is a higher-power view of the boxed area shown in Fig. 12.62. Arrows indicate the fenestrations (TEM; ×35,000).

two thin (8–10 μm in diameter) capillary ascending limbs and one or two postcapillary-sized venules. The crevicular capillary loops are separated from other more marginally situated loops in the gingival surface by a distinct gap and arise from a circular plexus, which is composed of between one and four intercommunicating vessels (6–30 μm in diameter) lying at the level of the junctional epithelium. The circular plexus anastomoses with both the gingival and periodontal ligament vessels. Species differences may occur in the pattern of the vasculature, which may also be affected by inflammation. More complex glomerular-like structures have also been described. The functional significance of the complex vasculature in this region is not fully understood, although it may be related to the provision of a dentogingival seal. It may provide a means for blood flow reversal and rapid redistribution of the blood under varying occlusal loads and as a reaction to pathological stimuli.

Fenestration of capillaries within the periodontal ligament (Figs. 12.62, 12.63) is unusual because fibrous connective tissues usually have continuous capillaries. The presence of fenestrated capillaries in large numbers (up to 40 × 10^6/mm^3 of tissue) is therefore a specialised feature of the periodontal ligament. Fenestrated capillary beds differ from continuous capillary beds in that the diffusion and filtration capacities are greatly increased. It is possible that the fenestrations are related to the high metabolic requirements of the periodontal ligament (high rate of turnover). Experimental evidence suggests that the number of fenestrations also relates to the stage of eruption.

Veins

The veins within the periodontal ligament do not usually accompany the arteries. Instead, they pass through the alveolar walls into intra-alveolar venous networks. Anastomoses with veins in the gingiva also occur. A dense venous network is particularly prominent around the apex of the alveolus.

The junctions between vascular endothelial cells in the periodontal ligament vary from close to tight to open. Open junctions are more permeable and provide pathways for fluid and molecular transport. These open junctions appear to be characteristic of the venous capillaries in the periodontal ligament.

Very few studies have investigated quantitatively and at the ultrastructural level the nature of vessels comprising the microvascular bed of the human periodontal ligament. One study that provides some data is illustrated in Fig. 12.64. The results give a total luminal volume of approximately 9.5%, with significant variation both across the width of the ligament and from coronal to apical parts. From this study, postcapillary venules are the predominant vessels.

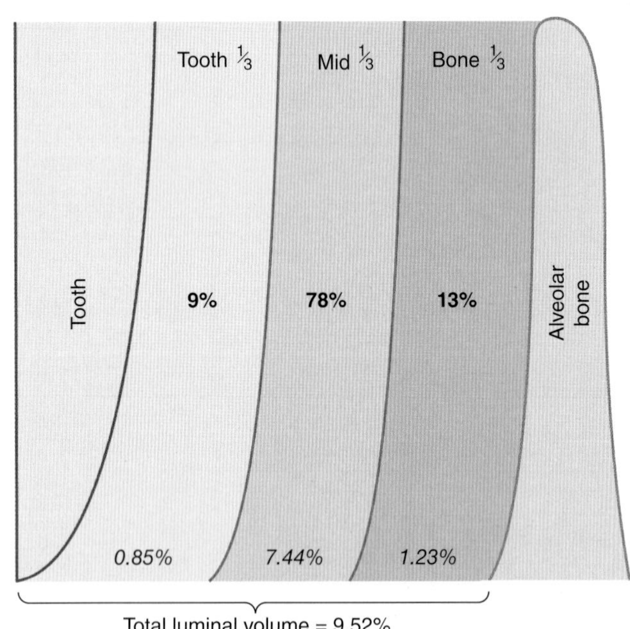

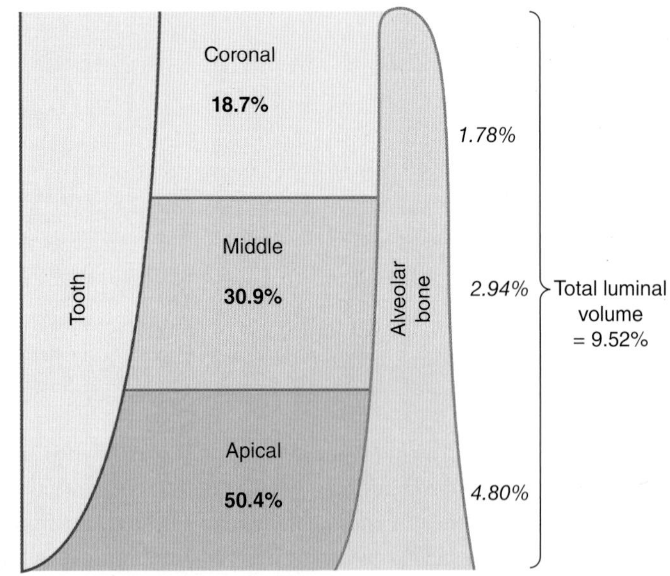

Fig. 12.64 The percentage distribution of the total luminal volume of the microvascular bed (A) across the circumferential thirds of the periodontal ligament and (B) in each vertical third of the periodontal ligament. The numbers in italics show the distribution of blood volume as a percentage of the total ligament volume. Redrawn from Foong, K., Sims, M.R., 1999. Blood volume in human bicuspid periodontal ligament determined by electron microscopy. Archives of Oral Biology 44, 465–474.

Nerves

The nerve fibres supplying the periodontal ligament are functionally of two types: sensory and autonomic. The sensory fibres are associated with nociception and mechanoreception. The autonomic fibres are associated mainly with the supply of the periodontal blood vessels. Compared with other dense fibrous connective tissues, the periodontal ligament is well innervated (Fig. 12.65).

Sensory nerves

The nerve fibres entering the periodontal ligament are derived from two sources. Some nerve bundles enter near the root apex and pass up through the periodontal ligament; others enter the middle and cervical portions of the ligament as finer branches through openings in the alveolar walls.

Periodontal nerve fibres are both myelinated and unmyelinated. The myelinated fibres are on average about 5 μm in diameter (although some are as large as 15 μm) and are sensory fibres only. The unmyelinated fibres are about 0.5 μm in diameter and are both sensory and autonomic.

At the light microscope level, a plethora of forms that are assumed to represent nerve endings have been described within the periodontal ligament. These forms vary from simple free endings to more elaborate arborising structures, although they still only mediate two sensory modalities – pain or pressure.

Mechanoreceptors

Most attention has been paid to the periodontal mechanoreceptors. These perform a major role in the transmission of touch and textural information when eating (smoothness, crunchiness, crispiness and chewiness). They also provide afferent feedback essential in the control of salivation, mastication and swallowing (see Chapter 6). They can be activated with loads as low as 0.01 N.

If recordings are made from afferent nerve fibres from periodontal ligament mechanoreceptors, the responses seem to vary according to the direction and amplitude of the displacing force, and the response properties range from very rapidly adapting to very slowly adapting (Fig. 12.66). Many studies have attributed the response properties to the variety of morphological types of receptors described in other tissues. However, there is

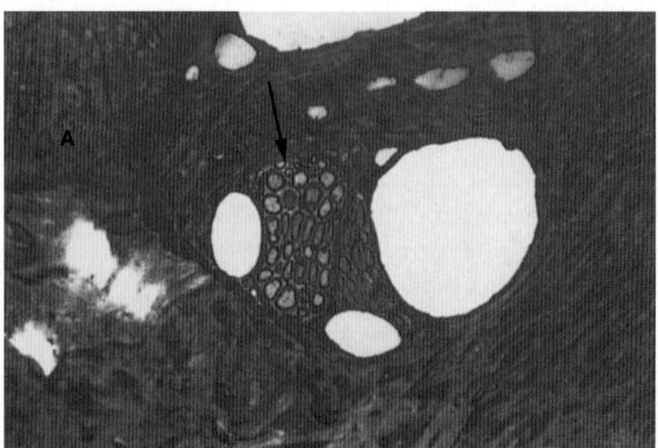

Fig. 12.65 The rich nerve supply (arrow) to the periodontal ligament. A = alveolar bone (decalcified, transverse section through a tooth and its periodontal ligament; toluidine blue; ×150).

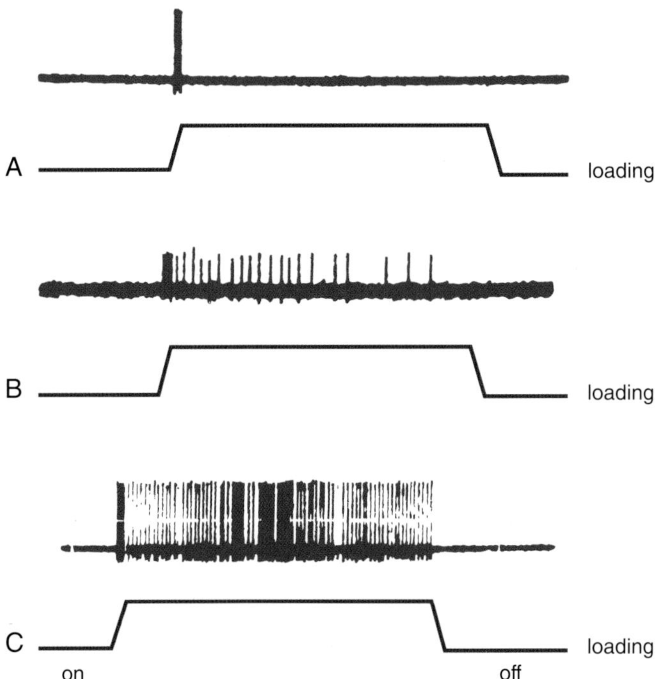

Fig. 12.66 The responses of three periodontal ligament mechanoreceptors to suprathreshold ramp-plateau stimuli of 1 N (duration 3 s; rise time 50 ms). (A) Rapidly adapting response. (B) Intermediate adapting response. (C) Slowly adapting response. The receptors were located in the same tooth: (A) 1.5 mm, (B) 3.0 mm, (C) 5.5 mm from the fulcrum. Courtesy Prof. R W A Linden.

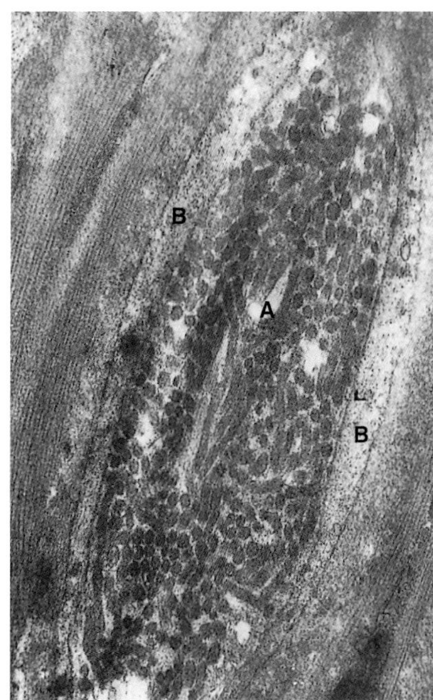

Fig. 12.67 The putative nerve endings (A) that may represent Ruffini-like mechanoreceptors in the periodontal ligament. B = ensheathing Schwann-type cell. Note the large number of mitochondria (TEM; ×5,700).

not a range of receptor types within the periodontal ligament – only one single type whose response characteristics depend on its position in the ligament in addition to the rate, magnitude and direction in which the stimulating force is applied to the tooth. Rapidly adapting responses are seen from receptors found close to the fulcrum of the tooth about which movement is taking place. Slowly adapting responses are seen from receptors close to the apex of the tooth. There appears to be a grading of adapting properties for receptors lying between these two locations. Furthermore, the thresholds of the receptors also appear to be related to their position in the ligament, with those located close to the fulcrum of the tooth having higher thresholds and those closer to the apex having very low thresholds. Evidence is also available to show that the responses of periodontal mechanoreceptors are temperature-dependent, with the activity peaking close to body temperature.

When morphological studies have been made on receptors, only Ruffini-like endings have been identified. These endings are branched and unencapsulated and are incompletely surrounded by terminal Schwann cells with extensions projecting towards the collagen bundles. The physiological response characteristics of the periodontal ligament mechanoreceptors are consistent with them being type II slowly adapting (SAII) receptors. Given optimal stimulation (i.e., those positioned at the apex rather than the fulcrum of the tooth), they exhibit typical SAII dynamic and static responses with a regular discharge of impulses. Those receptors located close to the fulcrum exhibit responses typical of a slowly adapting receptor receiving a just suprathreshold stimulus, in that they give what appears to be a rapidly adapting response. The lower thresholds exhibited by those closer to the apex can also be explained by the degree of stimulation being greater at the apex than at the fulcrum of the tooth. Periodontal ligament mechanoreceptors respond maximally when the area in which they lie is put into tension. They exhibit directional sensitivity in response to forces applied to the crown of the tooth, and this can be explained by their discrete receptive fields. Both the morphological and physiological evidence supports the view that periodontal ligament mechanoreceptors are Ruffini-type II mechanoreceptors.

Putative nerve endings, which may represent mechanoreceptors, are characterised by the very large concentrations of mitochondria in the unmyelinated terminations of myelinated nerves (Fig. 12.67). Unusually, the ensheathing Schwann cells contain the intermediate filament, nestin, which can be detected in neuroepithelial stem cells, though the significance of this awaits clarification. Periodontal Ruffini endings appear to be concentrated in the region where periodontal ligament fibres are most stretched, for example, around the root apex in a molar. Following removal of antagonist teeth, the ultrastructural features of the putative nerve endings are changed, including loss of organelles and changes in the location of the mitochondria. Occlusal loading may therefore be essential for maintaining the integrity of the periodontal mechanoreceptors. Unlike the cutaneous Ruffini endings, the periodontal Ruffini endings are devoid of a fibrous capsule.

Following nerve injury, the periodontal Ruffini endings may regenerate more rapidly than Ruffini endings in other tissues and may migrate into regions where they are not normally found. During regeneration, changes in the expression level of various bioactive substances occur in both axonal and Schwann cell elements in the endings.

More complex putative nerve endings have very occasionally been observed within the periodontal ligament (Fig. 12.68). These are characterised by numerous circularly arranged cell processes surrounding a central structure containing microfilaments, microtubules and mitochondria. This central structure is thought to represent a nerve terminal. The morphology of this lamellated structure is reminiscent of cutaneous mechanoreceptors of the Pacinian type. Because of their rarity, their significance in the periodontal ligament is unknown. Nevertheless, lamellated Pacinian corpuscles are associated with rapidly adapting type II (RAII) receptors. Such receptors signal information about vibration and acceleration of mechanical stimulation of the tissues. They can be stimulated by vibration of receptive fields with ill-defined borders, and they respond to step indentation with both an 'on' and an 'off' discharge of typically one (or maybe two) impulses. They have low mechanical thresholds with indentation thresholds of 7–10 μm. They also have low-frequency thresholds in the

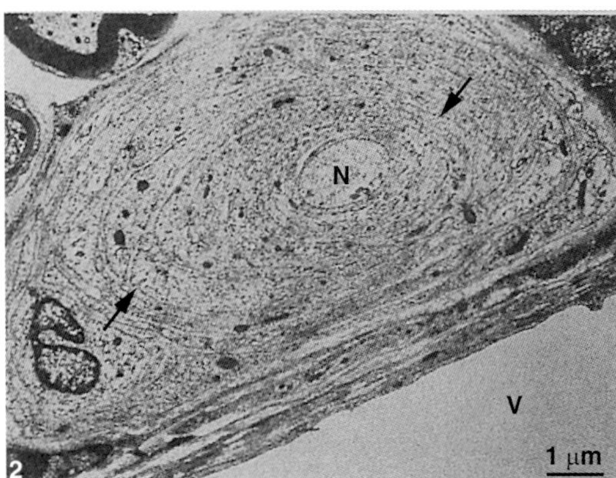

Fig. 12.68 Complex putative nerve ending in the periodontal ligament. Arrows indicate numerous circularly arranged cell processes. N = nerve terminal; V = blood vessel (TEM; ×4,500).

range of 80–300 Hz, but with higher strengths of stimuli, they can respond in a 'one-to-one fashion' to frequencies over the range 30–1000 Hz.

The surrounding process of the ensheathing Schwann-type cell is noteworthy, and this type of ending is regarded as being akin to a Ruffini-like nerve terminal. The cell bodies of the ensheathing Schwann-type cells contain rough endoplasmic reticulum, and the nucleus may be indented (Fig. 12.69). Numerous vesicles may be observed within, and forming on, both the inner and outer surfaces of the ensheathing cells. These vesicles may be associated with rapid transport of materials to and from the nerve terminal. The collagen in the immediate vicinity of the nerve ending appears to be arranged in a lamellar pattern.

Central pathways

The cell bodies of neurones innervating mechanoreceptors in the perioral tissues mostly lie within the trigeminal ganglion. Recordings have been made in the trigeminal ganglion from neurones that respond to mechanical stimulation of the periodontal ligament. The trigeminal mesencephalic nucleus also contains cell bodies of neurones that innervate structures within the oral cavity. Recordings have been made from neurones that innervate the ipsilateral maxillary and mandibular periodontal ligament mechanoreceptors and from receptors that respond to forces applied to all the teeth in the maxillary arch and to forces applied to the nose and hard palate. It has been suggested that these receptors lie in the palatomaxillary sutures. The mesencephalic nucleus also contains the cell bodies of the jaw elevator muscle spindles that are involved in signalling the changes in length of the extrafusal muscle fibres.

Within the trigeminal nuclei, neurones that respond to mechanical stimulation of the teeth have been found in the spinal trigeminal nucleus (comprising the subdivisions oralis, interpolaris and caudalis) and the main sensory nucleus. Recordings have also been made from the nucleus supratrigeminalis, although this is regarded as an extension of the main sensory nucleus. Neurones with varying properties can be observed in different parts of the trigeminal complex. Periodontal mechanoreceptive neurones in the oralis and interpolaris give sustained responses to forces applied to the teeth, similar to neurones in the trigeminal main sensory nucleus. In contrast, neurones in the subnucleus caudalis give transient responses. The receptive fields of neurones located in the trigeminal nuclear complex appear to be broader than those of the primary afferent neurones. Neurones that respond to forces applied to the teeth still exhibit directional sensitivity but may appear to respond to forces over a broader range of stimulus direction.

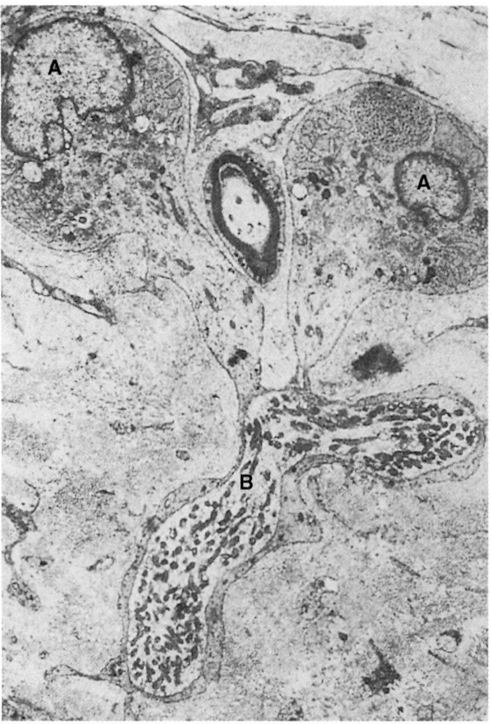

Fig. 12.69 The cell bodies of the ensheathing Schwann-type cells. A = indented nuclei; B = mitochondria-rich nerve terminal (TEM; ×5,000).

Recordings from first-order periodontal ligament mechanoreceptive neurones in the mesencephalic nucleus have shown receptors with intermediate adaptation properties and intermediate thresholds. It has been shown that these receptors are situated in a discrete area of the periodontal ligament and lie midway between the fulcrum and the apex of the tooth. The functional significance of this observation is presently unknown.

Neurones in some parts of the trigeminal nuclear complex respond to mechanical stimulation from several different structures. In the interpolaris and caudalis subnuclei, many neurones respond to forces applied to more than one tooth, although in the subnucleus oralis, most neurones respond to a single tooth. In the main sensory nucleus, approximately 25% of the neurones respond to forces applied to multiple teeth. In addition, some neurones are known to respond to mechanical stimulation of more than one type of tissue within the oral and perioral regions. Neurones in the main sensory nucleus respond to mechanical stimulation of the teeth and intraoral mucosa or facial hair. Similar observations have been made in the main sensory and spinal trigeminal nuclear complex on periodontal mechanoreceptive neurones that also respond to stimulation of receptors in the oral mucosa and facial regions.

Most fibres that arise in the trigeminal sensory nuclei (principally the main sensory and spinal nuclei) cross the midline and ascend in the trigeminal lemniscus to the nucleus ventralis posteromedialis of the thalamus. From the thalamus the fibres are relayed to the cortical postcentral gyrus (areas 3, 1 and 2). Some fibres from the trigeminal sensory nuclei ascend to the thalamus on the ipsilateral side (without crossing over). It is most likely that collateral branches of both primary and secondary afferent trigeminal neurones reach many other regions such as the reticular formation, tectum, cerebellum, subthalamus, hypothalamus and other cranial nerve nuclei.

Recordings have been made in the nucleus ventralis posteromedialis of the thalamus from neurones that respond to mechanical stimulation of the teeth. Most neurones receive contralateral inputs, and most neurones that respond to periodontal inputs also respond to mechanical stimulation of other oral and facial structures (such as hair [vibrissae], nose, lips, tongue and palate). These large receptive field areas of the thalamus, which are greater than those in the trigeminal nuclear complex, suggest there is a considerable amount of convergence of neurones.

Recordings have been made in the somatosensory cortex (S1) from neurones that respond to force applied to the teeth. As observed in the thalamus, periodontal ligament mechanoreceptors in the somatosensory cortex have receptive fields not only from multiple teeth but also from other oral structures such as gingivae, lips and tongue mucosa. Similarly, a range of adaptations has been observed. There is some evidence that many of the mechanosensitive neurones that respond to stimuli of the oral and facial regions can be modulated by tasks such as biting or tongue protrusion.

It appears that most periodontal mechanoreceptor neurones with their cell bodies in the mesencephalic nucleus have no functional role after tooth extraction. Indeed, the control of precisely directed, low biting forces is markedly disturbed in patients with osseo-integrated implants.

There is evidence that afferents from anterior teeth (the incisors and canines) convey information about the state of contact between the food and the teeth and thereby play an important role in the specification of the level of force needed to fold and manipulate the food between the teeth. Not only are the mechanoreceptors involved in masticatory reflexes but there is evidence that they are involved in salivatory reflexes, especially on the ipsilateral side. When the teeth are clenched in the absence of a food bolus, some parotid saliva is secreted. This is reduced if the intraoral nerves are anaesthetised. The periodontal mechanoreceptors also modulate the activity of the motor neurones of the hypoglossal cranial nerve, helping to control tongue position during mastication. In addition, activity of the neck musculature is probably modulated by periodontal mechanoreceptors, since pain and dysfunction of this musculature are frequently reported by patients suffering from occlusal or temporomandibular joint disorders.

Pain and autonomic fibres

Little is known about pain fibres within the periodontal ligament, but it is presumed that, as elsewhere in the body, they are represented by fine, unmyelinated fibres terminating as free nerve endings. A similar lack of information exists concerning the fine (0.2–1 μm diameter) autonomic fibres. These fibres are important in the control of regional blood flow, having vasoconstrictor activity. Thus, experiments affecting the sympathetic system are seen to produce changes in tooth position.

Neuropeptides

As for the dental pulp, sensory nerve endings in the periodontal ligament can release neuropeptides such as substance P, vasoactive intestinal peptide, neuropeptide Y and calcitonin gene–related peptide. These substances can have widespread effects on blood vessels and cells and must have an important, but as yet undetermined, role in the biology of the ligament in both health and the diseased state. Many of them are upregulated during orthodontic tooth movement.

Sensation following implants

The importance of maintaining the innervation of the periodontal ligament for ensuring proper functioning of the teeth has already been alluded to when considering the effects of tooth extraction. Indeed, the presence of osseo-integrated implants seems to improve orodental sensation and, even for badly damaged teeth, it could be clinically advantageous to retain tooth fragments or roots. Furthermore, some regeneration of periodontal mechanoreceptors occurs following reimplantation of teeth, although there will still be decreased neural activity.

Age changes in the periodontal ligament

Despite the obvious importance (both biologically and clinically) of investigating the effects of ageing on the periodontal ligament, our understanding of this subject needs more investigation than thitherto. There have been remarkably few studies concerned with the changing composition and functions of the periodontal ligament. Indeed, the effects of ageing upon the turnover rates of the extracellular matrix have yet to be assessed. Furthermore, most of the studies concerned with the structural aspects of the aged periodontal ligament have involved experimental animals, have been at the light microscope level and have been mainly qualitative. Any changes recorded must be shown to be related to ageing and not to disease processes. Changes are likely to be related to senescence in the stem cell population.

The width of the periodontal ligament space is said to reduce with age. This phenomenon can be explained by the accumulation of mineralised tissue and/or atrophy of structural elements within the ligament.

Concerning cellular age changes, a decrease in cellularity has often been reported within the human periodontal ligament, and this has been suggested as one cause for slower orthodontic movement in older patients. Cell density may decrease by more than 50% from young to aged individuals.

In addition to a reduction in cell density, a decrease in the mitotic index has also been described, and the suggestion has been made that the fibroblasts in the ageing periodontal tissues have longer 'lives' than those in younger tissues. Whether this cellular reduction affects stem cells awaits clarification. The decline of proliferative capacity by ageing ultimately leads to impaired wound healing and reduced tissue regeneration.

In terms of the cellular organelles, the fibroblasts of the aged periodontal ligament differ in three respects: the areas occupied by endoplasmic reticulum are significantly less, the areas occupied by intracellular collagen profiles are also less and both the numbers and sizes of intercellular contacts are significantly different (decreased numbers; increased size). Thus, the aged periodontal fibroblasts appear to have diminished protein synthesis and collagen degradative capabilities. Furthermore, the nature of cell–matrix and cell–cell interactions is markedly changed. Immunocytochemical investigation of the cytoskeletal components of periodontal ligament fibroblasts indicate that the aged cells express cytokeratin 19 in addition to vimentin (in younger tissues, only vimentin is expressed). Cytokeratin 19 intermediate filaments have also been seen during the most active phase of tooth eruption. Its appearance in the aged periodontal ligament may be related to the increased rates of eruption-like movements reported for aged teeth, or it may reflect the diminished cell–matrix and cell–cell interactions deduced from quantitative electron microscopy.

Other changes that have been reported with ageing of the periodontal ligament include a decrease in alkaline phosphatase activity and an increase in gene expression of MMP2, MMP8 and TIMP1 gene activity, with this gene activity suggesting that extracellular matrix might be more easily degraded with age. Aged periodontal ligament cells express a higher level of pro-inflammatory genes, including osteoprotegerin, IL-1 and IL-6. Considering that osteoclast activity is regulated by osteoprotegerin and RANKL, it is not surprising that bone turnover is increased with age. Aged periodontal ligament cells also show lower alkaline phosphatase activity, which means reduced osteogenesis and calcification. Consistently, osteoblastic gene expression gradually diminishes with age.

Periodontal ligament stem cells also undergo age changes. With age, their proliferation rates and osteogenic potential are decreased. Moreover, the immunosuppressive ability of stem cells is reduced, whereas apoptosis is increased. This suggests that stem cells from a younger age group are more appropriate in terms of periodontal regeneration.

It has been reported that fat cells appear within the aged human periodontal ligament. In addition, large, multinucleated fibroblastic cells have been seen in aged supracrestal periodontal connective tissues. Indeed, these cells accounted for more than 17% of the cells in this region. The multinucleated fibroblastic cells differ from osteoclasts in that they have considerable amounts of rough endoplasmic reticulum, a conspicuous Golgi apparatus and intracellular collagen profiles and also possess multiple centrioles. It can be concluded, therefore, that these cells arise by cell fusion. That the cells are fibroblastic is shown by their uptake of tritiated proline and by acid phosphatase activity associated with phagolysosomes. Unlike neighbouring (mononuclear) fibroblasts, the cell membranes do not show the presence of alkaline phosphatase.

Mohawk homeobox (Mkx) is a tendon-specific transcription factor that is specifically expressed in the periodontal ligament but not in the enamel, dentine or dental pulp. In young mice lacking this transcription factor, no changes in periodontal ligament are observed. However, in older mice, degenerative changes occur, such as expansion at the furcation area, abnormal collagen fibril structure, loss of periodontal ligament cell morphology, alveolar bone surface irregularity and the abnormal appearance of multinucleated cells. These results suggest a role of Mkx in periodontal homeostasis.

Differences have been observed in the distribution of epithelial cells according to site and age: during the first and second decades they are most prevalent in the apical zone; between the third and seventh decades the majority are located cervically in the gingiva above the alveolar crest.

For the extracellular matrix of the periodontal ligament, changes related to ageing have been reported for both the collagen fibres and the ground substance. The earliest studies suggested that the amounts of soluble collagen and 'acid mucopolysaccharides' decrease with age. From histological examination of the aged human periodontal ligament, results indicate that the main age change appears to be increased collagen fibrosis. More specifically, the principal collagen fibre bundles become thicker, the fibre groups seem to be broader and more highly organised, there are areas of hyalinisation and there is a reduction in areas staining positive with Alcian blue. Furthermore, some of the fibres may become mineralised. In contrast, the number of periodontal ligament fibres is said by other researchers to decrease with age, and there may be an age-dependent decrease in the rate of collagen synthesis. For the Sharpey's fibre insertions, it has been found that the alveolar bone surface changes from smooth and regular with evenly distributed insertions of principal fibres in younger tissue into jagged and uneven with irregular fibre insertions in aged tissue.

An important feature of the ageing of a connective tissue relates to the changes that occur in collagen fibril diameters. For the periodontal ligament, however, there is disagreement as to the fate of the collagen fibrils with age. It has been claimed that the mean fibril diameter decreases by nearly 50% over the life span. However, several findings from quantitative electron microscopy have shown that there is little change in fibril diameters with age. Although in many connective tissues ageing effects can be attributed to alterations in elastin (rather than to collagen), there is very little information concerning the effects of ageing on the elastic network of the periodontal ligament (including oxytalan). Furthermore, little is known about the changes that occur in the neurovascular elements of the ligament, although it has been reported that degenerative vascular changes can be discerned.

Unfortunately, there is almost no information concerning the effects of age upon the functions of the periodontal ligament. Nevertheless, it has been shown that human teeth become less mobile with age. This change might be related to increases in length of the root or to changes in the number and diameters of the principal fibres of the periodontal ligament. It has also been reported that the eruption rates (of the rat incisor) are markedly increased with age, with the mechanism whereby the eruptive force is generated being a property of the periodontal ligament (see page 461).

Other studies on the effects of ageing on the periodontium have been concerned with the influence of inflammatory periodontal disease. Indeed, differentiation between age change and pathological change is imprecise and provides one of the fundamental problems in studying the pathogenesis of periodontal disease. It is well established that the prevalence of periodontitis increases with age. However, it is questionable whether periodontal changes are the result of a disease process or an ageing process. It has been found that periodontal age-related changes occur in gnotobiotic rats in the absence of inflammatory periodontal disease. In particular, gradual recession of alveolar bone occurs with increasing age. On the other hand, some clinicians are of the opinion that lack of oral hygiene is the most influential factor in periodontal destruction and that the effect of age is negligible when good oral hygiene is maintained. Nevertheless, it has been shown that many aged persons have considerable quantities of plaque yet do not develop periodontal destruction. On this basis there is probably a multifactorial aetiology to the disease such that the influence of ageing cannot be overruled. The ageing of the periodontal ligament may have a bearing on other clinical problems. For example, orthodontic treatment is most often undertaken within the dentitions of teenagers or young adults, and it is probable that age is influential in the response of the periodontium (including alveolar bone) to orthodontic loads.

Overall, the evidence suggests that there is some degeneration of the periodontal ligament with age. However, some features (e.g., the lack of change for collagen fibril diameters) indicate that the reactions and mechanisms of this degeneration may differ markedly from other fibrous connective tissues. The relative paucity of studies on this topic is therefore to be regretted.

The periodontal ligament as a specialised connective tissue

Although the periodontal ligament has the same components as other soft, fibrous adult connective tissues (i.e., it is composed essentially of an unmineralised collagen and proteoglycan stroma in which are found connective tissue cells), it has features that, in combination, imply that it can be considered a specialised tissue. These are listed in Box 12.3.

However, the mere listing of these specialised characteristics does not permit inference of the role of these features in the function and pathobiology of the tissue. To do this, we need to discover whether there are structural and/or biochemical analogues for the periodontal ligament elsewhere in the body.

Initially, an analogue for the periodontal ligament was sought in mature (adult) fibrous connective tissues with known mechanical demands (i.e., connective tissue placed under either tension or compression). However,

Box 12.3 Features of the periodontal ligament indicating it is a specialised adult connective tissue

- The principal collagen fibres have a characteristic orientation.
- The types (and amounts) of collagen (types I and III) and the variety of collagen cross-links are unlike those found within most other adult fibrous connective tissues.
- In some species, a pre-elastin-like fibre (oxytalan) is present within the periodontal ligament.
- The rate of turnover of the periodontal ligament is very rapid.
- The periodontal ligament is remarkably cellular and rich in ground substance.
- The type of proteoglycan in the periodontal ligament may be specific to this tissue.
- The tissue hydrostatic pressure is high.
- The periodontal ligament fibroblasts have features unusual for fibroblasts in adult fibrous connective tissues (e.g., many intercellular contacts, cilia).
- The periodontal ligament has cells concerned with the formation of dental tissues.
- The periodontal ligament has a rich vascular and nerve supply.
- The capillaries within the periodontal ligament are fenestrated.

Box 12.4 Features common to both the periodontal ligament and other fetal-like connective tissues

- High rates of turnover
- Sharp, unimodal size/frequency distributions of small collagen fibrils
- Significant amounts of type III collagen
- The major reducible collagen cross-link is dehydrodihydroxy lisinonorleucine
- Changes in collagen fibrils with lathyrogens
- Large volumes of ground substance
- High content of glucuronate-rich proteoglycans
- High content of the glycoproteins tenascin and fibronectin
- Presence of pre-elastin fibres (oxytalan in the periodontal ligament)
- High cellularity, with the fibroblast-like cells possessing numerous intercellular contacts
- Similar biomechanical properties

Table 12.2 Relationship between the ultrastructural features of the periodontal ligament and mechanical properties

Features of the periodontal ligament suggesting tension	Features of the periodontal ligament suggesting compression
Sharpey's fibre structure (Fig. 12.20)	Small collagen fibril diameters (Fig. 12.7)
The flattened disc shape of the fibroblasts	Unimodal collagen size/frequency distribution (Fig. 12.8)
Dermatan sulphate-rich composition of ground substance (page 235)	Distribution of Sharpey's fibres to socket (Fig. 12.21)
	Smooth surface of fibroblast membrane
	Large amounts of ground substance (page 234)

such comparisons showed that the periodontal ligament had some characteristics of a tissue under tension and others suggestive of compression (see Table 12.2). More recently, it has been shown that the periodontal ligament resembles immature, fetal-like connective tissues. The periodontal ligament and fetal connective tissues (mesenchyme) have many common features that are indicated in Box 12.4.

Dental stem cells, with fetal-like features that are multipotent, can be easily harvested from the periodontal ligaments of teeth that have either been naturally lost or surgically removed. These cells are highly proliferative and have a lineage from neural crest cells. The stem cells are similar to those that have been isolated from the dental pulp, from the dental follicle and from the apices of developing teeth roots. All of them have mesenchymal stem cell properties and express, both *in vitro* and in vivo, marker genes associated with chondrocytes and osteoblasts. Periodontal ligament stem cells can differentiate into these cells and also into cementoblasts and adipocytes. In addition, the periodontal ligament stem cells express the transcription factor scleraxis that is associated with tendon cells. It seems that periodontal ligament stem cells are better able to form periodontal connective tissues than other stem cells that are found in or around the tooth. In culture, the periodontal stem cells rapidly attach and express nestin and notch-1 (known stem cell markers). Unusually, the proportion of stem cells increases with passage. The periodontal ligament stem cells also express the mesenchymal stem cell markers STRO-1 and CD146/MUC18.

The functional significance of the periodontal ligament being fetal-like relates to the fact that the structural, ultrastructural and biochemical features of the tissue do not depend primarily upon mechanical demands. Indeed, the high rates of turnover may have a greater role in determining the characteristics of the periodontal ligament.

The fetal-like characteristics of the periodontal ligament also may aid our understanding of inflammatory periodontal disease. First, it is well known that the processes involved in wound healing in fetal connective tissues differ markedly from those in adult tissues; consequently, our understanding of repair/periodontal reattachment may benefit from an appreciation of the mode of repair of fetal wounds. Second, it has been proposed that periodontal defects produced by inflammatory periodontal disease may be corrected by tissue engineering procedures. Thus, stem cells cultured to produce viable cell sheets have been grafted into animals with periodontal defects and have generated periodontal ligament fibres and acellular cementum. To regenerate a true periodontal ligament, however, major obstacles would need to be overcome. Suitable stem cells must be seeded into a suitable matrix, with the intention of producing cementoblasts, osteoblasts and fibroblasts in the right places, with growth factors added to encourage the development and migration of the various cell types. A further aim would be to encourage vessels and nerves to develop into the engineered product and to avoid any ankylosis of the tooth to alveolar bone. The regenerated periodontal ligament would then need to function correctly in terms of tooth support and eruption, turnover and mechanoreception. Further consideration of this topic in terms of guided tissue regeneration is considered in Chapter 28.

In addition to the stem cells of the periodontal ligament having clinical benefits directly related to dentistry, there is interest in them being of potential use in the treatment of more general medical conditions. Research is therefore ongoing to see how useful they might be for the future of regenerative medicine.

Tooth support mechanism

The tooth support mechanism describes the manner whereby the periodontal ligament resists the axially directed intrusive loads that occur during biting.

The suspensory ligament hypothesis

It is still frequently stated that the periodontal ligament behaves as a 'suspensory ligament' during masticatory loading. Accordingly, loads on the tissue are dissipated to the alveolar bone primarily through the oblique principal fibres of the ligament, which, being placed in tension, are analogous to the guy ropes of a tent. On release of the load, there is elastic recoil of the tissue, which enables the tooth to recover its resting position. The essentially elastic responses of the periodontal ligament during both loading and recovery imply that the tissue obeys Hooke's law. However, tooth mobility studies, surgical studies and morphological and biochemical studies have provided evidence against the notion that the periodontal ligament is a suspensory ligament.

Physiological tooth studies

These studies provide information concerning the basic biomechanical properties of the periodontal ligament. They rely upon analysis of the patterns of mobility when loading teeth whose periodontal tissues have not been altered experimentally. These studies show that the ligament does not obey Hooke's law during loading and recovery (Fig. 12.70) and show the property of hysteresis and exhibit responses whose time dependency suggests that the tissue has viscoelastic properties (Fig. 12.71). Furthermore, the patterns of loading are not dependent on the direction of the load relative to the orientation of the principal fibres in the periodontal ligament, and, for loads of similar magnitude, the amount of displacement for an axially directed intrusive load is greater than for an extrusive load.

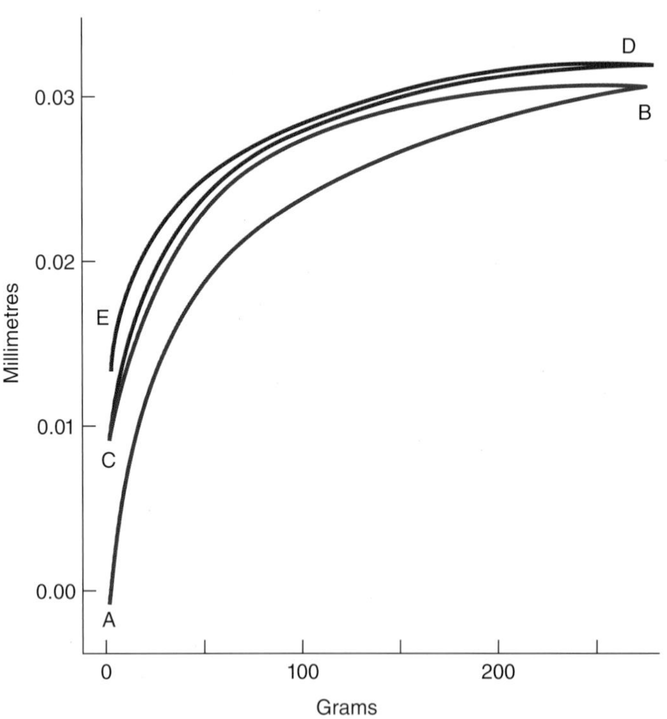

Fig. 12.70 Axial load/mobility curve for a human maxillary incisor to show hysteresis. A = initial position of tooth; B = position at peak force on the first application of load; C = return point on removal of load; D = position at peak force on second application; E = return point after second removal of load. Note the lack of straight-line relationship between load and displacement (expected for elastic responses) and also that successive loads and recovery cycles pass along different paths (i.e., there are hysteresis loops). From Parfitt, G.J., 1960. Measurement of the physiological mobility of individual teeth in an axial direction. Journal of Dental Research 39, 608–618.

Experimental tooth mobility: tension versus compression

These studies rely upon investigating the effects on the patterns of mobility obtained following alterations to a specific component of the periodontal ligament. Experiments with lathyrogens (drugs that specifically inhibit the formation of collagen cross-links and disrupt the fibrous network of the periodontal ligament; Fig. 12.72), with vasoactive drugs and following surgical disruption of the periodontal ligament indicate that both the periodontal collagen fibres and the periodontal vasculature are involved in tooth support.

In experiments where the apical half of the periodontal ligament is removed and the tooth was loaded to assess the effects on its mobility, no effects are observed; consequently it can be argued that the ligament does not behave as a compressive structure because it is presumed that only the tissue around the root apex can behave in this manner. However,

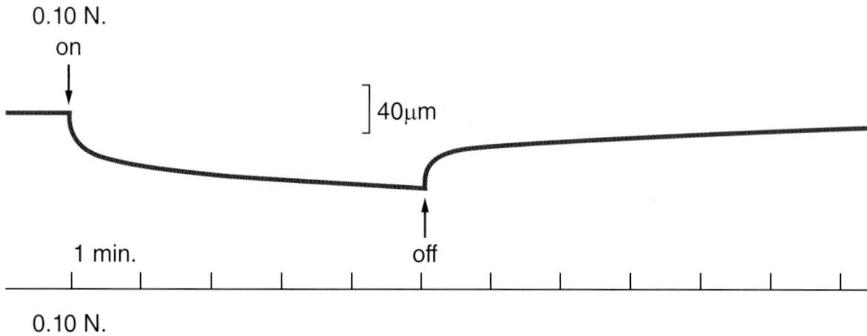

Fig. 12.71 The viscoelastic responses of a tooth observed with an axially directed intrusive load. This is a pen recorder trace of tooth position, which shows the effect of applying a load and then sustaining the load for a period of 5 minutes. Note the time dependency of the response, which is biphasic. The first phase is an elastic phase; the more gradual second phase is indicative of the property of creep (i.e., a viscous phase). The recovery responses are also biphasic and suggestive of viscoelasticity. From Coelho, A.J., Moxham, B.J., 1989. The intrusive mobility of the incisor tooth of the guinea pig. Archives of Oral Biology 34, 383–386.

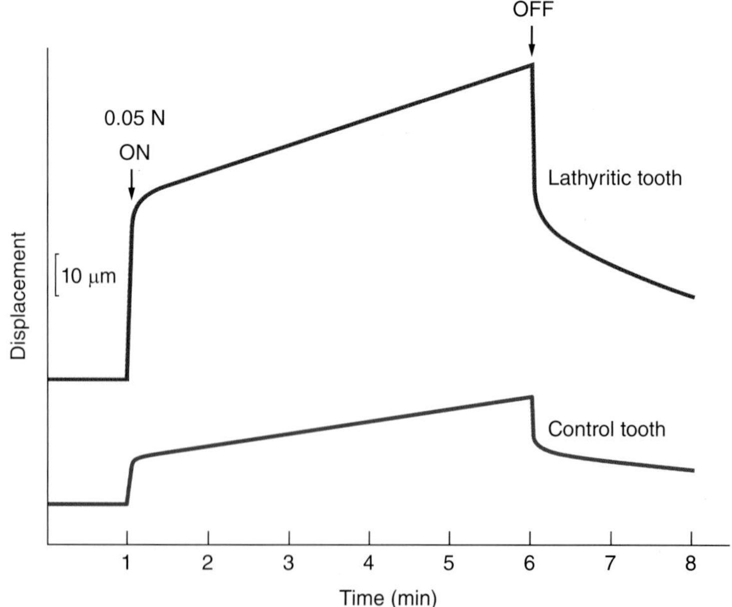

Fig. 12.72 The effects of lathyrogens on tooth support. This experiment assesses the effects of the drug on axially directed extrusive loads. Note the significant increase in mobility for the tooth in the lathyritic animal, which suggests a role for the periodontal collagen in tooth support. However, the precise mechanism of action remains elusive since the patterns of mobility are the same for normal and lathyritic animals. From Moxham, B.J., Berkovitz, B.K.B., 1984. The mobility of the lathyritic rabbit mandibular incisor in response to axially-directed extrusive loads. Archives of Oral Biology 29, 773–778.

subsequent experiments performed to assess the role of tension in the more cervically situated principal fibres of the ligament have shown that the periodontal ligament around the alveolar crest could also be removed without major changes in tooth mobility. These experiments therefore do not provide definitive evidence for or against tension or compression in the periodontal ligament, but do suggest that even where there is marked trauma to a region of the ligament, the remaining tissue can still perform a supporting function in the short term.

Some morphological evidence suggesting that the periodontal collagen is placed in tension during masticatory loading comes from study of the Sharpey's fibre attachments and from the collagen crimps. As mentioned previously (see Table 12.2), the Sharpey's fibres appear as mineralised stubs projecting into the periodontal ligament from the wall of the alveolus. The occurrence of mineralisation at approximately right angles to the long axes of the fibres has been adduced as evidence that the fibres are under tension. However, even if this were the case, the distribution of Sharpey's fibres along the alveolus indicates that they are limited mainly to the region of the alveolar crest (Fig. 12.21). The crimping of collagen in the periodontal ligament was described on page 232. Evidence from connective tissue elsewhere in the body (particularly from tendons) suggests that the crimps are involved in the initial stages of loading, allowing some degree of movement before the tissue is placed under tension.

Morphological and biochemical comparisons between the periodontal ligament and other connective tissues known to be under tension or compression have been undertaken to throw some light on the role of the periodontal ligament in tooth support. On the assumption that the structure of a connective tissue is dictated by the mechanical demands placed upon it, Table 12.2 shows the results of such a comparison. Whereas some features of the periodontal ligament suggest a tensional mode of activity, many of the features indicate a compressive mode. Indeed, experiments involving relatively long-term changes in the mechanical demands placed upon the tissue (e.g., pinning a tooth to completely prevent tooth movements) produce no major changes in the structure of the periodontal ligament and provide evidence for the view that the ligament is not as affected by the mechanical demands placed upon it as tissues elsewhere in the body.

Biochemical analysis of the proteoglycans within the periodontal ligament and under different loading regimens shows that the degree of aggregation/disaggregation of the ground substance may have a role in tooth support (Fig. 12.73). Where teeth are unloaded for a period of 3 hours, a high-molecular-weight fraction within the periodontal ligament is greatly increased. On the other hand, with loads between 0.25 N and 1 N, this fraction is greatly reduced. Loads of 4 N are associated with a further decrease, followed by an increase during a 3-hour undisturbed recovery phase.

There is thus evidence that the collagen fibres, vasculature and ground substance of the periodontal ligament are all involved in tooth support. Consequently, the mechanism of tooth support should not be regarded as a property of a single component of the periodontal ligament, but as a function of the tissue as a whole.

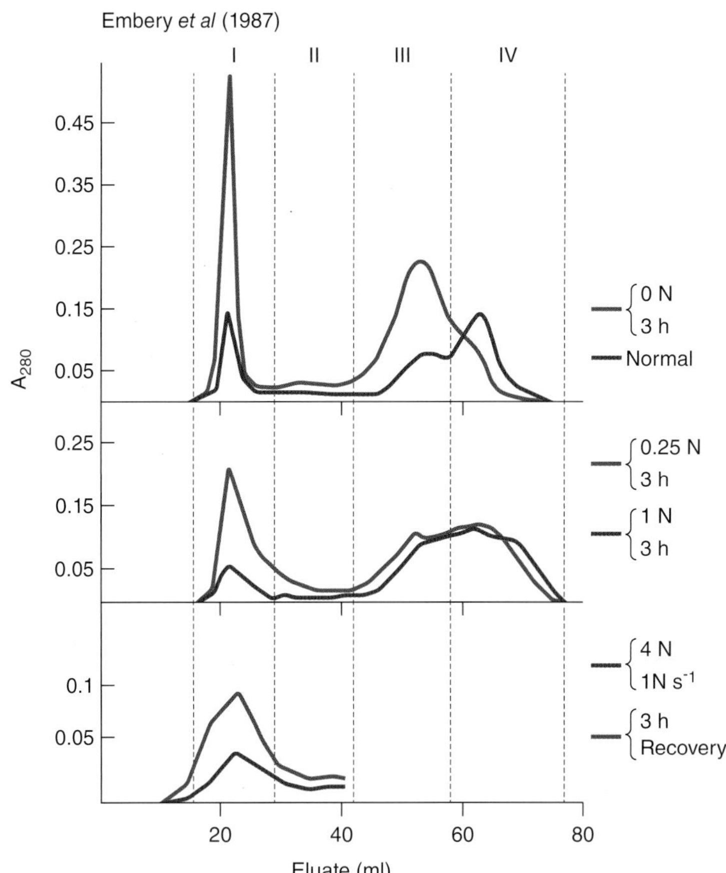

Fig. 12.73 Molecular size profiles of periodontal ligament proteoglycans following various degrees of intrusive loadings of macaque monkey teeth. Eluate resolved into four fractions (I–IV). (Top) High-molecular-weight fraction (peak I) increased when the periodontal ligament is undisturbed for 3 hours. (Middle) Decrease in peak I size between 0.25 N and 1 N loads. (Bottom) Further decrease in peak I size with 4 N loads followed by an increase during a 3-hour undisturbed recovery phase. From Embery, G., Picton, D.C., Stanbury, J.B., 1987. Biochemical changes in periodontal ligament ground substance associated with short-term intrusive loading in adult monkeys (*Macaca fascicularis*). Archives of Oral Biology 32, 545–549.

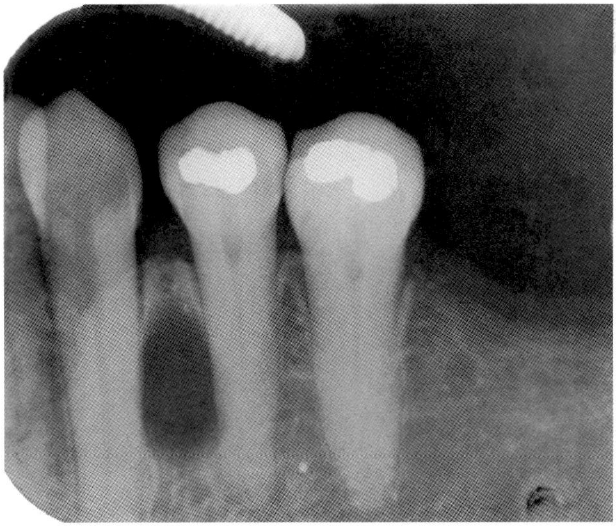

Fig. 12.74 Radiograph illustrating a lateral periodontal cyst located between the roots of a left mandibular canine and first premolar. Courtesy Dr. J Tankersley.

Clinical considerations

Lateral periodontal cysts

These cysts are seen in the mid-portion of the periodontal ligament of vital teeth. The teeth affected are usually the mandibular canine and premolar teeth (Fig. 12.74). Presumably arising from epithelial rests, they are lined by squamous or cuboidal epithelium.

Chronic inflammatory periodontal disease and regeneration

The most important clinical condition affecting the periodontal ligament is chronic inflammatory periodontal disease, when toxic products released by dental plaque (and the host's defence mechanisms) result in the destruction and loss of periodontal ligament tissue and adjacent alveolar bone (Figs. 12.75-12.77). The intensity and duration of inflammation in the periodontal tissues depend on a complex regulatory network involving neuropeptides, other inflammatory mediators and immune cells. Such a process often results in the formation of a deeper periodontal pocket, and the vicious circle continues. The loss of attachment tissue will expose the root of the tooth in the mouth, increasing tooth mobility, and the tooth may eventually be lost. When faced with such a condition, the dental surgeon may have two aims in mind: to repair the existing condition so that the disease process progresses no further (usually involving surgical removal of diseased tissue) and to regenerate the lost tissues, restore the bone and periodontal ligament to their original form and reattach new periodontal ligament fibres to the tooth and bone. One common problem after surgery is that the junctional epithelium proliferates rapidly downwards to cover the root surface, which will prevent periodontal ligament fibres from attaching to cementum. The diagnosis of periodontal disease by analysis of gingival crevicular fluid is considered further on pages 305 and 318.

After periodontal surgery (with the removal of diseased tissue and the possible application of various methods of conditioning the root surface, such as root planing or citric acid etching, to make it more likely to reattach periodontal ligament fibres), a blood clot will form. It is obvious that the connective tissue of the wound may be repopulated from stem cells derived from either the gingiva growing down or the periodontal ligament growing up (see also pages 450–454). There is a body of opinion that believes that the best result is achieved when most of the wound is repopulated by stem cells of the existing periodontal ligament (PDLSC). Although the tissues may appear to be similar, they differ in a number of features that may be important to the final outcome. For this reason, a particular surgical technique may be adopted to exclude the gingival tissues from the deeper part of the wound by placing some sort of tissue barrier over the alveolar crest to obtain 'guided-tissue regeneration'.

Bioactive molecules such as growth factors and cytokines may be important during the differentiation of PDLSC into osteoblasts, cementoblasts and fibroblasts and of bone itself. Such bioactive molecules (e.g., BMP) have been placed in suitable carriers within wounds and were claimed to help regenerate the periodontal tissues (bone, cementum and periodontal ligament). Periodontal regeneration is discussed further on pages 450–454 and Chapter 28. Unusually, the multipotent PDLSCs have also been induced to form retinal progenitors with competence for photoreceptor differentiation and may eventually provide a source of stem cells to treat retinal pathologies.

In the process of cementogenesis (see pages 442–449), enamel proteins may have an important role during the early stages. Evidence is accumulating that the application of such proteins to the root surface may be an aid to periodontal regeneration (see page 452).

Orthodontic loading

Important changes take place within the periodontal ligament with orthodontic loading. Should such a load act perpendicularly to the longitudinal axis of the tooth, wide areas of pressure on one side of the root and corresponding areas of tension on the other side are produced. Only if the

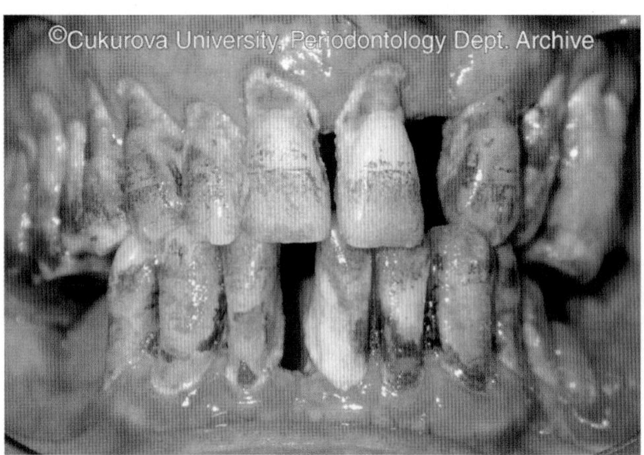

Fig. 12.75 Patient with advanced chronic periodontitis where dental plaque, subgingival calculus and poor oral hygiene have led to much loss of periodontal ligament and alveolar bone. Courtesy Drs. B.N. Lambrecht, H. Cheroutre, B. Kelsall, et al. From Essex, G., Laughter, L., Newman, M.G., et al. (Eds.), 2021. Newman and Carranza's Clinical Periodontology for the Dental Hygienist. Elsevier,Philadelphia).

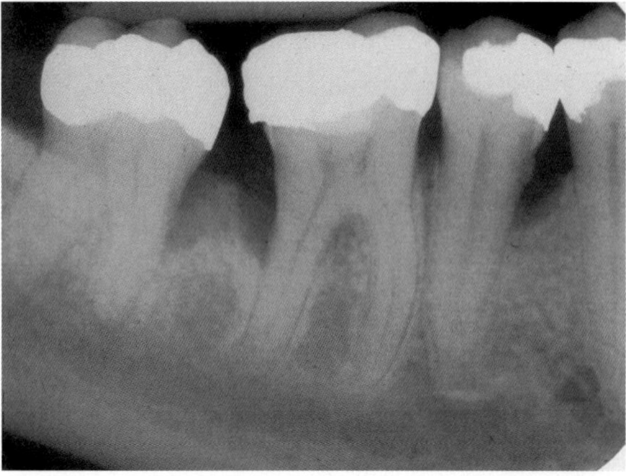

Fig. 12.76 Radiograph showing extensive bone loss around the cheek teeth of a patient with chronic periodontitis. Courtesy of Shirlaw, P.J., Thornhill, M.H., Challacombe, S.J. From Lambrecht, B.N., Cheroutre, H., Kelsall, B., et al. (Eds.), 2015. Mucosal Immunology, fourth ed. Elsevier,Philadelphia.

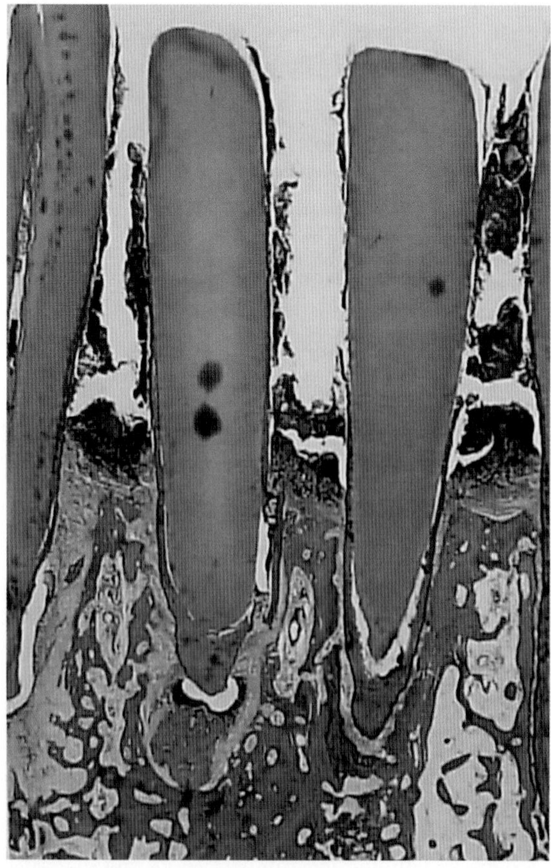

Fig. 12.77 Photomicrograph of mandibular incisor region exhibiting severe periodontitis, demonstrating loss of periodontal ligament and alveolar bone. (H & E stain.) From Odel, E.W. (Ed.), 2017. Cawson's Essentials of Oral Pathology and Medicine, ninth ed. Elsevier,London.

force is placed near the centre of the root (through its centre of resistance) could a translation (or bodily) movement of the tooth be produced, with essentially uniform distribution of pressures on one side of the root and of tension on the other. However, tipping can easily occur as a result of the application of an orthodontic load, with the point of rotation depending on the site of force application, the shape of the tooth and the nature of the periodontal tissues supporting the tooth. The result is that the crown and the root tip in opposite directions, producing pressure and tension zones on either side of the root and a varying distribution of stress such that the load is concentrated in localised areas of the periodontal ligament. In such areas, the fibrous part of the periodontal ligament will differ where the tooth is pressed against the alveolar wall and where it is drawn away from it. As the extracellular matrix binds to integrins, this will also result in strain of the periodontal ligament fibroblasts (PDLFs). In turn, this leads to a process known as *mechanotransduction*, which induces the production of various signalling molecules involved in tissue remodelling required for tooth movement. Leucocytes will be stimulated to produce signalling molecules, including chemokines, cytokines and growth factors, that stimulate PDLFs to further remodel their extracellular matrix. Orthodontic tooth movement induces dynamic changes in density and distribution of periodontal and pulpal nerve fibres, indicating their involvement in both early stages of periodontal remodelling and later in the regenerative processes of the periodontal ligament, generally occurring in concerted action with modulation of blood vessels.

Neuropeptides (e.g., CGRP and Substance P) may modulate bone remodelling during orthodontic tooth movement by their effects on RANKL and OPG 9 (see pages 272–275). Significant changes can also be detected in the distribution of growth factors (such as FGF and vascular endothelial growth factor [VEGF]) in the periodontal ligament during orthodontic movement.

Tension side

On the side under tension, the periodontal space will become wider where the tooth is drawn away from the alveolar bone following the application of a continuous orthodontic load. Bundles of fibres are stretched, and the alveolar crest is pulled in the same direction. There is an increase in connective tissue cell number, particularly near the socket wall. The periodontal fibroblasts appear spindle-shaped, although the cells near the alveolar wall are more spherical. The blood vessels also appear to be distended. Osteoid tissue is deposited on the socket wall and, where the fibrous bundles are thick, new bone is deposited along them. If the bundles are thin, a more uniform layer is deposited along the root surface. Calcification in the deeper layers of the osteoid starts shortly afterwards, while the superficial part remains uncalcified. New Sharpey's fibres are secreted simultaneously with new bone deposition. As the fibroblasts migrate with the bone, they may deposit either entirely new Sharpey's fibres or new fibrils, which are incorporated into existing fibres. While part of the newly synthesised collagen will be incorporated into the new osteoid, some will be incorporated into the periodontal ligament, perhaps associated with the increase in width on the tension side. Lengthening of fibres also seems to occur by incorporation of new fibrils into existing fibres (even at some distance from the alveolar bone wall).

Pressure side

On the side under pressure, the periodontal space becomes narrower and the crest of the alveolar bone is slightly deformed. Resorption of the alveolar bone surface occurs on the side towards which the tooth is moving by means of osteoclasts. Vascular activity is low, and few leukocytes and macrophages are seen. Changes on the pressure side can be categorised broadly into 'direct resorption', where the pressure is relatively light, and 'hyalinisation', where the pressure is large enough to produce degenerative changes. With 'direct resorption', osteoclastic activity is evident; with 'hyalinisation', osteoclasts are absent: there is oedema and obliteration of the blood vessels within the periodontal ligament. Degenerative changes in the fibroblasts are also seen. The term 'hyalinisation' comes from the 'glassy' appearance of the periodontal ligament in routine histological specimens. The necrotic hyalinised tissue is primarily removed by macrophages. In addition, multinucleated, tartrate-resistant acid phosphatase (TRAP)-positive cells lacking a ruffled border also appear to be involved in removing the necrotic tissue. When these multinucleated cells reach the cementum surface, they may continue their resorbing activity and initiate some root resorption.

An unwanted side effect of orthodontic treatment is resorption occurring at the root apex, with resultant loss in tooth length. This particularly affects permanent maxillary central incisors. In severe cases, there may be a 20% loss of root length (see Fig. 13.50). The factors that predispose teeth to root resorption are unknown, there being considerable individual variation. However, root resorption appears to be correlated with the size of the force and/or the total treatment time. Root morphology may be involved, as teeth with blunted roots can show more resorption. The development of new dental materials and designs for orthodontic wire (e.g., superelastic nickel–titanium) and brackets that have shape memory and are able to provide a constant force over the period of treatment (bioefficient therapy) should help reduce the amount of root resorption.

Further readings for this chapter can be found in the accompanying eBook. Explore online Self-assessment quiz to test and reinforce your understanding of the material in your free ebook. Follow instructions in the Inside Front Cover to unlock your access.

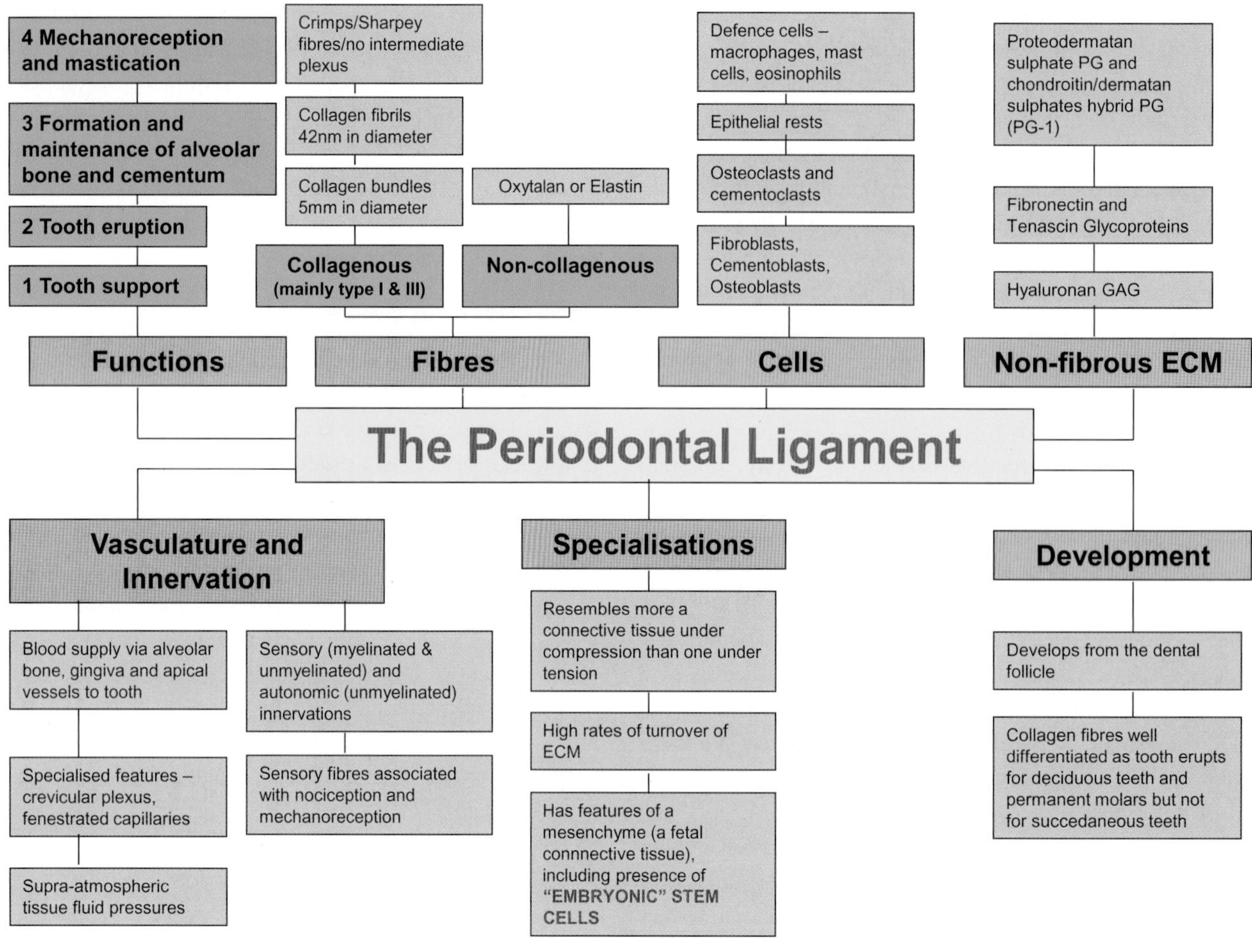

Mind Map 12.1 The periodontal ligament.

Sharpey fibre attachments dissipate loads into the alveolar bone; Hooke's law obeyed, suggesting PDL is an elastic tissue; Fibres placed under tension on loading

Being a function of the oblique principal fibres

The Periodontal Ligament as a "Suspensory Ligament"

Classical View

Tooth Support Mechanism

Experimental evidence against Classical View

Tooth Mobility Studies

Physiological studies to assess biophysical properties of PDL

Non-Hooke's Law (visco-elastic properties) with hysteresis

Experimental studies to assess biological aspects

Lathyrogens suggest role for principal fibres of PDL, not under tension but compression

Tooth support influenced by PDL vasculature

Morphological Studies

Although the "stub-like" appearance of the Sharpey fibres indicate they are placed under tension, there are few such fibres except at alveolar crest

Biochemical Studies

Changes in high molecular weight PDL ECM components with variety of loads

There is disaggregation of ECM PGs on loading and aggregation on recovery (and without

Summary

Much evidence to show that the classical view is simplistic and that the tooth support mechanism involves compression as well as tension of the PDL

All components of the PDL function in tooth support (multifactorial) – should take an "holistic" view.

Mind Map 12.2 Tooth support mechanism.

13 Alveolar bone

Introduction

The part of the maxilla or mandible that supports and protects the teeth is known as *alveolar bone*. An arbitrary boundary at the level of the root apices of the teeth separates the alveolar processes from the body of the mandible (Fig. 13.1) or the maxilla. To understand alveolar bone, it is necessary to appreciate bone biology in general. Like bone in other sites, alveolar bone functions as a mineralised supporting tissue, giving attachment to muscles, providing a framework for bone marrow and acting as a reservoir for ions (especially calcium). Apart from its obvious strength, one of the most important biological properties of bone is its 'plasticity', allowing it to model/remodel according to the functional demands placed upon it. In modelling, bone is formed at a different site from where resorption is occurring, leading to a change in the shape and/or size of a bone (as in growth). For remodelling (internal turnover), bone formation occurs at the same site following resorption, and there is no change in the overall shape of the bone (Fig. 13.2).

Bone depends on function (i.e., mechanical stimuli) to maintain its structure and mass, although the period of loading needs only be short to trigger an adaptive response. Such loading needs to be intermittent rather than static. Too little function may cause it to atrophy (including bone loss during space flight): increased stimuli, especially high-impact activities such as tennis, may cause it to thicken; excessive stimuli may cause it to fracture. Alveolar bone is dependent on the presence of teeth for its development and maintenance. Where teeth are congenitally absent (as in hypodontia/anodontia) or where a tooth is extracted, alveolar bone is poorly developed.

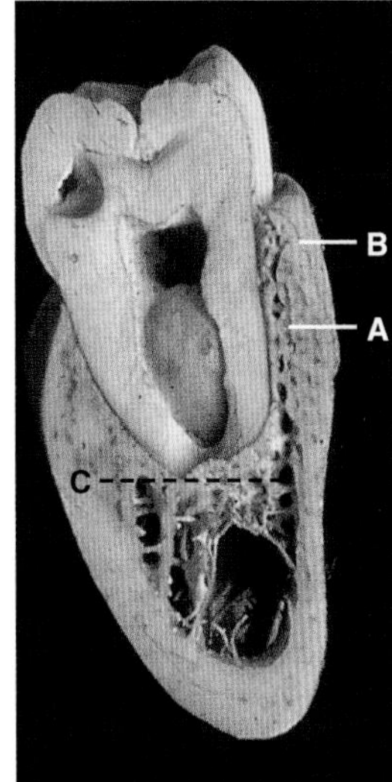

Fig. 13.1 Ground longitudinal section through the mandible showing the alveolar bone. A = inner layer of compact alveolar bone lining the tooth socket wall; B = outer layer of compact bone (note the cancellous bone lying between the two plates of alveolar bone); C = arbitrary boundary between the alveolar bone and the body of the jaw. Copyright the Royal College of Surgeons of England.

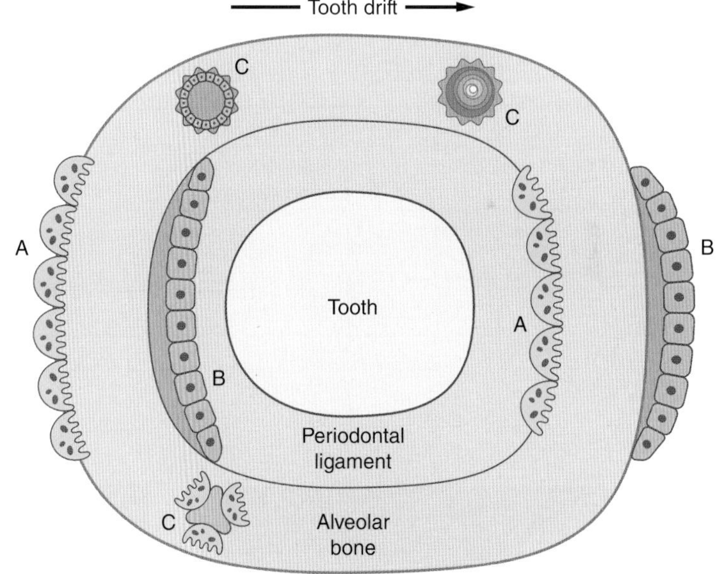

Fig. 13.2 Modelling of alveolar bone during physiological tooth drift in which resorption (A) and deposition (B) of bone take place at different sites, resulting in a change in bone morphology. Compare this with remodelling of bone (C), where resorption and deposition occur at the same site without any resulting change in bone morphology.

Classification of bone

Bone may be classified in several ways. Developmentally, there is endochondral bone (where bone is preceded by a cartilaginous model that is eventually replaced by bone in a process termed *endochondral ossification*) and intramembranous bone (where bone forms directly within a vascular "connective tissue). Although this vascular connective tissue is inappropriately termed a `membrane', the term *intramembraneous ossification* is employed. Histologically, and according to its density, mature bone may be categorised as compact (cortical) or cancellous according to its density. As the names suggest, compact bone forms a dense, solid mass, while if cancellous bone there is a lattice arrangement of the individual bony trabeculae that surrounds soft tissue.

Internally, a thin layer of compact bone lines the tooth socket and gives attachment to the principal fibres of the periodontal ligament. Externally, on the buccal/labial and lingual/palatal surfaces, are thicker layers of compact bone, forming the external and internal alveolar plates. Between these plates of compact bone are variable amounts of cancellous bone, depending on the site (Fig. 13.1; see also pages 12–13). This combination of compact and cancellous bone aims for maximum strength at minimum weight. In newly formed bone, its collagen fibres have a more variable diameter and lack a preferential orientation, giving the bone a matted (basket-weave) appearance when viewed in polarised light. This immature bone, termed *woven bone*, has larger and more numerous osteocytes that comprise about 30% of the volume of the tissue (compared with about 2% for adult bone). It is formed more rapidly and has a higher turnover rate. Woven bone is also seen initially at sites of fracture repair or in healing tooth sockets. It mineralises faster than adult bone, without an initial lag phase. Woven bone is subsequently replaced by fine-fibred adult lamellar bone.

One of the most important properties of bone concerns its ability to continuously remodel and adapt to changing functional situations. This relates to the different types of bone cell: one type having the property to form bone (osteoblasts), another type the ability to detect the mechanical stresses and strains to which the bone is subjected (osteoblasts and osteocytes) and a third type having the capacity to resorb bone (osteoclasts). Although bone under mechanical load will remodel, cementum is less readily resorbed than bone under similar loads. Although the reasons for this difference are unclear, it is a fundamental principle on which the basis of orthodontic tooth movement relies.

Table 13.1 compares immature (woven) and adult (lamellar) bone.

Gross morphology of bone

The alveolar, tooth-bearing portion of the jaws is composed of outer and inner alveolar plates. The individual sockets are separated by plates of bone, termed the *interdental septa*, while the roots of multirooted teeth are divided by *interradicular septa* (Fig. 13.3). The compact layer of bone lining the tooth socket has been given various names. It has been referred to as the *cribriform plate*, reflecting the sieve-like appearance produced by the numerous vascular canals (Volkmann's canals) passing from the alveolar bone into the periodontal ligament (Figs. 13.4, 13.5). It has also been called *bundle bone* because numerous bundles of Sharpey's fibres pass into it from the periodontal ligament. In clinical radiographs, the bone lining the alveolus commonly appears as a dense white line and is given the name *lamina dura* (see page 56). The radio-opaque appearance might give the false impression that it is denser than adjacent bone.

Table 13.1 Comparison of woven and adult (lamellar) bone

Woven bone (immature fracture repair)	Lamellar bone (mature adult)
Osteocytes larger and irregularly spaced	Osteocytes smaller, flattened and regularly spaced
Randomly oriented collagen fibres	Collagen fibres arranged in regular plywood orientation
Enriched in acid phosphoproteins and Bone sialoprotein	Enriched in osteocalcin
Rapid matrix mineralisation	Delayed matrix mineralisation (a few days)
Forms rapidly	Forms slowly
Rapid turnover	Slow turnover

However, the radiographic appearance derives from the X-ray beam passing tangentially through the socket wall and relates to the quantity of bone the beam passes through and not to any greater degree of mineralisation than adjacent bone. Superimposition also obscures the Volkmann's canals. The cribriform plate varies in thickness from 0.1 mm to 0.5 mm. The external alveolar plate is usually about 1.5 mm to 3 mm thick over posterior teeth but is highly variable around anterior teeth (depending on tooth position and inclination). The gross morphology and radiographic appearance of the alveolus and tooth sockets are described on pages 12, 13 and 56.

Chemical properties of bone

Some generalised features of bone are listed in Box 13.1.

Bone is a mineralised connective tissue. About 60% of its wet weight is inorganic material, about 25% organic material and about 15% water. By volume, about 36% is inorganic, 36% is organic and 28% is water. However, the composition can vary depending on site and age. For example, mineral comprises 98% dry weight of the stapes. The mineral phase provides the hardness and rigidity of bone and consists of hydroxyapatite with some carbonate. As with the other mineralised tissues, many trace elements are also present. The mineral is in the form of needle-like crystallites or thin plates about 50 nm wide, up to 8 nm thick and of variable length. The crystallites are distributed both within the spaces between and on the surfaces of the collagen fibrils. Although contributing little to the weight of bone, the cells, through their capacity for osteosynthesis and resorption, have a pivotal role in the maintenance of the matrix.

Organic matrix

The organic matrix of bone is about 90% collagen. Most of this can be regarded as intrinsic collagen secreted by osteoblasts. However, collagen inserted as Sharpey's fibres can be considered extrinsic collagen formed by adjacent fibroblasts. The dominant collagen in bone is type I, although small amounts of other types (e.g., type III and type V) may be present, particularly in immature or healing bone. The collagen contributes towards the important biomechanical properties of the tissue in terms of resisting loads and providing the necessary resilience that prevents fractures. It

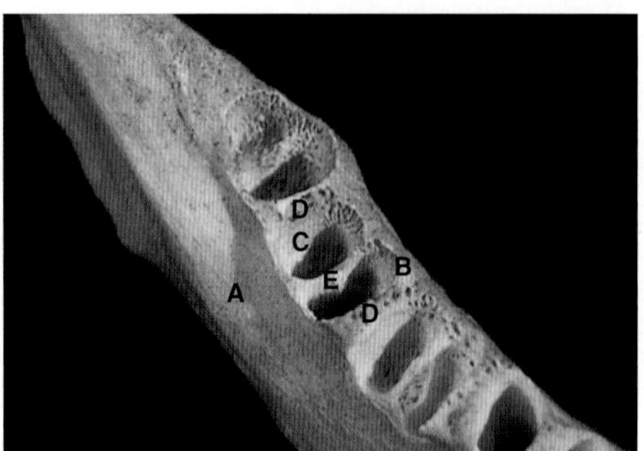

Fig. 13.3 Mandible with teeth removed to demonstrate the components of alveolar bone. A = outer alveolar plate; B = inner alveolar plate; C = cribriform plate lining the socket wall; D = interdental septum; E = interradicular septum.

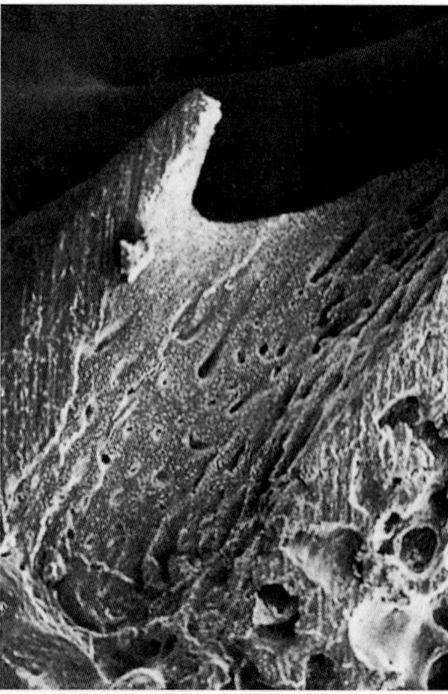

Fig. 13.4 A tooth socket showing the cribriform nature of the cribriform plate (SEM; ×5). Courtesy Prof. P Sloan.

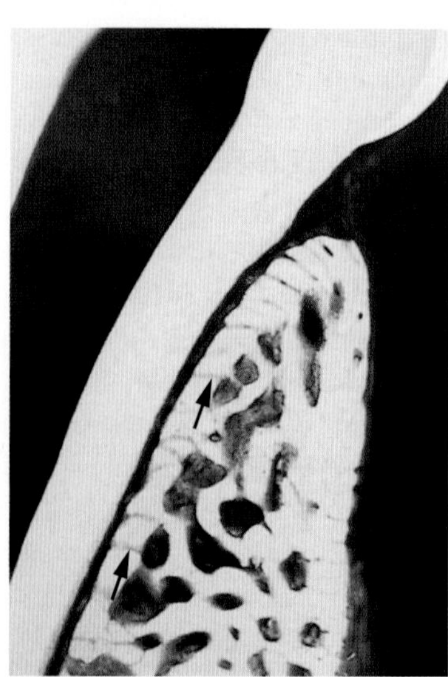

Fig. 13.5 Microradiograph of vascular canals in the cribriform plate (arrowed). Note the cancellous bone lying in the central part of the alveolar bone (×7).

> **Box 13.1 Basic features of bone**
>
> - Matrix of bone is a composite material of inorganic mineral and an organic matrix.
> - Inorganic component is hydroxyapatite – $Ca_{10}(PO_4)_6(OH)_2$. The tiny crystals that impregnate and surround collagen fibres provide rigidity and resistance to compression.
> - Organic component is ~90% type I collagen that provides strength and flexibility.
> - Remaining 10% of organic component is complex mixture of proteins, including growth factors, osteocalcin, osteonectin, osteopontin and glycoproteins. These proteins are all produced by osteoblasts, along with type I collagen.
> - Unmineralised matrix of bone is termed 'osteoid'.
> - Mineralisation of osteoid is dependent on the hormonally active form of vitamin D (1,25-dihydroxyvitamin D).

supports crystal mineralisation and binds other macromolecules. Mutation in the genes encoding the constituent peptides of the collagen type I triple helix are clinically important and may give rise to the inherited condition of osteogenesis imperfecta, where the assembly and structure of type I collagen molecules are disrupted, resulting in much reduced bone strength and spontaneous fracture.

Non-collagenous proteins

The non-collagenous proteins are a heterogeneous group of hundreds of proteins, most of whose functions are not understood. Collectively, they comprise about 5% of the total organic content of bone matrix. Most are endogenous proteins produced by the bone cells, while some, like albumin and immunoglobulins, are derived from other sources (such as the blood) and become incorporated into the bone matrix during bone formation. The main non-collagenous proteins comprise the proteoglycans (e.g., decorin, biglycan and versican), the glycoproteins (e.g., osteonectin, osteopontin, bone sialoprotein, thrombospondin and fibronectin), bone Gla-containing proteins (osteocalcin) and serum proteins (e.g., albumin). The biological function of individual glycoproteins awaits clarification. Some are presumably involved in the initial, formative aspects of bone, while others may play a role following their release during bone resorption. As the proteoglycans bind to collagen, they may help regulate collagen fibril diameters and/or play a role in mineralisation. Osteonectin, for example, has the ability to bind calcium and collagen, suggesting a role in mineralisation. The RGD-containing glycoproteins osteopontin, bone sialoprotein and fibronectin contain the specific tripeptide sequence arginine–glycine–aspartic acid (Arg–Gly–Asp). Bone cells have specific cell membrane receptors (e.g., integrins) binding to this sequence, allowing them to adhere to the matrix and, through secondary messengers, to modify their behaviour. If, for example, the tripeptide sequence is not available to the bone cell, this may result in its apoptosis. The bone Gla-containing protein osteocalcin (with the amino acid gamma-carboxyglutamic acid) is a calcium-binding protein synthesised only by osteoblasts and odontoblasts. This specificity means that recognition of osteocalcin in a cell characterises that cell as being of an osteoblastic or odontoblastic lineage.

Several non-collagenous proteins have been grouped together as the small integrin-binding ligand N-linked glycoproteins (SIBLING) family, including osteopontin, bone sialoprotein, dentine matrix protein-1 ((DMP-1), matrix extracellular phosphoglycoprotein and dentine sialophosphoprotein. The group members contain a large fraction of aspartic and glutamic acids and numerous serines that are 90% phosphorylated. They are therefore extremely acidic. They adopt an open and random configuration in solution, providing freedom for interaction with other molecules. Accumulating evidence has implicated the SIBLING proteins in matrix mineralisation of bone and dentine (see page 167). Clinically, they may play a role in cancer progression through malignant transformation, invasion and metastasis.

Some recently characterised molecules found in bone that may be associated with the regulation of local mineralisation are:

1) Dentine matrix acidic phosphoprotein-1 (DMP-1) (via its 57-kDa C-terminal fragment)
2) Phosphate-regulating neutral endopeptidase (PHEX)
3) Matrix extracellular phosphoglycoprotein (MEPE)

It is important to note that all three of these bioactive molecules can regulate the production of fibroblast growth factor 23 (FGF23) (see later).

Other exogenously derived proteins that may circulate in the blood and become locked up in the bone matrix include cytokines (such as interleukins, tumour necrosis factor and colony-stimulating factors) and growth factors (such as transforming growth factors [TGFs], fibroblast growth factors [FGFs], platelet-derived growth factors [PDGFs] and insulin-like growth factors [IGFs]). Such molecules have important biological activity in the life cycle of bone cells. When present within the bone itself, they are inactive but may become mobilised when bone is resorbed by osteoclasts. They may then play a determining role on the pattern of subsequent bone cell activity. Bone morphogenetic proteins (BMPs) are an important component of the bone matrix. They are so-named because, when first discovered, they had the ability to induce stem cells to differentiate into bone. However, they are now known to have much wider properties apart from being important in bone formation. They are important morphogens in general embryogenesis and development and regulate the maintenance of adult tissue homeostasis. They influence cell movement, cell division, cell differentiation and apoptosis. BMPs are part of the TGF-β superfamily, and about 30 have been identified, although their precise functions are not known.

Histology of bone

Osteoid

Any surface where active bone formation is occurring will be covered by a layer of newly deposited, unmineralised bone matrix called *osteoid* (see Fig. 13.9). This layer is analogous to predentine. The molecular ingredients of osteoid are secreted by osteoblasts that form a well-defined layer at its surface. Osteoid has a thickness of approximately 5–10 µm before reaching a level of maturity conducive to mineralisation. However, in certain pathological conditions where there is delayed mineralisation (e.g., osteomalacia) or increased bone formation (e.g., Paget's disease), this thickness may be increased (hyperosteoidosis).

The mineralising front of bone is relatively linear at the light microscope level, unlike that of dentine which reveal a calcospheritic pattern (see Fig. 23.14). In routine light microscopic demineralised sections, osteoid will stain differently from that of the matrix associated with mineralised bone, indicating that biochemical changes take place within the matrix at the

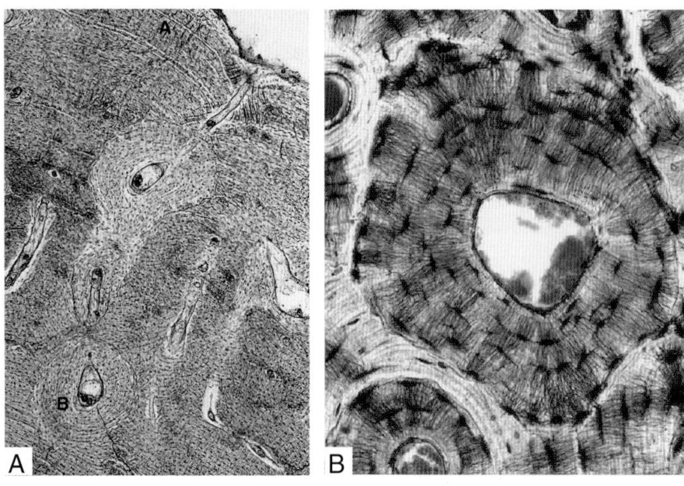

Fig. 13.6 (A) Horizontal ground section of alveolar bone showing circumferential lamellae (A) and Haversian systems (B) where a central vascular canal is surrounded by concentrically arranged bony lamellae (×80). (B) Ground cross-section of Haversian system, showing osteocyte lacunae with numerous interconnecting canaliculi surrounding central Haversian canal. (B) Courtesy Prof. T R Arnett.

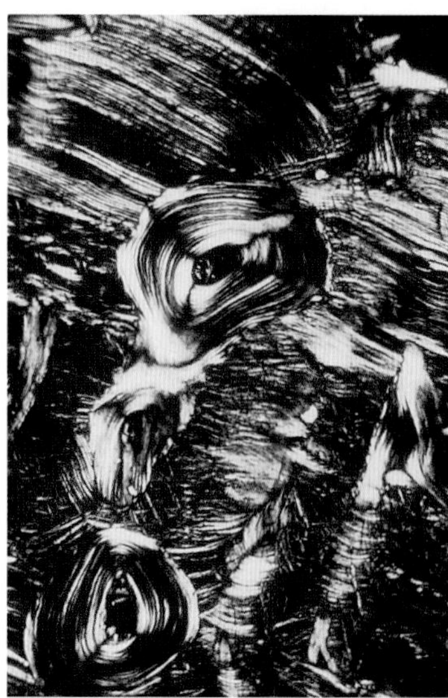

Fig. 13.7 Same section as Fig. 13.6A, viewed in polarised light. The alternating black and white bands indicate the different orientations of collagen in adjacent lamellae. Note the characteristic 'X' superimposed on the Haversian system (×80).

mineralising front to enable mineralisation to occur; some molecules may be added, and others may be degraded.

Osteoid consists of type I collagen fibrils arranged more or less parallel to the bone surface, embedded in a complex ground substance of proteoglycans, glycoproteins and other protein molecules. The biochemical changes occurring at the mineralising front are poorly understood. When alveolar bone is first formed, initial mineralisation may be controlled by osteoblasts from whose cell membrane matrix vesicles are budded off into the osteoid: the first crystals are formed within the matrix vesicles. The cell membrane of these matrix vesicles breaks down, and the first crystals form the seeds around which further mineralisation can occur by epitaxy. A similar process of initial mineralisation via matrix vesicles seems to occur in dentine (see page 426). However, whereas certain molecules involved in the mineralisation process may bypass the predentine by being transported via the odontoblast process directly to the mineralising front, this would not appear to be possible in osteoid. There is a lag phase before the deeper layer of the osteoid has matured sufficiently to undergo mineralisation.

Osteoid is resistant to the resorptive activity of osteoclasts. However, this can be overcome by the release of zinc proteases by osteoblasts.

Bone organisation

Adult bone is deposited in layers, or lamellae, each lamella being 3–5 µm thick. In compact bone the lamellae are arranged in two major patterns. At external (periosteal) and internal (endosteal) surfaces they are arranged in parallel layers completely surrounding the bony surfaces and are known as *circumferential lamellae* (Fig. 13.6A). Deep to the circumferential lamellae, the lamellae are arranged as small, concentric layers around a central neurovascular canal. The central (Haversian) canal (about 50 µm in diameter), together with the concentric lamellae, is known as a *Haversian system* or *osteon* (Fig. 13.6B). There may be up to about 20 concentric lamellae within each Haversian system, the number being limited by the ability of nutrients to diffuse from the central vessel to the cells in the outermost lamella. A cement line of mineralised matrix delineates each Haversian

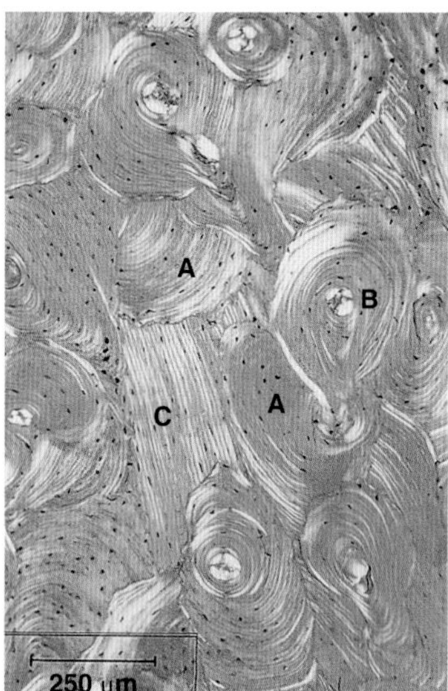

Fig. 13.8 Horizontal ground section of bone showing interstitial lamella (A), Haversian system surrounding a central canal (B) and original circumferential lamella lying deep within the bone following remodelling (C) (×60). Courtesy Prof. M M Smith.

system. The collagen fibrils within each lamella are parallel to one another and spiral along the length of the lamella but have a different orientation to those in the adjacent lamella. This change in orientation can be demonstrated by viewing bone in polarised light (Fig. 13.7). The longitudinally running Haversian canals are connected by a series of horizontal ones (interconnecting canals). As a consequence of remodelling, fragments of previous Haversian systems may be present (the interstitial lamellae) in addition to old circumferential lamellae (Fig. 13.8). This may cause confusion to the uninformed, who may misinterpret relocated Sharpey's fibres (which were originally in the circumferential lamellar bone but are now embedded deep within the bone in isolated islands among osteons) as 'unusual coarse fibres'. This is a common feature in growth with active cortical drift.

In cancellous bone, the lamellae are apposed to each other to form trabeculae up to about 50 µm thick. The trabeculae are not arranged randomly but are aligned along lines of stress so as to best withstand the forces applied to the bone while adding minimally to mass. The trabeculae surround the marrow spaces, from which they derive their nutrition by diffusion. The trabeculae present in alveolar bone appear to be thicker and more robust than in other sites such as vertebrae so that osteons are only occasionally encountered. In young bone, the marrow is red and haemopoietic. It contains stem cells of both the fibroblastic/mesenchymal type (capable of giving rise to fibroblasts, osteoblasts, adipocytes, chondroblasts and myoblasts) and blood cell lineage (capable of giving rise to osteoclasts). In old bone, the marrow is yellow, with loss of haemopoietic potential and increased accumulation of fat cells.

In the body as a whole, about 80% of bone is of the cortical variety while about 20% is cancellous. However, these figures are likely to vary according to site and age. Although it only occupies a small percentage of bone volume, cancellous bone has a far higher turnover rate than cortical bone; cortical bone is said to remodel about 3% of its mass each year, while cancellous bone remodels about 25%. The cortical bone functions mainly in a mechanical/protective role, while the cancellous (trabecular) plays a greater role in mineral metabolism, in addition to its structural function.

Cell types in bone

Several cell types are responsible for the synthesis, maintenance and resorption of bone (Fig. 13.9). They can be regarded as belonging to two main families, one mesenchymal and the other haemopoietic. The osteoblasts, osteocytes and bone-lining cells are derived from a mesenchymal (or ectomesenchymal) stem cell. These stem cells reside in the bone marrow and in a region of proliferating cells adjacent to the osteoblast layer in the periosteum. In the periodontal ligament and other bone-forming tissues, the osteogenic precursors may be associated with small blood vessels. The osteoclasts, however, belong to a different lineage. They form part of the haemopoietic system, being derived from the mononuclear/phagocyte system (including monocytes and macrophages).

Osteoblasts

Osteoblasts are specialised connective tissue cells of mesenchymal origin. A layer of these cells is prominent on bone surfaces where there is active bone formation (Fig. 13.10). Unlike cartilage, which grows interstitially, bone can be deposited (or resorbed) only at surfaces, called *appositional growth*. However, these surfaces are widespread and include the periosteal and endosteal surfaces, the linings of the Haversian canals and the surfaces of bony trabeculae in cancellous bone. Active osteoblasts appear cuboidal and exhibit a basophilic cytoplasm that is related to the conspicuous amounts of endoplasmic reticulum within the cells, reflecting a high level of protein (mainly collagen) synthesis. The cells are polarised, and the prominent, round nucleus tends to lie towards the basal end. Numerous cell contacts are seen between the cell membranes of adjacent cells. Osteoblasts are also in contact with underlying osteocytes.

Osteoblasts contact one another by means of adherens, gap and tight junctions. These are functionally connected to microfilaments and enzymes (such as protein kinases) associated with intracellular secondary messenger systems. This complex arrangement provides for intercellular adhesion and cell-to-cell communication, helping to ensure that the osteoblast layer completely covers the osteoid surface and that the osteoblasts function in a coordinated manner. At the ultrastructural level, active osteoblasts can be seen to contain an extensive rough endoplasmic reticulum (arranged in parallel stacks), a localised and extensive Golgi complex and numerous mitochondria and vesicles (Fig. 13.11, see also Fig. 12.44).

Osteoblasts secrete the organic matrix of bone that is initially represented by an unmineralised layer known as *osteoid*, about 5–10 μm thick (Figs. 13.9, 13.10). Some of the components of osteoid, such as collagen type I, are widely distributed and not unique to osteoblasts. Others are specific to cells of the osteoblast lineage and provide useful markers of the osteoblast phenotype.

Alkaline phosphatase activity, although not entirely specific to bone, is easy to identify and is a reliable indicator of osteoblastic differentiation. Although the precise role of this enzyme in osteoblasts is not known, it

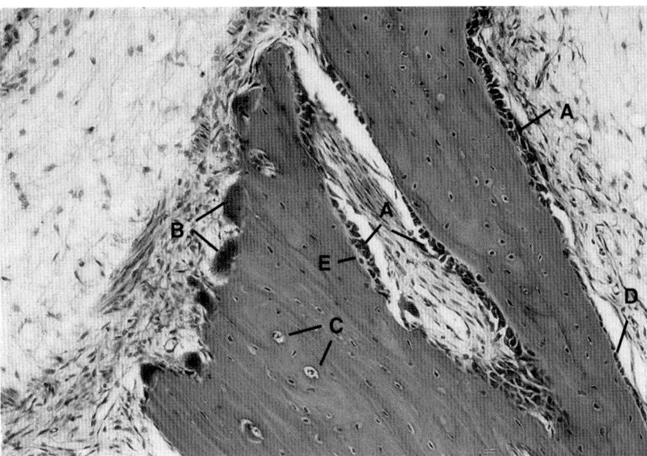

Fig. 13.9 Horizontal section of bone demonstrating a layer of osteoblasts (A) lining a surface where active bone formation is occurring (as indicated by the presence of a pale staining layer of osteoid), some large multinucleated osteoclasts (B) lying against Howship's lacunae in a region of bone undergoing resorption and large numbers of osteocytes (C) lying embedded within the bone matrix itself. D = bone-lining cells; E = pale-staining osteoid layer (decalcified section; H & E; ×80). Courtesy Prof. T R Arnett.

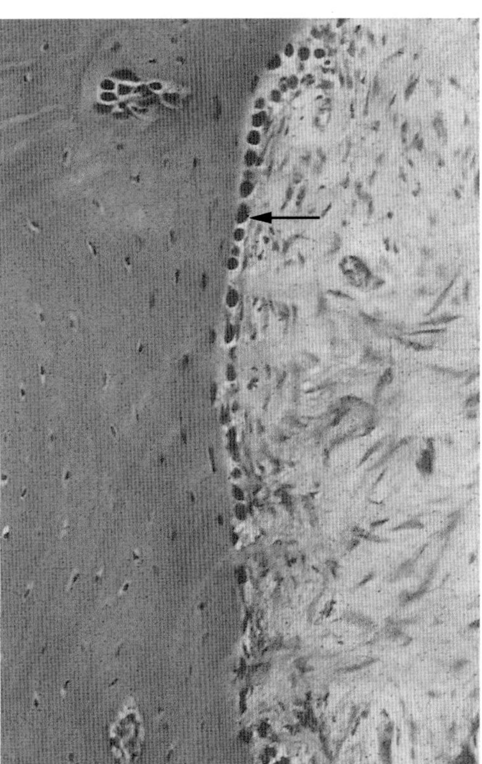

Fig. 13.10 Alveolar bone at the periodontal ligament surface showing a layer of osteoblasts (arrowed). Sharpey's fibres are seen passing into the bone, and there is a pale-staining osteoid layer. Within the bone itself are seen osteocytes, which, in routine demineralised sections, do not exhibit obvious canaliculi (decalcified section; H & E; ×400).

is thought to be involved in the mineralisation of the matrix. Alkaline phosphatase releases inorganic phosphate ions (PO_4^{3-}) from diverse molecules by hydrolysis, thus increasing the local concentration of inorganic phosphate ions. It also hydrolyses pyrophosphate, a key inhibitor of mineralisation in tissues, to generate more inorganic phosphate. The resulting increase in inorganic phosphate promotes mineralisation.

The secreted, intrinsic collagen fibrils lie parallel to the bone surface. At the surface of alveolar bone adjacent to the periodontal ligament, extrinsic Sharpey's fibres pass more or less perpendicularly into the osteoid layer (Fig. 13.10). Osteoblasts have a lifespan of the order of about 1 month. Up to 30% of osteoblasts become embedded in the organic matrix as osteocytes, while the remainder appear to flatten and become known as *lining cells*, or may sometimes undergo apoptosis.

In addition to secreting the formative components of bone, the osteoblast secretes molecules controlling its own activity (i.e., autocrine secretion), such as growth factors, cytokines and prostaglandins. The cell also possesses surface receptors to bind to such molecules. The osteoblast releases molecules that have a controlling influence in activating the bone-resorbing cells, the osteoclasts. This paracrine secretion involves molecules such as macrophage colony-stimulating factor (M-CSF) and receptor activator of nuclear factor kappa B (RANK) and its ligand (RANKL) (see pages 271–275). Osteoblasts also possess receptors for several hormones (e.g., parathyroid hormone, 1,25 dihydroxyvitamin D, sex steroids) that help regulate bone metabolism.

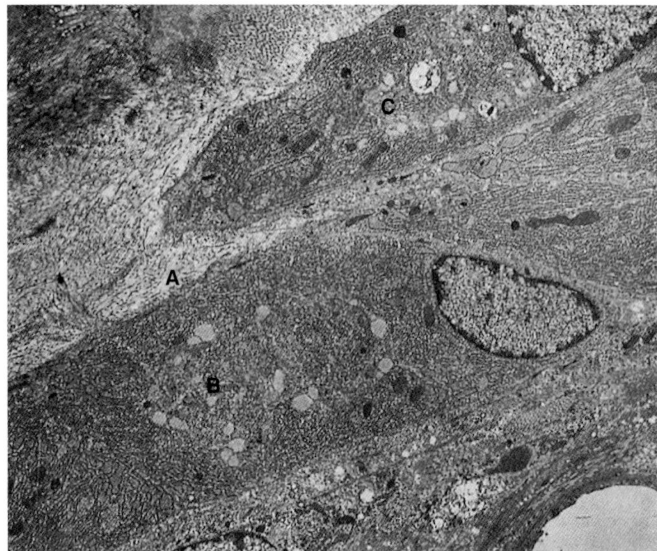

Fig. 13.11 Electron microscopic appearance of an active osteoblast. The cell contains an extensive rough endoplasmic reticulum and a conspicuous and localised Golgi apparatus (B) and is connected to adjacent cells by cell contacts. The cell surface adjacent to the demineralised bone (A) has many fine cytoplasmic processes, some of which contact underlying osteocytes. The flattened cell (C) immediately adjacent to the osteoblasts may be an osteoprogenitor cell (×6,000).

Osteoblasts lying on the surface of the alveolar bone have been seen possessing collagen-containing phagosomes. These intracellular collagen profiles have different appearances depending on various stages of degradation. The presence of acid phosphatase and cathepsin B activity are associated with the phagosomes and suggests that osteoblasts are capable of the phagocytosis and intracellular degradation of collagen.

Osteocytes

Osteocytes are the postmitotic cells lying within the bone itself. They are osteoblasts that have become trapped in the bone matrix. Although its entrapment may look passive, the osteocyte may play a more active role as it becomes entombed, such as releasing enzymes to cleave the surrounding collagen. They are by far the most numerous type of bone cell, comprising over 90% of bone cells compared with less than 5% for osteoblasts and less than 1% for osteoclasts. They also differ from osteoblasts and osteoclasts by being long-lived.

The number of osteocytes in bone may vary according to site and age, but they may number in the tens of thousands per cubic mm. In preparing ground sections of bone, the osteocytes themselves are lost, but the spaces or lacunae they occupy are filled with air or cell debris and appear black in routine transmitted light sections (Fig. 13.12A). The lacunae are regularly distributed in adult bone, and many narrow canals called *canaliculi* radiate from them in all directions. Numerous cell processes from the osteocytes run in the canaliculi in all directions, with more being directed perpendicularly to the bone surface than parallel to it (Fig. 13.12B). The processes of neighbouring osteocytes are linked by cell contacts called *gap junctions* (see later), and those of superficially situated osteocytes are in contact with cells lining the bone surface. In this manner, osteocytes are in constant communication with both osteoblasts and bone-lining cells. The cell processes in the canaliculi allow the diffusion of substances from adjacent blood vessels through the bone. Cell processes do not appear to cross cement lines and therefore are unlikely to allow osteocytes to make contacts with cells in adjacent osteons. Some osteocytes in interstitial lamellae may die and their lacunae may become filled in with mineral. In routine demineralised sections the osteocytes are retained, but the canaliculi are little in evidence. However, the canaliculi can be visualised in demineralised sections if perfused with a stain such as picrothionin (Fig. 13.13). It is possible to isolate and culture osteocytes, which retain their characteristic morphology (Fig. 13.14).

In comparison with cementocytes (see pages 215–216), osteocytes are more regularly distributed and do not show the more preferential orientation of cementocyte canaliculi (towards the periodontal ligament). It is not known what becomes of osteocytes that are released following bone

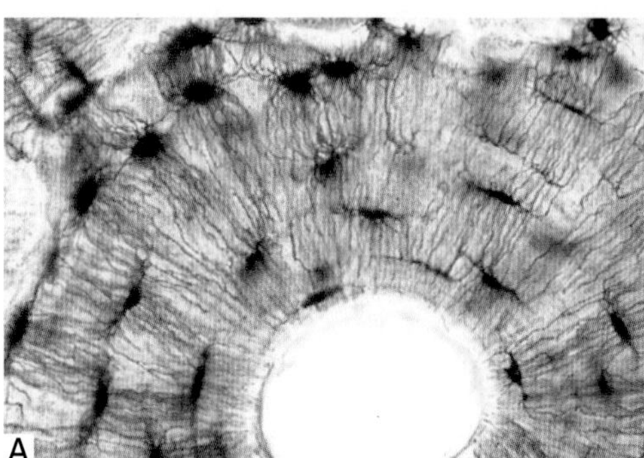

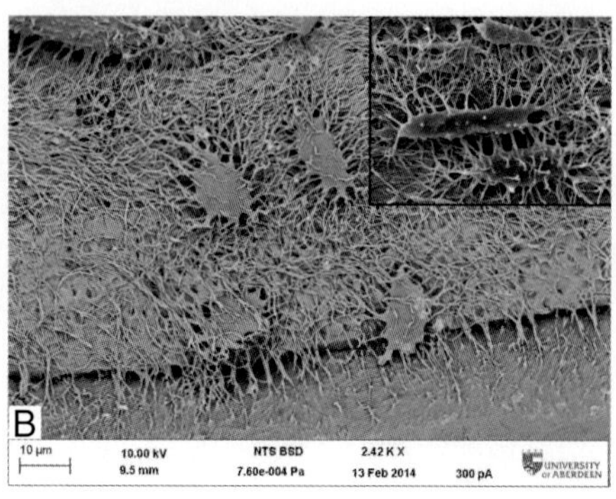

Fig. 13.12 (A) Ground section of part of an Haversian system cut horizontally to show osteocyte lacunae and associated canaliculi. Image width = 0.25 mm. (B) Demineralised bone showing the large number of processes passing out from osteocytes and linking up with similar processes from neighbouring osteocytes. Bone was fixed, dehydrated, embedded in resin, etched with 37% phosphoric acid and washed with bleach. (SEM) Inset: High-power view of osteocytes seen in Fig. 13.12B. (SEM) (A) Courtesy Prof. T R Arnett. (B) Courtesy K Mackenzie.

resorption activity by osteoclasts, but it is likely that most undergo apoptosis and are subsequently phagocytosed.

As they are derived from osteoblasts, it is not surprising that osteocytes share many common markers, such as the presence of osteopontin, osteocalcin, osteonectin, fibronectin, parathyroid hormone and oestrogen receptors, but osteocytes generally do not express alkaline phosphatase. However, osteocytes also express unique markers that have been discovered in recent years that are expressed sequentially as young osteocytes become first embedded in osteoid, during mineralisation and in mature osteocytes. These markers include E11/gp38, MEPE, DMP-1 and sclerostin, to mention but a few.

At the ultrastructural level, the appearance of osteocytes varies according to their position in relation to the surface layer. Osteocytes newly incorporated into bone matrix from the osteoblast layer have a high organelle content similar to osteoblasts. However, as they become more deeply situated with continued bone formation, they appear to be less active. The cells are then seen to have a nucleus and a thin ring of cytoplasm containing few organelles, reflecting the decreased cellular activity (Fig. 13.15). Some secretion is likely to be necessary for osteocyte function if, for example, the cells are involved in the reception and transduction of mechanosensory information.

Numerous slender processes containing bundles of actin filaments extend from the osteocyte into canaliculi in the matrix. The processes of one cell are joined to those of another by gap junctions, which allow cell-to-cell communication and coordination of activity. In this feature, they differ from chondrocytes, which are said to lack processes and are isolated from one another. A pericellular space (which might represent a shrinkage artefact) is usually seen to intervene between the cell membrane and the surrounding bone and contains unmineralised matrix, consisting of proteoglycans and a few collagen fibrils.

Unlike older views that the osteocyte was a relatively inactive cell, maintaining a level of homeostasis of bone, recent research has indicated it is a major controller of bone biology.

1) Osteocytes are inducers of osteoclast activation. In this context, osteocytes produce RANKL on their dendritic processes.

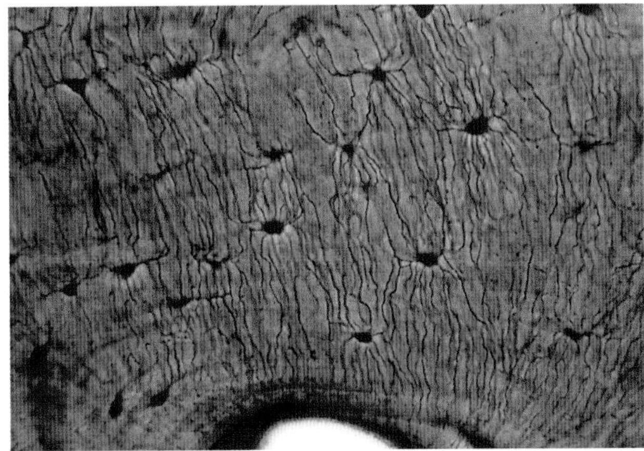

Fig. 13.13 Demineralised section of bone perfused with picrothionin to visualise the osteocyte lacunae and canaliculi (×280). Courtesy Prof. M M Smith.

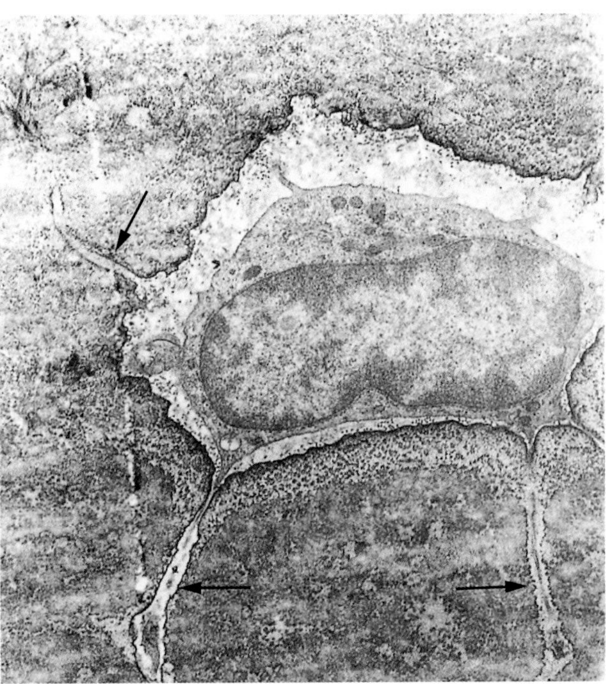

Fig. 13.15 Electron microscopic appearance of demineralised bone showing an osteocyte. The cell has few organelles and possesses cell processes (arrowed) extending into canaliculi. A pericellular space is seen between the cell membrane and the wall of the lacuna and is probably related to a shrinkage artefact (×5,300).

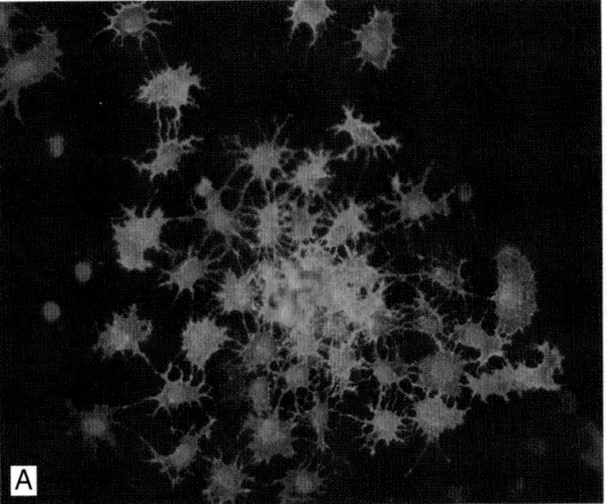

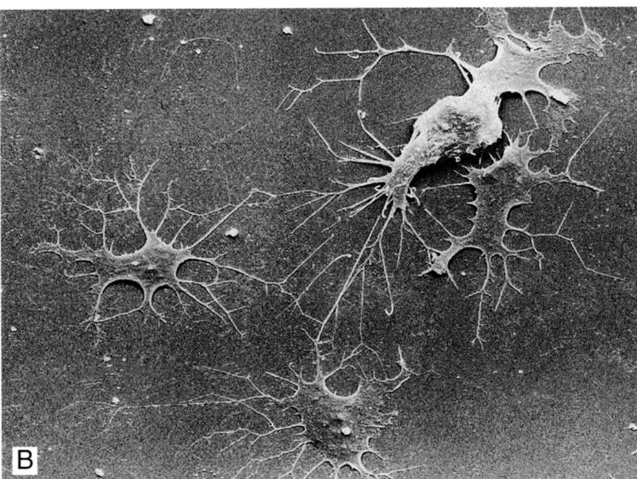

Fig. 13.14 Osteocytes in tissue culture. (A) A group of osteocytes isolated from bone and maintained for 24 hours in tissue culture on glass. The cytoplasm (green fluorescence) has been labelled with an osteocyte-specific monoclonal antibody (OB7.3), while the nuclei have been labelled using a blue fluorescence. A small number of osteoblasts (negative for the green osteocyte-specific antibody but with a blue-staining nucleus) can also be seen (×350). (B) SEM of cultured osteocytes. The cells are characterised by their positive staining with an osteocyte-specific antibody (OB7.3). Like osteocytes *in vivo*, the cells have long, slender, often branched cell processes by which they have contacted those of adjacent cells during culture (×1,000). From Van der Plas, A., Nijweide, P.J., 1992. Isolation and purification of osteocytes. Journal of Bone and Mineral Research 7, 389–396.

2) Osteocyte cell death/apoptosis can stimulate osteoclasis via a Wnt/beta catenin pathway. In this context, osteocytes have receptors for parathyroid hormone.
3) Osteocytes, via secretion of sclerostin (coded by the *SOST* gene), are thought to control the balance between bone formation and resorption. Sclerostin acts by inhibiting the Wnt pathway, through which it indirectly acts as an antagonist to BMP.
4) Osteocytes can cause localised remodelling of its lacunar wall, affecting both the mineral and organic matrix. By regulating this secondary mineralisation of bone, osteocytes may stop it becoming too brittle. Because of the huge surface area involved, the osteocyte is the key player in homeostasis of calcium and phosphate metabolism. With its production of FGF23, it has a wider role in kidney function. It regulates serum phosphate levels by acting on renal proximal tubules so that more phosphate is excreted, and by reducing the amount of phosphate absorption from the gut and bone.

As a result of their widespread distribution in bone and their interconnections, osteocytes are obvious candidates to detect load-induced strains in bone and are therefore regarded as the primary mechanosensors in bone. In support of this view is evidence of rapid changes in metabolism following intermittent loading of bone. How strain is detected is not known, but fluid flow through canaliculi and/or cell deformation is one possibility. In this context, the presence of cell adhesion molecules at the cell membrane (e.g., integrins): may be relevant.

Bone-lining cells

When bone surfaces are neither in the formative nor resorptive phase, with little or no osteoid present the bone surface is lined by a layer of flattened cells termed *bone-lining cells* (Fig. 13.9D). As for osteoblasts, the bone-lining cells are connected to underlying osteocytes. They show little sign of synthetic activity, as evidenced by their reduced organelle content, and may be regarded as postproliferative osteoblasts. By covering the surface of bone, they may: 1) play a role in calcium and phosphate metabolism, 2) protect the surface from any resorptive activity by osteoclasts or 3) participate in initiating bone remodelling. Bone-lining cells could also be a source of osteoprogenitor cells and be reactivated to form osteoblasts.

Osteoprogenitor cells

In order to generate osteoblasts throughout life, a stem cell population is required. Stem cells have the ability to maintain their numbers throughout life. When a stem cell divides, one of the daughter cells remains as a stem cell, while the other can differentiate into another cell type. This property of self-renewal is a unique feature of stem cells. In the case of alveolar bone, the cells derived from the initial stem cells that eventually give rise to osteoblasts are termed *osteoprogenitor cells*. They reside in the layer of cells beneath the osteoblast layer in the periosteal region, in the periodontal ligament or in the marrow spaces. Initially, the osteoprogenitor cells are fibroblast-like cells, with an elongated nucleus and few organelles (Fig. 13.11). Their life cycle may involve up to about eight cell divisions before reaching the osteoblast stage. There is a gradual acquirement of osteoblast-like features associated with an ordered increase in gene expression. Initially, genes related to cell growth are expressed (such as c-*myc*, c-*fos* and *Runx2*), followed by genes related to osteoblast products such as type I collagen, fibronectin, some growth factors and alkaline phosphatase. Finally, genes are expressed related to products associated with mineralisation (such as osteocalcin, osteopontin and bone sialoprotein).

Osteoclasts

Osteoclasts are the cells responsible for the resorption of mineralised tissue. Indeed, bone is a tissue that contains specialised cells dedicated to its own destruction. Osteoclasts are derived from haemopoietic cells of the monocyte/macrophage lineage by fusion of mononuclear precursors, giving rise to multinucleated cells. This cell fusion takes place close to the bone surface, so multinucleated osteoclasts are rarely seen at any distance from bone. The precise mechanism that guides osteoclasts to their sites of resorption is unknown but may involve chemotaxis. Resorbing surfaces of alveolar bone show typical resorption concavities (Howship's lacunae) in which the osteoclasts lie (Fig. 13.16). An osteoclast appears to undertake several resorption cycles before finally disappearing. Useful markers for osteoclasts are the enzyme tartrate-resistant acid phosphatase (TRAP) (Fig. 13.17), as well as the protease cathepsin K, which functions to remove the organic collagenous matrix during resorption.

Tissue culture studies indicate that osteoclasts are highly motile (Fig. 13.18A). Evidence from the presence of elongated 'snail track' resorption lacunae on bone surfaces (Figs. 13.18B, 13.19 and see Fig. 13.35) suggests that osteoclasts also move across the bone *in vivo*. Osteoclasts are recruited only when required, and consequently there is no significant reservoir of inactive osteoclasts. The lifespan of osteoclasts is not known with any certainty, although it is thought to be at least 10–14

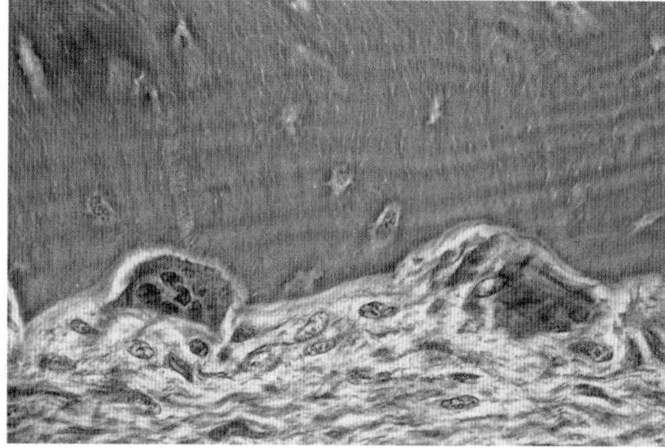

Fig. 13.16 Demineralised section of a resorbing alveolar bone showing two osteoclasts lying in Howship's lacunae (×350). Courtesy Prof. M M Smith.

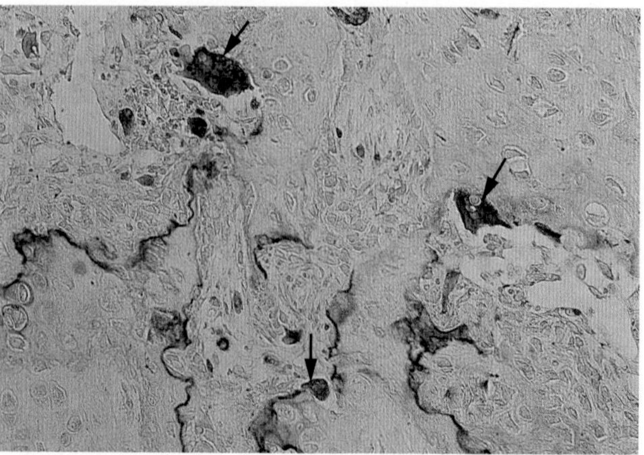

Fig. 13.17 Demineralised section of bone showing osteoclasts staining positively (red) for tartrate-resistant acid phosphatase (arrows) (×240). Courtesy Dr. A Grigoriadis.

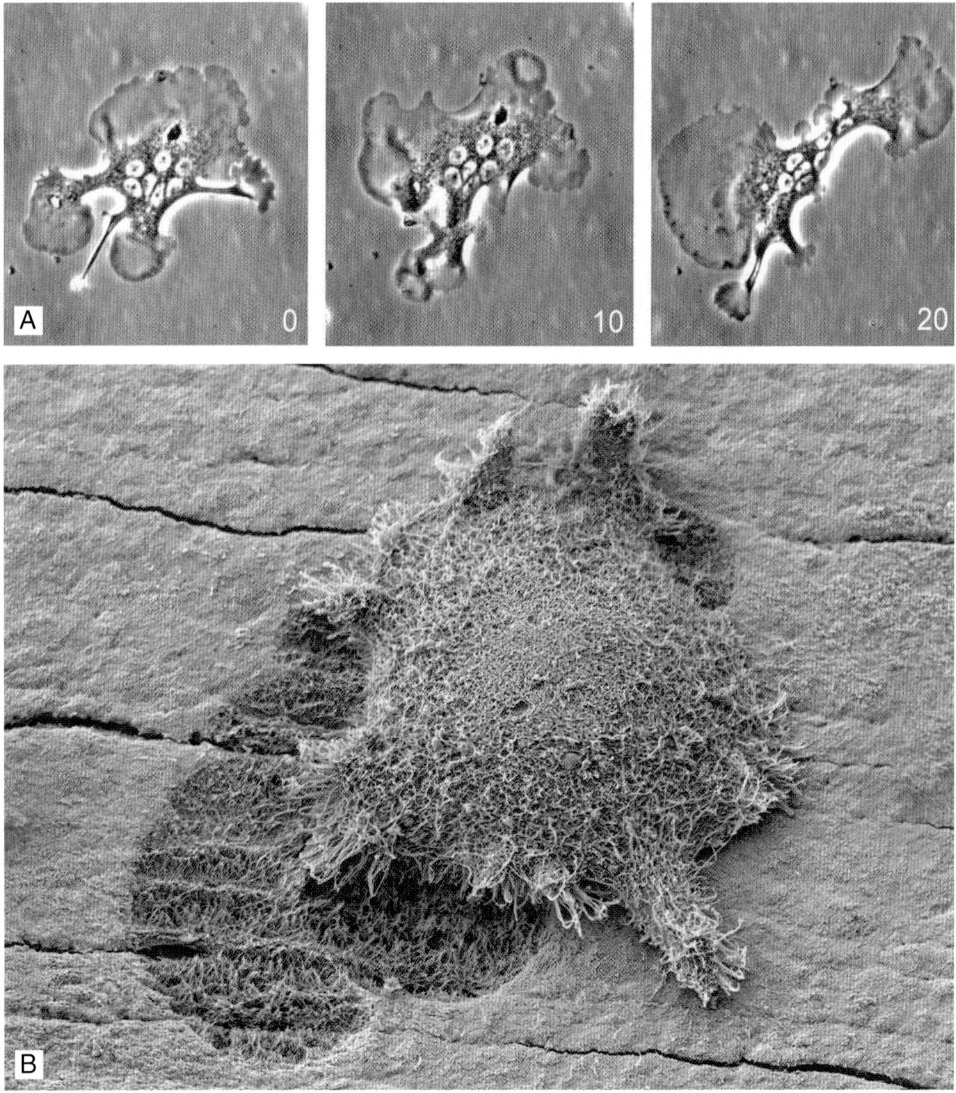

Fig 13.18 Osteoclasts in tissue culture. (A) Phase contrast, time lapse sequence of a living osteoclast (0, 10, 20 min), showing rapid cell motility. (B) Scanning electron micrograph of an osteoclast (blue) which has excavated a typical, scalloped resorption pit (pink) on a slice of dentine; exposed, demineralised collagen fibres are clearly visible in the pit. Image width: 120 microns (A), 150 microns (B). Courtesy Dr. T R Arnett, UCL.

days, after which the cells finally undergo apoptosis. Different nuclei within the osteoclast are often of different ages. The possibility exists that additional fusion of new cells may prolong the activity of osteoclasts.

Osteoclasts show considerable variation in size and shape, ranging from small mononuclear cells to very large cells with many nuclei. Characteristically, human osteoclasts may be up to 100 µm in diameter and have on average 10–20 nuclei, but there may be species variation in size (Fig. 13.20). When actively resorbing, osteoclasts are highly polarised cells and exhibit four main different membrane domains (Fig. 13.21): the ruffled border and the sealing zone in contact with bone and the basolateral and functional secretory domains away from the bone.

The ruffled border is that part of the cell that lies adjacent to bone and where resorption occurs. More than one ruffled border may be present at any one time. At the light microscope level it often has a foamy or striated appearance. At the ultrastructural level, the ruffled border is composed of many tightly packed microvilli adjacent to the bone surface, providing a large surface area for the resorptive process. It is now well established that products from the osteoclast, such as protons (H^+) and chloride ions (Cl^-), are secreted at the lateral aspects of the ruffled border, resulting in acidification of the cellular space and subsequent dissolving of the hydroxyapatite mineral. The resulting degraded matrix is absorbed (endocytosed) in the central region of the ruffled border, is transported to the basolateral surface and excreted (see later). Together with the secretion of proteases such as cathepsin K, this allows for efficient resorptive activity of both the inorganic and organic components of bone matrix.

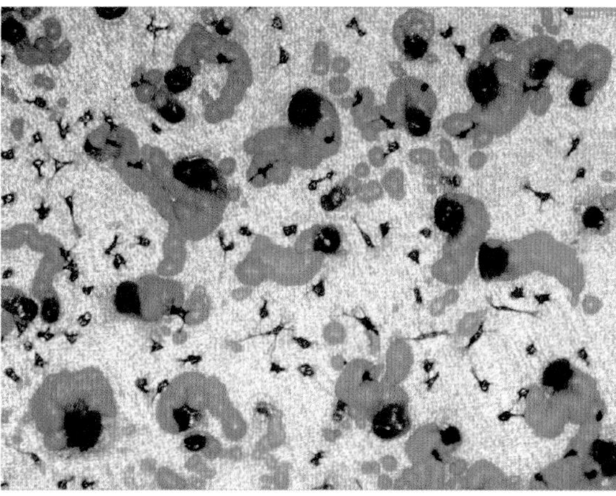

Fig. 13.19 Osteoclasts (red) cultured on dentine showing dark snail-track resorption areas. Image width = 1 mm. Courtesy Dr. T R Arnett.

The sealing zone (also referred to as the *annular* or *clear zone*) at the periphery of the ruffled border separates the ruffled border from the basolateral membrane. Here, the plasma membrane tends to become smooth and the organelle-free cytoplasm beneath it contains numerous contractile actin microfilaments (surrounded by two vinculin rings)

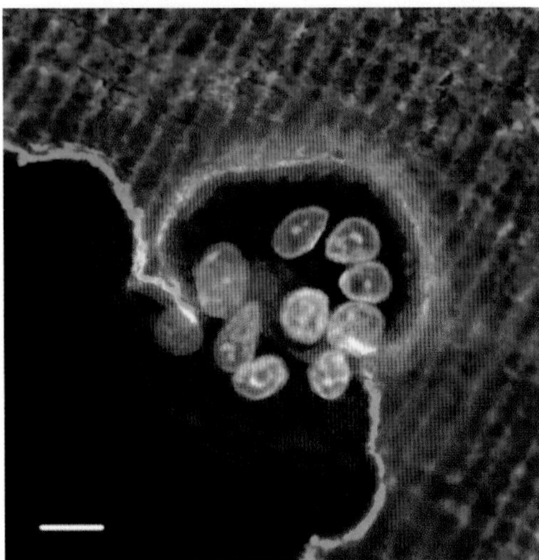

Fig. 13.20 Rabbit osteoclast cultured on dentine *in vitro*. The dentine is labelled with a fluorescent bisphosphonate (green), F-actin stained with TRITC-phalloidin (red), nuclei with DAPI (white) and the membrane with an antibody to the vitronectin receptor (blue). Image captured by laser scanning confocal microscopy, displayed as two merged optical sections taken at the surface of the dentine and the midpoint of the nuclei to demonstrate both the actin ring and multinuclearity. (Bar = 10 μm.) Courtesy Dr. F Coxon.

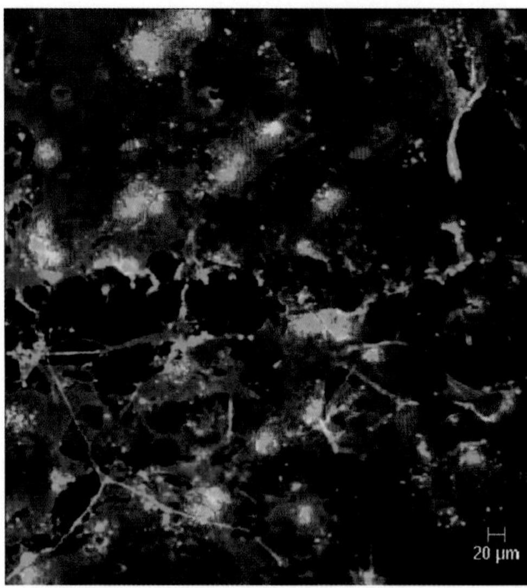

Fig. 13.23 Confocal image of human osteoclasts cultured on bone to show resorption areas enclosed by actin (red label). Cells are labelled for the osteoclast cell surface marker, integrin alpha-V beta-3 (green label). Courtesy Dr. G Stenbeck.

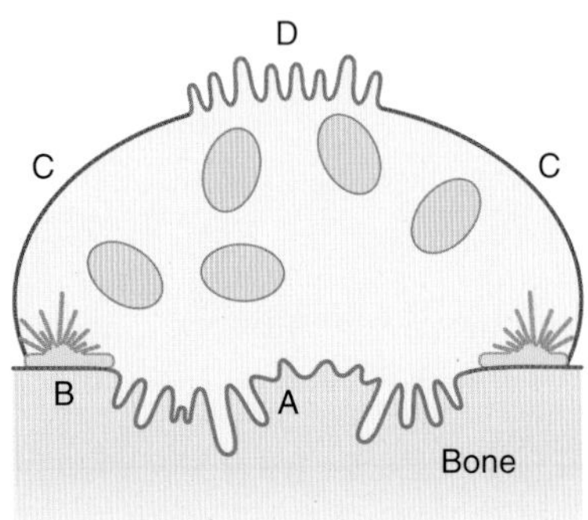

Fig. 13.21 Diagram showing the four domains of an osteoclast. A = ruffled border; B = sealing zone; C = basolateral zone; D = functional secretory domain.

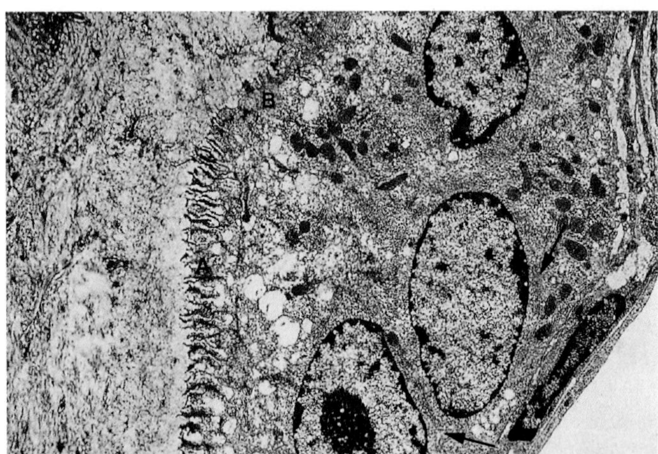

Fig. 13.22 Electron microscopic appearance of demineralised bone showing part of an osteoclast. The brush border (A) comprises numerous microvilli adjacent to the bone surface. At the circumference of the brush border, the annular zone (B) contains numerous microfilaments. There are numerous vesicles and mitochondria, and three nuclei are evident (×3,600). From Berkovitz, B.K.B., Shore, R.C., 1995. Cells of the periodontal ligament. In: Berkovitz, B.K.B., Moxham, B.J., Newman, H.J. (Eds.), The Periodontal Ligament in Health and Disease, second ed. Mosby–Wolfe, London, pp 9–33.

(Figs. 13.22, 13.23). The attachment of the osteoclast cell membrane to the bone matrix at the sealing zone is mainly owing to the presence of cell membrane adhesion proteins known as *integrins* (mainly $\alpha_v\beta_3$, but also $\alpha_v\beta_1$ and $\alpha_2\beta_1$), as well as non-integrin membrane receptors such as CD44. The integrins bind to specific amino acid sequences present in proteins of the bone matrix, namely Arg–Gly–Asp (RGD). Interference with the formation of such integrins, or the administration of competing synthetic RGD peptides that prevent osteoclasts from attaching to bone, will inhibit bone resorption. The sealing zone may serve to attach the cell very closely to the surface of the bone, thus creating an isolated micro-environment in which resorption of bone can take place without diffusion of the protons and proteases produced by the cell into adjacent soft tissue. This isolated micro-environment can be considered a specialised 'extracellular' lysosome.

The membrane regions of the osteoclast away from the bone are subdivided into functional secretory and basolateral domains. The functional secretory domain opposite the ruffled border is a collection site of vesicles. It is believed that bone matrix, degraded at the ruffled border, passes across the cell in these vesicles to be exocytosed here (transcytosis) (Fig. 13.21). The basolateral surface may be a regulatory surface for receiving messages from neighbouring cells.

The osteoclast contains numerous mitochondria distributed throughout the cytoplasm (except for the region immediately beneath the ruffled border). The remaining cytoplasm contains large numbers of vesicles of different sizes and types (Fig. 13.22), some containing lysosomal enzymes such as cysteine proteinases (e.g., cathepsins) and matrix metalloproteinases capable of degrading the organic matrix of bone. In addition, there are considerable amounts of F-actin and microtubules (Fig. 13.24).

Although under the control of osteoblasts, the osteoclast is responsive to many factors, the most important of which is RANKL (see pages 272–274). Although not widely mentioned in the literature, osteoclasts, like osteoblasts, also express receptors for parathyroid hormone at low levels. This allows for the possibility of a different action for this hormone on the two cell types.

Once the osteoclast has been activated, bone resorption occurs in two stages. Initially, the mineral is removed and, later, the remaining organic matrix (Fig. 13.25). To provide a low pH for dissolving the mineral, the osteoclast secretes protons across the ruffled border by means of a V-type ATPase proton pump: the enzyme carbonic anhydrase II is involved in generating protons by catabolising the reaction of carbon dioxide with water to form carbonic acid. Secretion of anions balances the pumping

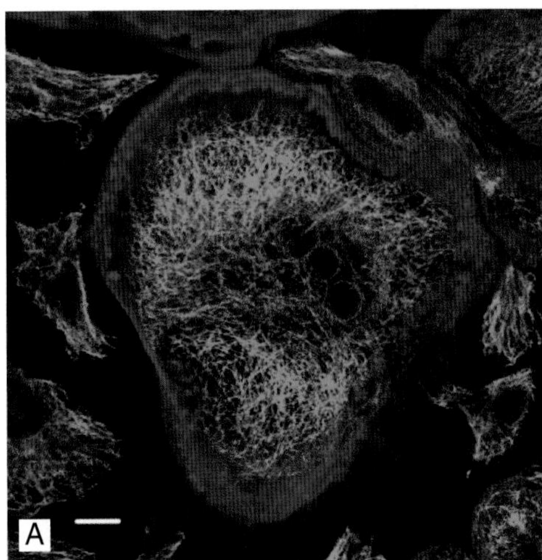

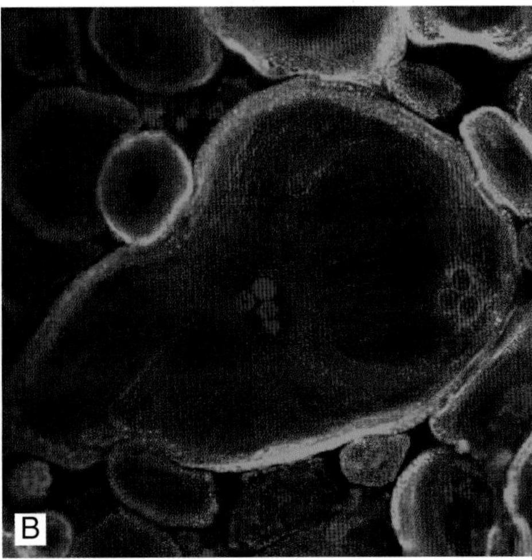

Fig. 13.24 (A) Rabbit osteoclast cultured on glass showing distribution of some constituents. Microtubules (green) labelled with antibody to alpha tubulin, F-actin (blue) stained with TRITC-phalloidin and circumnuclear Golgi apparatus (red) stained with wheat germ agglutinin-AF633. Laser scanning confocal microscopy. Bar = 10 μm. (B) Rabbit osteoclast cultured on glass showing distribution of some constituents. F-actin (green), microtubules (red) and nuclei (blue). Courtesy Dr. F Coxon.

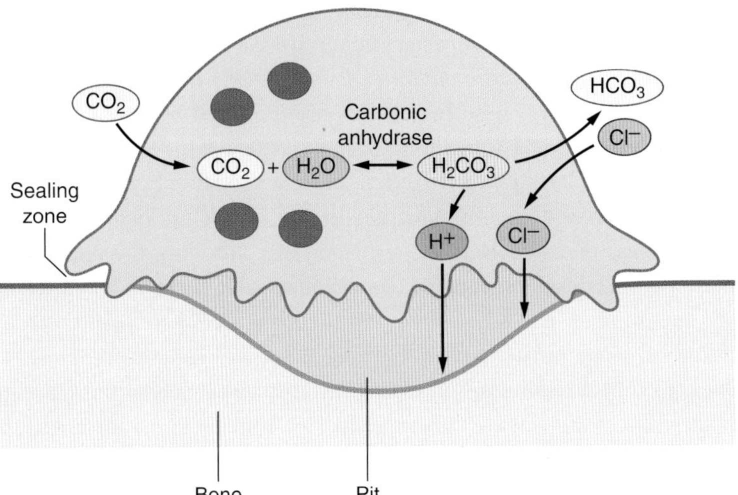

Fig. 13.25 Diagram showing action of osteoclast in resorbing bone. Courtesy Prof. T R Arnett.

of protons, accounting for the large number of chloride channels in the ruffled border.

The organic matrix exposed in the resorbing lacuna (Fig. 13.18B) is then degraded by enzymes, principally cathepsin K. It is not known how much of this organic degradation takes place extracellularly and how much intracellularly. Compared with the fibroblasts of the periodontal ligament (Fig. 12.35), intracellular collagen profiles have rarely been reported within osteoclasts.

Box 13.2 compares the main features of osteoblasts, osteocytes and osteoclasts.

Box 13.2 Comparison of the main features of osteoblasts, osteocytes and osteoclasts

Osteoblasts

Mesenchymal in origin

Lie on surface of forming bone

Secrete and mineralise organic matrix

Incorporated into bone matrix as osteocytes

Rich in alkaline phosphatase

Early expression of the nuclear transcription factor core binding factor 1 Cbfa1 (also called Runx2)

Rich in endoplasmic reticulum and Golgi apparatus

Osteocytes

Mesenchymal in origin

Lie within bone and surrounded by bone matrix

Most abundant cells in bone

Mesenchymal in origin

Communicate with each other and with osteoblasts via numerous fine canaliculi

Fewer intracellular organelles compared with osteoblasts

Detect strain in bone

May prevent hypermineralisation by releasing pyrophosphate

Endocrine/paracrine regulators of bone and mineral metabolism (FGF23, sclerostin, RANK ligand)

Osteoclasts

Haemopoietic in origin

Multinucleated giant cells that resorb bone

Motile

Specialised organ of resorption (ruffled border) adjacent to bone surface

Rich in acid phosphatase.

Ruffled border pumps acid (via H^+-ATPase) to dissolve bone mineral and enzymes (mainly cathepsin K) to degrade collagenous matrix

Early expression of the nuclear transcription factor c-Fos

Cell kinetics

Formation of osteoblasts

Much research on the life cycle of osteoblasts has been undertaken using stromal cells removed from bone marrow, where it has been demonstrated that stem cells are multipotential and can give rise to osteoblasts as well as fibroblasts, chondroblasts, adipoblasts and myofibroblasts. These are commonly referred to as bone marrow stromal cells (BMSCs), mesenchymal stem cells (MSCs) and, more recently, skeletal stem cells (SSCs). Stem cells for osteoblasts in the periodontal ligament may be derived from perivascular cells in the ligament as well as from the adjacent bone marrow. From a stem cell, intermediate progenitor cell forms have been described leading to postmitotic osteoblasts. These forms include osteoprogenitors (immature and mature forms) and preosteoblasts and involve about eight cell divisions. As cells generally increase in size during differentiation, the

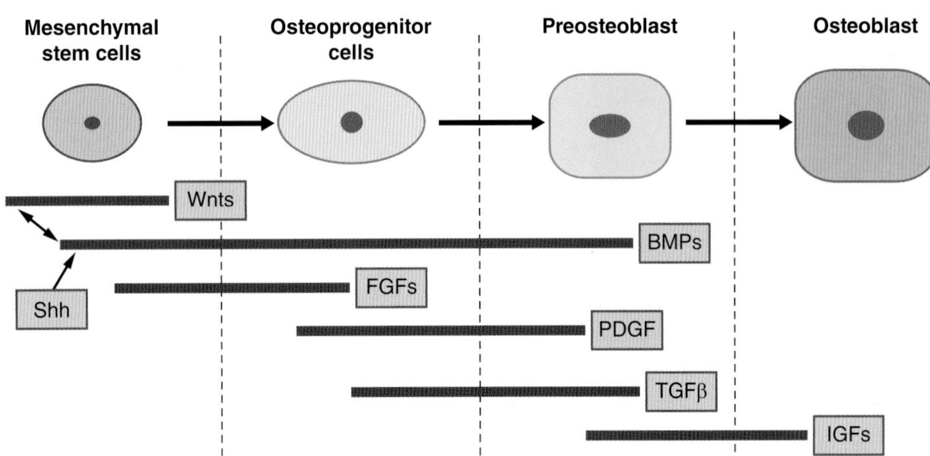

Fig. 13.26 The main stages of growth factor activity during osteoblast differentiation. BMPs = bone morphogenetic proteins; FGFs = fibroblast growth factors; IGFs = insulin-like growth factors; PDGF = platelet-derived growth factor; Shh = sonic hedgehog; TGF-β = transforming growth factor-β; Wnts = Wnt proteins. Redrawn after Hughes, F.J., Turner, W., Belibasakis, G., et al., 2006. Effects of growth factors and cytokines on osteoblast differentiation. *Periodontology* 2000 41, 48–72.

size of the cell has been used in an attempt to distinguish osteoblasts and their precursors. The process of bone formation requires

1) Cell proliferation
2) The synthesis and secretion of an extracellular matrix
3) Mineralisation of the matrix

The process is characterised by a decreasing proliferative capacity and an increasing degree of differentiation of the cells.

Among the earliest markers to indicate that a stem cell is progressing along an osteogenic phenotype is the expression of the nuclear transcription factor core-binding factor 1 (Cbfa1, more commonly called *Runx2*), which is responsible for regulating the production of some important protein products in bone matrix and specific cell surface markers (e.g., STRO-1). Supporting the importance of Runx2 is the observation that knockout mice without this gene lack osteoblasts and therefore lack bone. The induction of Runx2 involves the action of growth factors such as TGF-β and BMP-2.

Osteoprogenitor cells can be identified by the progressive expression of molecules such as type I collagen and osteopontin and by the appearance of specific receptors such as PTH1R. In the preosteoblast, the concentration of many of the osteogenic markers seen in the osteoprogenitor cells increases and there is still some limited proliferation. The cell is relatively undifferentiated, and there is little roughened endoplasmic reticulum. In the postmitotic osteoblast, even more activity of the markers first seen in preosteoblasts is present. In addition, new molecules related to mineralisation (e.g., osteocalcin) and cell adhesion molecules make their appearance.

The differentiation of osteoblasts and their subsequent life cycle is regulated by numerous factors, among which will be transcription factors (e.g., Runx2, TAZ, Msx2, Dlx5 and Osterix), growth factors and cytokines (e.g., BMP, TGF-β, IGF, interleukin [IL]-1) (Fig. 13.26) and hormones (e.g., glucocorticoids, oestrogen, parathyroid hormone, vitamin D_3). The actions of such molecules may differ according to the stage of differentiation and concentration (Table 13.2). The final stage of the osteoblast concerns its entrapment in bone matrix, where it becomes the osteocyte.

Formation of osteoclasts

Unlike the other cells associated with bone (e.g., osteoblasts, osteocytes, bone-lining cells), osteoclasts are derived not from stromal cells but from blood cells. The pluripotent stem cell is the haemopoietic stem cell, and the osteoclast arises specifically from the monocyte/macrophage lineage. Early important transcription factors indicative of its eventual fate are PU-1, c-Fos, nuclear factor kappa B (NFκB) and nuclear factor of activated T cells 1 (NFATc1). Differentiation from the myeloid progenitor to the mononuclear osteoclast precursor involves the activity of many factors, two of the most important being M-CSF and RANKL, formerly known as *osteoclast differentiation factor* (ODF) and *osteoprotegerin* (OPG) respectively. These two factors are produced by osteoblast/stromal cells. As osteoclast progenitors have a receptor for M-CSF (c-Fms) and a receptor (RANK) for RANKL, close association between the two cell types drives the differentiation of the osteoclast precursors into mononuclear preosteoclasts. As a method of controlling the rate of formation of osteoclast precursors, the osteoblast also secretes OPG, which acts as a soluble 'decoy' molecule by binding with RANKL and thereby inhibiting osteoclast formation. Preosteoclasts also contain receptors for calcitonin. Factors controlling osteoblast–osteoclast interactions during bone remodelling, including the role of osteocytes, are shown in Fig. 13.27. Some factors inhibiting and stimulating the activity of osteoclasts are presented in Table 13.3.

Fusion of mononuclear osteoclasts into multinucleated osteoclasts and their subsequent activation are also driven by the RANKL/RANK system. Many complex membrane interactions must occur when cells are undergoing fusion to become multinucleated. Initially, the cell is nonpolarized, and it is only on attaching to bone by cell–matrix interactions (involving transmembrane receptors such as integrins and matrix components such as collagen and osteopontin) that the osteoclast becomes polarised and develops the ruffled border, sealing zone and systems to successfully demineralise bone and degrade its organic matrix. Following its resorptive phase, osteoclasts are thought to be eliminated by apoptosis.

Two additional important factors involved in the activation of osteoclasts are acidification and hypoxia.

Acidification

In appropriate media, osteoclasts cultured on bone at pH 7.4 (physiological or blood pH) are virtually inactive. However, when the pH is lowered to 7.0, there is a marked increase in resorption. This reduction in pH also acts synergistically with osteolytic agents such as RANKL. As has been seen, RANKL is an important agent driving the development, activation and survival of osteoclasts. In this respect, it is worth noting that the activity of some cytokines and growth factors results in the release of hydrogen ions from the affected cells.

Hypoxia

There is evidence to suggest that a reduction in oxygen levels in the microenvironment of bone tissue provides a stimulus for osteoclasis, although

Table 13.2 Key natural regulators of bone remodelling and mineral metabolism

Regulator	Action	Produced by
Systematic hormones		
Parathyroid hormone	↑ Blood calcium ↑ Bone resorption ↑ Bone formation	Parathyroid glands
1,25 dihydroxyvitamin D	↑ Blood calcium and mineralisation ↑ Bone resorption	Skin (UV light)/liver/kidney
Glucocorticoids	↓ Bone formation	Adrenal glands
Oestrogen (and testosterone)	↓ Bone resorption ↑ Bone formation (smaller effect)	Ovaries (and testes); adrenals
Locally acting factors		
RANK ligand (RANKL)	↑↑ Bone resorption (forms osteoclasts)	Osteoblasts; osteocytes
OPG	↓ Bone resorption (blocks RANKL)	Osteoblasts; osteocytes
Inflammatory cytokines (interleukins 1 and 6; TNF-α)	↑ Bone resorption	Osteoblasts; immune cells
Sclerostin	↓Bone formation (blocks Wnt signalling)	Osteocytes
BMPs	↑ Bone formation	Osteoblasts; mesenchymal cells
VEGF	↑ Bone formation (via growth of new blood vessels)	Osteoblasts; many other cells
'Fundamental' (inorganic) agents		
Nitric oxide	↑ Bone formation (dilates blood vessels)	Blood vessel lining cells; nerves
Hypoxia (low oxygen)	↑ Bone resorption (forms osteoclasts) ↓ bone formation (blocks osteoblasts)	Ischaemia
Acidosis (low pH)	↑ Bone resorption (activates osteoclasts)	Kidney disease; tumours; diabetes; ischaemia
Pyrophosphate	↓ Bone mineralisation	Breakdown of ATP
Mechanical		
Strain/deformation	↑ Bone formation	Mechanical loading

From Arnett, T.R., 2015. Basics of bone biology. Osteoporosis Review 23, 12–16.

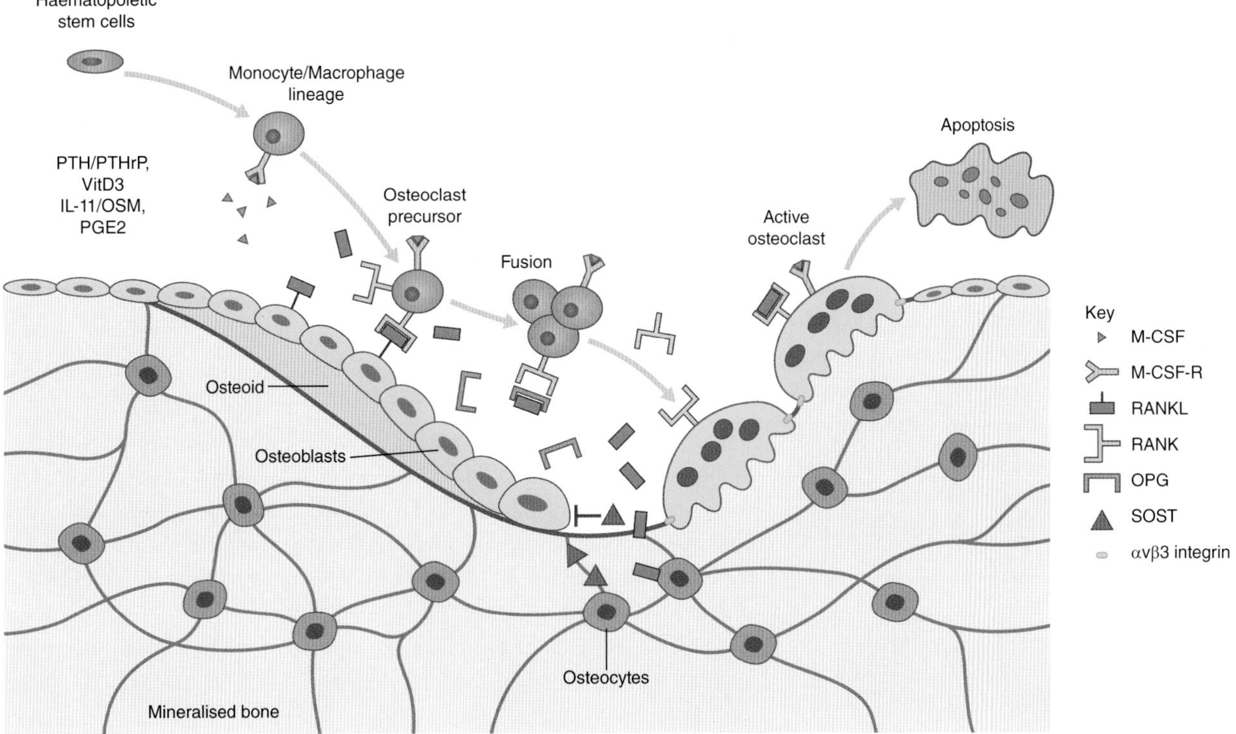

Fig. 13.27 Factors controlling osteoblast–osteoclast interactions during bone remodelling. In response to calciotropic factors (e.g., PTH/PTHrP, IL-11/OSM, VitD3, PGE2), osteoblasts secrete M-CSF and RANKL, which bind to M-CSF-R and RANKL, respectively. This results in increased osteoclast differentiation, fusion, activity and survival. Osteoblasts also produce OPG, which inhibits RANKL signalling. RANKL is also synthesised by osteocytes that can inhibit osteoblastic bone formation via SOST. cAMP = cyclic adenosine monophosphate; gp130 = glycoprotein 130; IL-11 = interleukin-11; M-CSF = macrophage colony-stimulating factor; M-CSF-R = M-CSF receptor; OPG = osteoprotegerin; OSM = oncostatin M; PGE2 = prostaglandin E2; PTH = parathyroid hormone; PTHrP = PTH-related protein; RANK = receptor activator of nuclear factor kappa B; RANKL = RANK ligand; SOST = sclerostin; VitD3 = 1,25-dihydroxyvitamin D3. Courtesy Dr. N W A McGowan, Dr. A Grigoriadis and Prof. T R Arnett.

Table 13.3 Some factors inhibiting and stimulating osteoclasts

	Differentiation	Resorption	Apoptosis
RANKL	↑	↑	↓
OPG	↓	↓	
Oestrogen	↓		
Calcitonin		↓	
High pH		↓	
Low pH		↑	
Bisphosphonates			↑

OPG = osteoprotegerin; RANKL = receptor activator of nuclear factor kappa B ligand.
Courtesy Dr. A Grigoriadis.

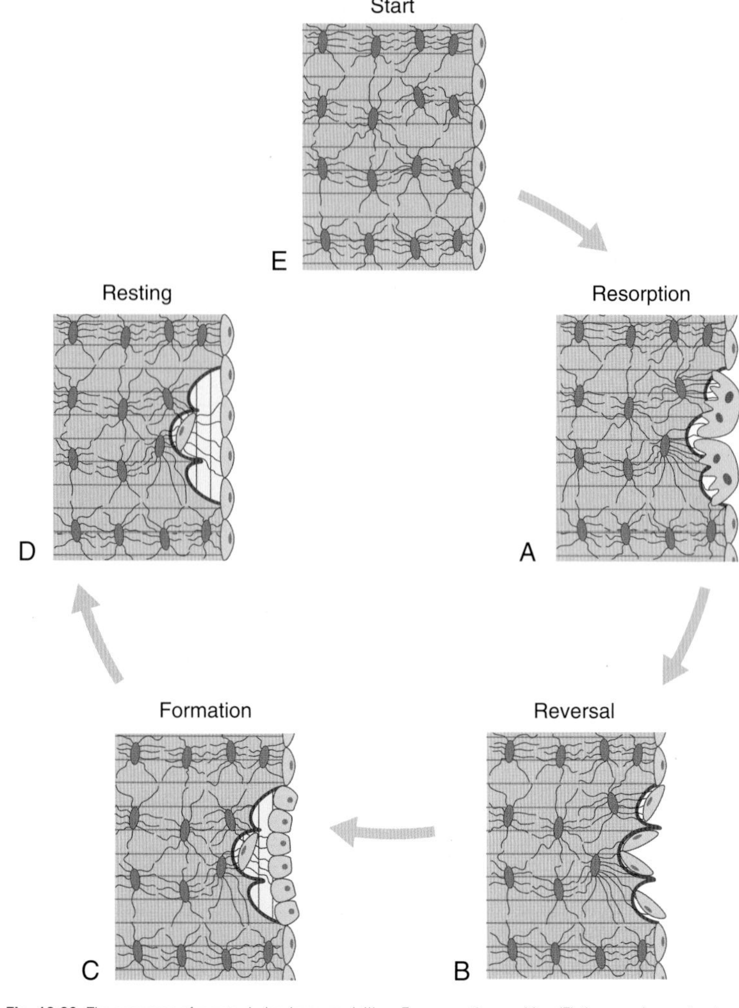

Fig. 13.28 The sequence of events during bone modelling. From a resting position (E) there are four main stages (A-D). A reversal line is indicated in red. See text for description.

the mechanism is poorly understood. The hypoxia may be associated with acidification, or it may cause the release of factors such as prostaglandins and vascular endothelial growth factor.

The importance of the factors listed earlier in association with the formation and activity of osteoclasts has been deduced from studies designed to produce deficiencies or overexpression of the factor. Thus, mice lacking the ability to produce M-CSF, RANKL or RANK do not develop osteoclasts. They are therefore unable to resorb bone, and thick bone is produced (osteopetrosis). Their teeth may be prevented from erupting (because of the inability to resorb bone overlying the erupting teeth), but this can be corrected by restoring the missing factor. In contrast, mice lacking the ability to produce OPG (the osteoclast inhibitor) have increased numbers of osteoclasts and develop osteoporosis.

Resorption and formation of bone during remodelling

The processes of bone resorption and formation at sites of remodelling do not occur randomly. Clearly, there must be tight control to ensure a balance between the two processes, as any disruption of this balance can lead to metabolic bone disease. This is referred to as *coupling*. However, it is important to realise that osteoclasts work much faster than osteoblasts. From a resting state (Fig. 13.28E), the sequence of remodelling consists of four main phases that occur in a remodelling cycle:

- **Resorption:** recruitment, migration and activation of osteoclasts causing bone resorption (Fig. 13.28A)
- **Reversal:** cessation of resorption and disappearance of osteoclasts by apoptosis or migration; the site becomes occupied by mononuclear cells (Fig. 13.28B)
- **Formation:** osteoblast recruitment, migration, differentiation and formation of new bone in the resorption site (Fig. 13.28C)
- **Resting:** formation of bone ceases following mineralisation and the surface is lined by a flattened layer of cells (Fig. 13.28D)

In this manner, an initial 'cutting cone' of osteoclastic resorption moves along the central canal of an osteon in cortical bone at about 50 μm/day, followed by a 'closing zone' of osteoblastic activity (Fig. 13.29). The changeover from resorption to deposition is characterised by a reversal (cement) line (Fig. 13.30; Fig. 13.46). This reversal line is rich in osteopontin and acid phosphatase (Fig. 13.30).

Many of the biological molecules capable of causing bone resorption, such as parathyroid hormone, interleukins (IL-11) and vitamin D_3, have their primary effect on osteoblasts, driving the production of RANKL, OPG and M-CSF. However, each may drive the production via a different route (Fig. 13.27). Thus, osteoblasts are generally essential for osteoclast differentiation and function. A close association of these cells with osteoclasts and their precursors is a further requirement necessary for the activation of bone

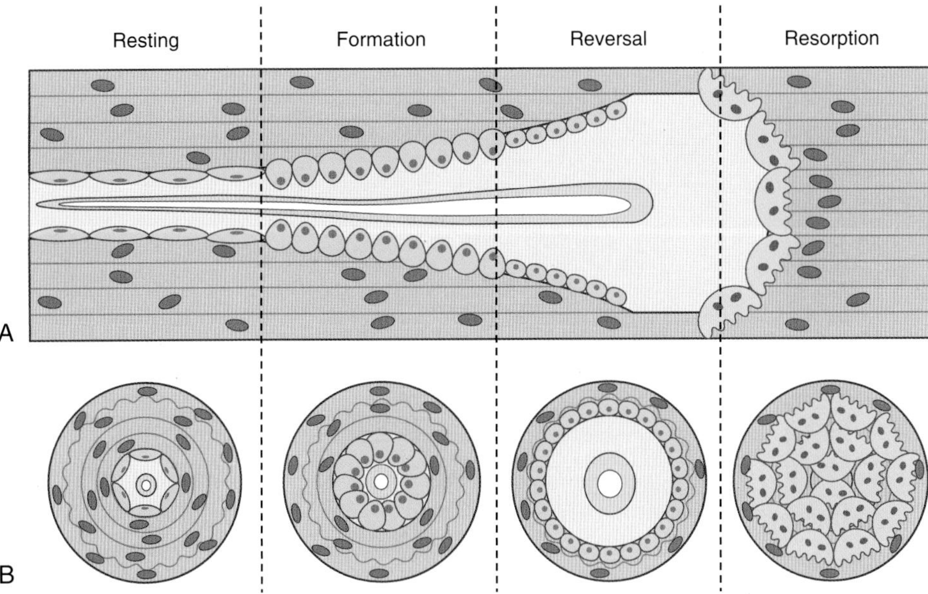

Fig. 13.29 A cutting cone. (A) Longitudinal section along an Haversian system showing the four main phases of the remodelling cycle. (B) Cross-sections of the Haversian system showing the corresponding appearance of each of the four main phases of the remodelling cycle.

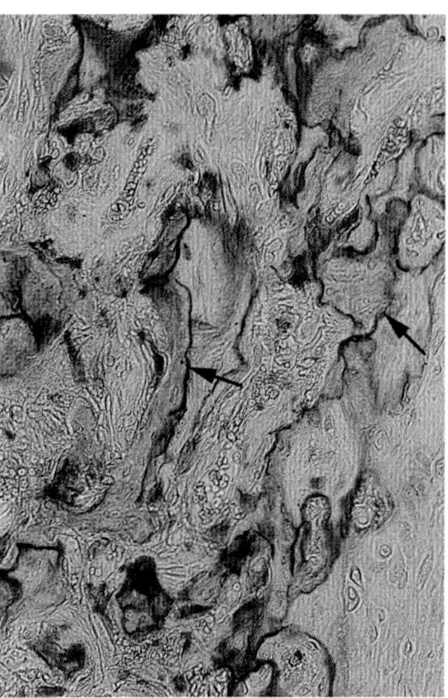

Fig. 13.30 Portion of bone showing the scalloped outline of a reversal line staining positively (red) for acid phosphatase (arrows) (×100). Courtesy Dr. A Grigoriadis.

resorption. As previously mentioned (see pages 272–273), ambient pH and levels of oxygen are also important factors affecting resorption. Not only do osteoblasts control osteoclast formation, but osteoclasts themselves can also secrete products that are important for stimulating osteoblast recruitment and differentiation to the resorption site during the remodelling cycle.

There is evidence that osteoclasts can be activated, and begin resorption, when they contact the mineralised surface of bone. Initially, therefore, any bone-lining cells or osteoblasts will have to retract or migrate away from the surface in order to expose the bone surface. Following this, any covering of osteoid will need to be removed. Osteoblasts/bone-lining cells have been implicated in this removal, possibly releasing enzymes such as matrix metalloproteinases (MMPs) to degrade the osteoid. Molecules in this milieu may then be chemotactic to osteoclasts.

The precise signals responsible for causing the cessation of resorption and a reversal to osteoblast differentiation and activation of bone formation are not known. However, the release of molecules such as growth factors initially bound up in the bone matrix but exposed and activated by the resorption process may be involved. For example, BMPs and IGF released from bone may stimulate bone formation (osteoblasis).

As a reduction in the mechanical loads impinging on bone is associated with bone loss, it can be assumed that such loading is normally required to stimulate the modelling/remodelling processes of bone necessary to maintain normal bone structure. Strains need to be intermittent (rather than continuous), and the osteogenic response is dependent upon the size of the load and the frequency and rate of application. To maintain bone mass may only require the application of relatively few loading cycles, as occurs in alveolar bone during mastication.

The molecular mechanisms whereby forces impinging on the bone are transduced into bone resorption or deposition remain elusive, although many theories have been proposed. Osteocytes, together with the surface layer of osteoblasts/bone-lining cells, appear to be the most obvious candidates for detecting strain within bone, as

1) they are present throughout bone
2) they maintain contact with neighbouring osteocytes and with osteoblasts/bone-lining cells via gap junctions
3) they are able to modify their volume, which in turn alters their sensitivity to loading

A widely held view envisages that deformation of bone following loading deforms the cell processes/cell membranes either directly or indirectly through movement of tissue fluid residing in the lacunocanalicular system. Signals are then transduced via the cell membrane at the surface (e.g., involving K^+ and Ca^{2+} ion channels and integrins) to cytoskeletal elements within the cell, with stimulation of secondary messengers. These changes eventually lead to the production and release of molecules that initiate an osteogenic response. Among the important molecules whose activity is upregulated in osteocytes (and osteoblasts) following the application of mechanical strain are prostaglandins, ILs, nitric oxide and certain growth factors (e.g., IGFs). However, it is the discovery of sclerostin that has provided a key osteocyte-derived factor that can control bone formation. Sclerostin normally *inhibits* osteoblasts, and mechanical loading decreases sclerostin expression in osteocytes, leading to upregulation of growth factors that stimulate osteoblasts. Changes in the micro-environment need to be considered, such as pH, oxygen tension, electric potential and concentration of ions such as calcium and sodium. Finally, it is also now thought that osteocytes themselves can produce RANKL, thus providing an additional level of control of osteoclast differentiation and activation during remodelling.

Radiographic techniques readily demonstrate that bone is continually remodelling to adapt to the different functional regimens impinging on it. In this context, newly formed bone is less dense (and therefore more radiolucent) than mature bone (Figs. 13.31, 13.32). As mentioned previously, cancellous bone remodels about 25% of its mass each year, compared with only about 3% for cortical bone.

A considerable number of factors can influence bone remodelling, with some of the more common being listed in Table 13.2. An idea of the complexity of the topic is given by the fact that some reagents can affect both formation and resorption of bone, while others can produce opposite effects, depending on concentration. Synergism must also be taken into account.

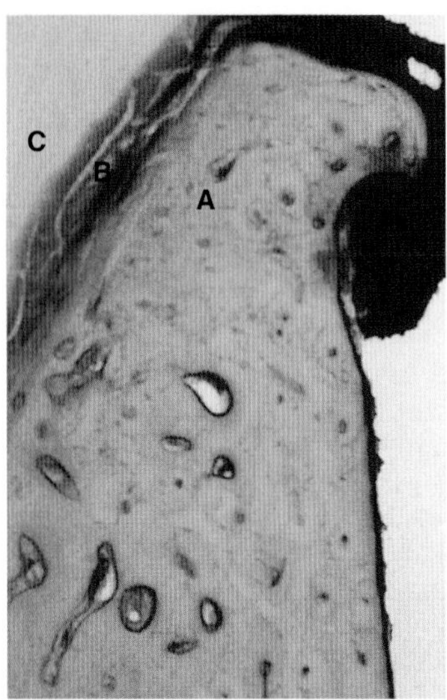

Fig. 13.31 Ground longitudinal section of alveolar bone at the alveolar crest. A = alveolar bone; B = periodontal space; C = root (×16). Courtesy R V Hawkins.

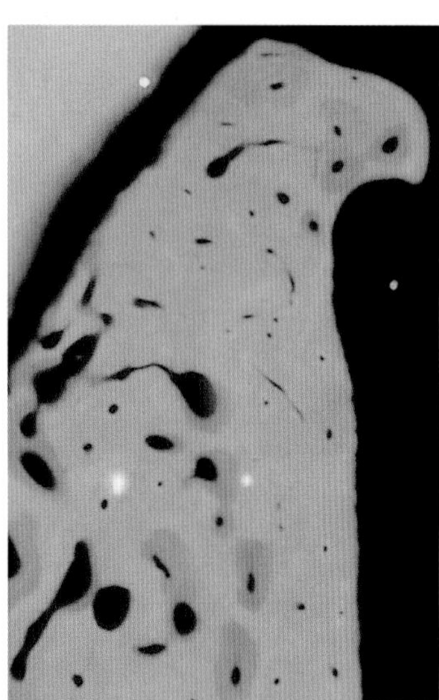

Fig. 13.32 Microradiograph of section shown in Fig. 13.31. The varying densities of alveolar bone indicate its active remodelling, with the darker, radiolucent areas being most recently formed and less mineralised. Courtesy R V Hawkins.

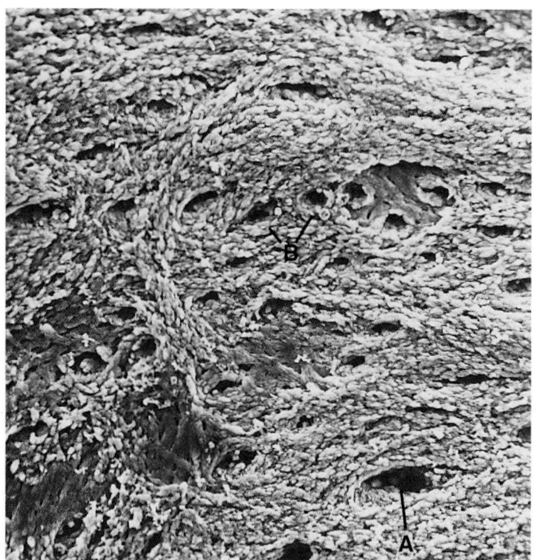

Fig. 13.33 SEM appearance of alveolar bone surface where bone formation is occurring. This is characterised by numerous small calcific nodules in partly mineralised intrinsic collagen that masks the underlying collagen fibrils. The larger, dark, elongated areas represent the lacunae of osteoblasts becoming entombed as osteocytes (A), while the smaller circular dark areas (B) represent the unmineralised cores of the Sharpey's fibres (anorganic preparation; ×550). Courtesy Prof. S J Jones.

Microdamage in bone

Microdamage within bone may result from the cumulative effects of mechanical stress or loading and takes the form of microcracks/microfractures, only visible under the microscope. A major difficulty related to studying this subject concerns the ability of distinguishing real bone microcracks from artefacts created during specimen preparation for microscopy. The development of such features results in the death (or apoptosis) of local osteocytes. Signals from the apoptosing cells or from living adjacent osteocytes may stimulate remodelling of the affected bone, primarily to repair the crack and presumably also to redistribute the functional loads more appropriately throughout the skeleton. Some authorities suggest that any remodelling involves initial resorption of the affected bone, while others claim that small cracks are removed by infilling with new mineral alone, without prior resorption. This latter view is consistent with the observation that, when osteocytes die, their lacunae and canaliculi may also ossify without resorting to prior resorption.

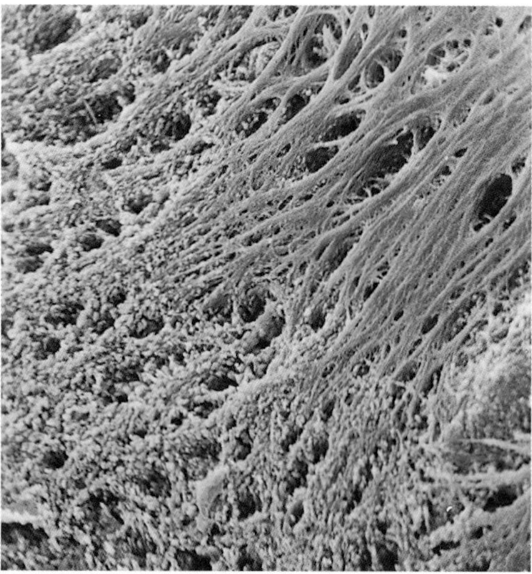

Fig. 13.34 SEM appearance of alveolar bone surface where bone formation is occurring, as evidenced by the numerous small nodules in the lower and left part of the field. However, the surface has been rendered only partly anorganic to show the collagen fibres of the extracellular matrix (partial anorganic preparation; ×550). Courtesy Prof. S J Jones.

Scanning electron microscope appearances of the alveolar bone surface

Scanning electron microscopy provides a useful technique for visualising the appearance of large areas of bone surfaces at high magnification. Cells and the organic material in any covering osteoid layer are removed by substances such as sodium hypochlorite, producing an anorganic preparation and revealing the underlying mineralised or mineralising surface layer.

An alveolar bone surface on which bone formation is occurring is characterised by the presence of numerous small, calcified nodules within and around collagen fibrils. Sharpey's fibres with a central unmineralised core may be encountered as small, dark, circular areas, and larger ovoid areas represent lacunae occupied *in vivo* by osteocytes becoming entombed in bone (Fig. 13.33). If the forming alveolar bone surface is rendered only partially anorganic, the smallest calcified nodules of bone may be seen depositing on the intrinsic collagen fibrils, and the orientation of the collagen parallel to the bone surface is also visualised (Fig. 13.34).

An alveolar bone surface on which bone resorption is occurring is characterised by the presence of Howship's resorption lacunae (Fig. 13.35). If a periosteal surface is examined, no Sharpey's fibres may be present. In addition to localised, pitlike resorption lacunae, bone may also exhibit longer 'snail-track' resorption lacunae. In contrast to a periosteal surface, the appearance of an area of resorption in bundle bone (periodontal surface) shows the presence of Sharpey's fibres in the resorbing areas (Fig. 13.36).

When neither bone deposition nor resorption is occurring, the surface of the bone is described as a resting surface. The resting surface may be characterised by projections marking the sites of extrinsic mineralised Sharpey's fibres, separated by smooth areas containing intrinsic mineralised collagen fibres. This contrasts with the granular appearance of the mineral of the intrinsic fibres of any adjacent forming surface (Fig. 13.37).

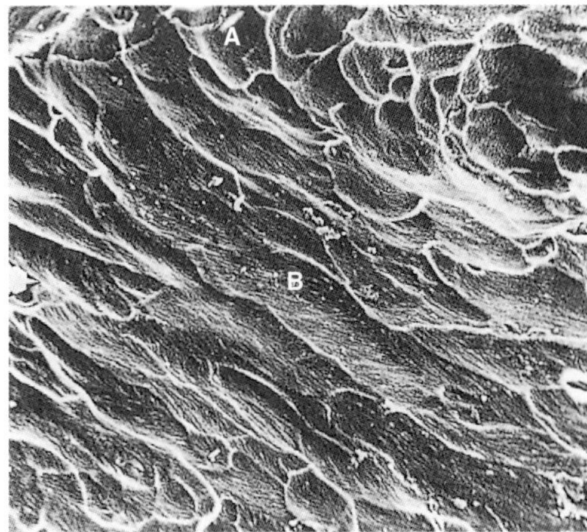

Fig. 13.35 SEM of periosteal surface of bone (lacking Sharpey's fibres) undergoing resorption. In addition to pitlike resorption lacunae (A), elongated 'snail-track' resorption lacunae are evident (B) (anorganic preparation; ×300). Courtesy Prof. S J Jones.

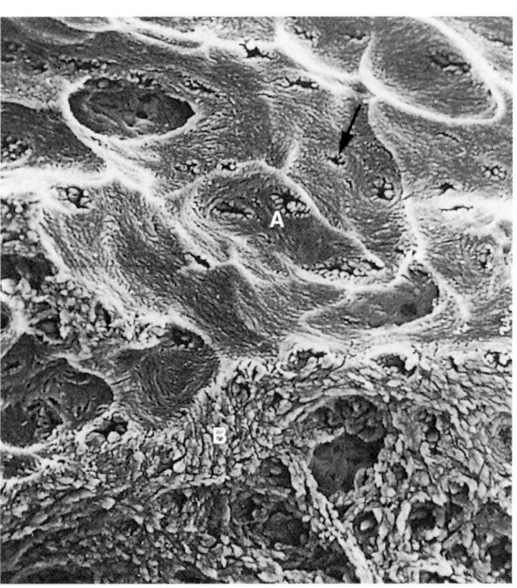

Fig. 13.36 SEM of alveolar bone surface contrasting the appearance of an area of bone resorption (A) with an adjacent area of bone formation (B). Note the presence of Sharpey's fibres with unmineralised cores in the resorbing areas (arrowed) (anorganic preparation; ×300). Courtesy Prof. S J Jones.

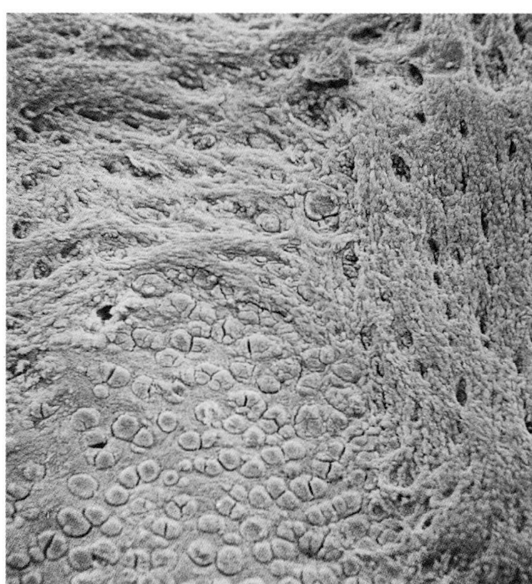

Fig. 13.37 SEM of resting alveolar bone surface (lower left part of field) characterised by projections marking the sites of mineralised extrinsic Sharpey's fibres separated by smooth areas. This contrasts with the granular appearance of the forming bone surface in the upper right part of the field, where the Sharpey's fibres whose cores have not yet fully mineralised are seen as holes (anorganic preparation; ×500). Courtesy Prof. S J Jones.

Sharpey's fibres

In addition to intrinsic fibres secreted by osteoblasts, which are aligned parallel to the bone surface, alveolar bone contains extrinsic Sharpey's fibres that enter bone perpendicular to the surface (Fig. 13.38). Extrinsic fibres, inserting into the cribriform plate as Sharpey's fibres, are derived from the principal fibres of the periodontal ligament. Sharpey's fibres are particularly prominent in the cervical portion (alveolar crest region) of the cribriform plate. Sharpey's fibres entering alveolar bone are less numerous but thicker than those at the cementum surface (Fig. 13.39). There is evidence that traces of type III collagen are found at the periphery of Sharpey's fibres (Fig. 13.40). Because of the attachments of numerous bundles of collagen fibres, the cribriform plate has also been called *bundle bone*. Bundle bone usually comprises thin lamellae running parallel to each other and to the root surface.

Scanning electron micrographs of anorganic preparations of the periodontal surfaces of alveolar bone show that the Sharpey's fibres have two main appearances, depending upon the degree of mineralisation. In one, the embedded fibres may remain unmineralised at their centres, and removal of their organic material results in a series of hollow centres (Fig. 13.41). Conversely, the inserting fibres may be fully mineralised and project beyond the surface of the bone as small, calcified prominences into the periodontal ligament (Fig. 13.42).

In the cervical part of the interdental septum, where the bone type is mainly compact, Sharpey's fibres entering the bone in the mesiodistal plane may pass straight through to become continuous with similar fibres from the root of the adjacent tooth. These are called *transalveolar fibres* (Fig. 13.43). A similar pattern exists in the interradicular bone, although in this situation the fibres link roots of the same tooth. Transalveolar fibres also pass through the entire thickness of the alveolar bone in the buccal and lingual planes, intermingling with the overlying periosteum or with the lamina propria of the gingiva (Fig. 13.44). However, where the alveolar bone is cancellous, no transalveolar fibres are seen.

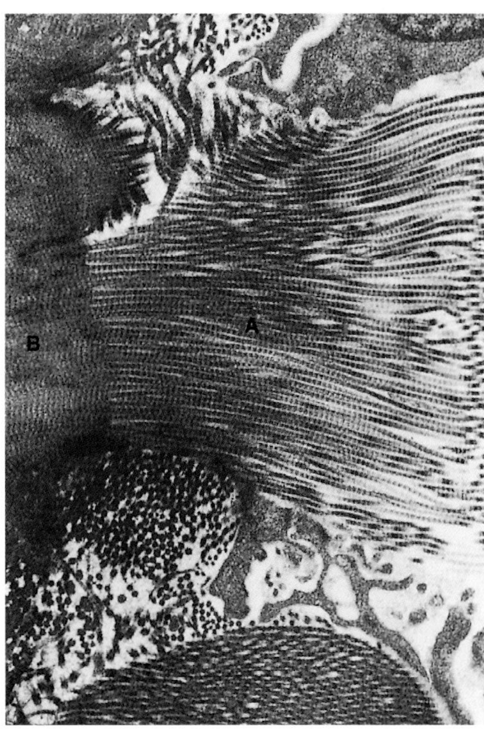

Fig. 13.38 TEM of a Sharpey's fibre (A) entering the surface of alveolar bone (B). Note the periodicity evident on the collagen fibrils (decalcified section; ×10,500).

Structural lines in bone

Bone is laid down rhythmically, which results in the formation of regular parallel lines that, because they are formed in periods of relative quiescence, are termed *resting lines*. Such resting lines differ biochemically from adjacent bone. These lines are prominent in bundle bone on the distal surface of the socket wall during physiological mesial drift of the teeth (Fig. 13.45). Bone will also contain reversal lines, representing the site of change from bone resorption to bone deposition (see Fig. 13.28).

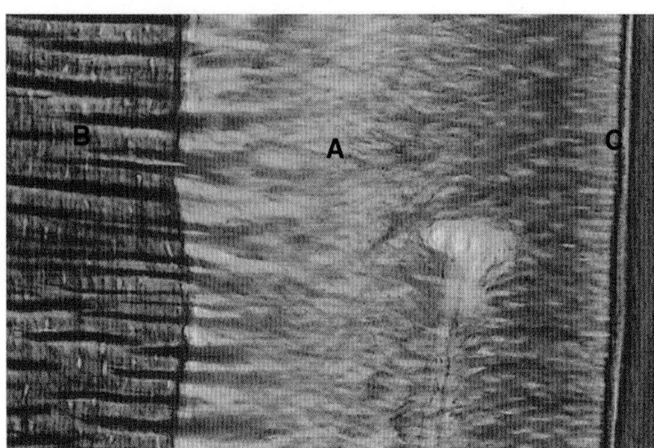

Fig. 13.39 Section of a root of a tooth showing Sharpey's fibres from the periodontal ligament (A) entering alveolar bone (B). The Sharpey's fibres in bone are seen to be thicker but less numerous than those entering the cementum on the tooth surface (C) (decalcified section; aldehyde fuchsin and van Gieson; ×250). Courtesy Prof. S J Jones.

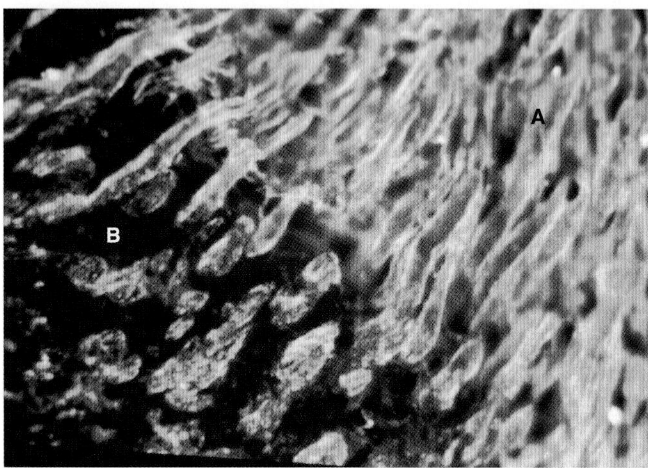

Fig. 13.40 Sharpey's fibre insertion from the periodontal ligament (A) into alveolar bone (B), showing peripheral labelling of inserting collagen bundles with immunofluorescent label for collagen type III (×350). From Sloan, P., Carter, D.H., 1995. Structural organisation of the fibres of the periodontal ligament. In: Berkovitz, B.K.B., Moxham, B.J., Newman, H. (Eds.), The Periodontal Ligament in Health and Disease, second ed. Mosby–Wolfe, London, pp 35–53.

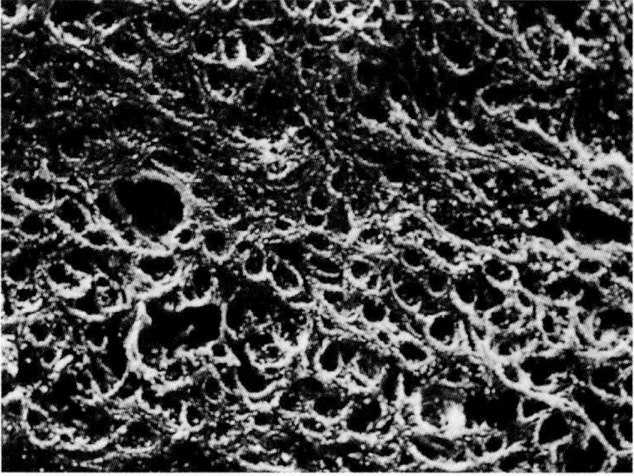

Fig. 13.41 SEM of Sharpey's fibres in alveolar bone with unmineralised centres, which are removed by the hypochlorite used to prepare this anorganic specimen (×300). Courtesy Prof. P Sloan.

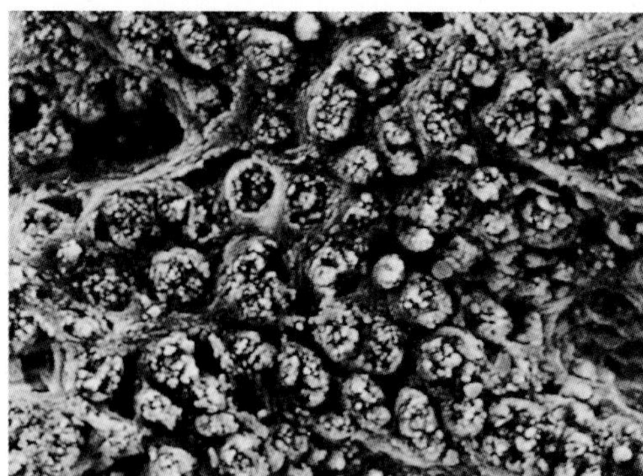

Fig. 13.42 SEM of Sharpey's fibres in alveolar bone, which are mineralised beyond the surface of the bone and remain as small, calcified projections into the periodontal ligament (anorganic preparation; ×300). Courtesy Prof. P Sloan.

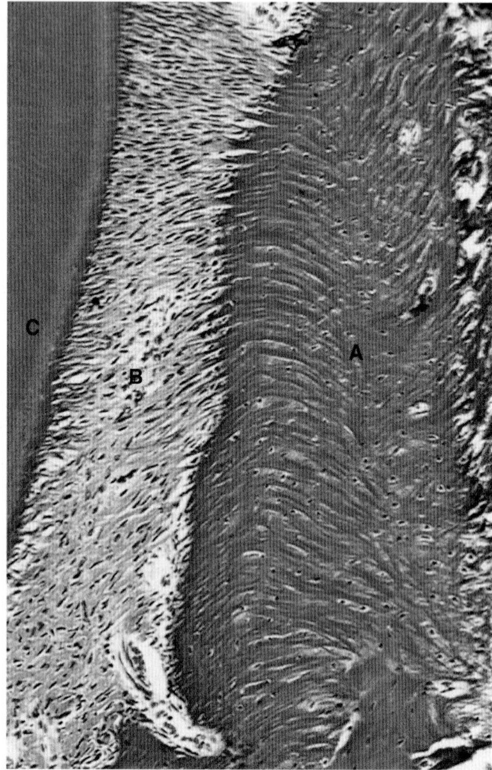

Fig. 13.43 Mesiodistal section of interdental bone (A), showing Sharpey's fibres from the periodontal ligament (B) appearing to pass more or less completely through the full thickness of bone between two adjacent teeth. C = root (decalcified longitudinal section; Masson's trichrome; ×100).

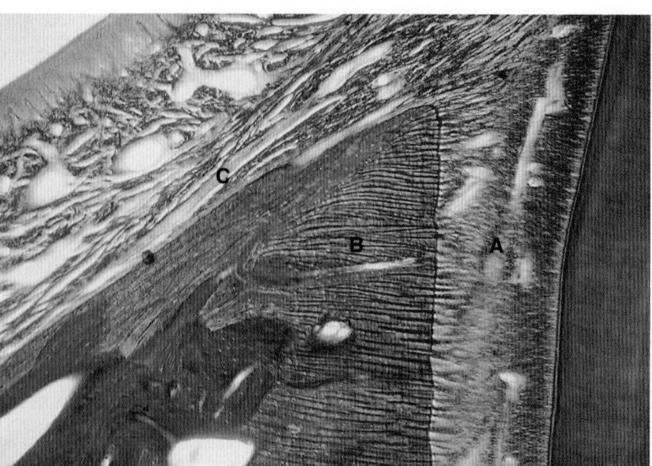

Fig. 13.44 Buccolingual section of tooth *in situ* appearing to show Sharpey's fibres passing from the periodontal ligament (A) through the compact alveolar bone (B) in the cervical region to reach the lamina propria of the attached gingiva (C) (decalcified longitudinal section; van Gieson; ×80). Courtesy Prof. S J Jones.

Such reversal lines will show evidence of a scalloped outline, reflecting the position of Howship's lacunae (Figs. 13.28, 13.30 and 13.46).

Age changes in alveolar bone

The most clinically important age change in bones is osteoporosis – the loss of cancellous bone in the hip and vertebrae predisposing towards fracture. The lack of significant amounts of cancellous bone in the jaws

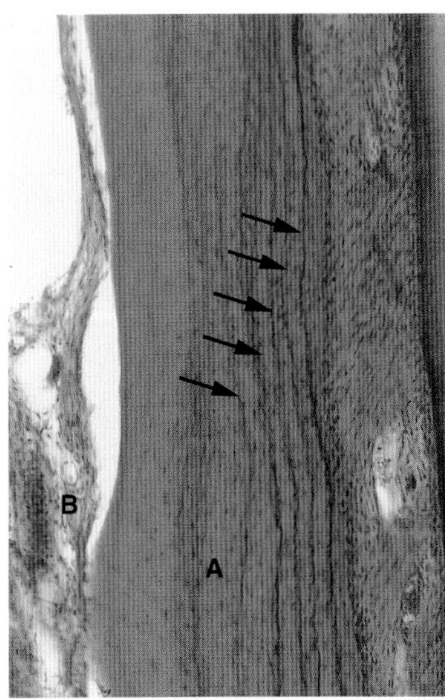

Fig. 13.45 Alveolar bone (A) on the distal wall of a tooth socket undergoing mesial drift, showing many vertical resting lines (arrows) resulting from the rhythmic deposition of bone with periods of quiescence. Together with Sharpey fibres inserting from periodontal ligament (B), this can be termed bundle bone. (H & E ×40).

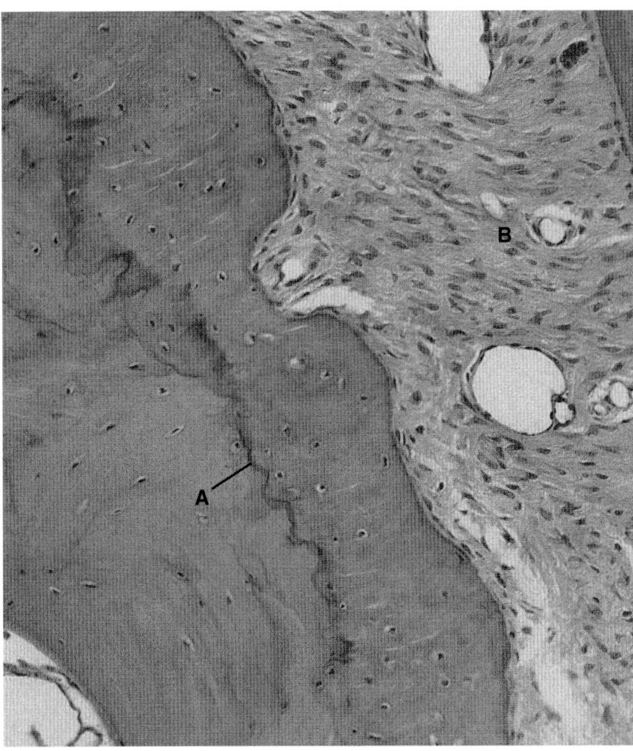

Fig. 13.46 Alveolar bone showing scalloped outline of a reversal line (A). B = periodontal ligament (H & E; ×250).

has not allowed for osteoporotic changes to be established in these sites. As alveolar bone is maintained by the presence of teeth, tooth loss will be accompanied by atrophy of the associated alveolar bone.

When measurements are taken on radiographs to determine the distance from the cementum–enamel junction to the alveolar bone crest, the results indicate a loss of crestal bone ageing, with the general state of oral hygiene contributing only slightly to the effect. Aging seems to reduce the height and width of the alveolar bone in the upper jaw rather than the lower, with the greatest effect on height. As the baseline alveolar bone height and width for a successful dental implant should approximate to 12 mm and 6 mm respectively, this indicates that older adults may not be able to receive implant treatment without also receiving a bone graft.

The degree of mineralisation of the mandible has been shown to be greater than that of other postcranial bones. There is also evidence of an increase in mandibular mineralisation density with age. The aged mandible also exhibits highly mineralised cement lines and pockets containing dead mineralised osteocytes. This increased mineralisation density may account for the clinical perception that tooth extraction is more difficult in the elderly: better-mineralised bone is more resistant to bending. As no relationship can be established between the overall degree of tissue mineralisation and the number, size or percentage of the tissue occupied by vascular (Haversian) canals, the possibility has been raised that bone tissue at different sites may be regulated by intrinsically distinct local and systemic factors.

It is often stated that the healing rate of fractures is slower in the elderly. This could possibly be related to a reduction in the number of stem cells available in the aged population. Aspects of treatment using tissue engineering principles are discussed on pages 282–283.

Clinical considerations

Localised bone loss

As maintenance of bone mass is dependent on suitable functional stimuli, alveolar bone tends to atrophy when tensile functional occlusal loading (transmitted via the periodontal ligament) is decreased. Thus following tooth extraction, alveolar bone will resorb unless the remaining ridge is loaded. Even the placement of a denture over the remaining alveolar ridge may retard total bone loss. However, if the prosthesis produces excessive compression, the denture-bearing area may show accelerated resorption.

The ability of alveolar bone to remodel throughout life allows teeth to be repositioned during orthodontic treatment, with resorption of bone in front of the moving tooth matched by deposition of bone behind. However, as osteoclasts cannot fully differentiate between dentine, cementum and bone, excessive orthodontic forces can cause root resorption, ranging from blunting the apices in minor cases up to destruction of a considerable portion of the root (see Fig. 13.50). As a consequence, many techniques are being examined to enhance orthodontic treatment and limit damage, including electrical pulses (note that this may stimulate the surrounding striated muscles, in turn deforming the bone), magnetic pulses and local injections of mediators of the inflammatory response. As yet, no technique has been shown to consistently enhance tooth movement or longevity.

The possible role of oxygen tension on osteoclast activity may help provide an explanation for the loss of bone that accompanies many clinical conditions where the blood supply is compromised and hypoxia is encountered (e.g., following inflammation, radiation damage, fractures and ageing).

Localised alveolar bone loss is found in periodontal disease (and in periapical abscesses) in response to the inflammatory process associated with the chronic presence of dental plaque and calculus at the cervical margins (see Figs 12.75-12.77). Bone loss is also associated with apical granulomas following inflammation of the pulp and cyst formation. In addition to dental cysts, there may be bone cysts related to the bone itself. If these cysts are present around the roots of teeth (Fig. 13.47), the teeth remain vital. Bone cysts may be lined by thin connective tissue. The cysts may be empty or contain a small amount of fluid. Among important bioactive molecules implicated in this resorption process are inflammatory cytokines and prostaglandins, as well as protons (as inflamed tissue is generally acidic). Differences exist between the collagen and the ground substance of bone and periodontal ligament. Analysis of their breakdown products in the local serum exudates contributing to gingival crevicular

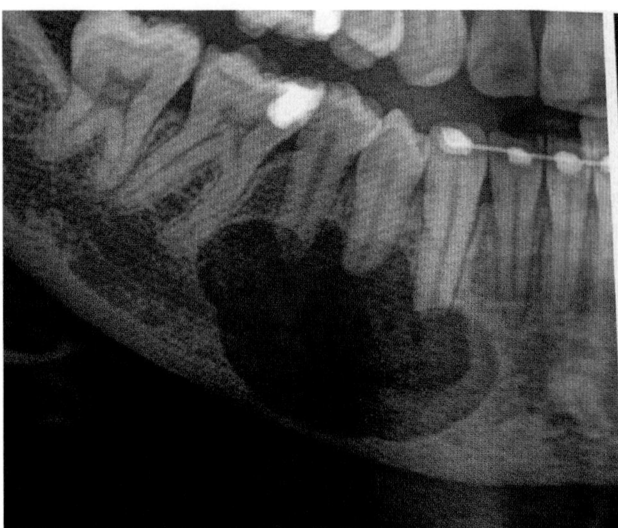

Fig. 13.47 Radiograph showing a solitary bone cyst developing around the root apices of a mandibular canine and the premolars. Some resorption of the root apices has occurred. From Odell, E.W. (Ed.), 2017. Cawson's Essentials of Oral Pathology and Medicine, ninth ed. Elsevier, 2017, London. 12.33A.

fluid may provide a marker to distinguish those patients who are more at risk of losing alveolar bone. Levels of such molecules will also be found to increase when crevicular fluid is analysed in patients undergoing orthodontic tooth movement.

Malignant tumours of bone

A primary osteosarcoma can occasionally occur in the maxilla and mandible. This condition will present as a rapidly growing, painful, firm swelling of the jaws (Fig. 13.48). A radiograph will reveal an irregular calcific mass (Fig. 13.49).

Jaw metastases are relatively uncommon and signify a late-stage disease. They may present as a small or large lesion. They may derive from a carcinoma whose primary site may be the breast, bronchus, prostate, thyroid gland or kidney.

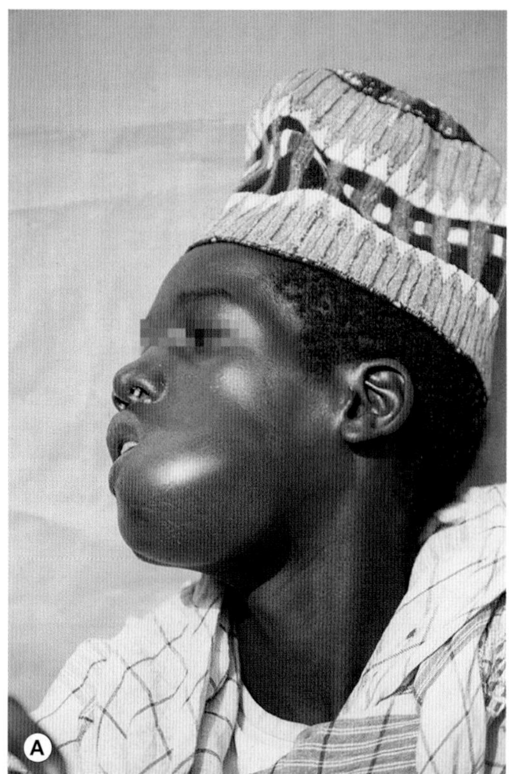

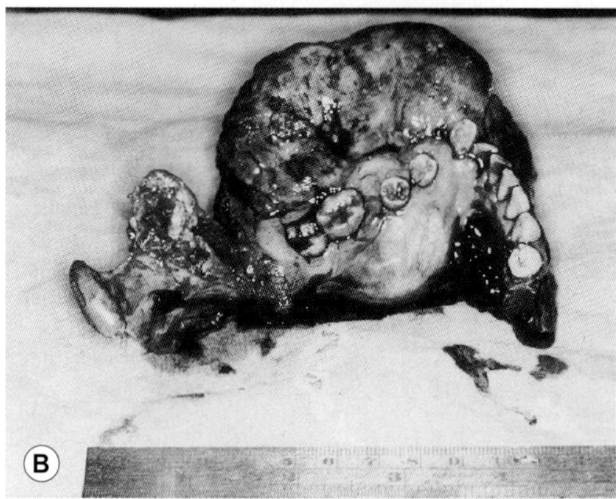

Fig 13.48 (A) 16-year-old boy presenting with a swelling of the left side of the mandible caused by an osteosarcoma. (B) Resection specimen shows 3 cm–plus margins. From Kaban, L.B., Troulis, M.J. (Eds.), 2004. Pediatric Oral and Maxillofacial Surgery. Elsevier, Philadelphia.

Osteoporosis

Apart from localised inflammation, more generalised conditions exist where the normal balance between bone formation and bone resorption is disturbed. A knowledge of the normal histological and radiological appearance of bone helps in diagnosing disease. For example, osteopetrosis is a heterogeneous disorder characterised by impaired osteoclast function. In one type, there is a deficiency of the enzyme carbonic anhydrase type II, and although bone formation occurs, the defective osteoclasts lose their ability to resorb normally formed bone, which becomes increasingly thickened. An analogous condition in rodents prevents teeth from erupting because of the inability of osteoclasts to resorb the overlying bone. The cause of one such condition is a lack of production of M-CSF. If the missing factor is replaced, osteoclasts can be formed to allow alveolar bone resorption and normal eruption.

Several different strategies can be considered to combat the reverse situation that follows when uncoupling results in more resorption than formation (primarily in cancellous bone), eventually leading to osteoporosis. This is a bone disorder characterised by a low bone mass but of normal constitution. It particularly affects trabecular bone, which has

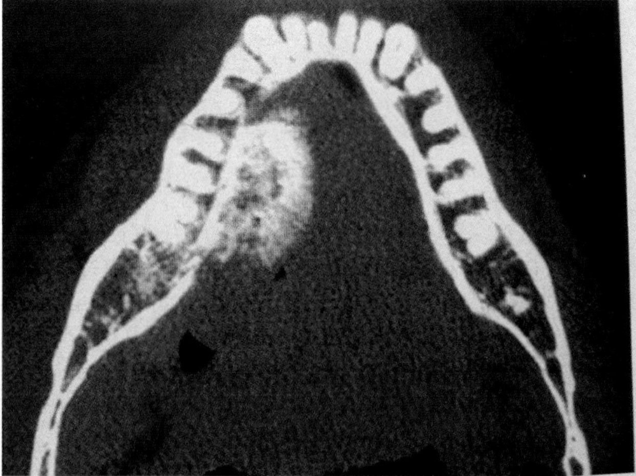

Fig 13.49 Computed tomography radiograph of an osteosarcoma revealing the mass to contain bone, which has a radiating 'sun-ray' appearance (arrow). Fernandes, R., et al., 2007. *Osteogenic sarcoma of the jaw: a 10-year experience*. J. Oral Maxillofac. Surg. 65 (7), 1286–1291.

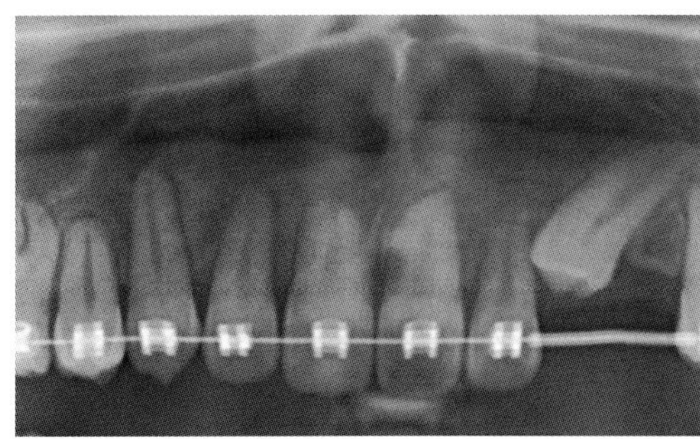

Fig. 13.50 Radiograph showing patient with fixed appliance attached to maxillary anterior teeth that has resulted in significant root resorption. Courtesy Dr J Makdissi.

a higher turnover rate than compact bone, and predisposes the patient to spontaneous or low trauma energy level fractures, as, once lost, the bone mass is not usually replaced. Vulnerable sites include the neck of the femur and the lumbar vertebrae. Osteoporosis can be age related and particularly affects postmenopausal women, but is of less importance for the jaws, which have comparatively small amounts of cancellous bone and therefore more mineralised tissue per unit volume than many other parts of the skeleton. The precise cause of osteoporosis is not known, although several factors, including sex hormone (particularly oestrogen) deficiency, lack of mechanical loading and glucocorticoid excess, have been identified (Table 13.2). From a knowledge of the different stages in the life cycle of the osteoclast (Fig. 13.27), various therapeutic strategies can be adopted to counteract bone resorption by administering drugs that might:

- enhance the OPG:RANKL ratio and interfere with the formation of osteoclasts (e.g., oestrogens)
- interfere with the attachment mechanisms of osteoclasts (e.g., calcitonin)
- speed up apoptosis in osteoclasts (e.g., bisphosphonates, OPG, denosumab)[a] and block the activity of degradative enzymes (e.g., odanacatib, a drug that blocks the activity of cathepsin K)

As sclerostin is localised specifically to bone, antibodies are being developed that, on injection, may increase the rate of bone formation. Thus, it is a potential form of treatment for osteoporosis.

A side effect of patients receiving bisphosphonates for treatment of bone cancer or osteoporosis is necrosis of bone in the jaws.

Analyses of various molecules in the blood and/or urine are also of importance in diagnosing conditions affecting the turnover rate of bone. These molecules include calcium, parathyroid hormone, acid phosphatase and alkaline phosphatase. In addition, collagen type I cross-linked N-terminals result from the proteolytic cleavage caused by osteoclasts, and their levels in serum or urine are indicative of turnover rates, as are the levels of hydroxyproline and hydroxylysine.

In a wider sphere, as osteocytes produce FGF23 and therefore help to regulate phosphate metabolism, a fuller understanding of these cells may provide a deeper insight into diseases of hypophosphatemia and hyperphosphatemia, such as chronic kidney disease and cardiovascular disorders.

[a]Denosumab is a drug that represents the first fully monoclonal antibody to treat osteoporosis in postmenopausal women. This drug is an inhibitor of RANKL and thus has a similar action to that of osteoprotegerin (which is present in decreasing concentrations in osteoporotic patients).

Dental implants

Implantology is a clinical area where knowledge of the biology of bone is important. Whereas a foreign material placed into bone is normally regarded as 'non-self' and becomes surrounded by a capsule of fibrous tissue running parallel to the foreign material surface, some materials allow for a direct structural osseous union. When inserted into the jaw to provide the basis of support for a crown, denture or orthodontic appliance, this union between the dental implant and adjacent living bone is termed *osseointegration*. The principal features of the two-stage placement of a dental implant are shown in Fig. 13.51. The materials most commonly used in the jaws are based on titanium or its aluminium/vanadium alloys, the spontaneously formed metal oxide (ceramic) surfaces being critical to integration. Although the earliest implants had a smooth surface, modifications of the surface texture provide a more successful outcome. A narrow interface (20–40 nm) between the bone and implant contains non-collagenous bone matrix proteins such as osteopontin and bone sialoprotein. The successful long-term retention of an implant depends on:

1) correct surgical technique to ensure minimum trauma, heating and infection at the implant site
2) absence of excessive micromotion following implantation
3) factors related to the implant (such as shape, topography, stiffness, composition and surface chemistry)

The host responses essential for a successful clinical outcome include blood clot formation in which the necessary factors for successful osteogenesis, such as cytokines, growth factors and osteoprogenitor cells, are present. If thermal control has not been optimal during placement, the bone immediately adjacent to the implant may be compromised.

Normally, adjacent to the implant, bone to a depth of 1 mm may necrose and be remodelled and replaced by new bone, with a period of about 17 weeks being required for the establishment of a suitable viable bone interface with the implant. Some modern implantation techniques can, however, allow immediate function if the implant is rigidly held in good-quality dense cortical bone. From a knowledge of basic bone biology, implants are being used that are coated with materials thought likely to encourage osseointegration, such as cell adhesion molecules and hydroxyapatite crystals, although delamination of material layers in such a hostile environment can cause long-term problems.

Of clinical importance is the fact that, following the insertion of a dental implant, the junctional epithelium regenerates and attaches to the implant surface and the implant abutment surface by a basal lamina and hemidesmosomes.

Despite the absence of a periodontal ligament, patients with dental implants have reported improved tactile and motor function when compared with patients wearing complete dentures. The development of tactile sensibility through osseointegrated dental implants is called *osseoperception*.

Despite the obvious success of osseointegration of dental implants, this does not allow for micromovements and shock absorption that occur in the presence of a periodontal ligament. Hence, some researchers are employing tissue engineering principles to manufacture a periodontal ligament around a dental implant. This necessitates the generation of a periodontal ligament whose fibres can attach on one side to the surface of the implant via a layer of cementum-like material and on the other side to the surface of the bony socket. This will necessitate coating the implant with tissue-cultured periodontal ligament–like stem cells seeded on a suitable extracellular matrix

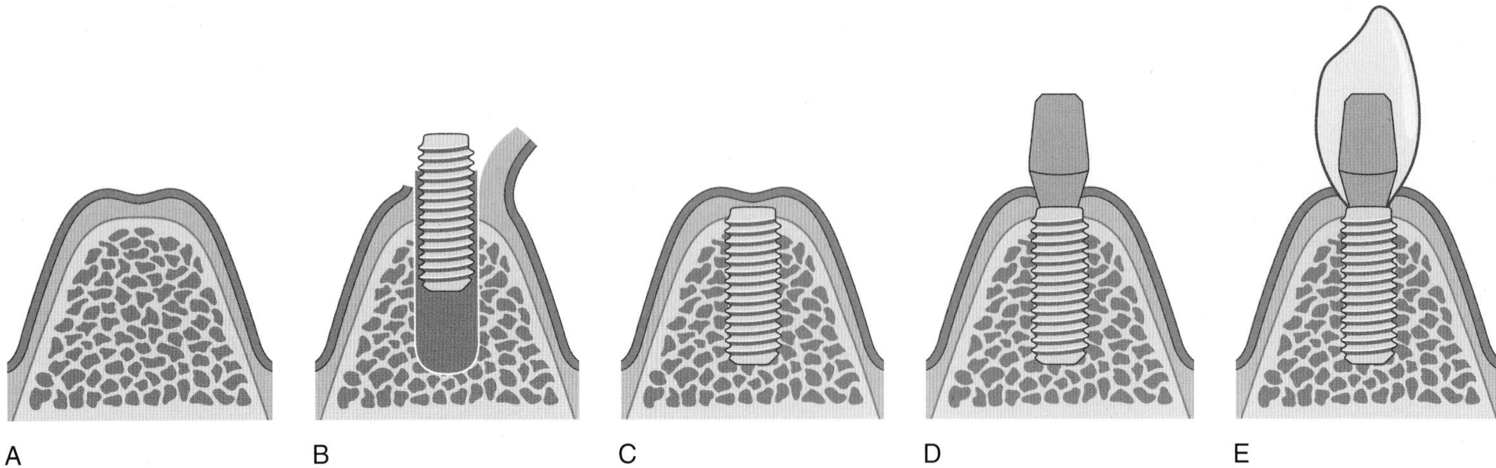

Fig. 13.51 Basic features of dental implant surgery in a two-stage operation. (A) Region of jaw where tooth has been lost. (B) Exposure of bone of jaw, drilling of channel and fitting of a cylindrical titanium screw-thread implant inserted into the jaw bone. The overlying gum is then replaced and sutured and the implant left to heal for about 3 months free from loading forces. (C) After 3 months, wound healing results in the implant becoming firmly bonded (osseointegrated) to the adjacent bone. (D) Implant re-exposed and a post (abutment) inserted into a channel at the top of the implant. (E) Crown fitted to the abutment. From Berkovitz, B.K.B., 2013. Nothing But the Tooth. Elsevier, London. Redrawn from Branemark, P.-I., Hansson, B.O., Adell, R., Breine, U., et al., 1977. Osseointegrated implants in the treatment of the edentulous jaws. Experience from a 10-year period. Scandinavian Journal of Plastic and Reconstructive Surgery 16, 1–132.

and including any relevant bioactive molecules such as growth factors. When this happens, it will then be possible to determine whether such an implant will be an improvement on the osseointegrated implant.

An alternative strategy for replacing a tooth is to use tissue engineering to develop a new one. Although this might be regarded as `the gold standard', the problems to be overcome to successful achieve this are considerable. If a crown is to be engineered, how does one produce enamel of such thickness and complexity within a reasonable timescale, apart from the present difficulties in obtaining epithelial stem cells? Similarly, how does one produce a root that will attach to the crown and function in tooth movement and support? One approach to this problem is to concentrate on just producing a root to which a synthetic crown can be attached, as for an implant. As a step towards this approach, it has been shown that stem cells that provide pulpal tissue can be derived from the apical region of teeth extracted for orthodontic reasons and from impacted third molars, both having incompletely formed roots. These stem cells from root apical papilla (SCAP) can then be tissue cultured in the laboratory to increase numbers. Similarly, periodontal ligament stem cells (PDLSCs) can be scraped off the root surfaces of an extracted tooth. A root-shaped matrix of tricalcium-phosphate/hydroxyapatite (TCP-HA) bone is then prepared to be of a correct size to fit into the socket to be filled. This matrix is designed with an inner post channel to allow for subsequent installation of a porcelain crown. The SCAP are placed in the central cavity of the matrix, while the PDLSCs are coated over the external surface of the matrix, which is then placed in the socket to be filled and sutured to prevent significant forces displacing it. After a few months it is envisaged that the tissue-engineered root may have developed a viable periodontal ligament and dental pulp tissue. If this results, then a crown can be placed in the channel of the post.

Fractures, tooth extraction and bone grafts

As fractures involving the face and jaws are common, an understanding of the principles involved in bone healing is essential. Similarly, after tooth extraction, the empty socket will initially fill with a blood clot. In this clot, granulation tissue will form and stem cells and osteoprogenitor cells will soon appear. These cells will eventually differentiate into osteoblasts, this process involving cell–matrix interactions. The initial immature (woven) bone will ultimately be remodelled to form mature, fine-fibred bone, having served its purpose by achieving an initial rapid fracture repair.

In some clinical situations, in particular the replacement of bone lost to trauma or to malignant disease, there is a need for larger amounts of bone to aid healing. Requirements may be met by bone grafting, sourcing material from either autologous bone (taken from the patient), allografts (taken from another person) or xenografts (taken from a different species, an example being Bio-Oss bovine bone chips, Fig. 13.52). One advantage of autologous grafting is that if large sites are chosen, such as the radius, a soft tissue flap can accompany the bone and be kept alive by uniting the microvascular circulation of the moved tissue to the host site circulation (a free flap with microvascular anastomoses). Bone transferred as allografts or as xenografts tends to be dead stored tissue, utilised as a scaffold for repair only.

However, major advances are being made to apply tissue engineering techniques to produce laboratory-based materials. There are significant advantages for donor site morbidity, chemical purity and cross-infection risks in the synthetic approach. Such materials can either substitute for bone or provide scaffolds and deliver stimuli to promote more rapid bony healing in both adverse sites and those too large to heal by themselves (critical-sized defects).

The three components to be considered in tissue engineering are 1) the scaffold, 2) the cells and 3) additional molecules to drive osteogenesis:

1) The scaffold must clearly be biocompatible and must have a specific configuration that allows osteogenic cells to migrate across, differentiate and then mineralise the artificial matrix. It must also allow for angiogenesis to maintain the newly colonised graft and for the possibility of being resorbed as new bone is formed and remodelled. It is an advantage if ultimately no residual foreign body remains as a long-term hazard. Among the materials under investigation are organic compounds such as collagen matrices and synthetic polymers (polylactic/polyglycolic acid fibres), inorganic osteoconductive ceramic materials (such as deproteinated corals and synthetic hydroxyapatites) and soluble bioactive glasses (Fig. 13.53). The latter's ionic dissolution products (including silicon) and their gel-like surface accrete hydroxyapatite, stimulate osteoprogenitor cells and accelerate mature functioning osteoblast production within a wound, stimulate angiogenic and inflammatory

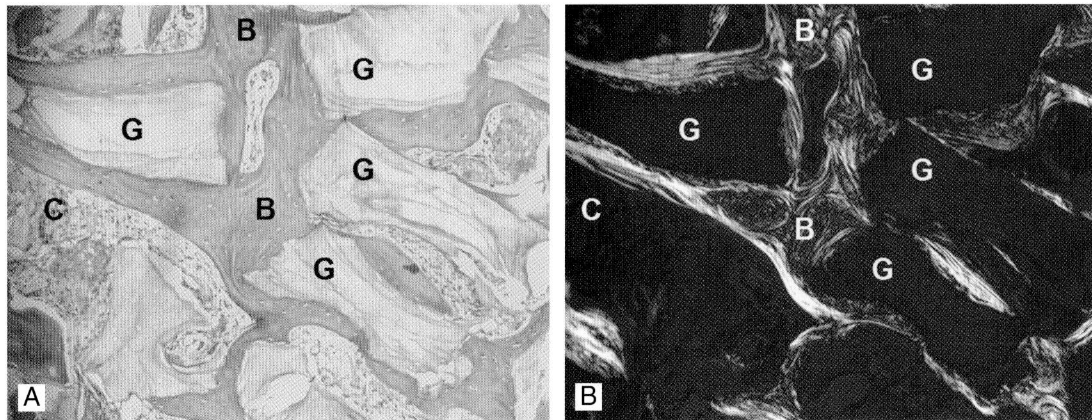

Fig. 13.52 (A) Demineralised section showing a well-healed, granular bovine xenograft (G) placed in an extraction socket to augment the alveolar bone prior to implant placement. New compact lamellar bone (B) and supporting connective tissue (C) have grown through the deproteinated, mineral graft (H & E; ×90). (B) Same section as in (A) but viewed under polarised light. Unlike the ordered collagen fibres of the new lamellar bone, the deproteinated graft does not show the birefringence patterns in polarised light and remains black (H & E; ×90). Courtesy Dr. R J Cook.

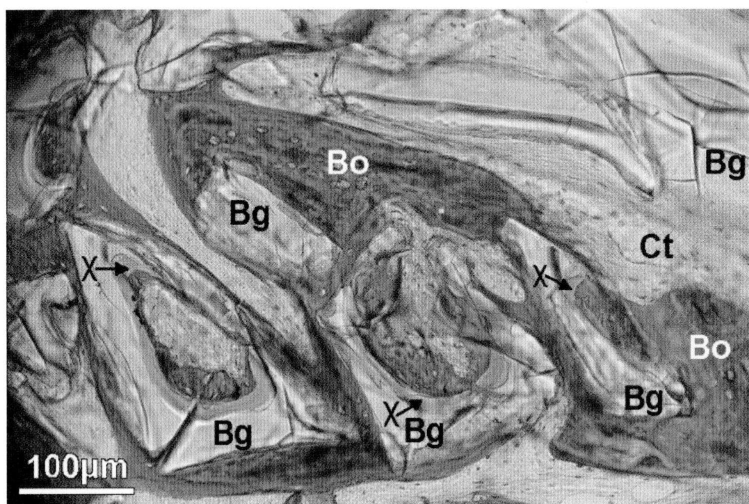

Fig. 13.53 Plastic-embedded ground section showing fully integrated soluble bioactive glass granules (Bg) placed in a human mandible to augment an extraction socket prior to implant placement. New bone (Bo) and connective tissue (Ct) have grown into and bonded directly to the new hydroxyapatite surfaces, formed on the outer silica gel layer (X) of the reacted glass particles (Sanderson's rapid bone stain). Courtesy Dr. R J Cook.

responses and provide an osteoconductive surface over which new bone may grow.

2) Stem cells and those able to divert to an osteogenic phenotype are the most important to enter the graft material or scaffold. These may be derived from the patient's own cells by two processes. Either they migrate to the wound sites directly or they can be delivered in concentrated form, having been isolated, selected, expanded in culture and then seeded into the scaffold *in vitro* or *in vivo*. Another approach is to develop lines of stem cells from embryos that have osteogenic potential and that may be safely seeded into a scaffold without fear of rejection by the immune system of the patient.
3) A large number of molecules such as cytokines, growth factors and cell–matrix adhesion factors are required for successful differentiation of stem cells into functional osteoblasts. It is not surprising, therefore, that much experimental work has been devoted to integration of these molecules into graft matrices in the hope of improving the properties of such artificial scaffolds. However, much work is still required to identify the best method of delivery of such molecules. For example, if BMPs are beneficial to the development of active osteoblasts, is it better to adsorb this protein to the material before implantation or to genetically manipulate stem cells used to seed the matrix to produce more of this factor themselves?

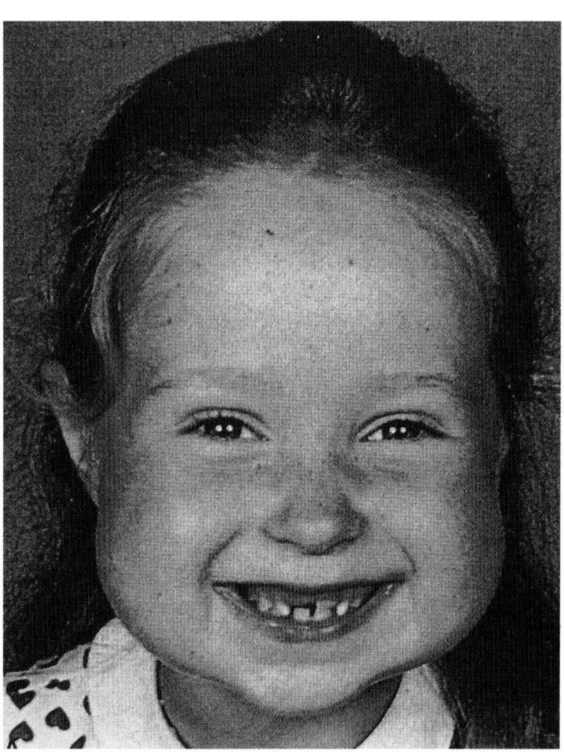

Fig. 13.54 A young child with cherubism. Note the rounded outline of the face due to multiple multilocular bone lesions in the mandible and maxillae. From Cawson, R.A., Binnie, W.H., Barrett, A.W., et al., 2001. Oral disease. third ed. Mosby, St. Louis.

The rate of fracture repair appears to slow down with age, the precise reason for which remains to be clarified. It may be that there is a reduction in the number of viable stem cells in bone with age. An approach to speed up fracture repair in older patients is to isolate some stem cells from the patient's bone, culture them to increase their numbers and then seed them in a suitable framework that is then placed in the fracture site.

Cherubism

Cherubism is a rare autosomal condition that arises in childhood and is believed to result from a mutation of the gene *SH3BP2*. The normal bone of the maxilla and mandible is lost and replaced by numerous cysts, which give the face a characteristic rounded "cherub-like" outline (Fig. 13.54).

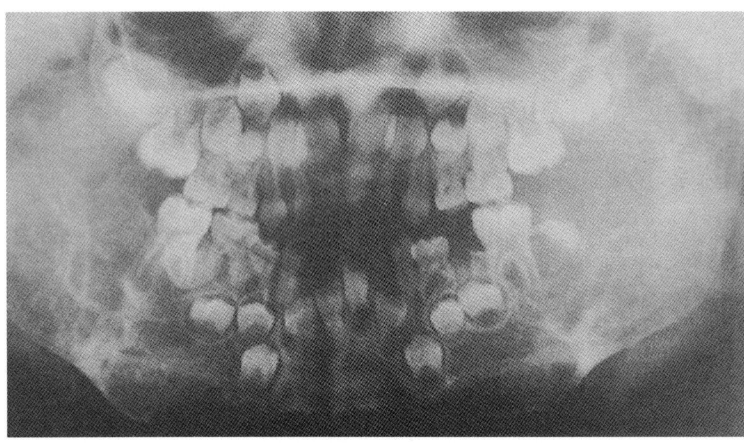

Fig. 13.55 Radiograph of young child with cherubism. The jaws are expanded by multilocular radiolucent lesions that have displaced and destroyed developing permanent teeth. From Odell, E.W. (Ed.), 2017. Cawson's Essentials of Oral Pathology and Medicine, ninth ed. Elsevier.

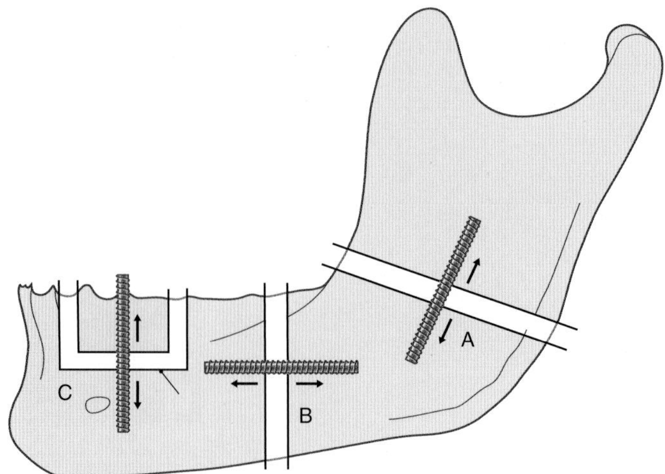

Fig. 13.56 Schematic diagram of the mandible showing osteotomy sites for distraction osteogenesis allowing for increase in height of ramus (A), increase in length of body of mandible (B) and increase in height of alveolus to allow for implants (C). A cut across the mandibular symphysis would allow for increase in width.

There is an associated displacement and premature loss of deciduous teeth and a lack of eruption of permanent teeth (Fig. 13.55).

Distraction osteogenesis

Distraction osteogenesis refers to the technique whereby a bone is sectioned (an osteotomy) and, after an initial interval of 5–7 days, a slow, controlled separation (about 0.5–1 mm/day) of the two bone fragments is undertaken to allow length augmentation by the sustained addition of new woven bone at the fracture site, formed under tension. When adequate length has been achieved, the two bone ends are immobilised for some weeks to allow the woven bone callus to be reinforced and ultimately replaced by mature dense lamellar bone. For success, the original periosteum and blood supply must be retained. Although this technique was initially developed to increase the length of long bones, it has been adapted for use in craniofacial situations where there is marked bony underdevelopment, such as the small mandible of micrognathia. The mandible can be increased in length and height, depending on the orientation of the preplanned osteotomies (Fig. 13.56).

When teeth have been extracted, the alveolar bone atrophies. In such cases, distraction osteogenesis may allow for an increased alveolar height to render the site suitable for implants. There is some evidence that, during the early phase of bone remodelling in the distraction site, there is a marked level of osteoclastic activity that may be reflected in root resorption of teeth being orthodontically moved into the distraction site.

Further readings for this chapter can be found in the accompanying eBook. Explore online Self-assessment quiz to test and reinforce your understanding of the material in your free ebook. Follow instructions in the Inside Front Cover to unlock your access.

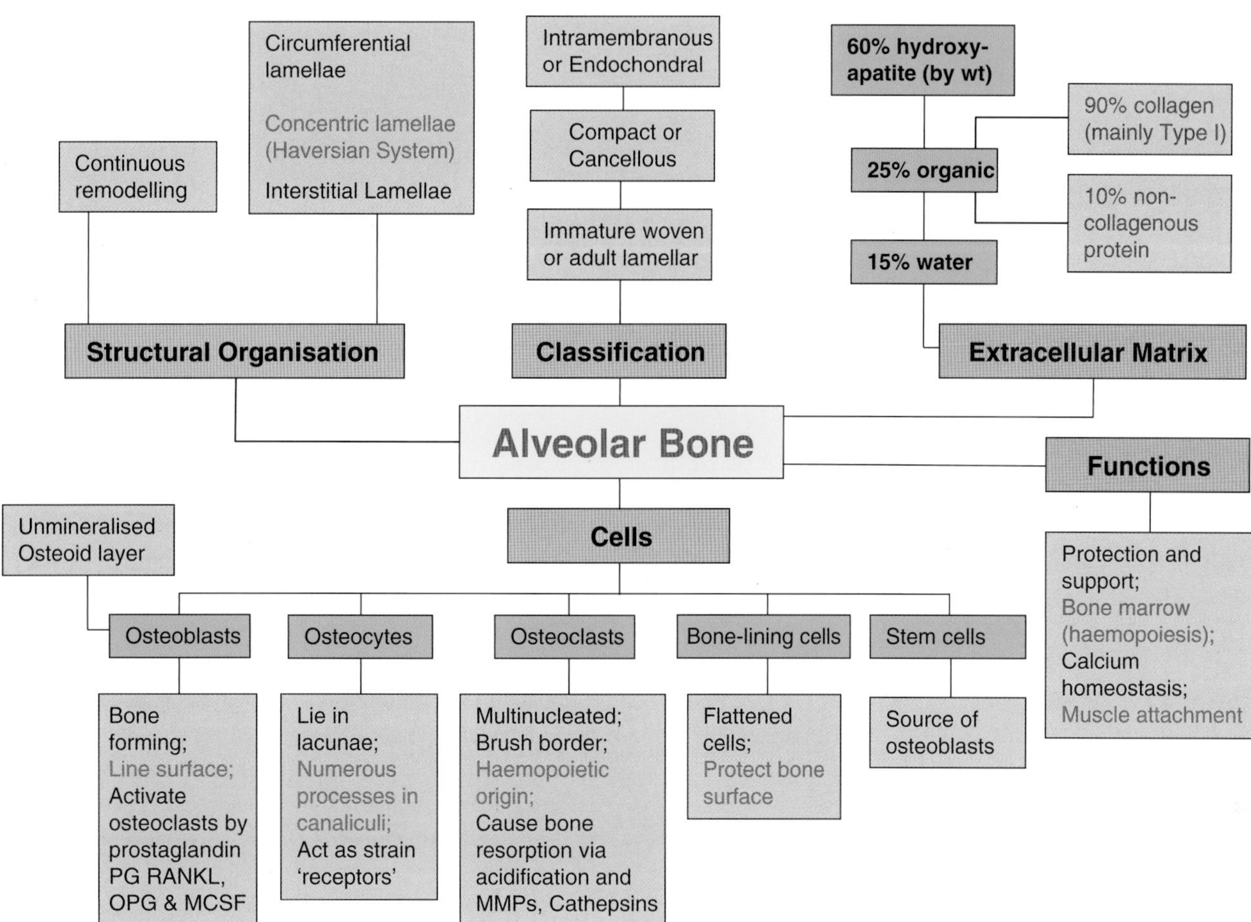
Circumferential lamellae
Concentric lamellae (Haversian System)
Interstitial Lamellae
Intramembranous or Endochondral
Compact or Cancellous
Immature woven or adult lamellar
60% hydroxy-apatite (by wt)
25% organic
90% collagen (mainly Type I)
10% non-collagenous protein
15% water
Continuous remodelling
Structural Organisation
Classification
Extracellular Matrix
Alveolar Bone
Functions
Unmineralised Osteoid layer
Cells
Osteoblasts
Osteocytes
Osteoclasts
Bone-lining cells
Stem cells
Protection and support;
Bone marrow (haemopoiesis);
Calcium homeostasis;
Muscle attachment
Bone forming;
Line surface;
Activate osteoclasts by prostaglandin PG RANKL, OPG & MCSF
Lie in lacunae;
Numerous processes in canaliculi;
Act as strain 'receptors'
Multinucleated;
Brush border;
Haemopoietic origin;
Cause bone resorption via acidification and MMPs, Cathepsins
Flattened cells;
Protect bone surface
Source of osteoblasts

Mind Map 13.1 Alveolar Bone.

14 Oral mucosa

Whereas the skin is dry and provides the covering for the external surface of the body, the alimentary tract is lined with a moist mucosa (mucous membrane). The mucosa is specialised in each region of the alimentary tract, but the basic pattern of an epithelium with an underlying connective tissue (the lamina propria) is maintained and is analogous to the epidermis and dermis of the skin, respectively. In many regions, a third layer (the submucosa) is found between the lamina propria and the underlying bone (palate) or muscle (cheeks and lips).

The oral mucosa shows specialisations that allow it to fulfil several roles:

- It is protective mechanically against both compressive and shearing forces.
- It provides a barrier to micro-organisms, toxins and various antigens.
- It is involved in immunological defence, both humoral and cell-mediated.
- Minor glands within the oral mucosa provide lubrication and buffering as well as secretion of some antibodies. The viscoelastic mucous film also acts as a barrier, helping to retain water and electrolytes.
- The mucosa is richly innervated, providing input for touch, proprioception, pain and taste.

Two distinct layers are readily recognised in the oral mucosa for all regions of the mouth (Fig. 14.1). The outer layer is a stratified squamous epithelium that in areas subjected to masticatory forces (e.g., gingiva, palate and dorsum of tongue) is keratinised. The epithelium is derived embryologically from either ectoderm or endoderm. Beneath the epithelium is the connective tissue comprising the lamina propria. The submucosa consists of a looser connective tissue containing fat deposits and glands. Larger nerves and blood vessels run in the submucosa. The boundary between the connective tissues of the lamina propria and the submucosa is often indistinct.

The oral mucosa may be classified into three types: masticatory, lining and specialised mucosa. Masticatory mucosa is found where there is high compression and friction and is characterised by a keratinised epithelium and a thick lamina propria, which is usually bound down directly and tightly to underlying bone (mucoperiosteum).

Epithelium

Several layers of cells of distinct morphologies may be recognised in the stratified squamous epithelium covering the oral cavity (Fig. 14.2):

- Basal layer (stratum germinativum or stratum basale)
- Prickle cell layer (stratum spinosum)
- Granular layer (stratum granulosum)
- Keratinised (cornified) layer (stratum corneum)

All four layers are present in masticatory mucosa and, as the end product is a covering layer of cells filled with cytokeratins (CKs), the cells are termed *keratinocytes*. Other proteins related to the cell membrane, such as loricrin, involucrin and filaggrin, are synthesised as the cells differentiate. In the case of lining mucosa, the outer two layers (granular and keratinised layers) are absent and replaced by a nonkeratinising superficial layer. Epithelial cells exhibit endocytosis and therefore have the capacity to internalise small particles.

Unlike skin, the oral mucosa does not have a clear layer (stratum lucidum) between the granular and keratinised layers.

The different layers of the oral epithelium represent a progressive maturation process. Cells from the most superficial layer are continuously. Turnover time is fastest immediately adjacent to the tooth surface (about 5 days) for the junctional and crevicular epithelia. This is about twice as fast as the turnover time in lining mucosa such as the cheek. Turnover time in masticatory mucosa appears to be a little slower than that in nonmasticatory (lining) mucosa.

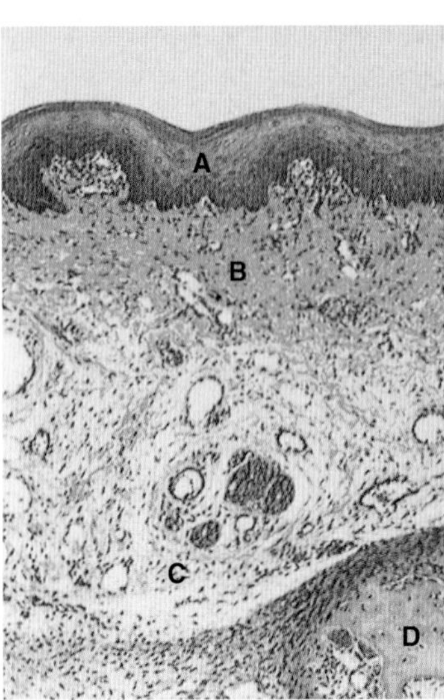

Fig. 14.1 Section showing regions of oral mucosa. A = stratified squamous epithelium; B = lamina propria; C = submucosa; D = bone (Masson's trichrome; ×35).

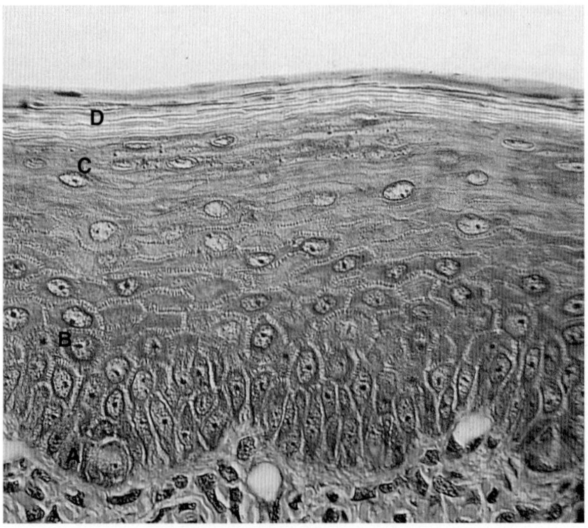

Fig. 14.2 Section showing layers of keratinised oral epithelium. A = basal layer; B = prickle cell layer; C = granular layer; D = keratinised layer (×180).

Basal layer

The basal layer is the single cell layer adjacent to the lamina propria and demarcated from it by a basal lamina (see pages 295–296). It consists of cuboidal cells, among which is a population of stem cells. Stem cells on mitosis give rise to two daughter cells, one of which at least remains a stem cell. Stem cells generate transit-amplifying cells that will undergo several further cell divisions, migrate from the basal cell layer and differentiate to give rise to replacement keratinocytes in the epithelial layers above. The stem cells within the basal layer are found mainly at the base of the epithelial ridges (rete) that project into the lamina propria. Not all cells dividing in the basal layer are true stem cells. Stem cells appear to express anti-apoptotic proteins (e.g., Bcl2 protein), and it has been claimed that this allows them to remain stem cells. Mitotic figures can occasionally be seen with routine staining (Fig. 14.3). However, all cells with mitotic potential can be seen with special stains (Fig. 14.4).

The cells of the basal layer are the least differentiated within the oral epithelium, and this is reflected in their ultrastructural appearance. They contain a limited amount of the intracellular organelles associated with secretion of proteins for the formation of components of the basal lamina (e.g., endoplasmic reticulum, Golgi apparatus and mitochondria). Some tonofilaments of keratin reflect their (Fig. 14.5). Cell contacts in the form of desmosomes, hemidesmosomes, intermediate and gap junctions are present, allowing for adhesion, cell signalling and other functions.

It is not known what triggers the start of differentiation in the basal layer, but it does not appear to be simply a matter of displacement away from the basal layer, as tissue culture studies indicate that, if cells are prevented from migrating away from the basal lamina, differentiation still occurs. Rather, the onset of differentiation seems to change the adhesive properties of the cell, perhaps involving the nature of its integrins, and leads to its ‘expulsion’ from the basal layer. Further movement upwards towards the surface and final desquamation will involve much activity relating to the development, quality, turnover and breakdown of cell attachments and adhesion molecules.

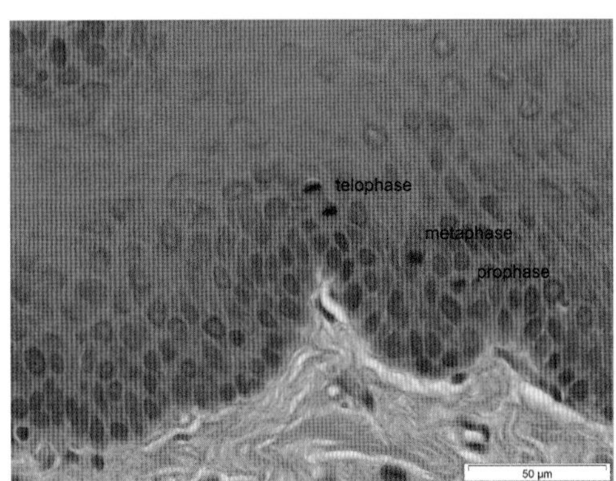

Fig. 14.3 Section of oral epithelium showing three mitotic figures and their stages (H & E). Courtesy Prof. P R Morgan.

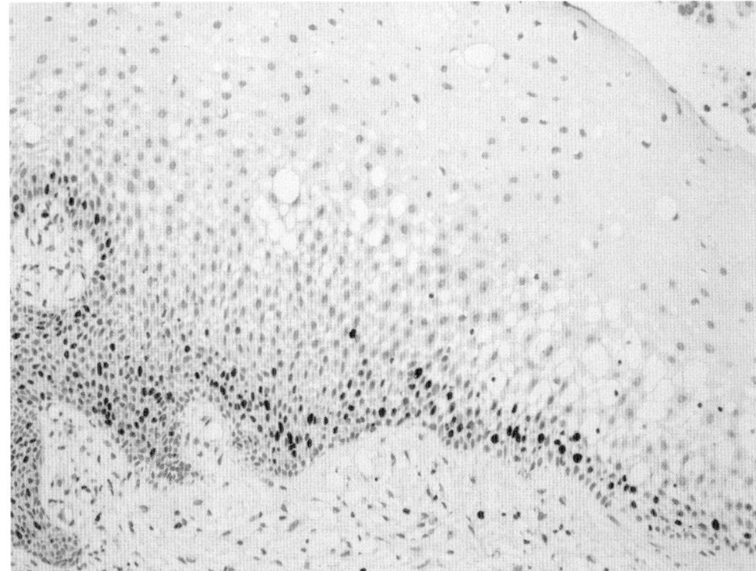

Fig. 14.4 Section of oral epithelium showing cells undergoing cell replication (red stain) (stained with MIB1 and counterstained with haematoxylin ×100). Courtesy Prof. P R Morgan.

Prickle cell layer

Above the basal layer round or ovoid cells form a layer several cells thick called the *prickle cell layer* (Fig. 14.2). These cells show the first stages of maturation, being larger and rounder than those in the basal layer. The transition from basal to prickle cell layer is characterised by the appearance of new CK types (see pages 290–291). They contribute to the formation of the tonofilaments, which become thicker and more conspicuous. Involucrin (the soluble precursor protein of the cornified envelope eventually found in the cornified layer) appears first in the prickle cell layer. There is a progressive decrease in synthetic activity through the layer.

In the upper part of the prickle cell layer small, intracellular membrane-coating granules (approximately 0.25 µm in length) appear. These granules are rich in phospholipids and, in keratinised epithelium, consist of a series of parallel lamellae. They probably originate from the Golgi apparatus. In the more superficial layers of the stratum spinosum the granules come to lie close to the cell membrane.

Within the prickle cell layer, desmosomes increase in number and become more obvious than in the basal layer (Figs. 14.6, 14.7). The slight

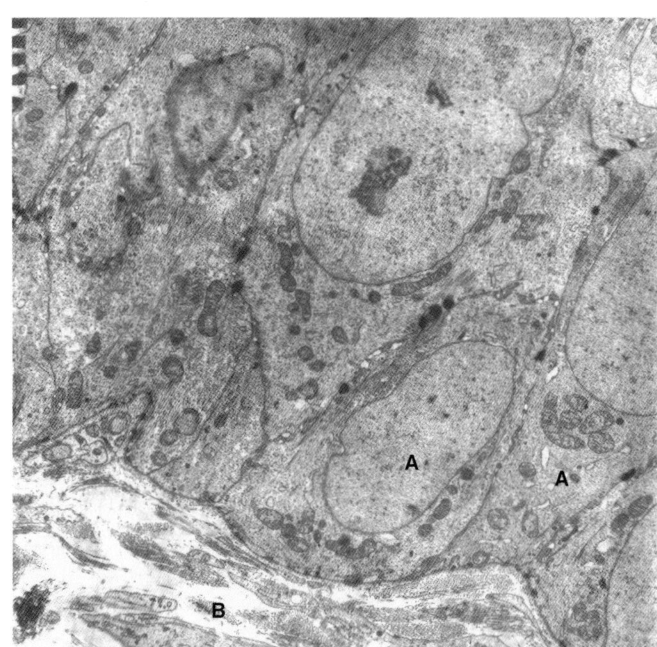

Fig. 14.5 Electron micrograph of basal layer of keratinised stratified squamous epithelium. The cells (A) are undifferentiated; contain various intracellular organelles such as mitochondria, free ribosomes and microfilaments; and rest on a basal lamina. B = lamina propria (×4,000). Courtesy Prof. M M Smith.

shrinkage that occurs in most histological preparations causes the cells to separate at all points where desmosomes do not anchor them together. This gives the cells their 'spiny' appearance. Desmosomes eventually come to occupy about 50% of the intercellular space.

The term 'parabasal' is used to refer to the deepest layer of cells of the prickle cell layer that lies next to the basal layer. Parabasal cells may show features similar to those of the basal layer in that they may be elongated and undergo proliferation.

Granular layer

The cells of the granular layer (Fig. 14.2) show a further increase in maturation compared with those of the basal and prickle cell layers. Many organelles are reduced or lost, such that the cytoplasm is predominantly occupied by the tonofilaments and tonofibrils. The cells are larger and flatter (Figs. 14.8, 14.9) but, most significantly, now contain large numbers of small granules, 0.5–1.0 µm in length, called *keratohyaline granules* (Fig. 14.10). These contain profilaggrin, the precursor to the protein filaggrin that eventually binds the keratin filaments together into a stable network. The membrane-coating granules first seen in the prickle cell layer move towards the superficial surface of the keratinocyte and discharge their lipid-rich contents into the intercellular space. This intercellular discharge 'cements' together with the cell contents (especially tight junctions in the upper region of the granular layer) and helps limit the permeability of the layer and prevents water loss. Synthesis of additional proteins, loricrin and involucrin, that will help form a more resistant cell wall (envelope) is evident in the granular layer.

Keratinised layer

In keratinised epithelium the final stage in the maturation of the epithelial cells results in the loss of all organelles (including nuclei and keratohyaline granules) (Figs. 14.8, 14.9, 14.11). This autolysis is probably the result of the release of proteases within the cell. The cells of the keratinised layer become filled entirely with closely packed tonofilaments

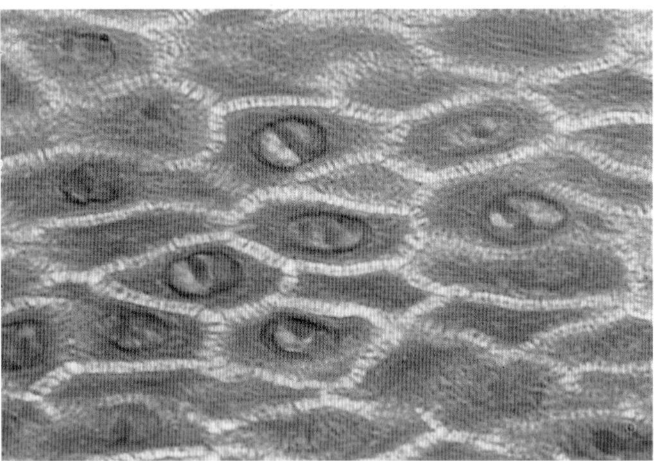

Fig. 14.6 Prickle cell layer at high power showing 'spiky' desmosomes connecting adjacent cells (H & E; ×1,000). Courtesy Prof. M M Smith.

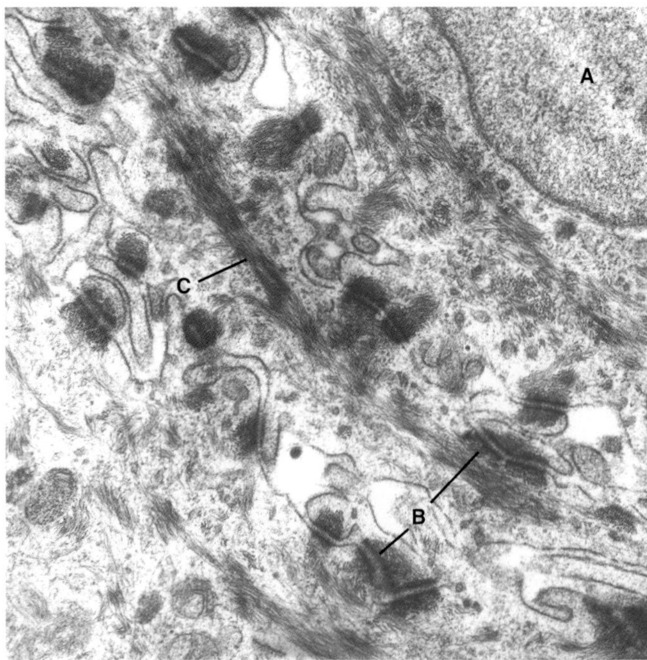

Fig. 14.7 Electron micrograph of the prickle cell layer. A = nucleus; B = desmosome surrounded by inserting tonofilaments; C = tonofilaments of keratin (×20,000). Courtesy Prof. M M Smith.

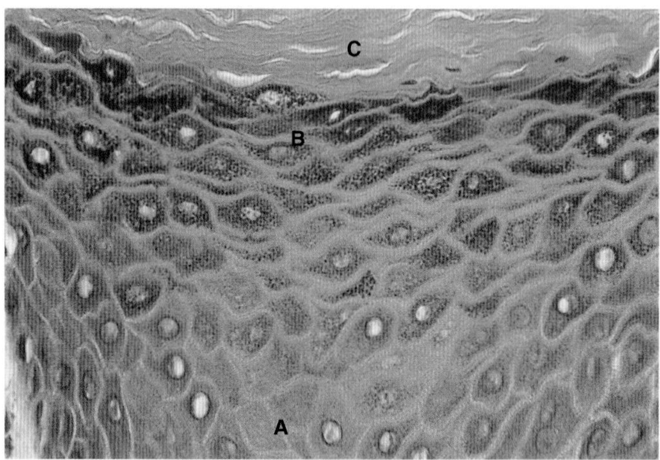

Fig. 14.8 Section showing upper part of prickle cell layer (A), the granular layer (B) and the keratinised layer (C). Note the granular nature of the cells in the granular layer (H & E; ×350). Courtesy Prof. M M Smith.

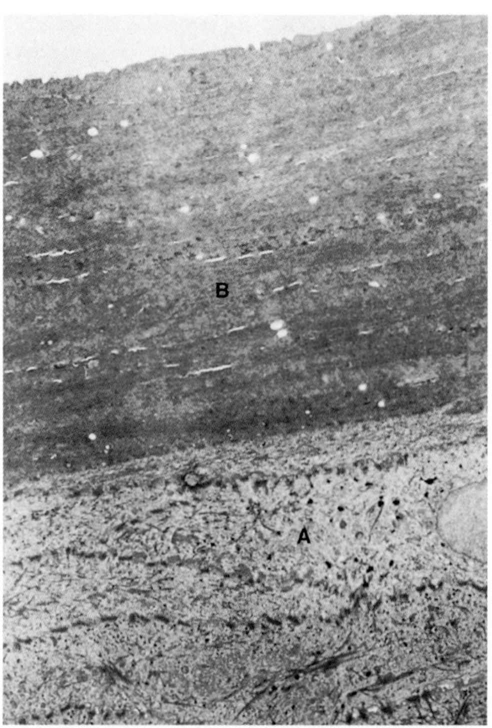

Fig. 14.9 Electron micrograph showing granular (A) and keratinised (B) layers. Within the cells of the granular layer can be seen the keratohyalin granules, while the cells of the keratin layer lack nuclei and other organelles (×2,800). Courtesy Prof. C A Squier.

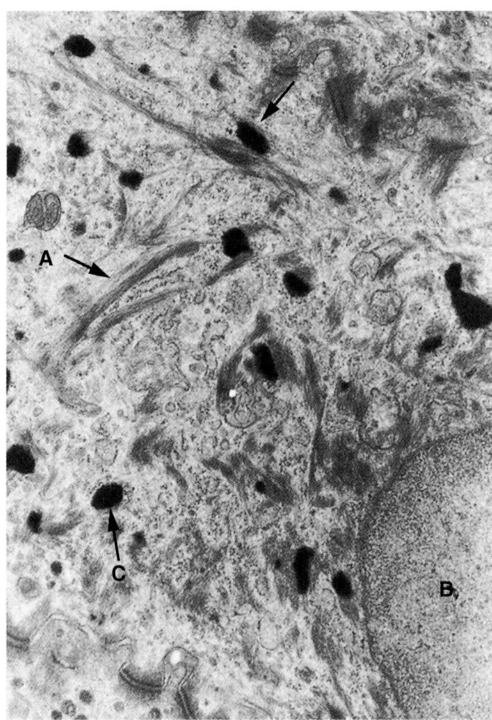

Fig. 14.10 Higher-power electron micrograph of a cell of the granular layer. A = tonofibril; B = nucleus. C=keratohyaline granule. (x12,000.). Courtesy Prof. C A Squier.

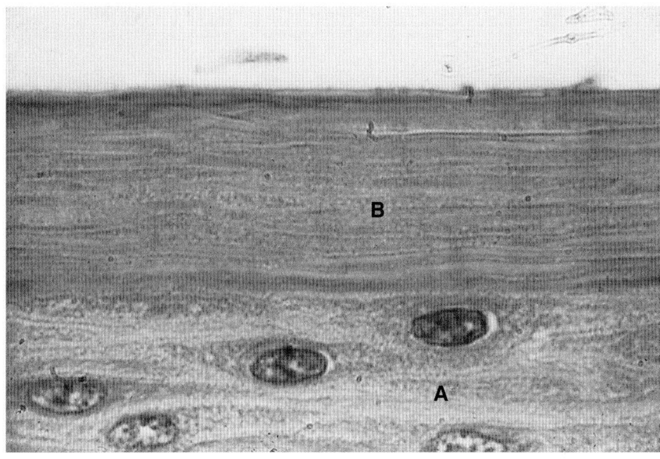

Fig. 14.11 Section showing the granular (A) and keratinised layers (B) (H & E; ×1,000). Courtesy Dr. D Adams.

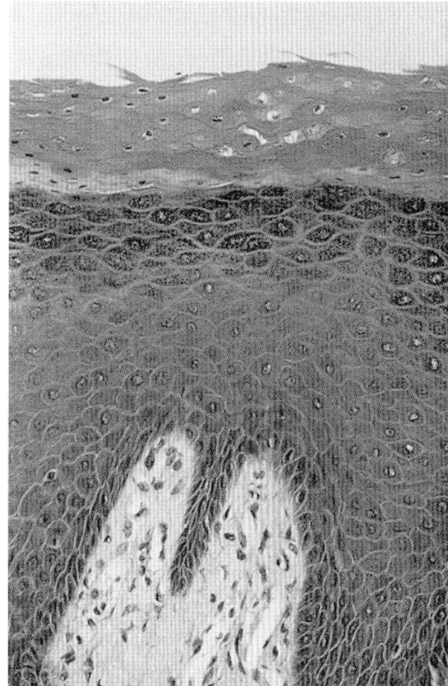

Fig. 14.12 Section of parakeratinised oral epithelium from the gingiva. The superficial layer stains more heavily for keratin, but nuclei are retained (H & E; ×100). Courtesy Dr. A W Barrett.

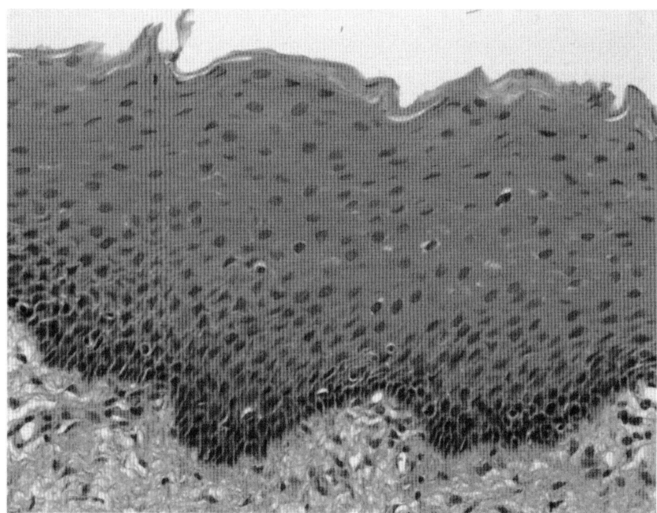

Fig. 14.13 Section of lining oral epithelium from the floor of the mouth. There is an absence of keratin in the superficial layer (H & E; ×150). Courtesy Prof. P R Morgan.

surrounded by the matrix protein filaggrin. This mixture of proteins is collectively called *keratin*. The keratin is also strongly cross-linked by disulphide bonds, contributing to the mechanical and chemical resistance of the layer.

In the cornified layer involucrin becomes cross-linked by the enzyme transglutaminase to form a thin (10nm), highly resistant, electron-dense, cornified envelope just beneath the plasma membrane. The trigger for this is probably cell death and the influx of calcium ions. Approximately 75% of the cornified envelope is loricrin. Although only constituting 5% of the cell envelope, involucrin is an important component on the internal aspect, acting as a binding site for lipids that are extruded to form a water-insoluble barrier.

The cells of the superficial layer may be termed *epithelial squames*; it is these cells that are shed (the process of desquamation) necessitating the constant turnover of epithelial cells. Desmosomes weaken and disappear to allow for this desquamation.

The keratinised layer provides the mechanical protective function to the mucosa. It varies in thickness (up to 20 cells) and is thicker for the oral mucosa than for most areas of skin (except for the palms of the hands and the soles of the feet). In some areas, such as the gingiva, the nuclei may be retained, although small and shrunken. These cells are described as parakeratinised (in contrast to the more usual orthokeratinised cells without nuclei) (Fig. 14.12).

Lining epithelium

In lining epithelium the cells are nonkeratinised at the surface (Fig. 14.13). As for the cells in keratinised epithelia, those in lining epithelium enlarge and flatten as they shift towards the surface. Ultrastructurally, the surface layers differ from the cells of keratinised epithelia in that they lack keratohyaline granules. This absence of filaggrin accounts for the less developed and dispersed tonofilaments present in lining epithelium. There are also more organelles in the surface layers compared with those in keratinised cells, although there are still considerably fewer than in the basal layer. Above the prickle cell layer, the layers are not as clearly defined as in a keratinised epithelium. The outer layer is termed the *superficial layer* (stratum superficiale). Nuclei persist as far as the surface within the superficial layer (Fig. 14.14). The membrane-coating granules are smaller and lack the lipid-rich lamellar structure of those in keratinising epithelia. This is thought to account for the greater permeability of lining epithelium compared to keratinised epithelium. Lining epithelium generally lacks filaggrin (Fig. 14.15A) and loricrin, but contains involucrin (Fig. 14.15B).

Cell kinetics

Although the processes involved in controlling the proliferation and maturation of keratinocytes are not fully known, many growth factors (e.g., epidermal growth factor, platelet-derived growth factor, transforming growth factor [TGF] and keratinocyte growth factor) and cytokines (e.g., interleukins [ILs]) produced by either the keratinocyte or adjacent fibroblasts can affect the rate of proliferation and differentiation. The nature of adjacent adhesion molecules and their interaction with integrins are also of importance. Epithelial cells themselves will have numerous cell-surface receptors and molecules important in regulating cell behaviour. The precise mechanisms are still being elucidated, but as the mitotic rate shows diurnal variation, systemic factors may be implicated.

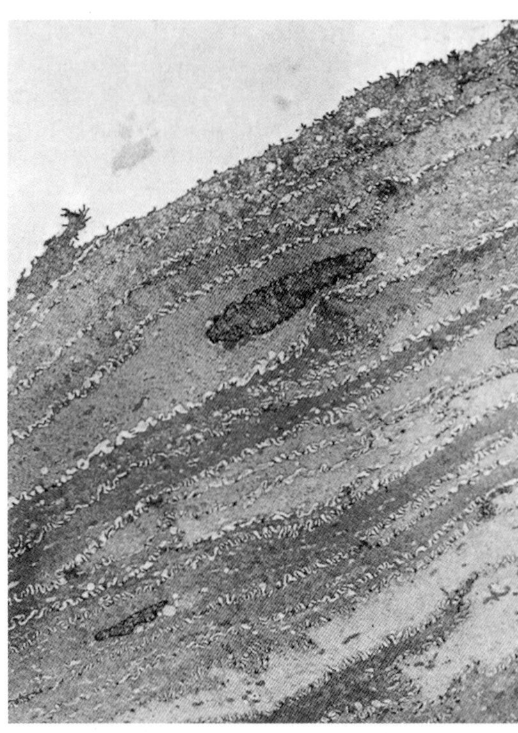

Fig. 14.14 Electron micrograph of surface layers in nonkeratinised lining epithelium. Note the retention of nuclei (×2,000). Courtesy Prof. C A Squier.

Cytokeratins (CKs)

In all cell types, the cytoskeleton is composed of microfilaments, microtubules and intermediate filaments. Microfilaments are approximately 4–6 nm in diameter and have a molecular weight of the order of 43 kDa. By contrast, microtubules are 25 nm in diameter with a molecular weight of 55 kDa. Although intermediate in terms of diameter (7–11 nm), the intermediate filaments have a molecular weight ranging from 40 kDa to as high as 200 kDa. In contrast to microfilaments and microtubules, which are ubiquitous proteins, intermediate filaments have a high degree of tissue specificity. Six major classes of intermediate filament have been identified, including the cytokeratins (CK), which have a high specificity for epithelial cells. 'Moll' numbers were assigned to the CK proteins, which are the products of two gene families and translate into around 30 individual cytokeratins. Each keratin is characterised by a chain of amino acids as the primary structure, which varies in their number and sequence. As for different collagens, this sequence influences the properties and therefore the functions of the particular keratin. Soft keratins with fewer cysteine–disulphide cross-links are found in the oral epithelium, while hard keratins possessing many cysteine disulphide cross-links are found in nails and hairs.

The products of each CK gene family are divided into the neutral or basic type II CK (numbered 1–8) and the acidic type I CK (numbered 9–20). They occur in pairs. The type I CK is the smaller of each pair, ranging between 40 and 56.5 kDa and always about 8 kDa smaller than its type II counterpart, which has a molecular weight of 53–67 kDa (Table 14.1).

Table 14.1 Distribution of cytokeratins in human stratified squamous epithelium (SSE)

	CK pair	
	Type II, basic, higher MW	**Type I, acidic, lower MW**
Suprabasal, keratinised SSE	1 and 2	10 and 11
Cornea	3	12
Suprabasal, nonkeratinised SSE	4	13
Basal keratinocytes (all SSE)	5	14
Hyperproliferative epithelia	6	16
Simple epithelia	8	18
Some simple epithelia, pilosebaceous tracts, basal cell carcinomas	5?	17
Basal keratinocytes in nonkeratinised SSE, some simple or 'plastic' epithelia (e.g., odontogenic)	5?	19

CK, Cytokeratins; *MW*, Molecular Weight.

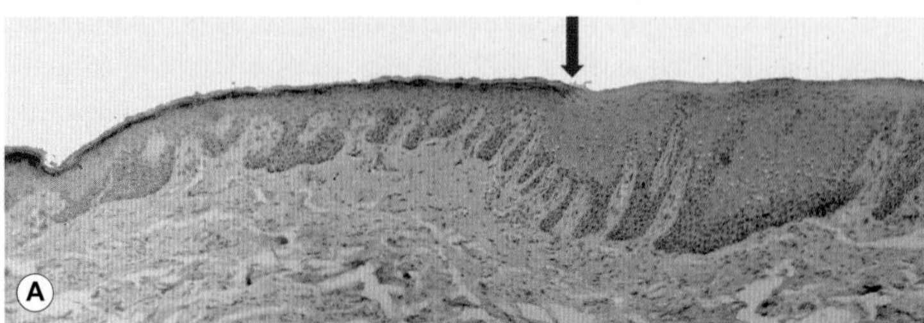

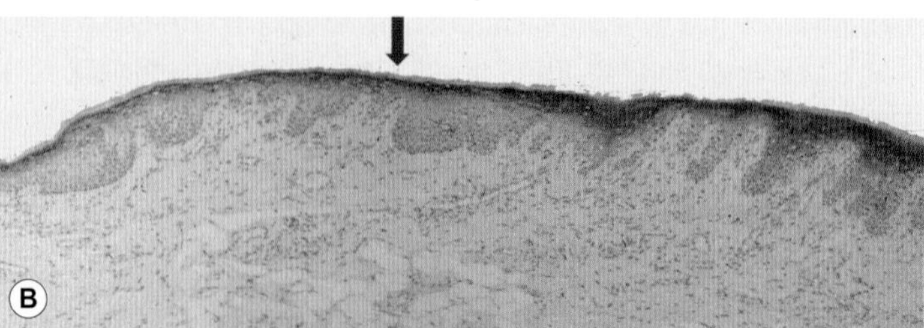

Fig. 14.15 (A) Section across lip stained immunohistochemically for filaggrin, showing its positive (brown) staining at the surface of the keratinised vermilion layer (left of arrow) and its absence over the nonkeratinised labial mucosa (right of arrow). (B) Section across lip stained immunohistologically for involucrin, showing positive staining (brown) at the surface of the keratinised vermilion (left of arrow) and the labial mucosa (right of arrow) (streptavidin-biotinylated immunoperoxidase stain; ×20). With permission from Barrett, A.W., Morgan, M., Nwaeze, G., et al., 2005. The differentiation profile of epithelium of the human lip. Archives of Oral Biology 50, 431–438.

CK expression conforms to several 'rules', with each epithelial cell expressing at least one CK pair comprising one type I and one type II. The ultimate CK phenotype reflects the differentiation pathway the cell has followed. Because they are only expressed in simple epithelia, such as ductal luminal cells, CKs 7, 8 and 18 are designated 'simple'. The best-characterised CKs associated with epithelial stratification are pairs 5 and 14, 4 and 13, and 1 and 10.

Within epithelial cells CK filaments function as components of the cytoskeleton and cell contacts (desmosomes and hemidesmosomes). However, the physiological reason for the large number of CKs remains obscure. Some insight into their functional significance can be obtained from analysis of congenital or experimental CK abnormalities. For example, in some forms of epidermolysis bullosa (a group of mucocutaneous lesions, all of which produce subepithelial blistering), there is a mutant form of CK14. Defects in CK4 and CK13 are associated with the presence of white sponge nevus (see page 315). Some CKs may be important in maintaining the metabolic homeostasis of the cell.

Apart from their structural role in the cytoskeleton, there is evidence for other roles for CKs, possibly related to their location. For example, CK14 is most strongly positive in the basal layer. The fact that CK14-positive basal cells in palatal and lingual epithelium synthesise neurogenic peptides may be related to the innervation of the superficial oral mucosa. This view is supported by work that showed that denervation of rodent taste buds causes loss of CK expression and is consistent with a possible role for CK in signal transduction.

Major distribution patterns of cytokeratins in oral epithelium (Table 14.1)

CK5 and 14 are usually restricted to the basal and parabasal layers (Fig. 14.16), although CK14 may also be expressed by suprabasal keratinocytes (Table 14.1). CK1 and 10 (or CK2 and 11) are characteristically found in the suprabasal layers of masticatory mucosa and are associated with terminal differentiation and keratinisation (Fig. 14.17). The keratin layer stains variably. In lining mucosa, the suprabasal keratinocytes stain primarily for CK4 (Figs. 14.18) and 13 rather than the CK1 and 10 found in masticatory mucosa. There is variable expression of other cytokeratins. CK6 and 16 are associated with rapid turnover epithelia. CK19 may also be a marker for basal keratinocytes in lining mucosa, but reports concerning its presence are inconsistent. Suprabasal epithelial cells of the hard palate and gingiva have been reported to express CK6, CK16 and the recently discovered CK76. CK17 occurs in myoepithelial cells (see pages 340–341). Variations in the CK distribution of nonkeratinised oral epithelium at different anatomical sites have been reported. The epithelium lining the ventral surface of the tongue may be distinguished from other lining oral epithelium by its increased expression of CK5, 6 and 14. However, most unusual is the epithelium covering the soft palate, which apparently expresses the simple cytokeratins (CK7, 8 and 18) as well as high levels of CK19.

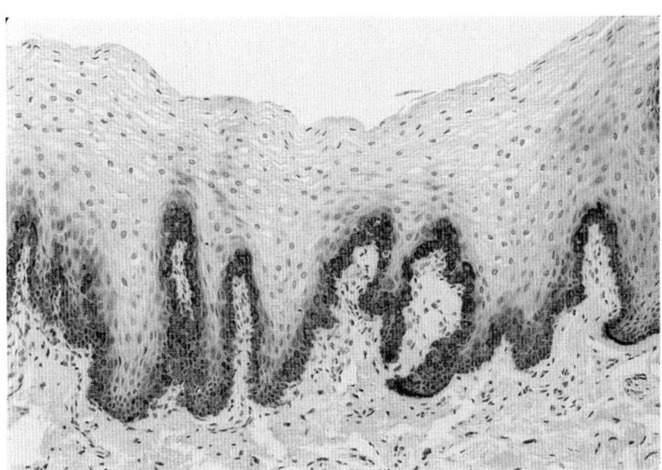

Fig. 14.16 Oral epithelium stained for cytokeratin 14, showing positive staining (purple) restricted to the basal cell layer (streptavidin-biotinylated immunoperoxidase alkaline phosphatase stain; ×100). Courtesy Dr. A W Barrett.

Other secretory products of keratinocytes

In addition to synthesising cytokeratins that remain inside the cell, keratinocytes can produce bioactive molecules such as interleukins, tumour necrosis factor-α and colony-stimulating factors. Such molecules can influence the biology of both the epithelium and the underlying connective tissue of the lamina propria.

Factors controlling the oral epithelial phenotype

In reviewing the nature of the oral epithelium, it has been shown that regional specificity exists throughout life, even though there is a continuous and rapid replacement of the components. This poses questions as to the nature of the factors determining such specificity. The specificity may

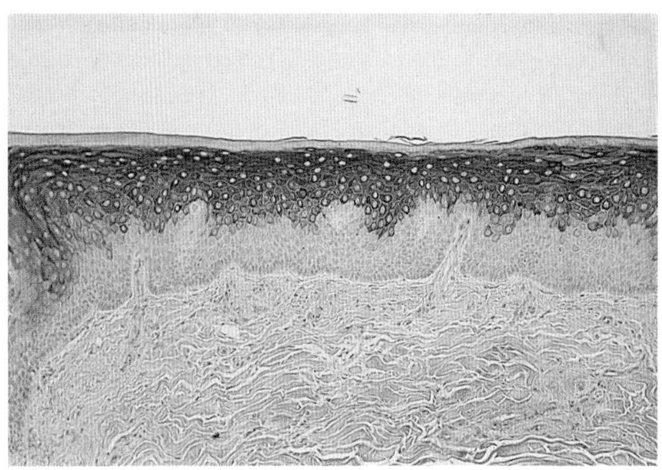

Fig. 14.17 Section of orthokeratinised epithelium from the hard palate stained for cytokeratin 10, showing positive suprabasal staining (brown) (streptavidin-biotinylated immunoperoxidase stain; ×50). Courtesy Dr. A W Barrett.

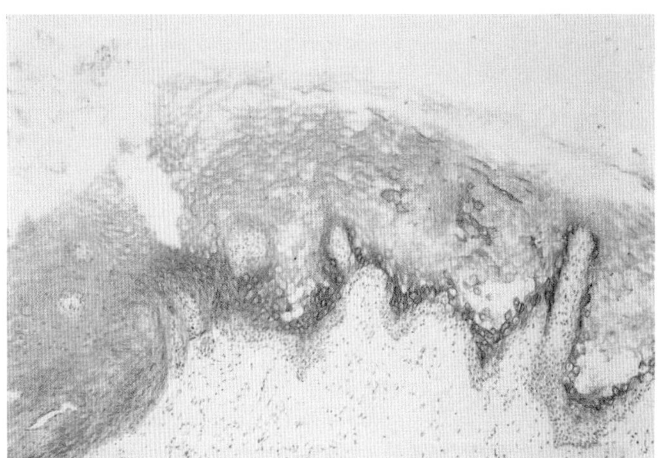

Fig. 14.18 Section of nonkeratinised epithelium from the cheek stained for cytokeratin 4, showing positive staining (brown) throughout except for the basal layer (streptavidin-biotinylated immunoperoxidase stain; ×60). Courtesy Dr. A W Barrett.

be considered as being the result of extrinsic inductive stimuli from the underlying lamina propria or an intrinsic property of the basal layer of the epithelium. Although nowadays little practised, knowledge of the underlying mechanisms has clinical relevance as, following surgical removal of the dentogingival tissues, the three distinctive epithelia of the oral gingiva, sulcular epithelium and junctional epithelium do regenerate, presumably from the remaining oral gingival epithelium. Furthermore, conditions exist where nonkeratinised zones of epithelia are encountered in regions of masticatory epithelia, and treatment may be geared towards attempting to replace these zones with the appropriate keratinised epithelium.

With regard to the view that specificity is the result of epithelial–mesenchymal interactions, this has been well established during tooth development (see pages 388–394). The role of mesenchyme in determining the phenotype of the overlying epithelium, and its ability to maintain this property and therefore redirect patterns of epithelial morphogenesis in the adult, has been investigated. Researchers use classical methods in which portions of oral mucosa are transplanted to different regions or are separated into their epithelial and connective tissue components and then homotypically and heterotypically recombined and transplanted. Such studies support the view that the underlying lamina propria is primarily responsible for the specificity of the overlying epithelia in terms of both morphology and CK content. Thus, lining oral epithelium combined with lamina propria from masticatory mucosa takes on the features of a masticatory mucosa, while masticatory epithelium combined with lamina propria from lining mucosa modulates to lining epithelium. Such modulation does not appear to require a vital lamina propria, as a similar effect is seen even after the connective tissue is frozen. These fundamental changes are not only seen in subcutaneous sites in animal experiments but have also been reported in clinical situations. Deep connective tissue, however, is not able to facilitate such changes. In this context, gingival fibroblasts also produce substances, such as keratinocyte growth factor and scatter factor, that are important in the growth and maintenance of the overlying epithelium, and these factors themselves are influenced by other growth factors and cytokines (such as TGF-β and IL-1β). This relationship may be of clinical significance when considering the junctional epithelium in health and disease (see pages 257–258).

Other evidence confirming the existence of epithelial–mesenchymal interactions is shown from experiments in which normal epithelium is combined with carcinogen-treated (and transformed) mesenchyme, when the epithelium is seen to show an increased mitotic activity and irregular nuclei. However, although there is considerable evidence for the importance of the underlying mesenchyme in specifying the form and phenotype of the overlying epithelium, both during development and in the adult, there is also evidence for some regionally related variations in the competence of epithelia to respond to these influences.

Nonkeratinocytes

As much as 10% of the cells in the oral epithelium are nonkeratinocytes and include melanocytes, Langerhans cells and Merkel cells. They lack the tonofilaments and desmosomes characteristic of keratinocytes (except for the Merkel cell). Nonkeratinocytes may appear as clear cells in sections stained routinely with haematoxylin and eosin (Fig. 14.19). Lacking the typical cytokeratins associated with normal keratinocytes, they remain unstained in sections of epithelium stained for cytokeratins (Fig. 14.20) except for Merkel cells. Some nonkeratinocytes are inflammatory cells that have migrated through the epithelium. Lymphocytes are the most common type of inflammatory cell, though polymorphonuclear leukocytes and plasma cells are also encountered. Lymphocytes are retained within the epithelial layer by binding to integrins that may increase in disease. The greater degree of permeability of nonkeratinised epithelium may account for the larger number of inflammatory cells there compared with masticatory epithelium.

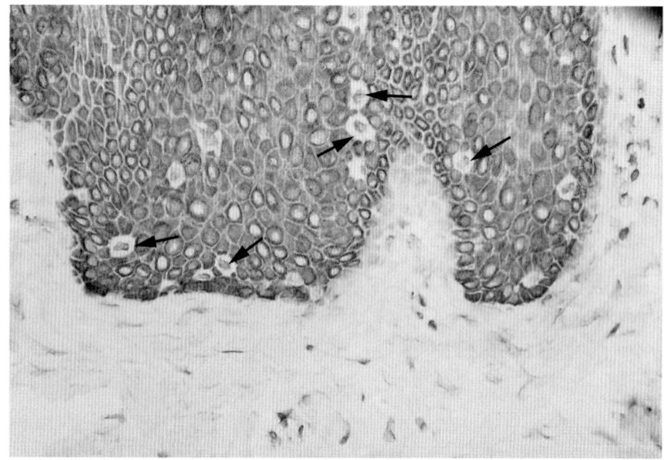

Fig. 14.20 Basal region of oral epithelium stained for cytokeratin 14 (brown) and illustrating clear cells (arrows) lacking cytokeratin and representing mainly melanocytes (×200). Courtesy Prof. P R Morgan.

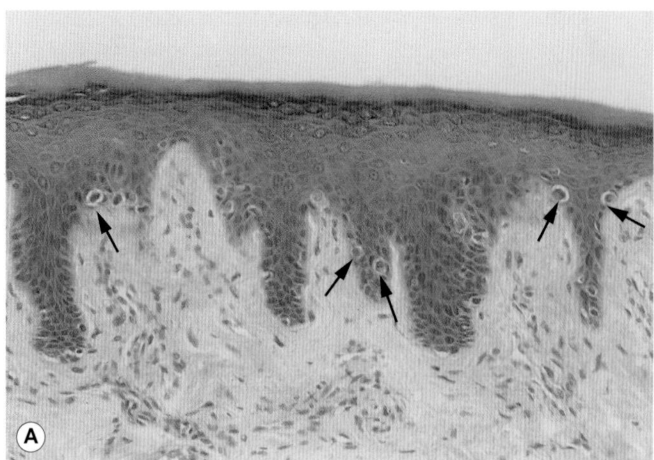

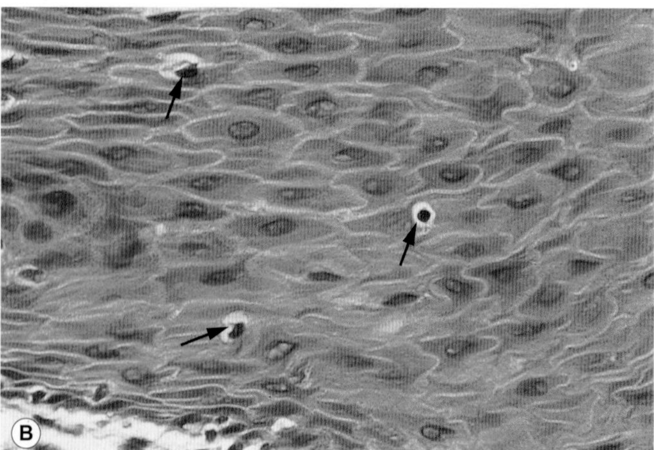

Fig. 14.19 (A) Section of the vermilion of lip showing clear cells (arrows) in the basal layer, representing mainly melanocytes (×80). (B) Clear cells in the upper layers of the epithelium (arrowed), mainly representing Langerhans cells (H & E; ×350). Courtesy Prof. M M Smith.

Melanocytes

Melanocytes are pigment-producing cells located in the basal layer. They are derived from the neural crest and are present in the skin at about 8 weeks of intra-uterine life. Once located in the epithelium, they are assumed to be long-lived, but with some powers of self-replication, and are seen to divide in vitro. Melanocytes have long processes that extend in several directions and across several epithelial layers. As suggested by their name, melanocytes produce the pigment melanin, using the enzyme tyrosinase (which is lacking in albinos). They can be identified by special staining (Fig. 14.21).

Ultrastructurally, in addition to mitochondria, endoplasmic reticulum and Golgi apparatus, the cytoplasm of melanocytes characteristically contains pigment that is packaged in small granules termed *melanosomes* (Fig. 14.22). The long processes of the melanocyte extend between adjacent keratinocytes, and each melanocyte establishes contact with about 30–40 keratinocytes. Indeed, keratinocytes release numerous mediators that are essential for normal melanocyte function. As the melanosomes mature under the activity of tyrosinase, their content of melanin increases. The pigment is passed to adjacent keratinocytes (and hair cortex cells) as the tips of the dendrites are actively phagocytosed by the keratinocytes. Melanin pigmentation is usually not pronounced in the buccal mucosa, tongue, hard palate or lip.

The number of melanocytes varies in different regions, but the difference in the degree of pigmentation between groups of different ancestral origin is the result of a combination of the size and degree of branching of the cells (rather than the absolute number), the size of the melanosomes, the number and degree of dispersion of the melanosomes, the degree of melanisation of the melanosomes and the rate of degradation of the pigment.

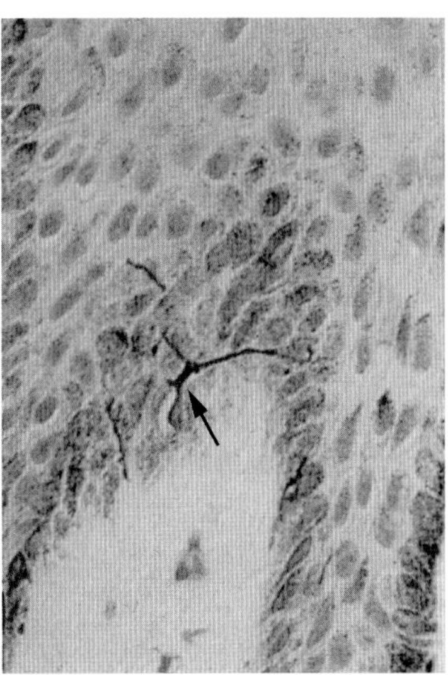

Fig. 14.21 Section of oral epithelium illustrating a melanocyte (arrowed) (Masson's Fontana stain; ×280). Courtesy Prof. I Mackenzie.

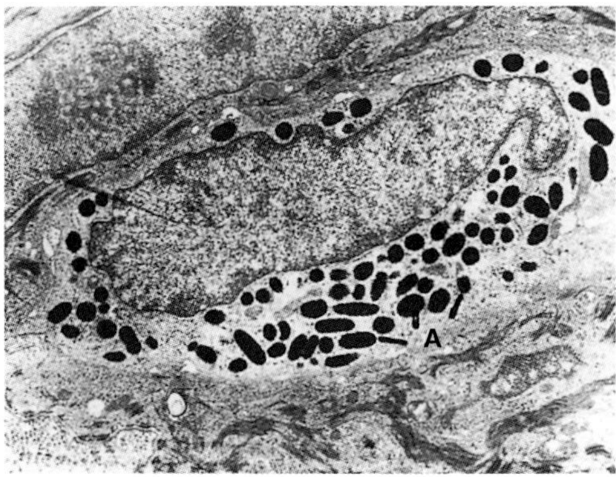

Fig. 14.22 Electron micrograph of a melanocyte packed with melanosomes (A) (×60,000). Courtesy Prof. C A Squier.

Langerhans cells

Langerhans cells are dendritic cells situated in the layers above the basal layer. They are derived from bone marrow precursors that are probably related to the monocyte lineage. They leave the bloodstream to enter the lamina propria before penetrating the basal lamina to reach the epithelium. Such migration may relate to certain chemokines released by keratinocytes with surface receptors on the Langerhans cells. Langerhans cells act as part of the immune system as antigen-presenting cells. To provide immediate protection against invading pathogens, dendritic cells (and other antigen-presenting cells) must quickly respond to bacterial structures. This is accomplished through a major class of signalling receptors called *toll-like receptors*. Immature dendritic cells are particularly well equipped to capture antigens through phagocytosis, pinocytosis and endocytosis via different groups of receptor families.

Dendritic cells express class II molecules of the major histocompatibility complex and Fc receptors and move back and forth from the epithelium via dermal lymphatics to local lymph nodes, presenting antigenic material to T lymphocytes. Indeed, lymphocytes present within the oral epithelium are commonly associated with Langerhans cells. Langerhans cells play an important role in skin in producing contact hypersensitivity reactions, in antitumour immunity and in graft rejection; they also react as propagators of human immunodeficiency virus (HIV)-1 transmission to T cells. The cells may be identified because of the presence of ATPase on the cell membrane (Fig. 14.23).

Ultrastructurally, the Langerhans cell contains characteristic trilaminar, rod-shaped granules called *Birbeck granules* (Fig. 14.24). These may be up to 50 nm long and 4 nm wide with a vesicular swelling at one end, resembling a tennis racquet. Foreign antigens penetrate the superficial layers and bind to dendritic antigen-presenting cells such as Langerhans cells, which stimulate helper T lymphocytes, and Granstein cells, which stimulate specific suppressor T lymphocytes. T cells also receive a signal in the form of a cytokine (IL-1) from both keratinocytes and dendritic cells, then secrete a lymphokine (IL-2) that causes the proliferation of T cells.

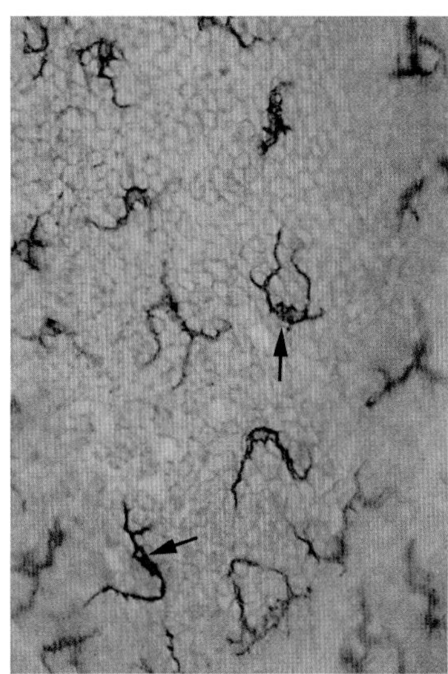

Fig. 14.23 Section of superficial layers of oral epithelium showing Langerhans cells (arrowed) (lead capture staining for ATPase; ×200). Courtesy Prof. I Mackenzie.

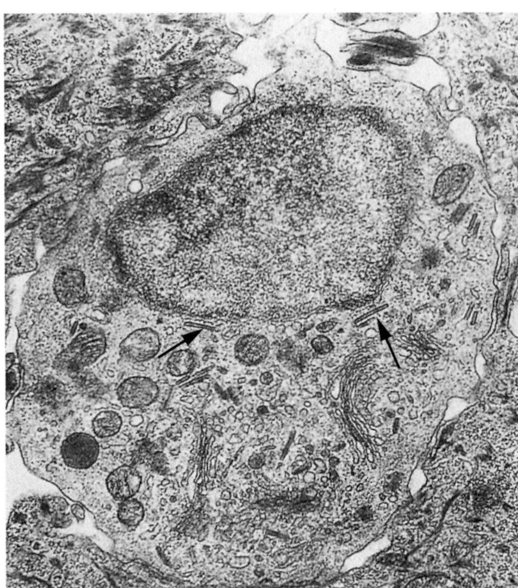

Fig. 14.24 Electron micrograph of Langerhans cell showing the characteristic Birbeck granules (arrows) (×15,000). Courtesy Dr. N G El-Labban.

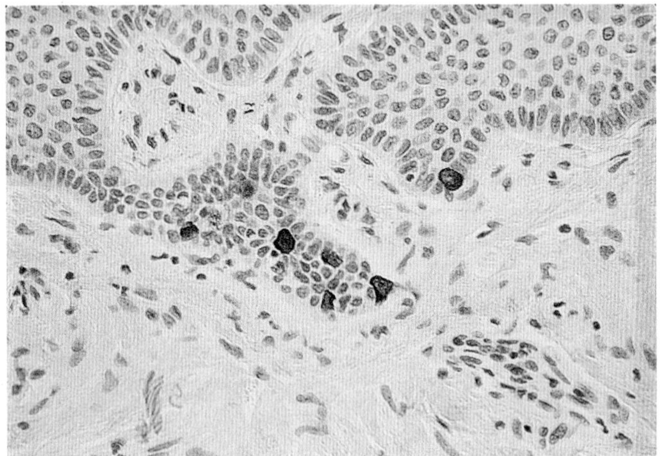

Fig. 14.25 Section showing Merkel cells in basal layer of epithelium staining positively (brown) for cytokeratin 18 (streptavidin-biotinylated immunoperoxidase stain; ×200). Courtesy Dr. W A Barrett.

The bacteria *Porphyromonas gingivalis*, implicated in the onset of periodontitis, is thought to be able to suppress the immune response in dendritic cells. During subsequent inflammation there is evidence that osteoclasts resorbing alveolar bone can be derived from dendritic cells.

Merkel cells

Merkel cells are slowly adapting sensory touch receptors, which reside in the basal layer of the stratified squamous epithelium covering the skin and oral mucosa. They can be identified immunohistochemically as they contain the 'simple' (CK) intermediate filaments CK 7, 8, 18, 19 and 20 (Fig. 14.25). In human oral epithelium they are almost entirely restricted to the keratinised mucosa of the hard palate, maxillary and mandibular gingivae. Merkel cell–neurite complexes are clustered in particularly large numbers in the lingual gingiva of humans and other primates, where they appear similar to the 'touch domes' of the skin. Their preferential distribution at sites of intimate contact with the tongue prompts the belief that they not only act as slowly adapting mechanoreceptors in the gingivae and palate, but their close association with sensory nerves may provide important somatosensory feedback on the position of the tongue.

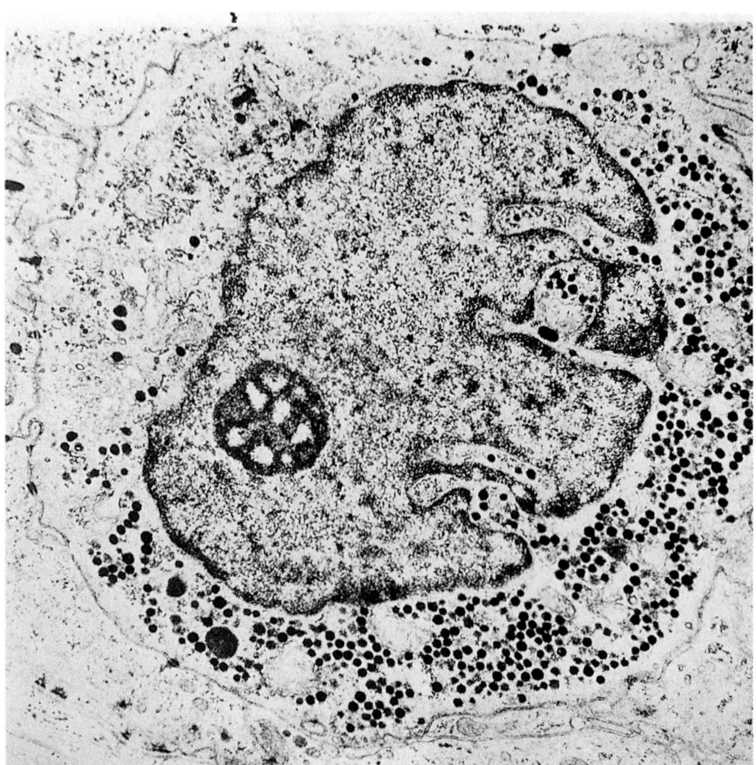

Fig. 14.26 Electron micrograph of Merkel cell. Note the indented nucleus and nuclear rodlet. The cytoplasm contains numerous characteristic dense granules 80–180 nm in diameter (×16,000). Courtesy Dr. S-Y Chen.

Ultrastructurally, the nucleus of the Merkel cell is often deeply invaginated and may contain a characteristic rodlet (Fig. 14.26). The cytoplasm contains numerous mitochondria, abundant free ribosomes and a collection of electron-dense granules (80–180 nm in diameter), the function of which is unknown. In addition, there are many small vesicles in the region adjacent to the nerve terminal. The granules may liberate a transmitter towards the terminal, giving the cell a sensory function. Desmosomes are associated with the cell membrane. Free nerve endings not associated with a Merkel cell are also found within the epithelium. These are nociceptors.

The number of Merkel cells has been found to be greater in complete denture wearers when compared with dentate patients and raises the possibility that reduced perception following loss of teeth may be compensated for by an increase in the local Merkel cell population.

Lamina propria

The connective tissue underlying the oral epithelium can be described as having two layers: a superficial, papillary layer between the epithelial ridges, in which the collagen fibres are thin and loosely arranged, and beneath this a deep, reticular layer dominated by thick, parallel bundles of collagen fibres. The lamina propria provides mechanical support for the epithelium as well as nutrition. Its nerves have a sensory function, while its blood cells and salivary glands have important defensive roles. Vascular concentration shows regional variation, and this, associated with the rate of blood flow, may account for the very small differences in temperature that are found (e.g., the temperature of the more vascularised alveolar mucosa is, on average, 0.67°C higher than that of the attached gingival mucosa). Furthermore, a similar slight temperature increase can be achieved following stimulation using an electric toothbrush.

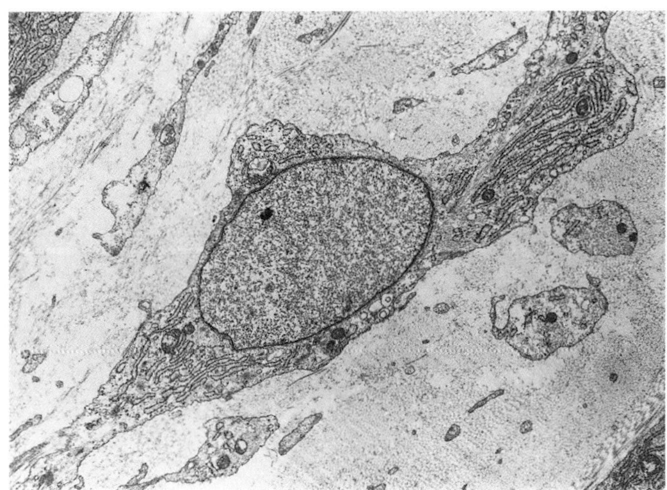

Fig. 14.27 Electron micrograph of fibroblast from lamina propria. The cell contains a full complement of all the intracellular organelles associated with collagen synthesis. Note the conspicuous rough endoplasmic reticulum (×11,000). Courtesy Prof. C A Squier.

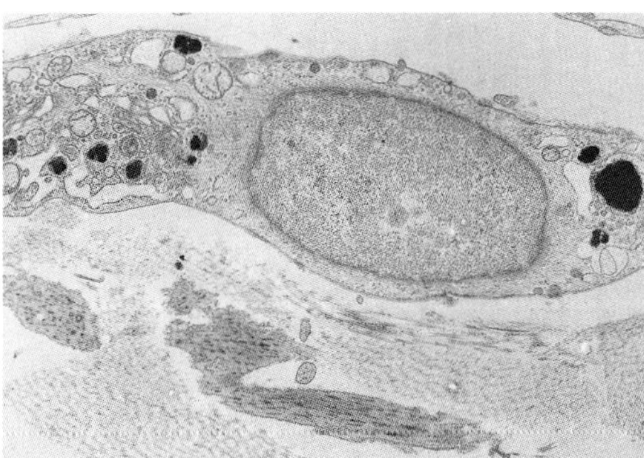

Fig. 14.28 Electron micrograph of macrophage in lamina propria. It contains many lysosomes but little endoplasmic reticulum (×10,000). Courtesy Prof. C A Squier.

As with other soft connective tissues, the principal cell of the lamina propria is the fibroblast. In outline, their shape varies, with many appearing spindle-shaped. They contain the full complement of synthetic organelles consistent with their role in the continuous production and secretion of extracellular fibres and ground substance for the lamina propria (Fig. 14.27). There is evidence of heterogeneity among the fibroblast-like cells. Tissue culture experiments have isolated clones of fibroblast-like cells that have different responses to the same bioactive molecule and that synthesise different ratios of extracellular matrix (ECM) molecules. Gingival fibroblasts also produce substances such as keratinocyte growth factor and scatter factor that are important in the growth and maintenance of the overlying epithelium. This relationship may be of considerable clinical significance when considering the junctional epithelium.

A population of stem cells exists in the lamina propria, characterised by the expression of embryonic and pluripotency markers Sox2 and Notch signalling pathways. They exhibit high proliferation rates in vitro and have the capacity to differentiate into several lineages, such as fat, bone and cartilage cells. They also demonstrate the feature of immunoprivilege, which may be important for tissue engineering.

The ECM of the lamina propria contains numerous collagen fibres. Most are type I (about 90%) with about 8% being type III. In addition there are small amounts of other types of collagen, including types IV and VII (associated with the presence of basement membranes) and types V and VI. Elastin fibres are also present, with their number dependent on site, while some oxytalan fibres have also been described in regions of the oral mucosa. The ground substance of the lamina propria consists of a hydrated gel of proteoglycans and glycoproteins. As with all general connective tissues, the usual defence cells are present. Macrophages are seen in the lamina propria. In their fixed, inactive stage, they are known as *histiocytes* and are difficult to distinguish from fibroblasts. They have a smaller, darker nucleus than fibroblasts and contain lysosomes but little endoplasmic reticulum (Fig. 14.28). In addition to having a phagocytic role, macrophages act as antigen-presenting cells. Mast cells are mononuclear, spherical or elliptical in shape and contain histamine and heparin intracellular granules (see page 245). They play a role in vascular homeostasis, in inflammation and in cell-mediated immunity and are responsible for anaphylactic (type 1) hypersensitivity. Lymphocytes are also found in small numbers in healthy mucosa, but increase dramatically in inflammation.

Epithelial–connective tissue interface

Basement membrane/basal lamina

A complex arrangement links the surface epithelium to the underlying lamina propria in the oral mucosa. In the light microscope, a layer 1–2 μm thick is seen on the lamina propria side of the junction. This is termed *the basement membrane*. Under the electron microscope, the layer appears much thinner and is then termed the basal lamina. The thicker appearance under the light microscope is probably owing to the inclusion of some of the subepithelial collagen fibres, which in this region have staining properties similar to those of the basal lamina. All the major products of the basal lamina appear to be synthesised by the epithelial cells.

Ultrastructurally, the cell membrane possesses specialised attachment plaques, the hemidesmosomes, along its length, where there is an increased density in structure. Cytoplasmic keratin filaments insert into the hemidesmosome. Immediately adjacent to the cell membrane is the basal lamina. In routine electron microscopy, the basal lamina is seen to consist of two layers (Fig. 14.29):

- An electron-lucent lamina lucida (20–40 nm thick) that lies immediately under the epithelium
- A thicker (20–120 nm) lamina densa

However, there is evidence that the lamina lucida is a preparation artefact.

The basal lamina is composed of a network of type IV (nonfibrillar) collagen in which is found several important proteoglycan and glycoprotein molecules. Among these are fibronectin, laminin and perlecan (heparin sulphate proteoglycan). Transmembrane molecules such as integrins and bullous pemphigoid antigens (BPAG-1 and BPAG-2) strengthen the link between the cell and the basal lamina. The bond is further strengthened by looping fibrils of type VII collagen that bind to the type IV collagen of the basal lamina and interdigitate with type I and type III collagen of the ECM.

Apart from providing a mechanism of attachment, the hemidesmosome/basal lamina complex allows for control of biological behaviour of the epithelial cells. The basal lamina acts as a molecular barrier and plays a role in the response to tissue injury. As will be seen when considering

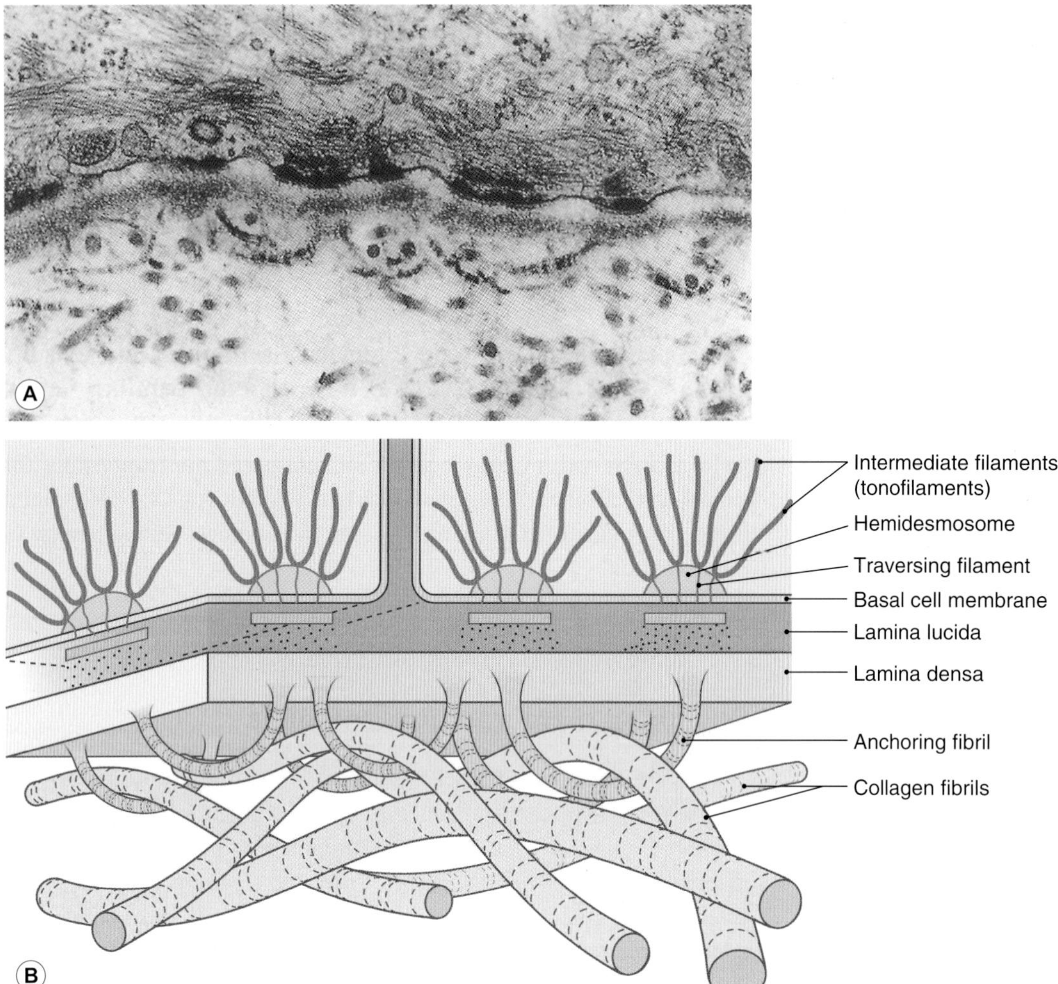

Fig. 14.29 Electron micrograph showing appearance of basal lamina (×34,000). Courtesy Prof. C A Squier.

the development of certain dental tissues, the basal lamina is important when considering epithelial/mesenchymal interactions. It is not surprising, therefore, to find that abnormalities resulting in defects in the composition of the hemidesmosomal/basal lamina complex are associated with pathologies (see pages 315–316).

Regional variations in the structure of the oral mucosa

In different parts of the mouth, the mucosa has different roles and experiences different degrees and types of stress during mastication, speech and facial expression. As a consequence, the structure of the oral mucosa varies in terms of the thickness of the epithelium, the degree of keratinisation, the complexity of the connective tissue–epithelium interface, the composition of the lamina propria and the presence or absence of the submucosa.

There are three types of oral mucosa: masticatory, lining and specialised mucosa. Masticatory mucosa is found where there is high compression and friction and is characterised by a keratinised epithelium and a thick lamina propria. The mucosa of the gingiva and palate is masticatory, the bulk of which is firmly bound down directly and tightly to underlying bone (mucoperiosteum), except for the region at the side of the palate, where a submucosa is present. Lining mucosa is not subject to high levels of friction but must be mobile and distensible. It is thus nonkeratinised and has a loose lamina propria. Within the lamina propria, the collagen fibres are arranged as a network to allow free movement, and the elastic fibres allow recoil to prevent the mucosa from being chewed. Commonly, lining mucosa also has a submucosa. The lips, cheeks, buccal and labial sulci, alveolar mucosa, floor of the mouth, ventral surface of the tongue and soft palate have a lining mucosa. Two areas of specialised mucosa occur: the specialised gustatory mucosa of the dorsum of the tongue and where the vermilion zone forms a transition between the skin and the oral mucosa.

Within the oral cavity about 60% of the mucosa is lining mucosa, about 25% of the mucosa is masticatory mucosa and the remaining 15% specialised mucosa.

Regional variations of the oral mucosa are summarised in Table 14.2.

Lip

The lip has skin on its outer surface and labial mucosa on its inner surface. Between these two tissues lies the vermilion zone (also known as the *red or transitional zone of the lip*) (Fig. 14.30). The lips have striated muscles in their core that are part of the muscles of facial expression. Substantial amounts of minor mucous salivary glands are present in the submucosa. The epithelial thickness gradually increases from the skin to the mucosal aspect.

The skin on the outer surface of the lip shows all the features of skin elsewhere (Fig. 14.31). A keratinised layer of epidermis lies on a bed of connective tissue, the dermis. The border between epidermis and dermis in this area is relatively flattened. The connective tissue contains sweat

Table 14.2 Principal features and regional variations of the oral mucosa

Region	Epithelium		Lamina propria		Submucosa		
	Thickness	Keratinisation	Papillae	Fibre types	Density	Attachment	Type of mucosa
Labial and buccal mucosa	Thick	Nonkeratinised	Short and irregular	Collagen and some elastin fibres	Dense	Firmly to underlying muscle	Lining
Vermilion (red) zone of lip	Thin	Keratinised	Long and narrow	Collagen and some elastin fibres	Dense	Firmly to underlying muscle	Specialised
Alveolar mucosa	Thin	Nonkeratinised	Short or absent	Many elastin fibres	Loose	Loose attachment to periosteum	Lining
Attached gingiva	Thick	Keratinised and parakeratinised	Long and narrow	Dense collagen firmly attached to underlying periosteum	No distinct submucosa		Masticatory
Floor of mouth	Thin	Nonkeratinised	Short and broad	Collagen and some elastin fibres	Loose	Loose attachment to underlying muscle	Lining
Ventral surface of tongue	Thin	Nonkeratinised	Short and numerous	Collagen and some elastin fibres	Not very distinct layer; attached to underlying muscle		Lining
Dorsum of tongue (anterior two-thirds)	Thick	Primarily keratinised	Long	Collagen and some elastin fibres	Not very distinct layer; attached to underlying muscle		Specialised gustatory
Dorsum of tongue (posterior one-third)	Variable	Generally nonkeratinised	Short or absent	Collagen and some elastin fibres	Not very distinct layer; attached to underlying muscle		Lining gustatory
Hard palate	Thick	Keratinised	Long	Dense collagen in submucosa laterally, but lamina propria firmly bound to periosteum without submucosa in midline			Masticatory
Soft palate	Thick	Nonkeratinised	Short	Many elastin fibres	Loose	Loose attachment to underlying tissues	Lining

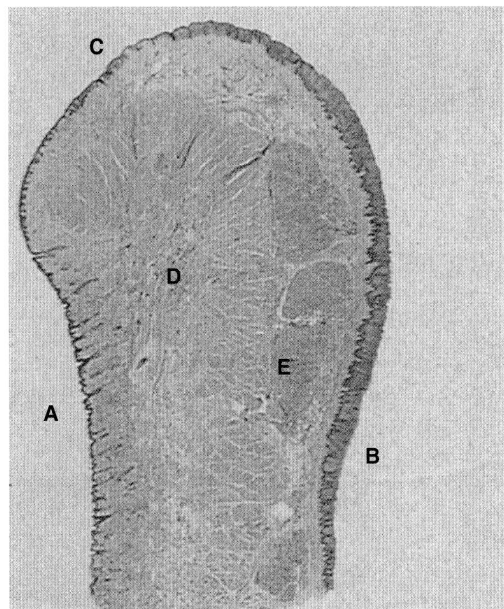

Fig. 14.30 Transverse section of the lip. A = skin on external surface; B = labial mucosa on inner surface; C = vermilion (red) zone; D = striated muscles of orbicularis oris; E = minor salivary glands (H & E; ×2). Courtesy S Kariyawasam.

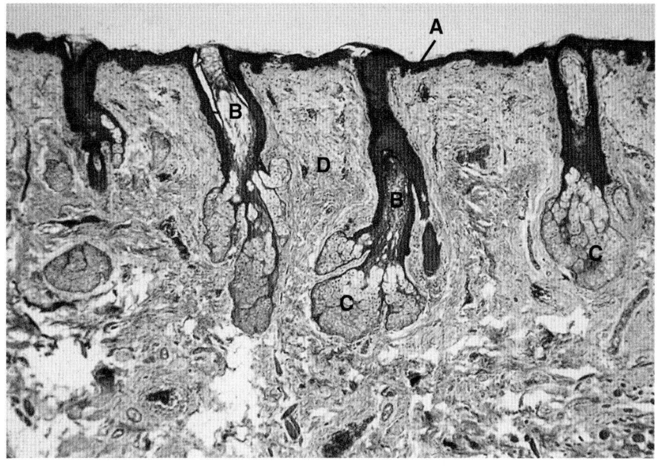

Fig. 14.31 Section of skin of lip. A = keratinised epidermis; B = shaft of hair; C = sebaceous gland; D = dermis (Masson's trichrome; ×30).

glands; sebaceous glands and the bases of hair follicles pass through the epithelium. The epidermis is continuous around the bases of the follicles and is responsible for producing the keratin of which the hair is formed. Sebaceous glands drain either into the hair follicles or occasionally directly on to the skin surface.

Vermilion (Red Zone)

The vermilion zone lacks the appendages of skin. However, very occasional sebaceous glands may be found, especially at the angles of the mouth. As the vermilion zone also lacks mucous glands, it requires constant moistening with saliva by the tongue to prevent drying. Moreover, transepithelial water loss is almost three times as high in the vermilion compared with the skin of the cheek, and decreases with age. The vermilion receives high exposure to solar radiation. The epithelium of the vermilion zone is keratinised, but thin and translucent. The connective tissue papillae of the lamina propria are relatively long and narrow and contain capillary loops (Fig. 14.32). The proximity of these vessels to the surface, combined with the translucency of the epithelium, gives the surface a red appearance – hence its name. This red appearance is a human characteristic. However, as stated in Chapter 1 (page 1) the term `vermilion' may require changing because persons of some ancestral origins do not have red lips. The junctional region between the vermilion zone and the labial mucosa is known as the *intermediate zone*. It lacks a granular layer and tends to have a thick parakeratinised layer. In infants this becomes thickened and forms the suckling pad.

Labial mucosa

The inner surface of the lip, the labial mucosa, is covered by a relatively thick, nonkeratinised epithelium. The lamina propria is also wide but the papillae are short and irregular. A submucosa containing many minor salivary glands is present (Fig. 14.33). Strands of dense connective tissue bind the mucosa down to the underlying orbicularis oris muscle.

As the vermilion and intermediate zones (when identifiable) separate the keratinised skin from the lining mucosa, the question arises as to their particular phenotype. From a study of the distribution of cytokeratins and other epithelial proteins, it has been concluded that a unique transitional phenotype with features of both epidermis and labial epithelium occurs across the vermilion and particularly the intermediate zone of the upper lip (Tables 14.3, 14.4).

Cheek

The buccal mucosa lining the cheeks is, as for the labial mucosa, a lining mucosa. The epithelium is nonkeratinised, and the lamina propria is dense with short, irregular papillae. A submucosa is present with many minor mucous salivary glands, beneath which lie fibres of the buccinator muscle (Fig. 14.34). The main collecting ducts of the minor salivary glands penetrate the overlying oral epithelium to drain into the vestibule of the mouth (Fig. 14.35). Sometimes, along a line coincident with the occlusal plane, the epithelium becomes keratinised, forming a white line: the linea alba (see Fig. 1.25). Sebaceous glands are sometimes present and seem to become more obvious after puberty in the male and after menopause in the female, when they appear as small yellow patches. These patches are termed *Fordyce spots* (see page 4). The role, if any, of sebaceous glands in this location is unknown, although it is important to differentiate them from pathological changes.

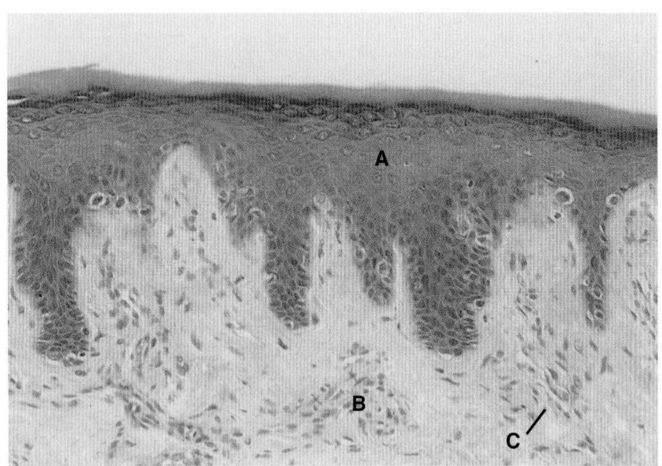

Fig. 14.32 Section of red zone of lip. A = keratinised epithelium; B = lamina propria. Note the folded interface between epithelium and lamina propria bringing blood vessels (C) close to the surface (×80).

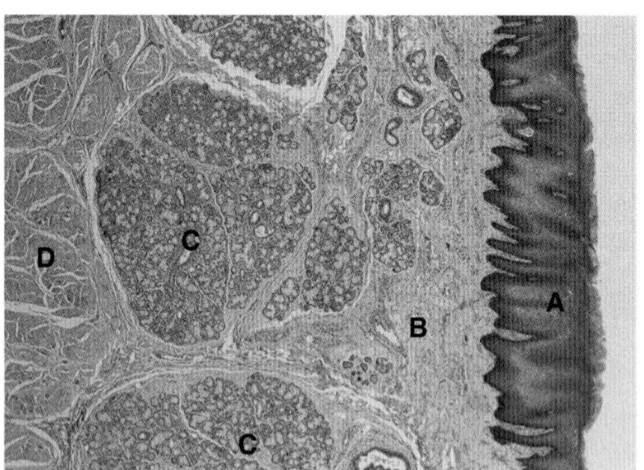

Fig. 14.33 Section of labial mucosa. A = nonkeratinised oral epithelium; B = lamina propria; C = minor salivary gland in submucosa; D = fibres of orbicularis oris (H & E; ×15). Courtesy S Kariyawasam.

Table 14.3 Staining patterns of principal cytokeratins in the stratified squamous epithelium of the lip

	Layer	CK1	CK10	CK4	CK13	CK5	CK14	CK19
Labial skin	Basal layer	–	–	–	–	+	+	–
	Prickle cell layer	+	+	–	–	±	–	–
	Granular layer	+	+	–	–	–	–	–
	Keratinised layer	–	–	–	–	–	–	–
Vermilion	Basal layer	–	–	–	–	+	+	–
	Prickle cell layer	+	+	–	–	±	±	–
	Granular layer	+	+	–	–	±	±	–
	Keratinised layer	–	–	–	–	–	–	–
Intermediate zone	Basal layer	–	–	–	–	+	+	±
	Prickle cell layer	±	±	±	±	±	±	±
	Keratinised layer	–	–	–	–	–	–	–
Labial mucosa	Basal layer	–	–	–	–	+	+	+
	Prickle cell layer	±	–	+	+	±	±	±

– = Negative staining; + = positive; ± = positive (with variable intensity of staining) or negative. Positive controls were cytokeratins (CK) 1 and 10 – suprabasal keratinocytes in abdominal epidermis and palatal mucosa; CK4 and CK13 – suprabasal keratinocytes in nonkeratinised cheek mucosal stratified squamous epithelium; CK5 and CK14 – basal keratinocytes; CK9 – basal keratinocytes of gingival and cheek mucosal stratified squamous epithelium, outer root sheath of hair follicles, luminal cells lining the ducts of sweat and minor salivary glands.

From Barrett, A.W., Morgan, M., Nwaeze, G., et al., 2005. The differentiation profile of epithelium of the human lip. Archives of Oral Biology 50, 431–438 and courtesy of the editors of Archives of Oral Biology.

Table 14.4 Staining patterns of filaggrin, loricrin and involucrin in the stratified squamous epithelium of the lip

	Layer	Profilaggrin/filaggrin	Loricrin	Involucrin
Labial skin	Basal layer	–	–	–
	Prickle cell layer	–	–	–
	Granular layer	+	+	+
	Keratinised layer	–	–	–
Vermilion	Basal layer	–	–	–
	Prickle cell layer	–	±	±
	Granular layer	+	+	+
	Keratinised layer	–	–	–
Intermediate zone	Basal layer	–	–	–
	Prickle cell layer	–	±	±
	Keratinised layer	–	–	–
Labial mucosa	Basal layer	–	–	–
	Prickle cell layer	+		+

– = Negative staining; + = positive staining; ± = positive or negative staining. Positive control was granular layer of epidermis.
From Barrett, A.W., Morgan, M., Nwaeze, G., et al., 2005. The differentiation profile of epithelium of the human lip. Archives of Oral Biology 50, 431–438 and courtesy of the editors of Archives of Oral Biology.

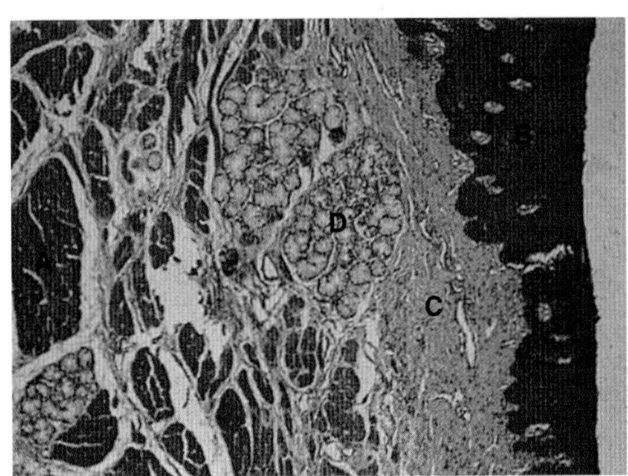

Fig. 14.34 Section of buccal mucosa. A = fibres of buccinator muscle; B = nonkeratinised oral epithelium; C = lamina propria; D = minor salivary gland in submucosa (H & E; ×15).

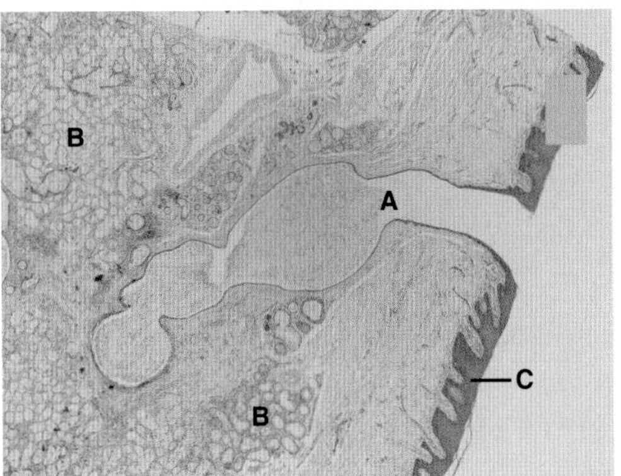

Fig. 14.35 Section of the buccal mucosa showing collecting duct (A) from a minor salivary gland (B) penetrating the overlying lining epithelium (C) (H & E; ×40).

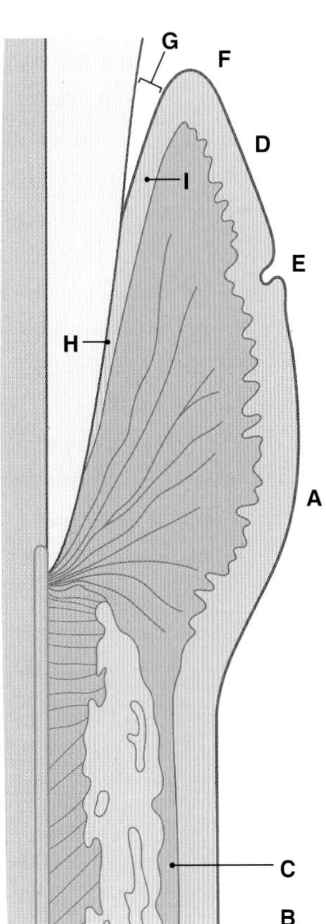

Fig. 14.36 Diagrammatic representation of gingiva. A = attached gingiva; B = alveolar mucosa; C = submucosa associated with alveolar mucosa; D = free gingiva; E = free gingival groove; F = gingival margin; G = gingival sulcus; H = junctional epithelium; I = crevicular epithelium.

Gingiva and alveolar mucosa

The gingiva is that portion of the oral mucosa that surrounds, and is attached to, the teeth and the alveolar bone. It has two recognised regions (Fig. 14.36). The main component is the attached gingiva, which is directly bound down to the underlying alveolar bone and tooth. Coronal to the attached gingiva is the free gingiva, which is the narrow rim of mucosa that is not bound down to underlying hard tissue. Its junction with the attached gingiva is sometimes demarcated by a shallow groove, the free gingival groove. Its coronal limit is the gingival margin. The unattached region between the free gingiva and the tooth is the gingival sulcus. The region apical to this, where the gingiva is bound to the underlying tooth, is the junctional epithelium.

Apically, the attached gingiva is demarcated from the alveolar mucosa (which is loosely attached to the lower part of the alveolar bone) by the mucogingival junction, which normally lies 3–5 mm below the level of the alveolar crest. The height of the gingiva above this junction is about 4–6 mm. The alveolar mucosa has a submucosa.

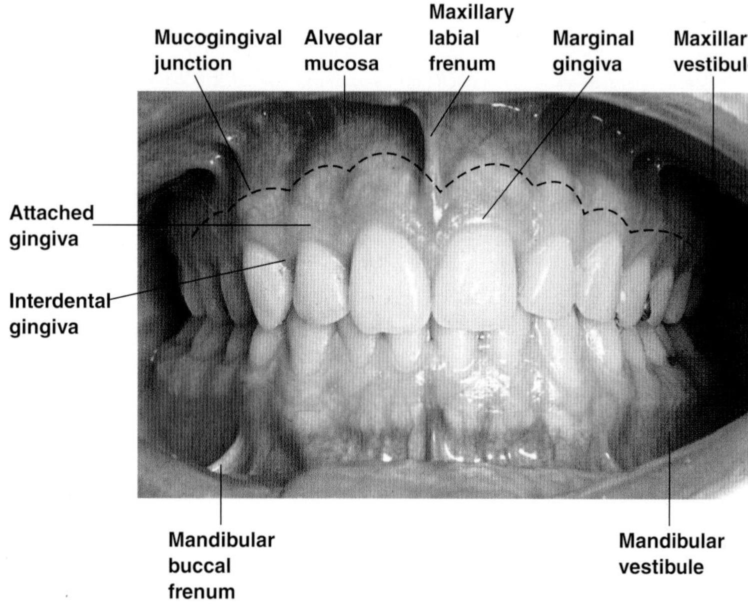

Fig. 14.37 Appearance of the gingiva. From Robinson, D., 2023. Essentials of dental assisting, seventh edition. Elsevier, Philadelphia.

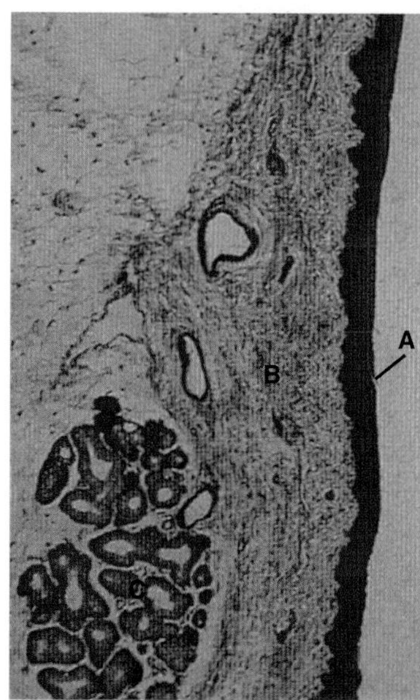

Fig. 14.38 Section of alveolar mucosa. A = nonkeratinised oral epithelium; B = lamina propria; C = minor salivary gland in submucosa (H & E; ×15).

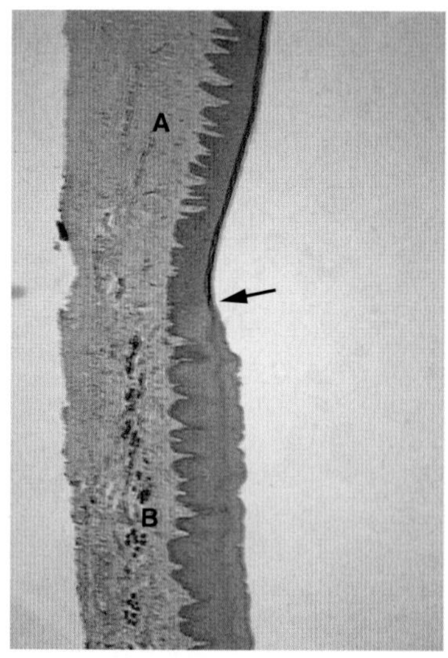

Fig. 14.39 Section of the attached gingiva (A) and alveolar (B) mucosa stripped off from underlying bone. The arrow points to the sharp demarcation site of the mucogingival junction. Note the keratinised epithelium covering the attached gingiva, the nonkeratinised epithelium covering the alveolar mucosa and the numerous blood vessels in the alveolar mucosa (Papanicolaou stain; ×20). Courtesy Prof. C A Squier.

The appearance of the gingiva and alveolar mucosa in the maxilla and mandible in vivo is seen in Fig. 14.37. The alveolar mucosa lines the lower part of the alveolus and is reflected over the buccal and labial sulcus to meet the buccal and labial mucosa, respectively. It has a loose submucosa that allows for wide degrees of movement. The submucosa on its deep aspect is firmly attached to the underlying periosteum. The mucogingival junction (or health line) demarcates the boundary between attached gingiva and alveolar mucosa. The difference in appearance between the alveolar mucosa and the attached gingiva is related to differences in keratinisation and translucency. The alveolar mucosa epithelium is translucent, and the blood vessels lie superficially. Small blood vessels are clearly seen. The mucogingival junction may be scalloped, paralleling the contours of the gingival margin. The free gingival groove that separates the attached gingiva from the free gingiva is apparent in only about 40% of teeth. It follows the contours of the cementum–enamel junction. The groove may be produced by the bundles of principal collagen fibres that run from the cervical cementum to the gingiva, or it may correspond to a heavy epithelial ridge. When present, the free gingival groove lies approximately at the level of the cementum–enamel junction. Healthy attached gingiva often shows surface stippling, which corresponds to sites of intersecting epithelial ridges. In some cases, when the free gingival groove is absent, an irregularly aligned line of stipples marks the junction between attached and free gingiva. The free gingiva is smooth. The widths of both the free and attached gingivae vary regionally. The interdental papilla (gingiva) is that part of the gingiva that fills the space between the teeth. Its shape in three dimensions, and its histological appearance, depend on the shape and nature of contact between the adjacent teeth.

On the palatal surface of the maxillary teeth, there is no alveolar mucosa. Here, the attached gingiva merges with the palatal mucosa, with no clearly demarcated boundary (see Fig. 1.11).

Alveolar mucosa

The alveolar mucosa comprises a thin, nonkeratinised epithelium overlying a lamina propria that shows poorly developed dermal papillae (Fig. 14.38). Underlying blood vessels lie near the surface (Fig. 14.39). The extensive submucosa houses many minor mucous salivary glands and, near the vestibular sulcus, is loosely attached with numerous elastin fibres, allowing for free movement. Where it adjoins the attached gingiva, the alveolar mucosa is thicker than elsewhere (and commonly thicker than the adjacent keratinised epithelium). The demarcation between keratinised and nonkeratinised epithelium (the mucogingival junction) is well-defined, and submucosal vessels and glands are limited to the alveolar mucosa (Fig. 14.39).

Gingiva

Attached gingiva (supracrestal tissue attachment)

The mucosa of the attached gingiva on its external surface (oral gingival epithelium) is a masticatory mucosa (Figs. 14.39, 14.40). It is keratinised, but the degree and extent vary considerably between and within individuals. Orthokeratinisation is the norm in mucosa unimpeded by inflammation; however, as much as 75% of the surface may be parakeratinised (i.e., the surface shows a strong pink stain with haematoxylin and eosin,

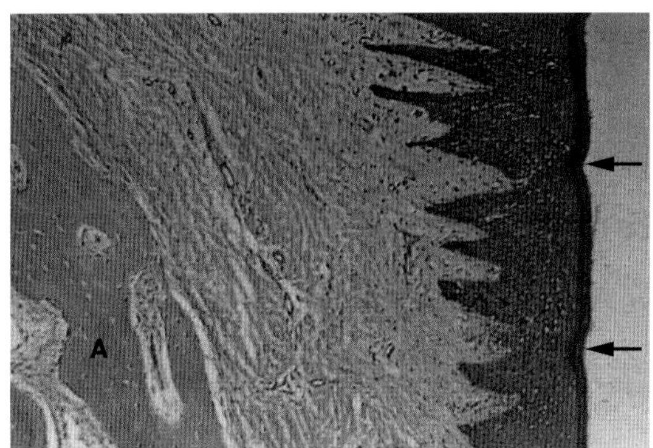

Fig. 14.40 Section of the attached gingiva. The epithelium is a keratinised stratified squamous epithelium. The lamina propria is dense and relatively avascular, and the interface with the epithelium is highly folded. The lamina propria is directly attached to the underlying alveolar bone (A), forming a mucoperiosteum. Arrows indicate surface stippling (H & E; ×75).

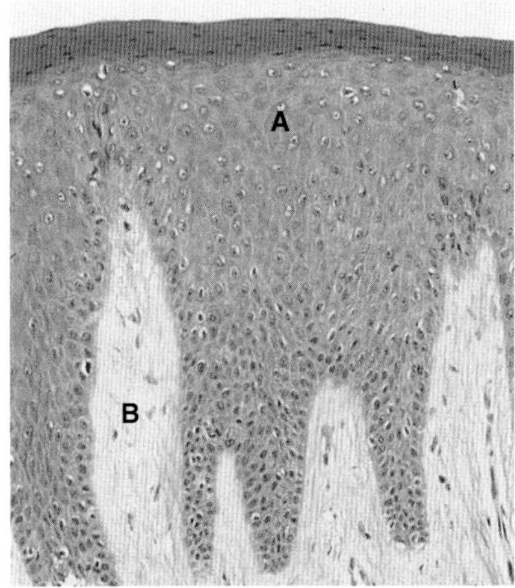

Fig. 14.41 Section of the gingival mucosa. The epithelium (A) is parakeratinised with nuclei being retained in the superficial keratinised layer. B = lamina propria (H & E; ×100). Courtesy Dr. A E Barrett.

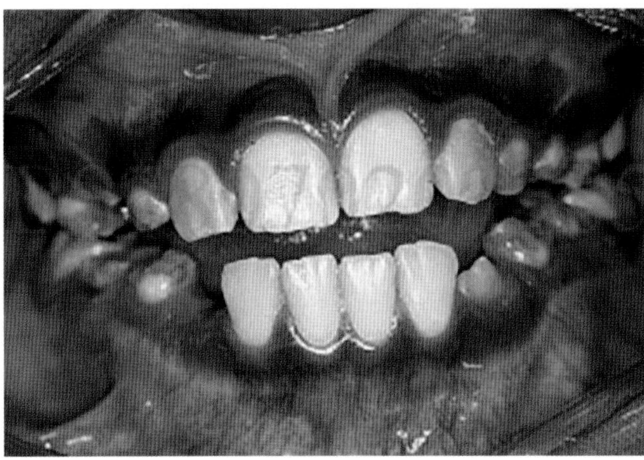

Fig. 14.42 Pigmentation of the attached gingiva owing to increased density of melanosomes in the melanocytes. Courtesy Georgiou, A., Widmer, R.P., Cameron, A.C., 2022. Handbook of pediatric dentistry, fifth edition, Elsevier, Philadelphia.

as for keratin, but nuclei are retained in the surface layer – Fig. 14.41) and as much as 10% nonkeratinised. Papillation is variable, with the papillae often being aligned in rows (especially at the margin). As little as 0.08 mm may separate the tips of some papillae from the surface. The surface is stippled, with the stipples arising from intersecting epithelial ridges. There may be varying degrees of pigmentation depending on the density of melanosomes within melanocytes (Fig. 14.42). There is no submucosa, with the lamina propria being bound directly to bone, forming a mucoperiosteum (Figs. 14.39, 14.40).

The width of the attached gingiva increases with age. This is associated with increasing alveolar bone growth, resulting in an increase in the distance between the cementum-enamel junction and the mucogingival junction. However, the distance from the mandibular border to the mucogingival junction did not change with age, suggesting that the lower border of the mandible may be a relatively fixed point for use in radiographic growth studies.

Free gingiva

The mucosa of the free gingiva is indistinguishable from that of the attached gingiva (Fig. 14.43), but may be demarcated from it by the free gingival groove (or a line of stipples). The gingival margin marks the boundary with the gingival crevice or sulcus. In germ-free animals, and in strictly healthy, plaque-free gingivae, the crevice is absent and the gingival margin corresponds to the coronal extent of the junctional epithelium. In clinically healthy mouths, the clinical crevice is 0.5–2.0 mm deep. Crevices deeper than 3 mm (measured clinically) are generally accepted as diseased and are described as 'periodontal pockets'. In routine decalcified sections the enamel will be lost, but its position must be envisaged in order to appreciate the approximate position of the gingival crevice and thus distinguish between the crevicular (sulcular) epithelium, which faces the gingival crevice, and the junctional epithelium, which is in direct contact with the enamel surface at the base of the crevice (Fig. 14.43).

Crevicular (sulcular) epithelium

The epithelium on the inner surface of the gingiva constitutes the crevicular epithelium and the junctional epithelium, both of which are nonkeratinised and therefore lack a granular layer. These form the so-called *gingival cuff* at the site where the oral mucosa meets the tooth. Histologically, the crevicular epithelium may be distinguished from the junctional epithelium by having a more folded interface with the underlying connective tissue. In addition, tags of an enamel cuticle may be seen at the interface between the two epithelia

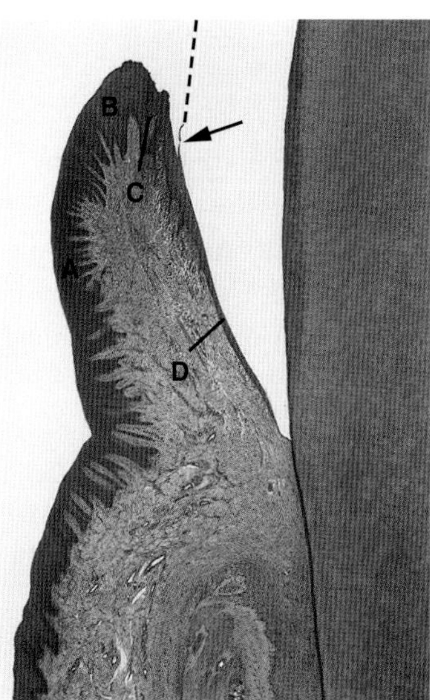

Fig. 14.43 Demineralised section showing the dentogingival junction. The outline of the original enamel surface is indicated by the broken black line. A = region of attached gingiva covered by masticatory epithelium; B = region of free gingiva covered externally by masticatory epithelium; C = nonkeratinised crevicular epithelium; D = nonkeratinised junctional epithelium. Note the tag of enamel cuticle (arrow) that helps to delineate the oral crevicular epithelium from the junctional epithelium (H & E; ×30). Courtesy Prof. H E Schroeder.

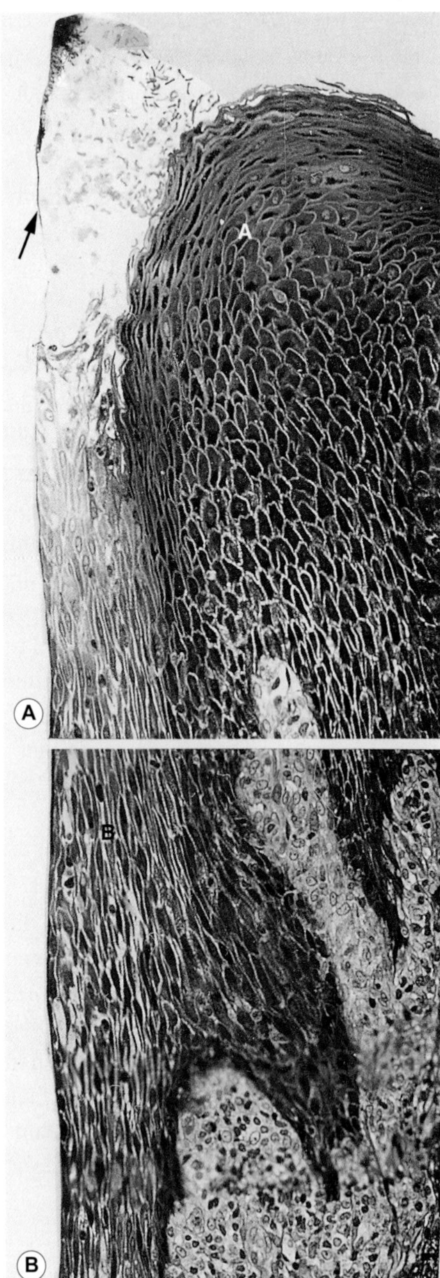

Fig. 14.44 Section of gingiva showing the crevicular epithelium (A) and the upper portion of the junctional epithelium (B). At this site the junctional epithelium may be 15–30 cells thick. Note the tag of enamel cuticle (arrow) helping to delineate the two types of epithelia (×200). Courtesy Prof. H E Schroeder.

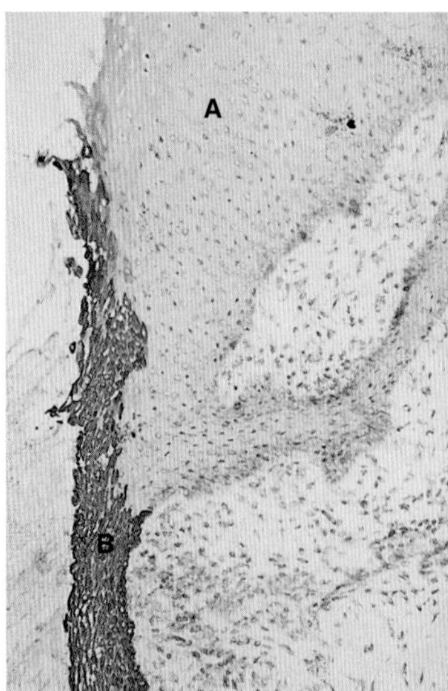

Fig. 14.45 Demineralised section of gingiva showing crevicular (A) and junctional epithelium (B) staining for cytokeratin 19. The junctional epithelium stains positively (brown) (×150). Courtesy Prof. P R Morgan.

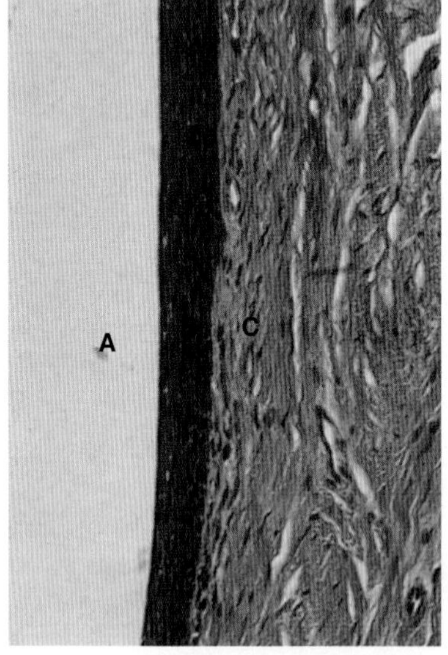

Fig. 14.46 Demineralised section of gingiva showing nonkeratinised stratified squamous epithelium forming junctional epithelium (B). Note the smooth interface with the underlying lamina propria (C). A = enamel space (H & E; ×150).

(Figs. 14.43, 14.44). The two epithelia can also be distinguished by their different cytokeratin profiles. As is to be expected, the superficial layers of the crevicular epithelium stain positive for CK4, typical of lining epithelium. However, junctional epithelium not only lacks CK4 (even though it can be considered a lining mucosa) but characteristically expresses the basal keratinocyte markers CK5, 14 and 19 throughout all its layers (Fig. 14.45), indicating that it is a nondifferentiating tissue. This CK profile is similar to that of the reduced enamel epithelium from which it is derived. Unlike the oral crevicular epithelium, the junctional epithelium also has receptors for, and expresses, epidermal growth factor.

The gingival crevice (Figs. 14.36, 14.43) is bounded by the gingival margin above and the junctional epithelium below. The epithelium is nonkeratinised and thinner. The crevicular epithelium merges with the junctional epithelium, and a distinct boundary is not usually seen. Externally, the base of the gingival crevice corresponds approximately with the free gingival groove, when present.

Junctional epithelium

The junctional epithelium is an epithelial collar that surrounds the tooth and extends from the region of the cementum–enamel junction to the bottom of the gingival crevice (Figs. 14.43–14.46). It may extend for up to 2 mm. Coronally the junctional epithelium may be 15–30 cells thick (up to 100 μm; Fig. 14.44), while apically it narrows to only 1–3 cells thick. It consists of two zones: a single cell layer of cuboidal cells (the stratum germinativum) overlying several layers of flattened cells equivalent to a stratum spinosum. There is no stratum granulosum or corneum. The junctional epithelium has a high rate of turnover (in the order of 5–6 days), and its cells are exfoliated coronally into the gingival crevice. It is derived from the rapidly replaced reduced enamel epithelium (probably from the stratum intermedium component of that tissue), and this may explain why its CK profile resembles odontogenic epithelium rather than the lining stratified squamous epithelium typical of oral mucosa (Fig. 14.45). The cells of the stratum germinativum rest on a typical lamina propria, which shows many capillaries and appears to be more cellular than other parts of the gingiva. The connective tissue interface is smooth (Fig. 14.46).

The principal features of the junctional epithelium are shown diagrammatically in Fig. 14.47. The cells of the junctional epithelium immediately adjacent to the tooth attach themselves to the tooth by hemidesmosomes and a basal lamina. The combination of the hemidesmosomes and basal lamina is known as the *attachment apparatus* or *epithelial attachment*. The basal lamina in contact with the tooth is termed the *internal basal lamina*. On the other surface of the junctional epithelium in contact with the lamina propria is the normal basal lamina (the external basal lamina). The junctional epithelium is therefore unique in having two basal laminae. However, differences exist between the two basal laminae (see later). Like epithelial cells elsewhere, the cells of the junctional epithelium are joined by desmosomes and gap junctions; tight junctions are rare. However, the desmosomes are fewer in number, and this is correlated with larger intercellular spaces that may comprise up to 5% of the volume of the tissue. This has profound clinical significance because not only crevicular fluid but also defence cells can pass across the junctional epithelium (Fig. 14.48). Indeed, even healthy gingival tissue may exhibit neutrophils in the intercellular spaces, indicative of its protective role. The lack of membrane-coating granules (see page 287) may also assist the permeability of the cell layer. In this context, cells of the junctional epithelium, together with underlying fibroblasts and endothelial cells, express intercellular adhesion molecule (ICAM)-1, which helps in the transmigration of neutrophils from the adjacent capillaries and through the junctional epithelium. The turnover rate for cells of the junctional epithelium is the highest of any oral mucosa. There is also evidence for a high turnover rate for the internal basal lamina.

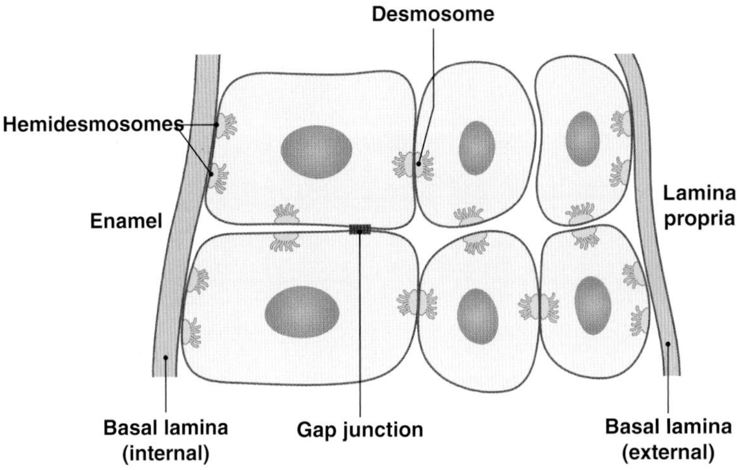

Fig. 14.47 Diagrammatic representation of junctional epithelium.

Ultrastructural examination of junctional epithelial cells interfacing with enamel shows that the attachment of the cell to the enamel is mediated by hemidesmosomes and a basal lamina (Fig. 14.49). The internal basal lamina, as elsewhere, is seen to contain two zones: an electron-lucent zone adjacent to the cell (which may represent a preparation artefact) and an electron-dense layer against the tooth surface. The pattern of a lamina densa and lamina lucida is apparently not as clear as in other basal laminae, with the lamina densa not always being clearly delineated. However, the combined thickness is similar (100–140 nm). The internal basal lamina also differs from the external basal lamina in lacking type IV collagen and anchoring fibrils. It is therefore not surprising that the composition of the internal basal lamina differs from the external basal lamina in lacking laminin. The basement membrane seen in light microscopy adjacent to the connective tissue would appear much thicker than in electron micrographs because of a reticular component derived from the connective tissue. The hemidesmosomes consist of thickenings of the inner leaflet of the plasma membrane (called the *attachment plaque*). Opposite the attachment plaque at the enamel surface there is a peripheral dense line comparable to that seen in the lamina lucida of the basal lamina between epithelium and connective tissue.

The nature of the adhesive mechanisms associated with the cells of the gingiva has been studied by observing the distribution of the integrins. Integrin α6β4, a transmembrane receptor glycoprotein component of hemidesmosomes, is present in both basal laminae of the junctional

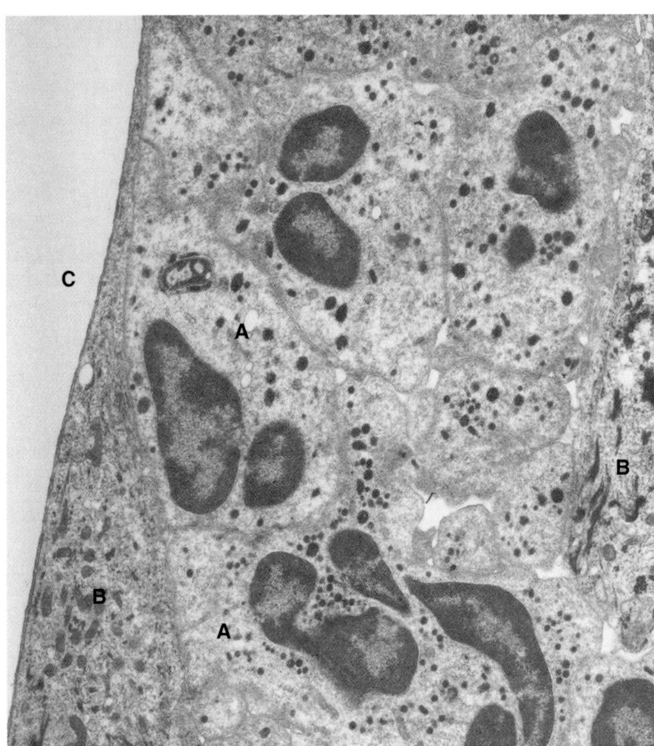

Fig. 14.48 Electron micrograph of demineralised section of junctional epithelium showing defence cells (leukocytes, A) migrating through junctional epithelial cells (B). C = enamel space (×10,000). Courtesy Prof. M M Smith.

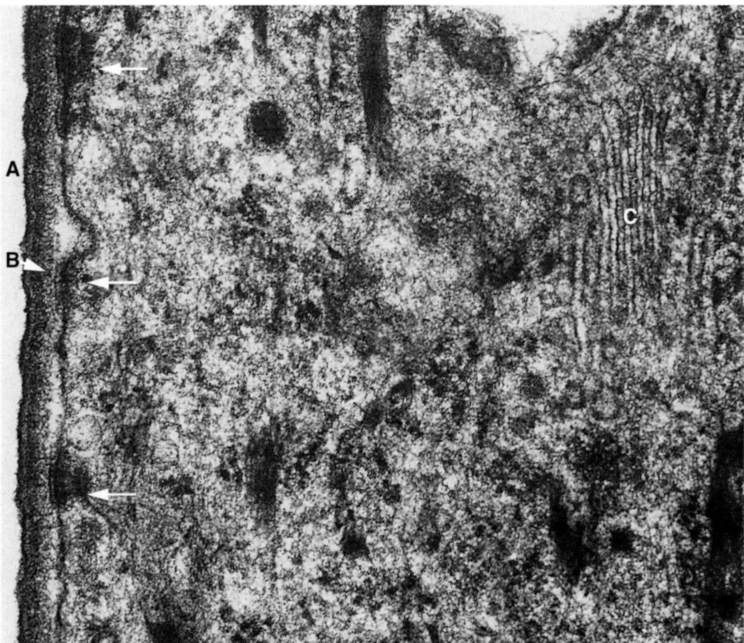

Fig. 14.49 Electron micrograph of demineralised section of part of junctional epithelial cell adjacent to enamel space (A). B = lamina lucida and lamina densa of basal lamina; C = Golgi apparatus; arrows indicate hemidesmosomes (×70,000). Courtesy Prof. J V Soames.

epithelium (compared with the crevicular epithelium, where it is only found in the single basal lamina). However, the α6 component is also associated with all the remaining cells of the junctional epithelium, allowing these cells to be distinguished from those of the crevicular epithelium. This, together with the distribution of CK19, implies a difference in adhesive mechanisms within the junctional and crevicular epithelia. The integrin αvβ6 has also been shown to be present in healthy junctional epithelial cells. However, in animals where the β6 component has been deleted, the early symptoms of periodontal disease (inflammation and bone loss) can be seen, suggesting that integrins play a central role in protection against inflammatory periodontal disease (probably through activation of TGF-1).

Expression of the odontogenic ameloblast-associated gene *(ODAM)* has been identified in the junctional epithelium, where it is believed to help maintain the integrity of the junctional epithelial attachment. From this, it has been speculated that mutations to *ODAM* may increase the risk of periodontal disease.

In addition, as the components of the basal lamina must also be synthesised, transported and secreted by junctional epithelial cells, the cytoplasm of the cells contains numerous free ribosomes, cisternae of rough endoplasmic reticulum and a prominent Golgi apparatus (Fig. 14.49). There is an absence of both membrane-coating granules and keratohyaline granules, and few CK filaments are present.

An element not visible in decalcified preparations is the enamel cuticle (see Chapter 8). This cuticle is a nonmineralised structure interposed between the junctional epithelium and the underlying hard tissue. It varies in extent and is not always present. When present, it is patchy and most prominent when filling depressions in the calcified surface. The cuticle is ultrastucturally amorphous and biochemically distinct from the basal lamina. It is probably proteinaceous and may be derived from an epithelial secretory product.

The length of the junctional epithelium attached to the enamel surface varies according to the stage of eruption (see Fig. 26.9). When the tooth first erupts into the oral cavity, most of the enamel will be covered by junctional epithelium. By the time the tooth reaches the occlusal plane, about one-quarter of the enamel surface is still covered by junctional epithelium. Eventually it will come to lie close to the cementum–enamel junction (Figs. 14.43, 14.50). In patients with exposure of the roots, the junctional epithelium proliferates apically and, as a consequence, may establish a firm union with the surface of the cementum (Fig. 14.51), also via a basal lamina (Fig. 14.52). When this occurs, and in the absence of obvious periodontal inflammatory disease, the question arises as to whether it is a physiological age change (passive eruption) or whether, as there must have been some associated loss of collagen fibres at the cervix of the tooth to allow for epithelial proliferation apically, it is the result of a disease process.

The lamina propria associated with the junctional epithelium has a rich blood supply arranged as a complex anastomosing network, with the major vessels representing postcapillary venules. This crevicular plexus is separated from the surrounding looping vessels that lie within the dermal papillae of the attached gingiva (see Fig. 12.61). The crevicular plexus is the obvious source of gingival crevicular fluid. The vessels of the plexus are very sensitive to stimulation and are likely to vasodilate under the slightest of insults. In response to dental plaque, they may become more permeable, increasing the production of crevicular fluid. The junctional epithelium has a rich plexus of nerves close to its basal layer, with many endings penetrating into the epithelium itself.

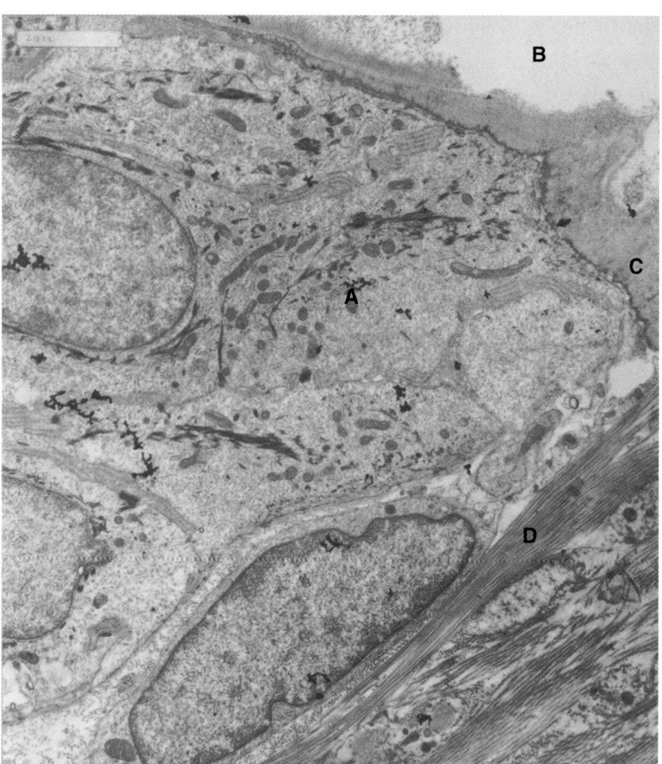

Fig. 14.50 Electron micrograph of demineralised section showing the apical limit of the junctional epithelial cells (A) at the cement–enamel junction; B = enamel space; C = cementum; D = collagen fibre of gingiva (×2,500). Courtesy Prof. M M Smith.

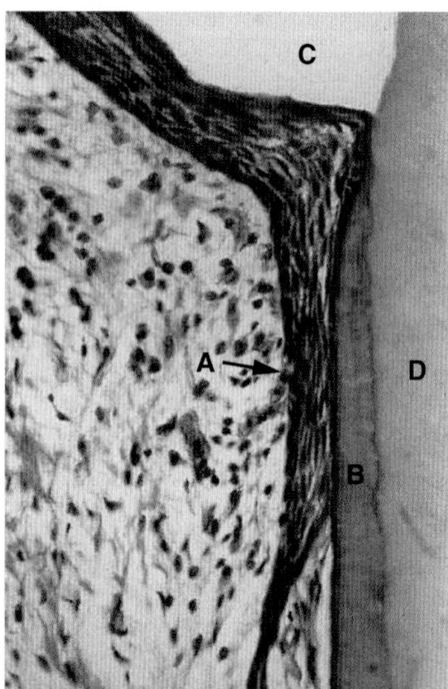

Fig. 14.51 Demineralised section showing junctional epithelium (A) having proliferated rootwards to lie on cemental surface of root (B). C = enamel space; D = dentine (H & E; ×120). Courtesy Dr D Adams.

The dentogingival junction seals the underlying connective tissue of the periodontium from the oral environment. The strength of the seal is thought to be dependent not only upon the attachment of the junctional epithelium to the tooth but also upon the pressure exerted by the fibres and tissue fluid of the underlying connective tissue. The weakness of the dentogingival junction derives from its situation, the enamel being a nonshedding surface, allowing persistent bacterial colonisation. The epithelium is therefore exposed to toxic products emanating from the consequent bacterial accumulation.

The turnover of the junctional epithelium is rapid. The epithelial cells migrate in a coronal direction, to be shed into the oral cavity via the gingival crevice. The continual breakdown and reformation of lamina densa, hemidesmosomes and desmosomes allow cells to alter their relationship

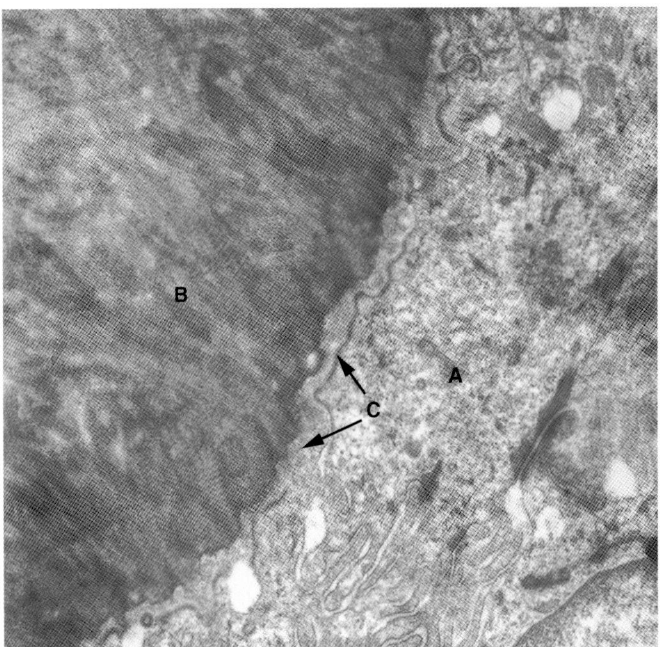

Fig. 14.52 Electron micrograph of demineralised section of junctional epithelium (A), which has proliferated rootwards to lie on cementum (B), the collagen fibrils of which are evident. The epithelial cells are attached to the cementum by a basal lamina/cuticle (C) (×20,000). Courtesy Prof. M M Smith.

as they migrate through the junctional epithelium. The rate of turnover is dependent on the demands placed upon the tissue and appears to be directly related to the degree of inflammation. Following the surgical removal of the gingiva, a new junctional epithelium rapidly forms that has all the original characteristics. As the newly formed dentogingival junction can only have been derived from the gingival epithelium (which is keratinised), it can be assumed that proliferating epithelial cells from this surface are modified by underlying connective tissue cells closer to the tooth surface to express a different phenotype (see pages 291–292).

Of clinical importance is the fact that, following the insertion of a dental implant (see page 281), the junctional epithelium regenerates and attaches to the implant surface and the implant abutment surface by a basal lamina and hemidesmosomes.

Gingival crevicular fluid

The junctional epithelium is permeable. Indeed, tissue fluid and cells (as well as experimental substances such as dyes, carbon particles and horseradish peroxidase) pass readily through the epithelium from the connective tissue into the gingival crevice. This is known as *gingival crevicular fluid* (GCF), and it can be collected using capillary tubing, gingival washing or absorbent paper strips. The GCF originates from the blood vessels of the gingival plexus.

In healthy tissues low levels of flow rates are present (0.05–0.2 μL/min). It is thought by some that fluid only passes into the crevice as a response to pathological stimuli and is absent from perfectly healthy gingiva.

The permeability of the junctional epithelium may be related to the presence of particularly wide intercellular spaces. GCF may be regarded as a transudate (exudate) of the periodontal tissues that reaches the gingival crevice through intercellular routes across the epithelial wall by osmosis. The basement membrane filters out large components. GCF contains material of low molecular weight that is said to pass continuously from the subepithelial tissue into the gingival crevice. Other oral epithelial surfaces do not show such exudation of tissue fluid. In addition to its fluid, GCF contains cells (polymorphonucleocytes and epithelial squames) and dental plaque bacteria. It is the toxins released by plaque bacteria that change the transudate into an exudate, increasing GCF flow rates. The complexity of the contents of GCF is shown by proteomics, which has revealed it contains hundreds of individual proteins.

In health, the composition of GCF is similar to plasma. It contains both inorganic and organic components. Inorganic components include sodium, potassium, calcium and magnesium. Indeed, calcium levels are higher than those in saliva, which has important implications for pellicle protein interaction, enhancing salivary protein precipitation, attachment of bacteria and ental calculus formation. In health, the concentration of organic components is similar to those in plasma. GCF contains immunoglobulins IgA, IgG and IgM; fibrinogen; complement; and protease inhibitors,

In terms of possible functions, GCF possesses leucocyte and antibody activity to protect the adjacent gingiva from antigens, and its flow will cleanse the gingival sulcus. It contains plasma proteins that may improve the adhesion of the epithelium to the tooth surface.

Once the immunological and phagocytic properties of the fluid undertake their defensive activity against the dental plaque, other inflammatory products will be present in the plaque, such as cytokines and metalloproteinases. The products of the protective inflammatory reaction, however, can then lead to damage of the host tissue. Flow rates of GCF will then increase, and the original transudate becomes an exudate. The depth of the gingival crevice will increase, allowing for a buildup of more dental plaque, setting up a vicious circle that may eventually lead to the formation of a periodontal pocket. With destruction of gingival tissue, this may result in gingivitis. If untreated, this may eventually extend more deeply to affect the periodontal ligament with loss of alveolar bone and the development of periodontitis.

The composition of the GCF provides an indicator of the state of health of the underlying periodontium, and this is discussed further on page 318.

Interdental gingiva

The interdental gingiva is the part of the gingiva between adjacent teeth. The shape and arrangement of the gingival tissues between the teeth depend on the shape of the contact between the teeth (although free and attached gingivae are always present). The interdental gingiva occupies the space between the teeth and conforms to its shape. From the buccal or lingual aspects, the interdental gingiva has a wedge-shaped appearance (Fig. 14.37). Between the anterior teeth (which contact only at a small point), it would appear similarly 'pointed' when viewed in a buccolingual plane. In the posterior cheek teeth, which have a broader area of contact, the appearance from the buccal or lingual side would show the typical wedge shape (Fig. 14.53), but across its buccolingual plane there are two peaks on the buccal and lingual aspects with a curved depression between them (the interdental col), which follows the contour around the contact point (Fig. 14.54).

The epithelium of the col is continuous with the junctional epithelium on each side. It is similarly nonkeratinised and initially derived from the reduced enamel epithelium. Its epithelium is thin and, as the region is not easy to keep dental plaque-free, inflammatory cells may be seen infiltrating the underlying lamina propria (Fig. 14.55). When teeth are spaced, the col does not exist and an often very flat gingiva is seen, which is covered by a keratinised epithelium.

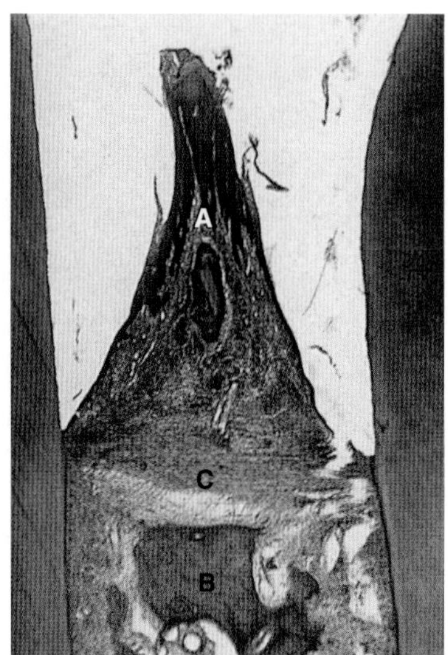

Fig. 14.53 Demineralised section showing the interdental gingiva (A) between two cheek teeth in the anteroposterior plane. B = alveolar crest; C = transseptal group of gingival fibres (H & E; ×20).

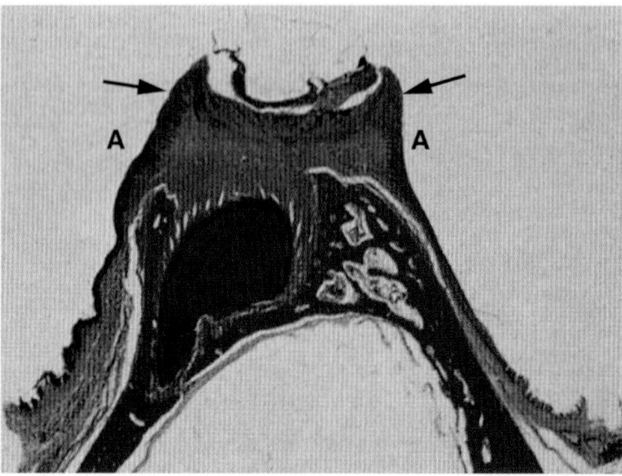

Fig. 14.54 Demineralised section of the interdental papilla cut in the buccolingual plane between two cheek teeth showing the 'interdental col'. The buccal and lingual margins (arrows) of the attached gingiva externally (A) are raised above the central concavity of the col, whose margin passes below the contact points of the teeth (H & E; ×4).

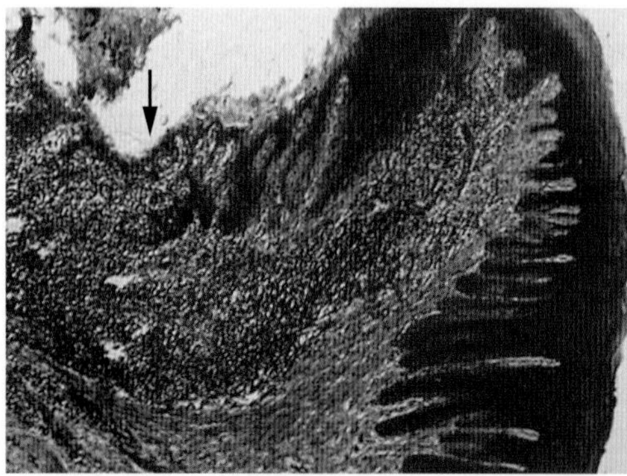

Fig. 14.55 Higher-power view of the thin, nonkeratinised epithelium of the interdental col (arrow). There is a substantial infiltrate of inflammatory cells in the area (H & E; ×40).

Most collagen fibres of the gingiva are composed of type I collagen. These are in the form of dense principal bundles, the functions of which include support of the free gingiva, binding of the attached gingiva to the alveolar bone and tooth (thereby resisting masticatory loads) and linkage of teeth one to another. These principal fibre groups have been given names based upon their orientation and attachments, although whether they always exist as such discrete and definable groups is debatable (Fig. 14.56). The turnover rate of gingival collagen appears to be faster than in other parts of the oral mucosa.

Dentogingival fibres arise from the root surface above the alveolar crest and radiate to insert into the lamina propria of the gingiva. The most superficial fibres lie beneath the crevicular epithelium, a middle group lies almost horizontally and the deepest group courses between the gingiva and the alveolar bone (Fig. 14.57).

Longitudinal fibres extend for long distances within the free gingiva, some possibly for the whole length of the arch.

Circular fibres encircle each tooth within the marginal and interdental gingiva. Some attach to cementum, some to alveolar bone. Some cross interdentally to join the fibre group of the adjacent tooth.

Alveologingival fibres run from the crest of the alveolar bone and interdental septum, radiating coronally into the overlying lamina propria of the gingiva.

Dentoperiosteal fibres occur only in labial/buccal and lingual gingiva. They arise from cementum and pass over the alveolar crest to insert into the periosteum.

Transseptal fibres pass horizontally from the root of one tooth, above the alveolar crest, to be inserted into the root of the adjacent tooth (Figs. 14.53, 14.58). Such fibres provide an anatomical basis for linking all the teeth in the dentition. They have been implicated in the mechanism of mesial drift (pages 472–473).

Semicircular fibres emanate from cementum near the cementum–enamel junction, cross the free marginal gingiva and insert into a similar position on the opposite side of the tooth.

Transgingival fibres reinforce the circular and semicircular fibres. The fibres arise from the cervical cementum and extend into the marginal gingiva of the adjacent tooth, merging with the circular fibres.

Interdental fibres pass through the coronal portion of the interdental gingiva in the buccolingual direction, connecting buccal and lingual papillae.

Vertical fibres arise in alveolar mucosa or attached gingiva and pass coronally towards the marginal gingiva and interdental papilla.

The lamina propria of the gingiva has properties that distinguish it from the connective tissue of the periodontal ligament. For example, the fibroblasts lack alkaline phosphatase, have less contractile proteins and can release more prostaglandin in response to histamine. The ECM has less ground substance and less type III collagen, is hyaluronan-rich and has a lower turnover rate. Such differences in properties may be relevant when considering periodontal regeneration (see pages 257–258).

The vasculature of the lamina propria of the gingiva is very rich and forms two plexuses, one beneath the oral gingival epithelium and the other beneath the oral crevicular epithelium. These plexuses allow the tissues to respond very quickly to stimuli. Each dermal papilla of the lamina propria beneath the oral gingival epithelium possesses an ascending arterial loop and a descending venous loop, between which lies a terminal capillary loop. Beneath the junctional epithelium lies a complex vascular plexus comprising postcapillary venules. From this region is derived the GCF. Specialisations also allow for the rapid passage of cells and molecules across the junctional epithelium.

Palate

Hard palate

The mucosa of the hard palate is a typical masticatory mucosa with part keratinised and part parakeratinised epithelia (Fig. 14.59). In much of the central region there is no submucosa and the dense lamina propria binds down directly to bone (mucoperiosteum; Fig. 14.60). The same

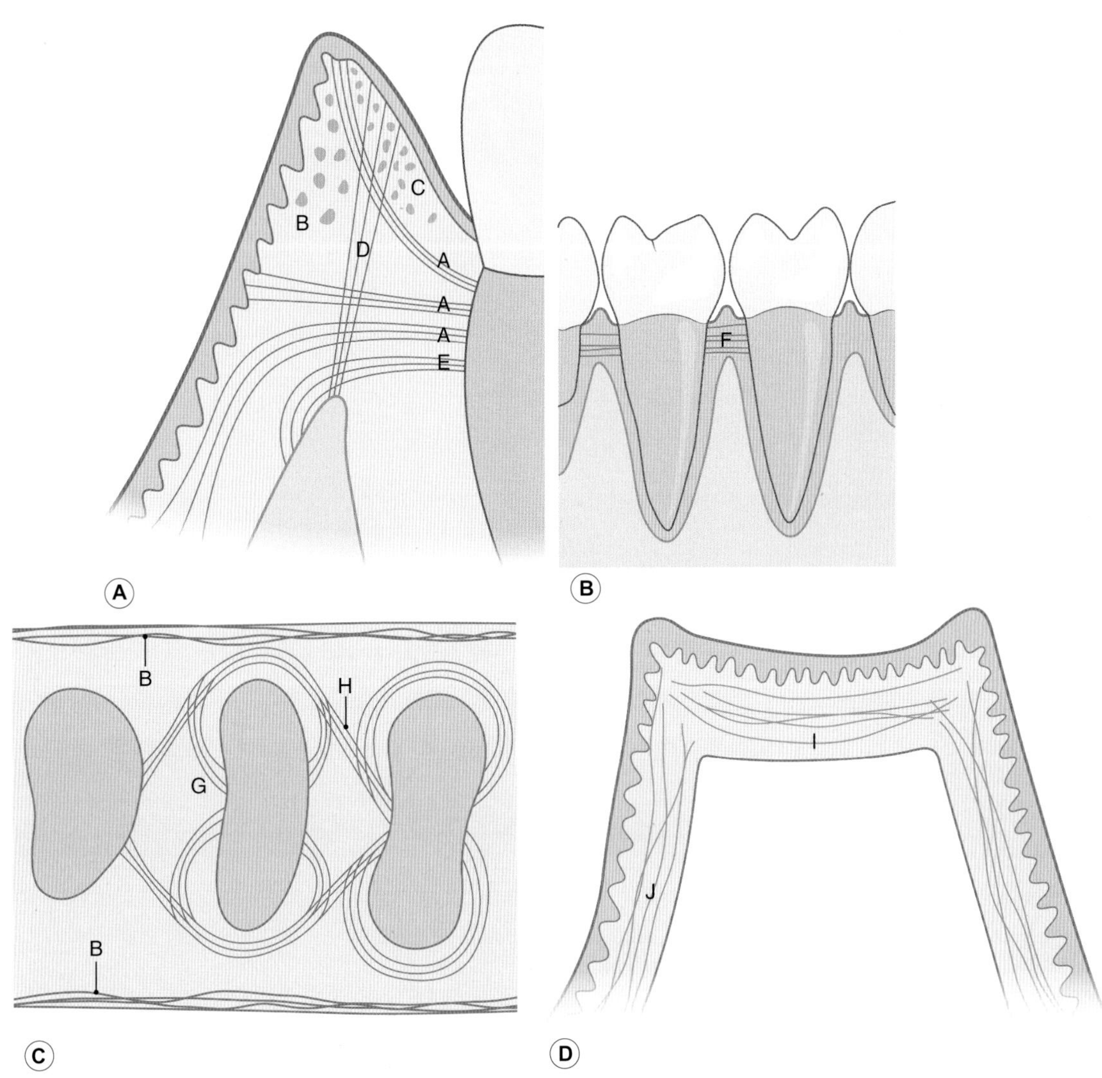

Fig. 14.56 Diagram showing arrangement of principal collagen fibre groups in the lamina propria of the gingiva. (A) Buccolingual section; (B) mesiodistal section; (C) horizontal section; (D) buccolingual section along interdental col. A = dentogingival fibres; B = longitudinal fibres; C = circular fibres; D = alveologingival fibres; E = dentoperiosteal fibres; F = transseptal fibres; G = semicircular fibres; H = transgingival fibres; I = interdental fibres; J = vertical fibres.

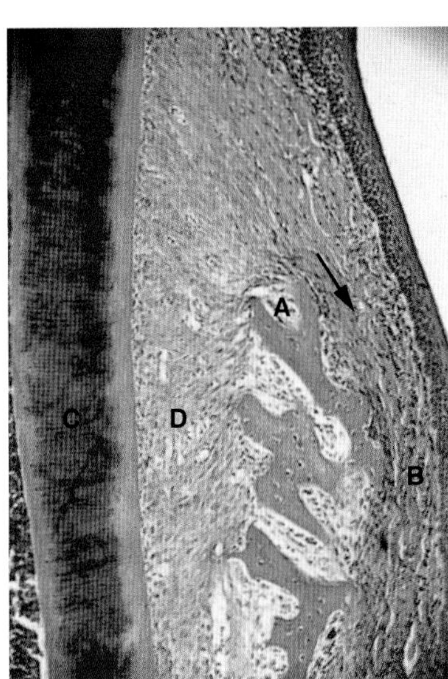

Fig. 14.57 Demineralised section showing direction of dentogingival fibres (arrowed) passing over the alveolar crest (A) and inserting into the lamina propria of the attached gingiva (B). C = root of tooth; D = periodontal ligament (Masson's trichrome; ×80).

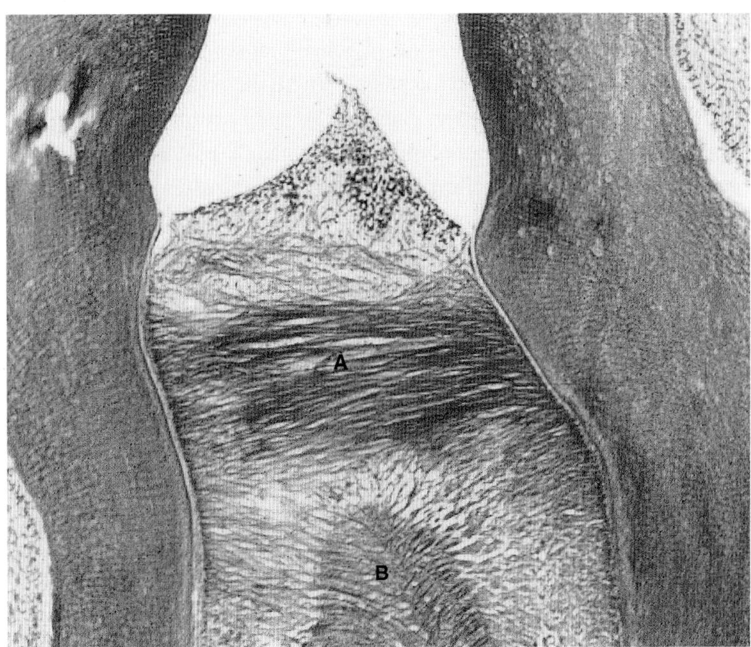

Fig. 14.58 Decalcified section of two cheek teeth sectioned in the anteroposterior plane showing transseptal fibres (A) passing from the cementum of one tooth over the alveolar crest (B) to attach into the cementum of the adjacent tooth (von Gieson; ×140). Courtesy Dr. M E Atkinson.

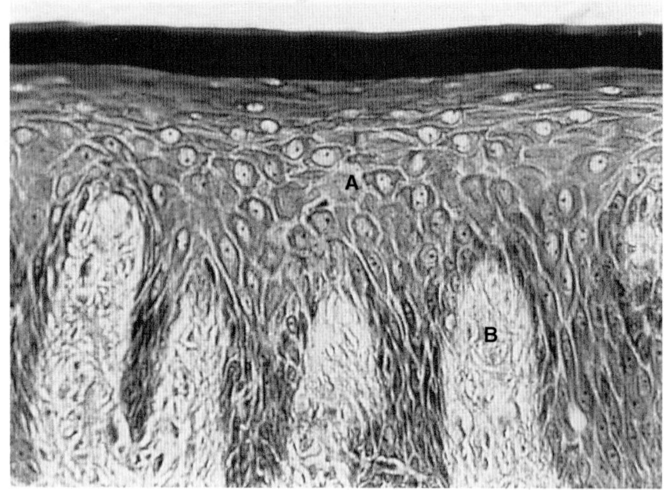

Fig. 14.59 Section of the masticatory keratinised epithelium (A) of the hard palate. Note the highly folded interface with the lamina propria (B) (H & E; ×250). Courtesy Dr. D Adams.

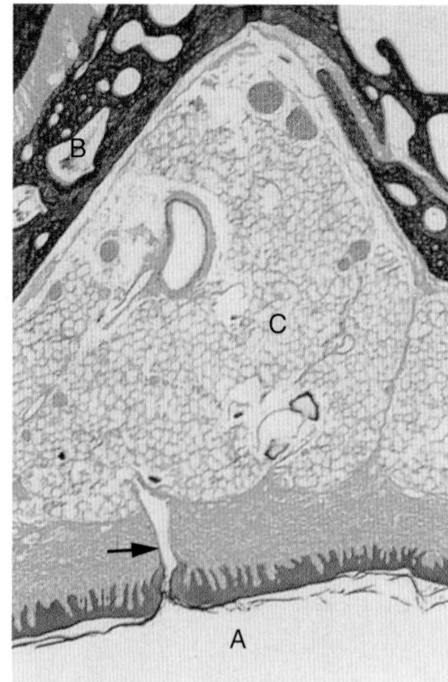

Fig. 14.61 Demineralised section of posterior part of the hard palate at its junction with the alveolar process showing the presence of a submucosa (C) containing minor mucous salivary glands with a duct (arrow) opening on to the surface. A = oral cavity; B = bone. Note the masticatory mucosa lining the surface (Masson's trichrome; ×15).

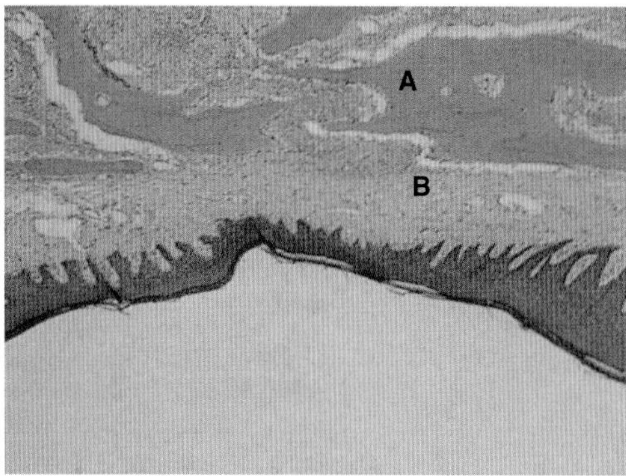

Fig. 14.60 Demineralised section of the hard palate. The keratinised epithelium exhibits deep epithelial rete. The dense lamina propria (B) is attached to the bone of the hard palate (A) in the absence of a submucosa, forming a mucoperiosteum (H & E; ×20).

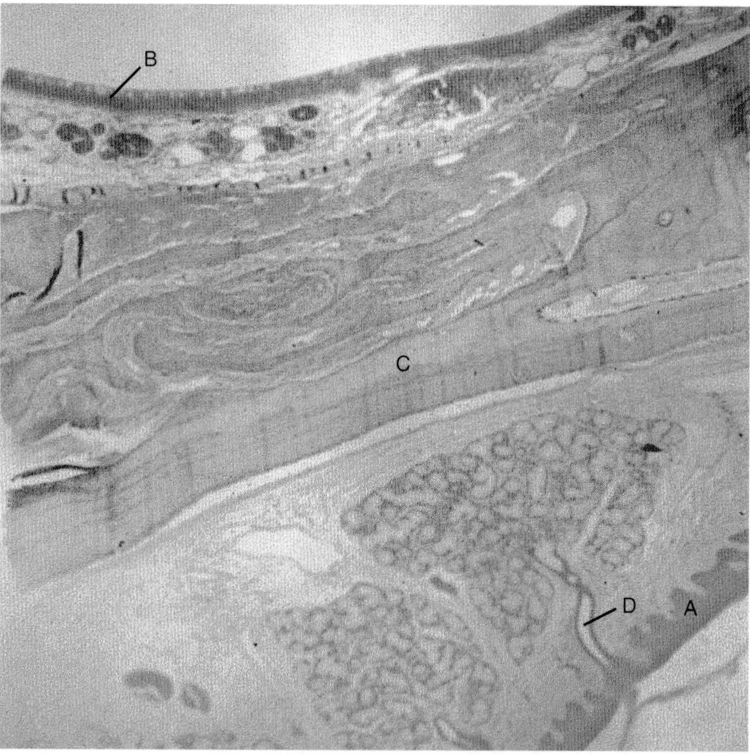

Fig. 14.62 Demineralised section of the hard palate showing the oral surface (A) lined by masticatory epithelium and the nasal surface (B) lined by a respiratory epithelium. C = bone of hard palate; D = duct from mucous gland opening onto surface (H & E; ×110). Courtesy Dr. M E Atkinson.

arrangement is seen in much of the attached gingiva (Fig. 14.40), but the epithelium is about twice the thickness. Where the palate joins the alveolus, a submucosa is present and contains the main neurovascular bundles. There are also minor mucous glands (predominantly posteriorly) that open onto the surface by ducts (Fig. 14.61) and adipose tissue (predominantly anteriorly).

While the oral surface of the hard palate is lined by masticatory epithelium, the nasal surface of the hard palate is lined by a respiratory mucosa (Fig. 14.62). The respiratory mucosa consists of ciliated columnar epithelial cells with many goblet cells (Fig. 14.63). The ciliated cells contain 'simple' cytokeratin types (i.e., 7, 8 and 18). In addition, there are proliferative basal cells characterised by cytokeratin types 5 and 14. Beneath the respiratory epithelium there is a vascular submucosa containing minor glands of both mucous and serous types.

Soft palate

The mucosa covering the oral surface of the soft palate is a nonkeratinised lining mucosa (Fig. 14.64). Thus, the connective tissue papillae are short and broad. The lamina propria contains many elastin fibres, and its collagen bundles are relatively thin. There is a broad submucosa containing many small mucous glands. The submucosa attaches into the palatal muscles. The nasal surface of the soft palate is lined by a respiratory mucosa of ciliated columnar epithelium.

Tongue and floor of the mouth

The ventral surface of the tongue and the floor of the mouth are covered by typical lining mucosa (Fig. 14.65). There is little wear and tear but a need for considerable mobility. The epithelium is thin, nonkeratinised and shows short papillae. The submucosa is extensive on the floor of the mouth but indistinct (if not absent) on the ventral surface of the tongue where the mucosa binds down to the tongue muscles. The thinness of the epithelium and the vascularity of the connective tissue make this a route by which some drugs can rapidly reach the bloodstream.

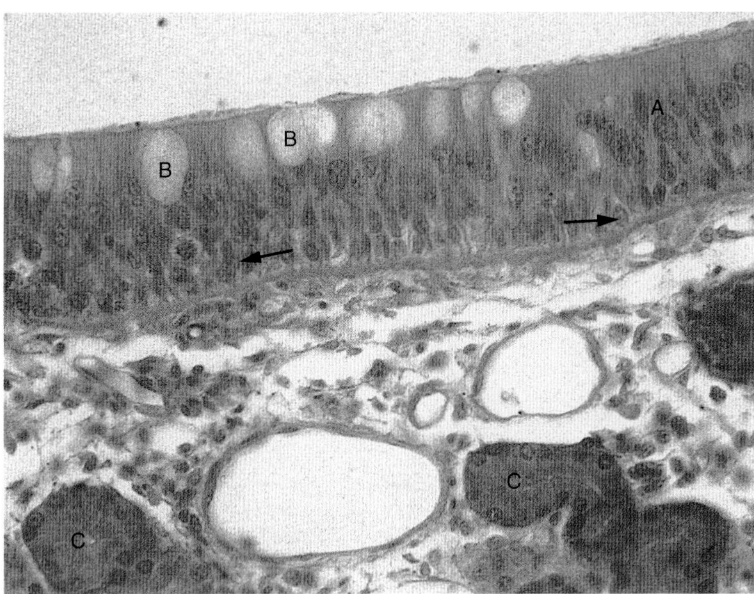

Fig. 14.63 Section of nasal surface of hard palate from Fig. 14.62. A = ciliated columnar epithelium; B = goblet cell; C = minor salivary gland; arrows indicate basal cells in epithelium (H & E; ×500). Courtesy Dr. M E Atkinson.

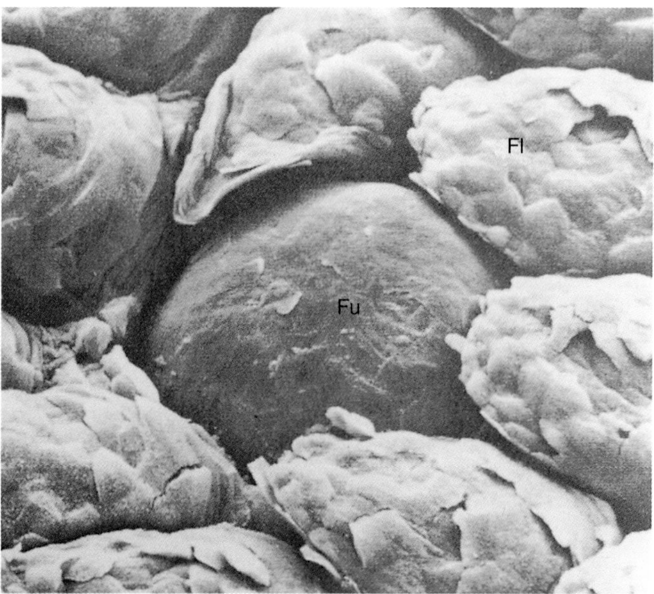

Fig. 14.66 Scanning electron micrograph showing filiform papillae (Fl) surrounding a fungiform papilla (Fu) (×90). Courtesy S Franey.

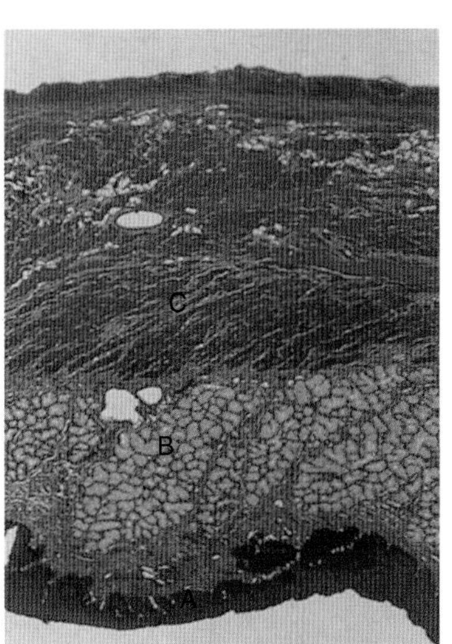

Fig. 14.64 Section of soft palate showing the oral surface being covered by a nonkeratinised lining mucosa (A). Numerous minor salivary glands lie in the submucosa (B), beneath which is seen the palatal musculature (C). The nasal surface is lined by a pseudostratified ciliated columnar epithelium (H & E; ×20).

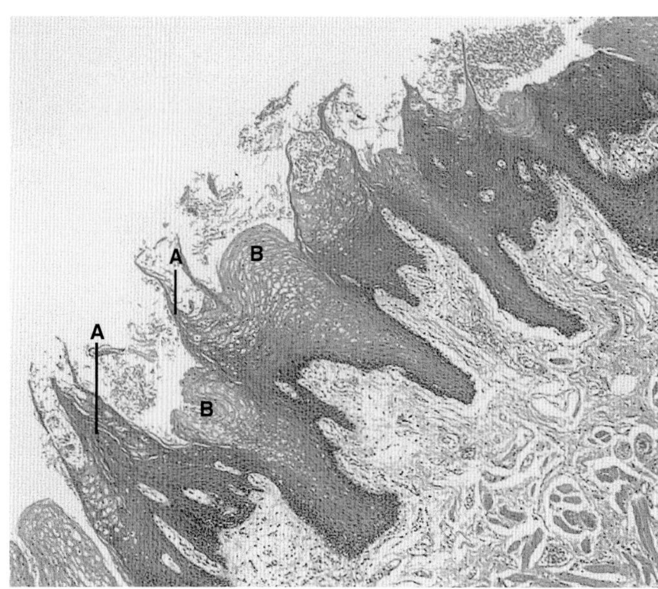

Fig. 14.67 Section showing dorsum of anterior two-thirds of tongue covered by keratinised filiform papillae (A) with nonkeratinised regions between (B) (H & E; ×35). Courtesy Prof. P R Morgan.

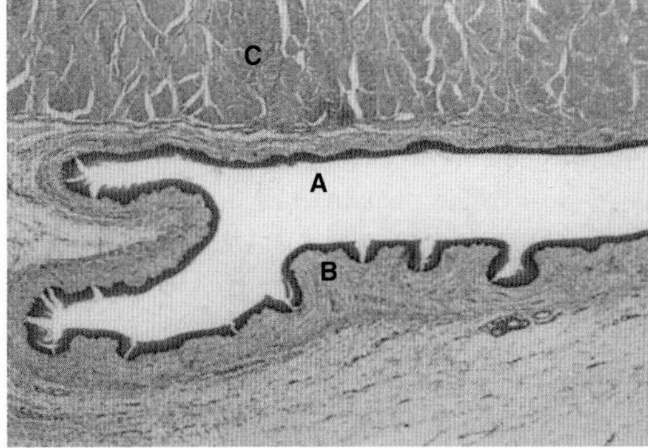

Fig. 14.65 Section showing the ventral surface of the tongue (A) and floor of mouth (B) being lined by nonkeratinised lining epithelium. The submucosa in the floor of the mouth is indistinct, with the thin lamina propria being bound to the underlying tongue musculature (C) (H & E; ×20).

An indistinct groove, the sulcus terminalis (see Fig. 1.14) divides the tongue into an anterior two-thirds (palatal surface) and a posterior one-third (pharyngeal surface). The anterior two-thirds of the tongue are covered with numerous papillae, which can be classified into four types: filiform, fungiform, foliate and circumvallate papillae (see Figs 1.16-1.18). The posterior one-third of the tongue is studded with small lymphoid nodules (or follicles). In addition to its mechanical functions, the tongue has important sensory functions (particularly taste) and is regarded as a specialised mucosa.

The mucosa on the dorsum of the anterior two-thirds of the tongue is classified as a masticatory mucosa, as a large part of it is covered by the numerous keratinised filiform papillae (Fig. 14.66). The overlying stratified squamous epithelium is keratinised and forms hairlike tufts, although the regions between the papillae are nonkeratinised (Fig. 14.67). Each filiform papilla consists of a central core of lamina propria with smaller, secondary papillae branching from it. The filiform papillae are highly abrasive during mastication when the bolus is compressed against the palate.

The simplest model of homeostasis in stratified epithelia is that all basal epithelial cells divide in a fairly homogeneous manner and that increased basal cell ‘pressure’ generated by dividing cells results in an upward random migration of keratinocytes destined for desquamation. However, it is now clear that many renewing tissues (including oral epithelium) are

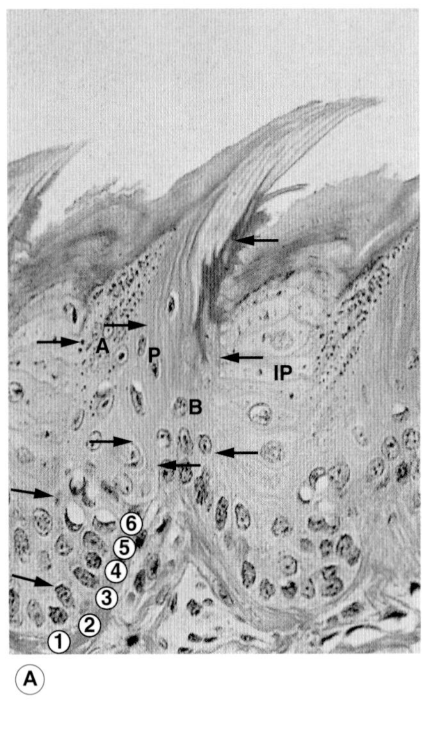

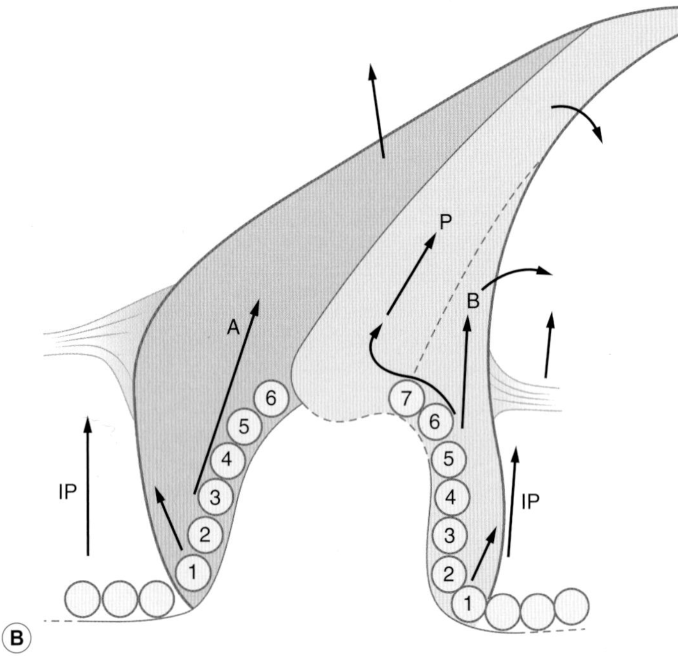

Fig. 14.68 (A) Section of mouse filiform papilla. (B) Schematic representation of column boundaries and cell migration patterns. A = anterior column; B = buttress column; IP = interpapillary epithelium; P = posterior column (Masson's trichrome ×120). Courtesy Prof. W J Hume.

organised in a much more complicated way, as reference to the mouse filiform papilla shows (Fig. 14.68A). Each mouse filiform papilla comprises several columns of cells around a central connective tissue core. The anterior column is two cells wide and has well-defined boundaries that result from the difference in cell size and differentiation on either side of each boundary. The posterior column of 16–20 cells piled one on top of another gradually inclines as cells move upwards so that the top cell desquamates backwards (towards the pharynx). The buttress column appears to fill in the rear of the papilla structure to 'buttress' the posterior column. Note the maturity of basal cells over the apex of the connective tissue core and the method used to number individual cell positions within each column. The posterior column shows keratinisation (its cytokeratin profile containing CK1 and 10), while the anterior column is nonkeratinised (its cytokeratin profile containing CK4 and 13).

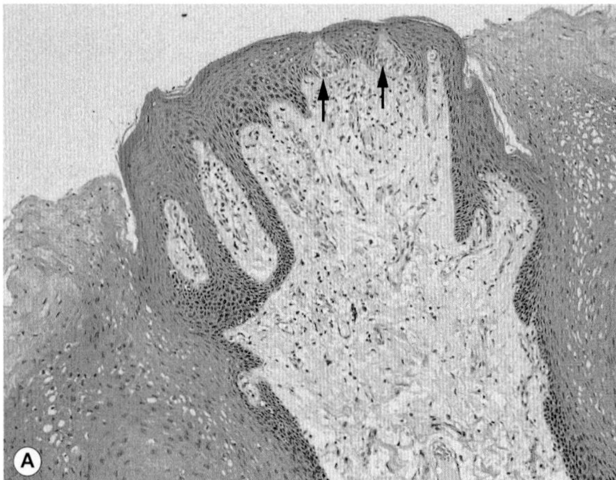

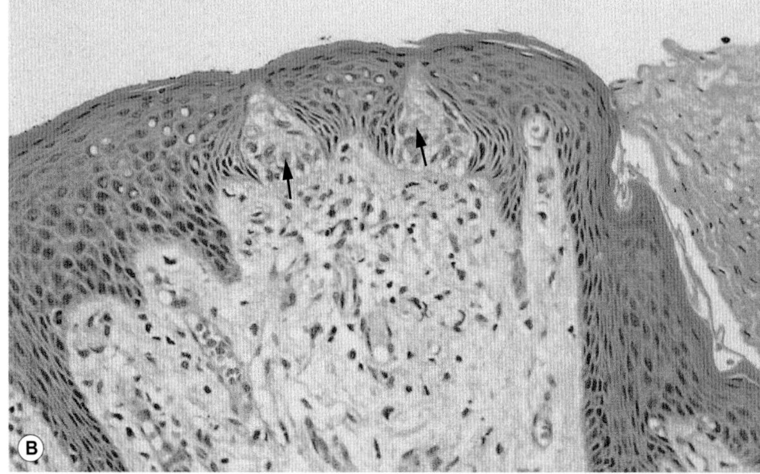

Fig. 14.69 (A) Section of fungiform papilla on dorsal surface of anterior part of tongue showing taste buds (arrowed). The papilla is keratinised (H & E; ×120). (B) High-power view of surface of fungiform papilla seen in (A), showing taste buds (arrows) (×240). Courtesy Prof. P R Morgan.

A schematic representation of column boundaries and cell migration patterns in the mouse filiform papilla is shown in Fig. 14.68B. The stem cell population is at position 1, next to column boundaries. As cells move bodily along the basement membrane (positions 1–6 or 6–7), their capacity for proliferation decreases so that, by the time they reach the highest cell position number, they are postmitotic, differentiating cells. This model implies that, because of rapid desquamation of cells, four or five cells per day in the posterior column are the stem cells. There is some suprabasal migration in the anterior column in addition to migration along the basement membrane. The posterior column is derived from lateral cell migration and the buttress column from suprabasal migration from the stem cell population at the rear of the papilla. Thus, each of these columns is one cell wide, whereas the anterior column is two cells wide.

Fungiform papillae are found as isolated, elevated, mushroom-shaped papillae scattered between the filiform papillae and are approximately 150–400 μm in diameter (Fig. 14.66). They are covered by a relatively thin epithelium that may or may not be keratinised and have a vascular core of lamina propria. Taste buds may be found on the surface (Figs. 14.69, 14.70).

Foliate papillae may be present as one or two longitudinal clefts at the side of the posterior part of the tongue (see Fig. 1.18). Taste buds may be found within the nonkeratinised epithelium of these papillae (Fig. 14.71).

Circumvallate papillae are large and rounded. They are surrounded by a trenchlike feature and do not project beyond the normal surface level of the tongue (Figs. 14.72, 14.73; see also Fig. 1.15). The circumvallate papilla is generally covered by a nonkeratinised epithelium. Taste buds predominate

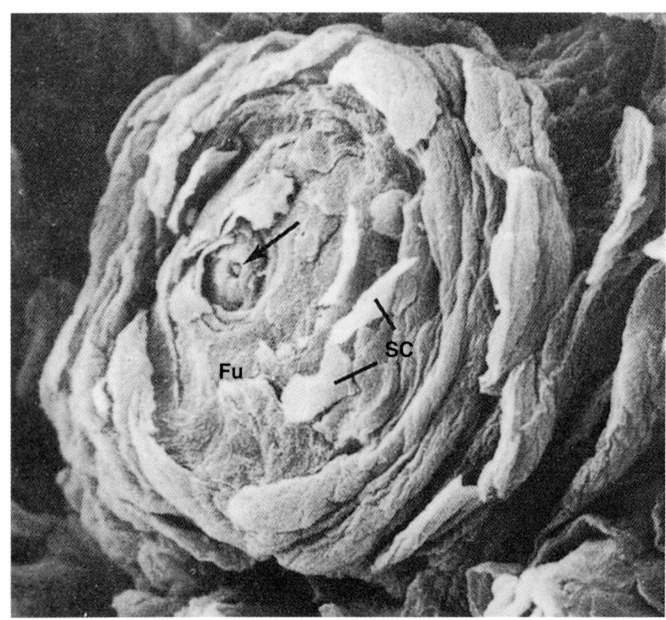

Fig. 14.70 Scanning electron micrograph of fungiform papilla (Fu) showing opening (pore) of taste bud on surface (arrow). SC = surface keratinocytes (×175). Courtesy S Franey.

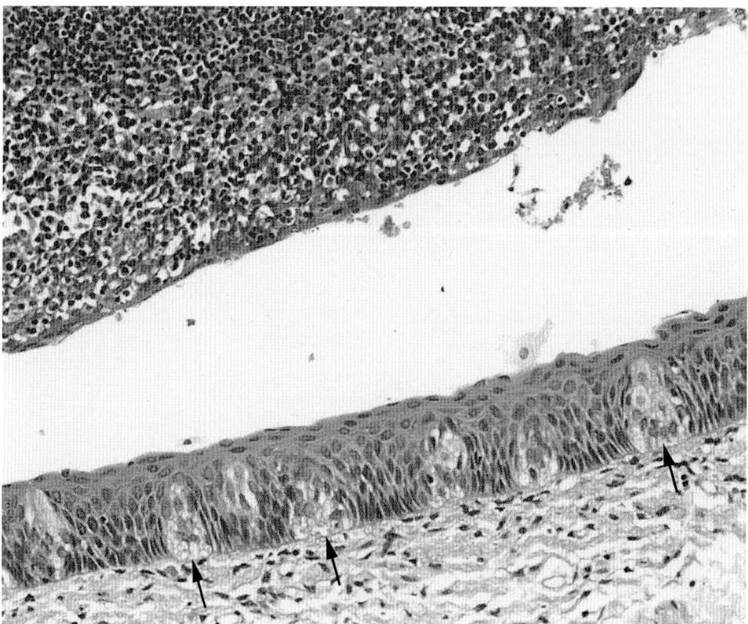

Fig. 14.71 Section of foliate papilla showing taste buds (arrowed). Note the adjacent lymphoid material characteristic of the posterior part of the tongue (×200).

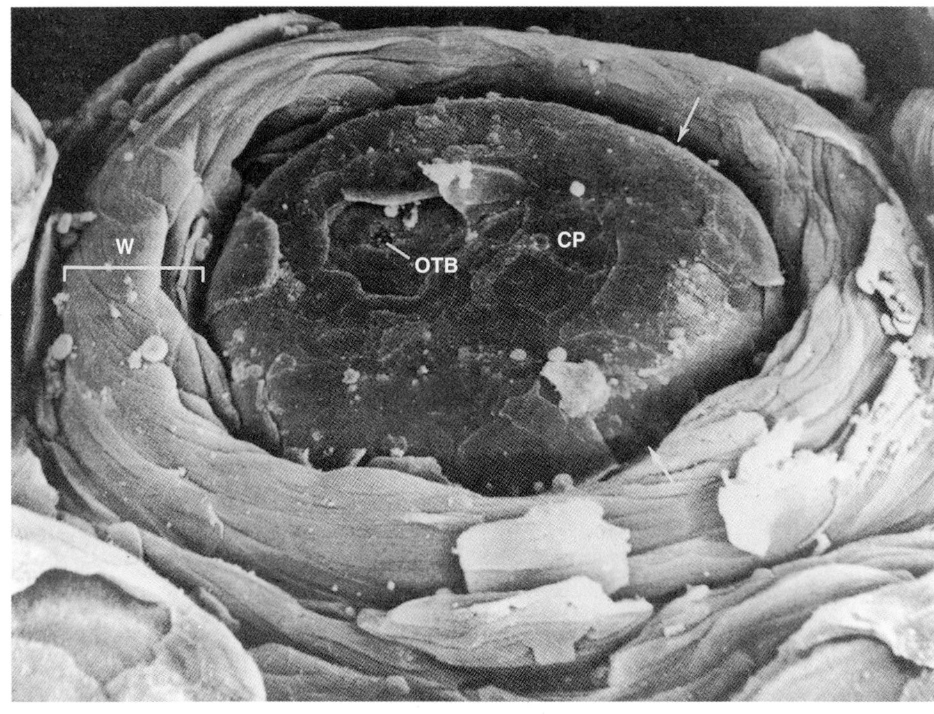

Fig. 14.72 Scanning electron micrograph showing a circumvallate papilla (CP), surrounded by a trench (arrow). OTB = opening pore of taste bud; W = wall of trench surrounding circumvallate papilla (×80). Courtesy S Franey.

on the internal wall of the trench in the epithelium. Small serous glands (of von Ebner) empty into the base of the trench (Fig. 14.74). Groups of mucous glands are also seen within the muscle of the tongue, particularly in the posterior part, and these are unencapsulated.

The taste buds, the special chemoreceptive organs responsible for taste, are located within the epithelium, particularly around the walls of the circumvallate papillae (Fig. 14.75) and also in small numbers on the upper surface of fungiform papillae (Fig. 14.69), in the lateral walls of foliate papillae, in the mucosa of the soft palate and in the epiglottis. Two types of cells are present in the taste bud: the supporting cell and the taste cell. A small pore opens from the surface into the taste bud (Fig. 14.76).

At the ultrastructural level the cells of the taste bud are clearly demarcated from the adjacent epithelial cells (Fig. 14.76). The morphology of a taste bud may vary according to species and site. Four distinct cell types have been described: the relatively undifferentiated type IV cells are distinguished by their basal position and the presence of intermediate filaments; type I cells have a dark appearance, while types II and III cells are lighter. Types I and III cells may form synapses with intragemmal nerves. The taste bud is separated from the underlying connective tissue by a basal lamina.

The collection of lymphoid follicles on the posterior one-third of the tongue is collectively known as the *lingual tonsil* and forms a component of Waldeyer's ring, which protects the opening into the pharynx (with the palatine tonsil and the tubal and pharyngeal tonsils within the nasopharynx). The follicles are deep crypts lined with epithelium and containing a mass of lymphoid material (Fig. 14.77). The follicles lie along shallow crypts

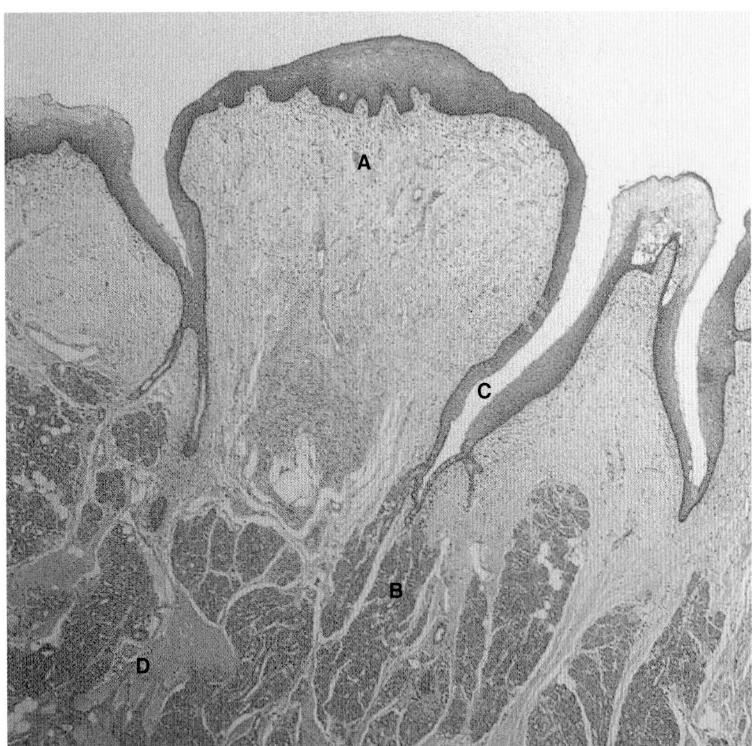

Fig. 14.73 Section of circumvallate papilla (A). Serous glands (B) of von Ebner empty via ducts into the base of the trench (C) surrounding the papilla, which is not raised above the surface of the tongue. D = muscle of tongue (H & E; ×35). Courtesy Prof. P R Morgan.

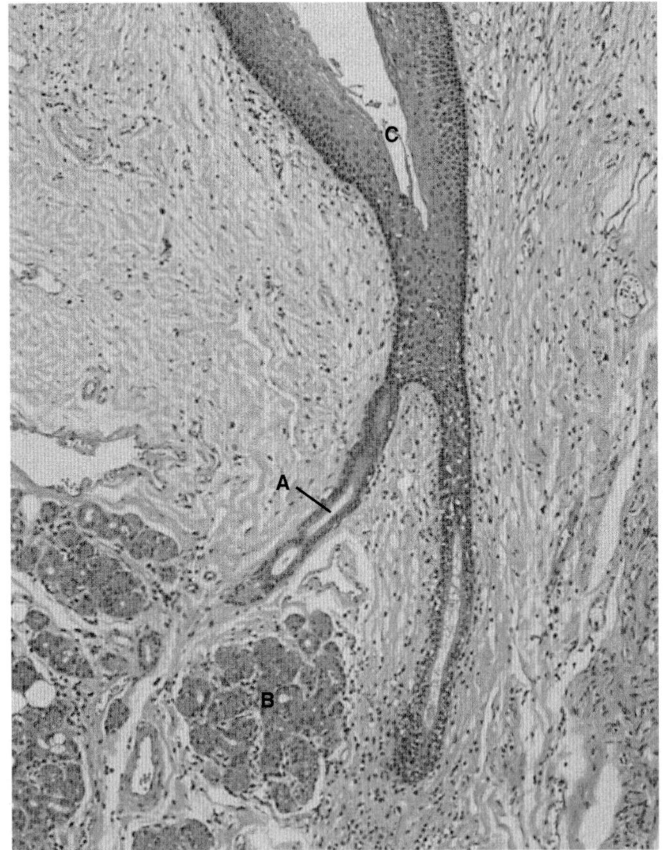

Fig. 14.74 Section of base of circumvallate papilla showing duct (A) from serous gland (B) emptying into the base of the trench (C) (H & E; ×90). Courtesy Prof. P R Morgan.

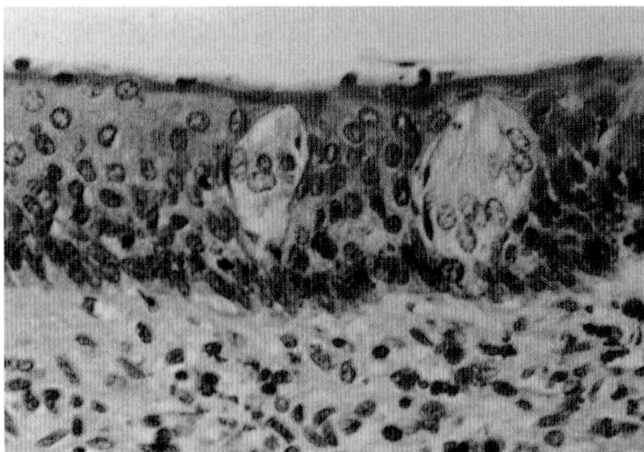

Fig. 14.75 Section of wall of circumvallate papilla showing two pale barrel-shaped areas representing two taste buds (Masson's trichrome; ×300).

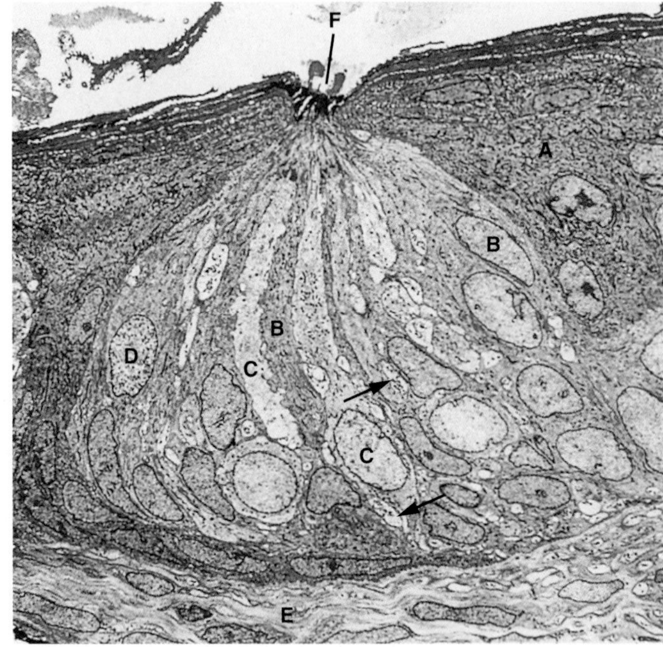

Fig. 14.76 Electron micrograph of a taste bud. A = epithelial cells adjacent to taste bud; B = darker type I cells; C = lighter type II cells; D = lighter type III cell; E = underlying connective tissue; F = taste pore; arrows indicate where type I and type III cells form synapses with intragemmal nerves (×11,000). Courtesy Dr. S M Royer and Dr J C Kinnamon.

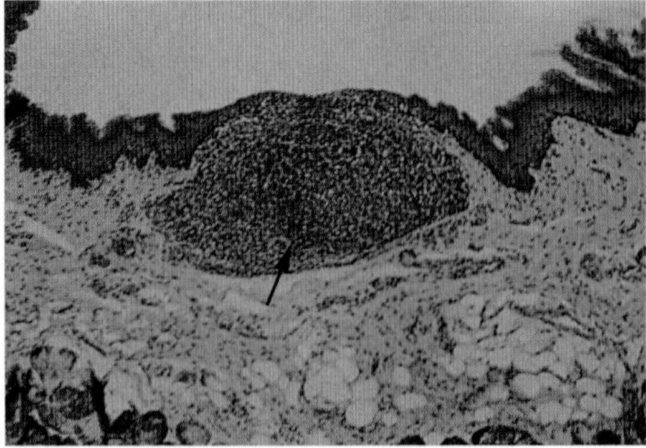

Fig. 14.77 Section of dorsal surface of posterior one-third of tongue containing a lymphoid follicle (arrow). This part of the tongue is covered by a nonkeratinised lining epithelium (H & E; ×40).

lined with epithelium and usually contain germinal centres (Fig. 14.77). The crypts usually open onto the surface of the tongue. The mucosa in this region also contains many mucous glands. Some small mucous glands also occasionally occur at the margin and tip of the anterior two-thirds of the tongue.

Simple cytokeratins are expressed by taste buds: most are positive for CK7, 8 and 19, with fewer expressing CK18.

Age changes in oral mucosa

Overall, the detailed changes with ageing that occur within the oral cavity have not been well established and, because of regionalisation, the findings for one type of oral mucosa may not necessarily be true for other regions.

With age, there is evidence of a thinning of the epithelium on the dorsal and lateral surfaces of the tongue, with less interdigitation at the epithelium–lamina propria interface. There is an increase in collagen content and a decrease in the number of taste buds.

Although gingival recession may be associated with age, it is difficult to determine whether this is a direct effect or whether it is secondary to lack of oral hygiene or other oral features such as incorrect tooth brushing. Although little change in the epithelium of the gingiva has been reported with age, there is some evidence of an increase in collagen content in the lamina propria.

There is an increasing susceptibility to the appearance of precancerous and cancerous conditions in the oral epithelium with age. As a possible contributing factor, it has been found that there is a raised level of p53, the protein associated with DNA repair.

As saliva contributes to the health of the oral mucosa, any possible age changes related to the salivary glands (see page 348), such as reduced output and salivary flow, may account for some of the age changes described in the oral mucosa.

Taste and smell perceptions diminish in older age, affecting quality of life and nutrition. For example, older age is associated with 15% lower umami taste and 26% lower menthol odour perception.

Clinical considerations

In dealing with the oral mucosa, one needs to be able to distinguish between conditions reflecting normal variation, benign conditions and those that may be premalignant. In addition, inflammation of the gingiva is one of the most common diseases.

Normal clinical variation and benign conditions of the tongue

As an example of variation in normal anatomy, lymphoid tissue exhibits considerable size variation, especially in the young. Lingual tonsils may show localised symmetrical swelling, being symptomless and without the presence of any observable underlying pathology (Fig. 14.78).

An example of a benign developmental condition is the lingual thyroid. The dorsum of the posterior one-third of the tongue may show a midline swelling that represents active thyroid gland tissue that has failed to migrate from its developmental situation at the site of the foramen caecum (Fig. 14.79; see also page 376). Remnants of the migrating thyroid gland may also form thyroglossal duct cysts in the neck. The diagnosis can be confirmed using a radioactive iodine test and by means of a biopsy that reveals the presence of thyroid tissue (Fig. 14.80).

Another example of a common benign condition is erythema migrans. This is an inflammatory condition of unknown cause characterised by the recurrence and disappearance of red areas on the tongue. It presents as smooth, red regions on the tongue related to atrophy of the filiform papillae that are surrounded by a grey-white, irregular boundary (Fig. 14.81A). The appearance has been likened to the outline of continents on a map, hence the more familiar name of 'geographic tongue'. A characteristic of the condition is that the outlines of the 'map' change, even from day to day, and the area covered may wax and wane (Fig. 14.81B). It may be symptomless, although some patients may complain of a burning sensation. Erythema migrans occurs in about 3% of the population and presents in adults more often than in children. The red colouration of affected areas coincides histologically with thickening of the epithelium and the presence of inflammatory cells in the region (Fig. 14.82A). In the grey-white borders, the epithelium contains the highest concentration of neutrophils (Fig. 14.82B).

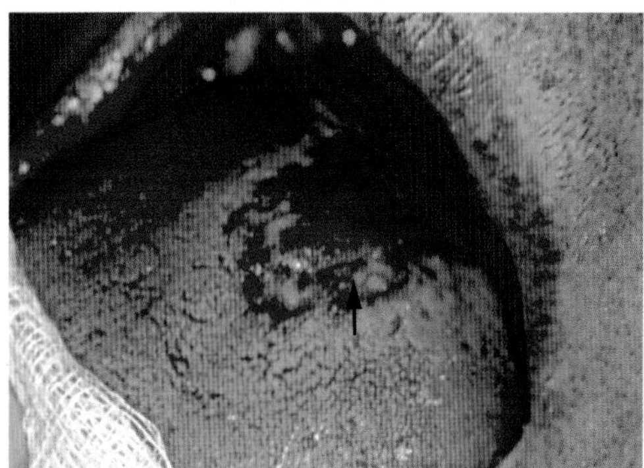

Fig. 14.79 View of back of tongue showing a lingual thyroid (arrow). Courtesy Prof. J D Langdon.

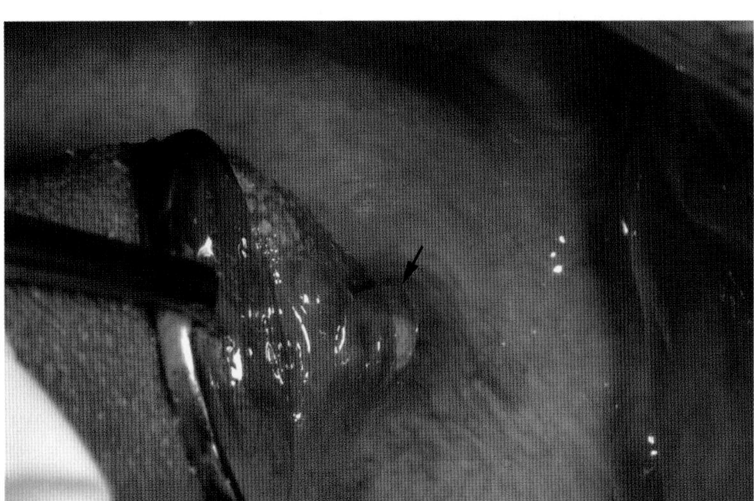

Fig. 14.78 Side view of tongue showing localised enlargement of a lingual follicle and foliate papillae (arrow). Courtesy Prof. P R Morgan.

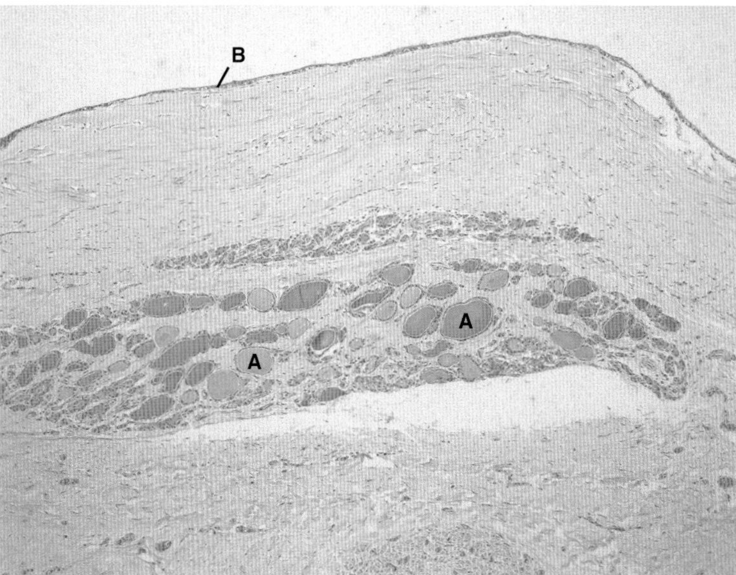

Fig. 14.80 Section taken from thyroglossal duct cyst removed from the back of the tongue showing the presence of thyroid tissue (A). B = epithelial lining of cyst cavity (H & E; ×50). Courtesy Prof. P R Morgan.

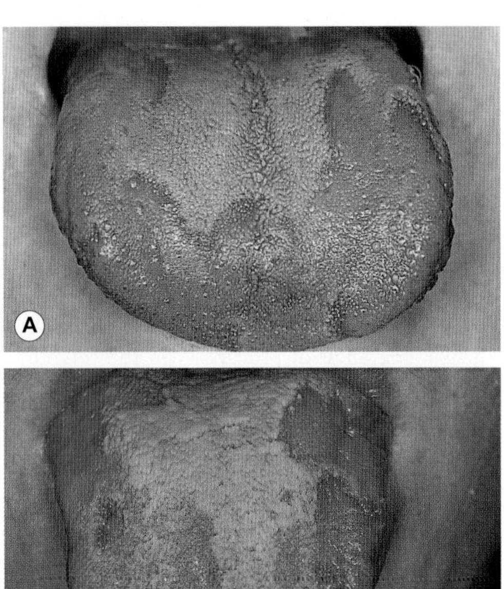

Fig. 14.81 (A) Typical appearance of erythema migrans (geographic tongue) showing irregular depapillated red patches centred on the lateral sides of the tongue, with each patch having a narrow red and white rim. (B) Tongue of the same patient shown in Fig. 14.81A but taken on a later occasion and showing a change in the pattern of red patches. From *Cawson's Essentials of Oral Pathology and Oral Medicine* eighth ed. 2008, Elsevier, London.

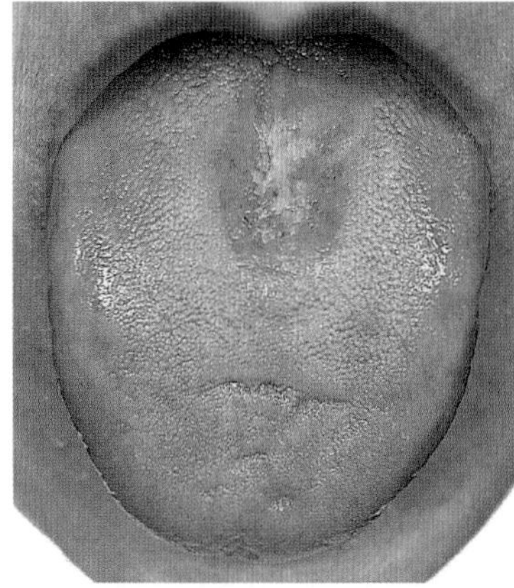

Fig. 14.83 The typical lozenge-shaped area of depapillation in the midline of the dorsum of the tongue representing median rhomboid glossitis. From Cawson's essentials of oral pathology and oral medicine, eighth ed. 2008.

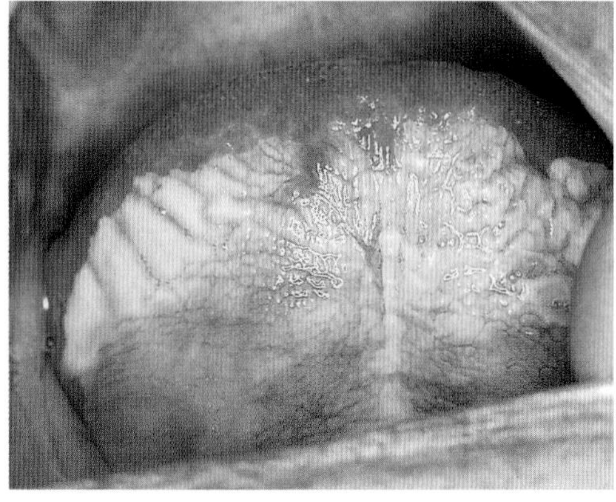

Fig. 14.84 White patch on the ventral tongue and floor of the mouth (sometimes referred to as sublingual keratosis) associated with smoking. From *Cawson's Essentials of Oral Pathology and Oral Medicine* eighth ed. 2008. Elsevier, London.

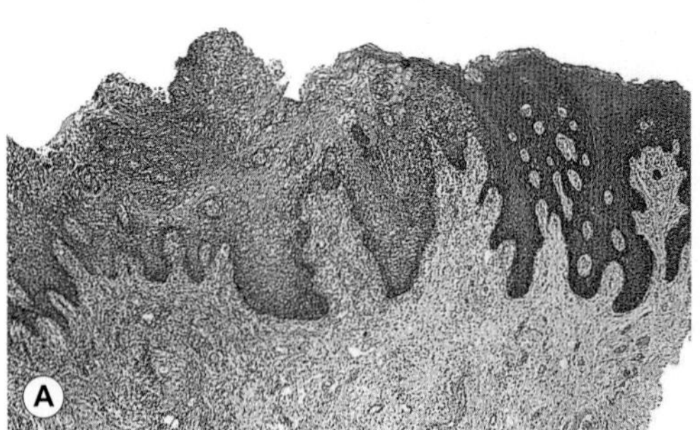

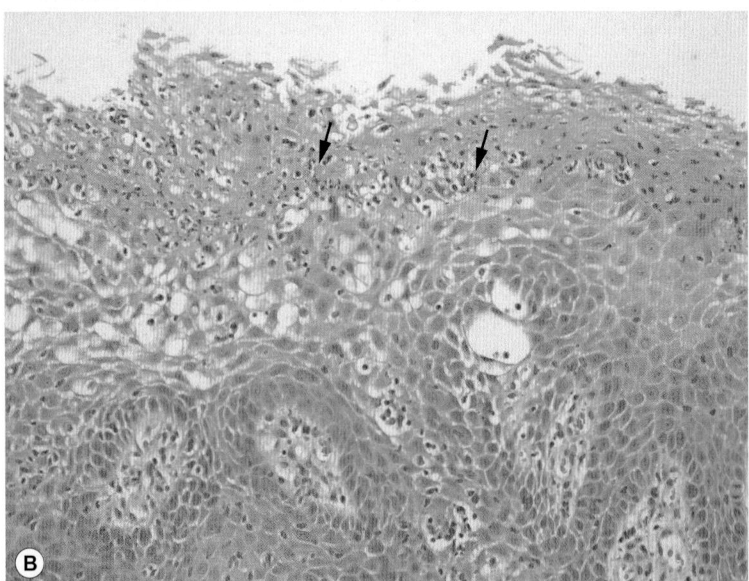

Fig. 14.82 Micrograph in grey-white area at the border of a lesion of migratory glossitis. (A) Low-power micrograph at the edge of a lesion of erythema migrans. The edge of the lesion on the right shows a normal mucosa, while to the left the affected epithelium is densely infiltrated with neutrophils and will be shed, leaving a depapillated red patch (H & E; ×30). (B) Higher-power view of affected epithelium, showing neutrophil infiltration of epithelium (arrows) (×125). A, From *Cawson's Essentials of Oral Pathology and Oral Medicine*, eighth ed. 2008. B, Courtesy Prof. P R Morgan, Elsevier, London.

Median rhomboid glossitis is a benign abnormality seen in the midline of the dorsum of the tongue at the junction between the anterior two-thirds and posterior third (Fig. 14.83). It appears as a nodular red or pink region devoid of papillae and showing infiltration of inflammatory cells. This harmless and symptomless condition can sometimes mistakenly be assessed as a carcinoma.

White lesions

White lesions are common in the oral cavity, being associated with areas of keratinisation in normally nonkeratinised lining mucosa. Of major significance is the need to differentiate those that are benign from those that may give rise to malignancies. At its mildest, in buccal mucosa and level with the occlusal plane, a linear, slightly raised whitish ridge may be seen – the linea alba (see Fig. 1.25) – commonly the result of low-grade, intermittent trauma upon folds of cheek mucosa trapped between the teeth. The constant irritation converts the surface epithelium from its normal nonkeratinised state into a parakeratinised layer (see page 289). One site in which a white patch is most conspicuous is the floor of the mouth and ventral surface of the tongue, here associated with smoking (Fig. 14.84). In one form a smooth-surfaced, white patch shows a characteristic rippling pattern, with the normal nonkeratinised lining epithelium alternating with areas of keratinised epithelium (Fig. 14.85).

A common chronic inflammatory disease that produces white, often striated lesions in the mouth, usually in the buccal mucosa, is lichen planus (Fig. 14.86), with the white appearance reflecting the presence of hyperkeratosis or parakeratosis.

Occasionally, white patch lesions do progress to malignancy (rather less than 1% by general consensus) and therefore they must be kept under observation. A change in form to a speckled appearance associated with a firmness on palpation (induration related to infiltration by tumour cells), ulceration and a rolled border may signify a malignant change (Fig. 14.87), producing a squamous cell carcinoma. Such a change can be confirmed by a biopsy showing invasion of the epithelium into the deeper tissues (Fig. 14.88). Metastasis from a carcinoma of the tongue may spread via the lymphatic vessels to the regional lymph nodes and may be unilateral or bilateral (see pages 101–102). Cancer of the tongue may also result in referred pain to the ear because of nerve fibres from the chorda tympani running with the lingual nerve.

White patches associated with infections caused by the fungus *Candida albicans* may also appear in lining mucosa (Fig. 14.89) and can be diagnosed with the aid of stains to reveal the causal organism within the epithelium (Fig. 14.90).

White patches are also a feature of white sponge naevus (a rare, benign, autosomal dominant condition). Here, areas of thick, white, soft plaques cover both sides of the nonkeratinised regions of the oral mucosa, particularly the tongue and cheek (Fig. 14.91). Histological features reveal a thickened epithelium showing parakeratinisation with widespread vacuolation of the suprabasal epithelium (Fig. 14.92). The underlying cause of this condition appears to be a mutation affecting the structure of CK13 and/or CK4.

The importance of the basement membrane complex in uniting the epithelium and the lamina propria is apparent when disorders in this region occur. The commonest example of such a disorder in the mouth is mucous membrane pemphigoid in which auto-antibodies are produced by the patient and directed against the transmembrane molecules bullous pemphigoid antigens (BP180 and BP230), important components in the hemidesmosomes of the basement membrane complex (see pages 295–296). This weakens the bond between the epithelium and lamina propria,

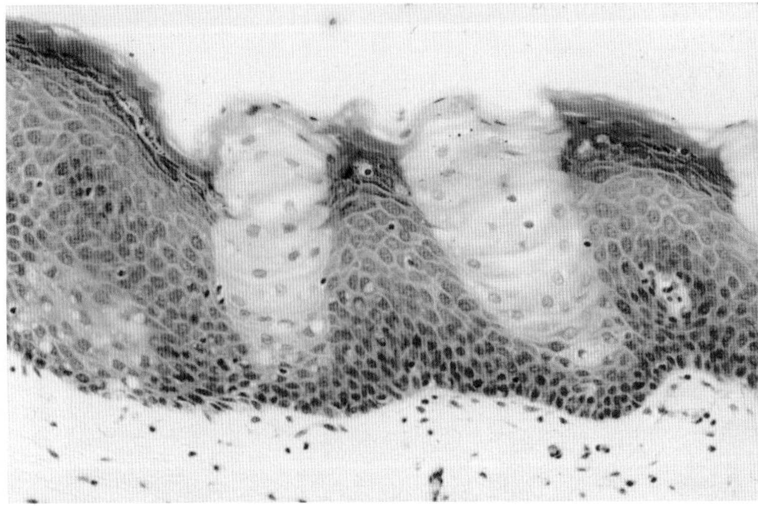

Fig. 14.85 Section of biopsy from sublingual keratosis from lesion with a rippling outline. The epithelium shows alternation of normal nonkeratinised and parakeratinised epithelium (H & E; ×150). Courtesy Prof. P R Morgan.

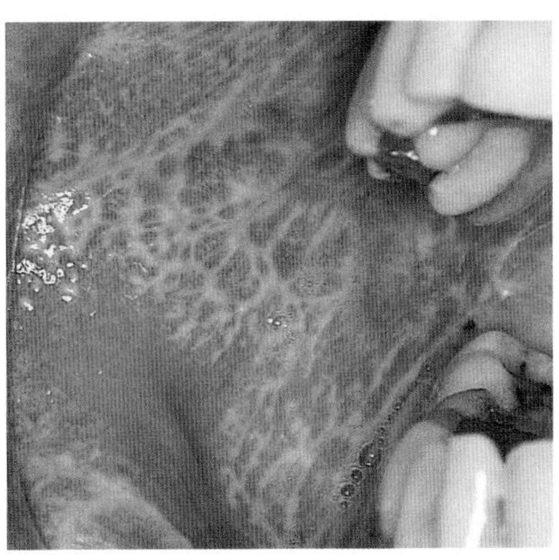

Fig. 14.86 Lichen planus in the buccal mucosa, producing a lacy network of white striae. From *Cawson's Essentials of Oral Pathology and Oral Medicine*, eighth ed. 2008. Elsevier, London.

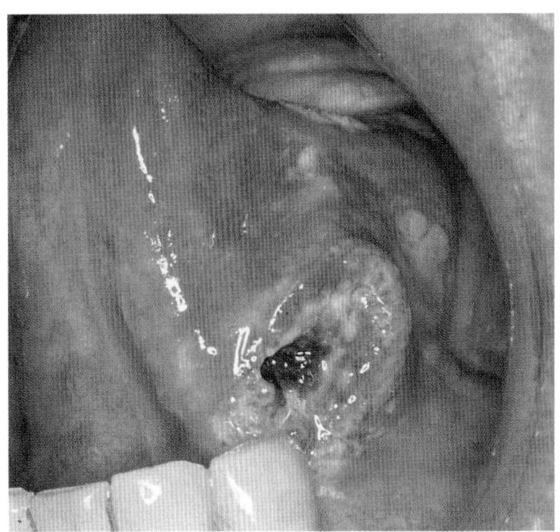

Fig. 14.87 Squamous cell carcinoma showing a speckled appearance, firmness on palpation (induration) and an ulcerated rolled margin. From *Cawson's Essentials of Oral Pathology and Oral Medicine*, eighth ed. 2008. Elsevier, London.

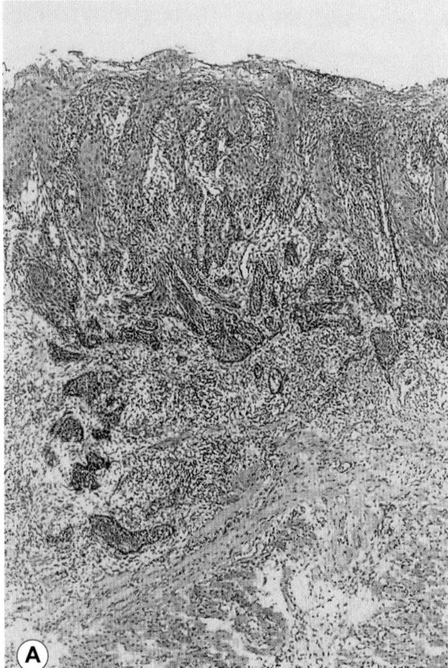

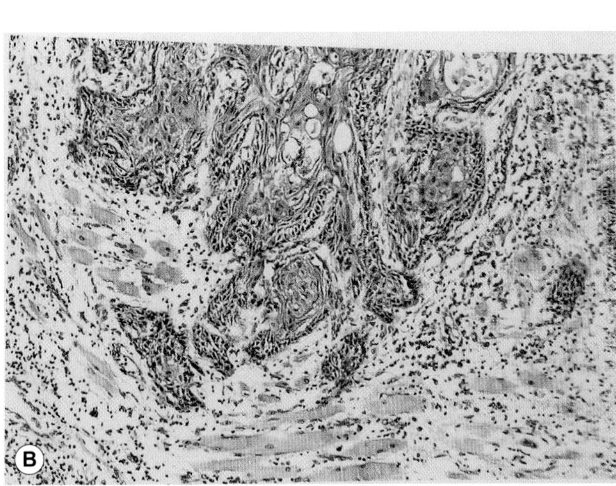

Fig. 14.88 Biopsy of squamous cell carcinoma from the lateral border of the tongue. (A) Low power shows very irregular overlying epithelium with rete processes penetrating deeply into underlying tissues. (B) Higher power of (A) showing darker epithelium invading underlying muscle tissue (H & E ×4). Banerjee, A., Thavaraj, S. (Eds.), 2020. Odell's Clinical Problem Solving in Dentistry, fourth ed. Elsevier, London.

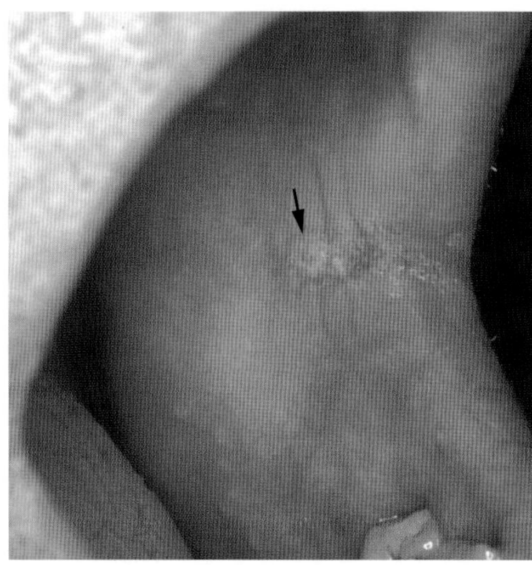

Fig. 14.89 White patch on cheek (arrow) resulting from infection with *Candida albicans*. Courtesy Prof. P R Morgan.

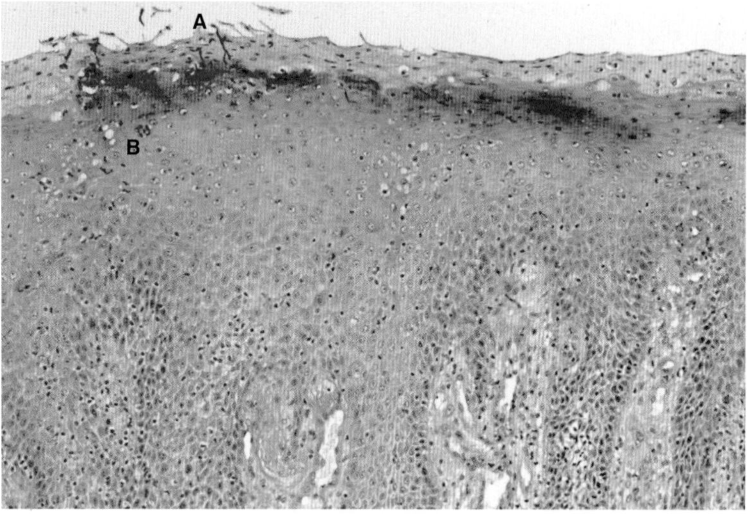

Fig. 14.90 Biopsy of lesion shown in Fig. 14.89 showing presence within the epithelial layer of red-staining fungal hyphae of *Candida albicans* filaments (A), while clusters of neutrophils (B) are present nearby (periodic-acid–Schiff stain; ×100). Courtesy Prof. P R Morgan.

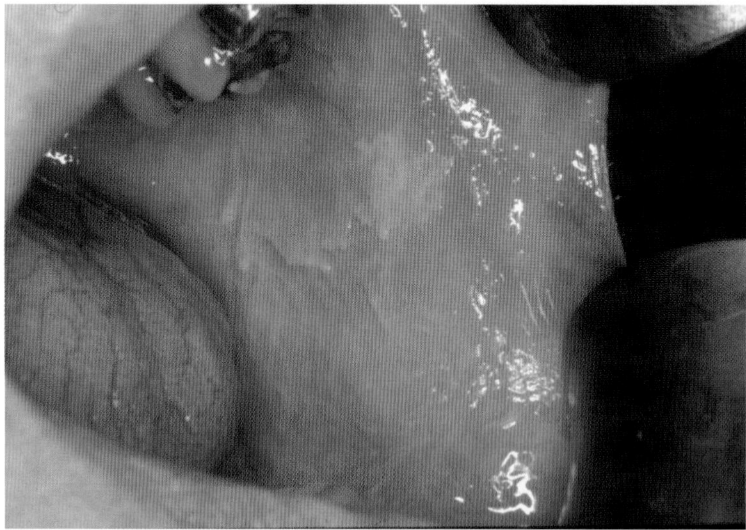

Fig. 14.91 White sponge naevus on the buccal mucosa. Courtesy Prof. P R Morgan.

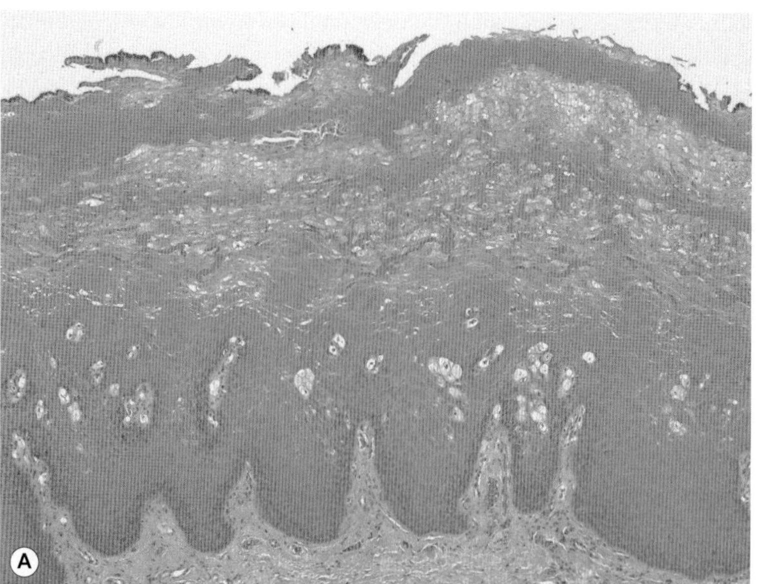

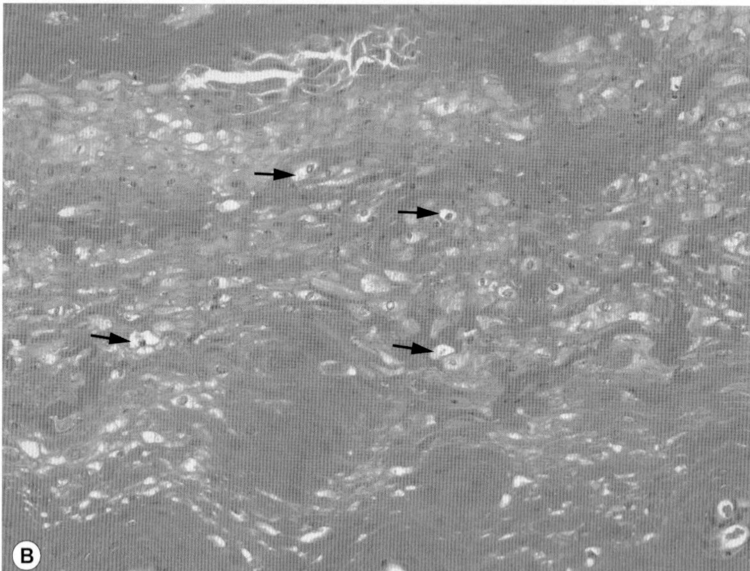

Fig. 14.92 (A) Low-power section of biopsy from a white sponge nevus showing the superficial layers of the epithelium parakeratinised (H & E; ×50). (B) Higher-power view of middle epithelial layers showing extensive vacuolisation of cells (arrows) and irregular keratinisation (darker red) (×125). Courtesy Prof. P R Morgan.

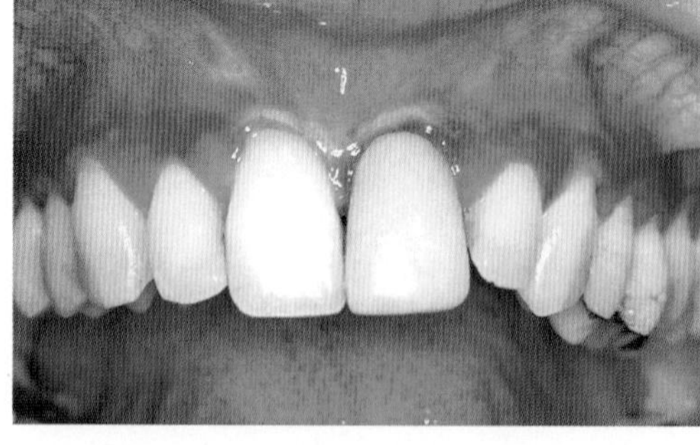

Fig. 14.93 Mucous membrane pemphigoid producing an inflamed appearance of the gingiva. From *Cawson's Essentials of Oral Pathology and Oral Medicine*, eighth ed. 2008. Elsevier, London.

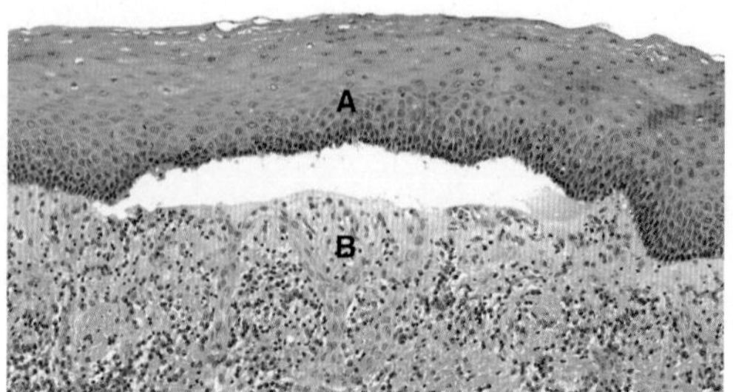

Fig. 14.94 Micrograph of biopsy from patient with mucous membrane pemphigoid, showing splitting between epithelium (A) and lamina propria (B) to form a microscopic fluid-filled bulla. Note the presence of inflammatory cells beneath the epithelium (H & E; ×50). From *Cawson's Essentials of Oral Pathology and Oral Medicine*, eighth ed. 2008. Elsevier, London.

resulting in splitting between them with associated inflammation producing blisters and ulcers within the mouth (Figs. 14.93, 14.94).

In pathological situations, the usual cytokeratin profiles of masticatory (e.g., CK1 and 10) and lining epithelium (e.g., CK4 and 13) may be altered. For example, some masticatory epithelium may show a reduction in, or even disappearance of, CK1 and 10 and an increased expression of CK4 and 13. This feature has been related to the presence of an underlying gingival inflammation (which may also produce CK19 expression in basal and parabasal layers).

Cytokeratins and malignancy

It has been recognised that there is potential to exploit the epithelial specificity of cytokeratins in diagnostic histopathology, principally in the determination of the tissue of origin of poorly differentiated neoplasms. A further possibility is that dysplastic lesions would 'declare' themselves by an alteration in cytokeratin profiles, thus enabling those with invasive potential to be identified early. In terms of the latter, these hopes have not yet reached fruition, but pancytokeratin antibodies helping to determine whether an anaplastic neoplasm is, for example, a poorly differentiated carcinoma or a lymphoma are now in widespread use (Fig. 14.95). It is to be remembered, however, that some malignancies are too poorly differentiated to synthesise appropriate intermediate filaments. Furthermore, other normal cell types (e.g., endothelial and mesenchymal cells) may express cytokeratins (usually at low levels), as may other malignant cell lineages which are expressing other abnormal phenotypes. It has been observed that there is an association in oral precancerous lesions and oral squamous cell carcinomas with a loss of CK76.

Gingival inflammation

Low-grade inflammation of the gingiva is known as *gingivitis*, when the gingivae becomes red and slightly swollen. The inflammation is related to the presence of dental plaque along the gingival margin (see Chapter 8). The inflammation may be restricted to the gingival margin (Fig. 14.96). However, once it extends into the periodontal ligament, the condition is known as *periodontitis* (see pages 257–258).

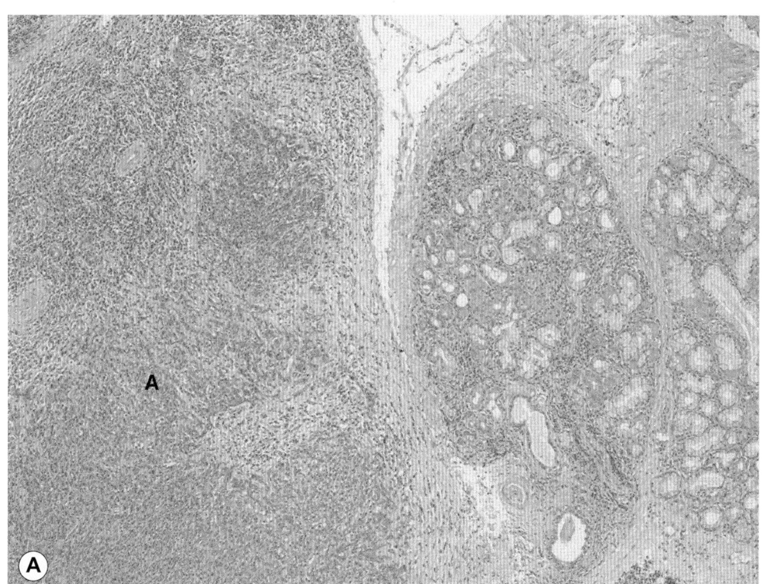

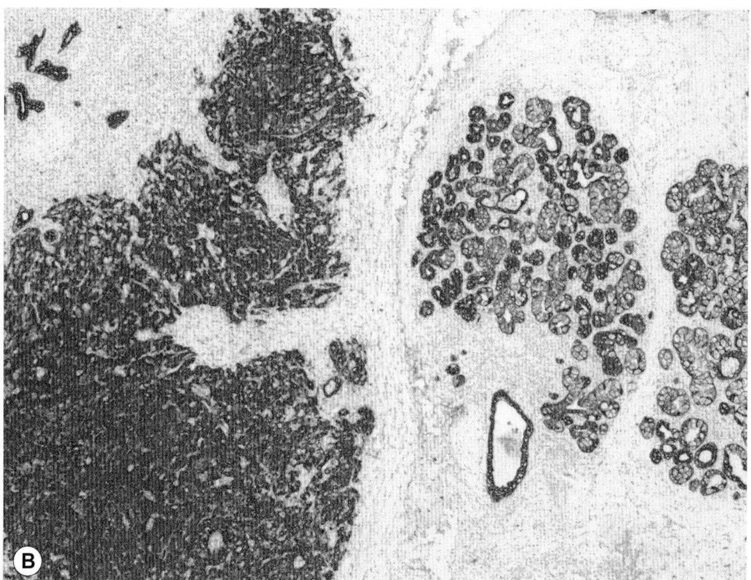

Fig. 14.95 (A) Section of a mass of poorly differentiated cells in the left part of the micrograph (A) representing an oral squamous cell carcinoma. The right part of the section represents an adjacent minor salivary gland (H & E; ×50). (B) Immunohistological staining of a section similar to (A) using a pankeratin antibody (AE1/3) that confirms the diagnosis of a squamous cell carcinoma by giving a positive response (brown stain) to many of the undifferentiated epithelial cells on the left side. Many of the unstained cells on the left represent lymphocytes. The normal salivary gland tissue on the right also stains positive (brown), acting as an internal control for the pancytokeratin antibody (streptavidin-biotinylated immunoperoxidase staining; haematoxylin counterstain; ×50). Courtesy Prof. P R Morgan.

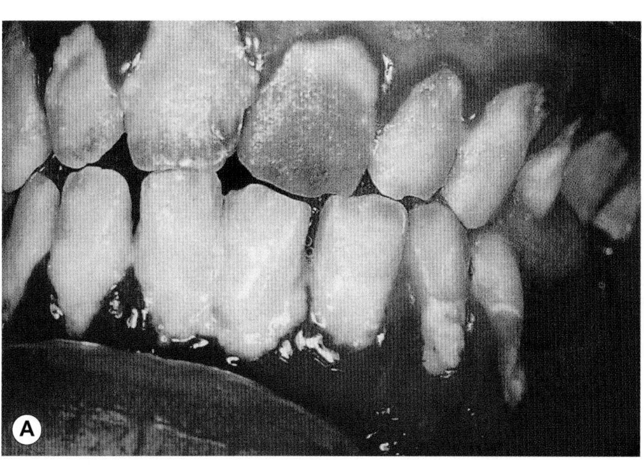

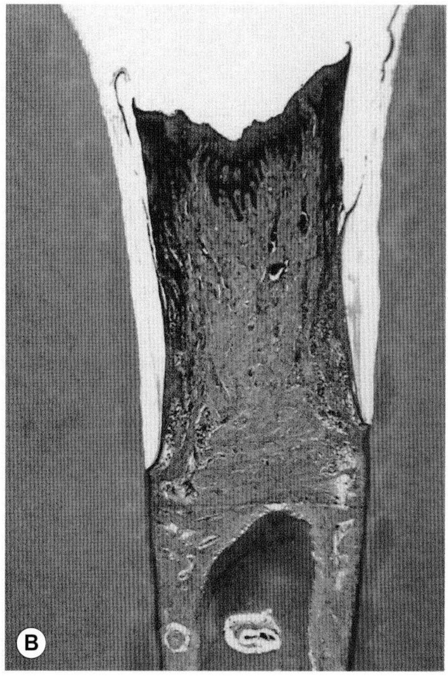

Fig. 14.96 (A) Left image shows a patient with gingivitis. The gingival margin is red and swollen in the presence of dental plaque. (B) The image represents a micrograph of the interdental region of a patient with gingivitis. The epithelial attachment remains at the level of the cementum-enamel junction. Inflammatory cells are present within the gingiva but do not invade the deeper periodontal ligament and there is no resorption of alveolar bone. From Odell, E.W., 2017. *Cawson's Essentials of Oral Pathology and Oral Medicine,* ninth ed. Elsevier, London.

Pigmented regions and melanomas

Zones of melanin pigment are common within the oral cavity and are part of normal variation (see Fig. 14.42). However, malignant change within melanocytes can occur, eventually giving rise to malignant melanomas. Melanomas are generally associated with the skin and are often related to exposure to the sun. Rarely, however, they occur in the mouth. On initial diagnosis they may have already spread to local lymph nodes and therefore have a poor prognosis. The most common sites are the palate and upper alveolar ridge (Fig. 14.97).

Analysis of gingival crevicular fluid (GCF)

It is to be expected that the composition of the GCF differs in terms of microbial composition, and the concentration and composition of molecular biomarkers will differ when comparing healthy with diseased sites. Therefore, the composition of the GCF provides an indicator of the state of health of the underlying periodontium, and a very large literature exists on the subject. Even in health, proteomics has revealed the presence of hundreds of proteins despite the flow rate of GCF being low. With inflammation, this will be accompanied by a significant increase in the flow of GCF, and the number of biomolecules will be greatly increased. About 100 different biomarkers have been used to assess periodontal health, and these can be divided into three main groups (Fig. 14.98):

1) Host-derived enzymes and their inhibitors (e.g., alkaline and acid phosphatases, cathepsins and serine proteinases)
2) Inflammatory mediators and host response modifiers (e.g., ILs, tumour necrosis factor alpha [TNF alpha], prostaglandins)
3) Tissue breakdown products (e.g., hyaluronan, collagen peptides, chondroitin-4-sulphate, osteonectin)

Different researchers use different biomarkers in their assessment of the degree of periodontal involvement and the response to treatment.

Cytokines as well as breakdown products of structural tissues (such as collagen and ground substance) are employed. Extension from a gingivitis to a periodontitis would also be distinguishable by the added appearance of biomarkers indicative of bone destruction. A biomarker is a chemically stable molecule that is readily quantifiable in a tissue or fluid sample from a patient and could be used to predict the onset, persistence, severity and

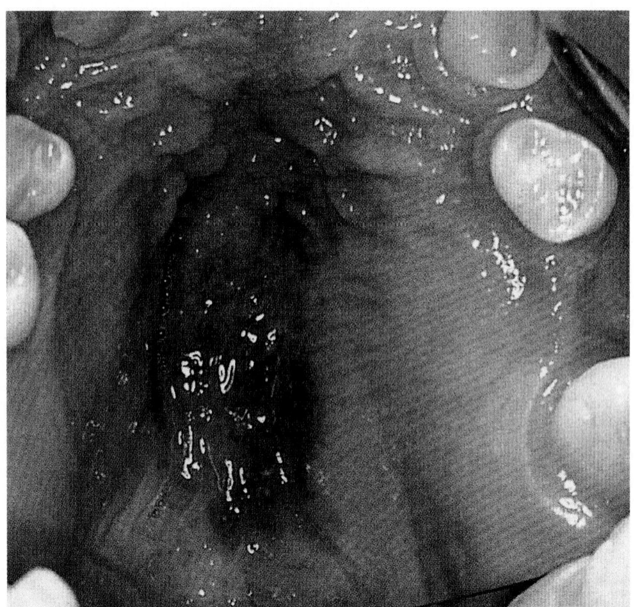

Fig. 14.97 (A) Large, poorly demarcated melanotic patch in the palate. All pigmented lesions such as this should be biopsied to confirm or exclude a melanoma. From. Odell, E.W., 2017. *Cawson's Essentials of Oral Pathology and Oral Medicine*, ninth ed. Elsevier, London.

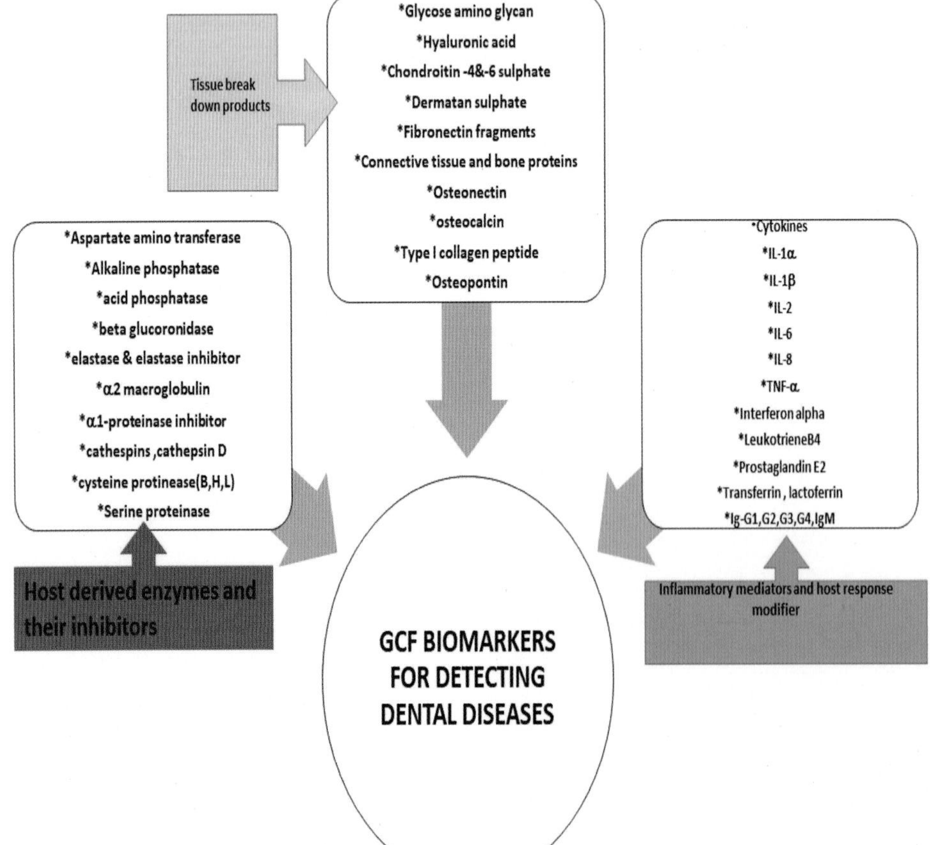

Fig. 14.98 Gingival crevicular fluid biomarkers for detecting dental diseases. From Bibi, T., Khurshid, Z., Rehman, A., et al., 2021. Gingival crevicular fluid (GCF): a diagnostic tool for the detection of periodontal health and diseases. Molecules 26, 1208.

prognosis of the patient's condition. Monitoring the composition of GCF allows an operator to assess the success or otherwise of treatment.

Following the application of orthodontic loads, GCF will reveal significant increases in the levels of molecules associated with remodelling of alveolar bone and the periodontal ligament, such as alkaline phosphatase, osteoprotegerin, cathepsin B, prostaglandins, ILs, TNF and epidermal growth factor. Breakdown products of the ECM of bone and periodontal ligament may be distinguishable in GCF because of known differences in composition between their ECMs. Breakdown products of basal lamina components in GCF may indicate the status of the junctional epithelium. Analysis of the GCF may eventually help indicate the severity of inflammatory periodontal disease and may allow for the development of markers to assist in identifying those in the general population who are most vulnerable to the spread of infection from a simple gingivitis into a periodontitis.

Further readings for this chapter can be found in the accompanying eBook. Explore online Self-assessment quiz to test and reinforce your understanding of the material in your free ebook. Follow instructions in the Inside Front Cover to unlock your access.

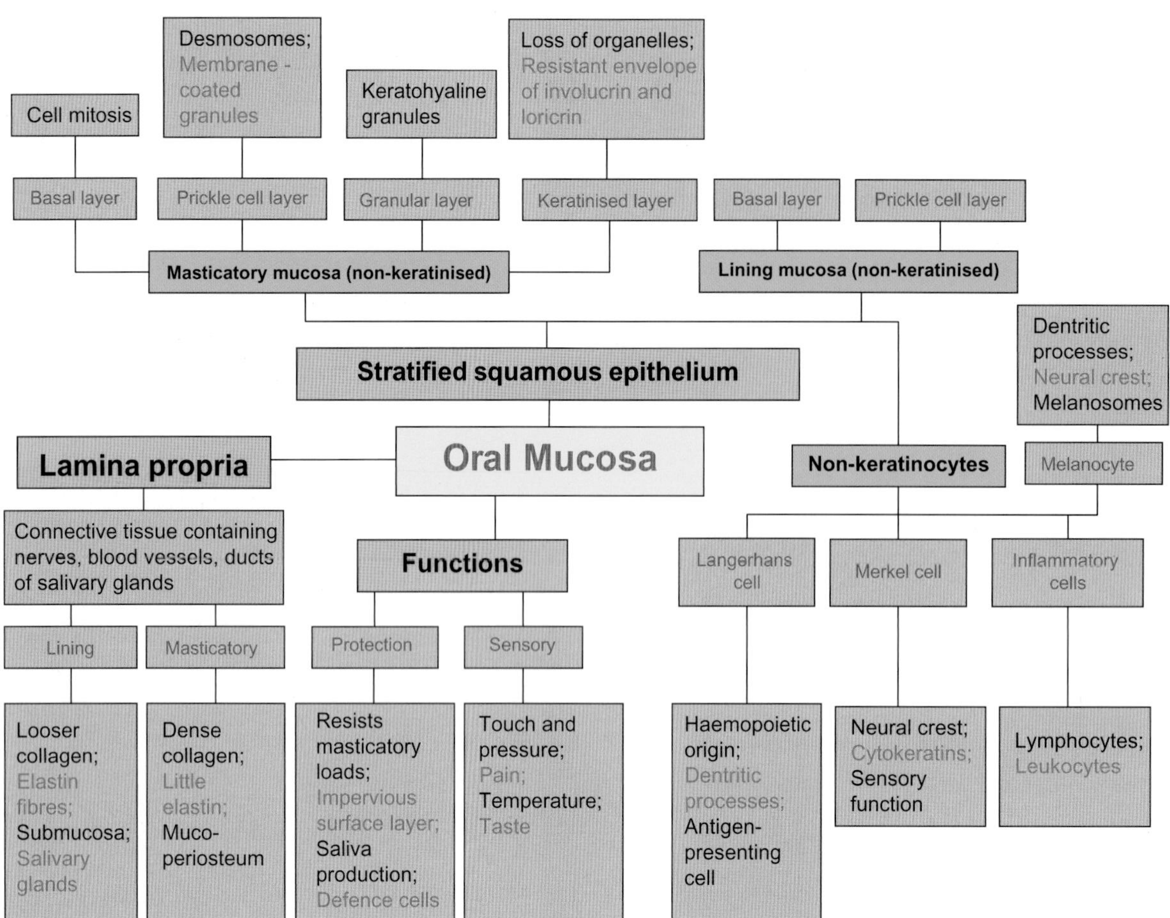

Mind Map 14.1 Oral mucosa.

Temporomandibular joint

15

The temporomandibular joint (TMJ) is the synovial articulation between the condyle of the mandible and the mandibular fossa of the temporal bone. It is also known as the *craniomandibular joint*. It is classified as a ginglymoarthrodial joint, having the form of both ginglymus and arthrodial, or hinge and sliding joints.

Being a synovial joint, the TMJ allows considerable movement and has a joint cavity filled with synovial fluid. The synovial membrane that secretes the synovial fluid lines the internal surface of the joint capsule. The gross anatomy of the TMJ is described on pages 77–81.

The TMJ has four special features:

- The joint space is divided into two joint cavities (upper and lower) by an intra-articular disc (Fig. 15.1); the upper joint cavity allows for gliding movements, the lower joint cavity for hinge movements.
- The articular surfaces are not composed of hyaline cartilage but of fibrous tissue (reflecting the joint's intramembranous development – see page 372).
- A secondary condylar cartilage is present in the head of the condyle until adolescence.
- Movements of the joint are influenced by the teeth and the two joints are unable to move independently, the mandible being a single bone. (see Box 3.1).

Articular surfaces of the temporomandibular joint

Four distinct layers have been described covering the bony head of the adult condyle (Fig. 15.2):

- The most superficial layer forms the articular surface and is composed of fibrous tissue. Although most of the fibres are collagenous, some elastin fibres are also present. The collagen fibres in the superficial layers are arranged parallel to the surface and, when viewed between crossed polars in a polarising microscope, show alternating light and dark bands that indicate the fibres are wavy or crimped (Figs. 15.3, 15.4). The collagen fibres in the deeper layers run more vertically. Fibroblasts/fibrocytes within the surface layer are sparsely distributed.
- Beneath the articular surface layer is a more cellular zone (cell-rich zone) in which proliferation occurs, providing a source of cells to replenish adjacent layers.
- Beneath the cell-rich zone is another fibrous layer that can have a variable appearance. However, as many of the cells are rounded and

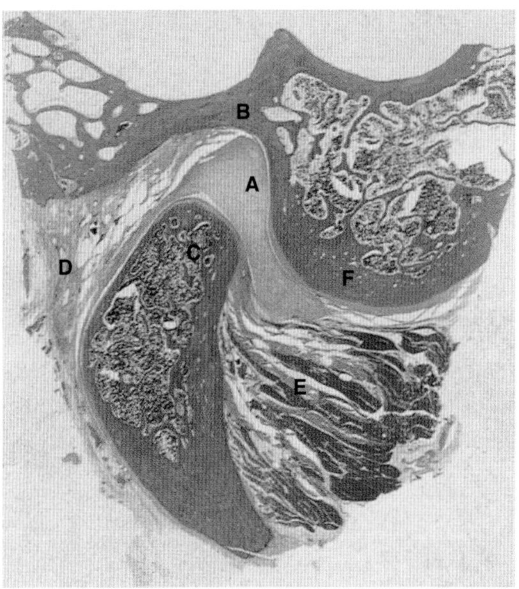

Fig. 15.1 Low-power sagittal section showing general distribution of tissues of the temporomandibular joint. A = intra-articular disc; B = mandibular (glenoid) fossa; C = condyle of mandible; D = capsule of joint; E = lateral pterygoid muscle; F = articular eminence (H & E; ×3). *Courtesy S Kariyawasam.*

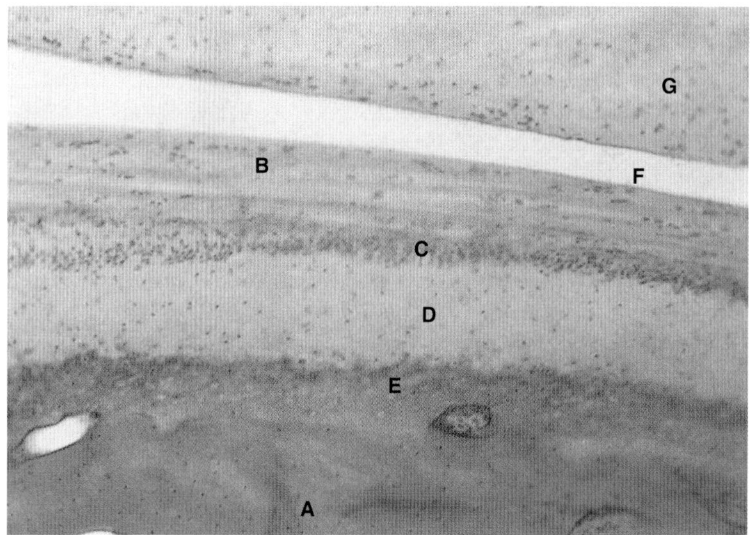

Fig. 15.2 Articular surface of adult condyle showing the four main layers covering the bone. A = bone of condylar head; B = fibrous articular surface layer; C = cell-rich layer; D = fibrocartilaginous layer; E = layer of calcified cartilage; F = lower joint space; G = intra-articular disc (H & E; ×100).

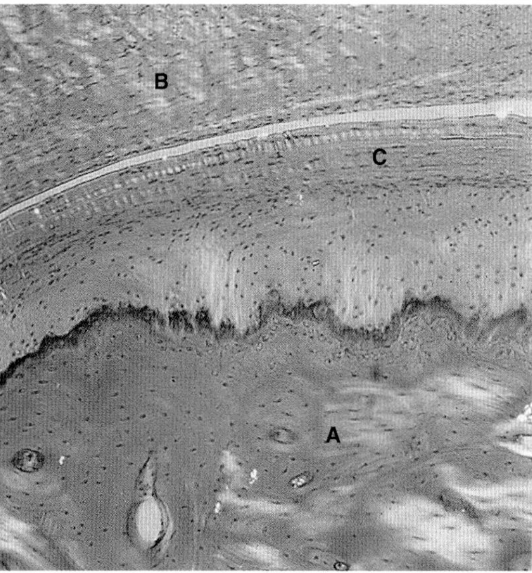

Fig. 15.3 Sagittal section of head of adult condyle (A) and lower part of intra-articular disc (B) viewed in partial polarised light. The alternating dark and light bands seen in the fibrous articular layer of the condyle (C) are indicative of the collagen being crimped. Crimping is also evident in the disc. Note that the bony surface is composed of compact bone (×75). *Courtesy Prof. M M Smith.*

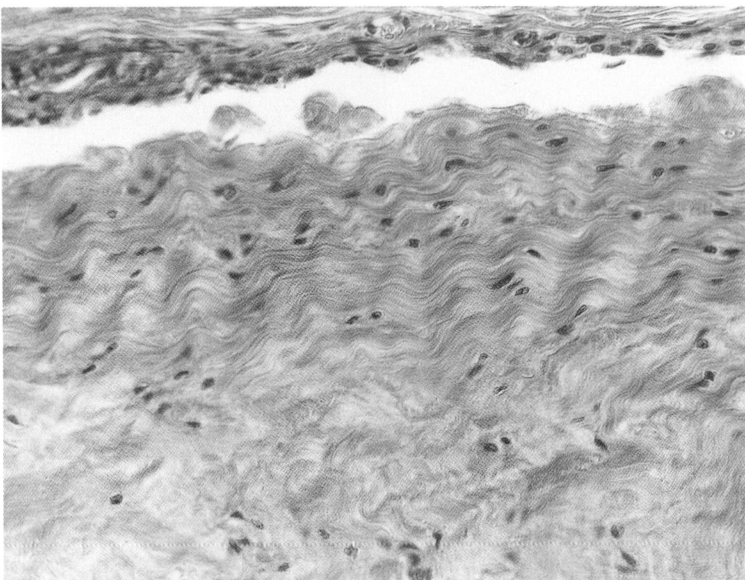

Fig. 15.4 Sagittal section of part of articular fibrous layer of condyle viewed with interference microscopy to directly demonstrate the crimped nature of the collagen fibres (×300). *From Berkovitz, B.K.B., 2000. Collagen crimping in the intra-articular disc and articular surfaces of the human temporomandibular joint. Archives of Oral Biology 45, 749–756.*

have an appearance reminiscent of cartilage-like cells, the layer is generally referred to as the fibrocartilaginous layer.

- Immediately covering the bone is a thin zone of calcified cartilage, distinguished from the bone by its different staining properties. This calcified cartilage is a remnant of the secondary condylar cartilage (see pages 372–373).

The articular surface covering the mandibular fossa of the temporal bone is similar to that of the condyle. Although generally thinner, it thickens as it passes over the articular eminence. It also shows crimping of the superficial collagen fibres.

Intra-articular disc

The gross anatomy of the intra-articular disc has been described on pages 79–81.

The disc is attached mediolaterally to the condylar head (through the collateral ligaments), anteriorly to the joint capsule and the lateral pterygoid muscle and posteriorly to the glenoid fossa as the retrodiscal tissue (bilaminar zone).

As for other soft, dense connective tissues, the intra-articular disc contains cells embedded in a matrix composed of fibres and ground substance. Most fibres consist of type I collagen, although traces of other types of collagen have been recorded. There is also a small quantity of elastin fibres present in the disc whose amount varies according to species. Up to 80% of the disc is composed of water (Box 15.1). The disc is an isotropic and non-homogeneous connective tissue.

Collagen fibres

In addition to the presence of type I collagen, which comprises about 80% (dry weight) of the disc, traces of other types of collagen (e.g., types III, VI, IX and XII) have also been reported within the intra-articular disc. The apparent presence of localised areas of fibrocartilage (see later) might also account for the presence of small amounts of type II collagen in some species.

Box 15.1 Composition of intra-articular disc

1) Water: 65–80%
2) Macromolecules: 20–35%
    - Collagen: 70–85%
    - Cells: 10%
    - Extracellular matrix components: 10% – proteoglycans, glycoproteins (fibronectin), glycosaminoglycans (chondroitin sulphate), elastin

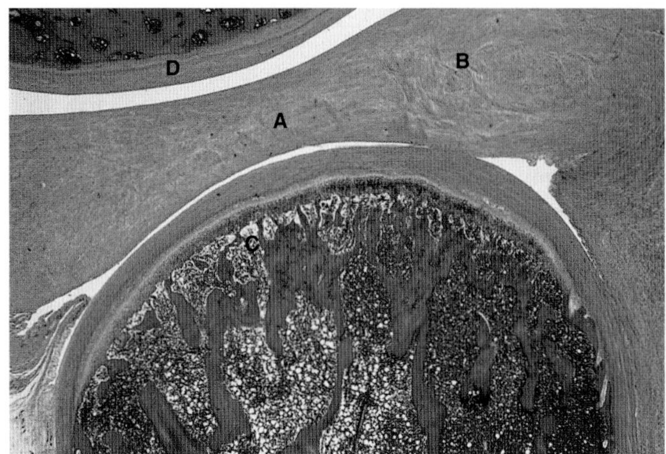

Fig. 15.5 Sagittal section of the temporomandibular joint of a child showing the collagen fibres of the central portion of the intra-articular disc (A) being more regularly aligned than at the periphery (B). Compare with Fig. 15.3 and note the larger marrow spaces and the lack of a layer of compact bone at the surface of the condyle (C). D = articular surface of mandibular fossa (×5). *Courtesy Prof. M M Smith.*

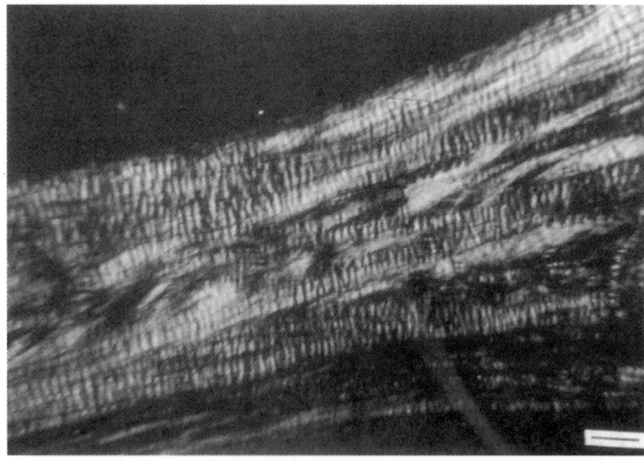

Fig. 15.6 Central (intermediate) zone of the intra-articular disc viewed between crossed polars to show that the main alignment of collagen fibres is anteroposterior. Banding indicates crimping of fibres. Marker bar = 100 microns. *From Berkovitz, B.K.B., 2000. Collagen crimping in the intra-articular disc and articular surfaces of the human temporomandibular joint. Archives of Oral Biology 45, 749–756.*

Collagen fibres in the thinner, central region of the intra-articular disc (also known as the *intermediate zone*) run mainly in an anteroposterior direction. In the thicker anterior and posterior portions (also known as the anterior and posterior bands, respectively), prominent fibre bundles also run transversely (mediolateral orientation) and supero-inferiorly, giving the fibres a much more convoluted appearance (Figs. 15.5, 15.6). Around the periphery of the disc, the collagen fibre bundles are arranged circumferentially (Fig. 15.7A). The arrangement of collagen fibres in the anterior and posterior bands is similar.

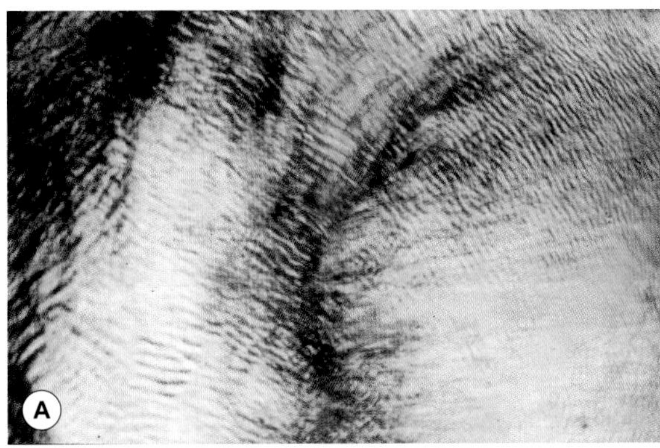

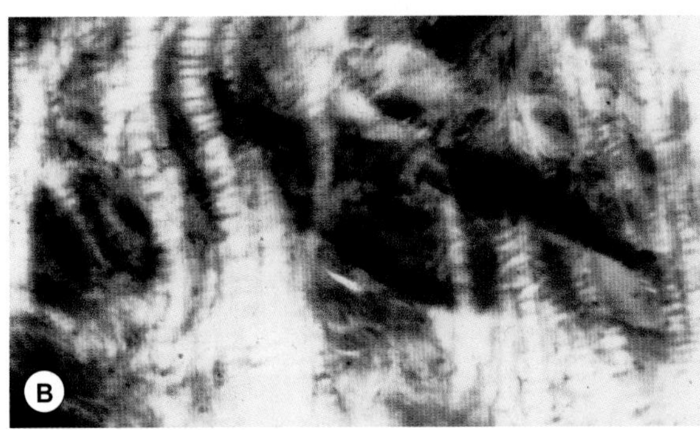

Fig. 15.7 (A) Intra-articular disc viewed between crossed polars. As indicated by the crimping of collagen (banded appearance), the peripheral fibres on the left side run circumferentially (top to bottom), while those more centrally (right side) run anteroposteriorly (right to left) (×35). (B) Posterior band of intra-articular disc showing vertically orientated collagen fibres, which are also crimped (banded) (×65). (A), *From Berkovitz, B.K.B., 2000. Crimping of collagen in the intra-articular disc of the temporomandibular joint: a comparative study. Journal of Oral Rehabilitation 27, 608–613.*

Fibre bundles in all regions decussate, branch and join with other fibre bundles. Although present in all regions, vertical fibres are more frequent in the posterior band and in the medial half of the disc (Fig. 15.7B).

Most of the collagen fibres of the intermediate zone extend into the band regions of the disc. A few fasciculi may be observed passing obliquely through the intermediate zone between the bands. The inferior fibre bundles at their junction with the posterior band form denser, more compact bundles than are seen adjacent to the superior surface. Fig. 15.8 diagrammatically illustrates the three-dimensional arrangement of fibre groups within the intra-articular disc.

Anteroposteriorly, the central region is significantly stiffer than medial and lateral regions. Mediolaterally, the posterior region is significantly stiffer than central and anterior regions. These findings indicate structure–function relationships between collagen fibre direction and organisation with biomechanical response to tensile loading.

When viewed in polarised light, the collagen fibres show alternating dark and light bands, indicating that they are wavy or crimped. Using specialised interference microscopy, the crimped nature of the collagen can be visualised directly (Fig. 15.9). Such crimping is seen in a wide variety of animal discs. It is unlikely to be the result of a fixation artefact, as it is evident even in fresh, unfixed material. As collagen crimping is a characteristic feature of the ligamentous attachment of muscles, it may be inferred that the intra-articular disc is similarly subjected to tensional loads. This does not preclude the presence of compressive loading falling on the intra-articular disc as well. In an intervertebral disc, for example, although the central portion is adapted to resist compressive loading, circumferential bundles of collagen at the periphery are crimped, presumably as an adaptation to tensional loads being generated at that site.

Ultrastructural studies show that collagen fibril diameters generally tend to be small (about 45 nm) with a unimodal distribution. This pattern is

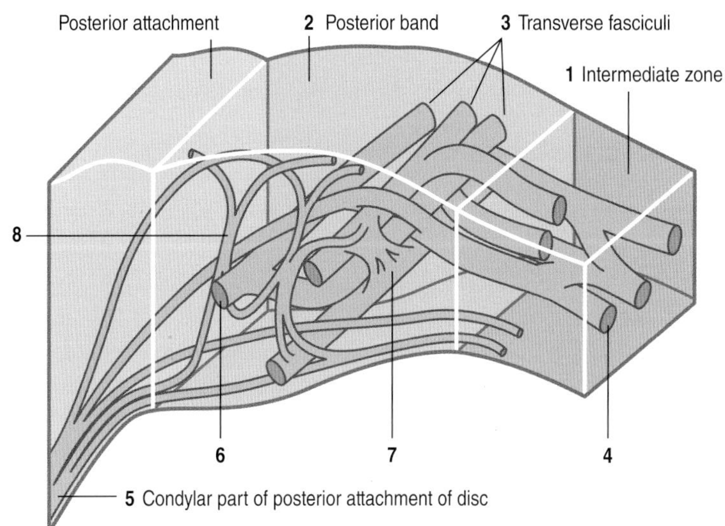

Fig. 15.8 Three-dimensional representation of collagen fibre bundle arrangement in intra-articular disc. Fibre bundles branch and join in the intermediate zone (1). On passing into the posterior band (2) some become continuous with transverse fasciculi (3); others (4) branch and join around the transverse bundle and join with bundles from the condylar part of the posterior attachment of disc (5). Some transverse bundles (6, 7) are joined by oblique or vertical fibre bundles. The vertical fibre bundles may extend between the surfaces, have continuity with fibres from the condylar part of the posterior attachment of the disc (5), branch and join around the transverse bundles (8) or become continuous with the latter in a mediolateral direction. *Redrawn after Scapino, R.P., Obrez, A., Greising, D., 2006. Organization and function of the collagen fiber system in the human temporomandibular joint disk and its attachments. Cells, Tissues, and Organs 182, 201–225.*

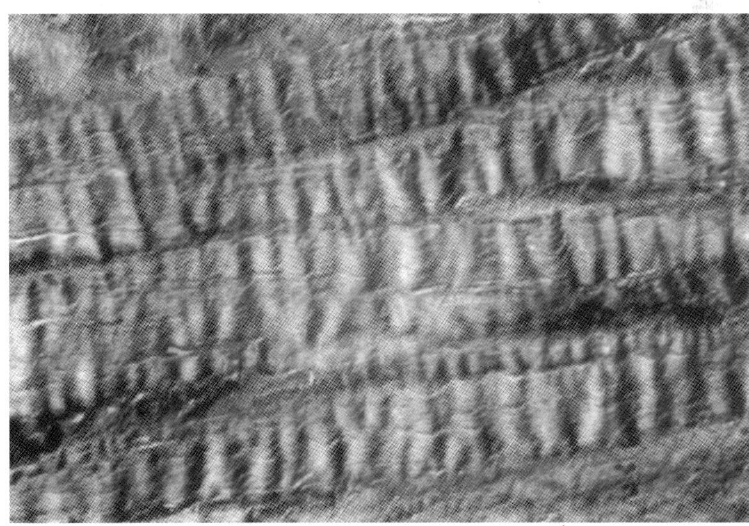

Fig. 15.9 Sagittal section of the intra-articular disc viewed with interference microscopy to directly demonstrate the crimped nature of the collagen fibres (×150).

often associated with connective tissues subjected to compression. Indeed, experiments in which collagen was disrupted by collagenase treatment undermined its resistance to compression. However, regional variation also exists, as collagen fibrils with larger diameters (mean of 70 nm, but with some fibrils reaching a diameter of 150 nm) and a non-unimodal distribution have also been reported. These dimensions are typically associated with a connective tissue subjected to tension (such as a ligament) (see page 229).

Elastin fibres

Elastin fibres are present throughout the intra-articular disc. They may comprise up to 5% of the dry weight of the disc and are said to decrease with age. They are conspicuous within the upper part of the bilaminar zone, with more laterally than medially. There are regional variations in the distribution of elastin. It has a complex and intertwined orientation in the anterior and posterior bands and a parallelism with the collagen fibres in the intermediate zone (with an anteroposterior orientation), which may contribute to the recovery of the disc tissues after deformation.

Ground substance

The ground substance of the disc comprises about 5% of its dry weight. There is species as well as regional variation. Most of the ground substance is located in the intermediate zone and the least in the posterior band. There is also more located medially than laterally. In addition, compositional changes may occur with age. The major glycosaminoglycans are chondroitin sulphate and dermatan sulphate, with additional traces of hyaluronan and heparin sulphate. Because of their anionic charge, these dominant glycosaminoglycans absorb water and adapt the intra-articular disc to resist compressive loading. Presumably, the compressive loading in one part of the disc will generate tensional loads elsewhere that can be resisted by the crimped collagen. Chondroitin sulphate is associated with proteins to form large-molecular-weight proteoglycans. These resemble aggrecan, an important component of the ground substance of cartilage. These proteoglycans are particularly localised at the periphery of the more rounded cartilage-like cells of the intra-articular disc (Fig. 15.10). Fibronectin and tenascin have also been located in the intra-articular disc.

Cells

Cells in the intra-articular disc seem to be more numerous at the time of birth (Fig. 15.11) and become more sparsely distributed in the adult (Fig. 15.12). The cells show an outline varying between flattened (fibroblast-like) and rounded (chondrocyte-like). The more rounded cells possess considerable amounts of cytoplasm. Cell kinetics are poorly understood. However, as the cells contain anti-apoptotic proteins (e.g., Bcl-2), this has suggested to some that the cells have a considerable life span. When the cells are isolated and placed in tissue culture medium, however, they show a rapid degree of cell proliferation.

At the ultrastructural level, the cells show moderate amounts of the intracellular organelles normally associated in fibroblasts with the synthesis and secretion of components of the extracellular matrix, such as endoplasmic reticulum, mitochondria, Golgi apparatus and vesicles (Fig. 15.13). This might indicate that there is reasonable turnover of the extracellular matrix (but see later). Some cells also exhibit considerable quantities of intermediate filaments (Fig. 15.14) whose diameter (approximately 9 nm) suggests the presence of vimentin. Cells differ in the types of intermediate filaments they contain. Ninety-nine percent of cells possess vimentin (type

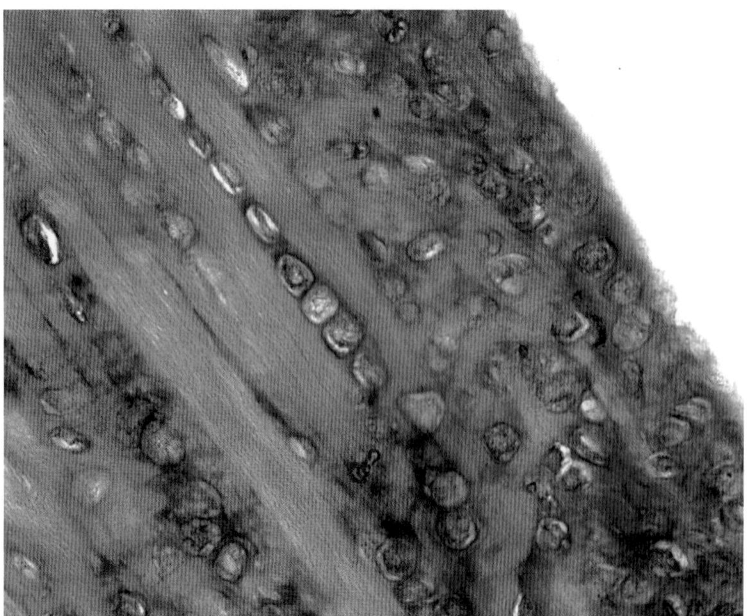

Fig. 15.10 Section of intra-articular disc. The blue staining surrounding the more rounded cells indicates the presence of chondroitin-sulphate–containing proteoglycans (Alcian blue/PAS stain; ×300). *Courtesy Prof. P R Morgan.*

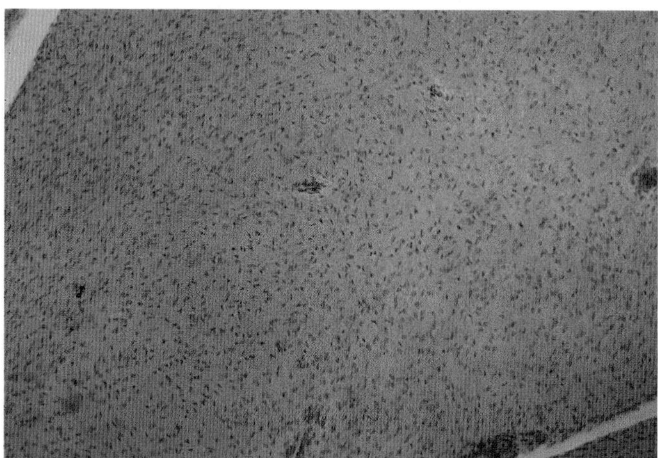

Fig. 15.11 Sagittal section of the intra-articular disc of a neonate showing the presence of numerous fibroblasts (H & E; ×100). *Courtesy Prof. M M Smith.*

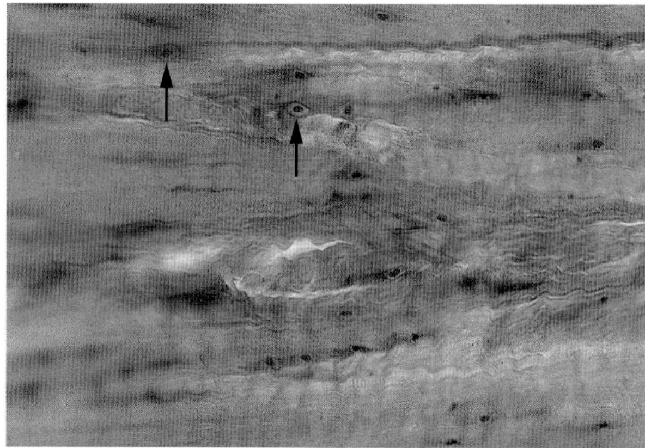

Fig. 15.12 Sagittal section of an adult intra-articular disc showing the sparse distribution of cells compared with Fig. 15.11. Note the rounded cartilage-like appearance of some cells (arrows) (H & E; ×150).

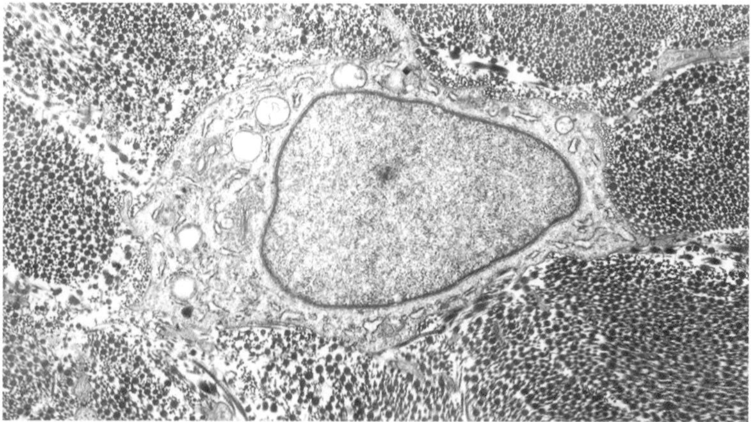

Fig. 15.13 Electron micrograph of fibroblast from the intra-articular disc showing moderate amounts of rough endoplasmic reticulum and mitochondria. The extracellular matrix shows collagen fibrils lying close to the cell membrane (×8,000). *From Berkovitz, B.K.B., Pacy, J., 2002. Ultrastructure of the human intra-articular disc of the temporomandibular joint. European Journal of Orthodontics 24, 151–158.*

III), 38% of cells possess glial fibrillary acidic protein (GFAP; type III), 5% of cells possess nestin (type II) and 1% of cells possess desmin (type III). The precise function of each of these intermediate filaments is unclear but is likely to involve cell communication, maintenance of cell shape and integrity, cell division and anchoring the position of organelles within the cytosol. The cell membrane is closely opposed to the collagen fibrils of the extracellular matrix (Figs. 15.13, 15.14).

The fluorescent marker phalloidin binds to the intracellular cytoskeletal filament F-actin within a cell and is small enough to penetrate the cell membrane in a thin block of tissue, thus highlighting the outline of the cell body and any processes. Studies using this technique have revealed new information about the cells in the intra-articular disc. When viewed in a confocal microscope that can optically section a cell and show its three-dimensional appearance, the cells are seen to possess numerous long, fine processes. These processes are present throughout the tissue (Figs. 15.15, 15.16), with some extending for distances of up to 100 µm or more. As the processes might be expected to contact those of other cells, the tissue has also been double-stained with both phalloidin and antibodies for the gap junction protein, connexin 43. The results reveal the presence of dense punctate staining for this gap junction protein throughout the numerous and extensive cell processes (Fig. 15.17).

The significance of the presence of a complex system of cell processes containing considerable quantities of gap junction protein is unclear. The precise route whereby the cells of the disc obtain their nutrition is not known, but the two sources are the local blood vessels and/or the synovial fluid. In the case of the blood vessels, these are situated at the periphery of the disc, with the bulk of the central part of the disc being avascular. As one of the functions of the connexin family of transmembrane proteins

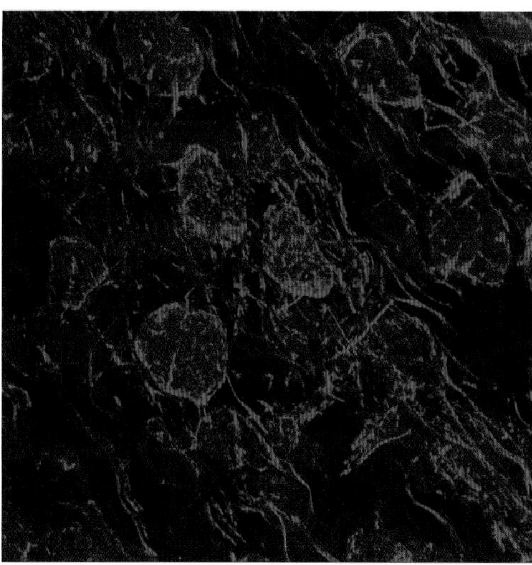

Fig. 15.16 Confocal micrograph representing a stacked series of 211 sections, each 0.2 µm thick, showing cells of the intra-articular disc labelled with phalloidin and showing a profusion of cell processes (×900). *From Berkovitz, B.K.B., Becker, D., 2002. The detailed morphology and distribution of gap junction protein associated with cells from the intra-articular disc of the rat temporomandibular joint. Connective Tissue Research 203, 12–18.*

Fig. 15.14 Electron micrograph of fibroblast from the intra-articular disc. The left part of the cell contains rough endoplasmic reticulum, while surrounding the nucleus and projecting into the right side of the cell is a clear zone containing microfilamentous material. The extracellular matrix shows transversely sectioned collagen fibrils (×8,000). *From Berkovitz, B.K.B., Pacy, J., 2002. Ultrastructure of the human intra-articular disc of the temporomandibular joint. European Journal of Orthodontics 24, 151–158.*

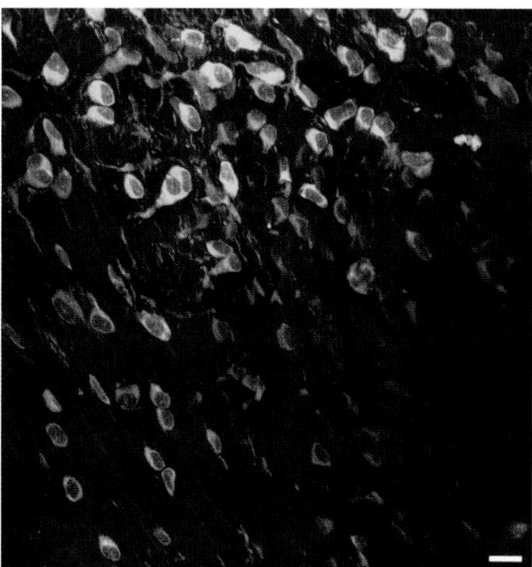

Fig. 15.17 Confocal image representing a stacked series of 14 sections, each 3 µm thick, showing cells of the intra-articular disc double-labelled with phalloidin (green) and an antibody to the gap junction protein connexin 43 (red). Note the rich concentrations of red stain in the cell processes (×250). *From Berkovitz, B.K.B., Becker, D., 2002. The detailed morphology and distribution of gap junction protein associated with cells from the intra-articular disc of the rat temporomandibular joint. Connective Tissue Research 203, 12–18.*

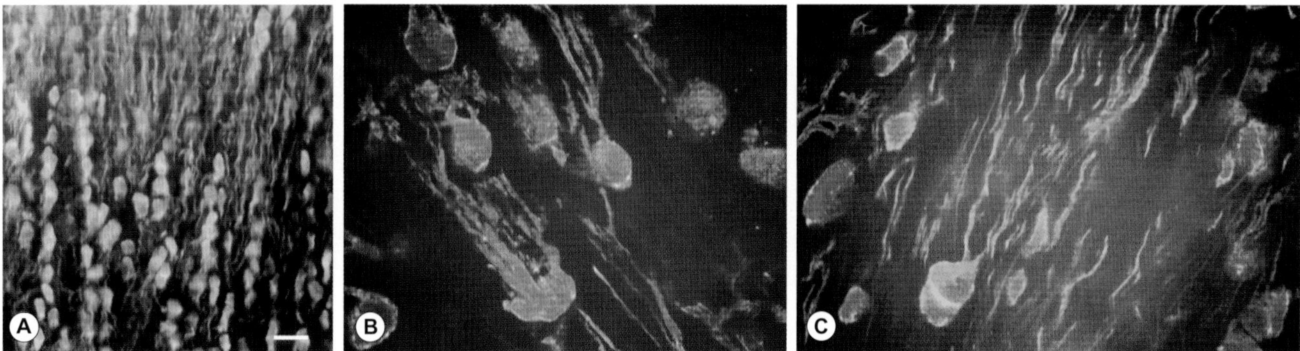

Fig. 15.15 (A) Confocal micrograph of intra-articular disc cells labelled with phalloidin. Note the numerous cell processes (×300). (B, C) Higher-power micrographs (×500). *From Berkovitz, B.K.B., Becker, D., 2002. The detailed morphology and distribution of gap junction protein associated with cells from the intra-articular disc of the rat temporomandibular joint. Connective Tissue Research 203, 12–18.*

is to permit the passage of small molecules between contacting cell processes, it could be suggested that the role of the cell processes in the intra-articular disc is to allow for the passage of nutrients and fluid from the peripheral blood vessels to the central avascular regions of the disc. That some diffusion of nutrients can occur at the surface of the disc seems evident from the observation that it is possible to maintain vital cells in thin intra-articular discs (e.g., rat) in tissue culture.

A characteristic feature of true cartilage cells is the presence at the ultrastructural level of a pericellular matrix intervening between the cell membrane and the adjacent type II collagen fibrils of the extracellular matrix. This pericellular matrix contains microfilamentous material and is delineated by a pericellular capsule. As the rounded cells in the intra-articular disc have been considered to be cartilage-like, electron microscopic studies have been undertaken to see whether these cells also possess a pericellular matrix. The results indicate that most cells do not (Figs. 15.13, 15.14). However, a pericellular matrix can be seen surrounding the cells of some older specimens (of the rat and marmoset) (Fig. 15.18), suggesting that their presence is related to age. Unlike the cells in hyaline cartilage, but like cells in fibrocartilage from other sites (e.g., at the insertion of tendons), cartilage-like cells in these older intra-articular discs lack a pericellular capsule at the periphery of the pericellular matrix. The presence of a pericellular matrix has yet to be confirmed in the cells of healthy intra-articular discs of humans.

A general question arises as to the terminology to be used for the cells of the intra-articular disc. If the intracellular organelles present in the cells of the disc are mainly associated with the secretion and turnover of extracellular matrix (collagen and ground substance), then the moderate amounts of such organelles would indicate that the cells are reasonably active and could be referred to as fibroblasts. However, if these organelles are more concerned with the synthesis of gap junction protein, and if collagen turnover is slow, then the cells could be termed fibrocytes. This is partly supported by the absence of intracellular collagen profiles, usually indicative of a rapid turnover rate of collagen (see pages 238–239). Future studies designed to determine the turnover rate of collagen in the disc should help clarify the situation.

The term *fibrocartilage* has been widely used to describe the tissue comprising the intra-articular disc. The features associated with cartilage can be seen in Box 15.2.

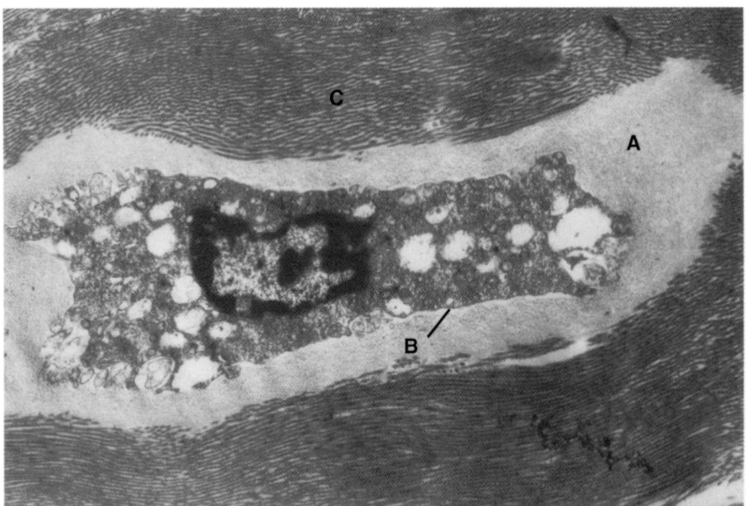

Fig. 15.18 Electron micrograph of a cell from an adult marmoset intra-articular disc. Note the presence of a pericellular matrix (A) between the cell membrane (B) and the collagen fibrils of the extracellular matrix (C) (×7,000).

With regard to these features, the intra-articular disc lacks blood vessels (especially in its central portion) and exhibits high-molecular-weight chondroitin-sulphate–containing proteoglycans. However, it may lack, or only have traces of, type II collagen, and its somewhat rounded cells are not surrounded by a pericellular matrix (except in relation to age) and possess numerous processes that form connections with adjacent cells. The term *fibrochondrocyte* has therefore been used by some to describe the rounded cells of the intra-articular disc.

To obtain further insight into the different populations of cells within the intra-articular disc, the transcriptomes of a large number of single cells isolated from the disc have been obtained. The expression of 21,340 genes was captured. The analysis allowed four main cell types to be identified. The most abundant cells were fibroblasts comprising about 80% of cells. In addition, different clusters of fibroblasts exhibited differentially expressed genes, indicating heterogenicity within the disc, with some being regarded as chondrogenic. The chondrogenesis-related fibroblasts were located around the intermedial zone of the TMJ disc, suggesting these terminally differentiated chondrocyte-like cells are functional for mechanical load bearing. In addition to fibroblast cell clusters, other cell clusters could be classified as macrophage clusters, endothelial cell clusters and mural cell clusters. The latter cells situated around blood vessels are thought to play an important role in regulating the growth and homeostasis of the vasculature of both the embryo and the adult.

Blood vessels

Although blood vessels are present in the intra-articular disc at the time of birth, most are soon lost, and the bulk of the intra-articular disc, especially the central region, becomes avascular (Fig. 15.5), with blood vessels being localised at the periphery of the disc. Perhaps this lack of blood vessels may explain the lack of regenerative capacity of a diseased disc. Similarly, there is a lack of lymphatics. However, posteriorly in the bilaminar zone where the disc divides into superior and inferior laminae (see page 80), the region of the superior lamella possesses numerous blood vascular spaces (Fig. 15.19). As the tendon of the lateral pterygoid muscle pulls the disc forwards during jaw opening, blood flows into the back part of the disc to fill the space behind the migrating mandibular condyle. The volume of this retrodiscal tissue appears to increase four to five times as a result of venous engorgement as the jaw is opened. This venous engorgement is not the result of the tissue having erectile properties, but more the result of continuity with the pterygoid venous plexus lying medial to the condyle. As the mandibular condyle moves backwards during jaw closure, blood leaves the retrodiscal tissues. Elastic tissue in the superior lamella has been regarded by some authors as providing elastic recoil, aiding the backward movement of the disc during jaw closure. Others believe that the return of the disc is entirely

Box 15.2 Features associated with cartilage

- The presence of type II collagen
- The presence of high-molecular-weight chondroitin-sulphate–containing proteoglycans
- The presence of a pericellular matrix surrounding the cells
- Chondrocyte-like cells that exhibit a rounded morphology with short, microvillus-like processes
- The absence of cell contacts
- The absence of blood vessels within the tissue

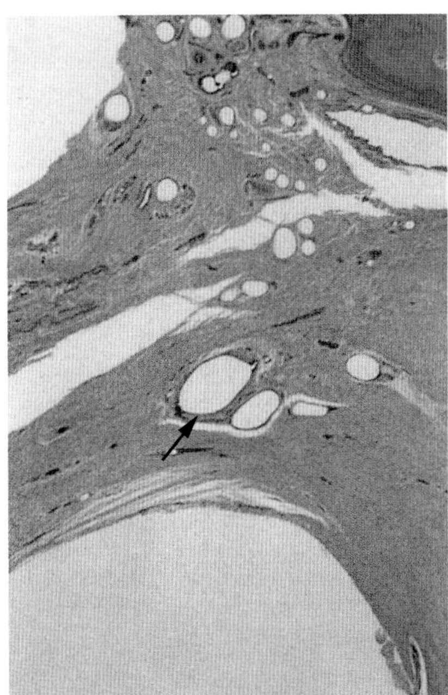

Fig. 15.19 Section of the superior lamella of the intra-articular disc showing considerable vascularity (arrowed) compared with the rest of the disc, which is relatively avascular (H & E; ×14).

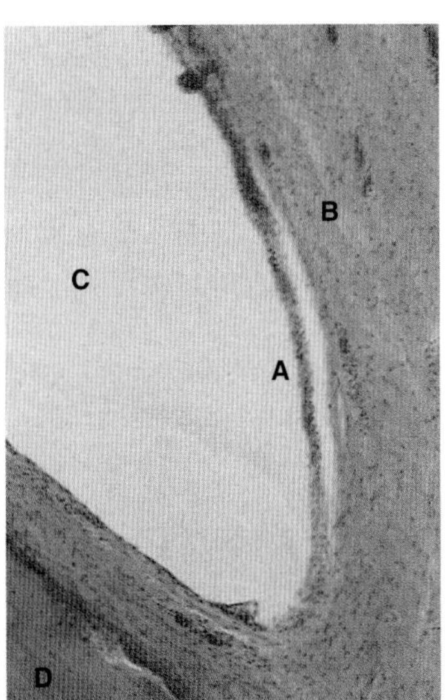

Fig. 15.20 Section showing the synovial membrane (A) lining the margins of the inferior joint cavity (C). B = articular disc; D = condyle (H & E; ×60).

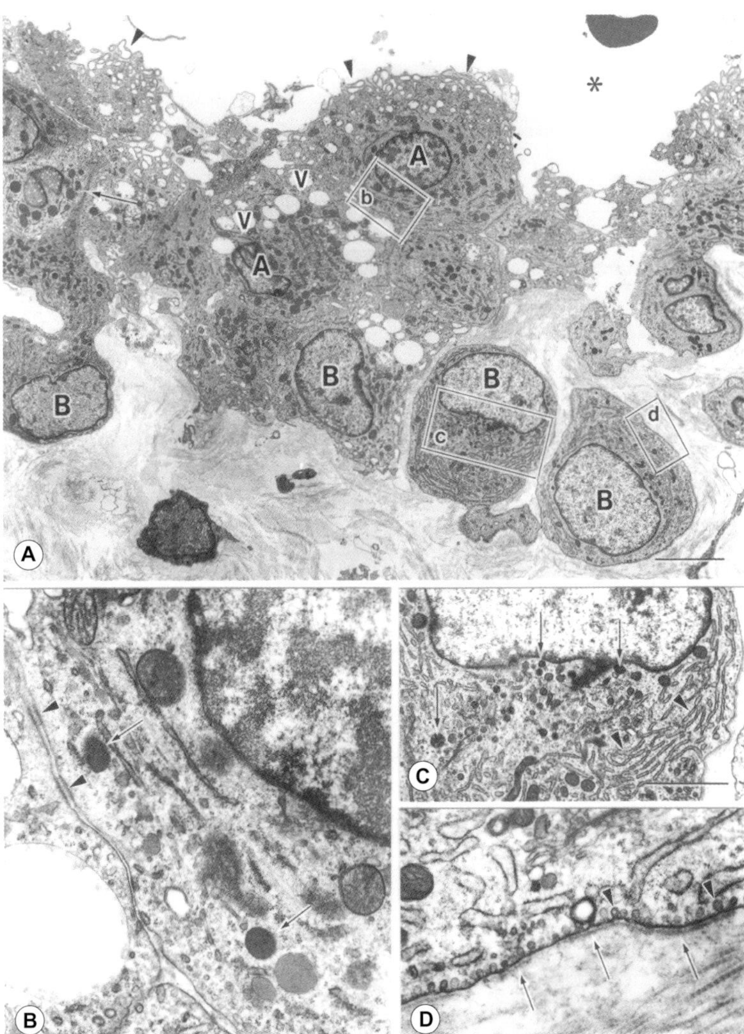

Fig. 15.21 Electron micrographs showing the synovial lining layer in the rat temporomandibular joint. Fig. 15.21A The synovial lining layer is composed mainly of macrophage-like type A (A) and fibroblast-type B (B) cells. The type A cell, which is exposed to the articular cavity (*), has numerous surface folds like filopodia (arrowheads) and many vacuoles (V). The nucleus contains rich heterochromatin. The fibroblast-like type B cell is located in the deeper portion of the lining layer. One of these cells extends long cytoplasmic processes, which often reach the articular cavity (arrow). Scale bar = 5 μm. Fig. 15.21B Magnification of boxed area b in Fig. 15.21A. The macrophage-like type A cell contains many lysosomes (arrows) in the cytoplasm. Note desmosome-like structures (arrowheads) between type A cells. Scale bar = 1 μm. Fig. 15.21C Magnified view of boxed area c in Fig. 15.21A. The fibroblast-like type B cell is characterised by a well-developed rough endoplasmic reticulum (arrowheads) and numerous secretory granules (arrows). Scale bar = 2 μm. Fig. 15.21D Magnification of boxed area d in Fig. 15.21A. An amorphous structure is seen around the type B cells (arrows). Note many caveolae (arrowheads) along the cell membrane. Scale bar = 1 μm. From Nozawa-Inoue, K., Amizuka, N., Ikeda, N., Suzuki, A., et al., 2003. Synovial membrane in the temporomandibular joint – its morphology, function and development. Archives of Histology and Cytology 66, 289–306.

passive. The inferior lamella is relatively avascular and inelastic. The posterior discal attachment tissues also appear to contain some type III collagen. This has been interpreted as providing increased distensibility and being an aetiological factor in eventual joint dysfunction.

Synovial membrane

The synovial membrane lines the inner surface of the fibrous capsule of the TMJ and the margins of the intra-articular disc (Fig. 15.20). It obviously does not cover the articular surfaces, where it would be rapidly worn away. The synovial membrane shows high metabolic activity and has considerable powers of regeneration. The synovial membrane may be folded at rest, with these folds flattening out during movements of the joint. With age, the number and size of the projections increase.

The synovial membrane consists of a superficial layer of flattened endothelial-like cells resting on a sublining connective tissue layer whose capillaries are fenestrated and which possess well-developed lymphatic vessels. The cells comprising the superficial layer are of two types: a macrophage-like type A cell and a fibroblast-like type B cell. The synovial membrane produces the synovial fluid that fills the joint spaces. The inferior joint cavity holds about 1 mL of synovial fluid, while the slightly larger superior joint cavity contains a little more.

Macrophage-like type A cell

This cell has a rounded appearance and, at the electron microscope level, is seen to possess filopodia-like surface folds and numerous vacuoles, vesicles and lysosomes (Fig. 15.21A). The macrophage-like cells are connected to each other by desmosome-like structures (Fig. 15.21B). As with other macrophage cells, the TMJ synovial cells participate in phagocytosis and the immune response. The cells can be identified through their staining with typical macrophage antibodies.

Fibroblast-like type B cell

Typical of a protein secretory cell, the fibroblast-like B cell contains a well-developed endoplasmic reticulum, dense secretory granules and few lysosomes (Fig. 15.21A and C). The cell membrane shows numerous small, smooth-walled invaginations (Fig. 15.21D). Fibroblast processes are seen to pass between the macrophage-like cells to connect with the synovial cavity. Unlike the macrophage-like cells, the fibroblast-like B cells lack cell contacts. The cell secretes connective tissue components such as collagen and molecules such as hyaluronan an important component in synovial fluid.

The lining layer of the synovial membrane maintains an epithelial-like layered appearance through the presence of an incomplete basement membrane containing laminin. In the absence of embryonically derived epithelial cells, it is assumed that the basement membrane is a product of the fibroblast-like B cells with which it is associated.

Synovial fluid

The synovial membrane secretes the synovial fluid that occupies the joint cavities. At rest, the hydrostatic pressure of the synovial fluid has been reported as being subatmospheric, but is greatly elevated during mastication. Raised fluid pressures may also be clinically relevant in patients who continually clench their teeth (bruxists).

Synovial fluid acts as a lubricant for the TMJ and is thought to provide a source of nutrition for the adjacent tissues of the articular disc and the lining articular surfaces. Although mainly composed of water, the molecule thought to play the most important role in lubrication is hyaluronan. Other molecules present, and thought to aid lubrication, are lubricin (proteoglycan 4) and surface-active phospholipids. In addition, trace amounts of other bioactive molecules will be present, reflecting the composition and turnover of the adjacent connective tissues, such as cytokines (e.g., transforming growth factor beta [TGF-β]), growth factors (e.g., vascular endothelial growth factor [VEGF]), collagenases (matrix metalloproteinases [MMPs] and their tissue inhibitors [TIMPs]), receptor activator of nuclear factor kappa-B ligand (RANKL) (see pages 271–275), reactive oxygen and nitrogen species and immunoglobulins (e.g., IgA and IgG).

Condyle of the child

The histological appearance of the mandibular condyle varies according to age. This is owing to the presence of the secondary condylar cartilage during childhood. This cartilage appears initially at about the 10th week of intra-uterine life (see page 372) and remains as a zone of proliferating cartilage until adolescence.

Four layers can be discerned in the growing condylar cartilage:

1) An outer fibrous cell layer
2) A proliferative cell layer
3) A chondrocytic cell layer
4) A hypertrophic cell layer

Unusually for a cartilaginous tissue, type I collagen is synthesised in all four layers, while type II collagen is restricted to the chondrogenic layers three and four.

As for that of the adult, the mandibular condyle of a child is lined by a layer of fibrous tissue containing flattened cells surrounded by dense collagen bundles. Beneath the outer fibrous layer is a layer of undifferentiated cells, with those in the upper part undergoing cell division. Cells from this proliferative layer divide to give rise to fibroblast-like cells that subsequently differentiate into chondrocytes, which form the secondary condylar cartilage (Fig. 15.22). As for cartilage elsewhere, the collagen is chiefly type II. Chondrocytes in the deep part of the condylar cartilage

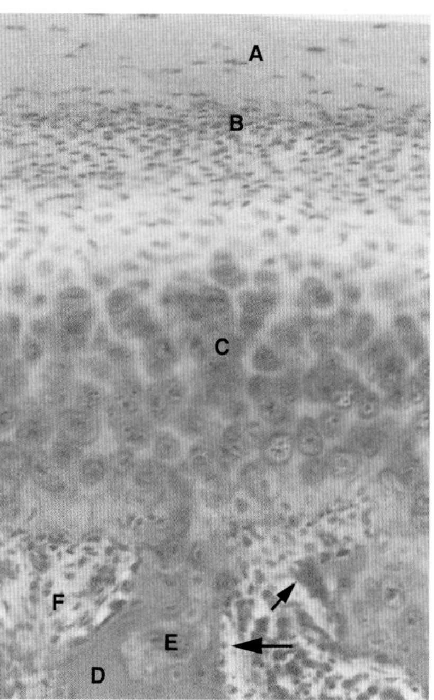

Fig. 15.22 Section through the condyle of a child. A = fibrous articular layer; B = cell-rich proliferative layer; C = hypertrophic chondrocytes of the secondary condylar cartilage; D = woven bone being deposited around a template of calcified cartilage (E); F = marrow space; small arrow = multinucleated osteoclast; large arrow = osteoblast layer depositing bone on calcified cartilage (×130). Courtesy Dr. D A Luke.

hypertrophy and synthesise type X collagen, following which the matrix undergoes endochondral ossification. In brief, this process involves mineralisation of the cartilage matrix and subsequent apoptosis of the hypertrophic chondrocytes. However, some have suggested that some hypertrophic cells can transform into osteogenic cells. Part of the calcified cartilage is resorbed by large, multinucleated osteoclasts. Subsequently, bone-forming cells, the osteoblasts, deposit woven bone around the template of calcified cartilage. Eventually, this area will be remodelled to produce mature bone. Unlike the chondrocytes in a typical growth plate, the chondrocytes of the condylar cartilage are not aligned into columns and do not secrete as much intercellular matrix. The possible role of the condylar cartilage in the growth of the mandible is controversial and is discussed on page 373. The condyle of the young child is not lined by a distinct layer of compact bone as for of the adult (compare Figs. 15.3 and 15.5).

The differentiation pathway in the growing condyle may be regulated by biomechanical force, as under nonfunctional conditions (e.g., *in vitro* organ culture), intramembranous bone may be formed.

Patches of bone newly formed beneath the condylar cartilage seem to be intermediate in form between cartilage and bone, showing an intense matrix reaction for type I collagen and only a faint pericellular reaction for type II collagen. Such bone has been termed *chondroid bone*.

Spheno-occipital synchondrosis

The spheno-occipital synchondrosis, an example of a primary cartilaginous joint, is described here to provide a comparison between a primary cartilage and a secondary cartilage, as exemplified by the condylar cartilage. Developmentally, the primary cartilage appears first and maps out the shape of the future bone. In the case of the condylar cartilage, the ramus has already formed in membrane before this secondary cartilage appears. Primary cartilages have inherent growth potential, as is evidenced when they are transferred to tissue culture. The condylar cartilage has little intrinsic growth potential when placed in tissue culture. In the spheno-occipital synchondrosis, proliferative zones lie on either side of the central region of the cartilage, and proliferation involves cartilage cells. This contrasts with the condylar cartilage, where it is undifferentiated fibroblast-like

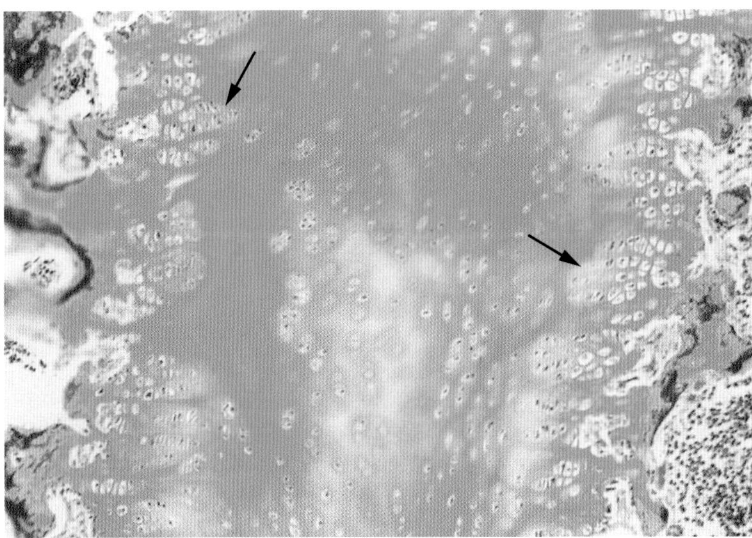

Fig. 15.23 Section through the spheno-occipital synchondrosis. Chondrocytes aligned in columns on each side of the cartilage (arrows). The reddish zones at both sides indicate the sites of endochondral ossification. Note the large amounts of extracellular matrix compared with that seen in Fig. 15.22.

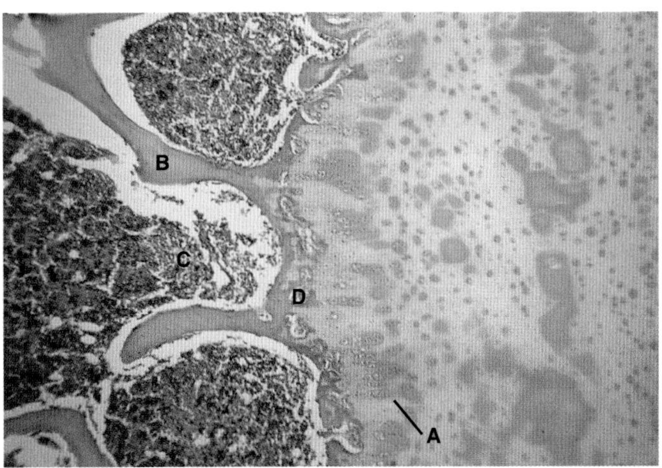

Fig. 15.24 Section at one surface of the spheno-occipital synchondrosis showing the alignment of chondrocytes into columns (A). B = bone; C = marrow space; D = endochondral ossification front (×80). Courtesy Dr. M E Atkinson.

cells that undergo proliferation. In the synchondrosis, the chondrocytes are aligned in columns in the direction of growth on both sides of the cartilage (Figs 15.23, 15.24), and there is considerable production of extracellular matrix which, together with the original cell proliferation and the absorption of water by the proteoglycans, is responsible for providing the growth force. In the secondary condylar cartilage, however, there is far less production of extracellular matrix and there is no alignment of the hypertrophic chondrocytes into columns. This might relate to the ability of the secondary cartilage to produce some growth in more than one direction. In the case of an epiphyseal growth plate (as opposed to a synchondrosis), columns of cartilage cells are produced only on one side of the cartilage.

Clinical considerations

Fractures of the temporomandibular joint

Fractures of the mandible frequently involve the mandibular condyle, and this is discussed on pages 58–61.

Temporomandibular joint disorder

Temporomandibular joint disorder (TMD) is a disorder of the masticatory system chiefly characterised by pain in the joint or face. It affects about 5–12% of the general population, although some studies report incidences as high as 25–40%. It is the second most common musculoskeletal pain condition after chronic back pain. Other symptoms include loss of function of one or both articulations, impairment of the masticatory system, clicking sounds in the joint, deviation or deflection upon mouth opening and limited mouth opening. Involvement of the discomalleolar ligament (see page 79) may also produce middle ear symptoms such as tinnitus.

TMD is multifactorial in origin, and amongst the various possible contributing factors are occlusal disturbances, para-function and psychological and/or emotional factors. Furthermore, changes in the shape of the articular eminence seem to predispose to progression of internal derangement of the TMJ. TMD is higher in to females compared with males (ratio 2:1). TMD may be divided into three categories: internal derangement (articular disc displacement), myogenic disorders and arthritis or arthrosis, with the first being the most common. Because of the heterogeneity of the disorder, diagnosis and treatment are difficult.

During movement at the TMJ, little friction is generated at the surface of the intra-articular disc because of the lubricating properties of the synovial fluid and the smoothness of the articular surfaces. Frictional forces on the disc are increased when synovial fluid is replaced with a less viscous substitute (e.g., phosphate-buffered saline). Like other synovial joints, the TMJ is prone to inflammatory and degenerative conditions such as rheumatoid arthritis and osteoarthritis. In these situations, damage to the articular surfaces will subject the articular disc to increased friction that may lead to degenerative changes within the disc. Experimental removal of the intra-articular disc results in degenerative changes being produced in the mandibular condyle.

The intra-articular disc may gradually become displaced from its normal position between the articular surfaces. With the more usual anteromedial displacement (see Fig. 3.12), the posterior part of the disc may end up between the bony articular surfaces and be subjected to abnormal loading. This may result in a loss of proteoglycans that, together with an increased water content, may affect the biomechanical properties of the tissues. Degenerative changes are seen in the disc with subsequent changes in its shape. The associated loss of structure may be accompanied by an invasion of blood vessels, with the disc eventually becoming perforated. The accompanying degenerative changes may also result in exposure of bone at the articular surfaces. Inflammatory changes and increased permeability of the vessels of the synovial membrane can raise the intra-articular fluid pressure and change the composition of the synovial fluid. Like gingival crevicular fluid in periodontal disease, the synovial fluid in TMD will also show an increased content in molecules such as proinflammatory cytokines (e.g., interleukin, tumour necrosis factor), MMPs and VEGF, which may aid in diagnosis. Furthermore, as pain is often a major symptom, biomarkers associated with pain may provide diagnostic help, such as neurotransmitters (glutamate and serotonin), neuropeptides (substance P and calcitonin gene–related peptide) and growth factors (nerve growth factor). Using a proteomics approach to analyse the proteins present in the synovial fluid and articular disc of three separate types of TMD, different proteins have been identified for each condition, giving hope that, in the future, this method of study may help with diagnosis and the evaluation of the response to any treatment.

TMJ disorders are not easily treated. Irrigating and aspirating the joint (arthrocentesis) can reduce symptoms and improve mobility. For those most severely affected, joint implants have been designed. As far as a damaged disc is concerned, part of the difficulty in treating the condition relates to its poor healing properties, perhaps related to the lack of blood vessels. For this reason, work is under way to attempt to construct replaceable substitute intra-articular discs using tissue engineering techniques, although attaching such a disc to the capsule is likely to provide a surgical challenge (see also Chapter 28).

Orthodontic considerations

During examination of children in their early teens, it may be evident that the mandible is developing at a greater or lesser rate than the maxilla and that this imbalance is likely to lead to a malocclusion and/or facial disharmony. Unlike some aspects of sutural growth in the upper jaw, which are amenable to intervention and improvement, growth is less easy to modulate in the mandible. Nevertheless, orthodontic appliances have been designed to try to modify any growth contributed by the condylar cartilage (although there is little evidence that the cartilage plays any significant role in the growth process). Thus, appliances that push the mandible back and compress the condylar cartilage against the mandibular fossa are used to try to retard mandibular growth. Conversely, in situations where the mandible is underdeveloped, appliances that relocate the condyle in a forward position have been used to enhance development of the condyle. However, the success of such procedures is not always predictable.

Further readings for this chapter can be found in the accompanying eBook. Explore online Self-assessment quiz to test and reinforce your understanding of the material in your free ebook. Follow instructions in the Inside Front Cover to unlock your access.

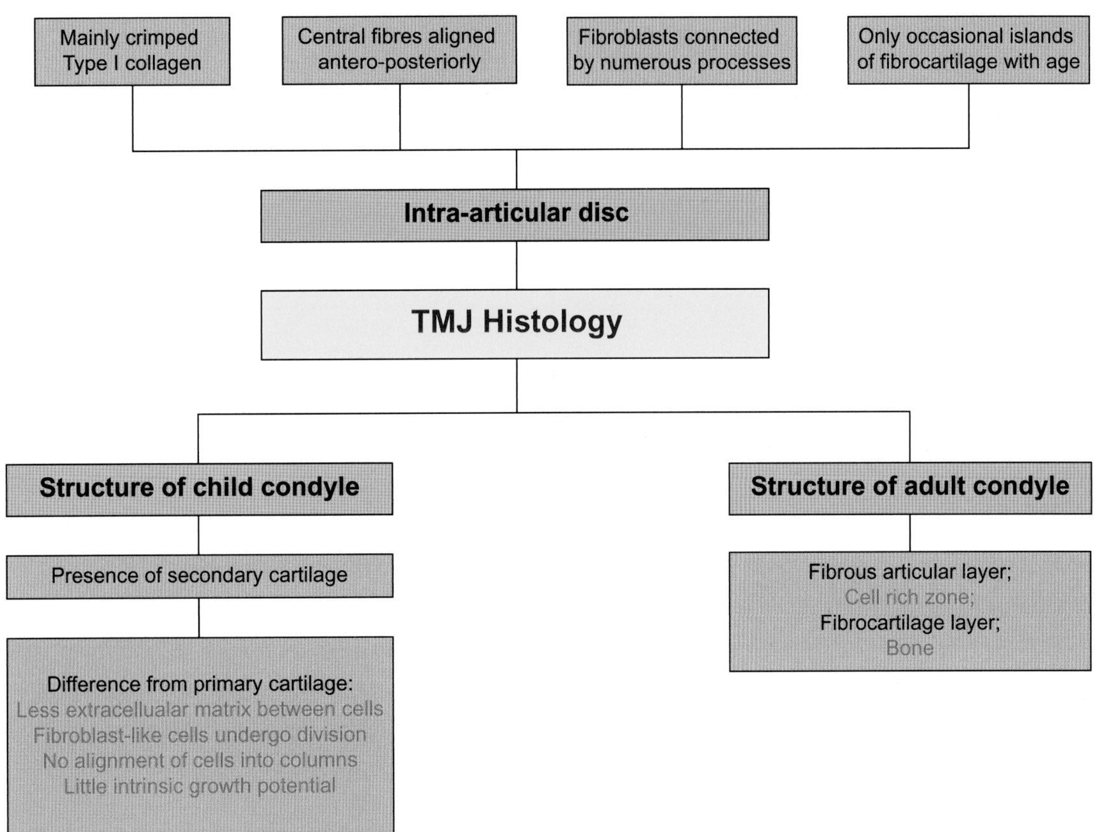

Mind Map 15.1 Temporomandibular Joint Histology.

16 Salivary glands

Introduction

Saliva is a complex solution which contains material from the following sources: salivary glands, oral mucosa cells, oral microbiota and viruses, blood vessels, gingival crevicular fluid and food (Fig. 16.1).

Salivary glands are compound, tubulo-acinar, merocrine, exocrine glands, the ducts of which open into the oral cavity. The term *compound* refers to the fact that a salivary gland has more than one tubule entering the main duct; *tubulo-acinar* describes the morphology of the secreting cells; *merocrine* indicates that only the secretion of the cell is released; *exocrine* describes a gland that secretes fluid on to a free surface. The main functions of saliva are to clear substances from the mouth; to buffer the pH; to maintain tooth mineralisation; to facilitate wound healing; to commence digestion of food; to assist with taste; to provide immunity; and to protect, lubricate and hydrate the oral mucosal surface.

Composition of saliva as secreted from salivary glands

The secretion of saliva is a reflex function emanating from salivary centres that is dependent on afferent stimulation (e.g., taste and mastication) and involves complex integration from salivary centres.

Saliva is over 99% water, but is crucial to oral homeostasis as it has properties very different from water owing to inorganic and organic compounds (such as proteins, glycoproteins and enzymes), which allows it to perform many important functions. Mucins play major roles, providing lubrication during mastication, swallowing and speech. Saliva containing high amounts of mucin tends to be viscoelastic, an important characteristic for the retention of saliva on oral mucosal surfaces. There is also an adherent layer (pellicle) of mainly salivary proteins that maintains enamel remineralisation and facilitates mucin interaction with oral mucosal surfaces. Saliva brings substances into solution so that they can be tasted. It also facilitates the presence of a commensal microbial

Box 16.1 Basic anatomy of salivary glands

- Salivary glands are exocrine glands.
- Main regulated secretion caused by reflex parasympathetic and sympathetic stimulation.
- Acinar secretory cells are either serous or mucous.
- Acinar cells produce primary secretion, which is modified as it passes down the ducts.
- Three pairs of major salivary glands are parotid, submandibular and sublingual glands.
- Numerous minor salivary glands (mainly mucous glands apart from von Ebner serous glands in tongue) are scattered throughout the oral mucosa.

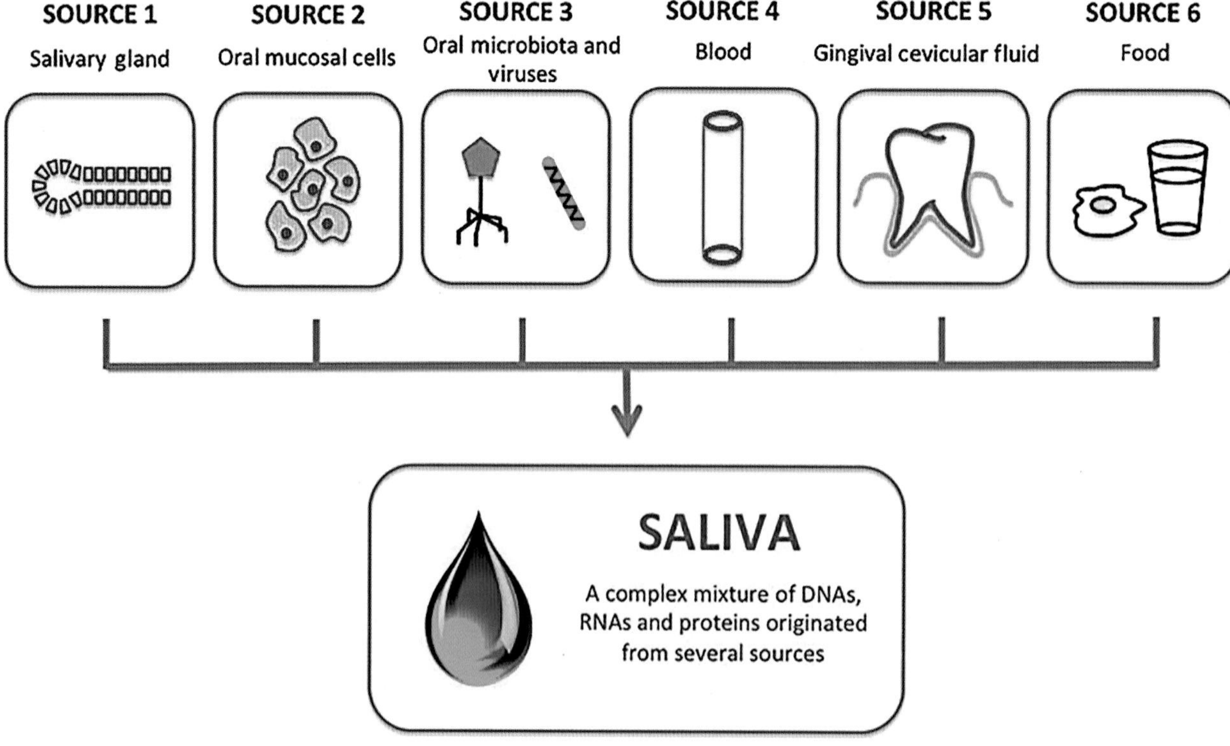

Fig. 16.1 Saliva is composed of biomolecules and fluids from different sources. Saliva is mainly secreted by salivary glands, and its informative biomolecules (DNA, RNA, proteins, metabolites and microbiota) are obtained from salivary glands, oral mucosa cells, oral microbiota and gingival crevicular fluid. From Zhang, Y., Sun, J., Lin, C.-C., et al. 2016. The emerging landscape of salivary diagnostics. *Periodontology* 2000 70, 38–52.

community (microbiome) and limits the activity of bacteria by causing their aggregation. Saliva contains minerals and acts as a buffer; both features help to maintain the integrity of the dental enamel. Peptide growth factors (e.g., epidermal growth factor, nerve growth factor) are produced by the submandibular gland. Their precise functions are not known, but epidermal growth factor may be involved in wound healing and (together with mucin) maintaining gastro-oesophageal epithelial integrity. Saliva contains numerous other proteins to which many different functions have been ascribed, such as lysozyme, histatin, lactoferrin and defensins (antibacterial agents); statherin (control of mineralisation); and carbonic anhydrase 6 (previously named gustin with a possible role in taste). Immunoglobulins (mainly IgA) are produced by plasma cells within the stroma of the salivary glands and are secreted into saliva to function as part of the mucosal immune system that also includes lymphoid tissue in the gut and bronchi. A starch-hydrolysing enzyme (alpha-amylase) is present in saliva to aid digestion, but there is uncertainty regarding the digestive function of lipase secreted by von Ebner's glands of the tongue. Salivary bicarbonate ions (HCO_3^-) are important in buffering plaque and dietary acid within the mouth, whilst the saturation of saliva with calcium and phosphate provides a remineralising potential following episodes of demineralisation.

The varied functions of saliva can be taken for granted, and it is only when salivary production and flow are disrupted, as in cases of dry mouth (xerostomia), that its true importance to the general well-being of the individual is realised (see pages 348–349).

Salivary glands consist of two main elements: the glandular secretory tissue (the parenchyma) and the supporting connective tissue (the stroma). From the stroma of the capsule surrounding and protecting the gland pass septa that subdivide the gland into major lobes; lobes are further subdivided into lobules. Each lobe contains numerous secretory units consisting of clusters of grape-like structures (the acini) positioned around a lumen (Fig. 16.2). A secretory acinus may be serous, mucous or mixed. Serous acini can be distinguished from mucous acini according to the nature of the secretion produced and, in structural terms, the morphology of their secretory granules. Serous cells secrete more protein and less carbohydrate than mucous cells. The acinus, via its lumen, empties into an intercalated duct lined with cuboidal epithelium, which in turn joins a larger striated duct formed of columnar cells. Both the intercalated and striated ducts are intralobular and affect the composition of the secretion passing through them. The striated ducts empty into the collecting ducts, which are mainly interlobular. Basal cells are present and are sparsely distributed in the striated ducts and more densely distributed in the collecting ducts. The collecting ducts join until the main duct is formed at the hilum. The main duct carries the saliva to the mucosal surface and may be lined near its termination by a layer of stratified squamous epithelial cells.

The connective tissue septa carry the blood and nerve supply into the parenchyma. Apart from fibroblasts and collagen, the connective tissue also contains fat cells, which show much variability in the case of the parotid gland. Plasma cells (which secrete the immunoglobulins) are found in the stroma of the gland around the intralobular ducts. With age, there is a decrease in the number of secretory cells. Unlike endocrine glands, the secretion of which is controlled by the activity of hormones, the secretion of saliva is under the control of the autonomic nervous system.

The acini of the parenchyma are responsible for the production of the primary secretion. Saliva is the product of an active secretory process and

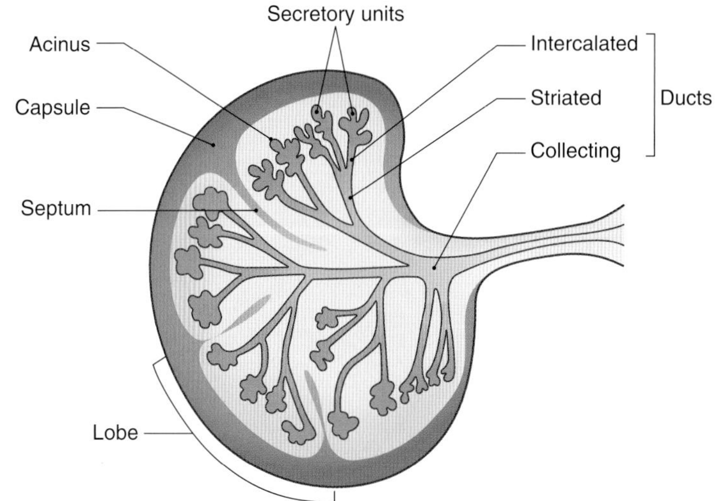

Fig. 16.2 The general organisation of a salivary gland.

is not an ultrafiltrate of blood. The serous cells produce a watery proteinaceous fluid and are the source of amylase. The secretory product of mucous cells contains proteins linked to a greater amount of carbohydrate, forming a more viscous, mucin-rich product. Both serous and mucous cells are arranged as acini, although groups of mucous cells may have a more tubular form. Acini may contain either serous or mucous cells, or they may be mixed. When mixed, the serous cells have been traditionally described as forming a cap or demilune outside the mucous cells (Fig. 16.3), although the results of recent studies have challenged this view (see page 342). Around the acini and intercalated ductal cells, contractile cells with several processes are present and represent the myoepithelial (basket) cells.

Salivary glands may be classified according to size (major and minor) and/or the types of secretion (mucous, serous or mixed). The three paired major salivary glands are the parotid, submandibular and sublingual glands. The numerous minor salivary glands are scattered throughout the oral mucosa and include the labial, buccal, palatoglossal, palatal and lingual glands. Salivary glands are not present in the gingiva or the dorsum of the anterior two-thirds of the tongue. In general, the parotid gland will synthesise more protein than glycoprotein. Consequently, parotid saliva has a lower carbohydrate content, whereas the submandibular and sublingual glands synthesise and secrete greater amounts of glycoprotein than protein. Furthermore, saliva from these two glands is higher in carbohydrate content.

There is a low level of secretion of saliva throughout the day, with periodic large additions from the major glands (e.g., at meal times). With an average salivary flow rate of 0.3 mL/min, it has been calculated that 500–750 mL of saliva are secreted each day (with about 90% derived from the major salivary glands). A very small contribution to the pooled saliva is derived from gingival fluid and from sebaceous glands. The sublingual gland and the minor salivary glands spontaneously secrete saliva, but the bulk of this secretion is nerve-mediated. The parotid and submandibular glands do not secrete saliva spontaneously, and their secretion is entirely nerve-mediated. Thus, secretion ceases during anaesthesia almost entirely. Salivary flow in females is about 70% that of males.

Just before swallowing, the volume of saliva in the mouth varies between subjects (0.5–2.1 mL), with a mean of 1.1 mL. Following a swallow, the residual volume of saliva in the mouth is reduced to 0.4–1.4 mL

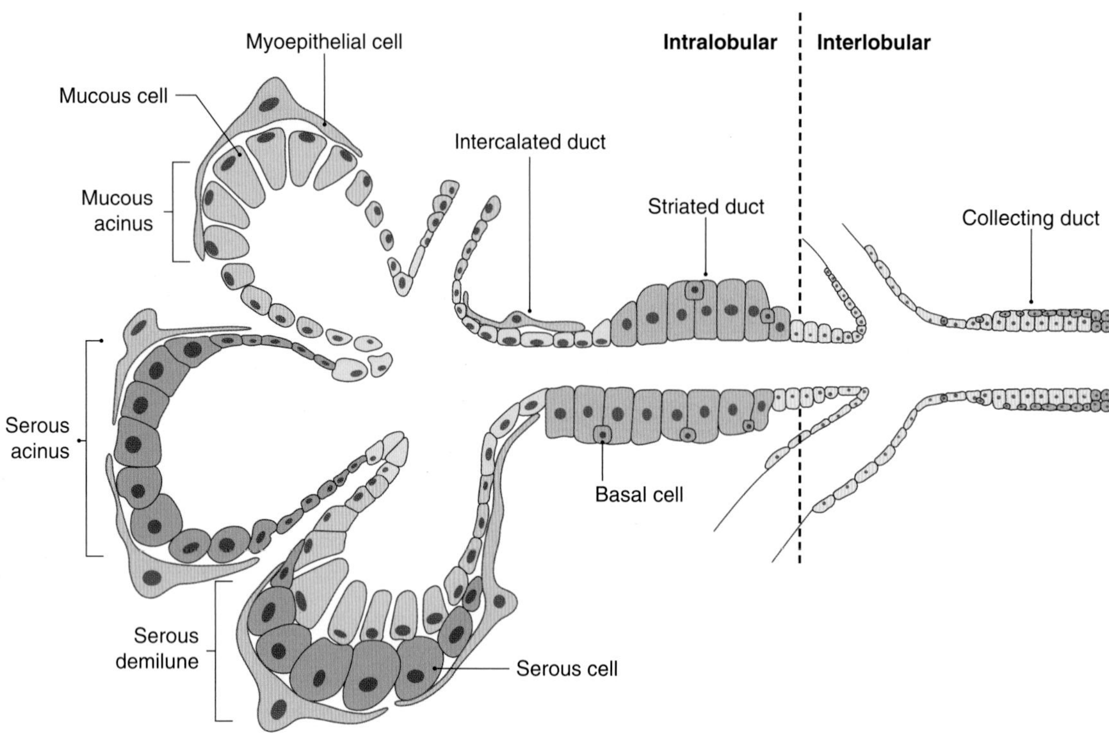

Fig. 16.3 The secretory and ductal elements in a mixed salivary gland. However, as discussed later, the serous demilunes are artefacts of preparation.

(mean of 0.8 mL), mainly in the form of a thin film of about 50 microns covering the mucosa and hard-tissue surfaces of the mouth.

The flow rates and composition of saliva are regulated by the autonomic nervous system and are dependent on signalling by neuropeptides and intracellular calcium (see pages 337–340). They are also affected by features such as age, circadian rhythm, psychological factors such as pain and stress, and types of medication and diseases influencing the physiology of the salivary glands.

Mechanisms of salivary secretion

Salivary acinar cells secrete the water, ions and most of the proteins present in saliva in response to nerve-mediated stimuli. Salivary fluid secretion is dependent on cell membrane transporter proteins (Fig.16.4), resulting in predominantly sodium and chloride secretion into the lumen of the acinus present, to be followed by water movement along the osmotic gradient. Protein secretion mainly involves protein storage granule exocytosis at the luminal membrane, releasing proteins synthesised by the acinar cells (Fig. 16.5). There are other protein-containing secretory vesicle pathways, one of which gives rise to the secretion of IgA across the cell from the basolateral to the apical membrane (polymeric immunoglobulin receptor–mediated transcytosis). Other minor vesicle pathways may be responsible for delivery of some of the blood and tissue proteins present in saliva.

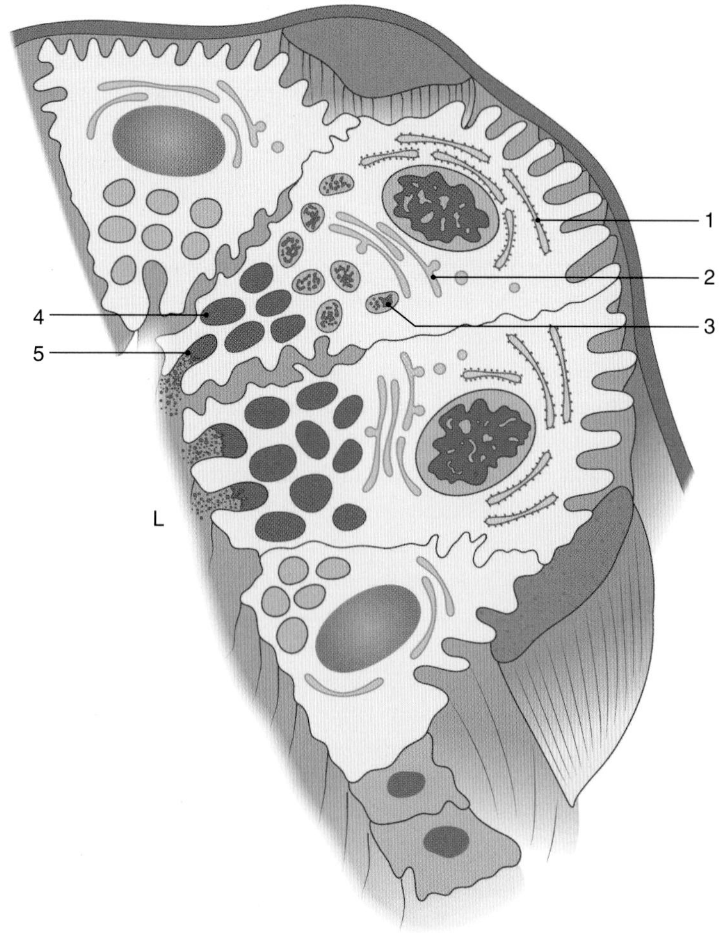

Fig. 16.4 The pathway in secretory protein synthesis, storage and stimulated exocytosis. 1 = protein synthesis in the rough endoplasmic reticulum; 2 = transport via the Golgi apparatus to the *trans*-face; 3 = initial storage within immature granules; 4 = concentration of secretory proteins in mature storage granules; 5 = exocytosis of stored proteins into the lumen of the acinus; L = lumen surface. Courtesy Prof. G B Proctor and Karger Press.

Parotid gland

Serous cells

The parotid gland is the largest of the salivary glands. It is enclosed within a well-defined capsule, the parotid capsule. The acini of the gland are

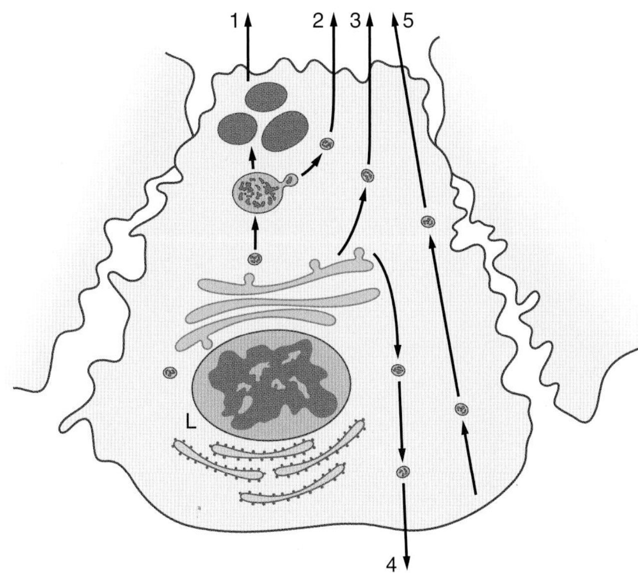

Fig. 16.5 The vesicular protein secretory pathways likely to be operating in parotid acinar cells. 1 = storage granule pathway; 2 = constitutive-like pathway; 3 = constitutive pathway to the apical membrane; 4 = constitutive pathway to the basolateral membrane; 5 = transcytosis from the basolateral to the apical membrane. L = nucleus. Courtesy Prof. G B Proctor and the Karger Press.

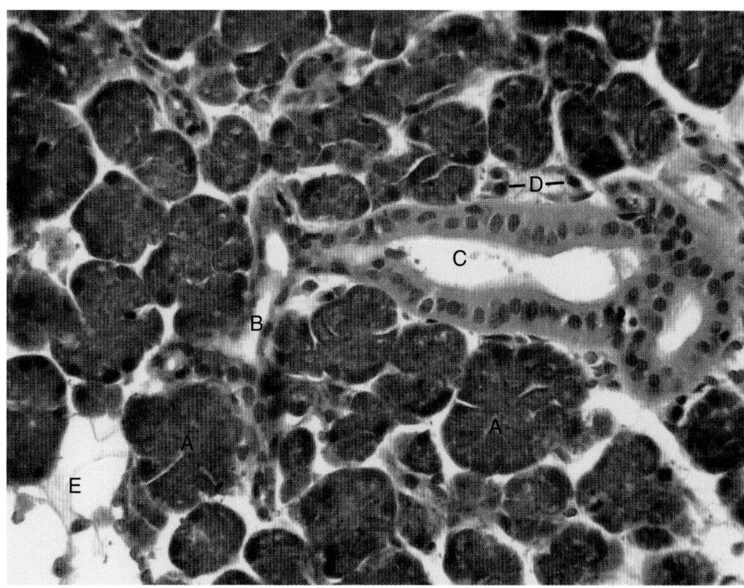

Fig. 16.7 Dark, granular appearance of cytoplasm of serous acini of parotid gland (A). B = intercalated duct; C = striated duct; D = plasma cells; E = fat cell (H & E; ×360). Courtesy Dr. J D Harrison.

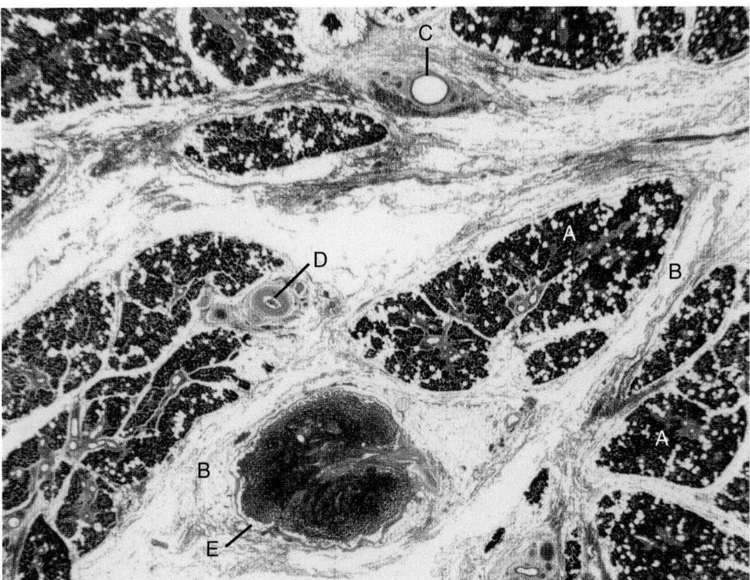

Fig. 16.6 The parotid gland showing the secretory parenchyma (A) being divided into lobules by septa of the stromal connective tissue (B). C = interlobular collecting duct; D = interlobular artery; E = lymph node (H & E; ×13). Courtesy Dr. J D Harrison.

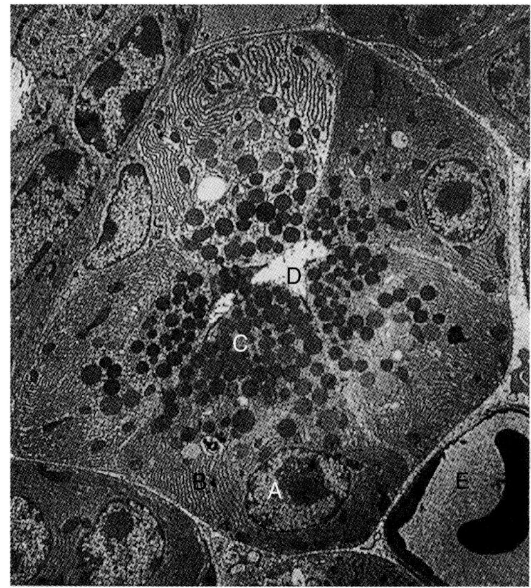

Fig. 16.8 TEM of serous acinus. A = nucleus in basal part of cell; B = rough endoplasmic reticulum; C = secretory granules in luminal part of cell; D = central lumen; E = capillary (×2,000). Courtesy Mr. P F Heap.

serous, although mucous cells are occasionally present. The cells produce a watery saliva and have a characteristic granular appearance with routine haematoxylin and eosin staining (Figs. 16.6 and 16.7), unlike mucin-producing glands that stain weakly with haematoxylin and eosin (see Fig. 16.38). Connective tissue septa can be seen subdividing the secretory parenchyma into lobes and then further into lobules. The connective tissue contains blood vessels, nerves and collecting ducts. The lumina of the acini are very small (Fig. 16.7). The cell nucleus is prominent and round and is located in the basal third of the cell, which is basophilic (because of the presence of rough endoplasmic reticulum). The granular appearance of the serous acinar cell results from the numerous refractile granules in the luminal portion of the cell (adjacent to the lumen). Intercalated ducts pass from the acini and open into striated ducts, which are well represented in the parotid gland.

The ultrastructural appearance of a serous acinus is illustrated in Fig. 16.8. The cells have a wedge-shaped outline surround the central lumen, with the basal surface being broader. The cell membranes show numerous microvilli and infoldings. The basal part of each serous cell is delineated from the surrounding connective tissue by a basal lamina. This region of the cell contains the nucleus and rough endoplasmic reticulum, and capillaries are seen in close proximity to this surface. The luminal part of the cell contains dense, round secretory granules. Many narrow canaliculi run between the cells and join the lumen. Both the canaliculi and the lumen are lined by short microvilli. Adjacent cell membranes contact at desmosomes, gap junctions and tight junctions.

Over 99% of saliva is water, which passes both across the cell membrane (transcellularly) and between adjacent cells (paracellularly) as a result of chloride secretion into the lumen. The proteinaceous components are packaged in granules for release into the luminal system by exocytosis at the luminal surface of the cells. For this reason, the cells are highly

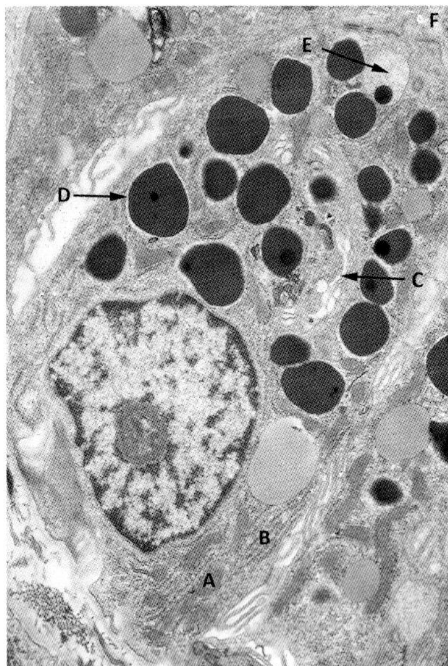

Fig. 16.9 TEM of parotid serous cell showing secretory pathway. A = mitochondria; B = rough endoplasmic reticulum; C = Golgi apparatus with small, irregularly shaped, nascent secretory granules of low electron density at the concave, trans part; D = mature secretory granules; E = secretory granule discharging by exocytosis into lumen; F = part of lumen (×6,000). Courtesy Dr. J D Harrison.

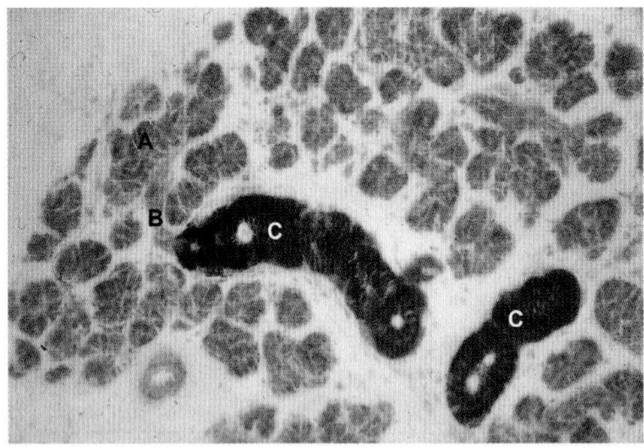

Fig. 16.10 Brown stain shows activity of the respiratory enzyme cytochrome oxidase in submandibular gland with moderate activity in serous acini (A) and intercalated ducts (B) and intense activity in striated ducts (C) (×130). Courtesy Dr. J D Harrison.

polarised. Like proteins in other cells, those in the serous cells of the parotid gland are assembled by the ribosomes of the rough endoplasmic reticulum and move into the cisternae of the rough endoplasmic reticulum and from there to the Golgi apparatus. At the trans face of the Golgi apparatus the proteins are glycosylated and packaged into small condensing vacuoles that are nascent secretory granules. They are initially of low electron density but increase in size and density as the protein is concentrated until they become mature secretory granules (Fig. 16.9). After this maturation period, the granules are discharged by exocytosis when required. Mitochondria within the cell supply the energy for the synthetic and secretory process, and associated moderate activity of respiratory enzymes can be demonstrated in the serous cells and in the submandibular gland (Fig. 16.10).

The appearance of serous cells will clearly vary with the levels of secretory activity. After the synthesis of secretory products, resting (unstimulated) serous cells will contain numerous secretory granules in the luminal parts of their cytoplasm (Fig. 16.11). With reflex stimulation of salivary flow during mastication at mealtimes, the number of granules will be severely depleted after being discharged into the lumen by exocytosis (Fig. 16.12).

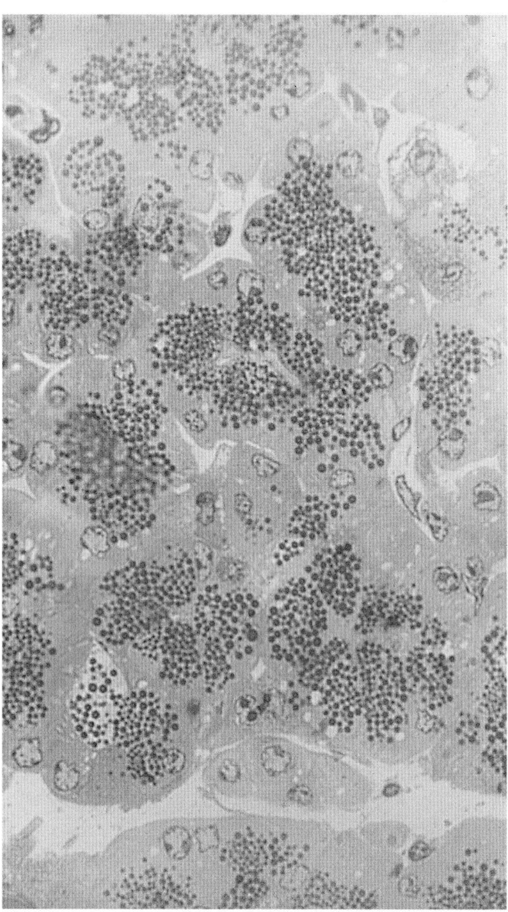

Fig. 16.11 After synthesis of secretory products, resting (unstimulated) serous cells contain numerous secretory granules (dark blue) in the distal parts of their cytoplasm (toluidine blue; ×600). Courtesy Mr. P F Heap.

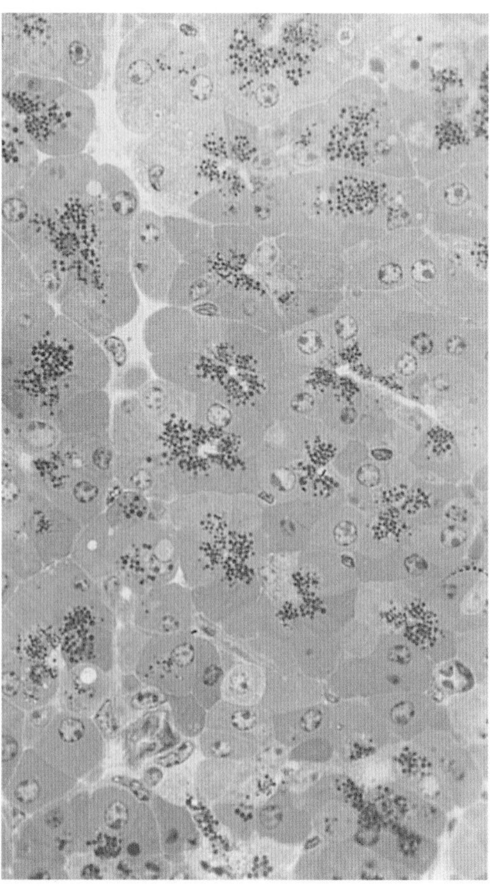

Fig. 16.12 Soon after stimulation, the secretory granules (dark blue) are depleted after being discharged into the lumen of the acini by exocytosis (compare with Fig. 16.11) (toluidine blue; ×600). Courtesy Mr. P F Heap.

Innervation of acini

Resting flows are present throughout the day and night, and this keeps the mouth and oropharynx moist, lubricated and protected. In human beings, however, large increases in secretion over short periods are seen during eating, and these increases are attributed, in varying degrees, to stimulation of several sensory receptors, including chemoreceptors involved in gustation and olfaction, mechanoreceptors and nociceptors.

Secretion from the major salivary glands is caused by the interaction of tastants with different receptors on taste buds mainly located on the dorsum of the tongue (see pages 310–311) and following activation of mechanoreceptors in the periodontal ligament (see pages 250–252) and mucosae. Secretion from minor salivary glands may also be increased in response to taste stimulation, but perhaps movement and tactile stimulation of the mucosa play a more important role in secretion from labial and palatine minor glands.

The control of salivation depends on reflex nerve impulses. These reflexes involve afferent limbs, salivary nuclei within the medulla oblongata and efferent limbs comprising both the sympathetic and parasympathetic secretomotor nerves supplying the various glands. Eating is the main cause of an increase of salivary flow above that of resting levels of flow. A variety of receptors are stimulated before, during and after the ingestion of food and drink; amongst these are gustatory, masticatory, olfactory, psychic, visual, thermoreceptive and possibly nociceptive. There are also several reflex responses in which salivary secretion occurs, which are not normally associated with eating (such as nausea, vomiting and pain).

Stimulation of gustatory receptors, mainly found in the taste buds, leads to the reflex secretion of saliva (gustatory-salivary reflex). All five basic tastes (salt, sour, sweet, bitter and umami) will cause a reflex salivary secretion. The volume and composition of saliva depend on the quality of the stimulus.

There is now considerable evidence that mastication causes a reflex salivary secretion (masticatory-salivary reflex). When chewing on one side of the mouth there is greater flow of saliva from the parotid gland on the same side than from the gland on the opposite non-chewing side. It appears that each gland seems to be most intimately associated with the receptors on its own side. It has been shown that the output of saliva from the parotid gland is directly proportional to the masticatory forces, and there is now substantial evidence that intraoral mechanoreceptors (and, in particular, periodontal ligament mechanoreceptors) contribute to this reflex.

It has been assumed that the smell of food causes salivation in human beings (olfactory-salivary reflex). This reflex involves the submandibular and sublingual glands and not the parotid glands. There is no convincing evidence that a non-conditioned salivary reflex exists in response to the sight or thought of food.

Both parasympathetic and sympathetic fibres innervate the acini and act collaboratively in the production of saliva during feeding. The main neurotransmitter for parasympathetic nerves is acetylcholine and that for sympathetic nerves is noradrenaline (norepinephrine). In addition to these substances, each axon contains arrays of neuropeptides (such as vasoactive intestinal polypeptide, substance P and calcitonin gene–related peptide). These neuropeptides are not necessarily uniform for each type of nerve, nor are all present within every nerve of the same type. Embryologically, the transmitters are likely to influence the genetic expression of the glandular cells and, conversely, the cell types are likely to influence the neuropeptides in the axons innervating them. Some neuroeffector sites occur beneath the basal lamina in direct contact with the plasma membrane (hypolemmal), whereas others remain outside the basal lamina (epilemmal) (Figs. 16.13–16.15). Neuroeffector sites of either type probably affect the cell if transmitter vesicles are present. In electron micrographs, the conventional neurotransmitters are contained in small vesicles, while the neuropeptides are contained in larger, dense-cored vesicles (Fig. 16.16). Parasympathetic drive causes formation and secretion of secretory granules and fluid by the secretory units; sympathetic drive usually increases the output of preformed components from the cells. Both pathways cause contraction of the myoepithelial cells, which helps direct fluid from the acinar lumen out along the duct system.

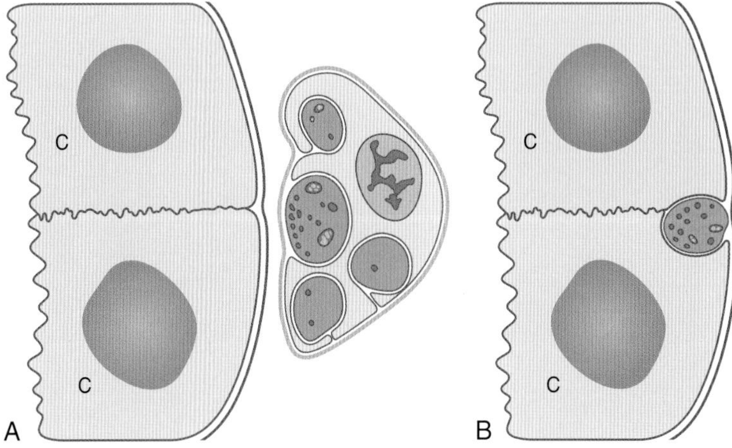

Fig. 16.13 Neuroeffector relationships in salivary glands. A = epilemmal; B = hypolemmal; C = parenchymal cells. Courtesy Prof. J R Garrett and Karger Press.

Salivary gland acinar cells make up a salt-secreting epithelium (i.e., sodium and chloride, bicarbonate and other less abundant anions are transported into acinar lumina). This process forms the basis of salivary secretion, as the generation of an environment in lumina that is hypertonic with respect to the adjacent blood capillaries and interstitial fluid enables the movement of water into lumina. Fig. 16.17 summarises the key events in this process. Anion channels in the apical acinar cell membrane, which are permeable to chloride and bicarbonate, are opened when acinar cells receive signals from autonomic nerves (principally acetylcholine from parasympathetic nerves). The electrochemical gradient created by chloride leads to sodium movement into the acinar lumen, and the osmotic gradient thus created leads to the movement of water into the lumen. The latter may occur by a transcellular route through aquaporin water channels. The isotonic saliva generated in the acinar lumen is rendered hypotonic by the removal of sodium, chloride and bicarbonate as it passes through striated ducts, which are impermeable to water.

Duct system

The smallest (and most distal) of the ducts is the intercalated duct. This leads from the serous acini into the striated duct and is usually compressed between the acini (Figs. 16.3, 16.7 and 16.18). It is lined by cuboidal epithelial cells. The nuclei in the duct cells appear prominent, owing to the relatively scanty cytoplasm. At the ultrastructural level, intercalated ducts are seen to consist of a simple cuboidal epithelial tube. Both luminal and basal surfaces of the duct cells are smooth, and desmosomes unite adjacent cells (Fig. 16.19). The cells sometimes contain apical secretory granules, and there are only small amounts of the organelles normally associated with protein synthesis. However, the intercalated ducts appear

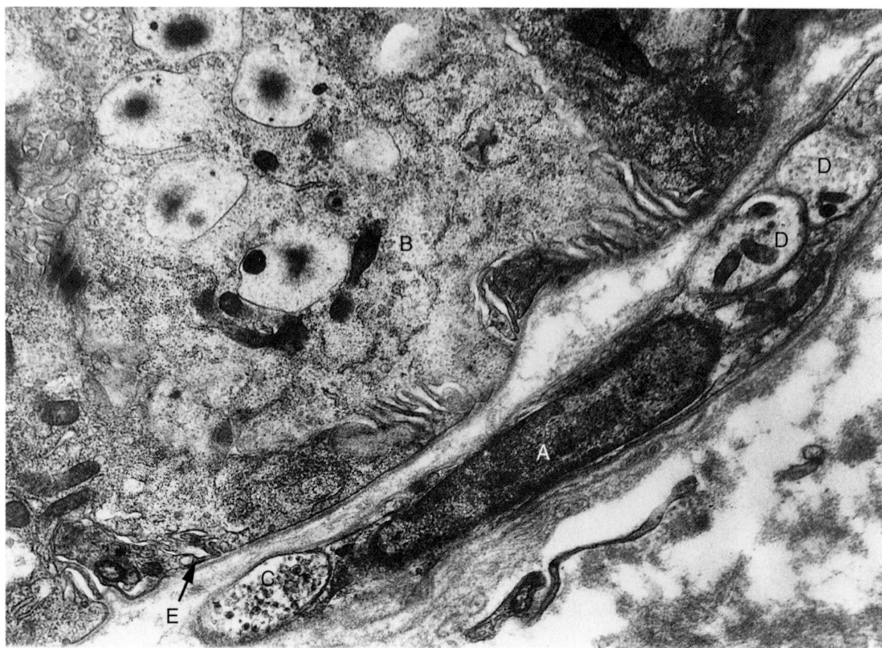

Fig. 16.14 TEM showing the Schwann cell nucleus (A) of an epilemmal nerve fibre in association with a parotid acinar cell (B). C = adrenergic axon; D = two cholinergic axons; E = basal lamina of acinus. Note the small translucent vesicles and the dense-cored vesicles (with neuropeptides) in the axons (×14,000). Courtesy Prof. J R Garrett and the editor of the *Archives of Oral Biology*.

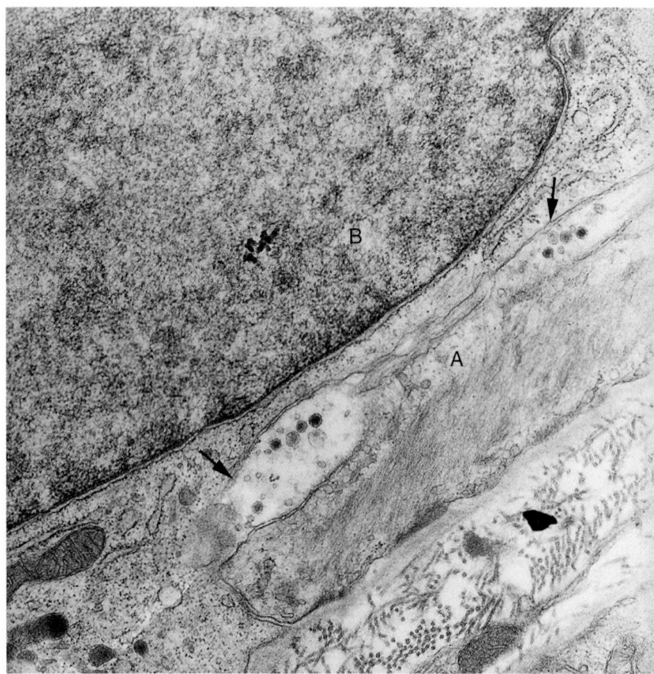

Fig. 16.15 TEM of submandibular gland showing hypolemmal axons (arrowed) containing many large dense-cored vesicles and lying between a myoepithelial cell (A) and a central acinar cell (B) (×15,000). Courtesy Prof. J R Garrett and the editor of *Microscopy Research and Technique*.

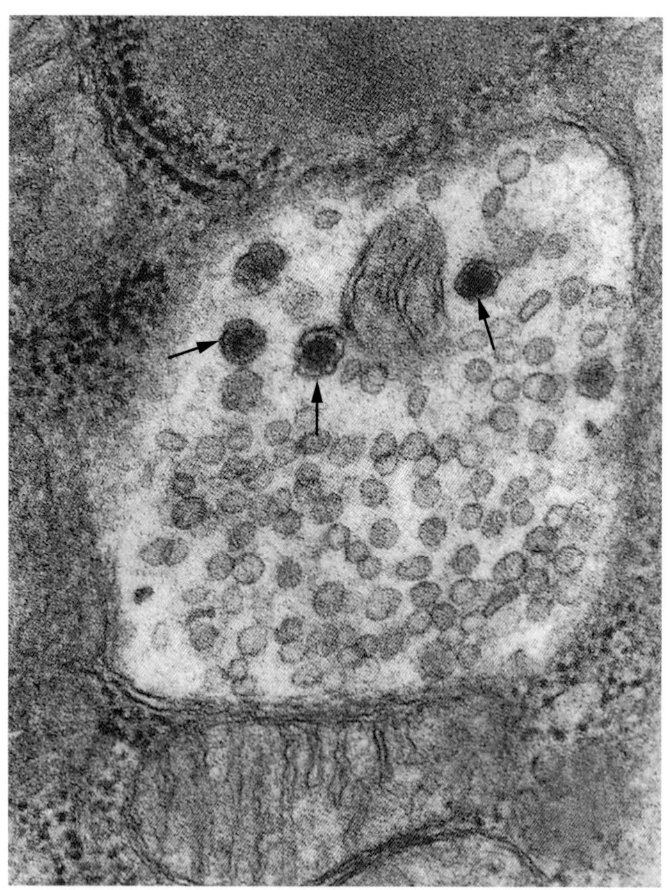

Fig. 16.16 TEM of neuroeffector part of a hypolemmal parasympathetic axon showing small agranular vesicles that contained acetylcholine and larger, dense-cored, granular vesicles (arrow) that contained neuropeptides (×60,000). Courtesy Prof. J R Garrett and the editor of *Microscopy Research and Technique*.

to contribute to the primary secretion. There is moderate activity of respiratory enzymes in the intercalated ducts, as in the acini and also the submandibular gland (Fig. 16.10). Several acini drain into each intercalated duct. In the parotid gland, intercalated ducts are characteristically long, narrow and branching.

The striated ducts are intralobular and form a much longer and more active component of the duct system than the intercalated ducts. The cell of a striated duct has a large amount of cytoplasm and a large, spherical, centrally positioned nucleus that makes the cell easy to identify. (Figs. 16.7, 16.18). The cells of the striated duct are highly polarised. Their luminal surfaces have short microvilli. The duct's basal (abluminal) surface, adjacent to the basal lamina separating it from the adjacent connective tissue, shows numerous striations under the light microscope. Ultrastructurally, the striations correspond to multiple infoldings of the plasma membrane at the bases of the cells (Fig. 16.20). Vertically aligned mitochondria are packed between the infoldings. Adjacent cells are intertwined in a complex pattern and anchored together by

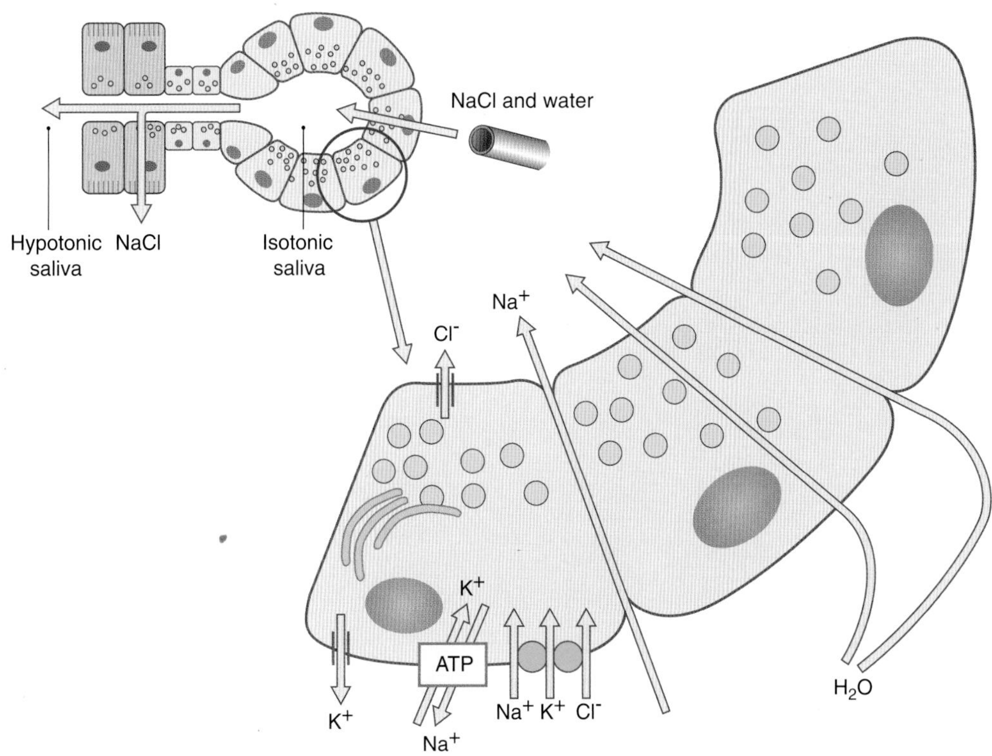

Fig. 16.17 Salivary fluid secretion by acinar cells and the resorption of salt in striated duct cells. See text for description. Courtesy Prof. G B Proctor.

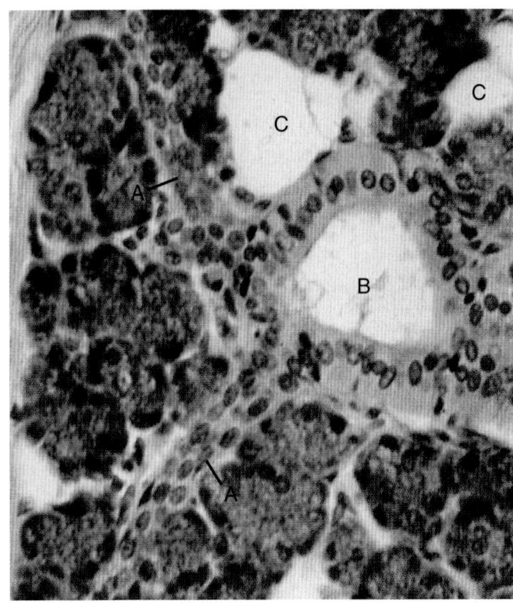

Fig. 16.18 Parotid gland showing intercalated ducts (A) leading from serous acini and into the striated duct (B). C = fat cell. Note the cuboidal epithelial cells lining the intercalated ducts have prominent nuclei due to their scanty cytoplasm. The nuclei in the striated ducts are more centrally positioned within the cells (H & E; ×360). Courtesy Dr E H Batten.

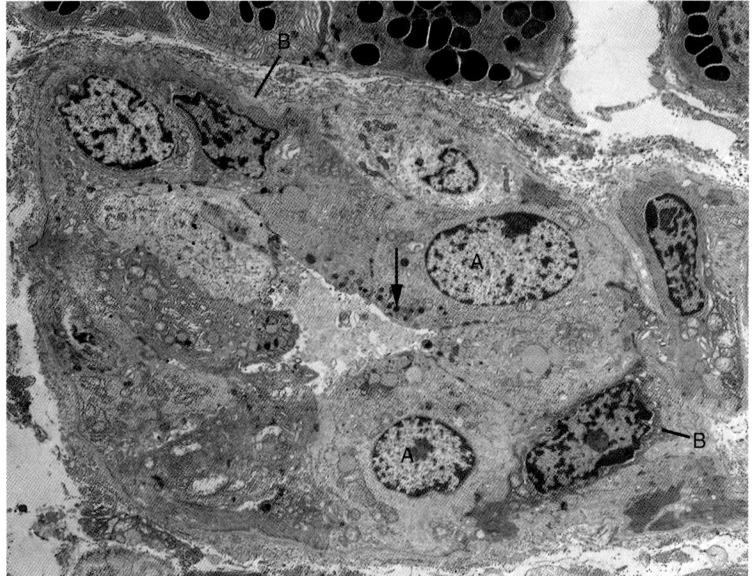

Fig. 16.19 TEM of an intercalated duct. The cuboidal lining cells of the duct (A) possess only small amounts of the intracellular organelles associated with protein synthesis. Some secretory granules are evident (arrow). The cells are united by desmosomes, and both the luminal and abluminal surfaces are smooth. Myoepithelial cells are present (B) (×2,520). Courtesy Dr. J D Harrison.

desmosomes. This large surface area, supplied with high levels of energy from the mitochondria, is clearly involved in active transport. The striated ducts are the site of electrolyte resorption (especially of sodium and chloride) and secretion (potassium and bicarbonate) without loss of water. As this resorption is against a concentration gradient, it requires substantial amounts of energy. The effect on the material in the lumen is to convert an isotonic or slightly hypertonic fluid (with concentrations similar to those in the plasma) into a hypotonic fluid. There is therefore intense activity of respiratory enzymes in the striated ducts in order to effect and maintain these concentration gradients and the hypotonicity of the fluid in the lumen, as in the submandibular gland (Fig. 16.10). The cells of the striated duct exhibit small secretory granules in the luminal region that may contain epidermal growth factor, lysozyme, kallikrein and secretory IgA. The granules are less abundant in humans than in many other species and less abundant in the parotid than in the submandibular gland.

The luminal cells of the intercalated, striated and collecting ducts contain the low-molecular-weight cytokeratin intermediate filaments 7, 8, 18 and 19 (Fig. 16.21).

The striated duct leads into the collecting duct (Fig. 16.22). Whereas the intercalated and striated ducts modify the composition of the saliva (as

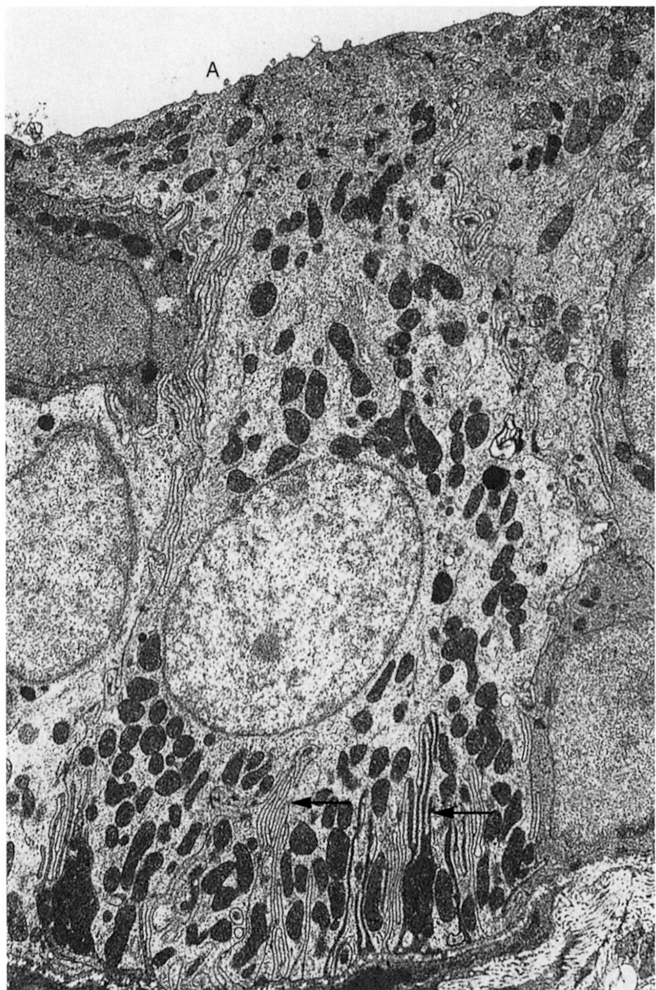

Fig. 16.20 TEM of striated duct cells. The nucleus is centrally positioned within the cell because of the large amount of cytoplasmic material. Adjacent cell membranes are intertwined in a complex pattern and united by numerous desmosomes. Note the multiple infoldings of the plasma membrane at the base of the cell (arrowed), between which are packed numerous mitochondria. A = luminal surface of duct (×12,000). Courtesy Mr. P F Heap.

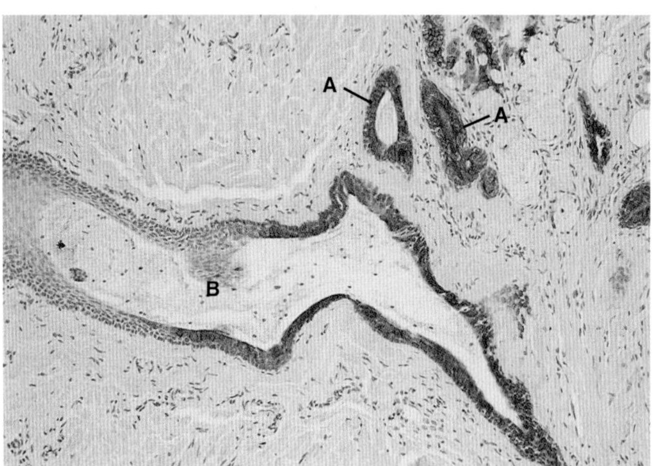

Fig. 16.21 Collecting ducts staining positive (brown) for cytokeratin 8 and 18 using immunohistochemical techniques (A), typical of the type of cytokeratin intermediate filaments associated with simple ducts. The positive stain is lost as the duct becomes stratified near the surface (B) (×80). Courtesy Dr. A W Barrett.

well as transport it) and may be termed *secretory ducts*, the main function of the collecting ducts is to transport it. In addition to the columnar layer (which now lacks striations), the collecting duct situated in the interlobular region may have a layer of basal cells. As it enlarges, the main parotid duct appears like many excretory passages and contains two layers: the mucosa and the outer connective tissue adventitia. Near its termination, the lining of the main duct becomes stratified as it merges with the stratified squamous epithelium of the surface oral epithelium. When stratified, the duct epithelium contains keratin intermediate filament types typical of stratified epithelium in the oral mucosa (see Table 14.1).

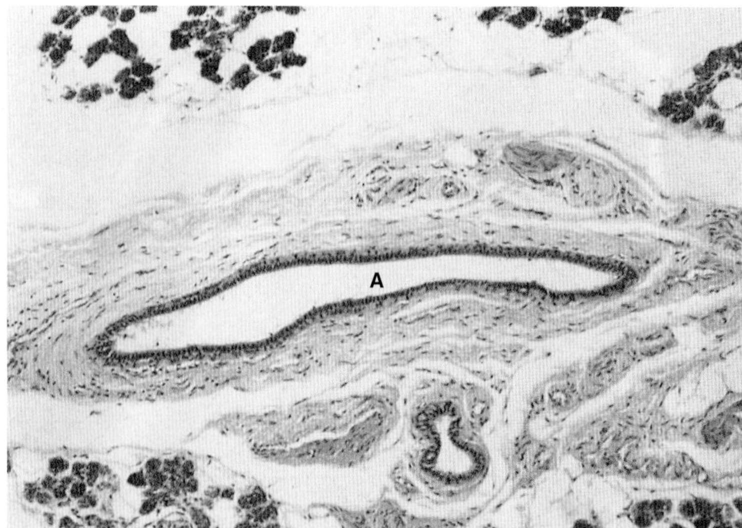

Fig. 16.22 A collecting duct (A) in the parotid gland. As illustrated here, the duct may have two layers of cells (H & E; ×60).

Unlike the tight junctions of acinar cells that allow the movement of some ions, water and small molecules (and may therefore be considered to be 'leaky' tight junctions), in the ductal system of salivary glands, the ductal epithelial cells are similarly polarised, but in this case the tight junctions are watertight, indicative of a greater number of tight junctional contacts between cells.

Because of its buffering capacity, salivary bicarbonate plays an important role in preventing dissolution of tooth mineral in the presence of acid. Although acinar cells secrete bicarbonate, ductal cells also play a major role in secretion of bicarbonate into saliva. As the bicarbonate concentration of stimulated saliva is many times higher than that of unstimulated saliva, ductal bicarbonate secretion is probably stimulated by autonomic nerves.

Myoepithelial cells

Myoepithelial cells lie between the basal lamina and the basal membrane of the acinar secretory cells and the intercalated duct cells. Myoepithelial cells around acini are dendritic cells. A myoepithelial cell has a stellate-shaped body containing the nucleus and some tapering processes radiating from it. A different arrangement exists around the intercalated ducts, where the myoepithelial cells are elongated, run longitudinally along the duct and have a few short processes. Around the acini, the processes lie in gutters on the surface of the secretory cells, so the outline of the acinus remains smooth; around the intercalated ducts, the cells lie more superficially and produce a bulge in the outline of the duct. Although salivary myoepithelial cells in some species stain positively for alkaline phosphatase, those in humans do not. Myoepithelial cells contain cytokeratin 17. Myoepithelial cells contract as a result of activity of both parasympathetic and sympathetic stimulation, supporting the view that the two autonomic divisions act in concert, not in conflict.

Ultrastructurally, the nucleus of a myoepithelial cell seems flattened and intracellular organelles associated with protein synthesis are not particularly abundant. However, the cell contains numerous contractile actin

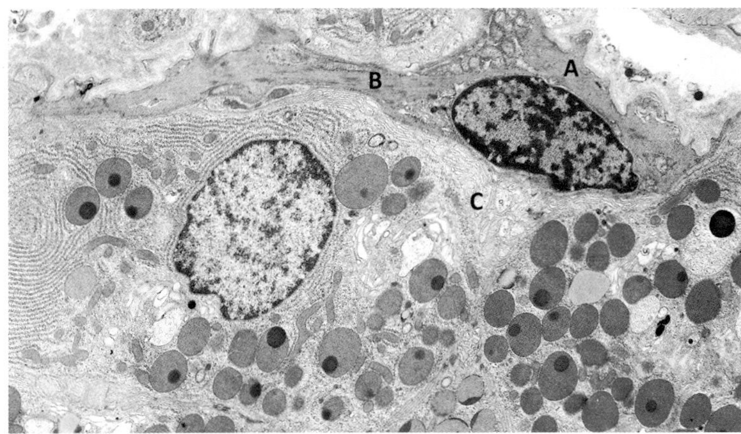

Fig. 16.23 TEM of part of acinus of submandibular gland showing a myoepithelial cell (A) with a dendritic process in which bundles of contractile myofilaments are seen (B). C = serous cell. The myoepithelial cell embraces the underlying serous cells, in which variation in the appearance and density of secretory granules is seen (× 4,700). Courtesy Dr. J D Harrison.

microfilaments about 7 nm in diameter (Figs. 16.15 and 16.23). Myoepithelial cells have desmosomal attachments with underlying parenchymal cells, gap junctions with adjacent myoepithelial cells and hemidesmosomal attachments with the basal lamina, the last suggesting that some of their activity is transmitted via the basal lamina. Myoepithelial cells (and the basal cells of double-layered ducts) also contain cytokeratin intermediate filaments (Figs. 16.24 and 16.25) and contractile actin filaments (Figs. 16.24 and 16.26), which can be used to help identify them using immunocytochemistry. The presence of cytokeratin confirms the epithelial origin of the myoepithelial cell. Pinocytotic vesicles and dense attachment areas are associated with that part of the plasma membrane of the myoepithelial cell covered by the basal lamina. At the cell membranes where myoepithelial cells contact serous acinar cells, CD44 is expressed in both cell types. As CD44 in other tissues is involved in many basic processes associated with cell proliferation and differentiation, it may play a similar role in salivary glands in both the normal and neoplastic state. Box 16.2 indicates what myoepithelial activity can produce.

Other possible functions include assistance for some parenchymal cells to expel their contents and a milking effect on any underlying extracellular fluid, assisting passage via parenchymal tight junctions.

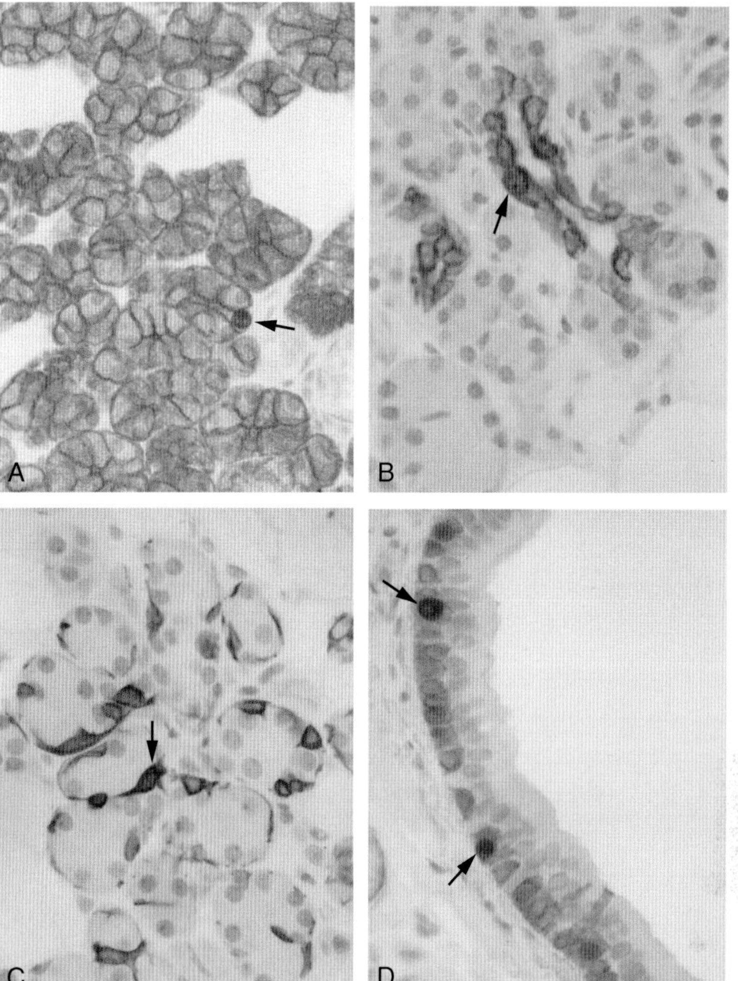

Fig. 16.24 Immunohistochemical double staining of parenchymal cells showing evidence of proliferation in normal parotid gland. Positive reaction of nuclei (red staining, indicated by arrows) for the cell proliferation marker Ki67 is seen (A) in acinar cells, the cytoplasm of which has been stained brown using an antibody to cytokeratin 18; (B) in an intercalated duct cell, the cytoplasm of which has been stained brown using an antibody to cytokeratin 7; (C) in a myoepithelial cell, the cytoplasm of which has been stained brown using an antibody to α-actin; (D) in basal cells of a collecting duct, the cytoplasm of which has been stained brown using an antibody to cytokeratin 14 (all ×300). Courtesy Prof. S Ihrler.

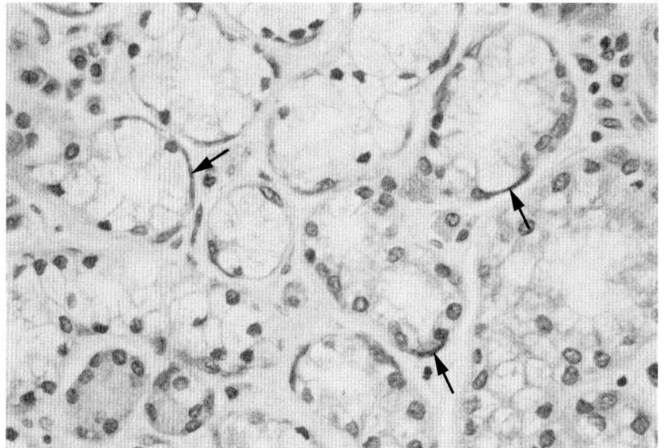

Fig. 16.25 Myoepithelial cells staining positively (brown) for the antibody to cytokeratin 14 using immunohistochemical techniques (arrows) (×240). Courtesy Dr. A W Barrett.

Basal cells

A population of basal cells is present in the striated and collecting ducts. They are sparsely distributed in the striated ducts and more densely distributed in the collecting ducts, in which they form a continuous layer as the ducts pass farther towards the hilum (Fig. 16.24D). These cells can be distinguished from other parenchymal cells by a combination of their morphology, their co-expression of cytokeratin 14, and the anti-apoptotic factor Bcl-2, and by a proliferative index of about 3% that is the highest of any cell in the region. Basal cells have been implicated as potential stem cells during turnover and/or cell regeneration in salivary glands and during metaplasia when oncocytes and sebaceous cells may appear. However, some cell division is seen in all parenchymal cell types, including myoepithelial cells (Fig. 16.24C), and all these cells may be involved in salivary gland regeneration.

Lymph nodes

Lymph nodes are situated both on the surface and within the parotid gland (Fig. 16.6) but are not found within the other salivary glands.

Submandibular gland

The second largest of the salivary glands, the submandibular gland, produces a mixed mucous/serous secretion. The overall mean of the

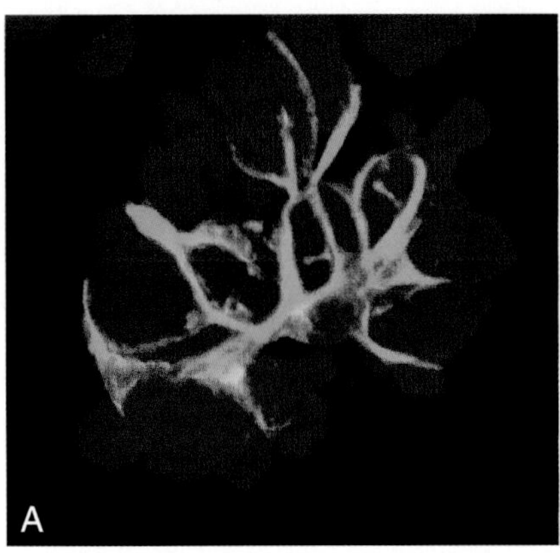

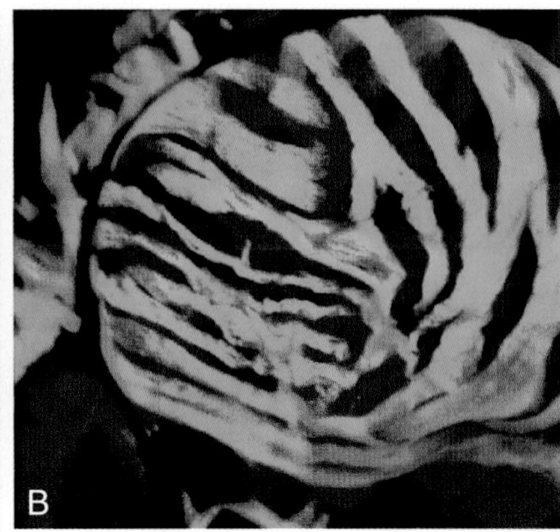

Fig. 16.26 Myoepithelial cells and their numerous dendritic processes staining positively (green) for antibody to F-actin (bodipy-phallacidin) around secretory acini (stained red with ethidium homodimer 1). (A) Submandibular gland. (B) Sublingual gland (×1,000). Courtesy Dr. Y Satoh.

Box 16.2 **Myoepithelial activity within salivary glands**

Myoepithelial activity can:

- Support the underlying parenchyma and reduce back-permeation of fluid
- Accelerate the initial outflow of saliva
- Reduce luminal volume
- Contribute to the secretory pressure
- Help salivary flow to overcome increases in peripheral resistance – but if this is excessive it may lead to sialectatic damage of striated ducts, thereby increasing overall permeability

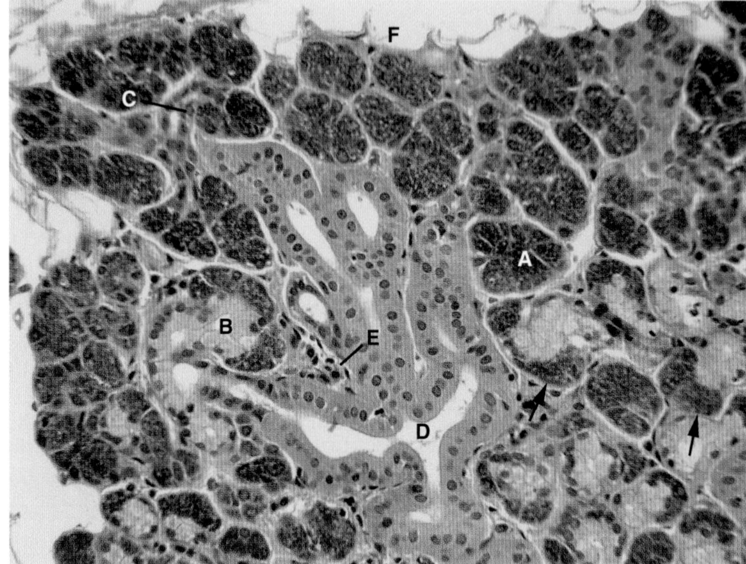

Fig. 16.27 Submandibular gland showing darker serous (A) and lighter mucous (B) acini. Crescent-shaped collections of serous cells form serous demilunes (arrows) (but see text). C = intercalated duct; D = striated duct; E = plasma cells; F = fat cells (H & E; ×245). Courtesy Dr. J D Harrison.

proportional volume of mucous cells is 8% of the total acinar volume, although it varies between 1% and 33%. The gland has a well-formed connective tissue capsule. The serous cells, duct system, myoepithelial cells and basal cells as described for the parotid gland also apply to the submandibular gland. The intercalated ducts are shorter, and the striated ducts are longer and more conspicuous.

Mucous cells

In routine microscopy, the collections of mucous acini within the submandibular gland are readily distinguished in the resting gland from the darker-staining and granular serous acini because the mucous acini are paler as their mucin content does not readily take up routine stains. In addition, their nuclei tend to be compressed into the basal parts of the cells. Small, crescent-shaped collections of serous cells may be found in routine sections at the most distal ends of the mucous acini; these are referred to as *serous demilunes* (Figs. 16.27, 16.28).

The traditional and widely held view relating to the disposition of serous demilunes and the ultrastructural morphology of the mucous cells has been challenged: it has been shown to be the result of an artefact of preparation. Using methods of rapid freezing and freeze substitution to obtain minimal distortion and dimensional changes during fixation, it has now been demonstrated that all the serous cells align with mucous cells to surround a common lumen, leaving no demilune structure (Fig. 16.29), whereas samples fixed by conventional methods result in distended mucous cells that displace the serous cells towards the basal portion of the acinus to form the demilune structure (Fig. 16.30). This has been confirmed using three-dimensional reconstruction techniques (Fig. 16.31).

The mucous cell can be readily distinguished from the serous cell at the ultrastructural level. In the early stages of synthesis of its secretory

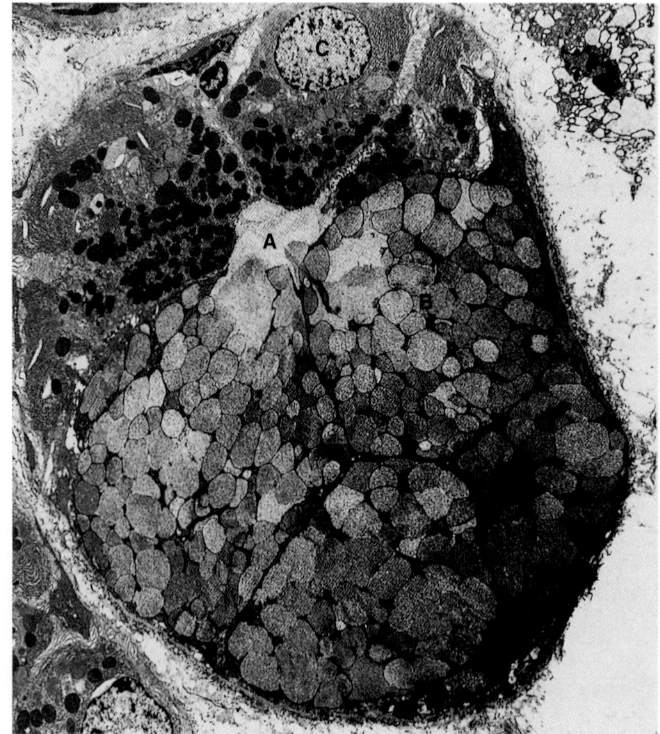

Fig. 16.28 TEM of the submandibular gland showing serous cells (C) forming a serous demilune capping mucous cells in which the secretory granules are packed together and of irregular size (B). A = lumen (×1,600). Courtesy Dr. J D Harrison.

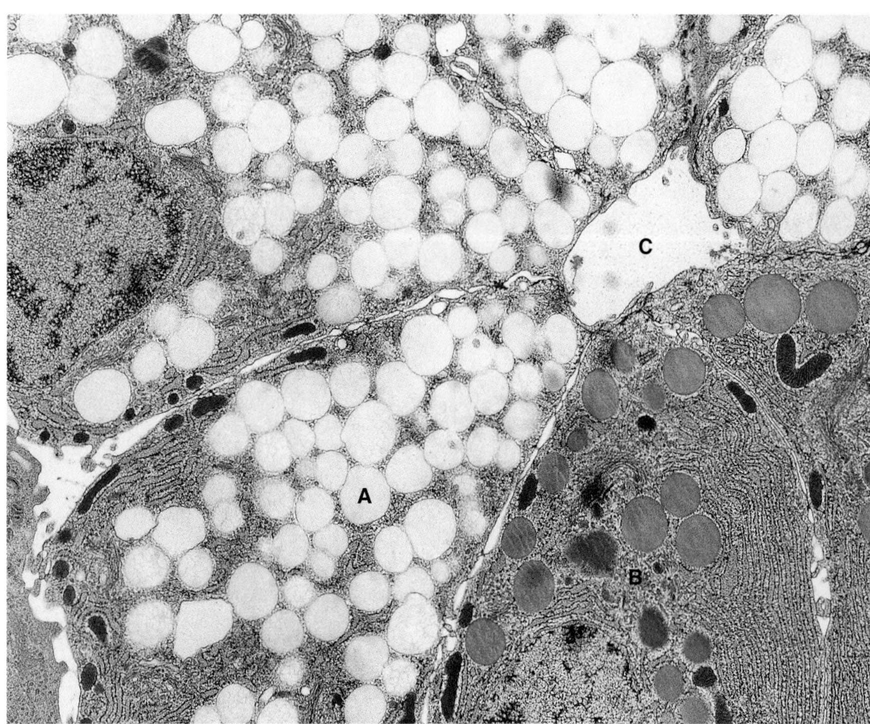

Fig. 16.29 TEM of the terminal portion of a mixed gland prepared by rapid freezing and freeze-substitution method. In the mucous cell (A) all secretory granules are round and discrete. The serous cell (B) is aligned to surround the common lumen (C), and no serous demilune could be detected (×10,000). Courtesy Dr. S Yamashina and the editor of *Archives of Histology and Cytology*.

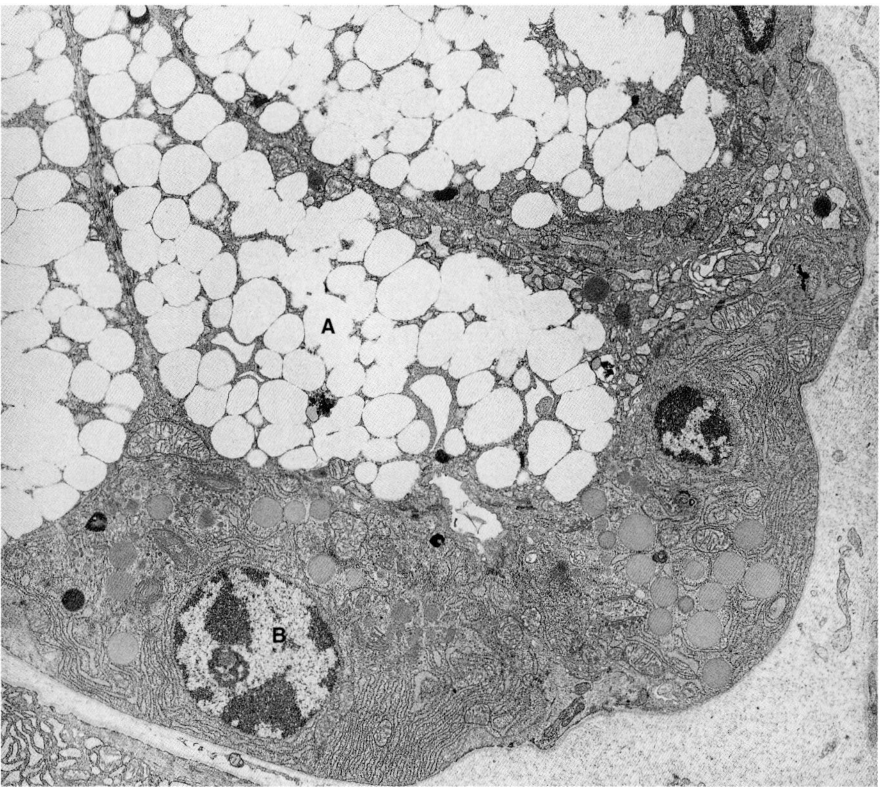

Fig. 16.30 TEM of the terminal portion of a mixed gland prepared by conventional immersion fixation in glutaraldehyde. Secretory granules of mucous cells (A) are enlarged, and some have coalesced because of the disruption of limiting membranes. Serous cells (B) are compressed by the distended mucous cells towards the peripheral portion of the acinus, forming the demilune structure (×5,500). Courtesy Dr. S Yamashina and the editor of *Archives of Histology and Cytology*.

products, large amounts of rough endoplasmic reticulum and a Golgi apparatus (conspicuous because of the amount of carbohydrate that is added to the secretory protein) are present in mucous cells, together with a few secretory granules. At a later phase of their secretory cycle, the mucous cells exhibit numerous secretory granules that are readily distinguished from those of serous cells by their pale appearance (Fig. 16.29). The cell membranes shows fewer microvilli and infoldings than those of serous cells. The nuclei of mucous cells are round and centrally located when the methods to obtain minimal distortion are used. In conventional fixation there is distension of the mucous secretory granules,

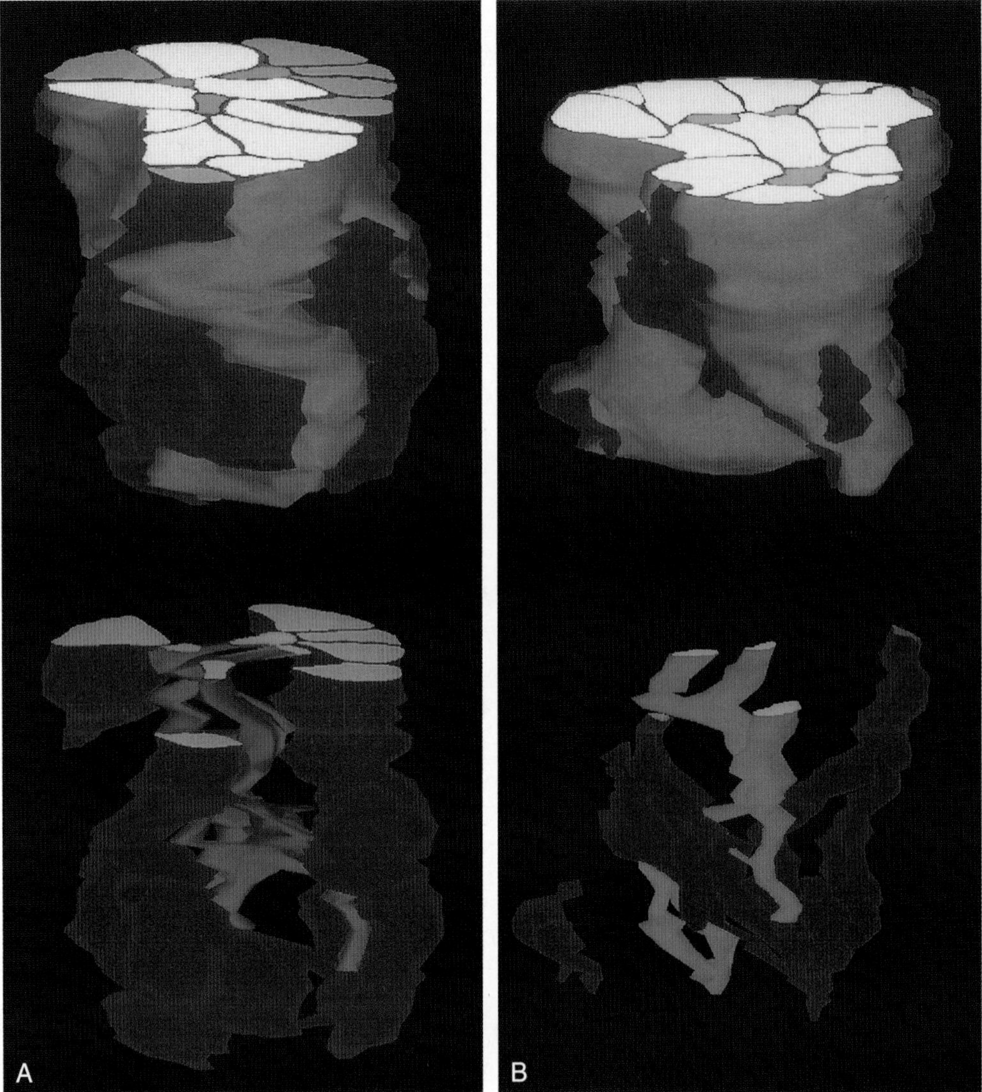

Fig. 16.31 Computer reconstruction of a terminal portion of the submandibular gland showing mucous (purple) and serous (red) cells and luminal space (green). (A) In the upper diagram, following rapid freezing, a surface view indicates that the terminal portion consists of mucous and serous cells distributed not only at the most fundal portion of the acinus but also in the portion nearest the duct. In the lower diagram, the mucous cells have been deleted from the reconstruction to show more clearly the relation of the serous cells to the luminal space. All serous cells prepared by the rapid freezing method are found to have a direct connection with the luminal space. (B) In the upper diagram, following conventional immersion fixation, the acinus illustrated is found to be branched, and serous cells appear attached to the outer wall of the acinus formed by mucous cells. In the lower diagram, the mucous cells have been deleted from the reconstruction to show more clearly the relation of the serous cells to the luminal space. The serous cells are found to be disconnected from the luminal space, giving a floating appearance. Courtesy Dr. S Yamashina and the editor of *Archives of Histology and Cytology*.

which show discontinuous limiting membranes and coalesce to form irregularly shaped secretory granules, and the nuclei are flattened and displaced into the basal parts of the cells (Figs. 16.28 and 16.32).

As for the serous cells, the granules discharge into the lumen by exocytosis. The depletion in granule content of mucous cells in recently stimulated and unstimulated cells is illustrated ultrastucturally in Figs. 16.33 and 16.34. Clearly, the nuclei will be less compressed against the basal surfaces of the cells following discharge of the mucous granules.

Salivary glycoproteins and calcium

The salivary glands contain a mixture of salivary glycoproteins that range from neutral to acidic. This is easily demonstrated by first staining with Alcian blue at pH 2.5, which stains any acidic groups present in the glycoproteins (e.g., carboxyl or sulphate groups), and then with periodic-acid–Schiff, which stains the glycol groups present in all glycoproteins. This technique has shown that:

1) Serous cells in the parotid gland contain neutral glycoproteins
2) Mucous cells in the submandibular, sublingual and minor salivary glands contain mainly acidic glycoproteins
3) Serous cells in the submandibular gland contain a mixture of neutral and acidic glycoproteins
4) Intercalated duct cells often contain glycoproteins that are a mixture of both neutral and acidic forms
5) Striated duct cells often contain neutral glycoproteins (Fig. 16.35)

Thus, although the division of salivary acinar cells into serous and mucous types in routine sections stained with haematoxylin and eosin is clear-cut, histochemical methods do not contribute further to the ease of identification. This is because serous cells can synthesise carbohydrates that are histochemically similar to those of mucous cells. This is reflected in the considerable variation seen among the secretory granules in serous acini (Figs. 16.23, 16.36).

Calcium is incorporated into the secretory granule during its formation in order for the negatively charged parts of the glycoprotein (which would normally repel each other) to be neutralised by the positive charge on the calcium. This allows the molecule to condense in the nascent secretory granule. The more acidic the glycoprotein, the more calcium is needed. Thus, the secretory granules of the mucous acini and the serous acini of

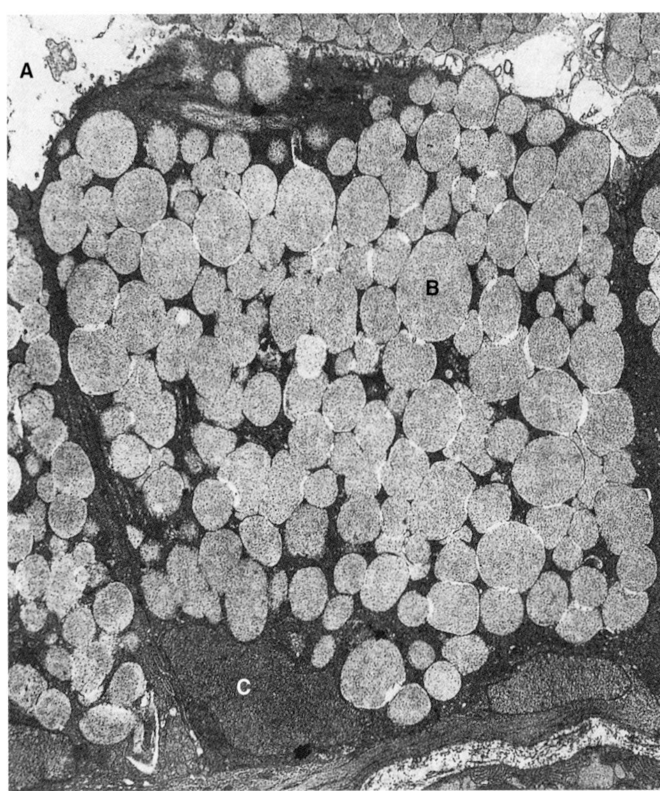

Fig. 16.32 TEM of mucous cell using conventional immersion fixation leading to swelling of the secretory granules. The cell illustrated is in a late secretory phase with numerous granules (B) of irregular size (owing to coalescence by the disruption of limiting membranes) occupying most of the cell and compressing the organelles and nucleus (C) to the periphery. The granules will discharge into the lumen (A) by exocytosis (×5,000). Courtesy Mr. P F Heap.

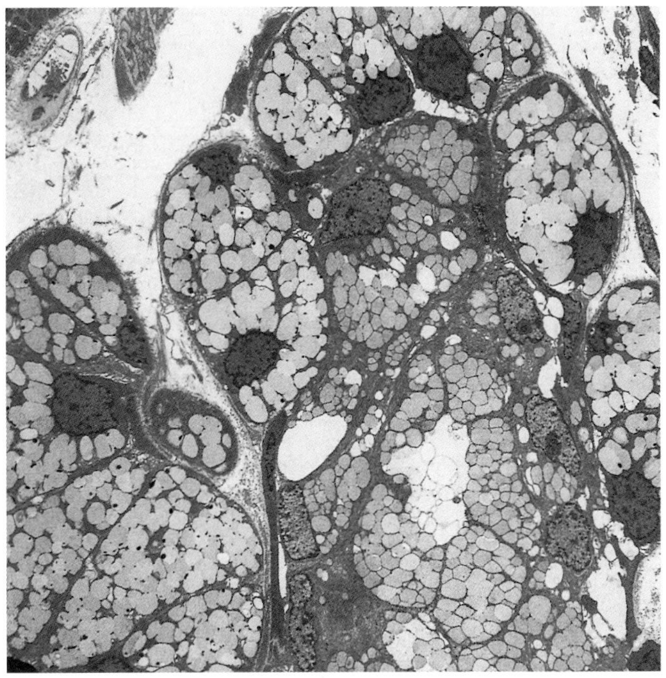

Fig. 16.33 Unstimulated mucous cells filled with secretory granules; consequently their nuclei are compressed into the basal parts of the cells (conventional immersion fixation; TEM; ×1,000).

the submandibular gland contain more calcium (Fig. 16.37) than those of the serous acini in the parotid gland, while the secretory granules of the striated ducts contain no demonstrable calcium. The calcium in the secretory granules, when released, may precipitate on exposed phospholipids of damaged membranes to form sialomicroliths (see page 351).

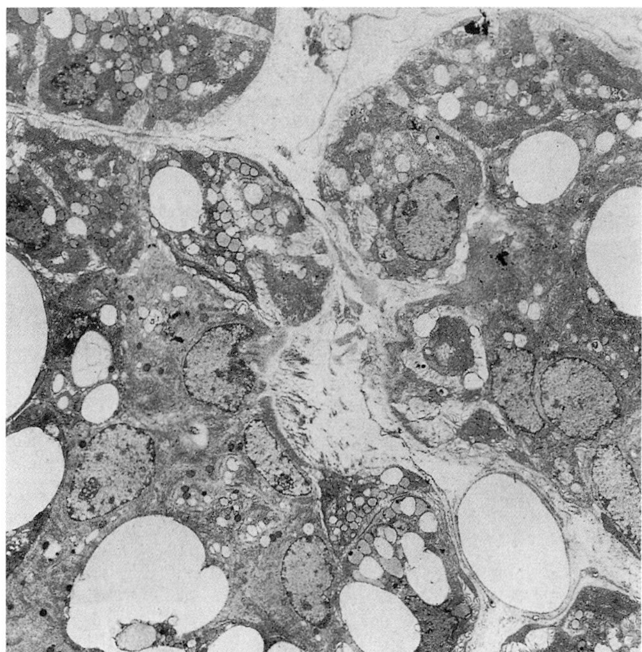

Fig. 16.34 TEM of mucous cells in a recently stimulated submandibular gland. The mucous cells have lost their secretory granules and consequently their nuclei are more prominent (×1,000).

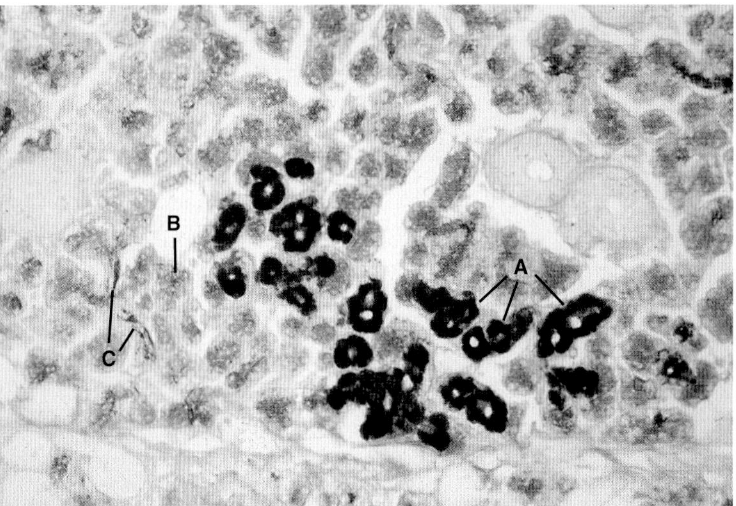

Fig. 16.35 Submandibular gland showing diffuse royal blue staining of acid glycoprotein in mucous cells (A) and discretely stained secretory granules in serous cells (B) and intercalated duct cells (C) that variously contain neutral glycoprotein stained red and acidic glycoprotein stained royal blue (Alcian blue at pH2.5 followed by periodic-acid–Schiff; ×190). Courtesy Dr. J D Harrison.

Sublingual gland

The human sublingual gland is not a single unit like the parotid and submandibular glands, but is made up of a posterior part (the greater sublingual gland) that is not always present and an anterior part (the lesser sublingual gland) that consists of 7–15 small salivary glands, each having its own duct system emptying into the sublingual fold.

The sublingual gland was conventionally considered to be a mixed gland with a preponderance of mucous elements. With routine staining at the light microscope level, it is seen to consist of many groups of pale-staining mucous cells with darker-staining so-called serous acini and demilunes (Fig. 16.38). However, recent research has shown that the so-called serous cells in this gland are immature mucous cells. The histological structure of the greater and lesser sublingual glands is identical to that of the mucous minor salivary glands.

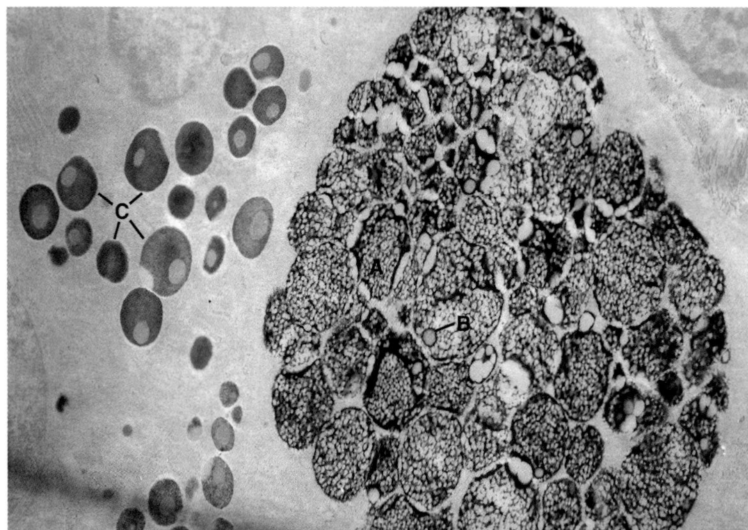

Fig. 16.36 TEM of mucous cell packed with secretory granules (A) that contain stained glycoprotein and small unstained spherules that contain protein (B). An adjacent serous cell shows scattered secretory granules (C) composed of stained glycoprotein and unstained spherules of protein (phosphotungstic acid stain; ×6,130). Courtesy Dr. J D Harrison.

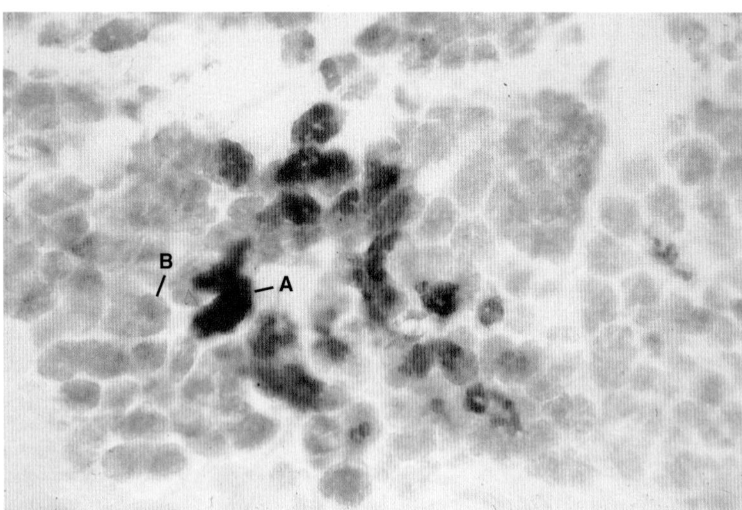

Fig. 16.37 Submandibular gland showing strong staining for calcium (orange) in mucous cells (A) and moderate to weak staining in serous cells (B) (Schäfer's modified GBHA technique; ×190). Courtesy Dr. J D Harrison.

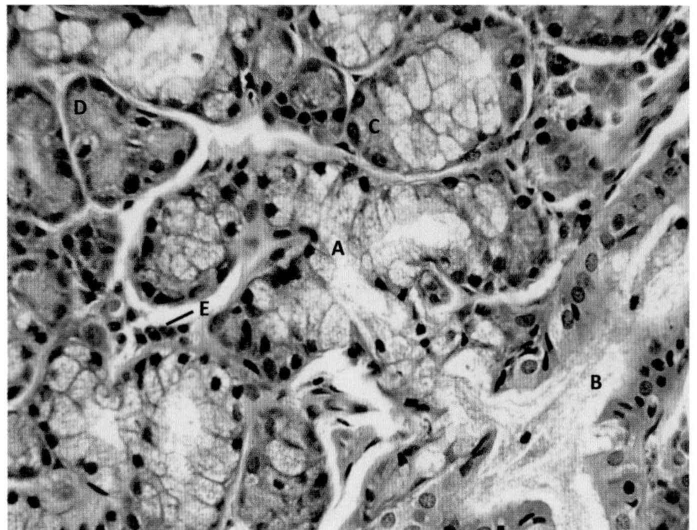

Fig. 16.38 Pale-staining mucous acini (A) of sublingual gland draining into a collecting duct (B). The appearance of serous demilunes (C) and acini (D) is caused by the scarcity of secretory granules in mucous cells at the beginning of the secretory cycle, although parts of these cells show pale areas as secretory granules accumulate. Plasma cells are seen interstitially (E) (H & E; ×350). Courtesy Dr. J D Harrison.

Table 16.1 Comparison of the three major salivary glands

Parotid gland	Submandibular gland	Sublingual gland
Largest	Intermediate	Smallest
Serous	Mixed, mainly serous	Mucous
Intercalated ducts	Intercalated ducts	Few intercalated ducts
Striated ducts present	Striated ducts present	No striated ducts
Collecting ducts end in single main duct	Collecting ducts end in single main duct	Collecting ducts end in many main ducts
Non-spontaneous secretor	Non-spontaneous secretor	Spontaneous secretor
Saliva hypotonic	Saliva hypotonic	Saliva isotonic

Duct system

The duct system is much less well developed than in the other major salivary glands, and striated ducts are usually absent. The acini sometimes lead to intercalated ducts, but these may be absent and the acini lead to collecting ducts, which lack the basal striations that characterise striated ducts. The sublingual saliva is therefore rich in sodium. The greater sublingual gland drains into a main duct, and the individual glands of the lesser sublingual gland drain independently through many smaller main ducts that open directly through the overlying oral mucosa. A comparison of the three major salivary glands is shown in Table 16.1.

Minor salivary glands

The minor salivary glands are classified by their anatomical location in the submucosa: buccal, labial, palatal, palatoglossal and lingual. It has been estimated that they may number between 450 and 1,000. They are mucous glands except for the serous glands of von Ebner, which drain into the trench of the circumvallate papillae (see Figs 14.73, 14.74). Labial and buccal glands are illustrated in Figs 14.33 and 14.34. The palatoglossal glands are located in the region of the pharyngeal isthmus. The palatal glands lie in both the soft and the hard palate (Fig. 16.39 and page 308). The anterior lingual glands are embedded within muscle near the ventral surface of the tongue and have short ducts opening near the lingual frenum. The posterior glands are located in the root of the tongue. Minor salivary glands have collecting ducts, but intercalated and striated ducts are usually absent. This duct system therefore does not usually remove salt, so the final saliva released from them is isotonic and rich in sodium. Whereas the sympathetic innervation appears to be important in evoking reflex protein secretion from major glands, such nerves sparsely innervate the secretory tissue of minor salivary glands, and so mucus secretion here is entirely mediated by parasympathetic nerve impulses. However, the minor salivary glands secrete spontaneously and continuously, as do the sublingual glands.

Sialomicroliths

Sialomicroliths are small, hard masses (concrements) that are only evident microscopically in the salivary glands and may occur in the parenchymal cells, in the lumina or in the stroma. They contain variable amounts of both mineral (in the form of calcium phosphates, including hydroxyapatite) and non-mineralised components in the form of condensed organic secretory material (Fig. 16.40). Sialomicroliths are often associated with atrophic foci (Fig. 16.41), and both increase in number with age. They remain small, as they are formed in small spaces.

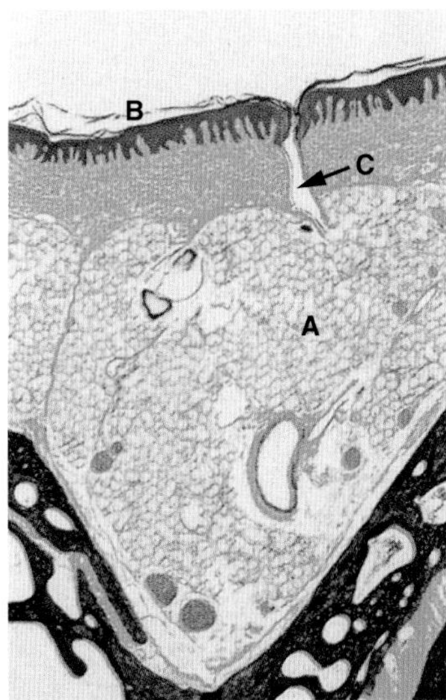

Fig. 16.39 Minor mucous gland (A) in hard palate. B = keratinised masticatory mucosa; C = duct of gland opening on to surface (Masson's trichrome; demineralised section; ×15).

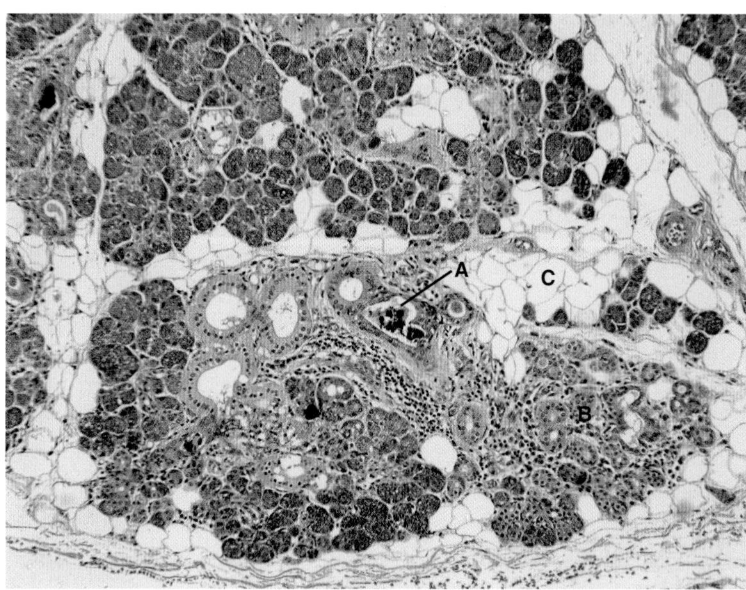

Fig. 16.41 Submandibular gland showing sialomicroliths (A) occluding the lumen of a striated duct that has led to the formation of an inflamed, atrophic focus (B). C = fat cells. Secretory inactivity leads to an increase in sialomicroliths and allows microbes to ascend the ducts and settle in the atrophic foci out of reach of microbicidal saliva (H & E; ×95). Courtesy Dr. J D Harrison.

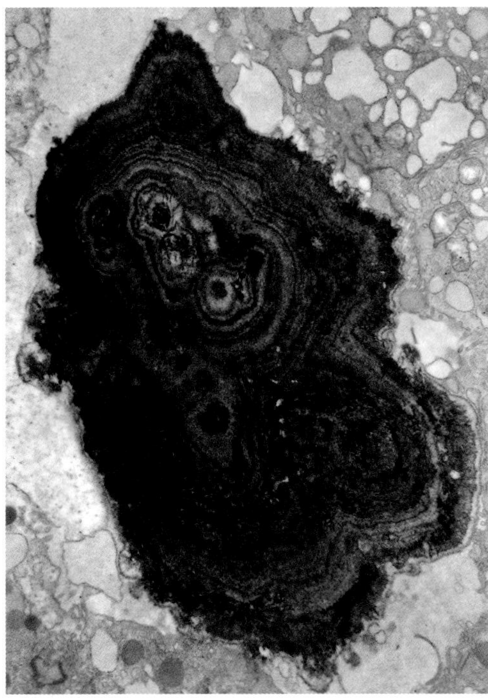

Fig. 16.40 TEM of a sialomicrolith in an acinar lumen. The presence of numerous cores and lamellae indicates that smaller sialomicroliths had accreted (fused together) to form this sialomicrolith (×5,100). Courtesy Dr. J D Harrison.

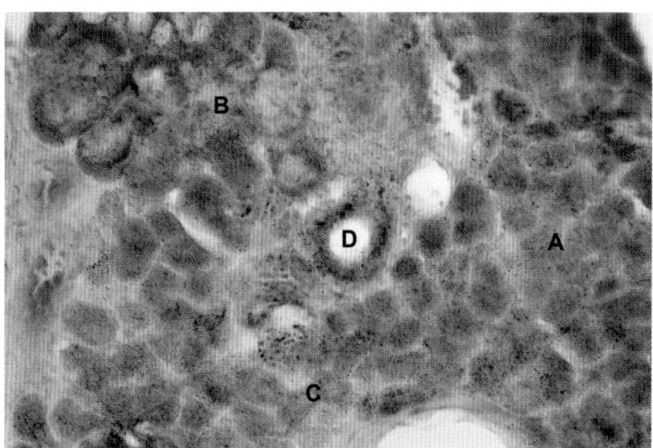

Fig. 16.42 Brown stain shows activity of the lysosomal enzyme acid phosphatase in submandibular gland with granules that represent lysosomes present throughout the parenchyma, including serous acini (A), mucous acini (B), intercalated ducts (C) and striated ducts (D) (×60). Courtesy Dr. J D Harrison.

Lysosomes are present throughout the parenchyma of the salivary glands (Fig. 16.42) and are involved in the degradation of superfluous secretory granules and other organelles during periods of secretory inactivity. These materials, which are rich in calcium, are degraded in autophagosomes, and calcium is released that may precipitate on remnants of membranes to form sialomicroliths (Fig. 16.43), which may pass from parenchymal cells into lumina. They may also form within lumina in the presence of stagnant secretory material. They remain small after their formation in small spaces and may be flushed away in saliva or scavenged by macrophages. Sialomicroliths therefore do not enlarge to become the bigger macroscopic salivary stones (sialoliths) seen in the large collecting ducts (see Figs. 16.51 and 16.52 and page 350).

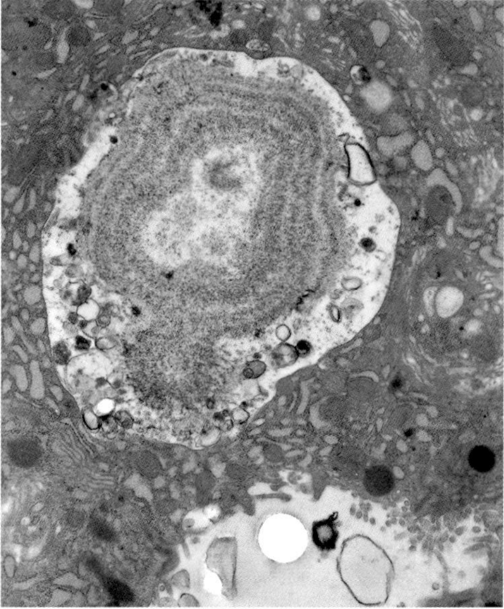

Fig. 16.43 TEM of an autophagosome in an acinar cell in which crystals of hydroxyapatite are being deposited in secretory material associated with membranous debris to form a sialomicrolith. The sialomicrolith will pass from the acinar cell into the lumen (×6,920). Courtesy Dr. J D Harrison.

Sialomicroliths are present in all normal submandibular glands and 20% of normal parotid glands. This frequency appears to relate to the higher concentration of calcium in the submandibular gland. Sialomicroliths are rare in sublingual glands and minor salivary glands, where secretion is continuous and stagnation is less likely.

Oncocytes

Oncocytes are epithelial cells occurring singly or in small groups in the acini and ducts of normal salivary glands (as well as in other tissues such as the thyroid and parathyroid glands, the kidneys and regions of the vocal tracts). They are acidophilic with haematoxylin and eosin staining (Fig. 16.44) and appear granular owing to a large increase in the number of mitochondria that, although initially having a normal morphology, subsequently display an abnormal morphology (Fig. 16.45) and are probably biochemically deficient. This increase in numbers of mitochondria is accompanied by a great reduction in other types of organelles (compare with normal cell, Fig. 16.20). Oncocytes increase with age and are thought to arise as the result of degeneration of normal cells.

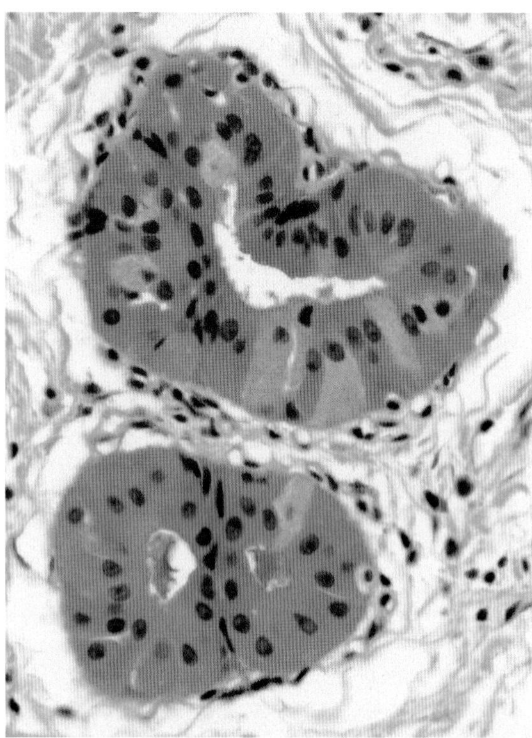

Fig. 16.44 Striated duct of parotid gland lined mainly by oncocytes. Compared with normal striated duct (see Fig. 16.18), the cells are larger and more eosinophilic. (H & E; ×375). Courtesy Dr. A W Barrett.

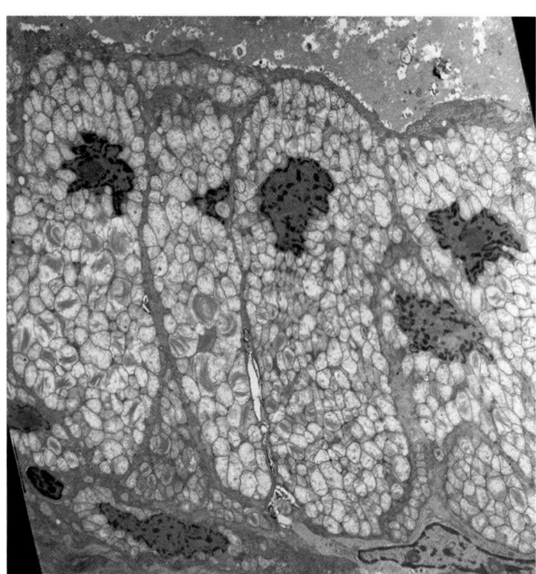

Fig. 16.45 TEM of oncocytes. Note that the cytoplasm is filled with mitochondria, many having an abnormal morphology (×2,250). Courtesy Dr. J D Harrison.

Age changes

A wide range of age changes has been documented in salivary glands. These include a decrease in the amount of glandular tissue (over 50 years) and an increase in the amount of fibrous tissue, fat cells, inflammatory cells and oncocytes. An increase in duct volume has also been described, although some of this increase may be due to shrinkage of acini, giving the appearance of duct-like forms.

Changes in the composition of saliva have been reported with age. Antioxidant enzymes in saliva decrease with age, including peroxidase, glutathione peroxidase and catalase. Mucins also decrease significantly with age, increasing the chance of inflammation and oral diseases. Sialin, a versatile anion transporter, is highly expressed in the striated and excretory ducts of salivary glands. Its expression is reduced with age and may be associated with changes in the physiological function of salivary glands with aging. The eating experience may also be decreased in quality by an age-related reduction in the number of olfactory and taste receptors

With such a significant loss of parenchyma (in both major and minor glands), it might be assumed that there would be a reduction in the amount of saliva produced in the aged population, giving rise to the clinical condition of xerostomia (dry mouth). On this matter, results are variable. Some authors report a reduction in both resting and stimulated salivary flow rates in older patients, while others report no differences in healthy, unmedicated individuals. This latter observation could be interpreted as being the result of salivary glands being able to produce more saliva than is needed. The increase in the incidence of xerostomia (see later) in the ageing population is more likely to be a secondary effect related to the increased use of medication (many drugs depress salivary production and are anticholinergic, e.g., antidepressants, antihistamines).

Age changes need to be taken into account when examining the salivary glands histologically in clinical diagnosis. This is particularly so when biopsies of lower labial salivary glands are examined in an attempt to diagnose Sjögren's syndrome, in which there are characteristic changes in the parotid and, to a lesser extent, other salivary glands that involve an infiltration by lymphocytes. However, there is an infiltration by lymphocytes to form lymphocytic foci in salivary glands that increases with age and may be as great as what has been considered to be diagnostic of Sjögren's syndrome in the lower labial glands.

Clinical considerations

Xerostomia

Older patients frequently complain of a dry mouth (xerostomia), with all the unpleasant symptoms one might expect from a consideration of the important functions of saliva. Xerostomia was once thought to be a reflection of decreased salivary production associated with the ageing process. However, this does not usually appear to be the case, and it is likely that many drugs depress salivary production, sometimes centrally as well as

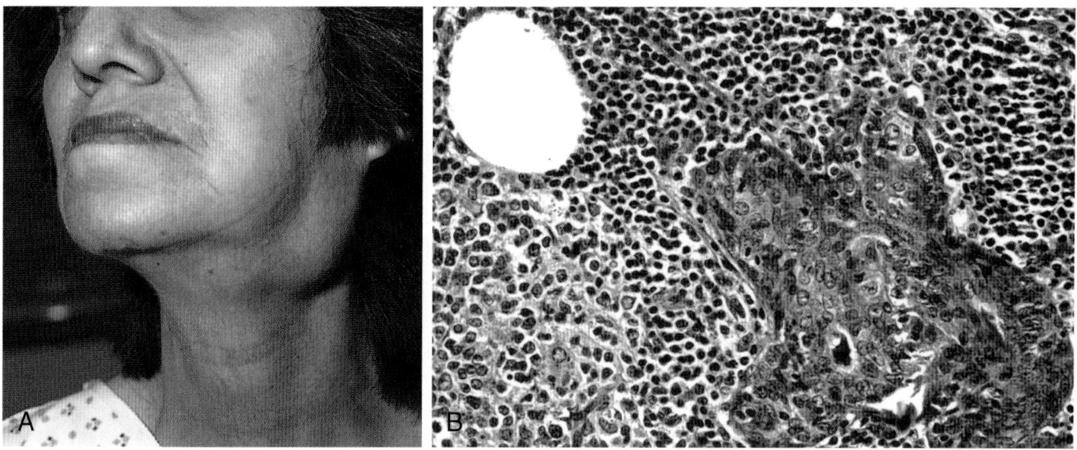

Fig. 16.46 (A) Courtesy Dr. Richard Sontheimer, Department of Dermatology, University of Texas Southwestern Medical School, Dallas, Tex. (B) Courtesy Dr. Dennis Burns, Department of Pathology, University of Texas Southwestern Medical School, Dallas, Tex.

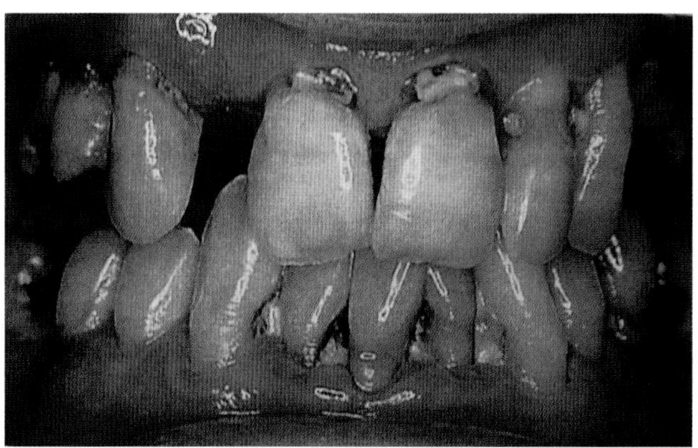

Fig. 16.47 Extensive cervical caries and periodontal disease in a patient suffering from Sjögren's syndrome. From Odell, E.W., 2017. *Cawson's Essentials of Oral Pathology and Medicine*, ninth ed. Elsevier.

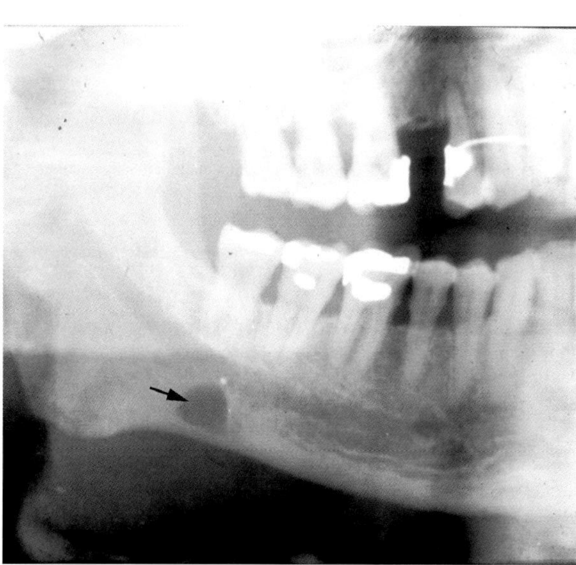

Fig. 16.48 Radiograph of a Staphne's cavity near the angle of the ramus of the mandible (arrowed). Courtesy Prof. N J D Smith.

peripherally, with unstimulated salivary flow rates falling from approximately 0.3 mL/min to less than half this value, and some are anticholinergic, such as some antidepressants and antihistamines.

Loss of salivary tissue is also a consequence of radiotherapy treatment for certain tumours in the region of the jaws or of Sjögren's syndrome. In this latter syndrome related to autoimmune disease, and also affecting the lacrimal gland, there is invasion and destruction of the parenchyma by lymphoid tissue, resulting in enlargement of the salivary glands (Fig. 16.46). As saliva is important in the maintenance of oral health, decreased secretion from the salivary glands results in an increased incidence of oral conditions such as periodontal disease, dental caries and candidal infections ('thrush') (Fig. 16.47). Partial relief may be obtained by the frequent administration of artificial saliva.

Gene therapy may also be attempted in order to increase the amount of saliva secreted. In this context, it is possible to infect a dysfunctional adult salivary gland with irradiated adenovirus expressing the water channel aquaporin-1 (AQP1) to increase the amount of saliva secreted.

Staphne's cavity (cyst)

A portion of the submandibular gland may invaginate into the lingual surface of the mandible, typically below the mandibular canal, near the angle of the ramus. On a radiograph this will give the appearance of a circumscribed, unilateral, radiolucent lesion with a radiopaque border (Fig. 16.48). It can be distinguished from other lesions by careful computed tomography imaging and by sialography, when a radiopaque dye injected in the submandibular duct will spread into the radiolucency. A similar but rarer radiolucency can occur in the anterior region of the mandible, where it is an invagination related to the sublingual gland.

Mucoceles and ranulas

Damage to the ducts of minor and sublingual salivary glands may result in the extravasation of mucus into the surrounding soft tissues (Fig. 16.49). When the extravasation persists, an extravasation mucocele is formed (Fig. 16.50). In the case of the sublingual gland, it is also termed a *ranula* because the swelling it causes to the floor of the mouth somewhat resembles the belly of a frog. When a ranula is situated above the mylohyoid muscle (oral ranula), it produces a painless swelling that may displace the tongue (Fig. 16.51). If it extends below the mylohyoid, either through a mylohyoid hiatus (page 88) or around the posterior margin of the mylohyoid, it produces a swelling in the neck (cervical or plunging ranula) (Fig. 16.52). Treatment of these conditions may necessitate the surgical removal of the affected sublingual gland.

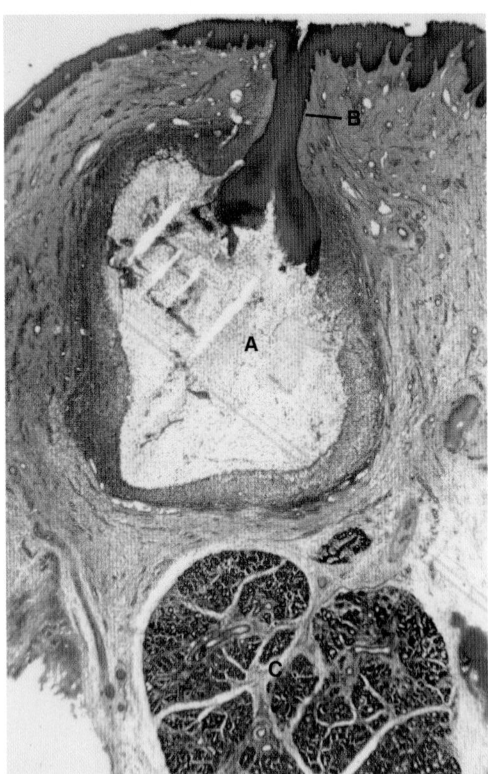

Fig. 16.49 Extravasation mucocele (A) caused by tearing of the main salivary duct (B). The affected minor salivary gland (C) may have to be surgically removed to prevent the continued extravasation of mucus (H & E; ×15). Courtesy Dr. J D Harrison.

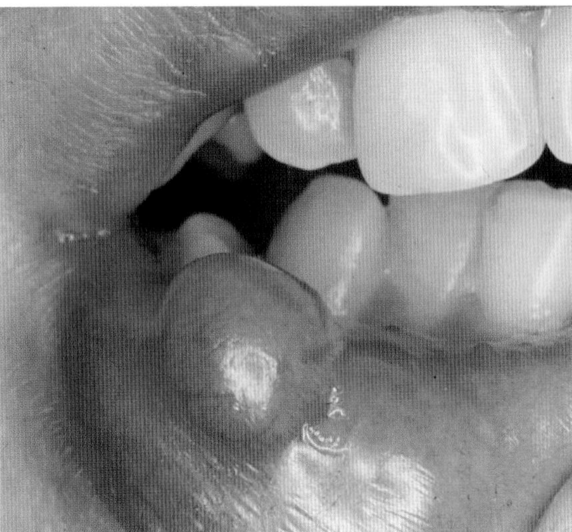

Fig. 16.50 Extravasation mucocele on the lower lip. Courtesy Dr. J D Harrison.

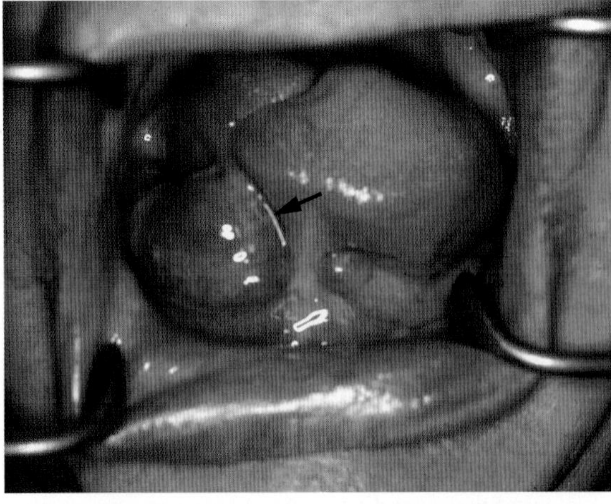

Fig. 16.51 Ranula (arrowed) in floor of mouth caused by trauma that damaged the floor of the mouth and also the tongue. Courtesy Dr. J D Harrison.

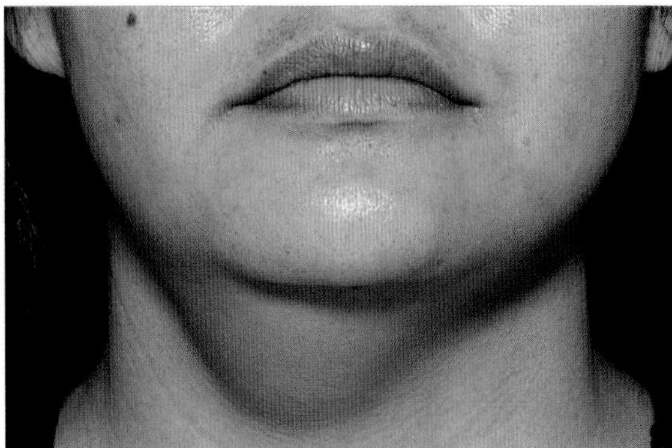

Fig. 16.52 Swelling in the right neck known clinically as a plunging ranula and caused by a damaged sublingual gland from which extravasated saliva is passing through a mylohyoid hiatus. Courtesy Prof. R P Morton and the editor of the European Archives of Oto-Rhino-Laryngology. From Samant, S., Morton, R.P., Ahmad, Z., 2011. Surgery for plunging ranula: the lesson not yet learned? *European Archives of Oto-Rhino-Laryngology* 268, 1513–1518.

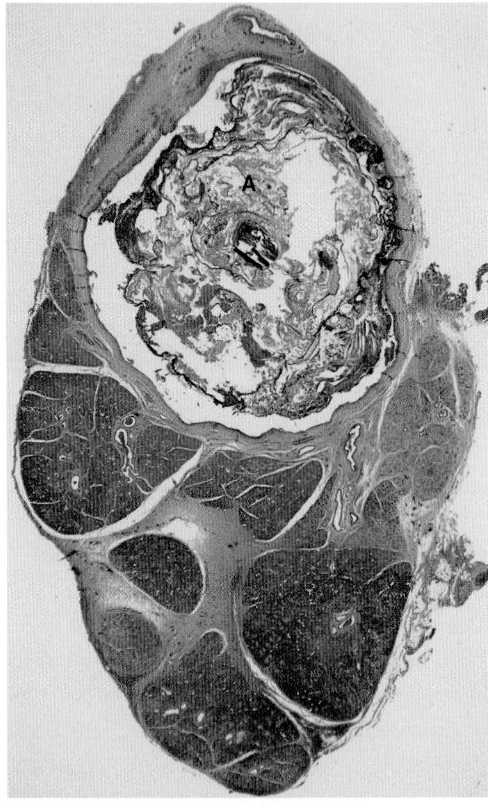

Fig. 16.53 Micrograph showing a sialolith (A) in a large, dilated duct at the hilum of the submandibular gland following chronic submandibular sialadenitis with associated inflammation, fibrosis and atrophy of normal parenchyma (H & E; ×5). Courtesy Dr. J D Harrison.

Sialoliths

Blockage may occur of the main collecting duct of a major salivary gland (usually the submandibular gland, but occasionally the parotid). The cause is usually a sialolith (stone or calculus) (Figs. 16.53, 16.54) but sometimes is a stricture or an inflammatory exudate. A sphincter near the opening of the submandibular duct has been described by some, but this was not supported by one study. The lack of access to the mouth caused by the blockage results in swelling of the gland at mealtimes, together with pain and subsequent discharge as saliva gradually flows past the obstruction.

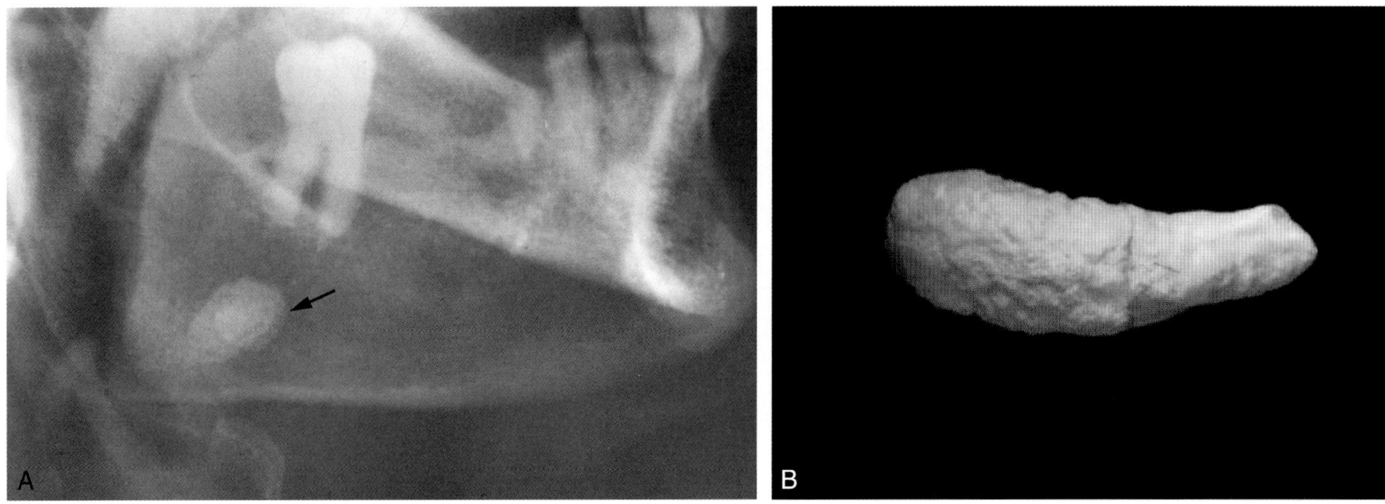

Fig. 16.54 (A) Radiograph showing the presence of a sialolith (arrow) at the proximal end of the submandibular duct at the hilum of the submandibular gland. (B) Sialolith removed from a submandibular duct. The length of this sialolith is 2.2 cm. Courtesy Dr. J D Harrison.

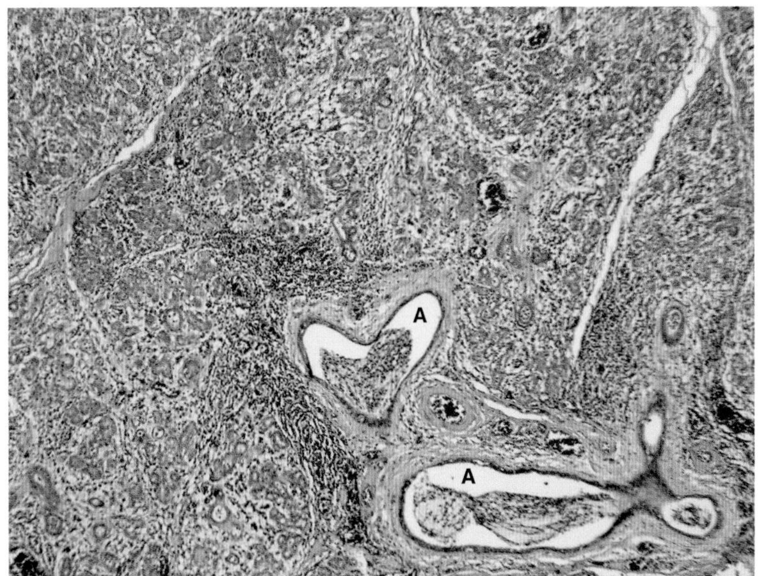

Fig. 16.55 Micrograph of a submandibular gland with chronic sialadenitis. There is widespread inflammation and atrophy of normal parenchymal tissue. The collecting ducts (A) are dilated and contain mucus and inflammatory cells resulting in the release of mucus into the mouth. The stroma around these ducts is fibrotic (H & E; ×60). Courtesy Dr. J D Harrison.

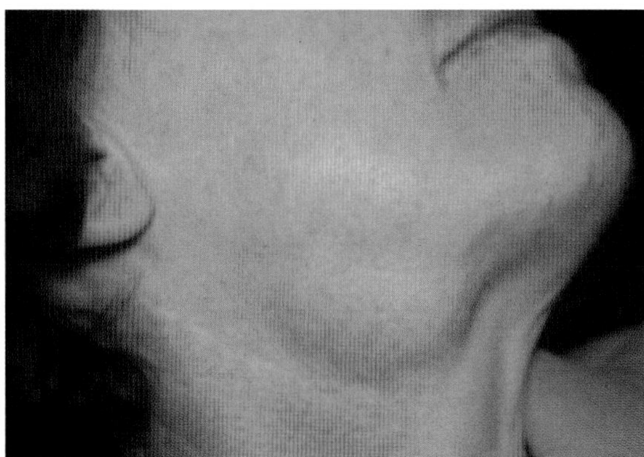

Fig. 16.56 Swelling in the neck produced by enlargement of the submandibular gland as a result of chronic obstructive submandibular sialadenitis. Courtesy Dr. J D Harrison.

Sialomicroliths and chronic submandibular sialadenitis

Though present in normal submandibular glands (and, less frequently, in normal parotid glands), sialomicroliths (Fig. 16.41) may be associated with chronic submandibular sialadenitis (inflammation of the submandibular gland; Fig. 16.55), which may produce symptoms of pain, swelling (Fig. 16.56) and discharge from the gland and sialolithiasis (sialolith or stone formation). The sequence of events is shown in Fig. 16.57.

Salivary gland regeneration

Radiation for the relatively common condition of head and neck cancer frequently destroys much of the sensitive salivary gland tissue, often resulting in irreversible hyposalivation. This has led to much research into the topic of salivary gland regeneration. Salivary glands have some capacity for regeneration, and multiple progenitor populations exist both in embryonic and adult salivary glands. Markers for identifying such cells include Sox-2.

There is considerable proliferation in the presence of noxious stimuli, as in chronic sialadenitis, which is the biological basis for the excellent results of the conservative treatment of this disease (rather than surgical removal of the gland). It has been assumed that this regeneration is essentially the property of the basal cell population associated with the striated and collecting ducts, these showing the highest proliferative index (approximately 3%). However, there is low baseline proliferation of mature acinar, ductal and myoepithelial cells (Fig. 16.24), indicating that these cells also have the capacity to contribute to parenchymal regeneration.

Three possible approaches are being investigated to repair damaged salivary tissue:

Gene therapy: Genes can be inserted into cells in the hope of stimulating acinar cell proliferation, the number of endothelial cells and saliva flow. The innervation could be targeted by neurotrophic factors such as neurturin.

Cell-based therapy: Cell therapy could involve isolating and expanding stem cells (preferably from the patient biopsy before radiation) and implanting the stem cells into the irradiated gland.

Tissue engineering therapy: As for other dental tissues, attempts to tissue engineer a salivary gland are under investigation. The stem cells in adult salivary glands may be less suitable than other types of stem cells (e.g., embryonic stem cells) for regenerating new salivary gland

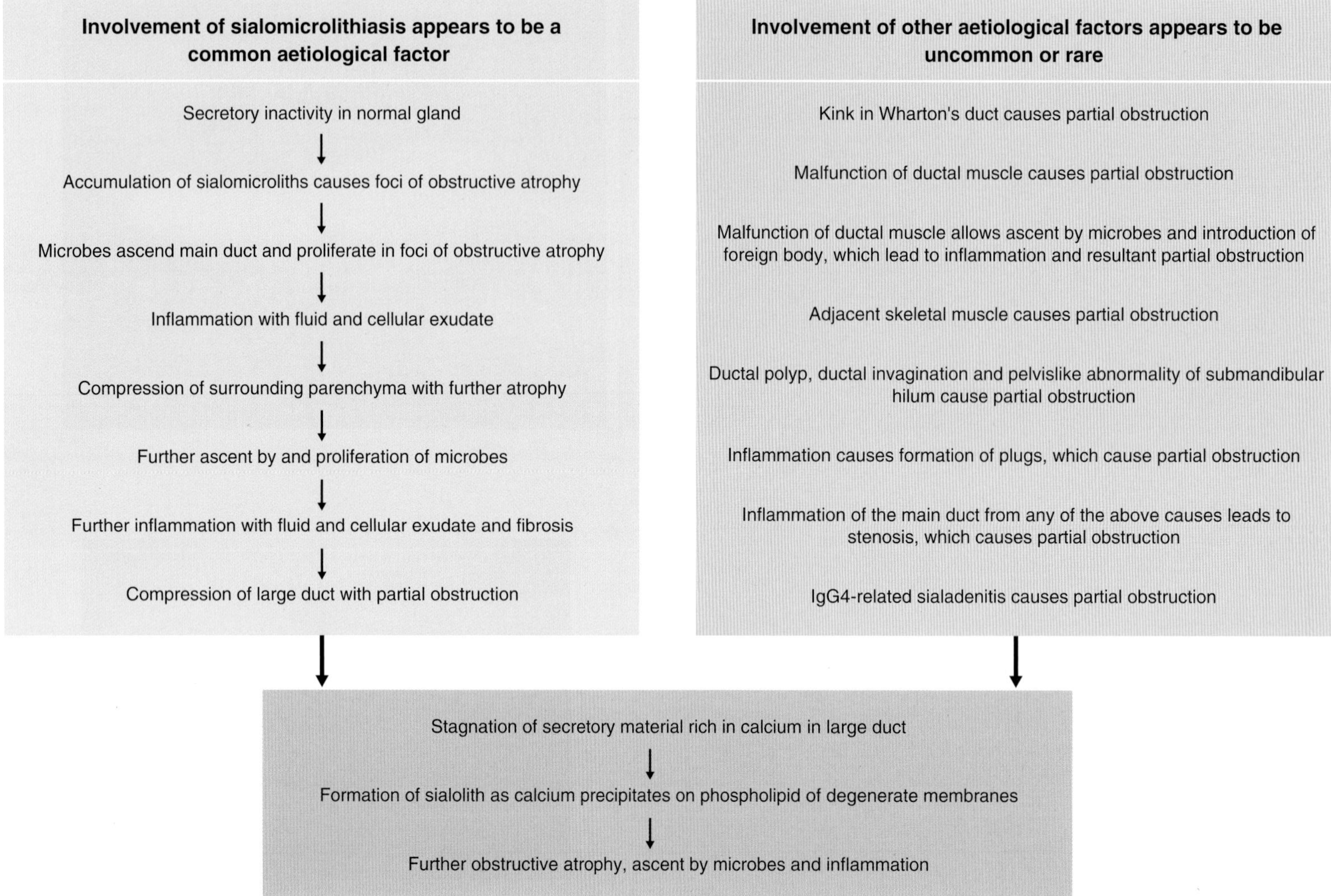

Fig. 16.57 Aetiology and pathogenesis of chronic sialadenitis and sialolithiasis. Courtesy Dr. J D Harrison and the editor of *Histopathology*. From Harrison J.D., Rodriguez-Justo, M., 2013. IgG4-related sialadenitis is rare: histopathological investigation of 129 cases of chronic submandibular sialadenitis. *Histopathology* 63, 96–102.

substance. To tissue engineer a salivary gland replacement, the usual obstacles will need to be overcome:

- Obtain a suitable epithelial stem cell population.
- Obtain a suitable stem cell population of mesenchymal stem cells.
- Obtain a suitable 3D scaffold suitable for the cells, being, amongst other things, nontoxic, permeable and biodegradable
- Define the ideal culture conditions that may require the provision of bioactive molecules such as growth factors and extracellular matrix molecules.
- Provide a functional blood supply and innervation.

Use in diagnosis

The use of saliva for diagnosis is known as **salivaomics**. Saliva is widely used because of its ease of collection, safety, non-invasiveness and accuracy. Biomarkers in saliva can help diagnose endocrine, immunological, infectious, inflammatory and numerous other conditions. However, in searching for such biomarkers, it must be remembered that whole saliva is derived from several different sources (Fig. 16.1), which must all be accounted for. The components of salivaomics include the salivary genome, the epigenome, the transcriptome, the proteome, the metabolome and the microbiome (Figs 16.58, 6.59):

1) The salivary **genome** consists of both human (70%) and microbial DNA (30%).
2) The **epigenome** consists of a record of the chemical changes to the DNA and histone proteins of an organism that can reflect abnormal pathological genetic processes.
3) The **transcriptome** relates mainly to messenger RNA (mRNA) and microRNA secreted from cells that enter the oral cavity from various sources, including salivary glands, gingival crevicular fluid and desquamated oral epithelial cells.
4) The salivary **proteome** is the entire set of proteins present in saliva and has been characterised following the development of new mass spectrometric–based methods of analysis and comparison with known gene sequences of proteins. Well over 2,000 proteins have been identified in saliva, a number of which are involved in many biological functions to maintain oral homeostasis.
5) The **metabolome** is the complete set of small molecules of different types found within a biological sample. The molecules may include both endogenous metabolites that are naturally produced by an organism (such as amino acids, organic acids, sugars and vitamins) as well as exogenous chemicals (such as drugs, environmental contaminants and food additives) that are not naturally produced by an organism

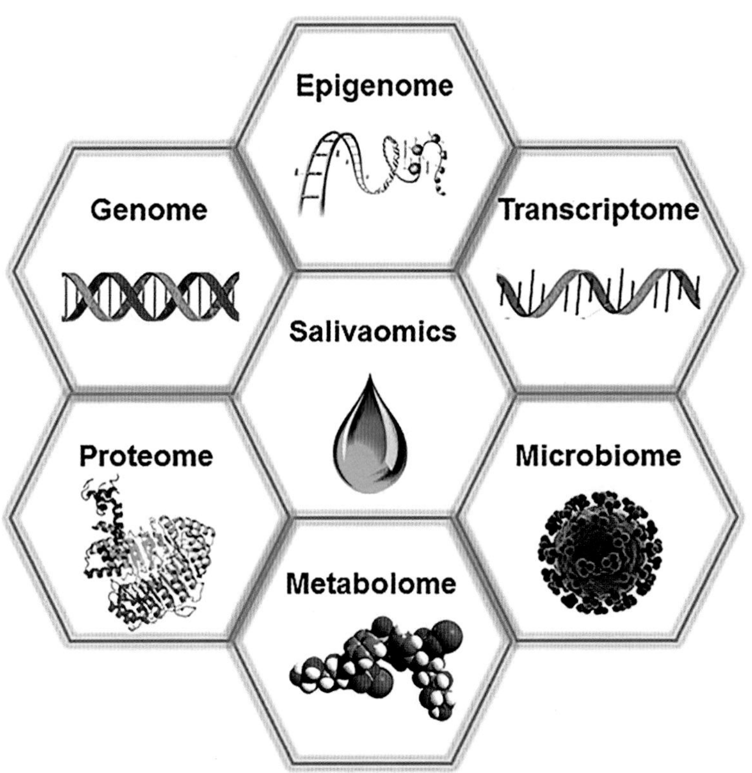

Fig. 16.58 The components of salivaomics. Salivaomics as the various '-omics' with constituents of saliva, including genomics (human and microbial), the oral microbiome, epigenome (DNA methylation), transcriptome (mRNA, microRNA and other noncoding RNAs), proteome and metabolome. From Zhang, Y., Sun, J., Lin, C-C., et al., 2016. The emerging landscape of salivary diagnostics. *Periodontology* 2000 70, 38–52.

6) The **microbiome** is the characteristic microbial community found in saliva based on gene sequencing and currently numbers over 700 species.

Interest has focussed on extracellular organelles found in large numbers in saliva that may have important functional and diagnostic significance. These are **exosomes** (30–120 nm) and **ectosomes** (100–350 nm) that contain nucleic acids and proteins, which they transport in body fluids (including blood, saliva, urine and breast milk). They are formed by exocytosis of multivesicular bodies formed in the cytoplasm (exosomes) or by direct budding from the plasma membrane and are secreted by most cell types. Although their functional significance awaits clarification, they have substantial biological functions, including intercellular communication and signalling.

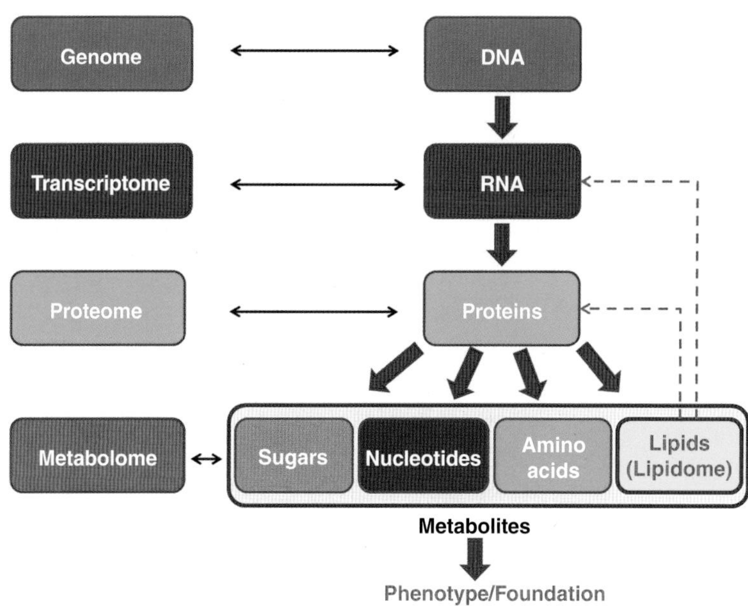

Fig. 16.59 The components of salivaomics. Courtesy Wikipedia.

Using a range of salivary biomarkers, it is possible to discriminate patients with oral and systemic diseases from subjects without such diseases. Thus, it is possible to detect and monitor periodontal disease (via the presence of gingival crevicular fluid; see page 305), Sjögren's syndrome and a range of oral cancers and viral diseases such as acquired immunodeficiency syndrome (AIDS) and SARS-CoV-2.

Biomarkers of diagnostic significance in oral cancer include interleukin 6, interleukin 8, endothelin 1 and cytokeratin fraction 21-1. Although the mechanisms of how diseases distant from the oral cavity lead to the appearance of discriminatory biomarkers in saliva are largely unclear, salivaomics can be used to aid the diagnosis of conditions such as type 2 diabetes, multiple sclerosis, lung and pancreatic cancers and Alzheimer's disease.

Further readings for this chapter can be found in the accompanying eBook. Explore online Self-assessment quiz to test and reinforce your understanding of the material in your free ebook. Follow instructions in the Inside Front Cover to unlock your access.

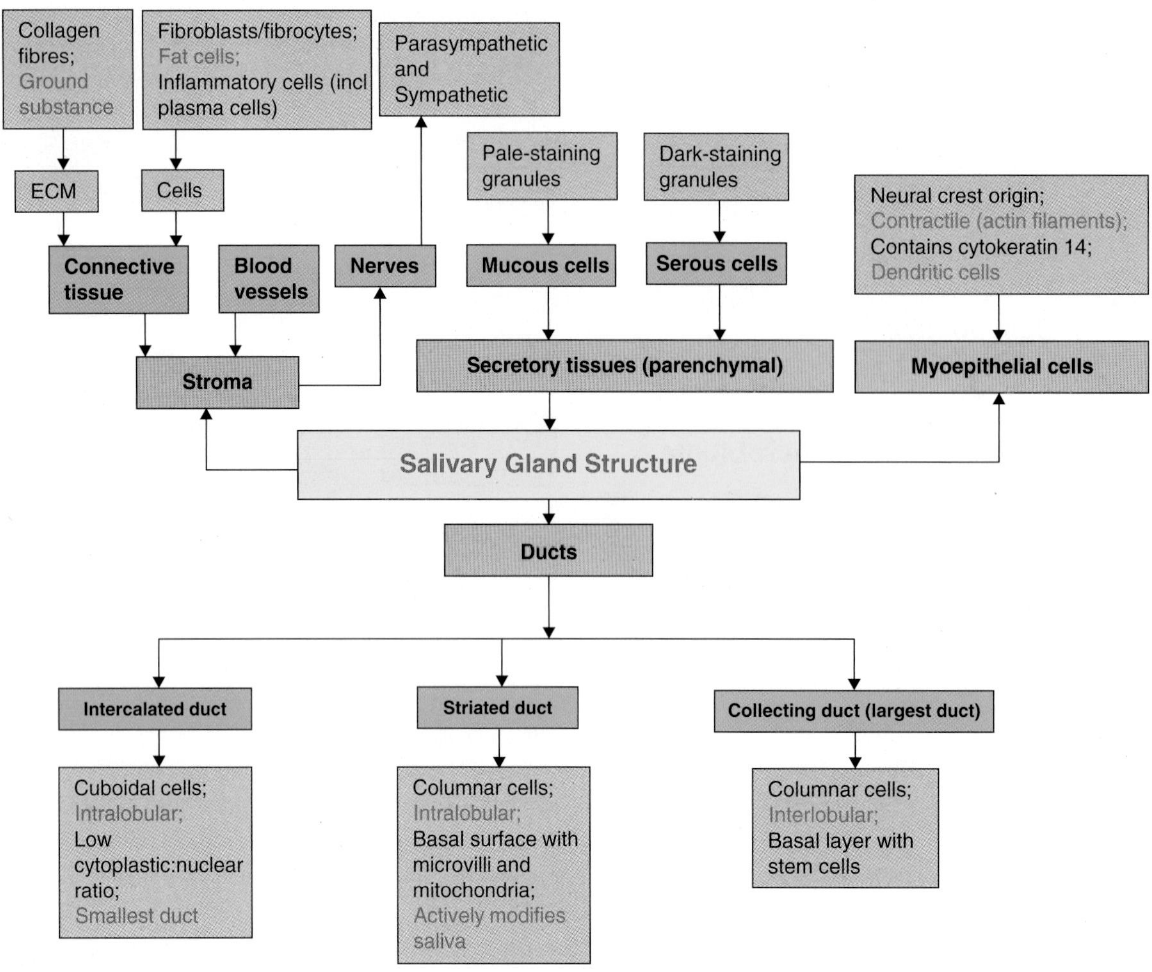

Mind Map 16.1 Salivary gland structure.

Development of the face

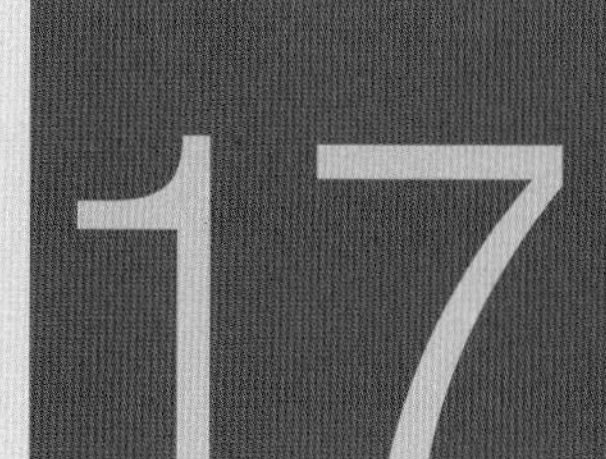

Facial development

Fourth week *in utero*

During the fourth week *in utero*, the primitive oral cavity (stomodeum) is bounded by five facial processes (sometimes referred to as swellings or primordia), produced by proliferating zones of mesenchyme lying beneath the surface ectoderm (Fig. 17.1). These are the unpaired frontonasal process and the paired mandibular and maxillary processes. The frontonasal process lies above, the two mandibular processes lie below and the two maxillary processes are located to the sides of the stomodeum. The frontonasal process is formed from the mesenchyme in front of the developing forebrain. The maxillary and mandibular processes are derived from the first pharyngeal (branchial) arches. The facial processes are demarcated by grooves that, in the course of normal development, become flattened out by the proliferative and migratory activity of the underlying mesenchyme. Although it was once believed that epithelial sheets partitioned the facial processes and that these sheets had to break down for facial development to proceed, such sheets do not exist, and facial clefts cannot therefore be related to such epithelial sheets and to their failure to break down. However, in this regard, some attention has been paid to an epithelial sheet termed the *nasal fin* that lies in the developing upper lip region (see later).

At an early stage of development (week 4), a membrane (the oropharyngeal membrane) separates the primitive oral cavity from the developing pharynx. This membrane is bilaminar, being composed of an outer ectodermal layer and an inner endodermal layer. The oropharyngeal membrane soon breaks down to establish continuity between the ectoderm-lined oral cavity and the endoderm-lined pharynx. Although not detectable in the adult, the demarcation zone between mucosa derived from ectoderm and endoderm is said to correspond to a region lying just behind the permanent third molar tooth.

Fifth week *in utero*

In a 5-week-old embryo (Fig. 17.2), localised thickenings of ectoderm give rise to the nasal and optic placodes. These placodes will form the olfactory epithelium and the lenses of the eyes, respectively (see page 357). The nasal placodes sink into the underlying mesenchyme, forming two blind-ended nasal pits (the primitive nasal cavities). Proliferation of mesenchyme from the frontonasal process around the openings of the nasal pits produces the medial and lateral nasal processes. In addition, the maxillary processes enlarge and grow forwards and medially.

Sixth week *in utero*

In the 6-week-old embryo (Fig. 17.3), the two mandibular processes fuse in the midline to form the tissues of the lower jaw. The mandibular processes and maxillary processes are continuous at the angle of the mouth, thus defining its outline. From the upper corners of the mouth, the maxillary processes grow below the lateral nasal processes and towards the medial nasal processes (Fig. 17.3B). Between the merging maxillary and the lateral nasal processes lie the naso-optic furrows (alternatively termed the *nasolacrimal grooves*). From each furrow, a solid ectodermal rod of cells sinks below the surface and canalises to form the nasolacrimal duct.

Intermaxillary segment

Two differing accounts have been given for the continued development of the upper lip beyond the sixth week of intrauterine life. One view suggests that the maxillary processes overgrow the medial nasal processes to meet in the midline and thus contribute all the tissue for the upper lip. A different slant on this view suggests that the mesenchyme of the maxillary processes entirely displaces the mesenchyme of the medial nasal processes. This idea of the development of the upper lip is based upon an appreciation of the innervation of the fully formed upper lip (i.e., the infraorbital branch of the maxillary division of the trigeminal nerve), the maxillary processes being supplied by the maxillary nerve and the frontonasal process by the ophthalmic nerve. Alternatively, it has been suggested that the maxillary processes meet the medial nasal processes without such overgrowth or mesenchyme invasion, the middle third of the upper lip (the intermaxillary segment) being therefore derived from the merged medial nasal processes of the frontonasal process. While histological evidence favours the latter explanation, at present too little is known about the behaviour of the mesenchyme of the facial processes after the initial fusion, thereby not excluding the possibility of subsequent migration of tissue derived from the maxillary processes towards the midline. The possible contributions to the adult face from the embryonic facial processes (based upon the suggestion that the middle third of the upper lip is derived from the frontonasal process) are described in Fig. 17.4. The facial derivatives shown are therefore at odds with the sensory distribution of the adult face, because (as previously mentioned) the fully developed lip is supplied only by the maxillary division of the trigeminal nerve and has no contribution from the ophthalmic division. The facial muscles are derived from mesenchyme of the second pharyngeal arches that migrates into the primitive lips and cheeks, and these muscles are therefore innervated by the facial nerve.

Some controversy persists concerning the so-called intermaxillary segment that is formed initially by the merged medial nasal processes. First, as mentioned earlier, there are different views concerning the contribution of the intermaxillary segment to the developing upper lip. Second, some embryologists persist with the notion of a 'premaxilla' at the site of development of the maxillary incisor teeth. While a premaxilla is seen in apes, where there are sutures between this region and the rest of the maxilla and where there is a separate centre of ossification, this does not apply to the human situation. As mentioned in Chapter 18, the primary palate is initially formed from the caudal aspect of the merged medial nasal processes of the frontonasal process.

Signalling mechanisms

The cells that make up the mesenchyme of the facial primordia are derived from two main sources: connective tissue cells migrating from the neural

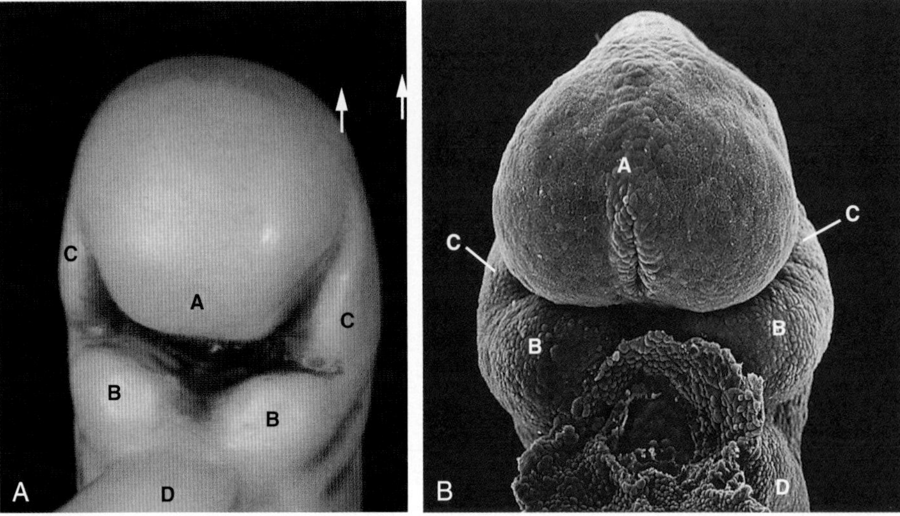

Fig. 17.1 (A) Model of a face of a 4-week-old human embryo (frontal aspect). (B) SEM of the face at an equivalent stage to 4 weeks in the rat (frontal aspect). A = frontonasal process; B = mandibular processes; C = maxillary processes; D = pericardial swelling. Courtesy Prof. A G S Lumsden.

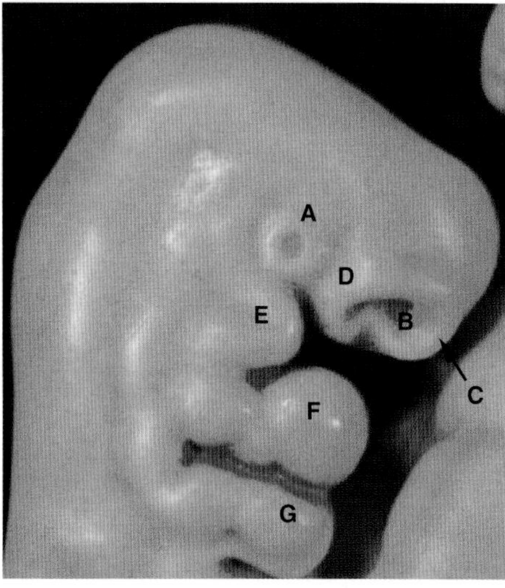

Fig. 17.2 Model of a face of a 5-week-old human embryo (lateral aspect). A = optic placode; B = nasal pit; C = medial nasal process; D = lateral nasal process; E = maxillary process; F = mandibular process; G = second pharyngeal arch.

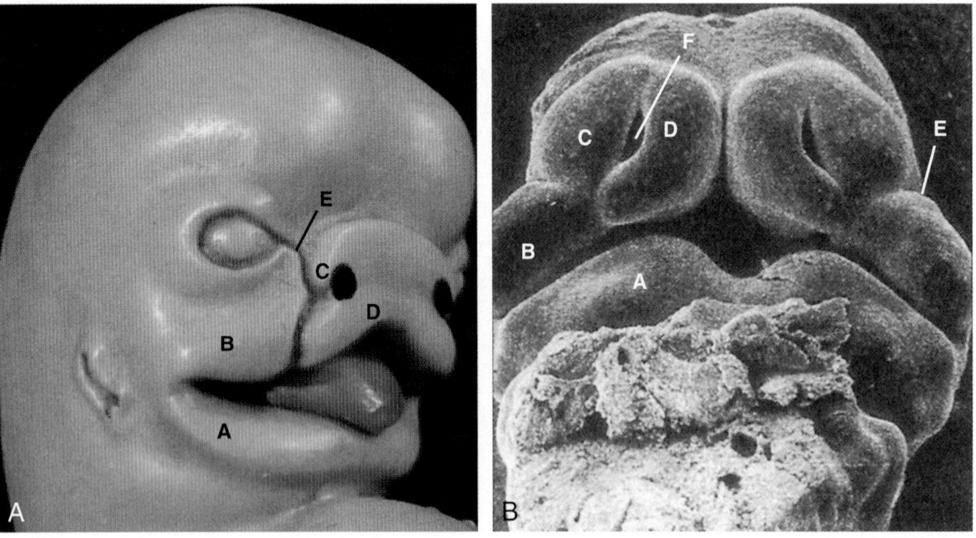

Fig. 17.3 (A) Model of a face of a 6-week-old human embryo (lateral aspect). A = mandibular process; B = maxillary process; C = lateral nasal process; D = medial nasal process; E = naso-optic furrow. (B) SEM of developing rat upper jaw and lip at an equivalent stage to 6 weeks showing the merging maxillary and medial nasal processes. Labelling as for Fig. 17.3A; F = nasal pit. Courtesy Prof. A G S Lumsden.

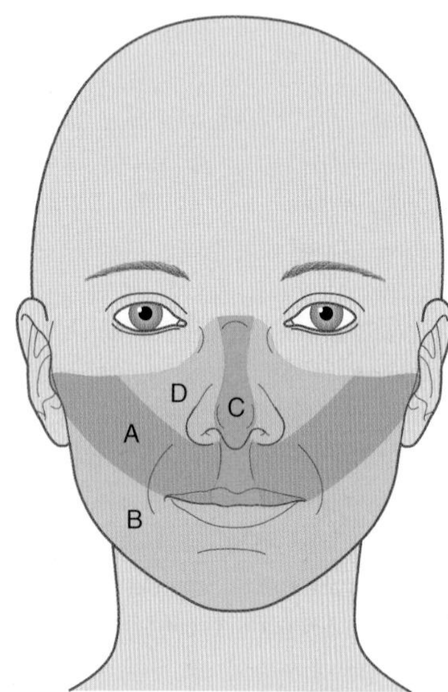

Fig. 17.4 The contributions to the adult face from the embryonic facial processes. A = maxillary processes; B = mandibular processes; C = medial nasal processes; D = lateral nasal processes.

crest and muscle cells from the paraxial mesenchyme. It has been reported that the mesenchyme of the frontonasal process is derived entirely from cranial neural crest, whereas the mesenchyme of the maxillary and mandibular processes originates from both cranial neural crest and mesoderm. However, fate mapping of the cells suggests that this notion is oversimplified. Although the two types of mesenchyme have distinct developmental histories, there are considerable and significant interactions between them. The signalling mechanisms are, however, as yet relatively poorly understood. The development of the craniofacial region involves the four fundamental mechanisms that underlie all embryonic development: growth, morphogenesis, cell differentiation and pattern formation. The last mechanism leads to the spatial ordering of cell differentiation. Present research into the development of the face is geared towards understanding the basis of all these mechanisms.

The size of the cell populations is of key importance and is controlled, at least in part, by growth factors. These may also be of significance in the epithelial–mesenchymal interactions known to induce cartilage, bone and tooth differentiation within facial primordia. Pattern formation in developing limbs is, in part, controlled by vitamin A derivatives (retinoids), which form morphogenetic gradients within the limb bud. While such gradients have not yet been demonstrated in the face, a similar mechanism seems likely, as the facial primordia are sensitive to exogenous retinoic acid and the mesenchymal cells contain specific retinoic acid receptors.

Quantitative electron microscopic studies (Fig. 17.5) show that, at the time of fusion of the facial processes, there is a marked increase in the number of small projections/processes from the mesenchymal cells. This increase is consistent with reports that changes within the epithelial cells occur and may be related to intercellular signalling between the mesenchymal cells at the time of fusion of the upper lip (i.e., just before the onset of major histiogenic events).

It is worth noting that the brain and facial mesenchyme have been shown to express particular genes at key times in their development.

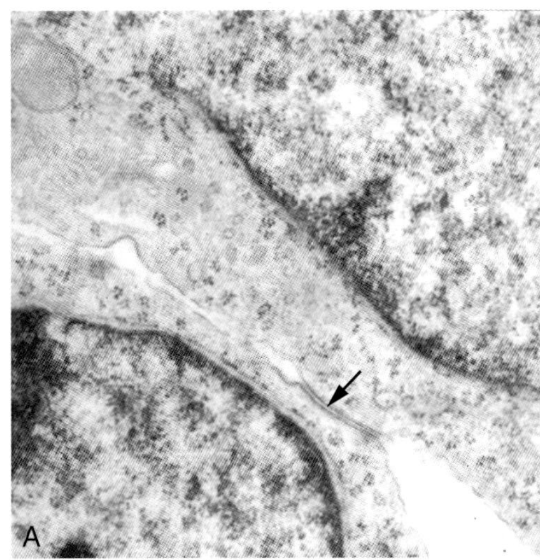

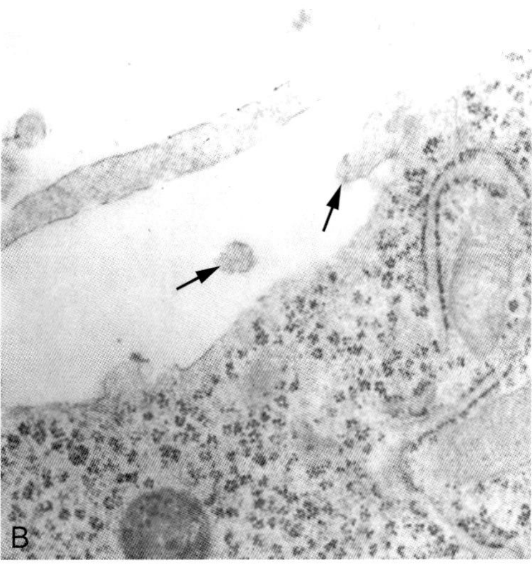

Fig. 17.5 Electron micrographs of the mesenchyme within the maxillary facial processes (TEM; ×15,000). (A) Shows cell junction (arrow). (B) Shows small cell processes (arrows). Courtesy D Symons.

These 'homeobox' (Hox) genes were discovered in embryos of the fruit fly *Drosophila* and are responsible for the spatial organisation of the developing *Drosophila* embryo. Similar genes are expected to be of major importance in mammalian development and are the subject of intensive research. It has been shown that neural crest cells that form the frontonasal process and the maxillary and mandibular primordium do not express *Hox* genes but express closely related factors such as the *Dlx* and *Msx* family. It has also been reported that *Hoxa2* is expressed in the second, but not the first, pharyngeal arch. Loss of *Hoxa2* function results in transformation of second arch structures into first arch elements. There is much evidence that the neural crest cells of the facial processes acquire significant patterning information from the surrounding epithelia and that the surface ectoderm plays an important role in initiating outgrowth of the frontonasal process. Patterning in the region requires integration of signals between the neural crest, ectoderm and endoderm, and it is noteworthy that neural crest transplantation experiments show that the neural crest can pattern the face. Studies have also highlighted the importance of *Dlx* genes in the development of the pharyngeal arches, including the mandibular and maxillary processes.

Sonic hedgehog (Shh) is a protein switched on by retinoic acid, which, along with fibroblast growth factor (FGF), has been located in the ectoderm of the frontonasal and maxillary processes in chick embryos. Their function is unclear, but it is possible that Shh may act as an organiser of morphogenesis, whereas FGF may be involved in the stimulation of the mesenchyme of the facial processes to produce growth. Indeed, Shh is a critical factor in regulating craniofacial development. Shh is expressed by the facial ectoderm, the pharyngeal endoderm and the mesoderm of the prechordal plate (underlying the forebrain). In this respect, there is a 'frontonasal–ectodermal zone' that is the junction between regions expressing FGF8 and Shh. This zone is the initial site of the outgrowth of the frontonasal process and, in avians, sets up the dorsoventral axis for development of the upper beak. When facial ectoderm not expressing Shh is removed, there is no effect, whereas removal of ectoderm expressing Shh results in the arrest of the outgrowth of the maxillary processes. Transgenic experiments have also shown that there are severe effects in craniofacial development in mice with mutations in *Shh*-expressing genes. Thus, there is ample evidence showing that there is 'cross-talk' between ectodermal, neural crest and endodermal tissues in the craniofacial region that relies upon Shh signalling pathways. Furthermore, there is evidence for signalling pathways involving FGF, wingless/integrated (Wnt) and bone morphogenetic protein (BMP).

Table 17.1 Signalling factors associated with lens, nasal and otic placodes

Signalling factor family	Lens placode	Nasal placode	Otic placode
FGF	FGFR	FGF	FGFR and FGF
PDGF	–	–	–
RA	–	–	–
Shh	–	–	–
TGF-β	BMP4 and BMP7	–	–
Wnt	–	–	Wnt

Three sets of facial placodes are seen on the developing face: nasal (olfactory) placodes optic (lens) placode (Fig. 17.2) and otic placodes. These placodes are thickenings of the surface ectoderm. They are sensory placodes that initially arise from a common 'preplacodal field' that lies close to the anterior neural crest border. Eventually, they have individual developmental fates under the influence of a variety of signalling factors (Table 17.1).

The nasal placodes are situated towards the front of the developing head (on either side of the frontonasal process) and give rise to the olfactory epithelia. The lens placodes invaginate and eventually become internalised to form the lens vesicles, which, as indicated by the name, become the lenses of the eyes. The otic placodes are the first part of the ears to develop. They appear over the regions of the developing hindbrain and, like the lens placodes, invaginate and become internalised to form the otic vesicles, which ultimately will develop into the internal ears (the primordium of the membranous labyrinths).

Development of nasal cavities

The nasal placodes invaginate from the surface by a combination of active growth of its epithelium and by proliferation of the mesenchyme at the edges of the placode. However, the nasal placodes do not become completely internalised and thus form two blind-ended pits, the nasal pits (Figs. 17.2 and Fig. 17.3, see page 355). They are separated in the midline by the primary nasal septum. The nasal pits continue to deepen (at least

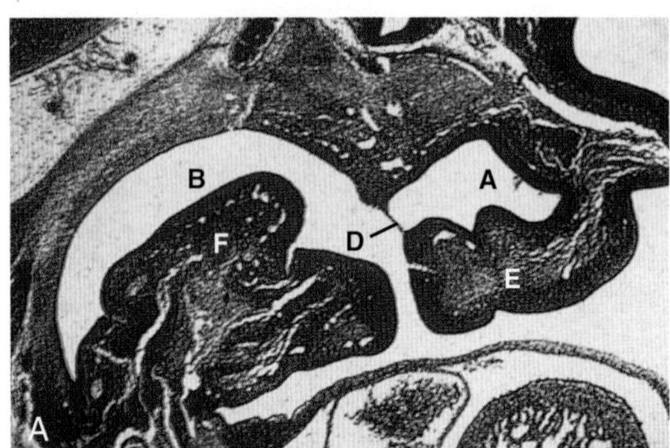

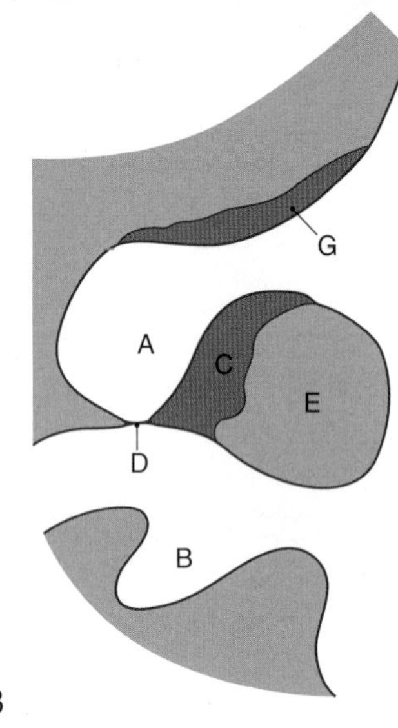

Fig. 17.6 Sagittal sections of the head illustrating aspects of the development of the nasal cavity. A = nasal pit; B = oral cavity; C = nasal fin; D = oronasal membrane; E = maxillary isthmus; F = developing tongue; G = nasal placode in root of nasal pit (A, toluidine blue; ×30). (A) Courtesy Prof. A G S Lumsden. (B) Courtesy Dr. D A Luke.

in part because of the growth of the surrounding medial and lateral nasal processes), and the nasal placodes come to lie in the roof of the nasal pits (Fig. 17.6B), where they will form the olfactory epithelium. Here, some of the cells become spindle-shaped olfactory cells or become basal and supporting cells. A vascular network appears in association with the olfactory epithelium, and the sensory epithelium sends out nerve processes that eventually will communicate with the olfactory region of the telencephalon of the developing brain.

The nasal pits continue to extend into the developing head of the embryo until the roof of the primitive oral cavity is partitioned from the floor of each nasal pit by a sheet of epithelium termed the *nasal fin*. The nasal fin thins to form an oronasal membrane separating the nasal pit from the developing oral cavity. By the end of the fifth week, the oronasal membrane ruptures to produce communication between oral and nasal cavities.

The nasal fin (the sheet of epithelium seen below each nasal pit) does not, as was once thought, form a complete epithelial partition between the maxillary and medial nasal processes. A bridge of mesenchyme, the maxillary isthmus, joins the two processes in front of the nasal fin. Fig. 17.6B shows a sagittal section through the developing nasal and oral cavities and the positions of the nasal fin, the oronasal membrane between the nasal pit and the developing oral cavity and the maxillary isthmus at the end of the fifth week of development. The nasal fin eventually becomes incorporated into the walls of the nasal pit and, at the roof of the developing oral cavity, thins to form the oronasal membrane. However, should the fin become enlarged, it may constitute a line of weakness between the mesenchyme of the maxillary and medial nasal processes and eventually lead to a cleft in this region.

The anterior openings of the primitive nasal cavities become filled with epithelial cells to form 'epithelial plugs'. Eventually, these plugs disintegrate so that the nasal passages become open again. The remains of the plugs contribute to the formation of the vestibule of the nose up to the ridge (the limen nasi) that marks the start of the nasal cavity proper.

Clinical considerations

Holoprosencephaly

This is a congenital abnormality in which the developing forebrain fails to divide into two separate hemispheres and ventricles. It occurs at a rate of 1:10,000 live births. The cause is unknown, although between 25% and 50% of affected individuals have either a numerical chromosomal abnormality (syndromic hydroprosencephaly) or a gene mutation (nonsyndromic hydroprosencephaly). Among environmental factors that may be relevant are maternal diabetes, infections during pregnancy (e.g., syphilis, rubella) and drugs during pregnancy (e.g., retinoic acid, alcohol, anticonvulsants). Factors associated with clefting of the lip/palate are described in Table 18.1 and pages 369–370.

Patients with holoprosencephaly display a spectrum of facial anomalies, especially of midline structures. In its severest form, there may be cyclopia (with a single or partially divided eye within a single midline orbit, Fig. 17.7), absence or severe reduction of nasal structures, microcephaly, cleft palate and cleft lip. Among dental abnormalities there may be a single first maxillary incisor.

Macrostomia, microstomia and astomia

Disturbances in the relationship between the mandibular and maxillary processes may give rise to macrostomia (enlarged oral orifice), microstomia (small oral orifice) or, rarely, astomia (lack of an oral orifice). Persistence of the naso-optic furrow (nasolacrimal groove) may produce an oblique facial cleft (Fig. 17.8C). Rarely, persistence of a midline groove between the two merging mandibular processes produces a mandibular cleft (Fig. 17.8E).

Facial clefts

Failure of fusion of the maxillary and medial nasal processes produces the common congenital malformation of cleft lip, which may be unilateral (Fig. 17.9) or bilateral (Figs. 17.8B, 17.10). Failure of the medial nasal processes to merge may be responsible for the formation of median cleft lip (Fig. 17.8A). Most clefts of the lip have a multifactorial aetiology, being associated with both genetic and environmental disturbances. The critical period for such disturbances is during the sixth and seventh weeks of intrauterine life. Candidate genes for clefts of the lip, with and without clefts of the palate, are now being recognised.

First arch syndromes

Most congenital abnormalities of the craniofacial region involve transformation of the pharyngeal arch apparatus. The so-called 'first arch syndromes/sequences', including Pierre Robin's sequence and Treacher Collins' syndrome, affect all or most of the structures derived from the first pharyngeal arch (i.e., the mandibular and maxillary processes). First arch syndromes/sequences are caused either by insufficient migration of neural crest cells into the region of the first pharyngeal arch during week 4 of

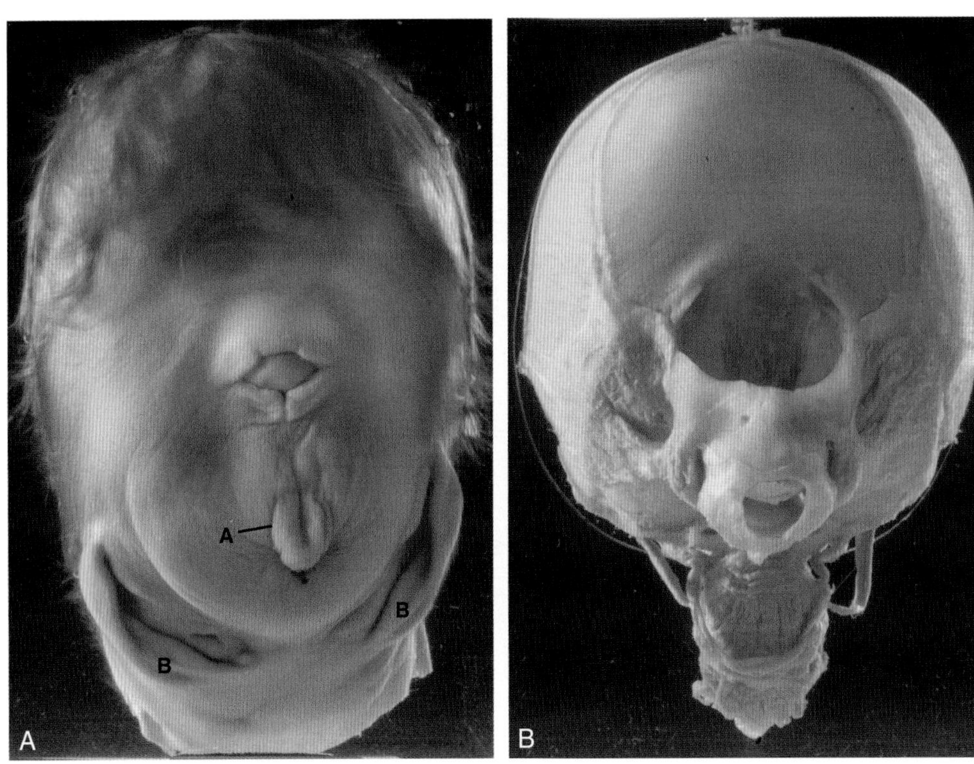

Fig. 17.7 Example of extreme holoprosencephaly in a human embryo exhibiting cyclopia. (A) External features. Note the appearance and position of the nose (A) and ears (B). (B) Skull exposed to reveal the central orbit. Copyright the Royal College of Surgeons of England.

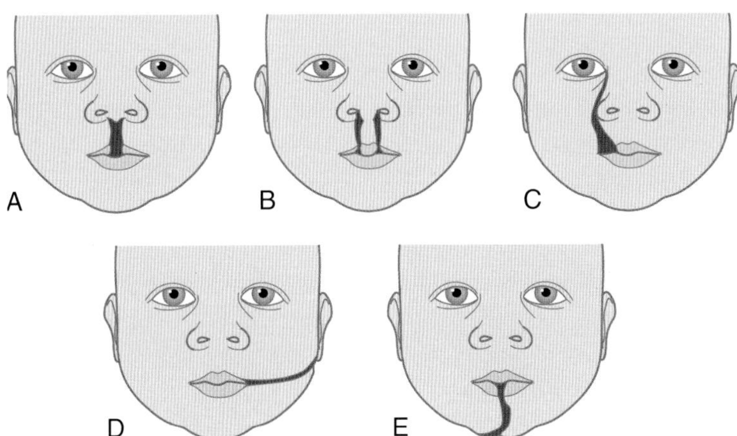

Fig. 17.8 Facial clefts. A = median cleft lip; B = bilateral cleft lip; C = oblique facial cleft; D = lateral facial cleft; E = median mandibular cleft.

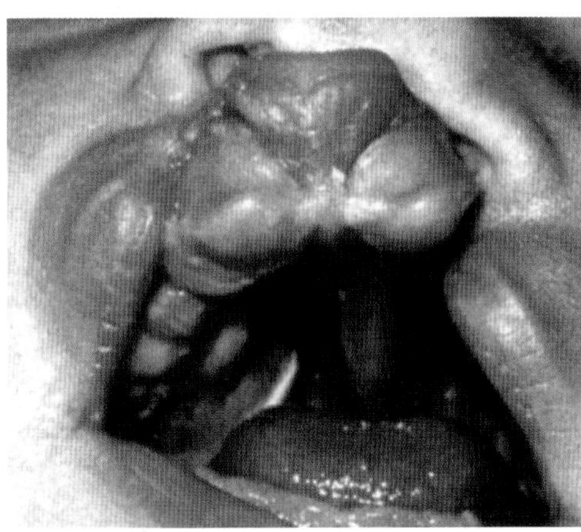

Fig. 17.10 Bilateral cleft lip.

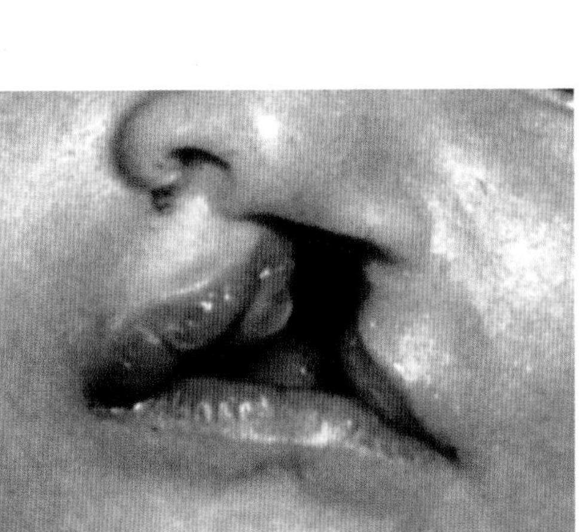

Fig. 17.9 Unilateral cleft lip.

intrauterine life, by decreased cell proliferation or by increased cell death.

Pierre Robin's sequence (Fig. 17.11) is a heterogeneous birth defect found in about 1:8,500 live births. In its usual manifestation, it is found equally in males and females. However, there is an X-linked form. Pierre Robin's sequence is characterised by micrognathia (underdeveloped mandible), glossoptosis (abnormal downward or backward placement of the tongue, which may produce respiratory distress and difficulty in feeding), ear defects, speech defects because of velopharyngeal insufficiency and clefts of the lips and palate. In its normal form, Pierre Robin's sequence is an autosomal recessive hereditary condition.

Treacher Collins' syndrome is found in 1:10,000 live births. Typically, the syndrome is characterised by downward-slanting eyes, coloboma of the eye (a notchlike defect with a keyhole appearance in the inferior part of the iris resulting from failure of closure of the retinal fissure of the

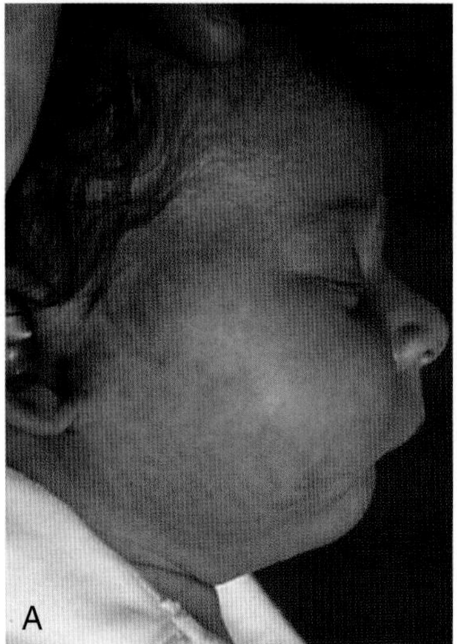

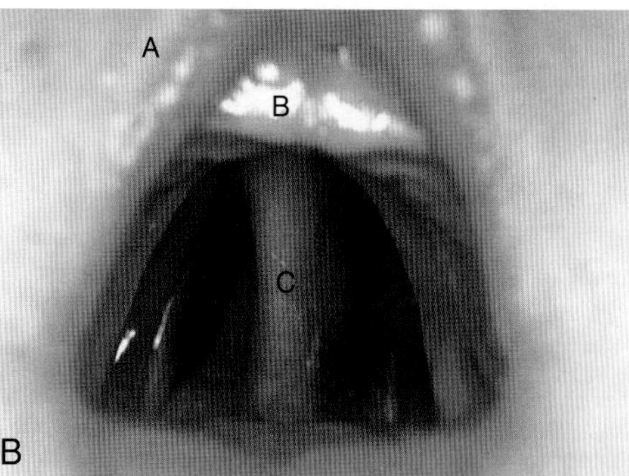

Fig. 17.11 Pierre Robin's sequence. (A) Neonate with a poorly developed mandible (micrognathia). (B) U-shaped palatal cleft viewed from the mouth. A = upper lip; B = maxillary alveolus; C = nasal septum. Courtesy Prof. R G Oliver; copyright Cardiff & Vale NHS Trust.

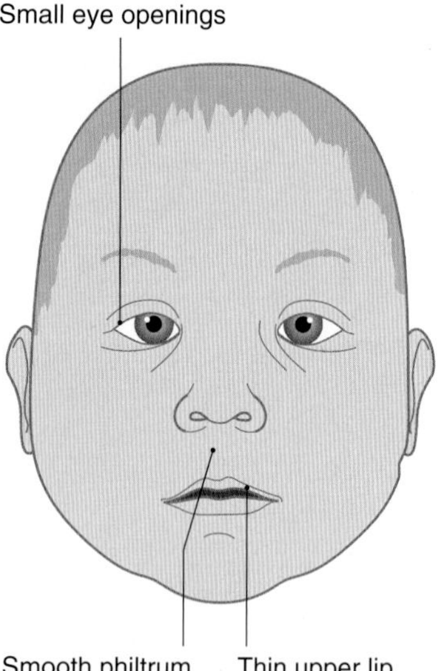

Fig. 17.12 Classic features of fetal alcohol spectrum disorder.

developing eye), micrognathia, absent or malformed ears and clefts of the lips and palate. Mutations in the *Tcof1* gene (at chromosome 5q32–q33.1) can cause this syndrome; the mutation results in disturbance in the synthesis of a protein called *treacle*, which is particularly important in craniofacial development for the survival of the neural crest progenitors and for neural crest proliferation. The disorder is an autosomal dominant condition.

Fetal alcohol spectrum disorder (FAS)

Caused by the mother drinking more than four standard units of alcohol per day during pregnancy, about 33% of children have FAS from alcoholic mothers, and it is one of the most important human teratogenic conditions known today. The effects of alcohol are, of course, dose dependent and related to the time when the fetus was exposed. The risk to the fetus relates to the fact that it does not have significant capacity for the detoxification of ethanol. FAS manifests itself in many different ways, from general appearance, height and weight problems to low intelligence and behavioural problems. Many changes affect the head and face. There may be problems of sight and hearing and head size, including microcephaly, a low bridge to the nose, micrognathia and the presence of epicanthal folds near the eyes. Three classic FAS facial features have been described (Fig. 17.12):

- Thin vermilion of the lips
- A smooth, flattened philtrum
- Small palpebral fissures giving the appearance of decreased eye width

These features are often measured by diagnosticians to provide assessment of the degree of severity of FAS. There is evidence that 'dental age' (determined by investigating stages of tooth formation) is also affected by FAS. A mind map that covers development of the face, together with the jaws, tongue and palate, is located at the end of Chapter 20, page 380.

Further readings for this chapter can be found in the accompanying eBook. Explore online Self-assessment quiz to test and reinforce your understanding of the material in your free ebook. Follow instructions in the Inside Front Cover to unlock your access.

Development of the palate

18

General development of palate

The definitive palate (or secondary palate) appears in the human foetus between the sixth and eighth weeks of intra-uterine life (1 week later for females). Palatogenesis is a complex event and is often disturbed, producing the congenital defect known as *cleft palate* (see pages 369–370). Consequently, the events and mechanisms responsible for the development of the palate have been much studied, although some controversy remains.

By the sixth week of development (Fig. 18.1), the primitive nasal cavities are separated by a primary nasal septum and are partitioned from the primitive oral cavity by a primary palate. Both the primary nasal septum and the primary palate are derived from the frontonasal process. The stomodeal chamber is divided at this stage into the small primitive oral cavity beneath the primary palate and the relatively large oronasal cavity behind the primary palate. As shown in Fig. 18.2, during the sixth week of development, two lateral palatal shelves develop behind the primary palate from the maxillary processes. A secondary nasal septum grows down from the roof of the stomodeum behind the primary nasal septum, thus dividing the nasal part of the oronasal cavity into two. Evidence suggests that the mesenchyme within the palatal shelves originates from the neural crest.

During the seventh week of development, the oral part of the oronasal cavity becomes completely filled by the developing tongue (Fig. 18.3). Growth of the palatal shelves continues such that they come to lie vertically. This orientation is characteristic of mammalians, but the reason for this is unknown. It has been suggested that the potential space in the oronasal cavity is insufficient because of the evolution of a large tongue in mammals. Two peaks of DNA synthesis occur as the palatal shelves are formed: during initial shelf outgrowth and during vertical shelf elongation.

During the eighth week of development (Fig. 18.4), the stomodeum enlarges, the tongue 'drops' and the vertically inclined palatal shelves become horizontal. It has been suggested that the descent of the tongue is related to mandibular growth and/or a change in the shape of the tongue. On becoming horizontal, the palatal shelves contact each other (and the secondary nasal septum) in the midline to form the definitive (or secondary) palate. The shelves contact the primary palate anteriorly so that the oronasal cavity becomes subdivided into its constituent oral and nasal cavities (Fig. 18.5). After contact, the medial edge epithelia of the two shelves fuse to form a midline epithelial seam. Subsequently, this seam degenerates so that mesenchymal continuity is established across the now intact and horizontal secondary palate. Fusion of the palatal processes is complete by the 12th week of development. Behind the secondary nasal septum, the palatal shelves fuse to form the soft palate and uvula.

Recent research on palatogenesis has concentrated on two main events: palatal shelf elevation and the initial stages of fusion of the shelves.

Palatal shelf elevation

Elevation of the palatal shelves from the vertical to the horizontal position takes place very rapidly. Several mechanisms have been proposed to account for the rapid movement of the palatal shelves. Although it was once thought that extrinsic forces might be responsible (e.g., from forces derived from the tongue or jaw movements or as a result of differential pressures above and below the palatal shelves), research has primarily focused on the search for a force intrinsic to the palatal shelf and within its mesenchyme. It has been proposed that the intrinsic shelf elevation force might develop as a result of hydration of extracellular matrix components (principally hyaluronan) in the shelf mesenchyme, or as a result of mesenchymal cell activity. The intrinsic shelf elevating force might be

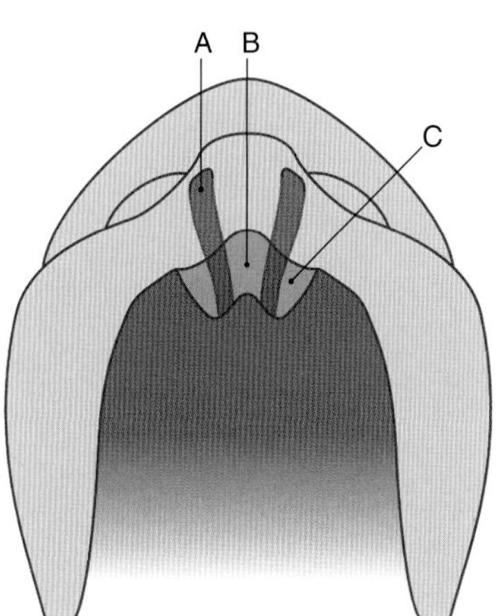

Fig. 18.1 The state of development of the palate by the sixth week of intra-uterine life. A = primitive nasal cavities; B = primary nasal septum; C = primary palate.

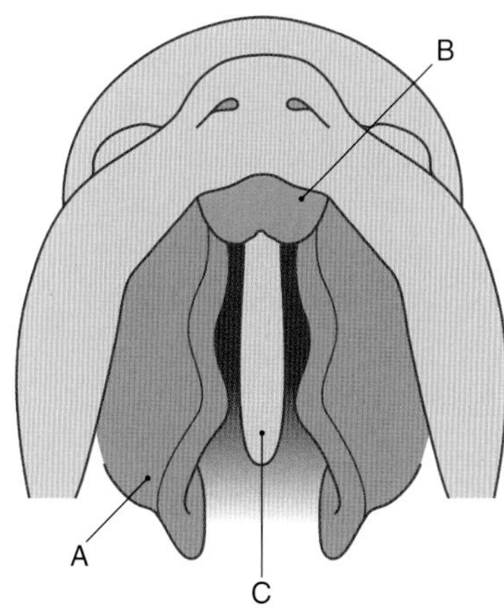

Fig. 18.2 The development of the palate during the sixth week of intra-uterine life. A = lateral palatal shelves; B = primary palate; C = secondary nasal septum.

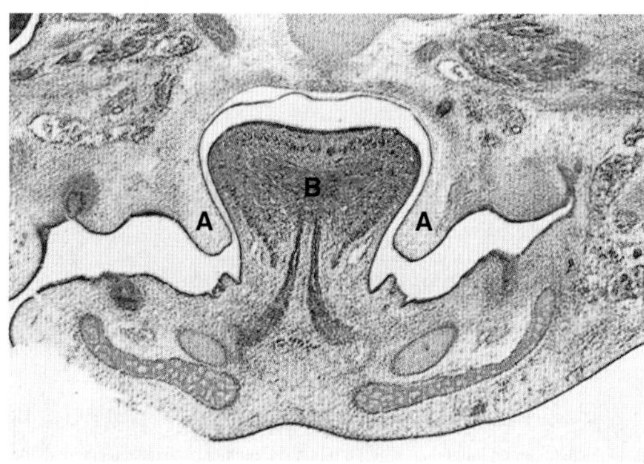

Fig. 18.3 Coronal section through the developing head during the seventh week of development showing the palatal shelves (A). B = developing tongue (Masson's trichrome; ×30).

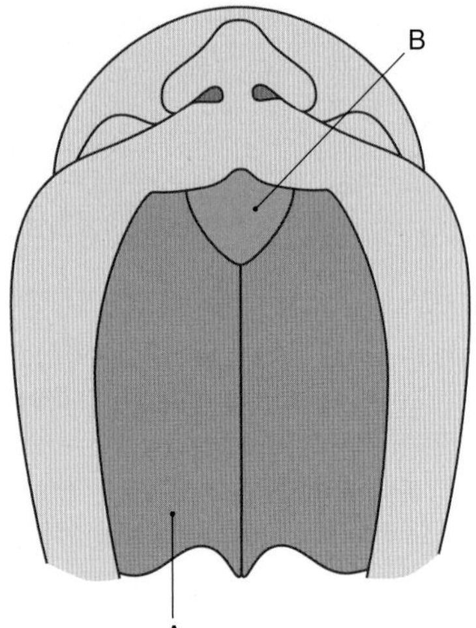

Fig. 18.4 The state of development of the palate during the eighth week of intra-uterine life. A = palatal shelves; B = primary palate.

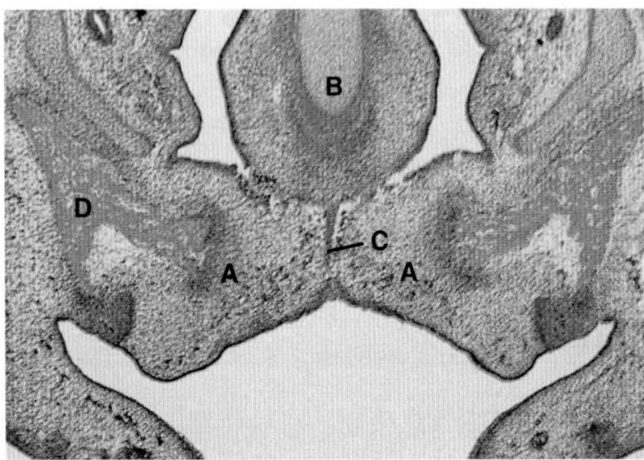

Fig. 18.5 Coronal section through developing oronasal regions following contact of the palatal shelves (A) and secondary nasal septum (B). C = midline epithelial seam; D = developing bone of maxilla (Masson's trichrome; ×30).

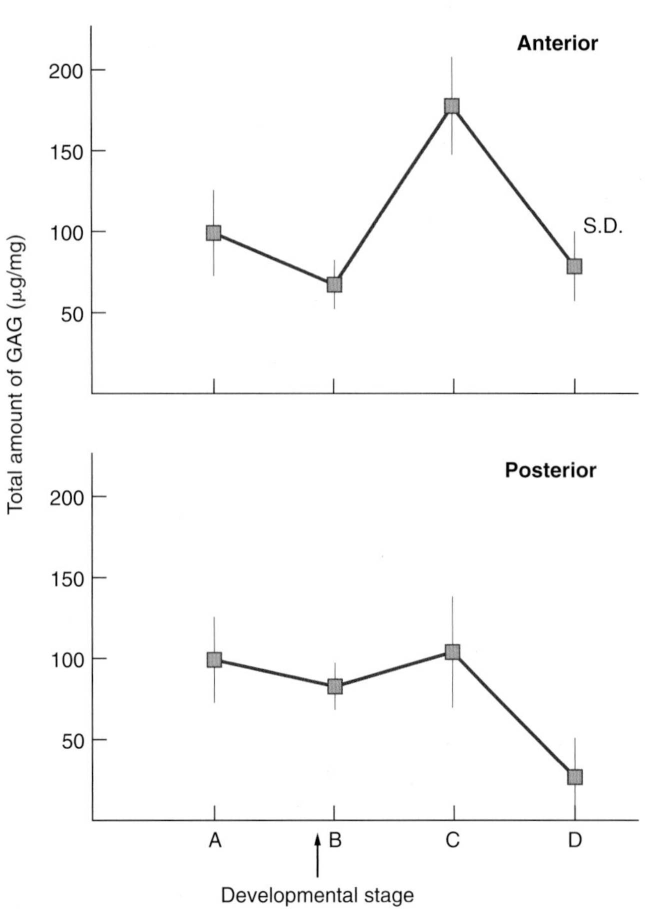

Fig. 18.6 Graphs illustrating the changing amounts of glycosaminoglycans (GAGs) during development of the anterior (presumptive hard) and posterior (presumptive soft) palates. Stage A = before shelf elevation; stage B = after shelf elevation; stage C = during shelf fusion and early histogenesis; stage D = a stage of marked histogenesis after fusion. Arrow indicates time of shelf elevation. Courtesy Dr. G D Singh and the editor of the *Archives of Oral Biology.*

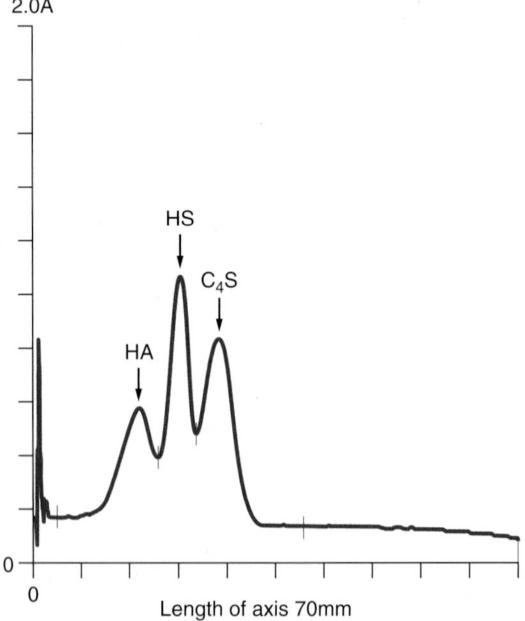

Fig. 18.7 Densitometric scan of electrophoretograms showing the GAGs within the palatal shelves *in vivo*. HA = hyaluronan; HS = heparan sulphate; C_4S = chondroitin 4-sulphate. Courtesy Dr. G D Singh and the editor of the *Archives of Oral Biology.*

multifactorial, although there is as yet no experimental evidence to support what otherwise might be considered this common-sense view.

The changing amounts of glycosaminoglycans (GAGs) during development of the anterior (presumptive hard) and posterior (presumptive soft) palates are illustrated in Fig. 18.6. Stage A occurs immediately before shelf elevation, stage B immediately after shelf elevation, stage C during shelf fusion and early histogenesis and stage D when there is marked histogenesis after fusion. The most significant changes occur after elevation: during the time of elevation, there are no differences between the anterior and posterior regions of the shelves even though, in the species studied in Fig. 18.6 (the rat), the posterior region of the shelf does not elevate but grows initially with a horizontal disposition. Three GAG types are found *in vivo*: hyaluronan, heparan sulphate and chondroitin 4-sulphate (Fig. 18.7). If palatal shelves are cultured *in vitro*, dermatan sulphate is also present, highlighting the difficulties of extrapolating from the findings of tissue culture to the *in vivo* situation.

A section through a vertical (pre-elevation) palatal shelf, stained using the hyaluronectin/antihyaluronectin technique, is shown in Fig. 18.8. Note the intense staining for hyaluronan within the palatal shelf mesenchyme. It has been proposed that hyaluronan is a GAG involved in shelf elevation because it is a highly electrostatically charged, open-coil molecule capable of binding up to 10 times its own weight in water. The changing concentrations of hyaluronan within the anterior and posterior regions of palatal shelves are illustrated in Fig. 18.9. The stages of palatogenesis (A–D) are the same as those described in Fig. 18.6. Note that, statistically, there is significantly more hyaluronan in the shelves immediately before elevation than immediately after; however, the data do not agree with some reports

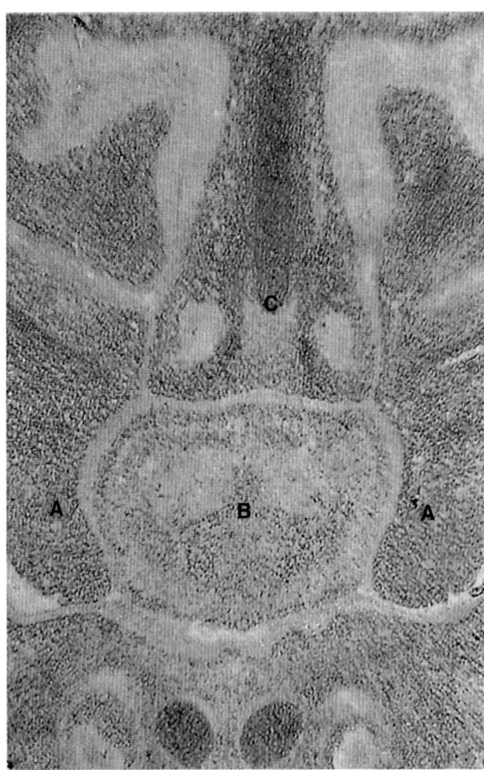

Fig. 18.8 Coronal section through a vertical (pre-elevation) palatal shelf (A) stained using the hyaluronectin/antihyaluronectin technique. Positive brown staining shows the presence of hyaluronan in shelf mesenchyme. B = tongue; C = nasal septum (×30). Courtesy Prof. M W J Fergusson.

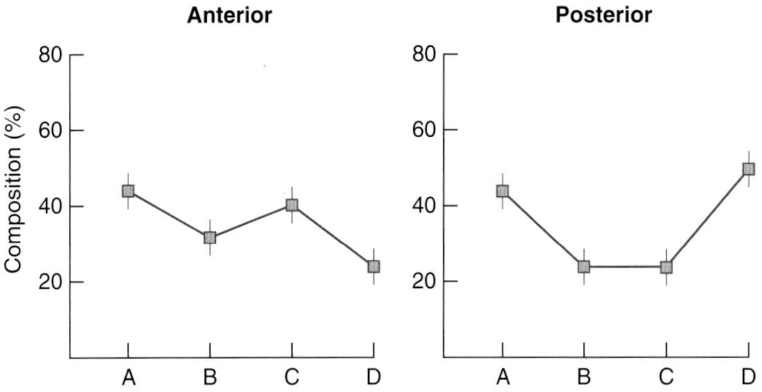

Fig. 18.9 Graphs showing the changing concentrations of hyaluronan within the anterior and posterior regions of palatal shelves. A–D = stages of palatogenesis described in Fig. 18.6. *From Singh, G.D., Moxham, B.J., Langley, M.S., Embery, G., 1994.* Changes in the composition of glycosaminoglycans during normal palatogenesis in the rat. *Archives of Oral Biology* 39, 401–407.

that there is less hyaluronan posteriorly than anteriorly, and again the pattern of change in hyaluronan is similar both anteriorly and posteriorly even though the posterior region does not undergo elevation to become horizontal.

Studies have revealed the presence during palatogenesis of enzymes associated with hyaluronan synthesis, of a cell-surface receptor associated with hyaluronan, of the hyaluronan-binding extracellular matrix components versican and hyaluronectin, and of hyaluronan binding sites (Fig. 18.10). Furthermore, using an organ-culture system (Figs. 18.11–18.14), palatogenesis is affected by agents that alter hyaluronan content or size, disrupt GAG substitution on proteoglycans or alter the balance of matrix molecules secreted via the Golgi apparatus and hyaluronan produced at the cell surface. However, while all agents prevent palatal fusion, there are variable effects on shelf elevation. For example, hyaluronidase digestion results in failure of elevation (Fig. 18.11), and treatment with a

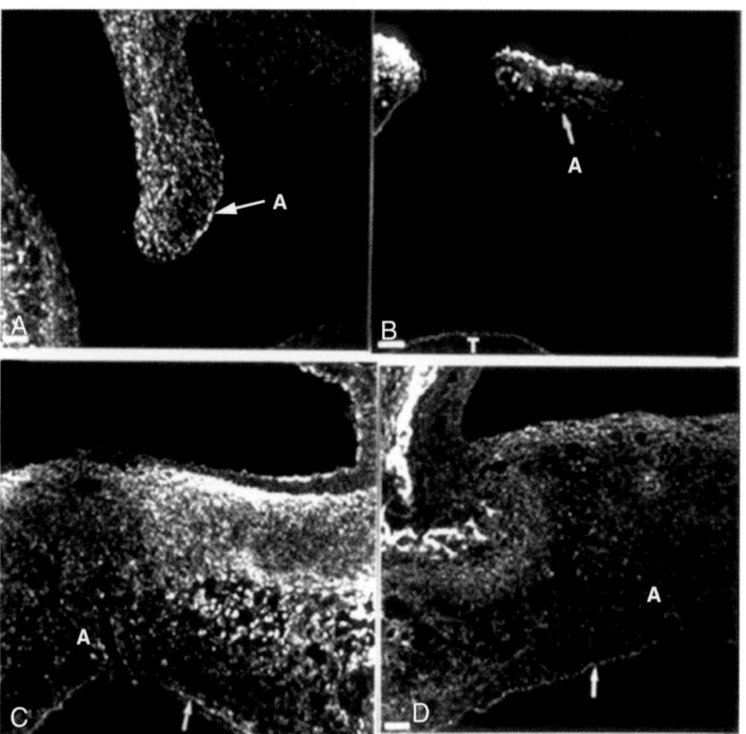

Fig. 18.10 The palatal shelves before (A) and after (B–D) elevation showing the presence of binding for the glycosaminoglycan hyaluronan (white label) using CD44 antibody immunohistochemistry. A = palatal shelves (fluorescent immunohistochemistry; ×80). Courtesy S Thomas, R Hall and B J Moxham.

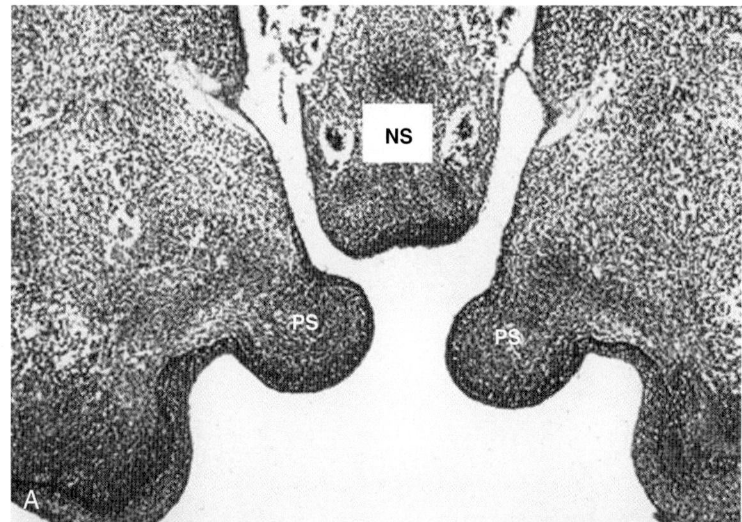

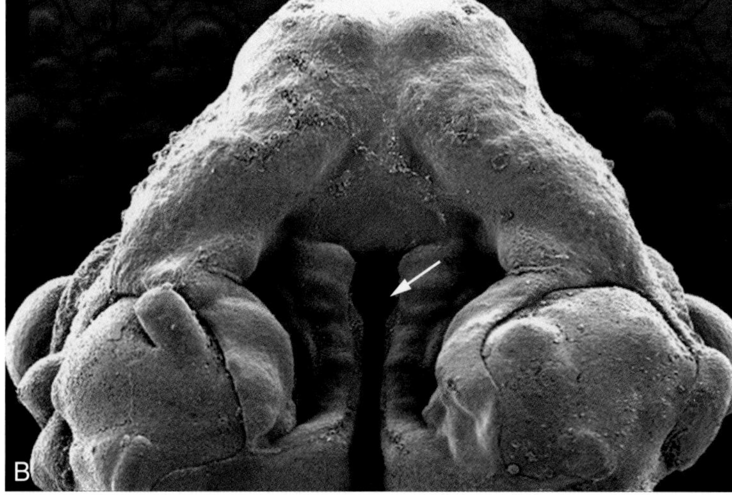

Fig. 18.11 The effects of *Streptomyces* hyaluronidase on the developing palate in organ culture. Clefts are produced, suggesting that palate development is disrupted in the absence of the glycosaminoglycan hyaluronan. (A) Section through a cleft palate resulting from hyaluronidase treatment. NS = nasal septum; PS = unfused palatal shelves (×60). (B) SEM showing the cleft (arrowed) (×30). Courtesy S Thomas, R Hall and B J Moxham.

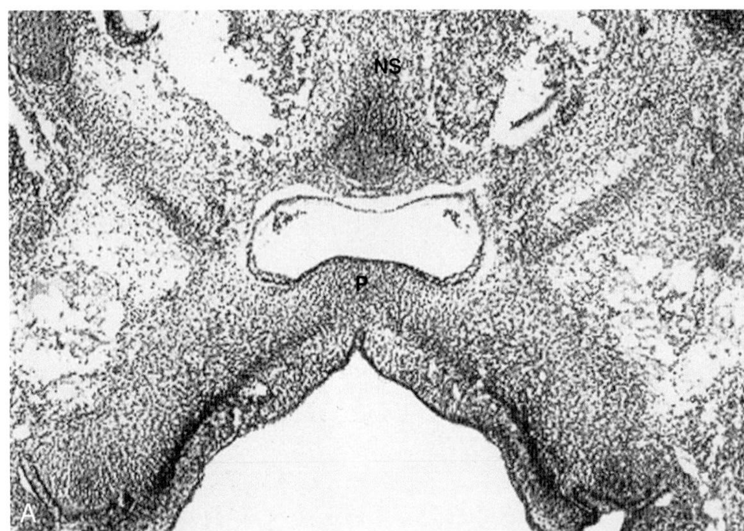

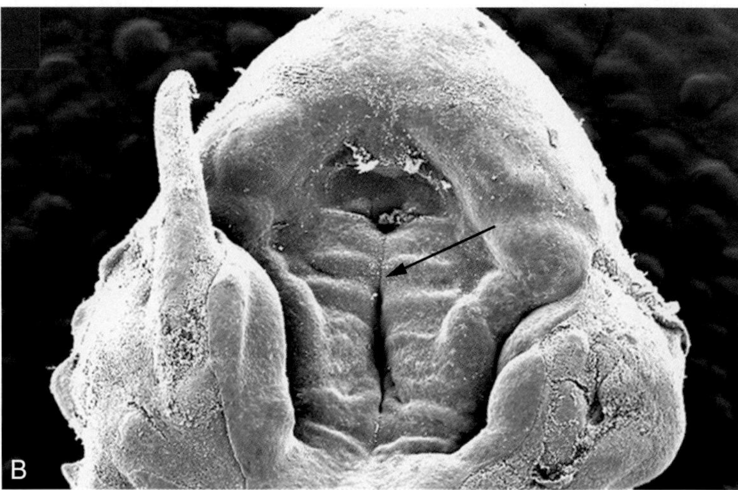

Fig. 18.12 The effects of UDP-xylose on the developing palate in organ culture. UDP-xylose is a natural inhibitor of UDPGD, the enzyme responsible for the conversion of UDP-glucose to UDP-glucuronic acid. Normal palatogenesis with UDP-xylose suggests that inhibition of UDPGD has no effect on palate development or that it may not be entering the tissue. (A) Section through a normally developing palate following UDP-xylose treatment. NS = nasal septum; P = fused palatal shelves (×50). (B) SEM showing normal palatogenesis (arrowed) (×25). Courtesy S Thomas, R Hall and B J Moxham.

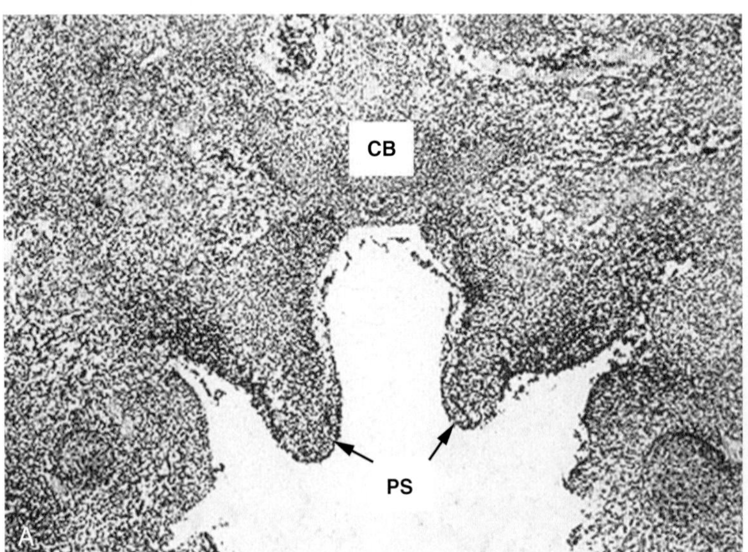

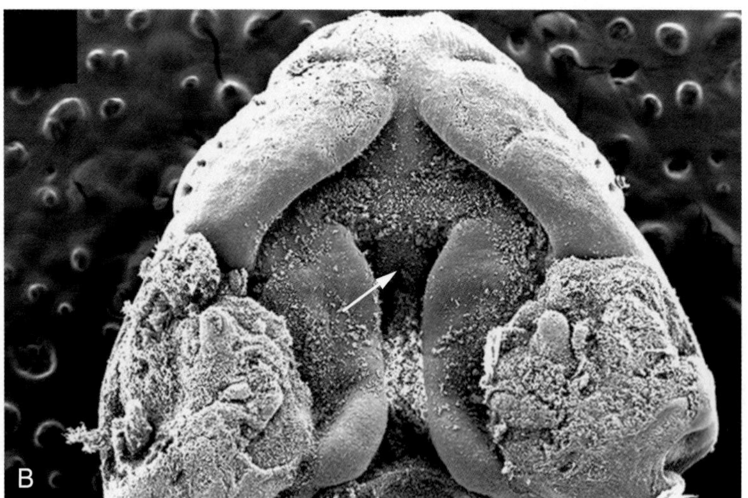

Fig. 18.13 The effects of chlorcyclizine (CHLR) on the developing palate in organ culture. CHLR enhances degradation of hyaluronan and chondroitin sulphate to lower-molecular-weight products, with little effect on their synthesis and on DNA synthesis. Clefts are produced, suggesting that the size of the glycosaminoglycan chain may influence palatogenesis. (A) Section through a cleft palate resulting from CHLR treatment. CB = cranial base; PS = unfused palatal shelves (×50). (B) SEM showing the cleft (arrowed) (×25). Courtesy S Thomas, R Hall and B J Moxham.

drug that blocks secretion from the Golgi apparatus, while still allowing hyaluronan production, also prevents elevation (Fig. 18.14). On the other hand, displacement of nascent hyaluronan with oligosaccharides allowed elevation (although the shelves were incorrectly oriented) (Fig. 18.12), and treatment with an agent that disrupts GAG assembly on proteoglycans resulted in abnormal elevation (Fig. 18.13). Overall, therefore, research indicates that hyaluronan is crucial to shelf elevation. To add to such findings, a reduced-molecular-weight hyaluronan leads to palate dysmorphogenesis (Fig. 18.13), suggesting that a minimum hyaluronan size is required to achieve normal palatogenesis.

Other matrix components, including proteoglycans, are of importance to shelf elevation. Versican and decorin have been identified at a range of molecular weights corresponding to various processed forms (Fig. 18.15). Link protein is absent within the mesenchyme of the palatal shelves (although present in other parts of the developing mouth) (Fig. 18.16). This could be important, since link protein 'stabilises' proteoglycans in the extracellular matrix, and its absence could mean that there is greater aggregation and disaggregation of the proteoglycans as palatogenesis proceeds. The role of collagen within the palatal shelves is disputed, although immunocytochemically, type I collagen can easily be identified (Fig. 18.17). Stout bundles of collagen can be seen running down the centre of the palatal shelf, oriented from the base towards the tip of the shelf. It has been suggested that the shelf elevation force is directed by these collagen fibres.

The role of the mesenchymal cells within the palatal shelves has also attracted some controversy. There is evidence that a critical number of cells is required for palatal shelf elevation to occur, but there is no reliable evidence that these cells, by their rapid division and proliferation and by migration or by contraction, can affect a palatal shelf elevation force (particularly in view of the rapidity of shelf elevation). Using a special silver staining technique, the degree of activity of the mesenchymal cells in the palatal shelf mesenchyme can be assessed. To determine whether cell activity changes at different stages of palatogenesis, the

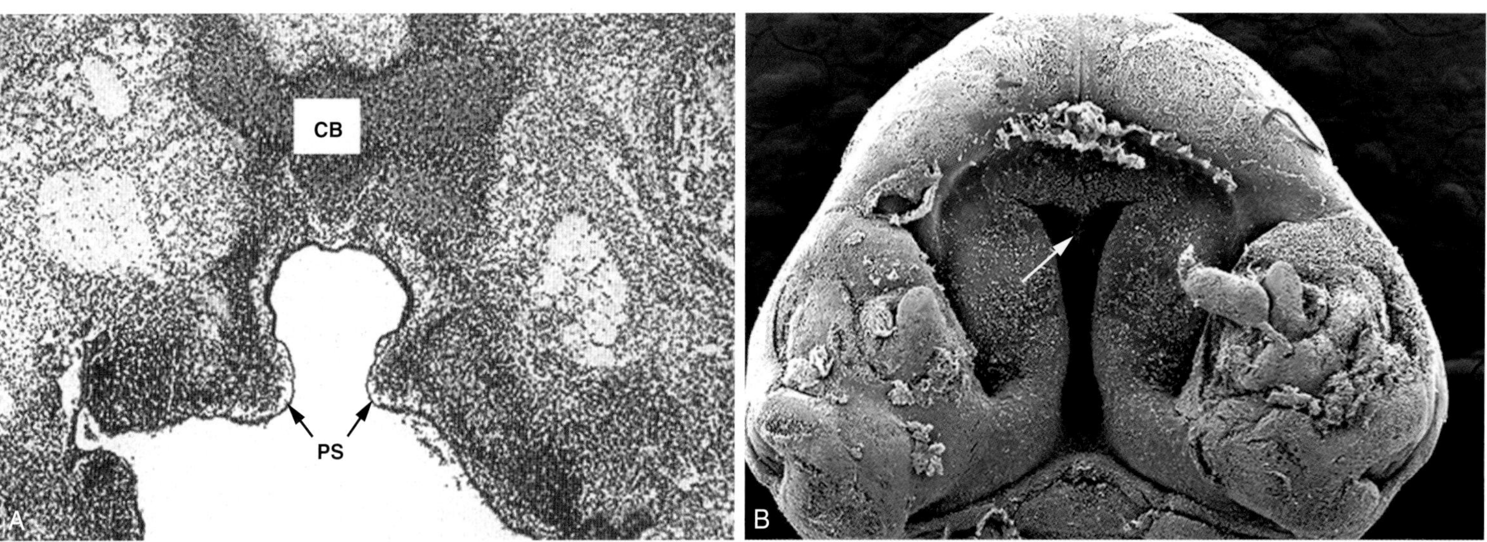

Fig. 18.14 The effects of brefeldin A (BFA) on the developing palate in organ culture. BFA inhibits vesicular transport through the Golgi apparatus. Hyaluronan synthesis is not affected, as this GAG, unlike other GAGs, undergoes a different synthetic pathway at or near the plasma membrane. Clefts are produced, suggesting that a set of macromolecules other than hyaluronan and synthesised in the Golgi play an important role in normal palatogenesis. (A) Coronal section through a cleft palate resulting from BFA treatment. CB = cranial base; PS = unfused palatal shelves (×50). (B) SEM showing the cleft (arrowed) (×25). Courtesy S Thomas, R Hall and B J Moxham.

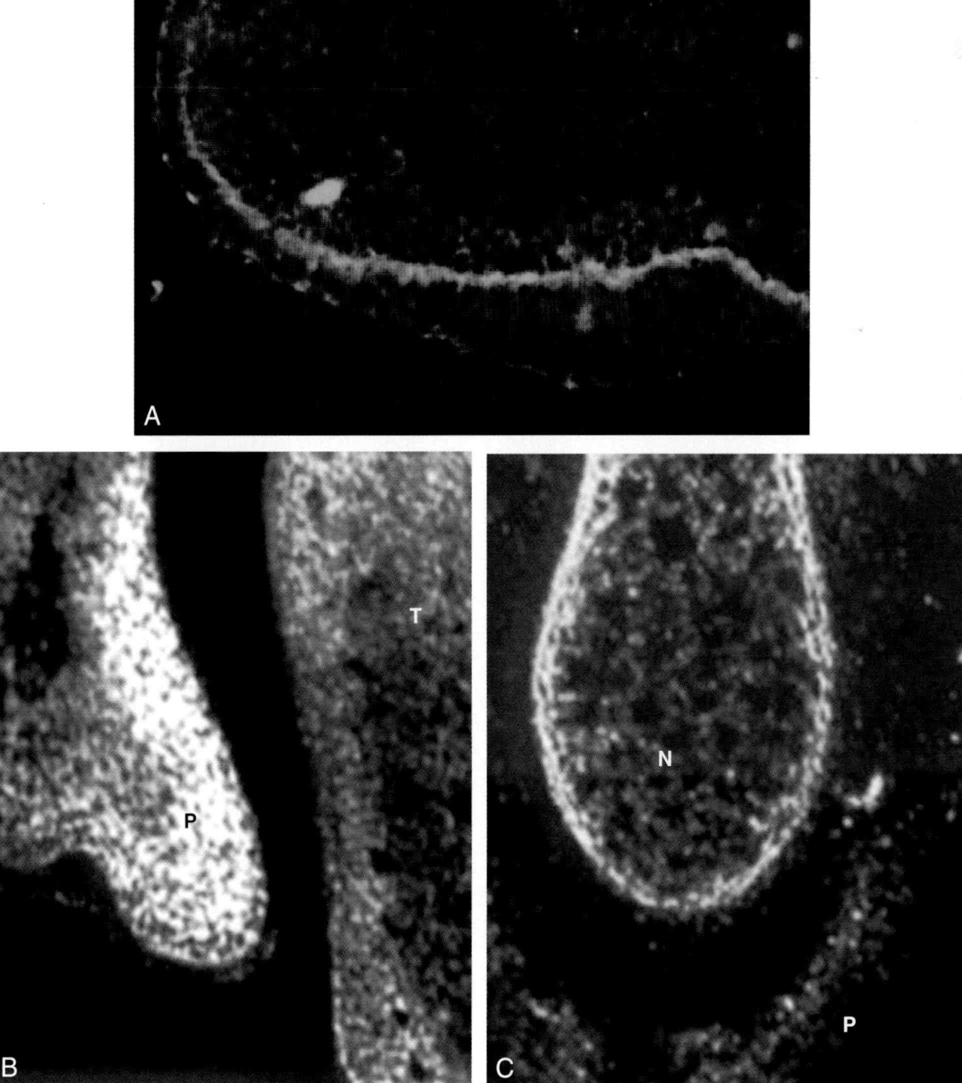

Fig. 18.15 The presence of some proteoglycans during normal palatogenesis. (A) Decorin (green labelling) beneath the lining epithelial cells of the palatal shelf pre-elevation (biglycan is not found). Note that decorin relocates to the centre of the shelf mesenchyme postelevation (fluorescence immunohistochemistry; ×240). (B) Versican (white labelling) in the palatal shelves (P); T = tongue (fluorescence immunohistochemistry; ×140). (C) Link protein (white labelling) found in the developing nasal septum (N) but absent in the palatal shelf (P), indicating that the proteoglycans within the shelf are 'labile' (fluorescence immunohistochemistry; ×60). Courtesy S Thomas, R Hall and B J Moxham.

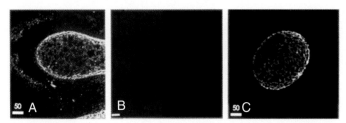

Fig. 18.16 Use of 8-A-4 antibodies to recognise link protein immunohistochemically. Immunopositivity (white labelling) is observed in the cartilages of the nasal septum (A) and Meckel's cartilage (C) but is absent from the developing palate, both before and after shelf elevation (B) (bar = 50 μm). Courtesy S Thomas, R Hall and B J Moxham.

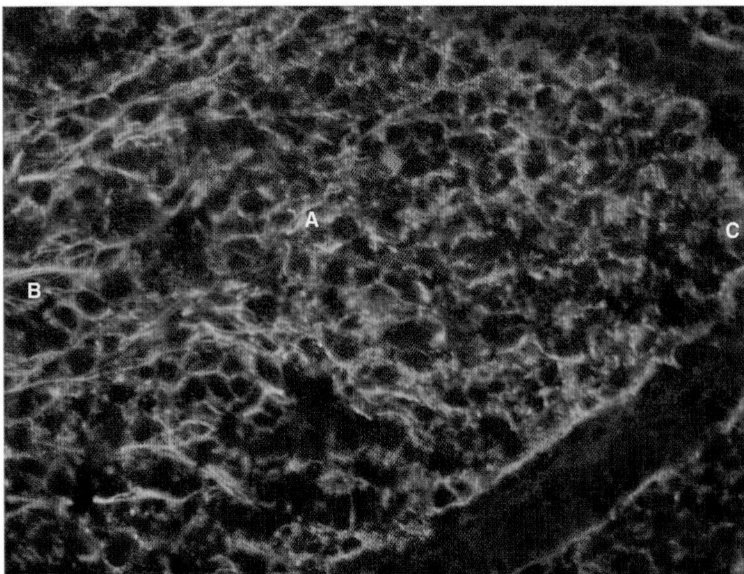

Fig. 18.17 Coronal section of a palatal shelf labelled immunocytochemically with antibodies against type I collagen showing positive green labelling throughout. A = collagen bundles; B = base of palatal shelf; C = tip of palatal shelf (×240). Courtesy Prof. M W J Fergusson.

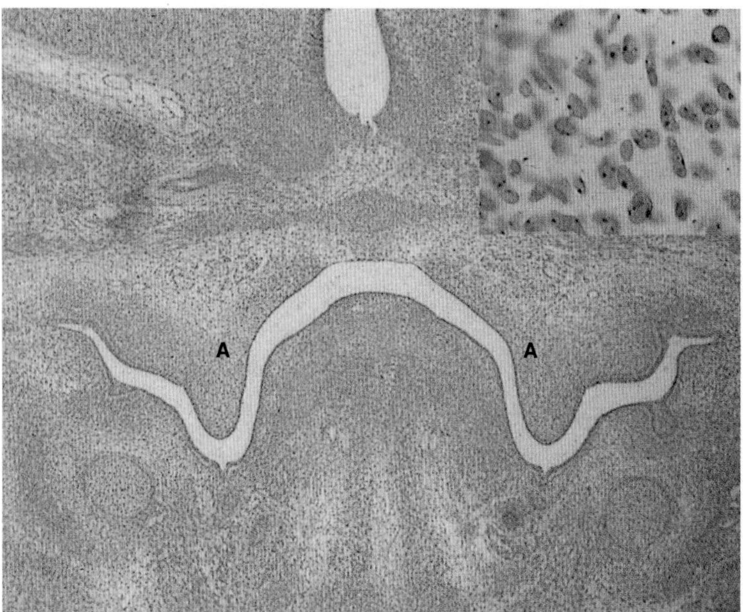

Fig. 18.18 Ag–NOR staining of the palatal shelves (A) to assess the degree of activity of the mesenchymal cells (silver stain; ×45). Inset shows black silver grains at higher power (×400).

silver-binding nucleolar organiser region (AgNOR) staining technique has been employed; this produces grains in the nucleolar region (Fig. 18.18). The number and configuration of these grains reflect the overall degree of protein synthesis by the cells. This staining procedure confirms that the rate of protein synthesis during palatogenesis is high, is higher pre-elevation than postelevation and is higher still during later stages of histogenesis. These results accord with the changes occurring in GAG synthesis at various stages of palatogenesis. The staining technique is, however, unable to demonstrate major differences between anterior and posterior regions within the rat foetus, where differences might have been expected. Quantitative electron microscopy of the cells within the palatal shelves has also not produced evidence that such cells can generate a shelf elevation force. Research has been undertaken to study the cell surface receptors for hyaluronan (CD44 receptors), and there is evidence that there is a transient and dynamic expression of CD44 splice variants during palatogenesis, particularly after shelf elevation. This suggests that although hyaluronan in the palatal shelves is most often associated with the development of a turgor pressure for shelf elevation via attraction of water molecules, this GAG might also influence cellular activity. For example, hyaluronan produces large intercellular spaces during early palatogenesis to prevent cell-to-cell and cell-to-matrix interactions, allowing assembly of extracellular constituents and presentation of growth factors that in turn influence cell growth and differentiation by altering the local concentration of intercellular signals. Following shelf elevation, there is a decline in hyaluronan shelf content, probably via CD44 receptor–mediated endocytosis of hyaluronan and via hyaluronidases that produce shorter hyaluronan chains. This enables the onset of palatal tissue differentiation. Hyaluronan that is taken up into cells can bind to intracellular hyaluronan binding proteins (e.g., receptor for hyaluronan-mediated motility [RHAMM]). Such binding induces cell signalling pathways that can, in turn, induce changes in the cytoskeleton. During differentiation, the intercellular matrix becomes denser where hyaluronan is replaced by proteoglycans, but the remaining hyaluronan binds to such proteoglycans (including hyaluronan-binding proteins such as versican, cell surface RHAMM and CD44) to form a stable extracellular matrix.

There have been many attempts to demonstrate active directional cell migration in the palatal shelves. Studies suggest that there are tissue and molecular heterogeneities in the shelves along the anteroposterior axis. Indeed, the mesenchymal cells in the anterior part of the palatal shelf migrate towards the lateral margins, whereas the cells in the posterior part migrate anteriorly. In this regard the Wnt family of genes may have a role, it being reported that *Wnt5a* mice have deformed palates that might result from aberrant cell migration. However, compelling as these studies are, they do not yet provide evidence that the cell migration produces a shelf elevation force.

Fusion of the palatal shelves

Once the palatal shelves have elevated, they contact each other (initially in the middle third of the palate) and adhere by means of a 'sticky' glycoprotein, which coats the surface of the medial edge epithelia of the shelves. The epithelial cells develop desmosomes, and consequently an epithelial seam is formed (Fig. 18.19). The adherence of the medial edge epithelia is specific, as palatal epithelia will not fuse with epithelia from other sites (e.g., the tongue). This may be related to the fact that the protein associated with the formation of desmosomes (desmoplakin) appears specifically on the cell membranes of the medial edge epithelia just before shelf contact.

Disruption of the epithelial seam, with penetration by mesenchymal cells, is shown in Fig. 18.20, although the signals that are responsible for

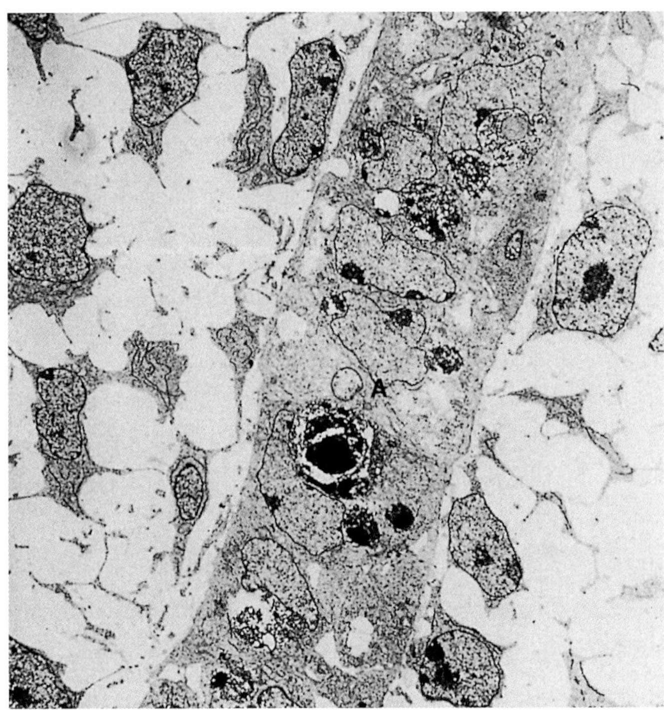

Fig. 18.19 TEM showing the midline epithelial seam for early fusing palatal shelves. An intact basal lamina lies on either side of the epithelial seam. A = epithelial cells (×3,900). Courtesy Prof. M W J Fergusson.

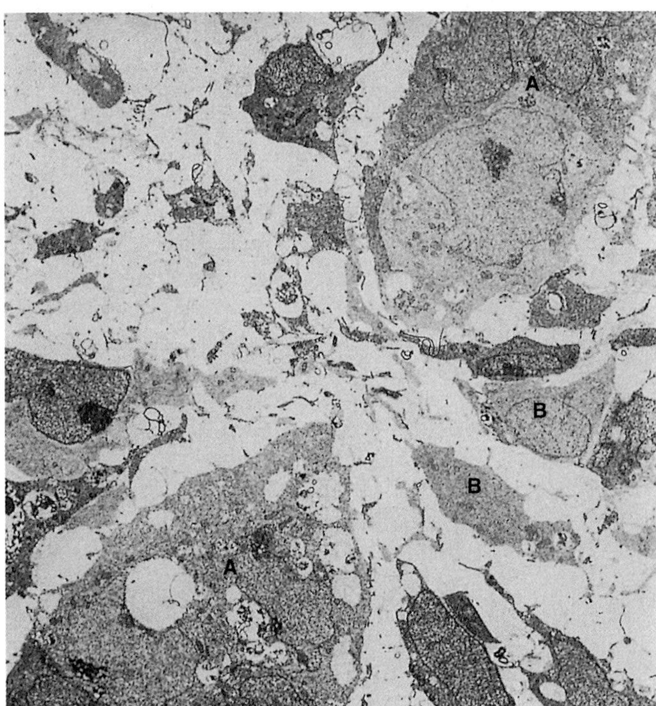

Fig. 18.20 TEM showing disruption of the epithelial seam (A) with penetration by mesenchymal cells (B) (×3,900). Courtesy Prof. M W J Fergusson.

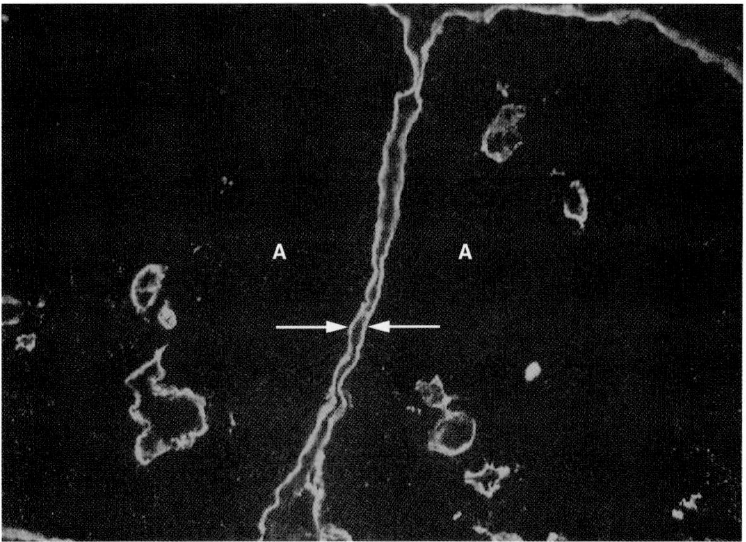

Fig. 18.21 Fusing palatal shelves (A) immunocytochemically labelled with antibodies against type IV collagen showing positive green labelling in basal lamina (arrowed) (×90). Courtesy Prof. M W J Fergusson.

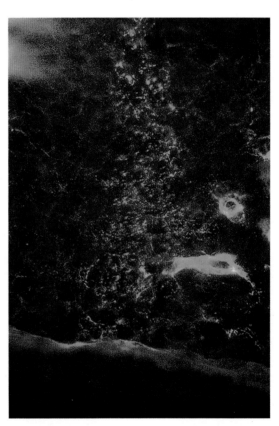

Fig. 18.22 Late stage of fusion of the palatal shelves immunocytochemically labelled for type IV collagen and showing disruption of the positively green-labelling midline epithelial seam; compare with Fig. 18.21 (×180). Courtesy Prof. M W J Fergusson.

such breakdown are not yet fully understood. Nevertheless, the breakdown of the basal lamina is likely to be a significant event. At this early stage of fusion (Fig. 18.21), the basal lamina remains intact. At a later stage of fusion (Fig. 18.22), with migration of the epithelial cells into the mesenchyme, the midline epithelial seam is disrupted and the migrating cells initially carry with them fragments of the disrupted basal lamina. Fibrils comprising tenascin and type III collagen have been shown to run at right angles to the basal lamina and may provide guiding pathways for the migrating epithelial cells. Evidence indicates that the events leading to the breakdown of the epithelial seam occur in single isolated palatal shelves and therefore do not depend upon shelf contact.

Almost as soon as the epithelial seam is formed, it thins to a layer two or three cells thick. This thinning may be the result of three processes:

1) The seam is thinned by growth of the palate (in terms of oronasal height) and by epithelial cell migration from the region of the seam onto the oral and nasal aspects of the palate.
2) There is programmed cell death (apoptosis) in the seam. This is shown by the finding that DNA synthesis ceases in the medial edge of epithelial cells 1 day before shelf contact. Furthermore, cyclic

adenosine monophosphate (cAMP) levels increase just before shelf fusion: exogenous cAMP is associated with precocious cell death in the medial edge epithelia. It has also been shown that epidermal growth factor (EGF) inhibits medial edge cell death and that this inhibition is blocked by exogenous cAMP. Care must be taken, however, when interpreting the effects of cAMP because physiologically it is an intracellular messenger and may therefore be mediating differential gene expression triggered by other events occurring at the cell surface.

3) There has been the suggestion that some of the epithelial cells migrate from the seam into the palatal shelf mesenchyme and differentiate into cells indistinguishable from the mesenchymal cells. Indeed, it is well known that epithelial cells can migrate and differentiate into mesenchymal-like cells in other situations during development. However, by using genetic markers for epithelial cells, it has been possible to identify the fate of the midline epithelial seam cells, and it has been shown conclusively that there are no epithelial–mesenchymal transformations.

There have been many experiments to help clarify the nature of the epithelial–mesenchymal interactions during fusion of the palatal shelves. In the main, these experiments have involved the separation and then the recombination in culture of the epithelial and mesenchymal components of the shelves. Overall, these experiments have shown that, as with epithelial–mesenchymal interactions for later tooth development (see pages 388–394), it is the mesenchyme that signals epithelial differentiation and behaviour. The nature of this signal is controversial. Although it was once proposed that the palatal mesenchyme could signal epithelial differentiation directly by cell-to-cell contact, mesenchymal–epithelial cell contacts are very rare during palatogenesis. Recent evidence indicates that extracellular matrix molecules may provide the signal, and work has been undertaken to assess the role of type IX collagen (Figs. 18.23, 18.24). At the earliest stages before shelf elevation, the medial edges of the palatal shelves label poorly for type IX collagen compared with floor of the mouth epithelia (Fig. 18.23). Note that at this stage of fusion, type IX collagen appears around the surfaces of the medial edge epithelial cells (Fig. 18.24). Present-day thinking suggests that the control of the synthesis of type IX collagen is influenced by growth factors.

Immunocytochemical labelling with antibodies against EGF receptors of the mesenchymal cells adjacent to the midline epithelial seam of fusing palatal shelves is shown in Fig. 18.25. EGF, or its embryonic homologue known as transforming growth factor (TGF)-α, inhibits palatal medial edge epithelial cell death in the presence of mesenchyme. Furthermore, it has been shown that the synthesis of extracellular matrix molecules (including type IX collagen) is stimulated by factors such as TGF-α and TGF-β and is inhibited by fibroblast growth factors (FGFs). When palatal shelves are organ-cultured with EGF, the medial edge of the palatal shelf shows a nipple-like bulge, medial edge epithelial cell death is absent and the mesenchyme possesses increased quantities of extracellular matrix molecules. It has been proposed, therefore, that the palatal shelf mesenchyme produces growth factors that either directly signal epithelial differentiation or, by stimulating extracellular matrix production, indirectly influence differentiation through this matrix. The photomicrograph in Fig. 18.25 suggests that EGF receptors show regional heterogeneity and that the receptors appear beneath the medial edge of the shelves only when the epithelial seam is degenerating.

Once fusion is complete, the hard palate ossifies intramembranously from four centres of ossification, one in each developing maxilla and one in each developing palatine bone. The maxillary ossification centre lies above the developing deciduous canine tooth germ and appears in the eighth week of development (Fig. 18.5). The palatine centres of ossification are situated in the region forming the future perpendicular plate and appear in the eighth week of development. Incomplete ossification of the palate from these centres defines the median and transverse palatine sutures. There does not appear to be a separate centre of ossification for the primary palate in humans (in other species, there being a separate

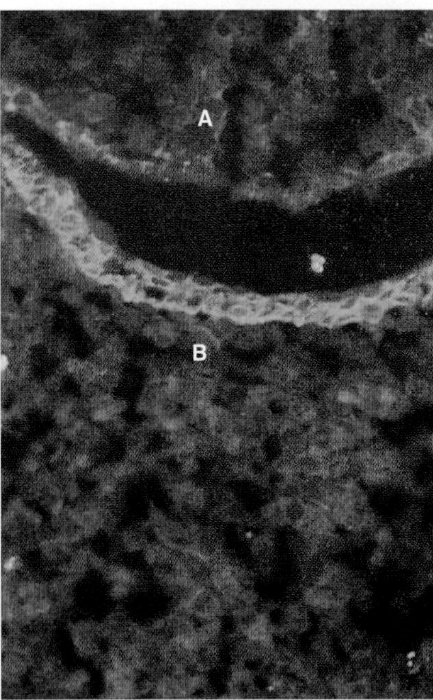

Fig. 18.23 The medial edge epithelia of palatal shelves (A) labelled immunocytochemically for type IX collagen before shelf elevation. Little positive green labelling is evident compared with the epithelium covering the floor of the mouth (B) (×280). Courtesy Prof. M W J Fergusson.

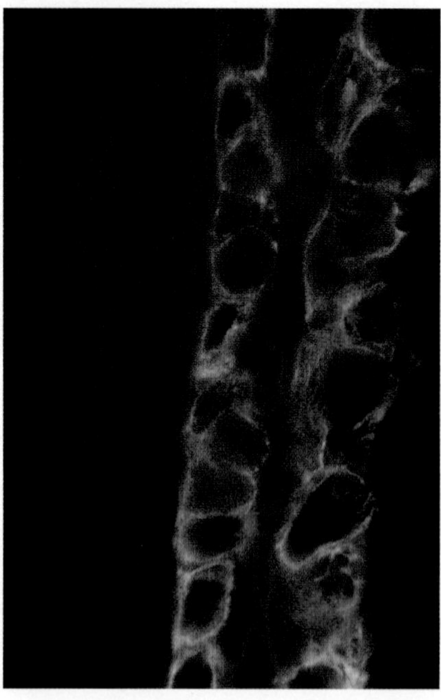

Fig. 18.24 The medial edge epithelia of palatal shelves labelled immunocytochemically for type IX collagen at a time when medial edge epithelial differentiation occurs. Compared with Fig. 18.23, positive green labelling is evident (×280). Courtesy Prof. M W J Fergusson.

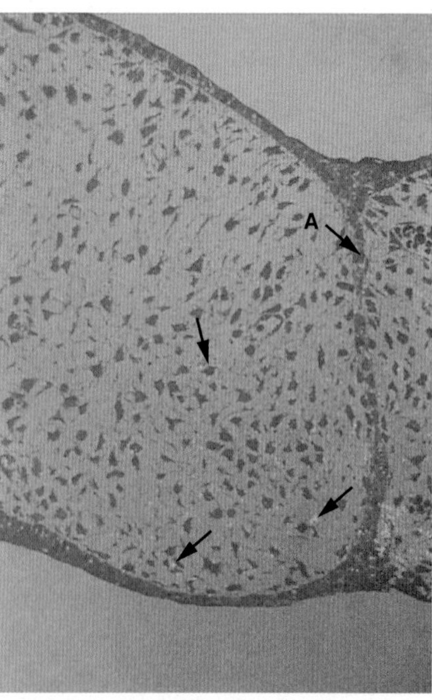

Fig. 18.25 Immunocytochemical labelling with antibodies against epidermal growth factor receptors of the mesenchymal cells adjacent to the midline epithelial seam of fusing palatal shelves. White dots indicate positive labelling (arrows). A = epithelial seam (×85). Courtesy Prof. M W J Fergusson and the editor of *Development*.

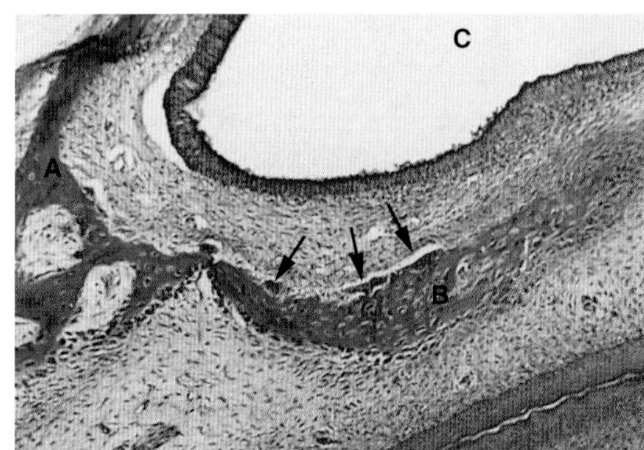

Fig. 18.26 Coronal section through the developing hard palate showing early ossification. A = developing body of maxilla; B = bone extending from body of maxilla into palate; C = nasal cavity. Note the osteoclasts on the nasal surface (arrowed) and osteoblasts on oral surface (Masson's trichrome; ×80).

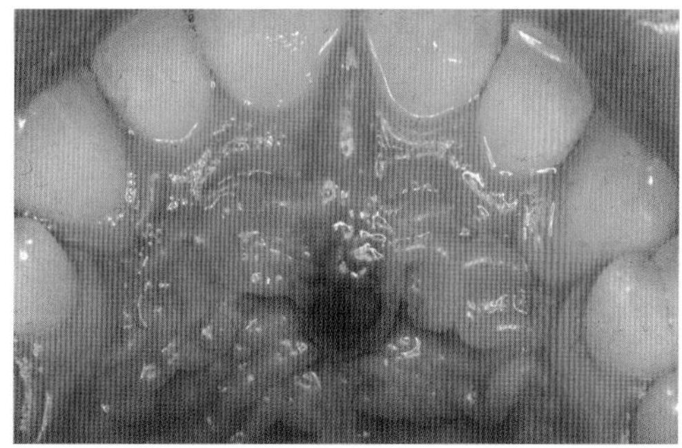

Fig. 18.27 Nasopalatine cyst evident as a bluish swelling in the anterior midline region of the palate. *Courtesy Dr. J Potts.*

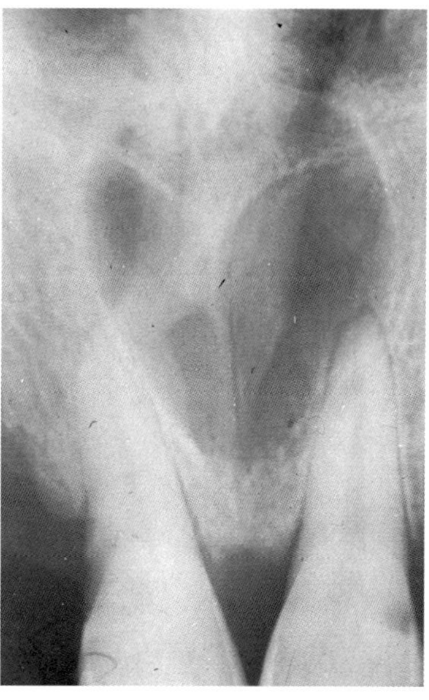

Fig. 18.28 Radiograph showing a heart-shaped radiolucent nasopalatine cyst in the anterior region of the maxillae. *Courtesy Dr. J Potts.*

'premaxilla'). Fig. 18.26 provides a coronal section through the developing hard palate to show early ossification.

Areas that remain unossified in the hard palate provide bony canals for the passage of nerves and vessels, namely the incisive canals combining to form an incisive fossa between the primary and secondary palate in the anterior midline and the greater and lesser palatine canals in the posterolateral region. During development, transient paired strands of epithelium are found in the region of the incisive canals termed *nasopalatine ducts*.

Clinical considerations

Palatal cysts

Remnants of the nasopalatine ducts may proliferate to give rise to non-neoplastic cysts that are considered to be the most common of the non-odontogenic cysts in the jaw region. Such cysts are found in the anterior midline region of the maxillae (Figs. 18.27, 18.28).

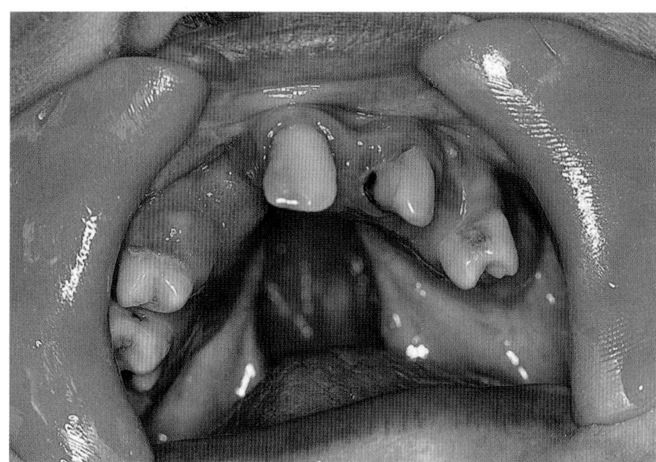

Fig. 18.29 Gross clefting of the palate. Courtesy Dr. B A W Brown.

Palatal clefts

Malformations of palatogenesis may result in the appearance of clefts. Palatal clefts are one of the most common congenital abnormalities (approximately 1:2,500 live births) and are more frequent in females (67%). Clefts may result from disturbances of any of the processes involved during palatogenesis (i.e., from defective palatal shelf growth, delayed shelf elevation or failure of elevation, defective shelf fusion or lack of degeneration of the midline epithelial seam or failure of mesenchymal consolidation and/or differentiation). The mildest form of cleft is that affecting only the uvula, with such a disturbance occurring relatively late in the process of palatal malfusion. Disturbances during the early phases of palatogenesis (e.g., during shelf elevation and early fusion) can result in a more extensive cleft involving most of the secondary palate. Should the cleft involve the primary palate, it may extend to the right and/or left of the incisive fossa to include the alveolus, passing between the lateral incisor and canine teeth. Cleft palate may be associated with cleft lip, although the two conditions are independently determined. Dental malformations are commonly associated with a cleft involving the alveolus. A submucous cleft describes a condition where the palatal mucosa is intact but the bone/musculature of the palate is deficient beneath the mucosa. Fig. 18.29 shows an extensive cleft of the palate, and Fig. 18.30 shows a cleft uvula. Less problematic than clefts (but more common) is the retention of epithelial remnants in the midline that may eventually become cystic (Fig. 18.31).

The most common problem experienced by people who have clefts of the palate is 'hypernasality' (a speech/resonance disorder caused by velopharyngeal [soft palate–pharyngeal] incompetence and characterised by air escaping through the nasal airway). Hypernasality can make speech incomprehensible and can severely affect quality of life and a person's self-esteem. Children with hypernasality can be 'judged' as unintelligent, unpleasant and unattractive and consequently as social outcasts.

Experiments have shown that clefts produced in animals are associated with the synthesis of much fewer GAGs than normally developing palates, although qualitatively the same types of GAG are still secreted, and the percentages of each of these GAGs are unaltered. The AgNOR staining technique referred to on page 366 further shows that protein synthesis is severely depressed during cleft formation.

Clefts of the palate, like those of the lip, are multifactorial malformations, involving both genetic (often polygenic) and environmental factors. The aetiology is not related to maternal age, and within a family with a child with a cleft, the probability of another child being affected is estimated as being 2%. Recent data show that clefts that are multifactorial are most common for clefts of the lip (67% of cases). Forty-one percent of cleft palates can be ascribed a multifactorial aetiology and 34% of submucous clefts are multifactorial in origin. Twenty percent of cleft

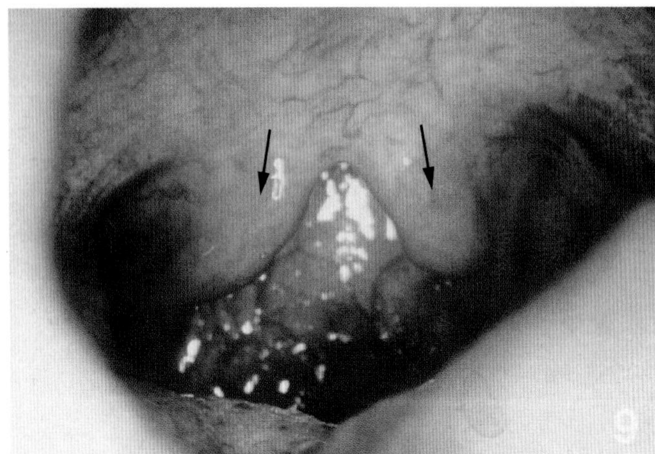

Fig. 18.30 A cleft uvula (arrows). Courtesy Dr. R W Pigott.

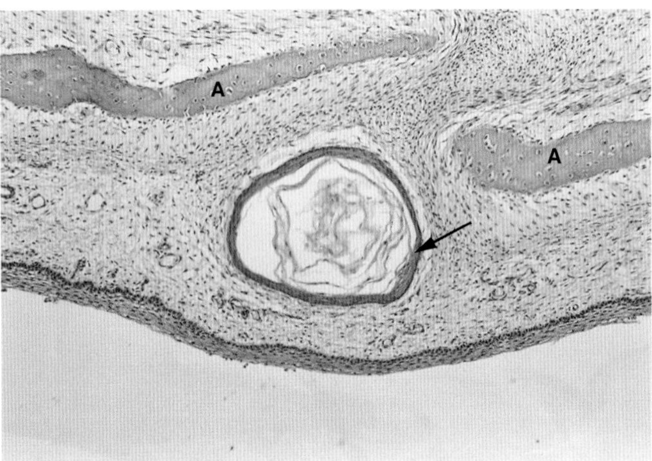

Fig. 18.31 Section through a developing midline palatine cyst (arrowed). A = bone of hard palate (H & E; ×40).

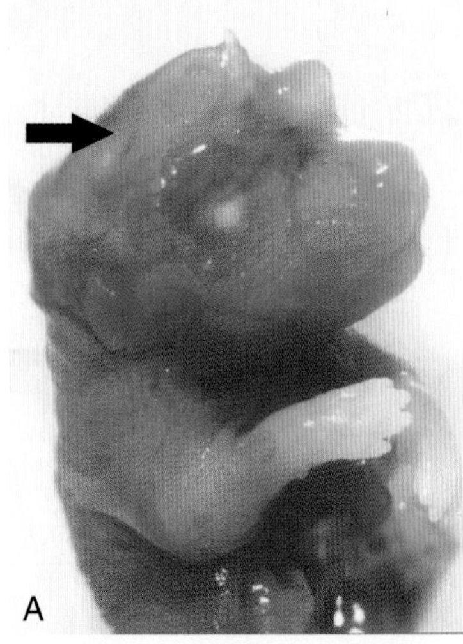

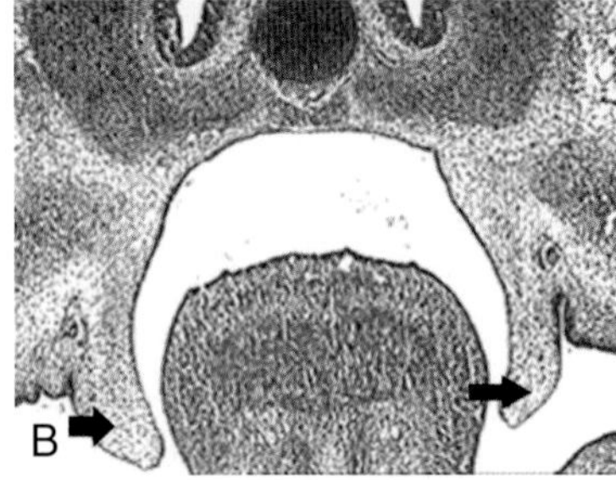

Fig. 18.32 The effects of high doses of all-*trans* retinoic acid on craniofacial development. (A) Fetal head showing exencephaly – the appearance of the brain close to the surface of the head (arrow). (B) Cleft of the palate produced by failure of elevation of the palatal shelves (arrows). Courtesy Gunston, E., Wise, M., Emmanouil-Nikoloussi, E.-N., Moxham, B.J., 2005. *European Journal of Anatomy* 9, 1–16.

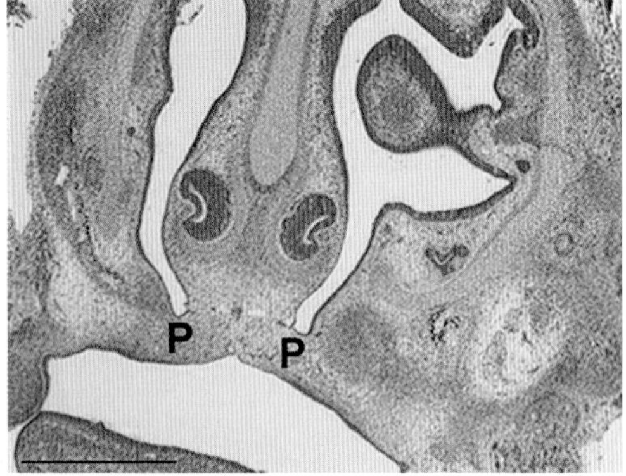

Fig. 18.33 Normally elevated and fused palatal shelves (P) resulting from supplementation of all-*trans* retinoic acid with calcium folinate. Note that, as shown in Fig. 18.32, all-*trans* retinoic acid alone would produce serious craniofacial abnormalities, including cleft palate. Courtesy L J Richardson, E-N Emmanouil-Nikoloussi and B J Moxham.

palates are monogenic, 5% are caused by teratogens, 1% are associated with chromosomal abnormalities and over 20% are of unknown aetiology. Concerning risk factors, smoking and alcohol abuse by the mother can increase the likelihood of clefting. Furthermore, drugs (both medical and recreational), some viruses and rubella infection can be associated with the development of a cleft. Some clefts may be caused by nutritional factors. For example, excessive vitamin A intake (retinoids) and deficiencies in folic acid can be related to clefting. Fig. 18.32 shows the effects on rat foetuss of large doses of all-*trans* retinoic acid, and Fig. 18.33 indicates that supplements of folinates can 'rescue' these disorders. Furthermore, a study of children in Greece suggests that, in terms of environmental influences on the development of palatal clefts, the occupation of the father (but not the mother) may be significant, particularly if he works with chemicals in heavy industry or in farming.

To date, there is a wealth of information concerning the molecular control of palatogenesis and therefore of the molecular influences on clefting. Overall, molecular control occurs by a complex series of epithelial–mesenchymal interactions. Cleft palate syndromes (as for cleft lip syndromes) seem to be associated in humans with polymorphisms in the *TGFA* gene that encodes TGF-α. Furthermore, EGF receptor inactivation produces clefts. Two relatively common syndromes involving clefts of the palate are Pierre Robin's sequence and Treacher Collins' syndrome (see pages 359–360).

Table 18.1 compares clefts of the upper lip and the palate.

Information regarding the development of the palate is available in Mind Map 20.1 (page 380).

Table 18.1 Clefts of the upper lip and of the palate

Cleft lip	Cleft palate
Unilateral or bilateral With or without cleft palate	Classification with reference to incisive fossa – anterior anomalies (primary palate) and posterior anomalies (secondary palate)
1:1,000 births	1:2,500 births
Mostly male infants	More common in females
67% with multifactorial aetiology	41% with multifactorial aetiology
Result of failure of fusion of mesenchymes in facial processes	Result of failure of elevation of palatal shelves (major clefts) or failure of fusion of shelves (minor clefts)

Further readings for this chapter can be found in the accompanying eBook. Explore online Self-assessment quiz to test and reinforce your understanding of the material in your free ebook. Follow instructions in the Inside Front Cover to unlock your access.

Development of the jaws

19

Introduction

Growth of the craniofacial skeleton influences jaw relationships, occlusal relationships and orofacial functions. Growth is both endochondral and intramembranous. While the mandible shows both types of growth, the maxilla is primarily intramembranous. The spheno-occipital synchondrosis contributes to the forward growth of the face and is mentioned on pages 328–329. A problem in studying growth occurring continuously in three dimensions is finding fixed points from which to measure, so that images taken at different times can be superimposed. One of the surest methods employed in human studies involved implanting small metal pins into cranial bones.

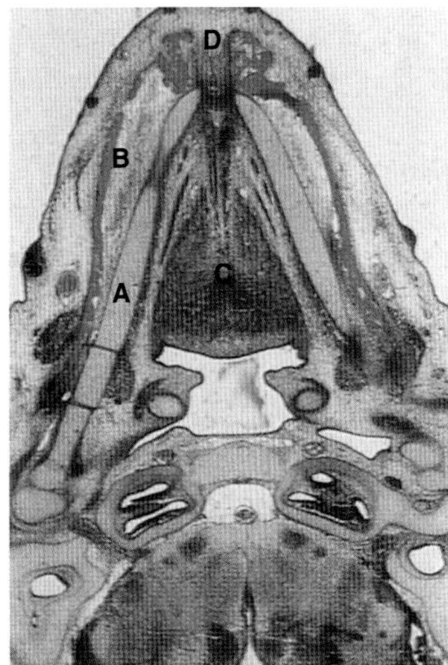

Fig. 19.1 Meckel's cartilage (A), around which the bone of the mandible (B) is forming in membrane. This is a horizontal section through the developing mandible during the eighth week of intrauterine life. Note that Meckel's cartilage extends from the cartilaginous otic capsule to the midline symphysis (D), where initially it is separated from its fellow of the opposite side by mesenchyme. C = tongue (Masson's trichrome; ×12).

The mandible

The mandible initially develops intramembranously, but its subsequent growth is related to the appearance of secondary cartilages (the condylar cartilage being the most important). The developing mandible is preceded by the appearance of a rod of cartilage belonging to the first pharyngeal arch. This is known as *Meckel's cartilage* (Figs. 19.1, 19.2), and it first appears at about the sixth week of intrauterine life. Meckel's cartilage extends from the cartilaginous otic capsule in the region of the developing ear to a midline symphysis. However, it makes little contribution to the adult mandible, merely providing a framework around which the bone of the mandible forms.

The mandible first appears as a band of dense fibrous tissue on the anterolateral aspect of Meckel's cartilage. During the seventh week of intrauterine life, a centre of ossification appears in this fibrous tissue at a site close to the future mental foramen. From this centre, bone formation spreads rapidly backwards, forwards and upwards and around the inferior alveolar nerve and its terminal branches (the incisive and mental nerves). Further spread of the developing bone in a forwards and backwards direction produces a plate of bone on the lateral side of Meckel's cartilage that corresponds to the future body of the mandible and extends towards the midline, where it comes to lie in close relationship with the bone forming on the opposite side. However, the two plates of bone remain separated by fibrous tissue to form the mandibular symphysis (Fig. 19.1). Experiments have shown that, in the absence of metalloproteinase activity, maturation and fusion of Meckel's cartilage segments are delayed (probably because of failure of the remodelling of the perichondrium that would allow cartilage elements to expand into the surrounding mesenchyme). Furthermore, where embryos lack epidermal growth factor (EGF) receptors, much lower amounts of metalloproteinases are expressed, and again there are developmental defects in the cartilage and mandible.

At a later stage in the development of the body of the mandible, continued bone formation markedly increases the size of the mandible, with development of the alveolar process occurring to surround the developing tooth germs (Fig. 19.3). At an even later stage, Meckel's cartilage resorbs (Fig. 19.4). The neurovascular bundle that initially was located with the developing tooth germs now becomes contained within its own bony canal, and there is considerable development of the alveolar process.

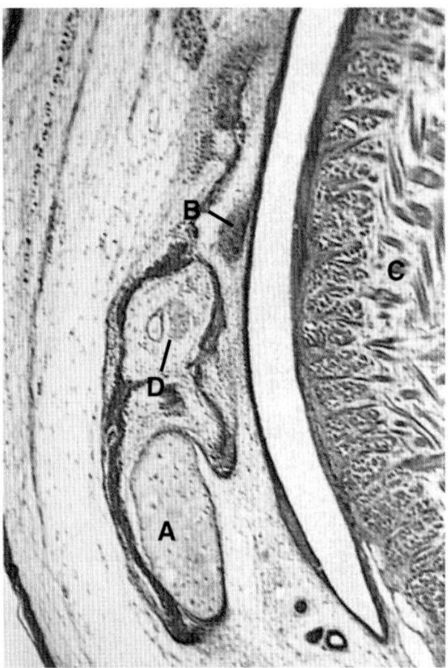

Fig. 19.2 Transverse section through the early developing mandible (eighth week of development). At this stage, only a small amount of mandibular bone has formed intramembranously on the lateral aspect of Meckel's cartilage (A). Note the beginnings of tooth development in this region as indicated by the dental lamina (B). C = tongue; D = neurovascular bundle (Masson's trichrome; ×60).

Although Meckel's cartilage contributes no significant tissue to the developing mandible, nodular remnants of cartilage may be seen in the region of the mandibular symphysis until birth and, in its most dorsal part, Meckel's cartilage ossifies to form ear ossicles (the malleus and incus). Behind the body of the mandible, the perichondrium of Meckel's cartilage persists as the sphenomandibular and sphenomalleolar ligaments. The sphenomandibular ligament ossifies at its sites of attachment to form the lingula of the mandible and the spine of the sphenoid bone.

As the developing tooth germs reach the bell stage (see pages 383–386), developing bone becomes closely related to them to form the alveolus (Figs. 19.4, 19.5). The size of the alveolus is dependent upon the size of the growing tooth germ. Resorption occurs on the inner wall of the alveolus (indicated by Howship's lacunae), while, on the outer wall of the alveolus, bone is deposited (indicated by osteoblasts lining an osteoid seam). The developing teeth therefore come to lie in a trough of bone. Later, the teeth become separated from each other by the development of interdental septa. With the onset of root formation, interradicular bone develops in multirooted teeth.

The ramus of the mandible is first mapped out as a condensation of fibrocellular tissue that, although continuous with the developing body of the mandible, is positioned some way laterally from Meckel's cartilage. Further development of the ramus is associated with a backward spread of ossification from the body and by the appearance of secondary cartilages. Between the 10th and 14th weeks *in utero*, three secondary cartilages develop within the growing mandible. The largest and most important of these is the condylar cartilage, which, as its name suggests, appears beneath the fibrous articular layer of the future condyle (see Figs. 15.22 and 19.7). Through proliferation and subsequent ossification, the cartilage is thought by some to serve as an important centre of growth for the mandible (functioning up to about the 16th year of life). The mandibular condyle in the child is discussed further on page 328. Less important, transitory, secondary cartilages are seen associated with the coronoid process and in the region of the mandibular symphysis. The appearance of the developing jaws of a human fetus at 14 weeks is shown in Fig. 19.6.

The temporomandibular joint (TMJ) develops from mesenchyme lying between the developing mandibular condyle below and the temporal bone above, which develops intramembranously. During the 12th week of intrauterine life, two clefts appear in the mesenchyme producing the upper and lower joint cavities. The remaining intervening mesenchyme becomes the intra-articular disc. The joint capsule develops from a condensation of mesenchyme surrounding the developing joint. At birth, the mandibular fossa is flat and there is no articular eminence; this eminence becomes prominent only following the eruption of the deciduous dentition. The early developing condylar cartilage and TMJ are shown in Fig. 19.7.

Fig. 19.8 illustrates the postnatal development of the mandible by lateral and occlusal views at birth, at 6 years and in an adult. The ratio of body to ramus is greater at birth than in the adult, indicating a proportional increase with time in the development of the ramus. At birth, there is no distinct chin and the two halves of the mandible are separated by the mandibular symphysis. Ossification of the symphysis is complete during the second year, with the two halves of the mandible uniting to form a single bone. The chin becomes most prominent after puberty (especially in the male). There is some evidence that the angle of the mandible decreases from birth to adulthood.

Some indication of the directions of growth of the mandible can be obtained by superimposing traces of neonatal and adult mandibles (Fig. 19.9). Indeed, there is some evidence that the region around the mental foramen is a 'fixed' point for such an endeavour.

Growth of the mandible occurs by the remodelling of bone. In general terms, increase in the height of the body occurs primarily by formation of alveolar bone, although some bone is also deposited along the lower border

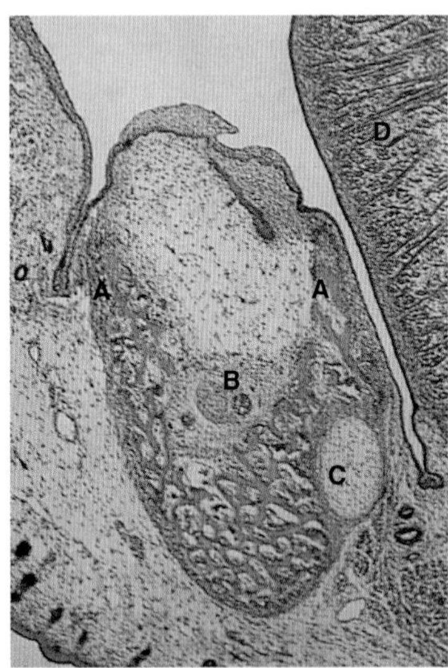

Fig. 19.3 A later stage in the development of the body of the mandible. Continued bone formation has increased the size of the mandible. The alveolar process (A) grows to surround the developing tooth germ. The developing teeth share the same common crypt as the neurovascular bundle (B). Note that Meckel's cartilage (C) is now comparatively small, although it still lies medial to the developing mandibular bone. D = developing tongue (Masson's trichrome; ×25).

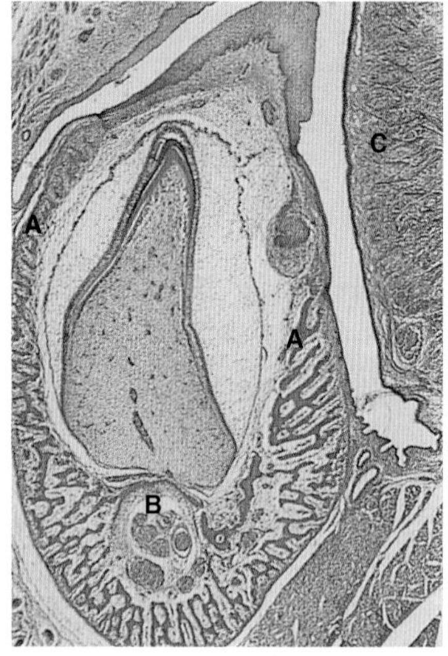

Fig. 19.4 An even later stage in the development of the body of the mandible. Meckel's cartilage has been resorbed. The neurovascular bundle (B) is now contained within its own bony canal, and there has been considerable development of the alveolar process (A). C = developing tongue (Masson's trichrome; ×25).

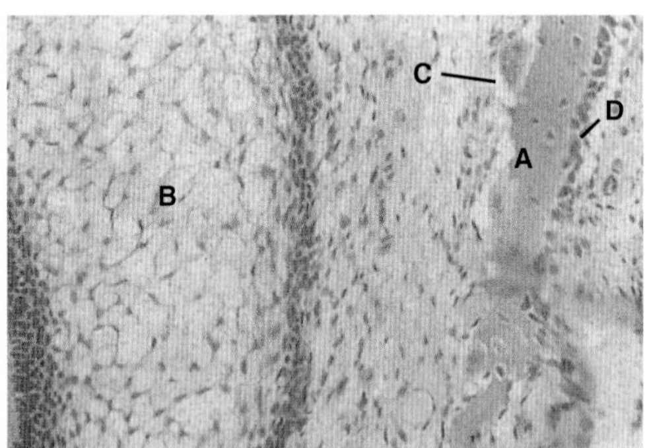

Fig. 19.5 Development of the mandibular alveolus (A) in the region of a developing tooth (B). Note that resorption is occurring on the inner wall of the alveolus, indicated by an osteoclast (C), while on the outer wall of the alveolus, bone is being deposited, indicated by osteoblasts (D) lining an osteoid seam (decalcified section; Masson's trichrome; ×110).

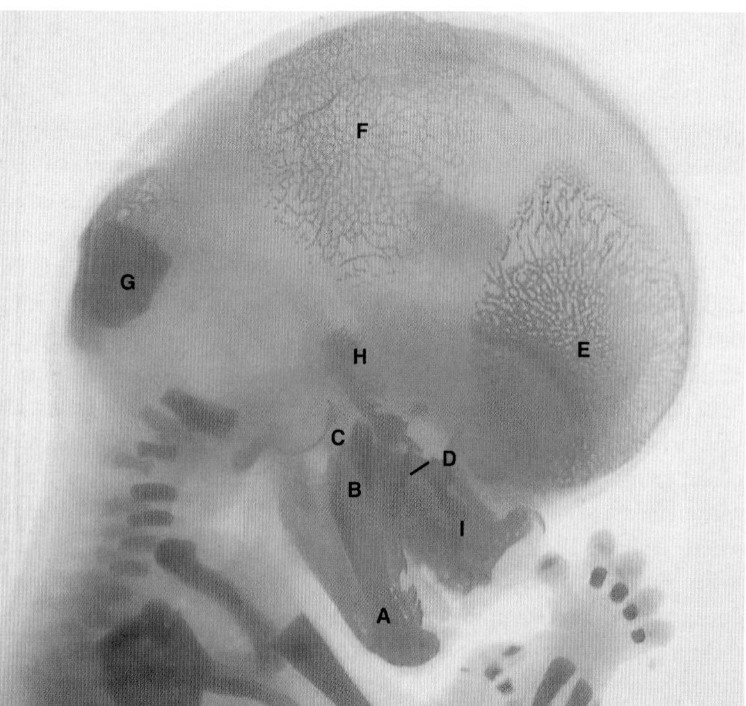

Fig. 19.6 The appearance of the developing jaws of a human fetus (14 weeks). A = body of mandible; B = ramus of mandible; C = secondary condylar cartilage; D = secondary coronoid cartilage; E = frontal bone; F = parietal bone; G = occipital bone; H = squamous portion of temporal bone; I = maxilla (cleared alizarin red preparation; ×5).

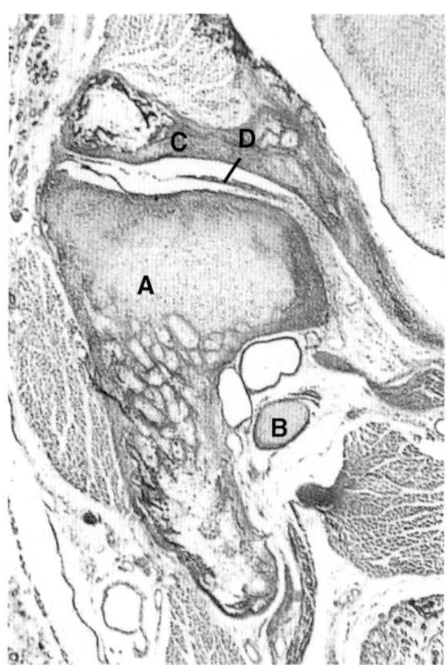

Fig. 19.7 The early developing condylar cartilage (A) and temporomandibular joint. B = Meckel's cartilage; C = developing bone of mandibular fossa; D = part of developing intra-articular disc of temporomandibular joint (decalcified section; Masson's trichrome: ×20).

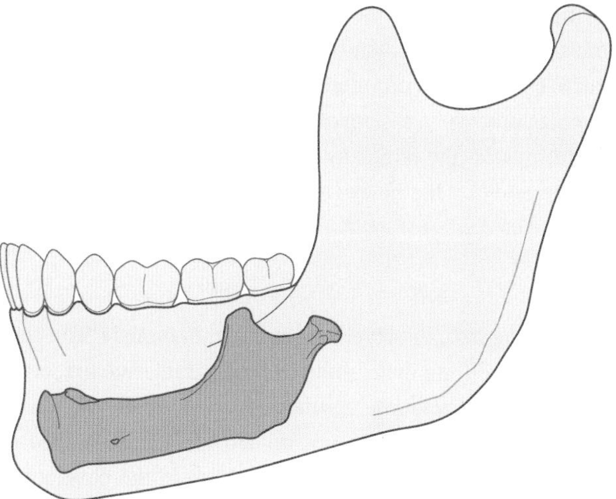

Fig. 19.9 Superimposed neonatal and adult mandibles. Note that growth of the mandible results in posterior relocation of the ramus of the mandible.

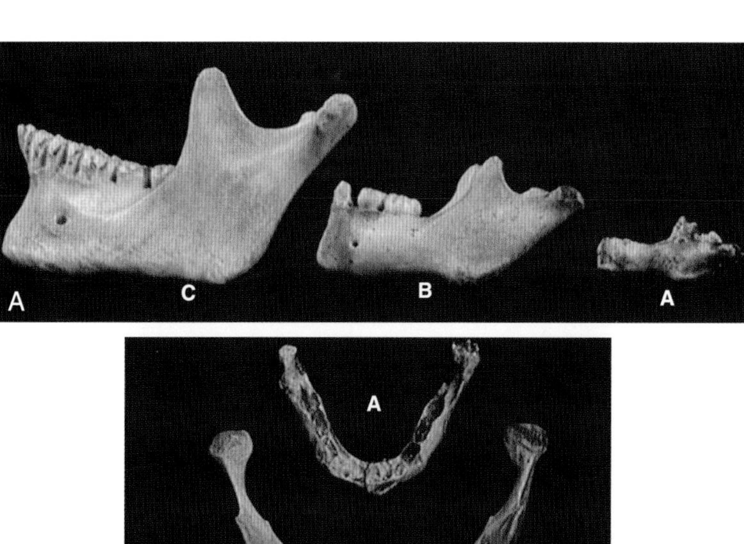

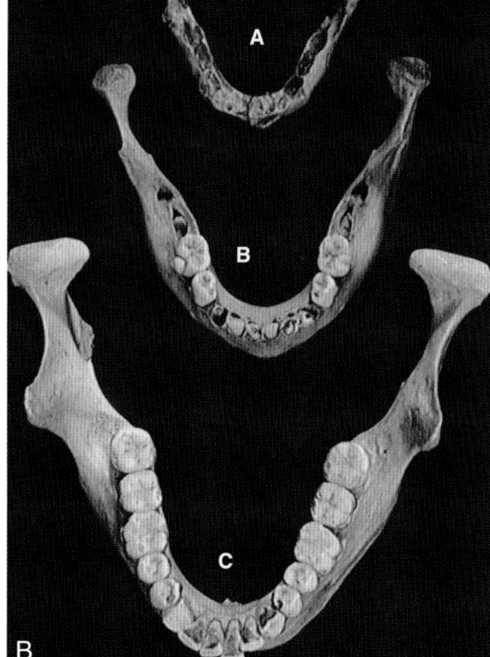

Fig. 19.8 The postnatal development of the mandible illustrated by lateral (A) and occlusal (B) views of the mandible at birth (A), at 6 years (B) and in an adult (C).

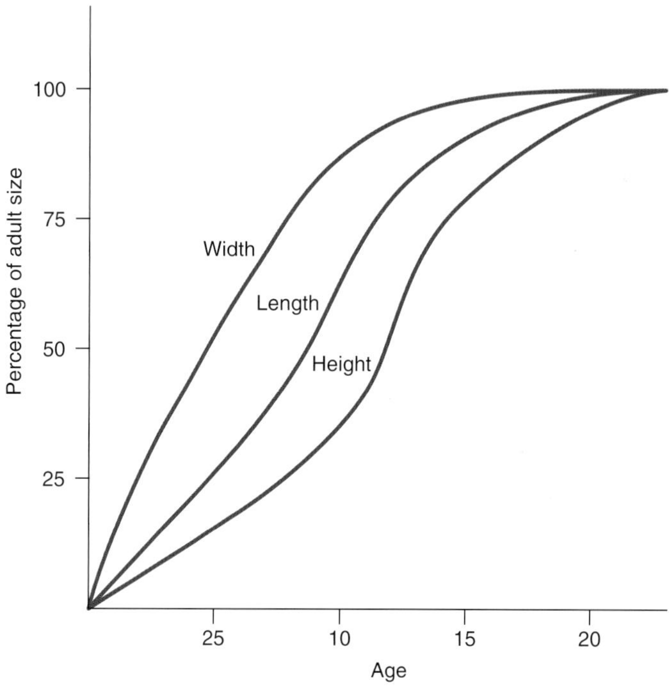

Fig. 19.10 Growth curves for attainment of adult width, length and height of the mandible. From Bell, W.H., Proffit, W.R., White, R.P., 1980. *Surgical Correction of Dentofacial Deformities*. W B Saunders, Philadelphia.

of the mandible. Increase in the length of the mandible is accomplished by bone deposition on the posterior surface of the ramus with compensatory resorption on its anterior surface, accompanied by deposition of bone on the posterior surface of the coronoid process and resorption on the anterior surface of the condyle. Increase in the width of the mandible is produced by deposition of bone on the outer surface of the mandible and resorption on the inner surface. Fig. 19.10 presents growth curves for attainment of adult width, length and height of the mandible.

There is some controversy concerning the role of the condylar cartilages in mandibular growth. One view states that continued proliferation of this cartilage is primarily responsible for the increase in both the mandibular length and the height of the ramus. Alternatively, it has been suggested that proliferation of the condylar cartilage is a response to growth and not its cause. The latter view has been supported by experiments showing that mandibular growth is relatively unaffected following condylectomy, provided that normal mandibular function is maintained.

Although the mandible is a single bone, it may be thought of as comprising several skeletal units, each associated with one or more soft tissue 'functional matrices'. The behaviour of these matrices primarily determines the growth of each skeletal unit. For example, the coronoid process forms a skeletal unit acted upon by the temporalis muscle. Sectioning of the temporalis muscle during early mandibular development may result in atrophy or complete absence of a coronoid process in the adult mandible. Similarly, the alveolar process is influenced by the teeth, the condyle by the lateral pterygoid muscle, the ramus by the medial pterygoid and masseter muscles and the body by the neurovascular bundle.

The maxilla

As with the mandible, the maxilla develops intramembranously. The centre of ossification appears during the eighth week of intrauterine life, close to the site of the developing deciduous canine tooth. Unlike the mandible, maxillary growth and development are not related to the appearance of secondary cartilages. Because of the maxilla's position in the developing skull, its growth is influenced by the development of the orbital, nasal and oral cavities.

From the region of the developing deciduous canine (Fig. 19.11), ossification spreads throughout the developing maxilla into its growing processes (palatine, zygomatic, frontal and alveolar). The appearance of the developing maxilla in a cleared alizarin red preparation may be seen in Fig. 19.6. The ossification of the palatine processes is described on pages 368–369.

At one time it was thought that the incisor-bearing part of the maxilla, which develops from the frontonasal process (see page 355), had a separate centre of ossification. It was consequently called the premaxilla. However, it is now clear that ossification spreads from the body of the maxilla into its incisor-bearing component.

Growth of the maxilla occurs by bone remodelling (i.e., surface deposition of bone with associated resorption) and by sutural growth. Among the agents that provide the forces separating the maxilla from the adjacent bones (thus permitting growth at the sutures) are the growing eyeballs, cartilaginous nasal septum and orbital pad of fat. Thus, growth of the maxilla is not an isolated phenomenon, but occurs in association with the development of the orbital, nasal and oral cavities. It has been suggested that the growing nasal septum pulls the maxilla forward by means of a septo-premaxillary ligament that runs from the anterior border of the nasal septum posteroinferiorly towards the anterior nasal spine and interpremaxillary suture. As in the lower jaw (pages 371–374), growth in height of the maxilla is related to the development of the alveolar process. It is difficult to determine how much of the adult alveolus is the result of bone deposition and how much results from bodily displacement of the maxilla. Studies using metal implants suggest that each method of growth contributes equal amounts. Increase in height of the nasal cavity is associated with resorption of bone on the upper surface of the palatine process of the maxilla and deposition of bone on the lower surface (see Fig. 18.26). Transverse growth of the maxilla occurs at the median palatine suture, but sutural separation is greater posteriorly than anteriorly.

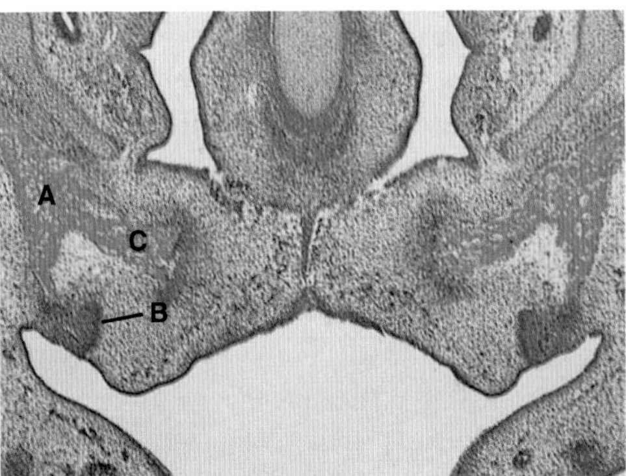

Fig. 19.11 The early developing maxilla (A) in the region of the developing deciduous canine (B). From this site, ossification spreads throughout the developing maxilla into its growing processes (e.g., palatine process; C) (decalcified section; Masson's trichrome; ×35).

The maxillary sinus appears as an outpocketing of the mucosa of the middle meatus of the nose at the beginning of the fourth month of intrauterine life. Although small at birth, the maxillary sinus is identifiable radiologically. After birth, the maxillary sinus enlarges with the growing maxilla, although it is only fully developed following the eruption of the permanent dentition. Forward growth of the whole face (including the maxillae) is dependent upon growth of the spheno-occipital synchondrosis (see Figs. 15.23 and 15.24). Although some have suggested that transverse facial skeletal growth is completed before either anteroposterior or vertical growth, this is not the case. Instead, a dramatic spread and an overlap of growth curves are observed throughout the developing years.

Clinical considerations

Orthodontics

The timing of orthodontic intervention is a challenge and requires a full understanding of facial growth and the ability to predict future growth potential. Because of the large amount of data built up concerning facial growth, it is possible to predict, with varying degrees of confidence, the amount of growth of various parameters between the ages of 6 and 12 years (Table 19.1). Where it is predicted that not enough growth or too much growth of the maxilla and mandible is likely, then orthodontic intervention to help increase or decrease jaw sizes may be considered. For example, if palatal width is inadequate and might lead to a crossbite (see page 46), an appliance may be fitted to act across the median palatine suture, whereas if the mandible is likely to have a deficient length, functional matrices/extraoral appliances may be considered.

Congenital abnormalities

Congenital abnormalities of the jaws are most often associated with 'first pharyngeal (branchial) arch syndromes'. Treacher Collins' syndrome and Pierre Robin's sequence are the two most common types of 'first arch syndrome' and have been described already in relation to the development of the face (see pages 359–360).

Table 19.1 Predictability for growth completion at ages 6 and 12

	Male		Female	
Transverse measurement	6 years	12 years	6 years	12 years
Cranial width	XXX	XXX	XXX	XXX
Facial width	XXX	XXX	XXX	XXX
Nasal width	XX	XXX	X	XX
Maxillary width	XX	XXX	XXX	XXX
Mandibular width	XXX	XXX	XXX	XXX
Maxillary intermolar width (6-6)	–	XXX	–	XXX
Mandibular intermolar width (6-6)	–	XXX	–	X

From Nanda, R., Snodell, S.F., Bollu, P., 2012. Transverse growth of maxilla and mandible. *Seminars in Orthodontics* 18, 100–117.

Cherubism

Cherubism is a rare autosomal condition that arises in childhood and is believed to result from a mutation of the gene *SH3BP2*, a gene encoding for a signalling protein. The normal bone of the maxilla and mandible is lost and replaced by numerous cysts, which give the face a characteristic, symmetrical, swollen, rounded 'cherub-like' outline (Fig. 19.12). There is an associated premature loss of deciduous teeth and a lack of eruption of permanent teeth (Fig. 19.13).

Temporomandibular disorders

Trauma and infection in the region of the TMJ may lead to an ankylosis of the condyle with the base of the skull. The most obvious sign of this condition would be limitation of jaw opening, as well as reduced growth of the ramus on that side, with resultant asymmetry. Although this might provide evidence in supporting a major role for the condylar cartilage as a growth centre for the mandible, the reduced growth may simply reflect the lack of function of the mandible.

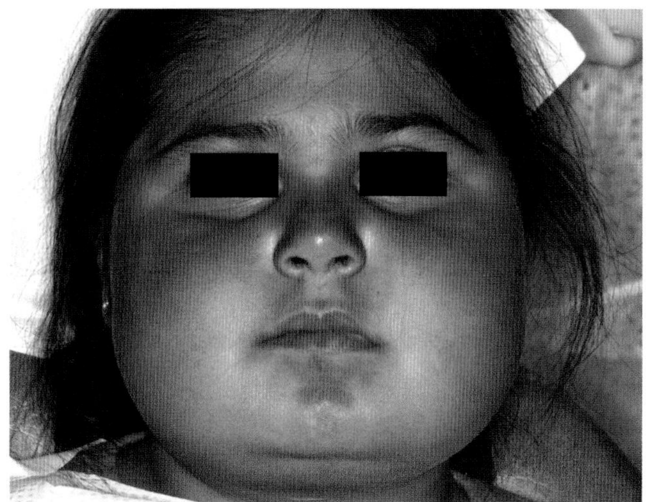

Fig. 19.12 A 7-year old female with painless, symmetrical enlargement of the mandible and maxilla typical of cherubism. Courtesy of Dr. P Sedghizadeh.

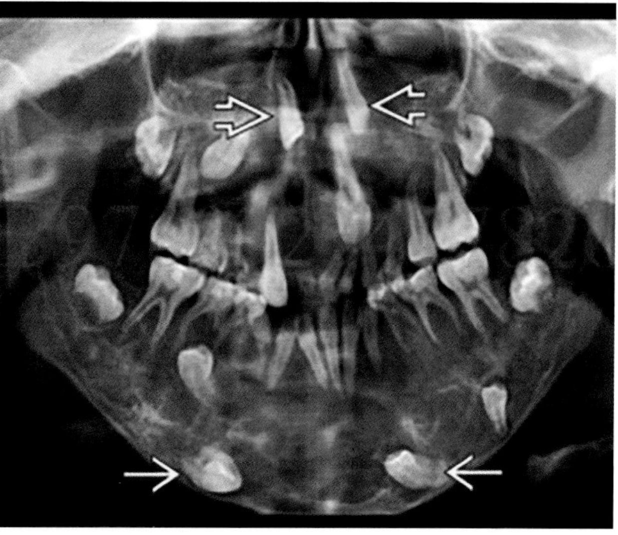

Fig. 19.13 Panoramic radiograph of an 11-year-old boy with cherubism showing expansion of the maxilla and mandible. There is significant displacement of the developing permanent teeth, and several are missing. The mandibular canines (lower arrow) are displaced to the inferior border of the mandible, and two maxillary anterior teeth (upper arrows) are displaced superiorly to the junction of the maxillary sinus and nasal cavity. From Tamimi, D., Koenig, L.J., Perschbacher, S.F., et al., 2017. *Diagnostic Imaging: Oral and Maxillofacial*, second edition. Elsevier, Philadelphia.

A mind map that covers development of the jaws, together with the face, tongue and palate, is located at the end of Chapter 20, page 380.

Further readings for this chapter can be found in the accompanying eBook. Explore online Self-assessment quiz to test and reinforce your understanding of the material in your free ebook. Follow instructions in the Inside Front Cover to unlock your access.

20 Development of the tongue and salivary glands

Development of the tongue

The anterior two-thirds of the tongue, the 'oral tongue', develops from three swellings: two distal tongue buds (lateral lingual swellings) and a median tongue bud (tuberculum impar) (Fig. 20.1). Each is formed by proliferation of mesenchyme beneath the endodermal lining of the first pharyngeal (branchial) arch. The caudal border of this part of the developing tongue is marked by the foramen caecum (the site of origin embryologically of the thyroid gland). The distal tongue buds (lateral lingual swellings) expand rapidly to overgrow the median tongue bud (tuberculum impar), and consequently this median swelling contributes little to the adult tongue.

The posterior third of the tongue, the 'pharyngeal tongue', develops from a single midline swelling, the hypopharyngeal eminence, which is derived mainly from the third pharyngeal (branchial) arch (with a small contribution from the fourth arch). The hypopharyngeal eminence rapidly overgrows the second arch (the copula) to merge with the first arch swellings.

The muscles of the tongue develop primarily from paraxial mesoderm of the occipital somites that migrates into the developing tongue. Evidence suggests that neural crest cells within the tongue buds have an 'instructive role' in guiding the development of the tongue musculature. Furthermore, Smad4-mediated transforming growth factor beta (TGF-β) signalling influences the development of the tongue musculature, probably through a signalling cascade that involves fibroblast growth factor 6 (FGF6). It also appears that metalloproteinases have an influence upon the tongue, since, in the absence of such enzymes, migration and proliferation of myoblasts in the tongue buds are greatly impaired.

The development and shape of various papillae on the tongue are also controlled by genes and growth factors. For example, bone morphogenetic proteins (BMPs) influence the shape of filiform papillae, as experimental changes in the distribution of BMPs caused by the presence of the BMP antagonist noggin can change the shape of these papillae.

Molecules such as sonic hedgehog (Shh), Wnt6, Lef1, Sox2 and epidermal growth factor (EGF) can be detected in the epithelium during development of fungiform papillae, with their distribution changing during ontogeny. Where Wnt signalling is reduced, fungiform papillae may be smaller and greatly reduced in number. In contrast, activating Wnt signalling causes an increase in the numbers of fungiform papillae. Reduced expression of Sox2 leads to an absence of fungiform papillae (although filiform papillae do develop). Overexpression of Sox2 results in atypical fungiform development (but filiform papillae do develop). With additional EGF, fewer fungiform papillae are present. The *Six* family genes encode homeobox transcription factors. *Six1* and *Six4* deficiencies are associated with a poorly developed tongue, there being severe deficiencies in many papillae.

The diverse embryological origin of the tongue explains its diverse sensory supply (see Fig. 4.12). General sensation to the anterior two-thirds of the tongue is supplied by the lingual nerve, a nerve of the first pharyngeal (branchial) arch. General sensation and taste to the posterior third of the tongue are supplied by the glossopharyngeal and superior laryngeal nerves, the nerves of the third and fourth arches. The perception of taste in the anterior two-thirds of the tongue is associated with the chorda tympani nerve, a branch of the facial nerve, the nerve of the second pharyngeal (branchial) arch. As this arch does not contribute tissue to the anterior part of the tongue, in this situation it is termed a 'pretrematic' nerve. Because the muscles of the tongue arise from occipital somites, as they migrate into the developing tongue, they carry their nerve supply, the hypoglossal nerve, with them.

For the development of the taste buds, Sox2 (whose expression lies downstream from Wnt signalling) is required, since, in its absence, mature taste buds do not develop.

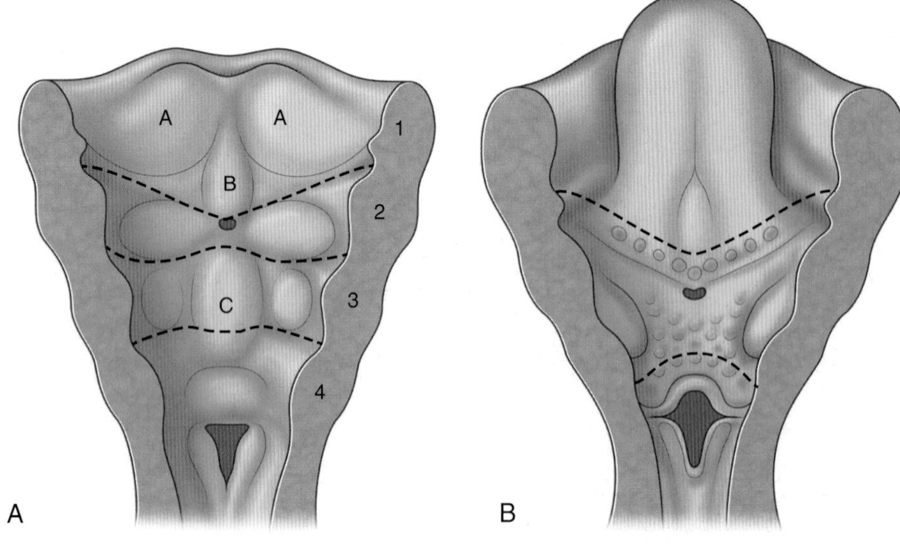

Fig. 20.1 The schema of tongue primordia. (A) The ventral wall of the pharynx in the fourth week of intra-uterine life. (B) The developing tongue at the fifth month. Numbers 1–4 indicate the positions of the pharyngeal (branchial) arches. Four swellings are seen: two distal tongue buds (lateral lingual swellings, A), the median tongue bud (tuberculum impar, B) and the hypopharyngeal eminence (C).

As previously mentioned, the thyroid gland develops between the median tongue bud (tuberculum impar) and the copula (on day 24 of intra-uterine life). It is the first endocrine gland to develop. On the fully formed tongue, the site of origin of the thyroid gland is demarcated by a small pit, the foramen caecum (see Fig. 1.15). The thyroid diverticulum remains connected to the embryonic tongue by a thyroglossal duct. This descends into the developing neck anterior to the hyoid bone and trachea. The definitive shape and position of the thyroid gland are complete by the seventh week of intra-uterine life.

Development of the salivary glands

The three main salivary glands initially form during the sixth and seventh weeks of intra-uterine life as solid epithelial buds extending from the developing mouth into the underlying mesenchyme. It is this oral epithelial-derived tissue that forms the ducts and secretory elements of a salivary gland. The surrounding mesenchymal connective tissues of salivary glands are derived from the neural crest.

The parotid gland is the first to be formed and appears near the angles of the developing mouth (stomodeum). The epithelial bud for the parotid gland extends towards the developing ear and initially branches to form solid cords. By week 10 the cords canalise to form the salivary ducts, and the rounded ends of the cords form the secretory acini. It is 8 weeks later that the acini become functional.

The submandibular gland is the second major salivary gland to develop (late in the sixth week of intra-uterine life). The epithelial bud grows posteriorly and laterally to the tongue and, during the 12th week, canalises to form the ducts and acini. The submandibular gland becomes functional in week 16 of intra-uterine life.

The sublingual glands appear late in the eighth week of intrauterine life. Part of the gland develops from multiple epithelial buds that appear in the paralingual sulcus of the forming mouth. They canalise to form up to 12 ducts that open independently into the floor of the mouth.

Epithelial–mesenchymal interactions

As for tooth germs (see Chapter 21) and hair follicles, salivary glands develop from a series of reciprocal epithelial–mesenchymal interactions as well as control from nerves and blood vessels.

The specific branching pattern of the different glands requires coordinated cell proliferation, clefting, differentiation, migration and apoptosis. The pattern of branching is controlled by signals primarily from the mesenchyme. This has been shown from experiments where the epithelium and mesenchyme of the early budding salivary gland have been separated and then recombined in different combinations. Thus, salivary gland mesenchyme recombined with epithelium from other areas will cause epithelial cells to take on a salivary gland–like branching pattern. Conversely, salivary gland epithelium from the initial bud stage combined with mesenchyme from other sites is unable to form its normal branching structure.

Although the branching pattern can be changed by the mesenchyme, the cytodifferentiation of the epithelial cells can not as easily be altered. When submandibular mesenchyme is combined with parotid epithelium, the epithelium continues to form serous rather than mucous acini.

The same genes, growth factors and their receptors that are essential for tooth development are also essential for normal salivary gland development. Thus animals lacking FGF, TGF-β, EGF, platelet-derived growth factor (PDGF), Pitx2 and Shh will show abnormalities or even absence of salivary glands.

Cavitation to form the salivary gland duct lumen requires apoptosis of the central-most cells of the duct in order to leave a lumen space. Interference of the pathways of apoptosis involving, for example, survivin, tumour necrosis factor (TNF) and Eda may also result in abnormal development.

The branching of the salivary glands is regulated by the extracellular matrix and the basement membrane. Changes in the nature of molecules, such as glycosaminoglycans (GAGs), collagens, fibronectin, integrins and in associated enzymes, will affect salivary gland development.

Following the completion of salivary gland development, adult tissue stem cells present in the excretory duct have the capacity to regenerate gland tissue (see pages 351–352).

Clinical considerations

Clinical considerations are also discussed on pages 348–353 in connection with the structure and function of the adult salivary glands.

Ankyloglossia

The tongue is prone to many abnormalities, a considerable number of which are congenital. For example, should the lingual frenum on the ventral surface of the tongue be short (less than 2 cm) and only extend from the sublingual papilla and across the floor of the mouth, there may be a 'tongue-tie' (ankyloglossia) (Fig. 20.2). This condition has a prevalence of between about 4% and 11%. It is associated with restricted movement of the tongue, which, if untreated, may cause problems with breastfeeding in the newborn and later with speech. A short lingual frenulum is also associated with various genetic syndromes, for example, dystrophic epidermolysis bullosa, oral-facial-digital syndrome type I and Van der Woude's syndrome.

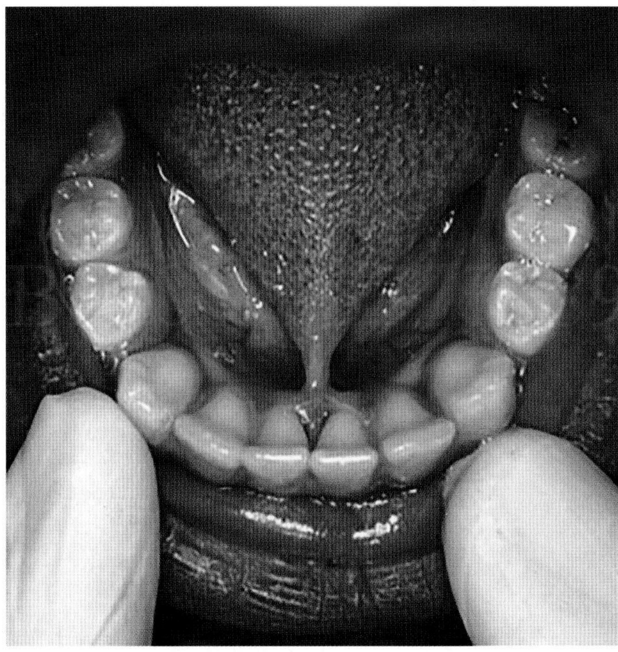

Fig. 20.2 Intraoral view of patient with ankyloglossia. There is a short lingual frenum extending across the floor of the mouth to become attached to the lingual alveolus behind the mandibular incisors, restricting the movement of the tongue. Courtesy Drs. M Chapman, A D'Alesio, K Woods, et al. From McIntire, S.C., Garrison, J., Zitelli, B.J., et al., 2023. *Zitelli and Davis' Atlas of Pediatric Physical Diagnosis*, eighth edition. Elsevier.

Microglossia and macroglossia

Microglossia refers to the presence of an abnormally small tongue. As cranial neural crest–derived fibroblasts appear to regulate the fate of mesoderm-derived myoblasts through TGF-β–mediated regulation of FGF and BMP signalling during tongue development, a microglossia may result from disturbances in such signalling.

Macroglossia refers to an abnormally large tongue (Fig. 20.3). Macroglossia is more common than microglossia and can be associated

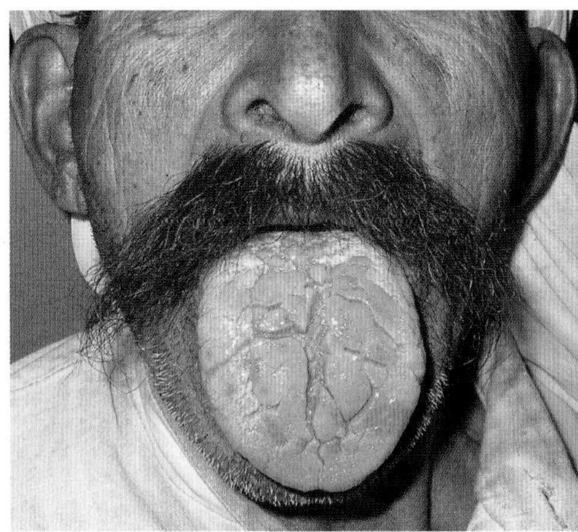

Fig. 20.3 A macroglossia. Courtesy Dr. S Saraf.

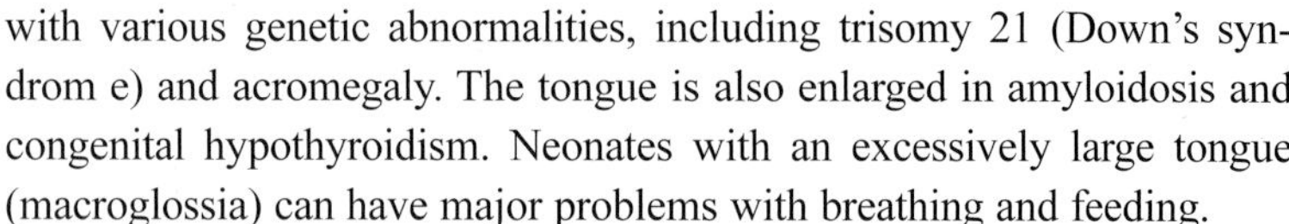

with various genetic abnormalities, including trisomy 21 (Down's syndrom e) and acromegaly. The tongue is also enlarged in amyloidosis and congenital hypothyroidism. Neonates with an excessively large tongue (macroglossia) can have major problems with breathing and feeding.

The tongue may also be enlarged as the result of the presence of a lymphangioma (Fig. 20.4) or haemangioma.

Fissured tongue and bifid tongue

Fissured tongue describes a situation where the surface of the tongue is deeply grooved (Fig. 20.5). As a result, the person with this condition may have to regularly clean the tongue in order to remove food debris within the fissures. Bifid tongue occurs when the right and left portions of the tongue do not merge during development. This is usually seen close to the tip of the tongue in the anterior two-thirds (oral tongue).

Medium rhomboid glossitis

Median rhomboid glossitis is a condition characterised by a nonpapillated, reddish region in the anterior two-thirds of the tongue in front of the sulcus terminalis and in the midline (Fig. 20.6). As the name suggests, it has a diamond-shaped outline and is usually asymptomatic. Although once thought to represent a congenital malformation, it is now thought to be associated with candidal infection, although the underlying reason for its specific location is not understood.

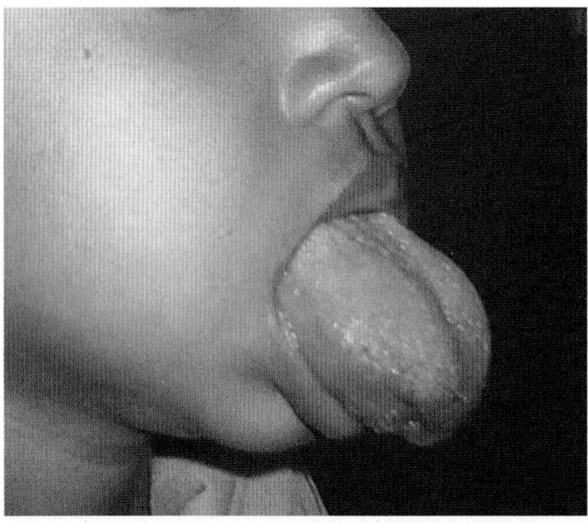

Fig. 20.4 An enlarged tongue in a child resulting from the presence of a lymphangioma in a child. Courtesy Dr. S Saraf.

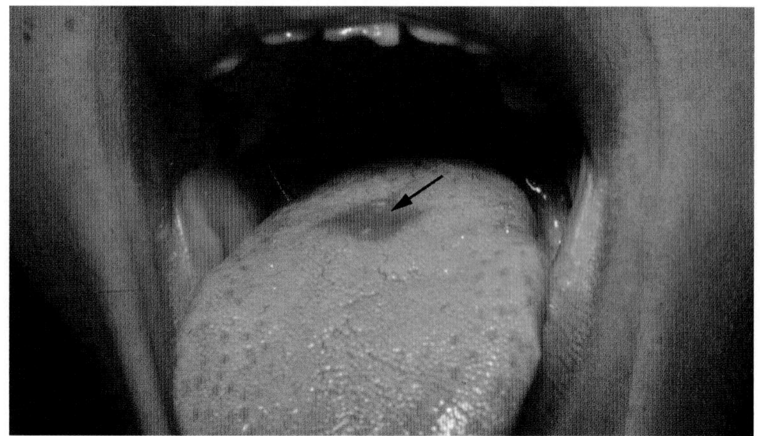

Fig. 20.6 A median rhomboid glossitis (arrow). Courtesy Dr. J D Harrison.

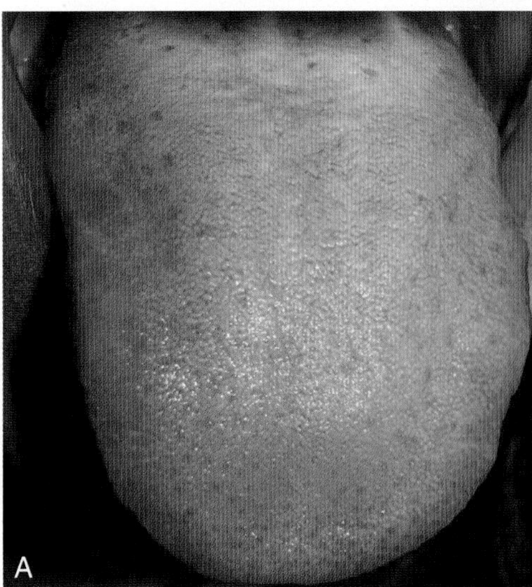

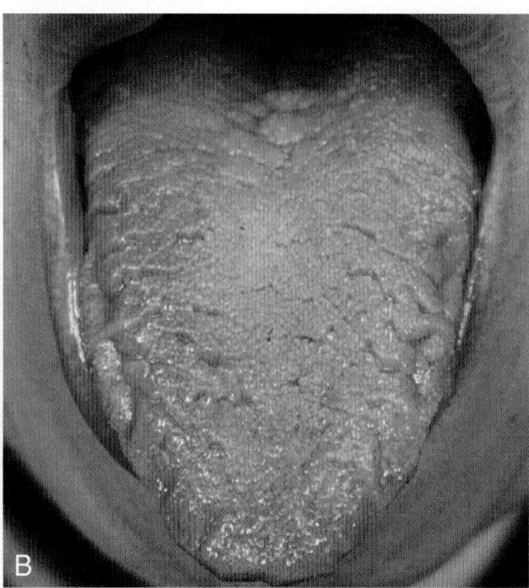

Fig. 20.5 (A) Normal tongue. The red spots represent fungiform papillae. (B) A fissured tongue where the dorsal surface is grooved. Courtesy Prof. P R Morgan.

Lingual thyroid

Although the only remains of the developing thyroid gland on the normal adult tongue is the foramen caecum, in some instances thyroid tissue can be retained at this site. When this occurs, it is referred to as a 'lingual thyroid' (see Fig. 14.79). It is possible for a lingual thyroid to secrete sufficient thyroxine hormone to satisfy the metabolic requirements of the individual. Indeed, technetium-99m pertechnetate scans can be employed to detect sites of secretion of the hormone. In this context, accessory thyroid tissue may be found along the midline of the neck in locations related to the track of the migrating thyroid gland during its development. Furthermore, thyroglossal duct cysts may be located along this pathway.

Further readings for this chapter can be found in the accompanying eBook. Explore online Self-assessment quiz to test and reinforce your understanding of the material in your free ebook. Follow instructions in the Inside Front Cover to unlock your access.

Key features:

5 facial processes appear around primitive mouth (stomodeum):

frontonasal process over prosencephalon, 2 mandibular processes from 1st phrayngeal arch (below stomodeum) and extending from these 2 maxillary processes.

Ectodermal placodes – nasal, lens and otic placodes

Frontonasal process around the nasal pits (from invaginating nasal placodes) – medial and lateral nasal processes. Upper lip is initially formed by the meeting of the 2 medial nasal processes centrally with the 2 maxillary processes laterally. Note that the upper lip seems to eventually be formed entirely by the maxillary processes that merge in the midline where the medial nasal processes initially are located.

Key features:

Initially there is a primary palate (rostral aspect of fontonasal process) and a common oro-nasal chamber. Subsequently, palatal shelves appear from maxillary processes. These processes are vertical and have to elevate to the horizontal position before fusing.

Elevation of the palate shelves is thought to occur because of rapid hydration of the mesenchymal ECM to produce a turgor pressure. Hyaluronan is involved in this process.

Fusion involves the initial formation of a midline epithelial seam that subsequently breaks down (with loss of the basement membrane) as a result of apoptosis and redifferentiation of the epithelial cells.

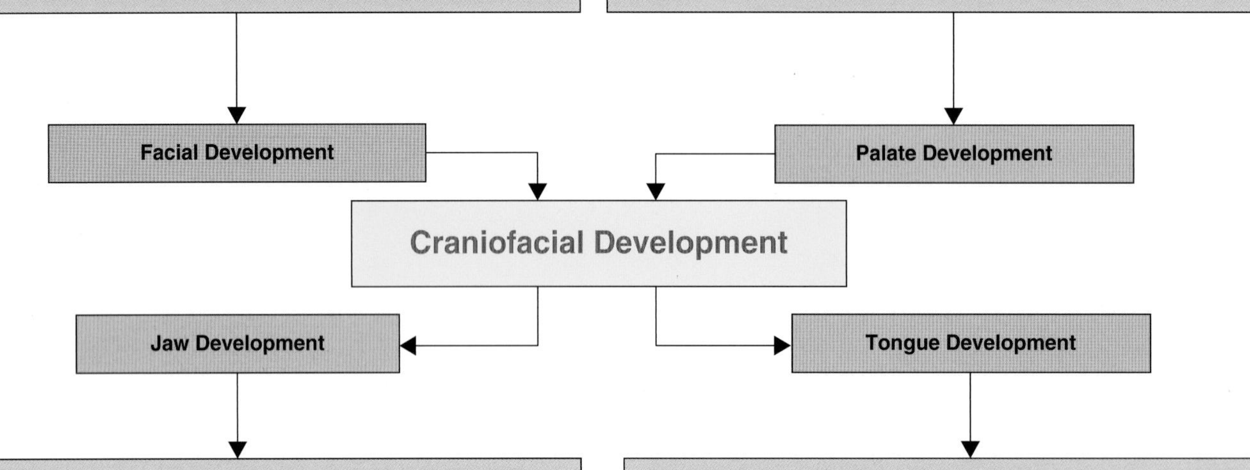

Key features:

Mandible – develops intramembranously around (not in) the cartilage of the 1st pharyngeal arch (Meckel's cartilage). Development of the ramus of the mandible is associated with the appearance of secondary cartilages (condylar and coronoid cartilages). There is also a secondary cartilage at the midline – mandibular symphysis.

Maxilla – develops intramembranously from centres of ossification located near the developing deciduous canine teeth. No secondary cartilages.

Growth of mandible by surface remodelling, with little contribution from condylar cartilage. Growth of maxilla by surface deposition plus sutural growth.

Key features:

Anterior $2/3^{rd}$ of tongue formed by lateral lingual swellings and a midline tuberculum impar (median lingual swelling) beneath the endoderm of the 1st pharyngeal arch. Thus the sensory innervation is derived from the mandibular division of the trigeminal nerve (with taste from the facial nerve – the nerve of the 2nd pharyngeal arch).

Posterior $1/3^{rd}$ formed by copula primarily from the 3rd and 4th pharyngeal arches. Thus, the sensory innervation is derived from the glossopharyngeal (and vagus) nerve.

The tongue musculature is derived from occipital myotomes that are therefore innervated by the hypoglossal nerve.

Note the origin of the thyroid gland from the developing tongue (remaining as the foramen caecum on the fully formed tongue).

Mind Map 20.1 Craniofacial development.

Early tooth development

21

Tooth development can be divided into three overlapping phases: initiation, morphogenesis and histogenesis. During initiation, the sites of the future teeth are established, with the appearance of tooth germs along an invagination of the oral epithelium called the *dental lamina*. During morphogenesis, the shape of the tooth is determined by a combination of cell proliferation and cell movement. During histogenesis, differentiation of cells (begun during morphogenesis) proceeds to give rise to the fully formed dental tissues, both mineralised (i.e., enamel, dentine and cementum) and soft tissues (i.e., dental pulp and periodontal ligament). Tooth development is characterised by complex interactions between epithelial and mesenchymal tissues.

In the oral epithelium, localised thickenings are the first signs of tooth development, sometimes referred to as 'dental placodes'. At this early stage of tooth development, the dental epithelium induces odontogenic fate in the underlying mesenchyme. Following the initial thickening, mesenchymal cells condense around the epithelial invagination. These ectomesenchymal cells are derived from the neural crest, which migrates into the jaws from the neural tube margins during the early stages of head development.

Research on amphibians suggests that, in addition to oral ectoderm and neural crest mesenchyme, foregut endoderm can play a role in tooth initiation. In amphibians and bony fish, the more posterior teeth form from endoderm rather than ectoderm.

By the sixth week of development in humans, the oral epithelium thickens and invaginates into the mesenchyme to form a primary epithelial band (Fig. 21.1). By the seventh week, the primary epithelial band divides into two processes: a buccally located vestibular lamina and a lingually situated dental lamina (Fig. 21.2). The vestibular lamina contributes to the development of the vestibule of the mouth, delineating the lips and cheeks from the tooth-bearing regions. The dental lamina contributes to the development of the teeth. To form the vestibule of the oral cavity, the cells of the vestibular lamina proliferate, with subsequent loss of cell adhesion and degeneration of the central cellular component cells, to produce the sulcus of the vestibule (Fig. 21.3). Further development of the dental lamina (Fig. 21.4) is characterised by an increase in length, owing to proliferation. By the eighth week, a series of swellings develops on the deep surface of the dental lamina (Fig. 21.5). The complete dental lamina of the lower jaw is shown in green on the model, and the epithelial swellings indicating early developing tooth germs are arrowed. It is important to appreciate that the dental lamina appears as an arch-shaped band of tissue, which follows the line of the vestibular fold. Although not shown on the model, each epithelial swelling is almost completely surrounded by a mesenchymal condensation.

For descriptive purposes, and based on 2D observations of histological sections, tooth germs are classified into bud, cap and bell stages according to the degree of morphodifferentiation and histodifferentiation of their epithelial components (enamel organs). Leading up to the late bell stage, the tooth germ changes rapidly both in its size and shape; the cells are dividing and morphogenetic processes are taking place. At the late bell stage, hard tissues are forming and further growth of the crown is related mainly to the deposition of enamel by the enamel-forming cells (ameloblasts), while the rate of cell division reduces.

Bud stage

The enamel organ at the bud stage (Fig. 21.6) appears as a simple, spherical to ovoid, epithelial condensation (swelling) that is poorly morphodifferentiated and histodifferentiated. It is surrounded by mesenchyme. The cells of the tooth bud have a higher RNA content than those of the overlying oral epithelium, a lower glycogen content and increased oxidative enzyme activity. It would appear that the epithelium is instructive in tooth initiation (see page 388). Nevertheless, the successful development of the tooth germ relies upon complex interactions by means of reciprocal exchange of signals between both mesenchymal and epithelial components. Should

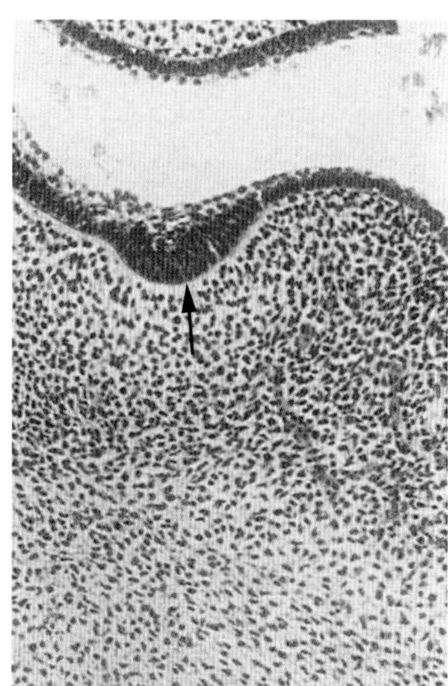

Fig. 21.1 Primary epithelial band (arrowed) at the sixth week of intra-uterine life (H & E; ×115).

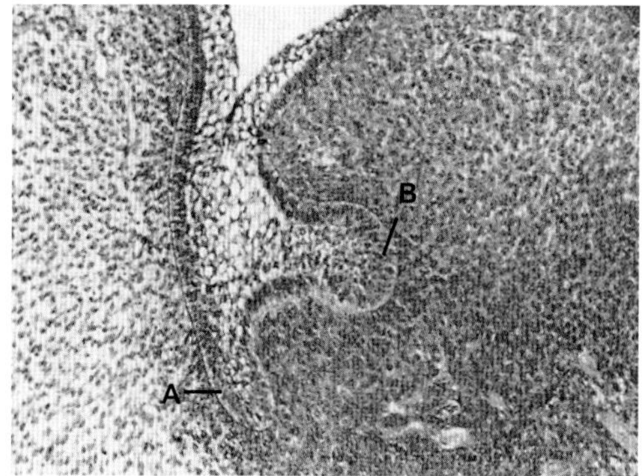

Fig. 21.2 The vestibular lamina (A) and dental lamina (B) seen at the seventh week of intra-uterine life (H & E; ×120). Courtesy Dr. D Adams.

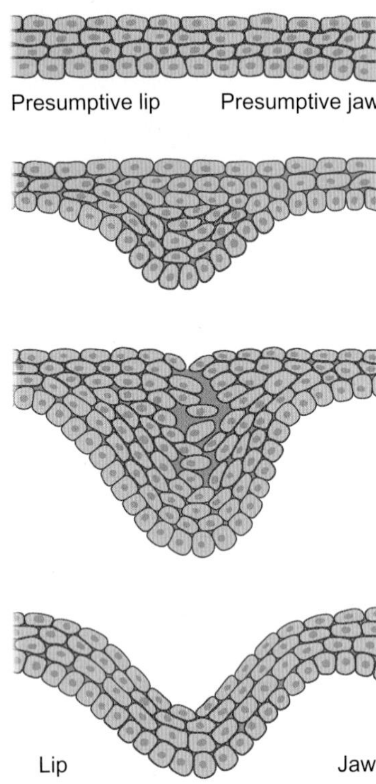

Fig. 21.3 Diagram illustrating the formation of the vestibule of the oral cavity.

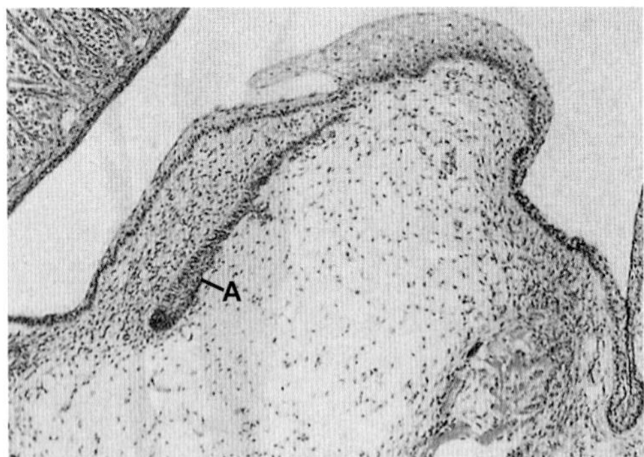

Fig. 21.4 The developing dental lamina (A) (Masson's trichrome; ×55).

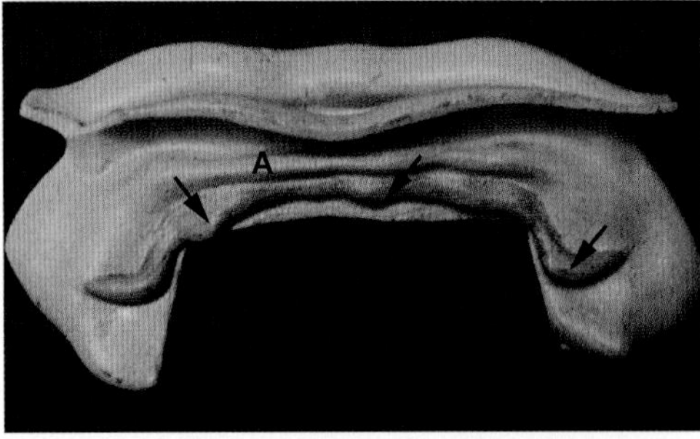

Fig. 21.5 Model showing the stage of tooth development by the eighth week of intra-uterine life when a series of swellings representing developing tooth germs (arrows) develops on the deep surface of the dental lamina. A = vestibular fold.

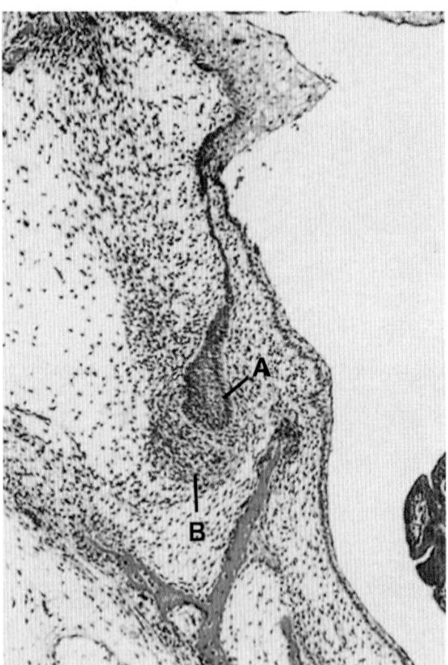

Fig. 21.6 Bud stage of tooth development. A = enamel organ; B = mesenchymal condensation (Masson's trichrome; ×60).

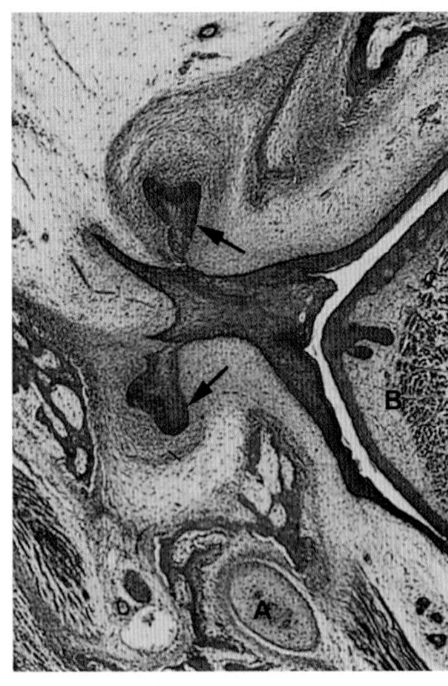

Fig. 21.7 Early cap stage of tooth development (arrows). A = Meckel's cartilage; B = developing tongue (Masson's trichrome; ×32).

these components be separated and cultured individually, neither will differentiate further. The epithelial component is separated from the adjacent mesenchyme by a basement membrane.

Cap stage

By the 11th week, morphogenesis has progressed, with the deeper surface of the enamel organ invaginating and the mesenchyme condensing to form a cap-shaped structure. In the section shown in Fig. 21.7, both maxillary and mandibular early cap stages are shown, with each enamel organ appearing relatively poorly histodifferentiated. However, a greater distinction develops between the more rounded cells in the central portion of the enamel organ and the peripheral cells, which are becoming arranged to form the external and internal enamel epithelia.

In the late cap stage of tooth development (Fig. 21.8), by about the 12th week, the central cells of the enlarging enamel organ have become separated (although maintaining contact by desmosomes), with the intercellular spaces containing significant quantities of glycosaminoglycans. The resulting tissue is termed the *stellate reticulum*, although it is not fully developed until the later bell stage. The cells of the external enamel epithelium remain cuboidal, whereas those of the internal enamel epithelium become more columnar. The latter show an increase in RNA content and hydrolytic and oxidative enzyme activity, while the adjacent mesenchymal cells continue to proliferate and surround the enamel organ. The part of the mesenchyme lying beneath the internal enamel epithelium is termed the *dental papilla*, while that surrounding the tooth germ forms the dental

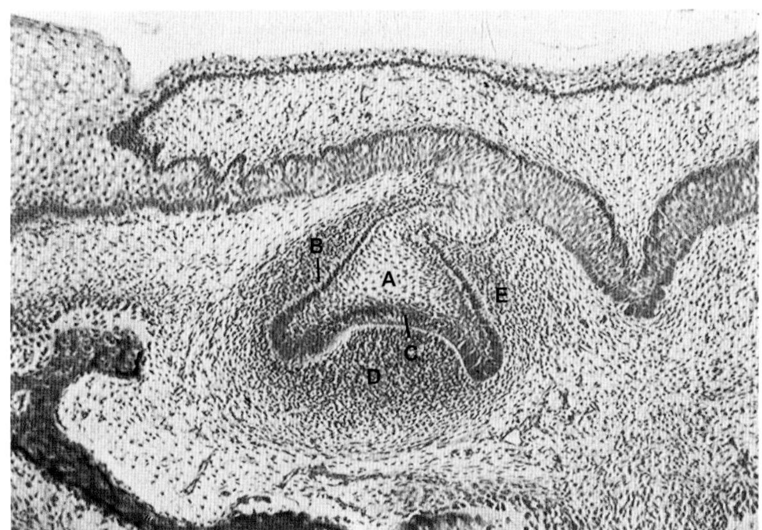

Fig. 21.8 Late cap stage of tooth development. A = stellate reticulum; B = external enamel epithelium; C = internal enamel epithelium; D = dental papilla; E = dental follicle (H & E; ×75).

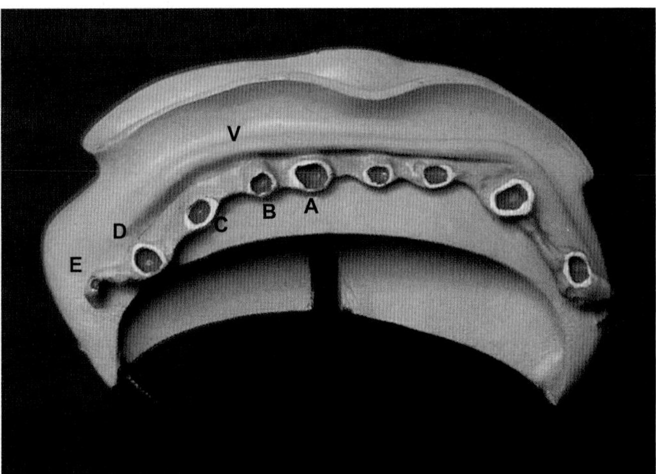

Fig. 21.9 Model illustrating the arrangement of deciduous tooth germs (identified by the Palmer-Zsigmondy system, A–E) at 13 weeks on the dental lamina of the lower jaw. V = vestibular fold.

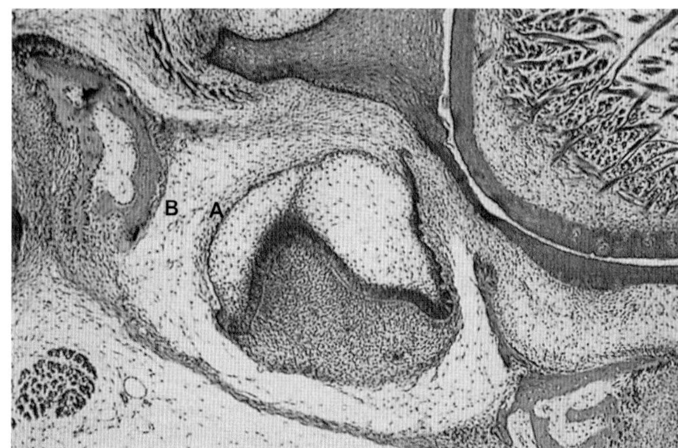

Fig. 21.10 Early bell stage of tooth development. A = inner investing layer of dental follicle; B = outer layer of dental follicle (Masson's trichrome; ×45).

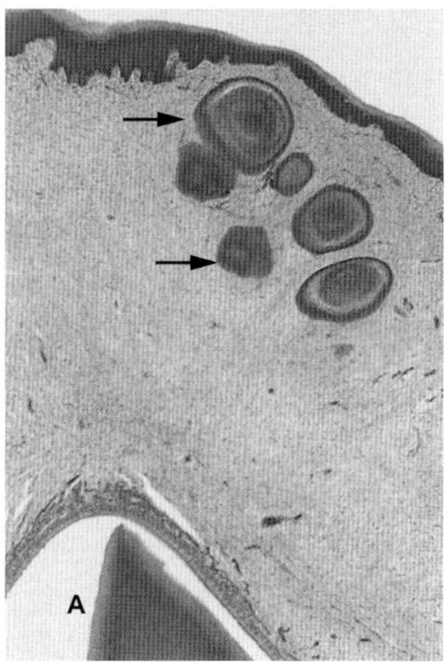

Fig. 21.11 Epithelial pearls (of Serres) (arrows). A = enamel space (H & E; ×8). Courtesy Dr. D A Luke.

follicle. A model describing the arrangement of deciduous tooth germs at 13 weeks on the dental lamina of the lower jaw is shown in Fig. 21.9.

Early bell stage

By the 14th week, further morphodifferentiation and histodifferentiation of the tooth germ lead to the early bell stage (Fig. 21.10). The configuration of the internal enamel epithelium broadly maps out the occlusal shape of the crown of the tooth. This folding is related to differential mitosis along the internal enamel epithelium. The future cusps and incisal margins are sites of precocious cell maturation associated with cessation of mitosis, while areas corresponding to the fissures and margins of the tooth remain mitotically active. Thus, cusp height is related more to continued downward growth at the margin and fissures than to upward extension of the cusps. During the bell stage, any bone resorption defects that restrict the space for development of the tooth germ may be associated with the increased folding pattern of the internal enamel epithelium, leading to changes in tooth shape. Consequently, spatial impediment, and the changing mechanical forces that ensue, may be a cofactor in dental morphogenesis.

It is during the bell stage of development that the dental lamina breaks down and the enamel organ loses connection with the oral epithelium. At the same time, the dental lamina between tooth germs also degenerates. Remnants of the dental lamina may remain in the adult mucosa (Fig. 21.11) as clumps of resting cells (epithelial pearls [of Serres]) that may contain keratin and can be involved in the aetiology of cysts.

Interposed between the enamel organ and the wall of the developing bony crypt is the mesenchymal tissue of the dental follicle, which is generally considered to have three layers (Fig. 21.10). The inner investing layer is a vascular, fibrocellular condensation, three to four cells thick, immediately surrounding the tooth germ; the nuclei of the cells tend to be elongated circumferentially. The outer layer of the dental follicle is a vascular mesenchymal layer that lines the developing alveolus. Between the two layers is loose connective tissue with no marked concentration of blood vessels. All layers of the dental follicle mesenchyme are derived from the neural crest.

A high degree of histodifferentiation is achieved in the early bell stage (Fig. 21.12). The enamel organ shows four distinct layers: external enamel epithelium, stellate reticulum, stratum intermedium and internal enamel epithelium.

The cervical loop at the margins of the enlarging bell-shaped enamel organ is a site of mitotic activity. Here, the central cells of the stellate reticulum/stratum intermedium may be the site of a stem cell niche providing

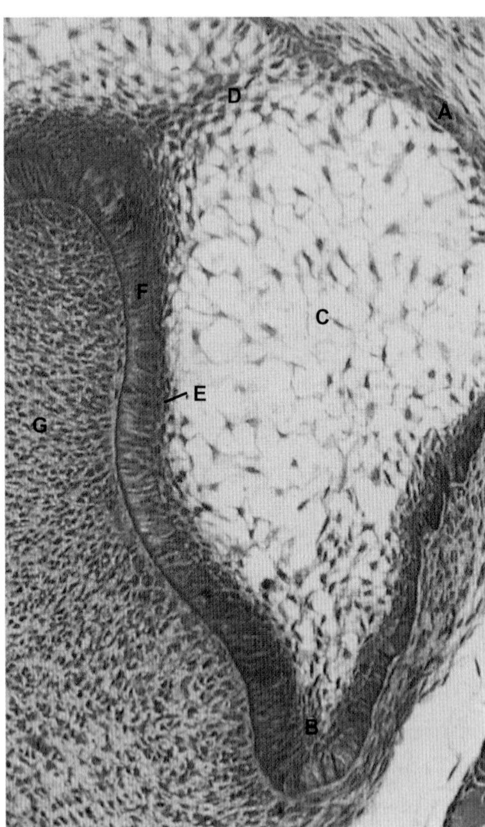

Fig. 21.12 A high-power view of the early bell. A = external enamel epithelium; B = cervical loop; C = stellate reticulum; D = enamel cord; E = stratum intermedium; F = internal enamel epithelium; G = dental papilla (Masson's trichrome; ×120).

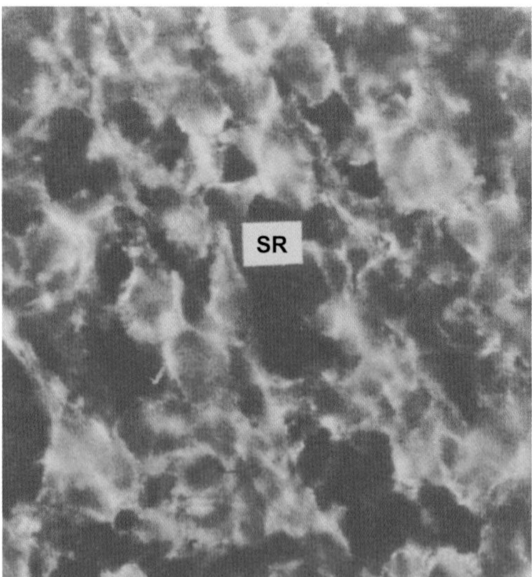

Fig. 21.13 Immunohistological labelling of type II collagen showing positive (white) labelling in the stellate reticulum (SR) (×350).

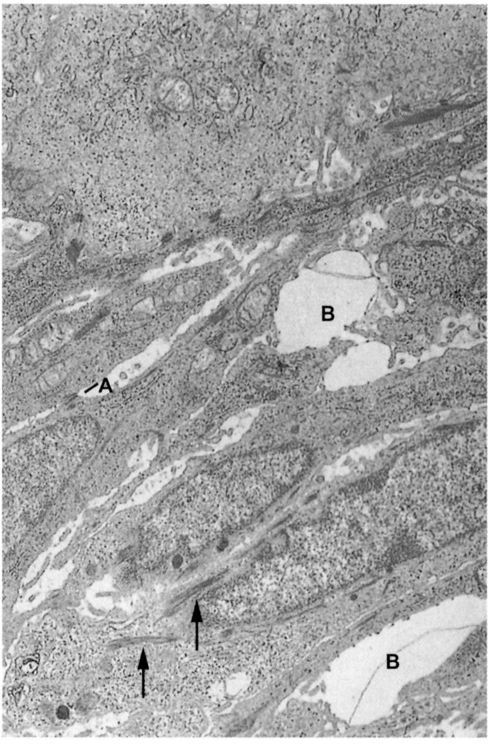

Fig. 21.14 Ultrastructural appearance of the stellate reticulum. A = desmosomes; B = intercellular space; arrows show tonofilaments (TEM; ×6,380). Courtesy Dr H Azawa and Dr H Nakamura.

cells that pass to the internal enamel epithelium and later form ameloblasts. This may be under the control of Notch protein in the epithelium and growth factors, such as bone morphogenetic protein-4 (BMP-4) and fibroblast growth factor-10 (FGF-10), in the adjacent dental mesenchyme (see page 388).

External enamel epithelium

As its name suggests, this forms the outer layer of cuboidal cells that limits the enamel organ. It is separated from the surrounding mesenchymal tissue by a basement membrane 1–2 μm thick, which, at the ultrastructural level, corresponds to the much narrower basal lamina with associated hemidesmosomes (see Fig. 14.29). The external enamel epithelial cells contain large, centrally placed nuclei. Ultrastructurally, they contain relatively small amounts of the intracellular organelles associated with protein synthesis (e.g., endoplasmic reticulum, Golgi material, mitochondria), and they contact each other via desmosomes and gap junctions. The external enamel epithelium is thought to be involved in the maintenance of the shape of the enamel organ and in the exchange of substances between the enamel organ and the environment. The cervical loop, at which there is considerable mitotic activity, lies at the growing margin of the enamel organ, where the external enamel epithelium is continuous with the internal enamel epithelium.

Stellate reticulum

This tissue is most fully developed at the bell stage. The intercellular spaces become filled with fluid, presumably related to osmotic effects arising from the high concentration of glycosaminoglycans. The cells are star-shaped with bodies containing conspicuous nuclei and many branching processes. In addition to glycosaminoglycans, the cells also contain alkaline phosphatase but have only small amounts of RNA and glycogen. The mesenchyme-like features of the stellate reticulum include the synthesis of collagens in the tissue. Collagen types I, II and III are expressed in the cells of the stellate reticulum, although their functional significance is unclear (Fig. 21.13).

The cells of this layer (Fig. 21.14) possess little endoplasmic reticulum and few mitochondria. However, there is a relatively well-developed Golgi apparatus, which, together with the presence of microvilli on the cell surface, has been interpreted as indicating that the cells contribute to the secretion of the extracellular material. Numerous tonofilaments are present within the cytoplasm, and desmosomes and gap junctions are present between the cells.

The main function ascribed to the stellate reticulum is a mechanical one. This relates to the protection of the underlying dental tissues against physical disturbance and to the maintenance of tooth shape. It has been suggested that the hydrostatic pressure generated within the stellate reticulum is in equilibrium with that of the dental papilla, allowing the proliferative pattern of the intervening internal enamel epithelium to determine crown morphogenesis. However, a change in either of these pressures might lead to a change in the outline of the internal enamel epithelium, and this could be important for crown morphogenesis.

The stellate reticulum also produces macrophage colony-stimulating factor (MCSF), transforming growth factor (TGF)-β_1 and parathyroid hormone–related protein (PTHrP). These molecules may be released into the dental follicle and help recruit, and activate, the osteoclasts necessary to resorb the adjacent alveolar bone as the developing tooth enlarges and erupts (see pages 457-458).

Stratum intermedium

This first appears at the bell stage and consists of two or three layers of flattened cells lying over the internal enamel epithelium (and its derivatives). The cells of the stratum intermedium resemble the cells of the stellate reticulum, although their intercellular spaces are smaller and the cells contain more alkaline phosphatase. It has been suggested that the stratum intermedium is concerned with the synthesis of proteins, the transport of materials to and from the enamel-forming cells (the ameloblasts) derived from the internal enamel epithelium and/or the concentration of materials.

Internal enamel epithelium

The cells of this layer are columnar at the bell stage, but, beginning at the regions associated with the future cusp tips (i.e., the sites of initial enamel formation), the cells become elongated. The internal enamel epithelial cells are rich in RNA but, unlike the stratum intermedium and stellate reticulum, do not contain alkaline phosphatase. Desmosomes connect the internal enamel epithelial cells and link this layer to the stratum intermedium. The internal enamel epithelium is separated from the peripheral cells of the dental papilla by a basement membrane and a cell-free zone 1–2 μm wide.

The differentiation of the dental papilla is less striking than that of the enamel organ. Until the late bell stage, the dental papilla consists of closely packed mesenchymal cells with only a few delicate extracellular fibrils. Histochemically, the dental papilla becomes rich in glycosaminoglycans.

Fig. 21.15 provides a model demonstrating the arrangement of deciduous tooth germs at 17 weeks on the dental lamina of a lower jaw quadrant. The dental lamina (green) is beginning to degenerate. Downgrowths on the lingual aspect of the enamel organs indicate the early development of the successional (permanent) teeth.

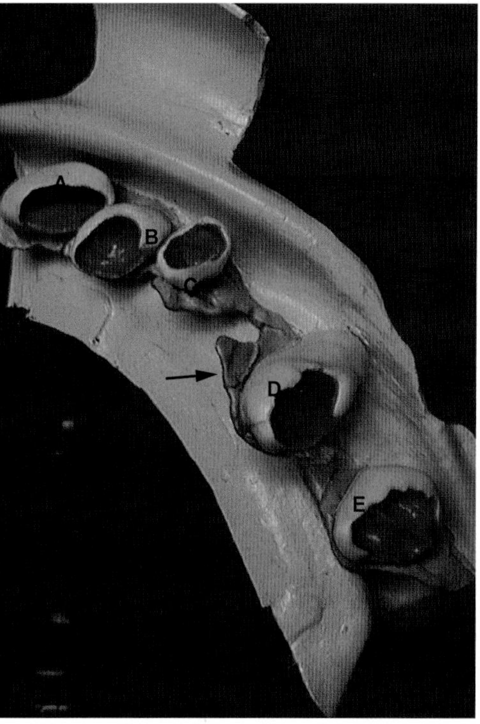

Fig. 21.15 The arrangement of deciduous enamel organs (identified by the Palmer-Zsigmondy system, A–E) at 17 weeks on the dental lamina of a lower jaw quadrant. Arrow indicates developing permanent tooth.

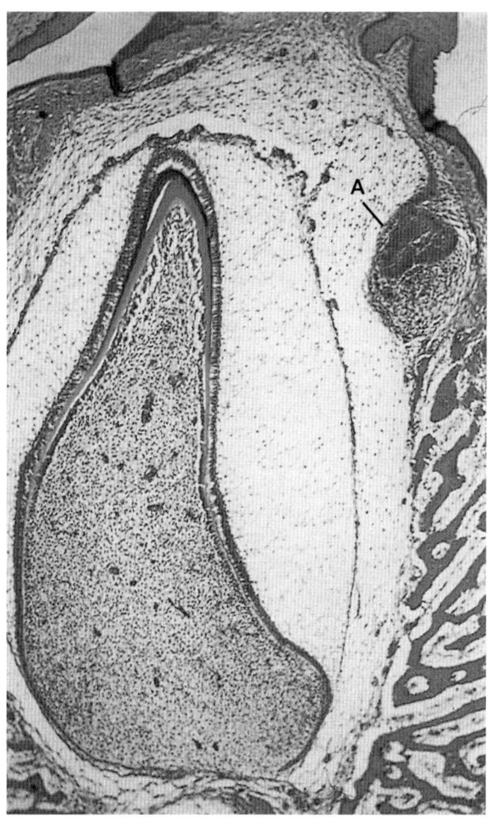

Fig. 21.16 Late bell stage (appositional stage) of tooth development. Dentine matrix stained blue; enamel matrix stained red. A = permanent tooth (Masson's trichrome; ×60).

Late bell stage

The late bell stage (appositional stage) of tooth development (Fig. 21.16) is associated with the formation of the dental hard tissues, commencing at about the 18th week. Dentine formation always precedes enamel formation. Detailed accounts of amelogenesis and dentinogenesis are given in Chapters 22 and 23. In the section shown in Fig. 21.16, downgrowths of the external enamel epithelium appear from the lingual sides of the enamel organs. In deciduous teeth, these lingual downgrowths give rise to the tooth germs of the permanent successors and first appear alongside the incisors at about 5 months *in utero*. In enamel organs of permanent teeth, however, these downgrowths eventually disappear. Behind the deciduous second molar, the dental lamina grows backwards to bud off successively to create the permanent molar teeth. The first permanent molar appears at about 4 months *in utero*, the tooth bud for the second permanent molar appears about 6 months after birth and that for the third permanent molar appears at about 4–5 years after birth.

Fig. 21.17 provides a high-power view of a region of a tooth germ at the late bell stage to show enamel and dentine formation commencing at

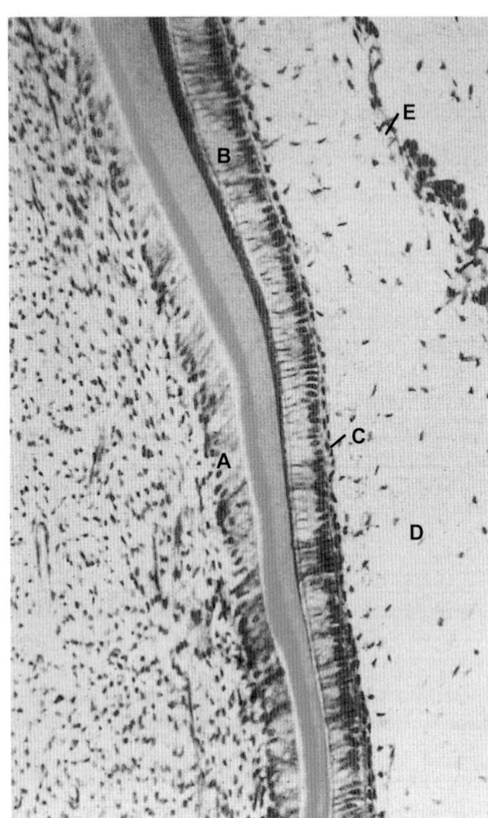

Fig. 21.17 High-power view of a region of a tooth germ at the late bell stage to show enamel and dentine formation. A = odontoblasts; B = ameloblasts; C = stratum intermedium; D = stellate reticulum; E = external enamel epithelium; dentine matrix stained green; enamel matrix stained red (Masson's trichrome; ×130).

the tips of future cusps (or incisal edges). Under the inductive influence of developing ameloblasts (preameloblasts), the adjacent mesenchymal cells of the dental papilla become columnar and differentiate into odontoblasts. The odontoblasts then become involved in the formation of predentine and dentine. The presence of dentine then induces the ameloblasts to secrete enamel.

Transitory structures

During the early stages of tooth development, three transitory structures may be seen: the enamel knot, enamel cord and enamel niche.

Enamel knot

An important development during the bud stage is the induction by the mesenchyme of the *primary enamel knot* (Fig. 21.18). This is a localised, non-proliferating cluster of cells at the centre of the inner dental epithelium, which is central to establishing the form of the tooth crown. Characteristically, the enamel knot forms a bulge into the dental papilla, at the centre of the enamel organ. The primary enamel knot is an important signalling centre expressing ten or more growth factors, including members of the BMP, FGF, Shh (sonic hedgehog) and Wnt families. The primary enamel knot is not a permanent feature of the tooth germ and is removed by apoptosis at the end of the cap stage. In monocuspid teeth (incisors, canines), the primary knot is the only one to form, and it marks the site of the tooth tip. However, in premolars and molars, additional *secondary enamel knots* are formed at the sites of the future cusps and in a sequence that matches the relative importance of the cusps in the mature tooth. Although the primary and secondary enamel knots consist of nondividing cells, they secrete mitogenic factors that diffuse outwards to stimulate proliferation and folding of the adjacent internal enamel epithelial and mesenchymal cells. This results in expansion of the epithelial cap and also infolding of the inner dental epithelium; downgrowths of the expanding dental epithelium on the flanks of the enamel knots result in the formation of cusps during the bell stage. Many mutations affecting signalling factors associated with enamel knots result in altered tooth morphology. As many genes participate in the signalling activities of the enamel knots, the system is capable of very fine control of crown morphology. Fig. 21.19A shows Shh in the primary enamel knot, and Fig. 21.19B shows BMP-2 expression in secondary enamel knots in molars at the sites of cusp formation. Fig. 21.20 demonstrates FGF-20 expression in the enamel knots of molars.

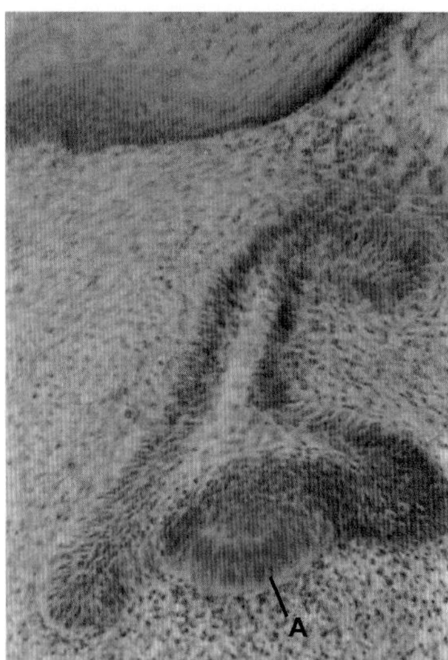

Fig. 21.18 The enamel knot (A) (H & E; ×120).

Enamel cord

The enamel cord (Fig. 21.21) is a strand of cells seen at the early bell stage of development that extends from the stratum intermedium into the stellate reticulum. When present, the enamel cord overlies the incisal margin of a tooth or the apex of the first cusp to develop (primary cusp). When it completely divides the stellate reticulum into two parts, reaching the external enamel epithelium, it is termed the *enamel septum*. Where the enamel cord meets the external enamel epithelium, a small invagination termed the *enamel navel* may be seen. The cells of the enamel cord are distinguished from their surrounding stellate reticulum cells by their elongated nuclei. It has been suggested that the enamel cord may be involved in the process by which the cap stage is transformed into the bell stage (acting as a mechanical tie) or that it is a focus for the origin of stellate reticulum cells.

Enamel niche

The enamel niche (Fig. 21.22) is seen where the tooth germ appears to have a double attachment to the dental lamina (the lateral and medial enamel strands). These strands enclose the enamel niche, which appears as a funnel-shaped depression containing connective tissue. The functional significance of the enamel niche is unknown. The enamel cord and the double attachment of the tooth germ around the enamel niche were once regarded as evidence supporting the view that the complex crown form of mammalian teeth evolved from fusion of several individual, simpler elements. However, this view is not now accepted.

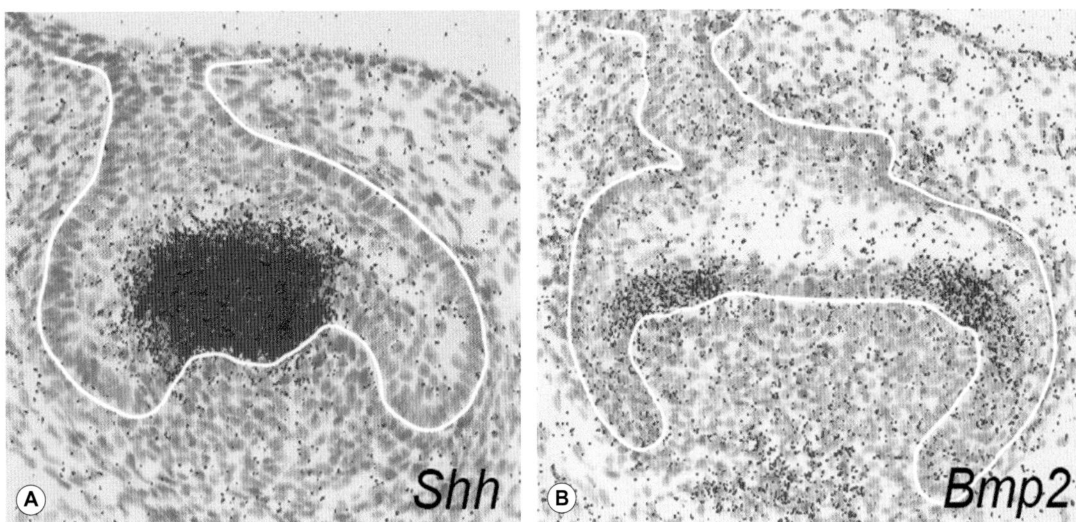

Fig. 21.19 (A) Staining for Shh (sonic hedgehog – red stain) in the primary enamel knot of a molar tooth by *in situ* hybridization (×140). (B) Staining for BMP-2 (red stain) in the secondary enamel knots of a molar tooth by *in situ* hybridization (×140). Courtesy Dr. M Jussila.

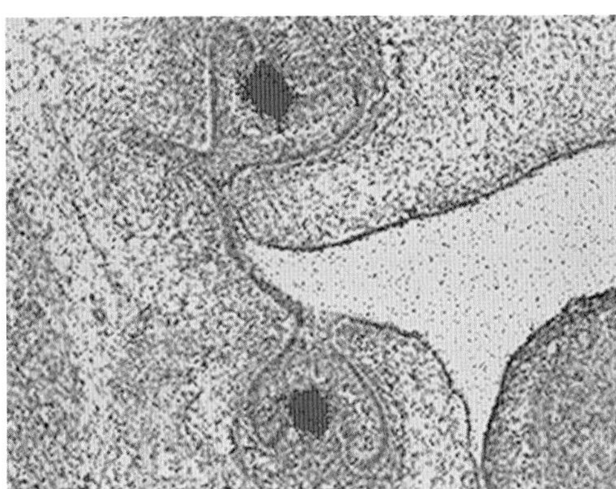

Fig. 21.20 Staining for FGF20 expression (red stain) in upper and lower molar tooth germs by *in situ* hybridization (×50). Courtesy Dr. M Jussila.

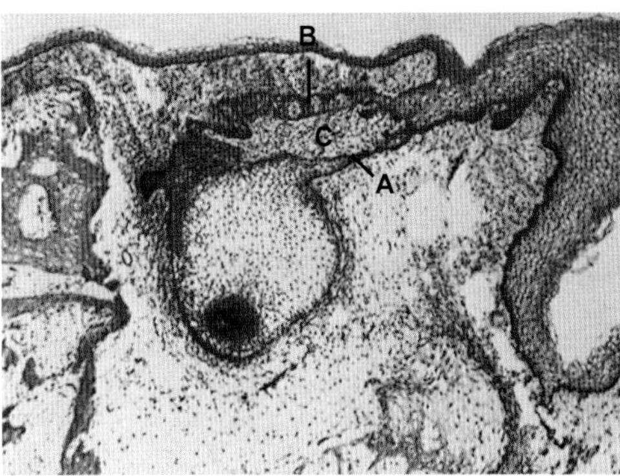

Fig. 21.22 The enamel niche (C). A = lateral enamel strand; B = medial enamel strand (H & E; ×40).

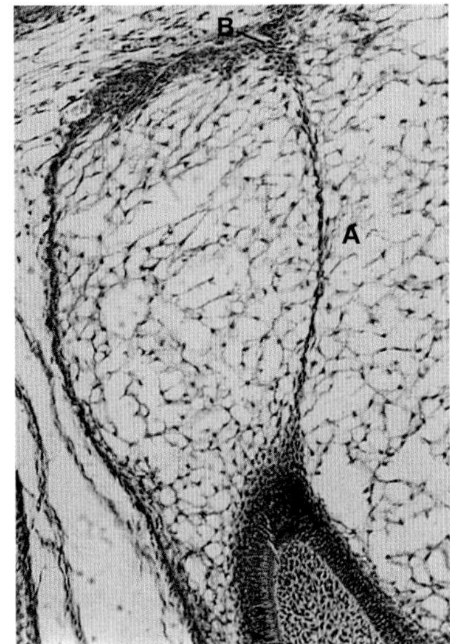

Fig. 21.21 The enamel cord (A). B = enamel navel (Masson's trichrome; ×120).

Nerve fibres

There is conflicting evidence as to when, and where, nerve fibres first appear during tooth development. It has been reported that nerve fibres are present in the immediate vicinity of presumptive dental epithelium at the very earliest stage of tooth induction and subsequently form a plexus below the dental papilla at the cap stage. From such plexuses, the nerves spread into the dental follicle as it develops. Penetration of nerves into the dental papilla occurs with the onset of dentinogenesis. The nerve fibres associated with blood vessels are presumed to be autonomic; others lying free within the papilla are assumed to be sensory. However, the innervation of the dental papilla remains rudimentary until after birth and may be fully developed only after the tooth has erupted. Controversy also remains concerning the role of neuronal cells and neurotrophins in tooth development. Recent work indicates that although nerve fibres are not required for odontogenesis, the pattern of localisation of neurotrophins (and their associated receptors) does suggest a role for neural-like cells – perhaps related to the neural crest derivation of the dental mesenchyme. However, in transgenic animals where neurotrophins and their receptors are not expressed, tooth development is not affected.

Blood supply

Small blood vessels invade the dental papilla at the early bell stage. They are also evident in the dental follicle in close association with the external enamel epithelium. Studies in both mice and humans have shown that the blood vessels penetrate the stellate reticulum from the outer enamel epithelium and reach the ameloblasts.

Epithelial–mesenchymal interactions during tooth development

During tooth development, the epithelial-mesenchymal 'conversation' is largely controlled by ligand-receptor interactions (signals), which trigger transcriptional changes to cause cell differentiation, histogenesis and morphogenesis. Mesenchymal and epithelial cells communicate through the basement membrane and exchange diffusible signal molecules throughout the developmental process. Different gene regulatory networks control this exchange during development in order to regulate complex spatiotemporal changes of the cells.

Initiation of tooth development

Direction of the odontogenic signal

There is evidence that the oral epithelium determines the location of prospective teeth and that neural crest cells migrating into the mandibular arch are tooth-unspecified before and during migration. Therefore, the epithelium is initially responsible for sending an inductive odontogenic signal to the mesenchyme. In response, the mesenchyme condenses and sends an inductive signal back towards the epithelium.

In 5-week-old human embryos, epithelial thickenings are already visible on unfused facial processes. As shown by 3D reconstruction studies of tooth development, the upper lateral incisor has a double origin, with thickenings both from the medial nasal and maxillary processes, making it more likely to disappear, duplicate or undergo hypoplasia, especially in patients with clefts.

The epithelium of the mouse first arch has been separated from mesenchyme and then recombined with non-dental ectomesenchyme, resulting in the formation of teeth. In the reciprocal experiment (at the same embryonic stage of development), when the second arch epithelium is combined with the first or second arch mesenchyme, bone and cartilage are formed instead of tooth germs. Only very early in odontogenesis can the epithelium of the first arch initiate tooth development. Following its induction from the epithelium, when first arch mesenchyme is then combined with second arch epithelium (which, as stated earlier, does not initiate odontogenesis), tooth germs are formed. This confirms that after initiation by the oral epithelium, the 'control' of tooth development passes to the mesenchyme.

Many investigations have been conducted into the role of neural crest cells (ectomesenchyme) in odontogenesis, and there is much evidence from both non-mammalian and mammalian vertebrates showing that the mesenchyme within a tooth germ is derived from the neural crest. Table 21.1 provides information regarding the derivatives of the cranial neural crest.

It has also been shown that cranial neural crest cells taken from their site of origin (near the developing neural tube), and before their migration into the pharyngeal arches, can produce tooth germs when combined with first arch epithelium but not when combined with second arch epithelium or epithelium from other sites. This confirms that, at this early stage, the neural crest cells are responding to the odontogenic signal from early, inductive dental epithelium.

During embryonic development, multiple growth factor–encoding genes are expressed in thickened dental epithelium. Among them are FGF-8, FGF-9, BMP-2, BMP-4, BMP-7, Shh, Wnt-10a and Wnt-10b. These epithelial signalling molecules are responsible for the induction of gene expression in the adjacent dental mesenchyme, including *Msx1, Msx2, Lef1, Dlx1, Dlx2, Barx1, Patched (Ptc), Gli1* and *syndecan-1*.

Table 21.1 Derivatives of the cranial neural crest cells

Ganglia	Skin	Carotid body cells	Craniofacial skeleton
Sensory cranial ganglia	Melanocytes	C cells of the ultimobranchial body and thyroid gland	Dermal bone-forming cells
Parasympathetic (ciliary) ganglia	Pigment cells of the inner ear		Endochondral osteocytes
Enteric ganglia			Chondrocytes
Satellite glial cells in ganglia			
Enteric glia			Myofibroblasts/ smooth muscle cells (conotruncus and aortic arch-derived arteries)
Schwann cells along PNS nerves			Pericytes in brain
Ensheathing and olfactory cells lining the olfactory nerve			Meninges (forebrain)
			Odontoblasts, cells in periodontal ligament and tooth papillae
			Adipocytes
			Dermal cells of the face
			Connective tissue cells of glands, muscles and tendons
			Corneal cells in endothelium and stroma
			Ciliary muscles

Recently identified within the epithelial layer of the embryonic mandible is a migratory population of FGF-8–expressing cells, which are progenitors of the epithelial component of the tooth germ. At early embryonic stages, these cells are arranged in a rosette and migrate as a group. FGF-8 is essential for the motility of the cells, but their migration is dependent on attraction by Shh-expressing cells located at the anterior margin of the dental lamina. The presence of both FGF- and Shh-expressing cells is essential for determining the site of tooth initiation and implies that tooth development involves interaction between these two groups of epithelial cells, as well as interactions between epithelium and mesenchyme.

In the mesenchyme, at the earliest stage, the position of the tooth germs involves the paired box gene *Pax9*. Expression of *Pax9* is restricted to the mesenchyme that underlies the sites of the future invaginations and presents the earliest mesenchymal marker of the position of the future tooth germs. *Pax9*, similarly to *Barx1*, is positively regulated by FGF-8 and negatively regulated by BMP-4.

Studies investigating the origins of the dental epithelium have compared the molecular characteristics of oral ectoderm with those of pharyngeal endoderm. It is found that Claudin6, Hnf3-β, α-fetoprotein, Rbm35a and *Sox2* are expressed in the endoderm where molars are developing. This suggests that molar teeth (but not more anterior teeth) in amphibians and pharyngeal teeth in teleosts are derived from epithelium of endodermal origin. This being the case, multicuspid teeth would evolve from 'externalisation' of pharyngeal tooth-like structures, while monocuspids would evolve from 'internalisation' of ectodermal structures (e.g., the ectodermal armour odontodes found in ancient fish).

The nature of the inductive message

The epithelium and mesenchyme exchange 'messages' during tooth development to produce changes of increasing complexity (i.e., differentiation). Induction is the process by which one cell type affects another. Several studies have shown that bioactive signalling molecules, usually proteins, pass between the epithelium and mesenchyme and interact with their receptors. A series of intracellular cascades are triggered by these interactions, which control gene expression and change cell behaviour. Inductive messages can still be understood by referring to early experiments. To explain how information leading to induction might be transferred between epithelium and mesenchyme, three main hypotheses have been proposed:

Chemical substances (diffusible signalling molecules) are produced by cells that diffuse across the narrow space to be taken up, and cause, induction in other cells.

Induction is governed by direct cell-to-cell contact and does not involve a diffusible molecule.

Induction results from the presence of the initial extracellular matrix, a thin layer situated between the epithelium and mesenchyme and comprising the basal lamina and adjacent region. This extracellular matrix has a complex composition, consisting of collagen (mainly type IV but possibly some types I and III), proteoglycans and glycoproteins.

To assess which of the three hypotheses is likely to provide the correct explanation for reciprocal control of differentiation, experiments have been undertaken in which the epithelial and mesenchymal components are dissected out and separated at the early bell stage, before any significant degree of cytodifferentiation. They are then recombined for tissue culture, but with a porous membrane placed between; the size of the pores in the membrane can be varied to ascertain the point at which both ameloblasts and odontoblasts differentiate. As molecules can readily diffuse through a pore size just less than 0.2 μm, and yet there is an absence of differentiation (Fig. 21.23), appears to argue against hypothesis 1 (a diffusible chemical substance). The lack of differentiation with pores less than 0.2 μm coincides with both the absence of the extracellular matrix and the absence of cell processes invading the porous membrane. Thus, either cell-to-cell contact or the extracellular matrix could be implicated in differentiation. Differentiation of the enamel organ and dental papilla is seen when pore size is 0.6 μm and cell processes are evident passing through the micropores (Fig. 21.24). However, as specialised cell contacts between differentiating odontoblasts and ameloblasts do not appear to occur *in vivo* (although the processes do come very close together), it is likely that the extracellular matrix has an important role in induction.

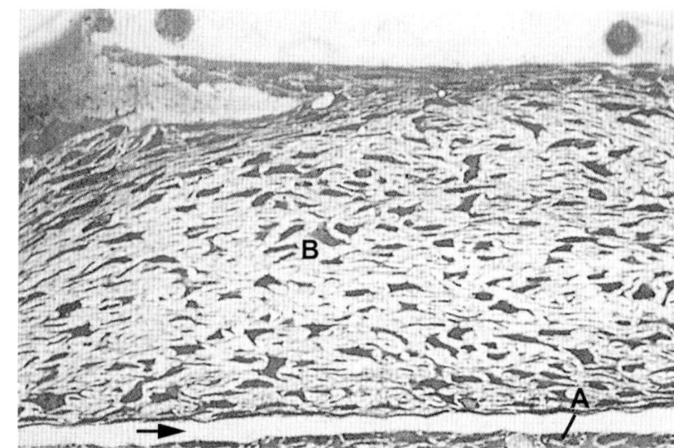

Fig. 21.23 The enamel organ (A) and dental papilla mesenchyme (B) cultured on either side of a porous membrane (pore size, 0.1 μm) (arrowed). No differentiation has occurred and cell processes do not pass through the membrane (toluidine blue; ×70). Courtesy Prof. I Thesleff and the editor of the *Journal of Embryology and Experimental Morphology*.

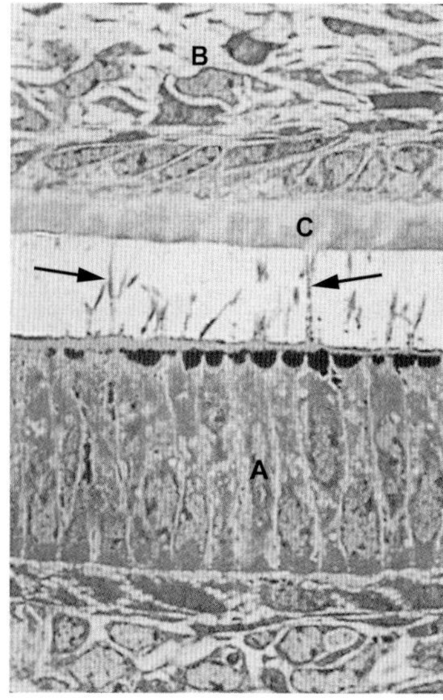

Fig. 21.24 The enamel organ (A) and dental papilla mesenchyme (B) cultured on either side of a porous membrane (pore size, 0.6 μm). C = predentine; cell processes from odontoblasts passing through pores are arrowed (Mallory's trichrome stain; ×45). Courtesy Prof. I Thesleff and the editor of the *Journal of Embryology and Experimental Morphology*.

The extracellular matrix itself is a product of both the epithelial and the mesenchymal cells.

Evidence indicating the importance of the extracellular matrix in the inductive process can also be obtained from the following experiments. First, drugs are available that can inhibit the formation of specific components of the extracellular matrix (e.g., lathyrogens interfere with cross-linking of collagen). When added to tissue culture medium, these drugs inhibit differentiation of the tooth germ. Second, isolated pieces of extracellular matrix will produce histological signs of differentiation in internal enamel epithelial cells of the enamel organ. It is conceivable that, in relation to the physical properties of the initial extracellular matrix, this matrix provides a surface for attachment of cells or enables interactions between bioactive molecules that induce early differentiation.

Mechanochemical control of mesenchymal condensation

Based on different hypotheses for reciprocal epithelial–mesenchymal induction, studies have suggested a complex mechanochemical control driving tooth development. FGF-8 and Sema3f are produced by the dental epithelium and are known to act in a repulsion or attraction mechanism that results in the condensation of mesenchymal cells. Mechanical compaction induces odontogenic transcription factors (*Pax9, Msx1*) and chemical cues such as

BMP-4. During the different stages of tooth development, the compression of mesenchyme causes the switch from one cell fate to another. This demonstrates that a mechanochemical control system is needed to regulate mesenchymal condensation. Research also indicates that mechanical stimulation causes odontogenic induction by signalling molecules (RhoA) that mediate cell compaction. These observations raise the possibility that physical alterations in the cells leading to cell compaction in the condensed mesenchyme also could have an active role in the differentiation process, along with the preservation of chemical factors (morphogens) that play an important role in the process. Regenerative approaches for engineering a biological replacement of teeth and organ engineering require *in vitro* systems that are capable of mimicking, and enabling, mechanochemical control of mesenchymal condensation (see Chapter 28).

Development of teeth from a spatiotemporal perspective

Much research has been undertaken on the molecular regulation of the cellular behaviours that drive tooth development. However, most studies focusing on tooth morphogenesis use static histological analyses. Although providing us with knowledge about the underlying mechanisms that drive morphogenesis, these studies often only offer a snapshot of cellular activities, limiting our understanding of tissue behaviour in a dynamic spatiotemporal environment where cellular activities are taking place. They are also based on 2D observations of the shape of the dental epithelium on histological sections such that the stages of tooth development are termed the ‘bud’, ‘cap’ and ‘bell’ stages. The spatial shape of the dental epithelium can never adequately be represented by such 2D terms, especially during the bud stage, as revealed by 3D reconstructions from 2D sections. Dental epithelium in the buccal region changes shape along the anteroposterior axis in response to the anteroposterior gradient. On frontal sections viewed anteroposteriorly, the dental epithelium seems to take on the appearance of several different ‘stages’, depending on its shape. Moreover, the anteroposterior growth gradient in the cheek region changes the shape of the dental epithelium along the axis.

3D reconstructions using a series of 2D sections reveal some important insights into tooth development, but there are still some drawbacks to using slides with tissue treatments that can introduce artifacts. For example, it has been reported that the molar epithelial progenitor cells initially form a rosette-like structure during tooth development. Owing to its sensitivity to formaldehyde, the structure can be disrupted by fixation during ‘tissue processing’ for histology. In order to overcome these problems, different research groups have begun studying cellular processes in conditions similar to those *in vivo*. These approaches use imaging techniques to model the development of tooth germs grown in laboratory conditions that mimic normal tissue growth, gene expression and differentiation markers during development. Consequently, it is possible to map events both spatially and temporally.

Mechanisms responsible for specifying the tooth-forming zones in the oral region and for controlling tooth number

The transcription factor Pitx2 is selectively expressed in the oral epithelium from the earliest stages of oral cavity formation, and its expression is thereafter restricted to dental epithelium. As with a broad range of other tissues, Shh is a major determinant of (or at least marks) the sites at which teeth develop. *Shh* gene expression is restricted to the dental epithelium at sites of tooth development and also appears to be involved in epithelial–mesenchymal interactions. During the initiation of tooth development, the *Shh* gene encodes a signalling peptide that is limited to localised thickenings of oral epithelium.

As Shh increases cell proliferation, restriction of expression to tooth-forming regions is important and seems to be accomplished by interactions with Wnt-signalling molecules. Indeed, Wnt helps maintain boundaries between tooth-forming areas and non-tooth-forming areas. The importance of Wnt/7b signalling can also be seen from experiments where its activity is inhibited, leading to the arrest of tooth morphogenesis at an early stage. Conversely, where Wnt signalling is stimulated (by stabilising beta-catenin) in the oral epithelium, it results in the production of dozens of extra teeth. In the molar region of mice, these supernumerary teeth are in the form of unicuspid cones (Fig. 21.25). In non-mammalian vertebrates with continuous tooth replacement (polyphodonty) Wnt signalling is maintained in the dental lamina.

The *Pax9* and *Msx1* genes appear to be required to enable the tooth germ to progress beyond the bud stage, as absence of the genes arrests the tooth germ at the bud stage.

Some important information concerning the mechanisms responsible for specifying tooth-forming zones has arisen from study of ‘hens’ teeth’. The absence of teeth in modern birds has given rise to the phrase ‘as rare as hens’ teeth’. However, the topic also provides a stimulus to research into epithelial–mesenchymal interactions. Because the ancestors of birds had teeth, the question arises as to whether there is any latent potential in either the epithelium or mesenchyme of modern birds to form teeth and whether this potential can be unlocked. Research has shown that several growth and transcription factors expressed during tooth development in mammals are present in the oral epithelial and mesenchymal tissues of chicks (e.g., *FGF-8, Pitx2, Barx1* and *Pax9*). However, other factors are missing, such as *Shh*, BMP-4, *Msx1* and *Msx2*. When BMP-4 protein is added exogenously to chick mandibles, it induces the expression of *Msx1* and *Msx2* in the mesenchyme. When chick epithelium is cultured with chick dorsal skin mesenchyme that does contain *BMP-4*, tooth bud–like structures are produced (Fig. 21.26).

Experiments have been undertaken in which chick neural crest is replaced by mouse neural crest (Fig. 21.27). The resulting mouse/chick chimaeras produce tooth germs (Fig. 21.28) up to the stage of the initial formation of organic matrix. This matrix is regarded as a dentine matrix, as the odontoblast-like cells produce dentine sialoprotein and nestin. This experiment indicates that mouse neural crest–derived mesenchymal cells with avian oral epithelium have the ability to induce the avian oral epithelium and thus initiate the avian tooth developmental programme. That the teeth fail to mineralise properly and produce enamel is not surprising, as the chick genome appears to lack the genes associated with the production of enamel matrix.

A recent experiment that sheds further light on why modern birds lack teeth relates to a chick mutant known as ‘talpid’ (ta^2). This is an autosomal recessive mutation that has serious consequences for the development of many organ systems. However, this mutant also uniquely exhibits the development of simple, unmineralised, tooth-like structures in the jaws. In explanation, from analysis of the distribution of growth and transcription factors (Fig. 21.29), it can be seen that a responsive mesenchyme is present in the normal (wild-type) situation but is displaced away from the responsive epithelium above, whereas in the mutant talpid, the responsive mesenchyme is displaced to lie directly beneath the responsive epithelium.

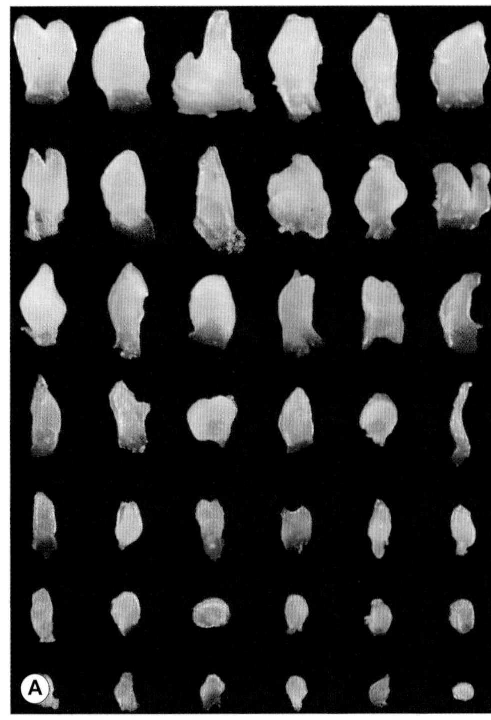

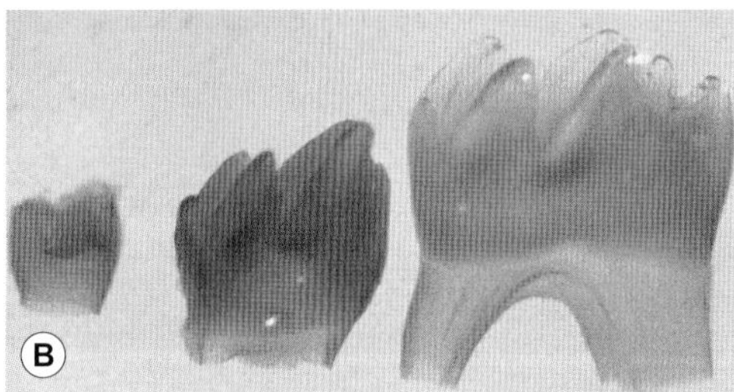

Fig. 21.25 (A) Forty-two mineralised teeth of various sizes collected from one developing molar tooth in a mouse in which Wnt signalling was sustained. (B) The three molars present in normal mouse controls (×13). From Jarvinen, E., et al., 2006. Continuous tooth generation in mouse is induced by activated epithelial Wnt/β-catenin signalling. Proceedings of the National Academy of Sciences of the United States of America 103, 18627–18632.

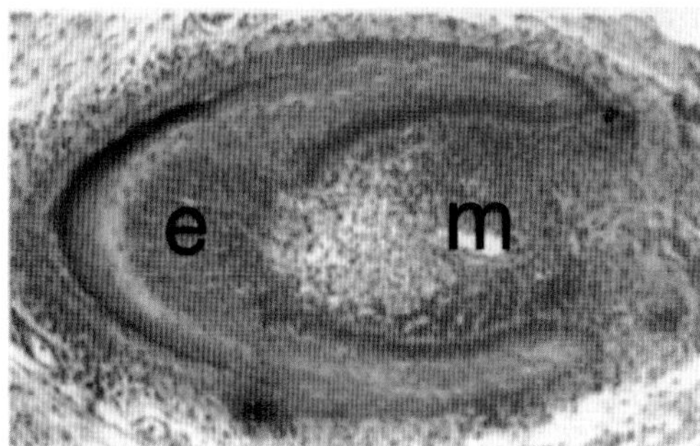

Fig. 21.26 Chick 'tooth-like structure' formed by recombining chick mandibular epithelium (E) with chick skin mesenchyme (M) and culturing for 2 days (×80). From Chen Y, et al., 2000. Conservation of early odontogenic signalling pathways in Aves. Proceedings of the National Academy of Sciences of the United States of America 97, 10044–10049.

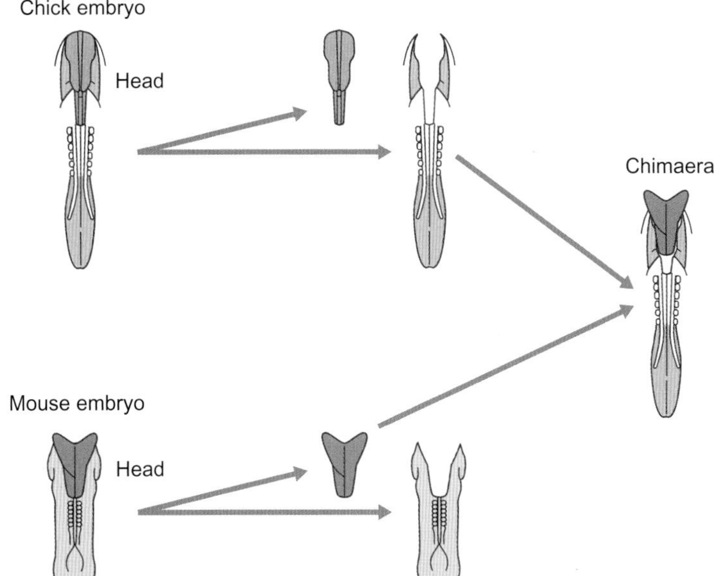

Fig. 21.27 Diagram of the experimental procedure of mouse neural tube transplantation into chick host embryos for the creation of a chick/mouse chimaera that has an abnormal head morphology. From Mitsiadis, T.A., Caton, J., Cobourne, M., 2006. Waking up the sleeping beauty: recovery of the ancestral bird odontogenic program. *Journal of Experimental Zoology (Molecular and Developmental Evolution)* 306B, 227–233.

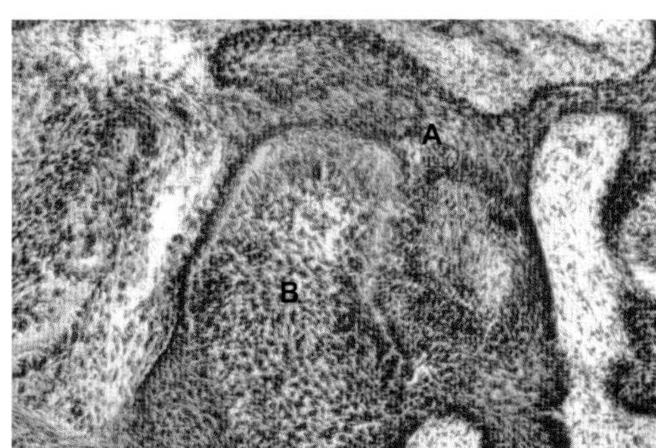

Fig. 21.28 'Chick tooth' derived from the chick/mouse chimaera experiments shown in Fig. 21.27 at the bell stage. The epithelial enamel organ (A) is chick-derived and the dental papilla (B) is mouse-derived. The blue staining represents initial dentine matrix (Masson's blue trichrome; ×63). Courtesy Dr. T A Mitsiadis.

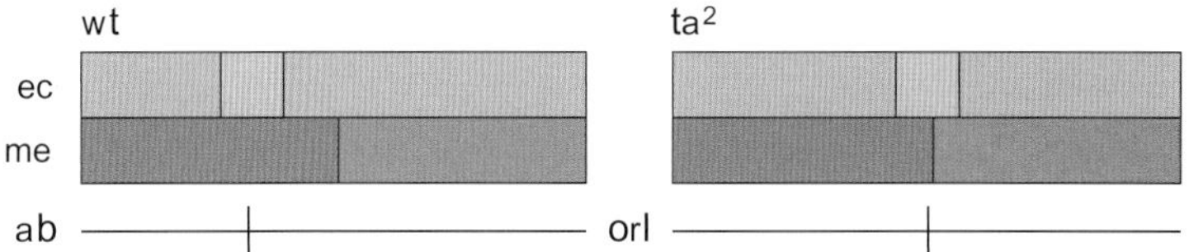

Fig. 21.29 Model of alteration in the inductive interactions in wild-type chicks (wt) and ta^2 jaw leading to the initiation of teeth in the ta^2 mutant. In the wild type, a regional signalling centre is localised in the epithelium (yellow) by the interaction between FGF-8, BMP-4 and Shh signalling. This signalling centre demarcates the boundary between the oral and aboral epithelium (vertical mark on horizontal ab–orl line). This epithelial signalling centre does not overlie oral mesenchyme (purple) competent to make appendage structures. In the ta^2 mutant, early changes in FGF-8, BMP-4 and Shh signalling lead to medial positioning of the forming oral/aboral boundary such that the signalling centre and underlying competent mesenchyme are juxtaposed, permitting initiation of tooth developmental programmes. ab = aboral; ec = ectoderm; me = mesenchyme; orl = oral epidermis. From Harris, M.P., Hasso, S.M., Ferguson, M.W.J., Fallon, J.F. 2006. The development of Archosaurian first-generation teeth in a chicken mutant. *Current Biology* 16, 371–377.

Mechanisms responsible for specifying tooth type and tooth shape (morphogenesis)

Early experiments were designed to answer the question posed by investigators: Which of the two components is more important for inducing morphogenesis and histogenesis – the enamel organ or the dental papilla? Such experiments involved interchanging the epithelial and mesenchymal

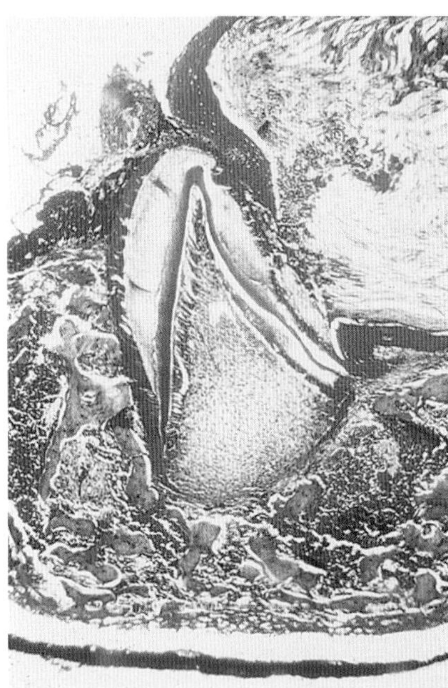

Fig. 21.30 The result of culturing dental papilla mesenchyme with epithelium from the developing foot pad. A normal tooth develops (Masson's trichrome; ×40). From Kollar, E.J., Baird, G.R., 1970. Tissue interactions in embryonic mouse tooth germs II. The inductive role of the dental papilla. *Journal of Embryology and Experimental Morphology* 24, 173–186.

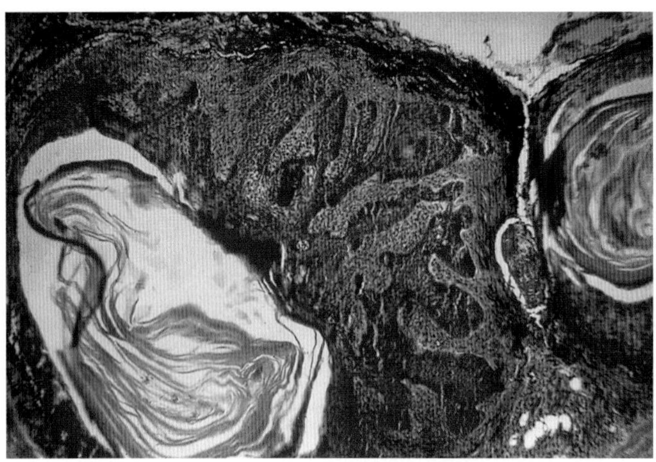

Fig. 21.31 The result of culturing the enamel organ of a tooth with mesenchyme from the developing foot pad. Note the absence of tooth development (Masson's trichrome; ×75). Courtesy Prof. E Kollar and the editor of the *Journal of Embryology and Experimental Morphology*.

components between different developing teeth (incisors and molars) and with tissues from nondental regions. The results indicated that, at the cap stage of tooth development, the principal organiser is the dental papilla in terms of both morphogenesis and histogenesis. The result of culturing dental papilla mesenchyme with epithelium from the developing foot pad (Fig. 21.30) is normal tooth development, illustrating the importance of the dental papilla. On the other hand, if the enamel organ of a tooth is cultured with mesenchyme from the developing foot pad (Fig. 21.31), tooth development does not occur. Similar experiments have been conducted to determine whether the enamel organ or the dental papilla determine tooth shape. Such experiments involve separating and recombining enamel organ and papilla at the cap stage between incisors and molars. Should an incisor enamel organ be combined with a molar papilla, the resulting tooth is molariform. Furthermore, if a molar enamel organ is combined with an incisor papilla, the resulting tooth is incisiform. Thus, as for histogenesis, the dental papilla is the dominant tissue determining tooth shape at the cap stage.

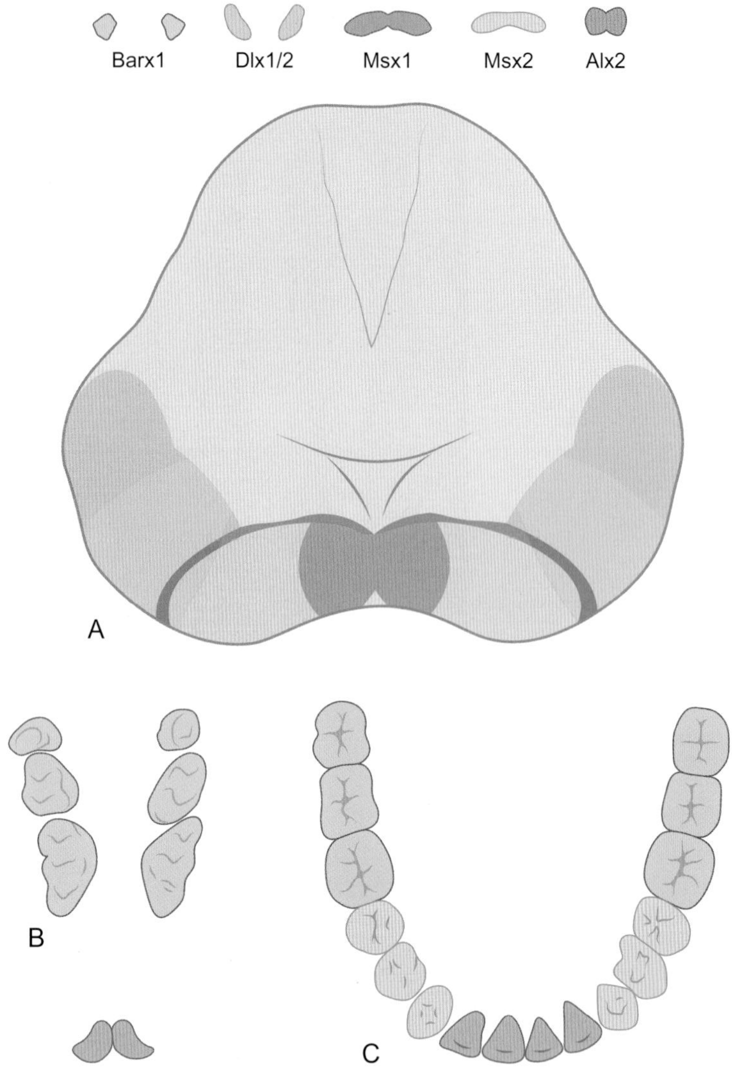

Fig. 21.32 Schematic diagrams to show the mesenchymal odontogenic homeobox gene code. (A) Diagram illustrating the lower jaw of the mouse. Note the overlap (orange) between the domains of *Msx1* (red) and *Msx2* (yellow). (B) Model representing the mouse dentition. Note that molars develop from cells expressing *Barx1* and incisors from cells expressing *Msx1*, *Msx2* and *Alx3*. (C) Model representing the human dentition, where it is predicted that incisors develop from cells expressing *Msx1*, *Msx2* and *Alx3*, canines and premolars from cells expressing *Msx1* and *Msx2* and molars from cells expressing *Barx1*. Courtesy Prof. P T Sharpe and the editor of *Bioessays*.

From these experiments, research has progressed to try to understand the molecular mechanisms involved in morphogenesis. The underlying control of such patterning is based upon the hypothesis that, as in other parts of the body (such as the vertebral column), patterning is related to the spatially restricted expression of homeobox genes in the ectomesenchyme of the developing jaws (referred to as the *odontogenic homeobox code*). These genes contain DNA-binding proteins that regulate gene transcription, thus controlling the expression of other genes necessary for the development of a particular structure, in this case a tooth. Accordingly, the group of homeobox genes expressed in the presumptive incisor region will dictate that incisiform teeth develop here, while the group of homeobox genes expressed at the back of the tooth row (in the presumptive molar region) will specify molariform teeth. For this hypothesis to be tenable, an important prerequisite is to establish that the presumptive incisor and molar regions do indeed contain some difference in their homeobox gene array, and this feature has been demonstrated. It is known that the neural crest cells for the mesenchyme of the first pharyngeal arch express non-Hox homeobox genes, including *Msx1, Msx2, Dlx1, Dlx2, Barx1* and *Alx3*. Different combinations of these homeobox genes appear to instruct the tooth germ with respect to its tooth type. Thus, the neural crest–derived

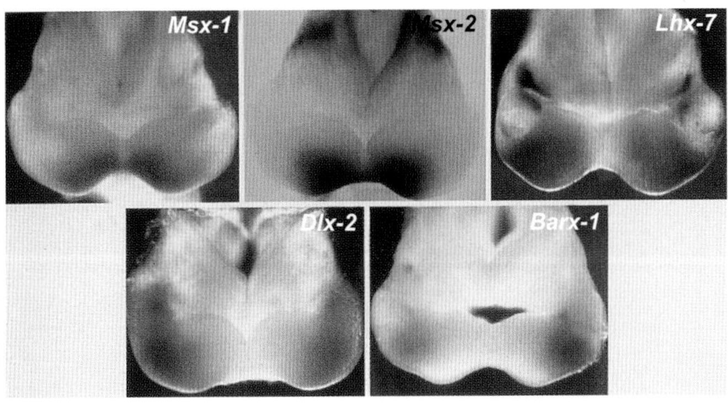

Fig. 21.33 Whole-mount *in situ* hybridisation to show localisation of homeobox genes (the darkly 'stained' regions) for the developing mandible. Courtesy Prof. PT Sharpe.

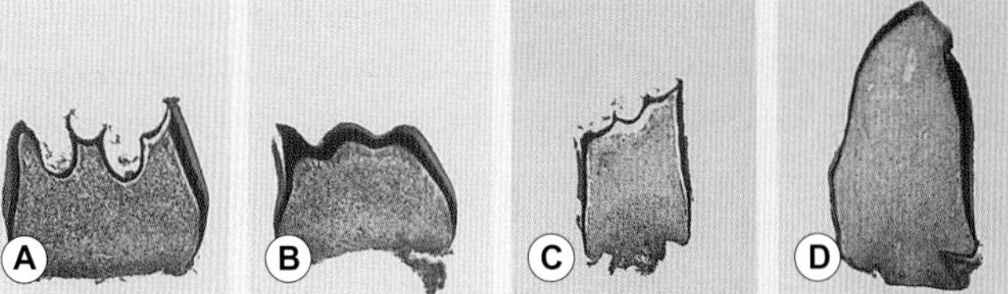

Fig. 21.34 The results of experiments to transform teeth from incisor to molar shape following downregulation of *Msx1* and upregulation of *Barx1* in incisors. (A) Control section of normal molar. (D) Control section of normal incisor. (B, C) Sections from incisor teeth showing change to molar shape following upregulation of *Barx1* in the mesenchyme (×25). From Tucker, A.S., Matthews, K.L., Sharpe, P.T., 1998. Transformation of tooth type induced by inhibition of BMP signaling. *Science* 282, 1136–1138.

mesenchyme in the incisor region expresses *Msx1* (but not *Barx1*), while neural crest–derived mesenchyme in the molar region expresses *Barx1* (but not *Msx1*) (Figs 21.32, 21.33). As with other systems of early development and differentiation, temporal factors mean that there is only a narrow window of opportunity to successfully manipulate the homeobox genes. The difference in distribution of homeobox genes between the incisor and molar regions is at least consistent with the odontogenic homeobox code hypothesis. Evidence to support the importance of such molecules in initiating tooth development can be seen in transgenic mice where, for example, an absence of the homeobox gene *Msx1* results in tooth development being arrested at the bud stage. Similarly, early mesenchyme isolated from the overlying epithelium can still continue to develop in tissue culture if molecules such as BMPs and FGFs are added to the medium.

The odontogenic homeobox code can be considered in the light of a 'field model hypothesis' where each tooth germ starts the same but different concentrations of morphogens (e.g., growth factors) in the local environment are responsible for producing different tooth types. The patterning of the dentition has been shown to be related to the polarity of the epithelium. This epithelial polarity is thought to be associated with expression of FGF-8 and BMP-4 growth factors. Accordingly, FGF-8 (with FGF-9) is expressed in the future molar region, whereas BMP-4 is expressed in the future incisor region. In relation to the homeobox genes, FGF-8 stimulates expression of *Barx1* and *Dlx2* and BMP4 stimulates *Msx1* and *Msx2* but inhibits *Barx1*.

One way of assessing the 'field model hypothesis' is to try to change the odontogenic homeobox code and determine whether the shape of a developing tooth can be altered. In this context, it is possible to culture early incisor tooth germs and absorb the BMP produced by the epithelium so that it does not switch on *Msx1* in the underlying mesenchyme cells. This is achieved by placing on the epithelial surface very small beads soaked in noggin protein, which is a BMP antagonist. In this situation, not only is *Msx1* downregulated in the mesenchyme but *Barx1* (normally only present in the molar region) is seen to be expressed. When such tooth germs are then transplanted *in vivo* to renal capsules and allowed to continue to develop, multicuspid teeth with a molariform rather than an incisiform morphology can be produced (Fig. 21.34). The odontogenic homeobox code therefore would explain the formation of different tooth homologies.

There is also evidence that the odontogenic homeobox code differs in the mandibular and maxillary regions. This is based upon the observation that when *Dlx1* and *Dlx2* gene expression is disrupted, mandibular molars still develope but not maxillary molars.

In contrast to the 'field model hypothesis', a 'clonal model hypothesis' has been put forward to explain tooth form. Accordingly, the tooth type is prespecified (probably at the original site of the neural crest cells) and is not dependent on the environment within the jaws. An experiment in which the possible contribution of the jaw environment was assessed required the removal of the dental lamina in the developing molar region, together with the surrounding mesenchyme. This very early, and undifferentiated, tooth germ (which would have given rise to the first molar) was then cultured in a site well away from the jaws. A tooth germ of the first molar at the cap stage of development removed from an embryo and transplanted for culture at a different site was seen to continue to develop normally, and the remaining second and third molars also developed. This finding is consistent with the idea that a series of related structures can form by budding off from a single precursor and that the differences between the individual structures (e.g., size and crown complexity) result from the increasing age of the tooth-budding region as it grows distally from the jaw (rather than from local environmental factors in the jaws). This 'clonal model hypothesis' could explain the successionary tooth formation of the second and third molars.

The formation of the specific shape of a tooth (including cusps) is signalled during the bud and cap stages of tooth development. Particular significance in morphogenesis has been placed on the presence of the enamel knot (Figs. 21.19 and 21.20). The shape of the enamel organ (producing the shape of the crown of the tooth) relates to the pattern of folding seen within the internal enamel epithelium and/or the forces present on either side of it. The enamel knot is thought to play a role in this morphogenesis, as it is associated with each main cusp that develops and as it possesses molecules seen in other patterning situations. The enamel knot is under the direction of signals emanating from the underlying mesenchyme, with BMP-4 stimulating the expression of *p21* (an inhibitor of cell proliferation) to produce the enamel knot. The enamel knot itself also expresses signalling molecules (FGF-4, Shh and BMPs and Wnt growth factors). Shh in particular is involved in the formation of the cap stage of the tooth germ, regulating cell survival at the tip of the enamel organ as it changes from the bud to the cap. Indeed, survival of the enamel knot is a balance between growth and apoptosis (FGF-4 for growth, BMP-4 for apoptosis).

Single-cell regulatory atlas shows neural crest lineage diversification during morphogenesis

Using transcriptomic analysis of the dental mesenchyme, research has revealed a spatiotemporal map for neural crest lineage diversification during tooth morphogenesis. Studies looked at postmigratory neural crest cells that commit to the dental mesenchymal lineage after arriving in the oral region of the first pharyngeal arch.

The cell fate diversification of postmigratory cranial neural crest cells that give rise to the dental mesenchyme has been investigated by profiling single cells from the mouse molar. Accordingly, transcriptional heterogeneity defines specific cellular domains that contribute to distinct molar mesenchymal tissues. Other studies have shown that Pax9+ cells in the mouse molar mesenchyme are located at the cap stage and are indeed progenitor cells, as they can contribute to all of the mesenchymal lineages of mouse molar development.

Further sub-clustering analysis of *Pax9+* cells reveals that two well-separated clusters (cell lineages) correspond to dental follicle and dental papilla cell populations. This study discovered previously unknown markers for these two lineages. Additionally, RNAscope *in situ* staining indicates that some marker genes (e.g., *Crym+/Egr3+/Fgf3+*) are expressed specifically in the dental papilla but are absent from the dental follicle, while others (e.g., *Epha3+/Fxyd7+/Foxf1+*) are found in the dental follicle cell domain surrounding the dental epithelium and dental papilla. In addition, the findings suggest that Foxp4 is essential for periodontal ligament differentiation.

Why permanent molars cannot be replaced

As for the deciduous incisors, canines and molars, the permanent molars at the bell stage also develop a successional dental lamina. However, unlike the deciduous teeth, the successional lamina of the permanent molars remain rudimentary and soon disappear without producing any replacement teeth. To shed light on why the transient rudimentary successional dental laminae (RSDL) by the sides of the permanent molars do not give rise to a further successional generation of teeth, genes known to be pivotal for the development of tooth germs in the RSDL of the mouse molar have been compared to the genes present in the RSDL of the primary dentition of the minipig, which do form successional teeth. It was observed that the RSDL in the minipig does not express *Sox2 or Sox9* at its tip but expresses high levels of nuclear β-catenin. However, the mouse RSDL houses *Sox2*-positive cells but no Wnt/β-catenin signalling. When Wnt/β-catenin signalling in the RSDL of the mouse was stabilised, formation of lingually positioned teeth occurred, suggesting that it is the lack of Wnt/β-catenin signalling in the RSDL that prevents the formation of a second generation of teeth (Fig. 21.35).

These findings support previous studies of the rudimentary laminas in monophyodont reptiles, which also lack Wnt/β-catenin signalling.

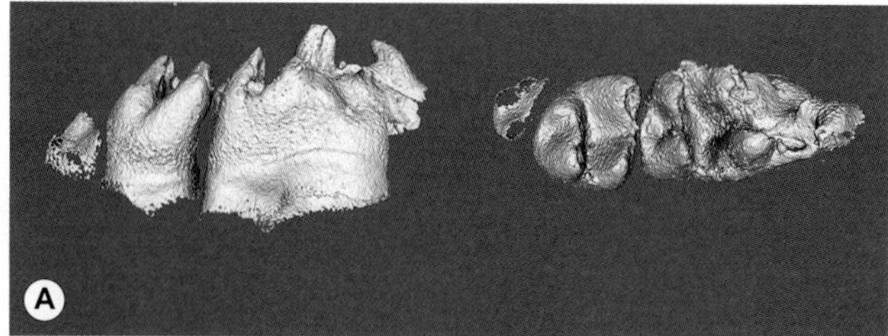

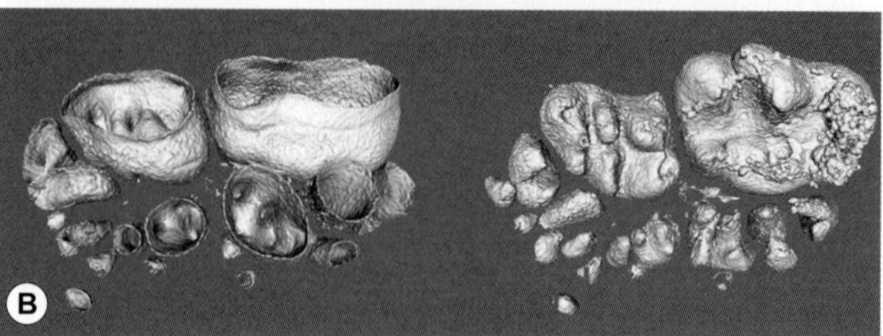

Fig. 21.35 (A) Dentition of control mouse teeth showing the normal development of the three molar teeth. Left image: lingual view; right image: occlusal view. In this situation, the expression of SOX2 in the rudimentary successional dental laminae (RSDL) inhibits Wnt/β-catenin signalling, preventing the development of a successional series of teeth. (B) Dentition of experimental mouse teeth where the RSDL has been allowed to develop in an environment where the inhibition of SOX2 has stabilised (activated) Wnt/β-catenin signalling (using the Cre-lox system). This has produced numerous supernumerary teeth on the lingual side, some with multiple cusps, that can be viewed as evidence of a successional series. Left image: lingual view; right image: occlusal view. This experiment supports the view that it is the lack of Wnt/β-catenin signalling in the RSDL that prevents the formation of a second generation of teeth. Scale bar = 0.5 mm for both images. From Popa, E.M., Buchtova, M., Tucker, A.S., 2019. Revitalising the rudimentary replacement dentition in the mouse. *Development* 146, dev171363.

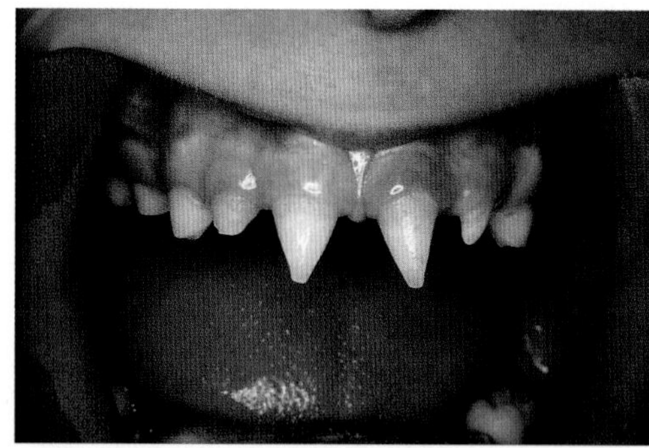

Fig. 21.36 Patient with ectodermal dysplasia showing several upper teeth present but with the characteristic peg shape. Cawson, R.A., Odell, E.W., 2008. *Cawson's Essentials of Oral Pathology and Oral Medicine*. Churchill Livingstone, Edinburgh.

Clinical considerations

Although much is known about normal tooth development, many details await investigation. It is hardly surprising, therefore, that we know relatively little about the changes in the tooth germ that lead to the range of congenital tooth abnormalities. Clearly, disturbance of the epithelial–mesenchymal interactions can markedly disturb tooth development and can result in the splitting of a tooth germ or the joining of adjacent germs to be responsible for some of the variations in tooth numbers and shape. Trauma and infection of the deciduous predecessors have also been implicated in the malformation of the permanent teeth. Malformations of teeth can occur in the deciduous or permanent dentition, although they are more common in the permanent dentition. This may reflect the stable environment of the child before birth.

Malformations of teeth can be related to variations in size, shape, number or structure, and many of these are illustrated on pages 61-65.

Anodontia and hypodontia (see also page 61)

Anodontia refers to a complete absence of teeth. This condition is very rare and may be found in some cases of ectodermal dysplasia. More commonly in ectodermal dysplasia a few teeth are present (Figs 21.36, 21.37). Areas where the teeth are absent lack an alveolar process, so there is little bone naturally available to receive an implant.

Where just one or two teeth are absent (hypodontia), the most frequently affected teeth are the permanent third molars, then the permanent maxillary second incisors, followed by the mandibular second premolars. Fig. 21.38 shows a patient with both maxillary lateral and mandibular central incisors missing. Knowing the important part played by certain transcription factors during tooth formation (pages 388-394), it is not surprising to find in both mice and humans that an absence of teeth has been associated with mutations in *Pax1, Pax9, Eda, Axin2* and *Msx1* genes.

Hyperdontia

Hyperdontia is an increase in tooth number, either by the appearance of supernumerary teeth (not having normal morphology – see page 61) or supplemental teeth (having normal morphology). A 'mesiodens' in the middle of the maxilla is an example of a supernumerary tooth (see Fig. 2.166). Supplemental teeth may be either single (Fig. 21.39) or multiple (Fig. 21.40). Fig. 21.41 illustrates a rare situation with a large number of supernumerary teeth and one supplemental tooth. In cleidocranial

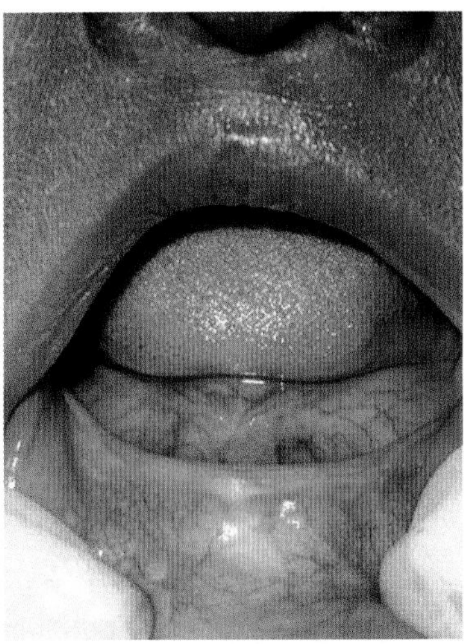

Fig. 21.37 Young patient with ectodermal dysplasia showing a complete absence of teeth. Courtesy Dr. S Saraf.

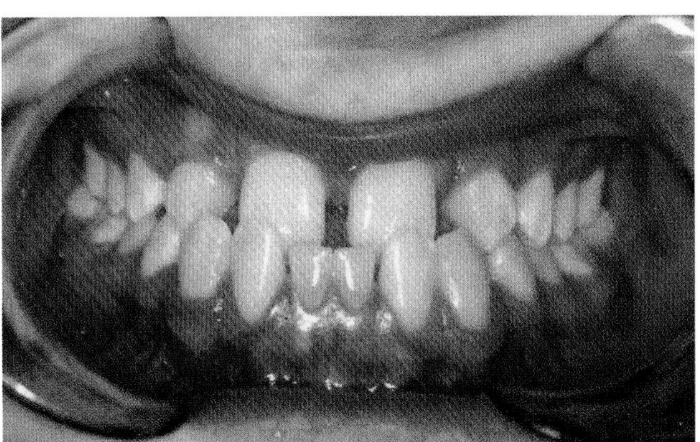

Fig. 21.38 Twelve-year-old patient presenting with missing maxillary lateral and mandibular central incisors. The incisor relationship is Class III. From Banerjee, A., Thavaraj, S. (Eds.), 2020. *Odell's clinical problem solving in dentistry*, fourth edition. Elsevier, London.

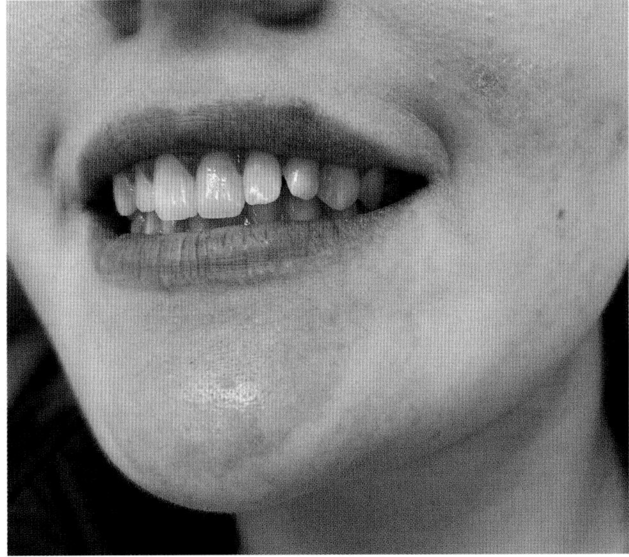

Fig. 21.39 Patient presenting with a supplemental maxillary second left incisor. Courtesy Dr. BJ Doherty.

dysplasia, a condition caused by mutations in *Cbfa1*, many of the teeth may remain unerupted (see Fig. 26.58). In addition, there may be several supernumerary teeth.

In humans, mutations of the *APC* gene, whose activity normally restricts Wnt pathway activity, may produce a variant known as Gardner's syndrome. In addition to familial adenomatous polyposis (FAP), there are associated dental features such as hyperdontia, unerupted supernumerary

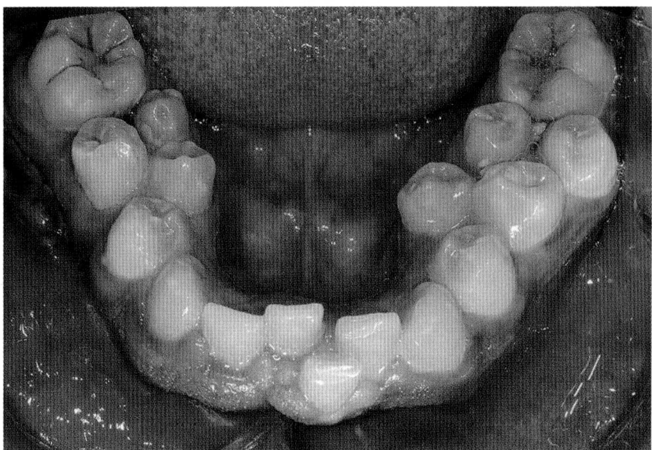

Fig. 21.40 Hyperdontia patient presenting with multiple supplemental bilateral mandibular premolars. From Chi, A.C., Damm, D.D., Allen, C.M., et al. (Eds.), 2019. *Color atlas of oral and maxillofacial diseases*. Elsevier, Philadelphia.

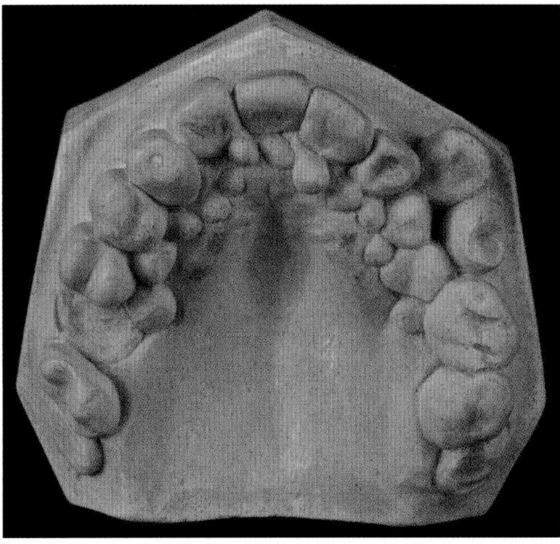

Fig. 21.41 Plaster cast of the maxilla of a 25-year-old male showing one supplemental premolar and 12 peg-shaped supernumerary teeth on the palatal side of the permanent teeth. Copyright the Royal College of Surgeons of England.

teeth, odontomas and osteomas (Fig 21.42). Early recognition of the syndrome from these dental features can save the patient's life from subsequent cancer of the colon.

Macrodontia and microdontia

Macrodontia refers to an enlarged tooth (see Fig. 2.168) and microdontia to a tooth very much reduced in size. Microdontia may accompany clefts of the lip or palate and be present in Ehlers–Danlos syndrome, hypopituitary disorders and ectodermal disorders. Microdontia usually affects a single tooth, especially the 'peg-shaped' permanent maxillary lateral incisor (see Fig. 2.167). Less frequently, multiple teeth may be affected (Fig. 21.43).

Gemination, fusion and concrescence of teeth

Gemination refers to a situation where there is partial cleavage of a tooth germ (see Figs 2.169, 2.170). Fusion occurs where there is union of two adjacent germs. In both gemination and fusion, the appearance can suggest a 'double' tooth. However, in fusion the total number of adjacent teeth is one less than normal (see Fig. 2.171). Concrescence is the fusion of adjacent teeth at the roots between adjacent teeth caused by hypercementosis. It is rarely noticed until one of the teeth is due for extraction, when it is found that the other tooth is displaced as well and surgical separation is necessary. Concrescence particularly affects permanent second and third molar teeth (Fig. 21.44; see also Fig. 2.179B).

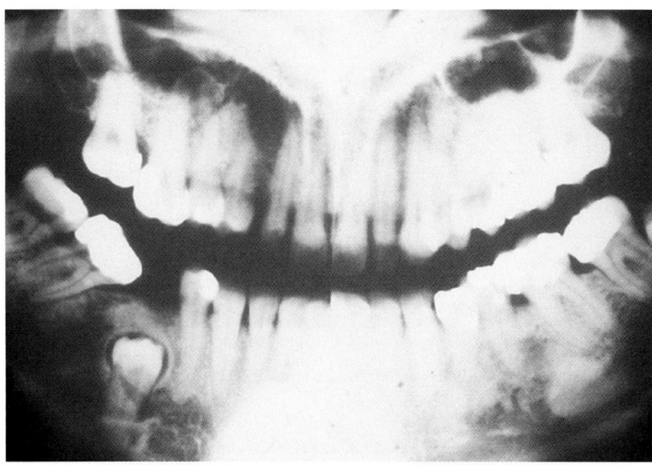

Fig. 21.42 Radiograph of patient suffering from Gardner's syndrome, resulting in the presence of a number of unerupted teeth. From Wysocki, G.P., Eversole, L.R., Sapp, J.P. (Eds.), 2004. *Contemporary oral and maxillofacial pathology*, second edition. Mosby, Philadelphia.

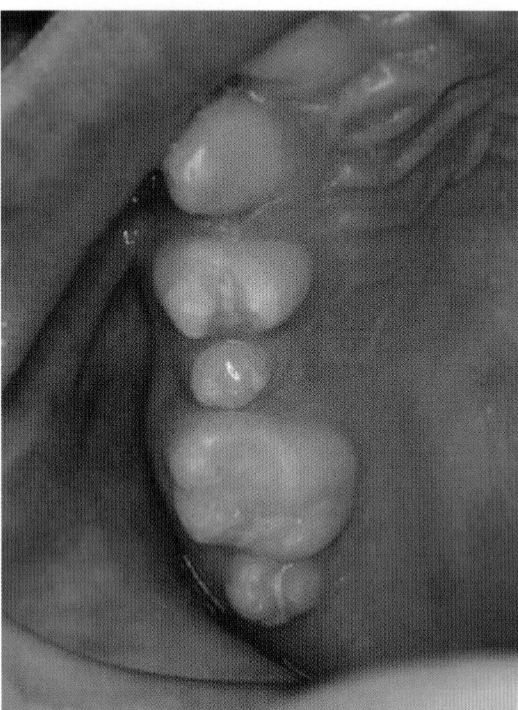

Fig. 21.43 Patient with microdontia affecting two teeth, namely the maxillary second premolar and maxillary second molar. Courtesy Drs. RP Widmer, AC Cameron and M Harrison. From Cameron, A., Widmer, R. (Eds.), *Elsevier handbook of pediatric dentistry*, fifth edition. Elsevier, London.

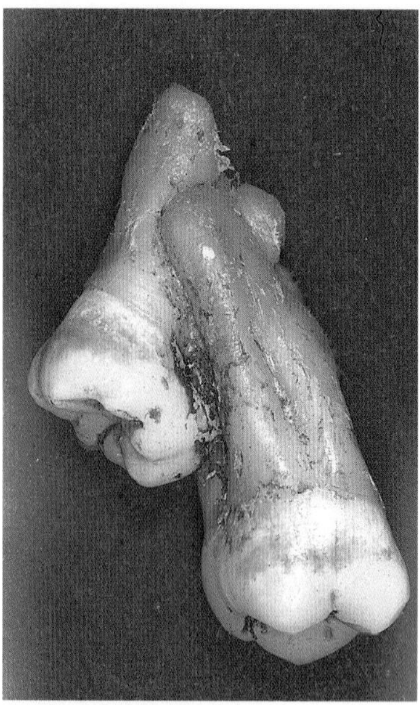

Fig. 21.44 Two upper molar teeth being bound together by cementum (concrescence). From Cawson, R.A., Odell, E.W., 2008. *Cawson's Essentials of Oral Pathology and Oral Medicine*. Churchill Livingstone, Edinburgh.

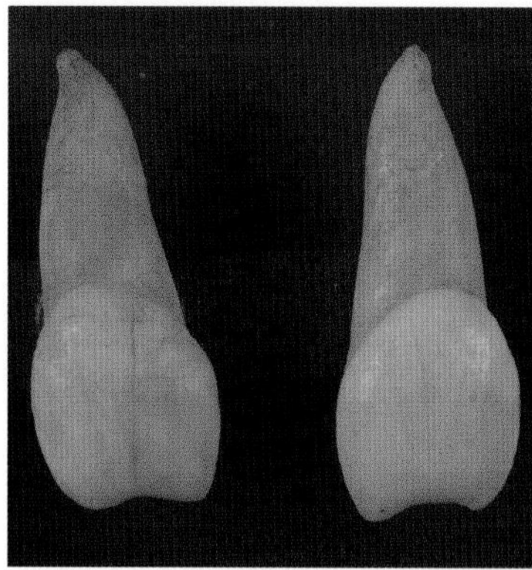

Fig. 21.45 Maxillary permanent first incisors from a patient with congenital syphilis, showing a barrel-shaped outline and notched edge ('Hutchinson's incisors'). Copyright the Royal College of Surgeons of England.

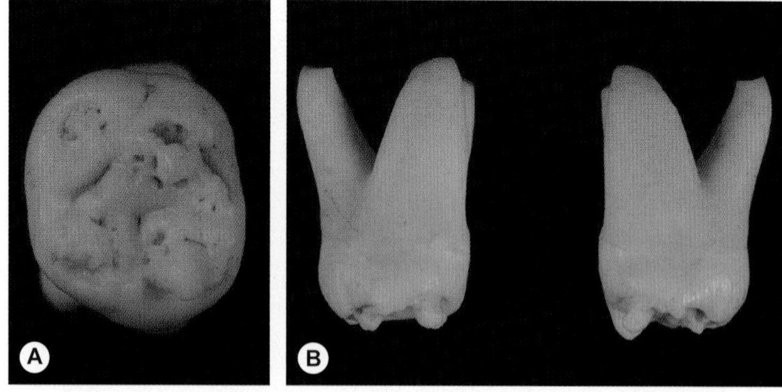

Fig. 21.46 Maxillary permanent molar teeth from a patient with congenital syphilis. (A) Occlusal view and (B) side view, both showing projections on the crown surface ('mulberry molars'). Copyright the Royal College of Surgeons of England.

Abnormal shapes

Abnormal tooth shapes (e.g., Hutchinson's incisors and mulberry molars) can result from congenital syphilis (Figs. 21.45, 21.46). Recent studies suggested a role for calcium signalling in both cusp and root organisation, affecting cell dynamics in the dental epithelium and resulting in formation of 'mulberry molars'.

It has been shown that some molar crown and root dysmorphologies are caused by Wnt10 defects. The severity of tooth agenesis is correlated with the number of defective Wnt10A alleles present.

An anomaly of root shape associated with Wnt10 defects is 'taurodontism', in which the pulp chamber of multirooted teeth is enlarged (see Fig. 2.189). In addition, the pulp floor is apically displaced and the roots are bifurcated.

There has been an increase in susceptibility to taurodontism in human patients with mutations in the Eda pathway (EDA-A1). A taurodont tooth is formed when the most extensive area of proliferation of the neighbouring root mesenchyme occurs in the direction of the extension of the epithelial root sheet from the crown, accompanied by defects in the direction of the root sheath's extension from the crown.

Cysts, ameloblastomas and odontomes

Remnants of the enamel organ and epithelial root sheath may remain and become cystic. These may form dentigerous cysts, preventing the eruption of a tooth (see Fig. 26.54), lateral periodontal cysts (see Fig. 12.74), radicular cysts below non-vital teeth (see Fig. 10.48) and dental lamina cysts found on the alveolar ridge and usually occurring singly (Fig. 21.47).

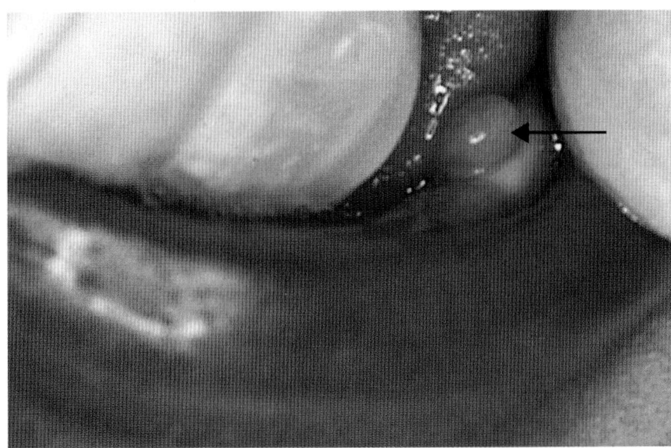

Fig. 21.47 A dental lamina cyst (arrow) on the alveolar ridge formed from remnants of the dental lamina. Courtesy Drs. B Martin, A D'Alesio, H Baumhardt, K Woods. From Zitelli, BJ., Nowalk, A.J., McIntire, S.C. (Eds.), 2018. *Zitelli and Davis' atlas of pediatric physical diagnosis*, seventh edition. Elsevier, Philadelphia.

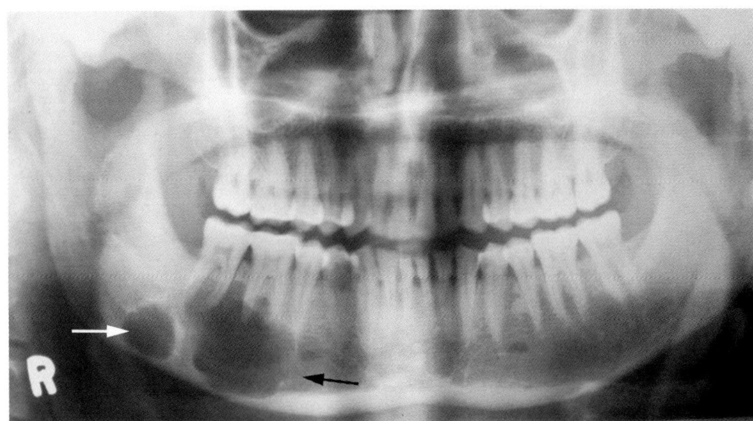

Fig. 21.48 A radiograph showing the presence of an ameloblastoma in the right quadrant of the mandible of a 35-year-old male patient. It may present as a multilocular cyst or as multiple cystic cavities (arrows). Courtesy Dr. S Saraf.

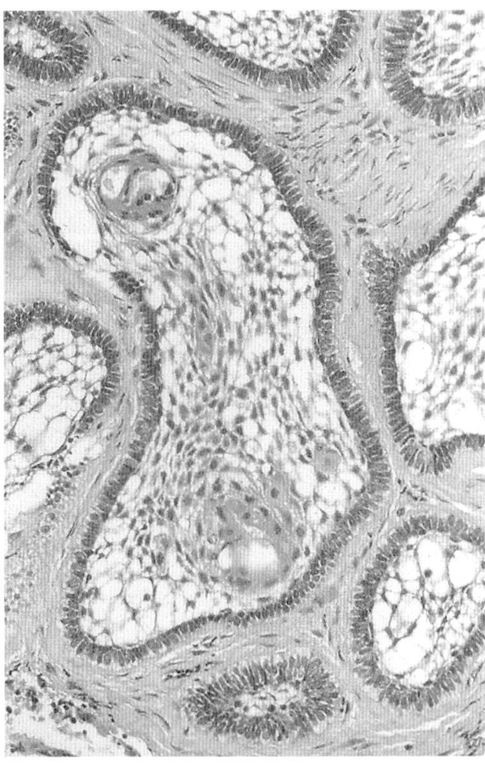

Fig. 21.49 Histological appearance of an ameloblastoma, showing islands comprising cells with a stellate reticulum appearance and a peripheral layer of elongated, ameloblast-like cells (H & E stain). From *Cawson's essentials of oral pathology and oral medicine*, eighth ed. 2008. Churchill Livingstone, London.

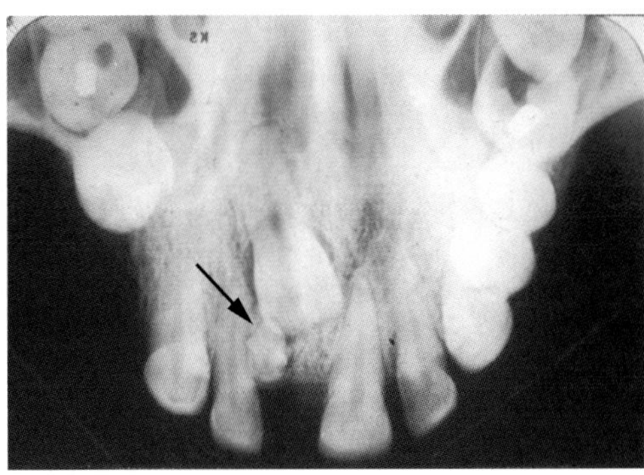

Fig. 21.50 Maxillary occlusal radiograph showing the presence of an odontome (arrow) that has prevented the eruption of the underlying permanent first incisor. Courtesy Prof. D Smith.

During tooth development, components of the enamel organ may undergo abnormal proliferation. In its simplest form, the odontogenic tumour known as an ameloblastoma may appear as a benign cyst, often multilocular, that is most commonly seen in the mandible between the ages of 30 and 50 years (Fig. 21.48). Histologically, its main component comprises strands of epithelial tissue that may resemble preameloblasts, with the nuclei showing a reversal of polarity (Fig. 21.49).

The tooth germ may also form a tumour-like mass of hard tissue called an *odontome*. An odontome may be symptomless or be associated with a localised swelling. It can be found in the anterior region of the maxilla, where its presence may prevent eruption of an anterior tooth (Fig. 21.50), or it can also be encountered in the posterior region of the jaws, where it may prevent a posterior tooth from erupting (Fig. 21.51). When the odontome is composed of many small, discrete, simple, tooth-like structures (denticles), each containing the normal arrangement of dental tissues, it is referred to as a *compound odontome* (Figs 21.52, 21.53). Where the calcified mass bears no resemblance to rudimentary teeth and the dental tissues are arranged haphazardly, it is termed a *complex odontoma* (Figs 21.54, 21.55). Complex odontomes are said to be more common in the molar region of the mandible.

An invaginated odontome also occurs and has been originally termed 'dens in dente' ('tooth within a tooth') (Fig. 21.56). This results either from downward proliferation of a portion of the internal enamel epithelium of the enamel organ into the dental papilla or from retarded growth of part of the tooth germ. It presents on the fully erupted tooth as an extremely deep pit and most commonly affects the permanent maxillary second incisor. The full range of dental tissues (including cementum and bone from incorporation of the dental follicle) may be associated with the 'infolded' organ.

Conditions producing abnormalities in enamel and dentine, such as amelogenesis imperfecta, dentinogenesis imperfecta and hypomineralised teeth, are covered in the chapters concerned with the development of enamel and dentine (Chapters 22 and 23).

Concluding remarks

The experiments described earlier indicate that successful tooth development depends on complex reciprocal interactions between the dental epithelium and the underlying mesenchyme in a spatiotemporal setting. They also show that, initially, the epithelium from the first pharyngeal arch is instructive on the underlying neural crest–derived ectomesenchyme. At a later stage, however, this instructive capacity is transferred to the mesenchyme. Signals involving bioactive molecules (such as transcription factors, growth factors and cytokines) are produced in a specific spatial and temporal sequence, and the cascade of events results in a tooth consisting of the appropriate tissues and of an appropriate shape.

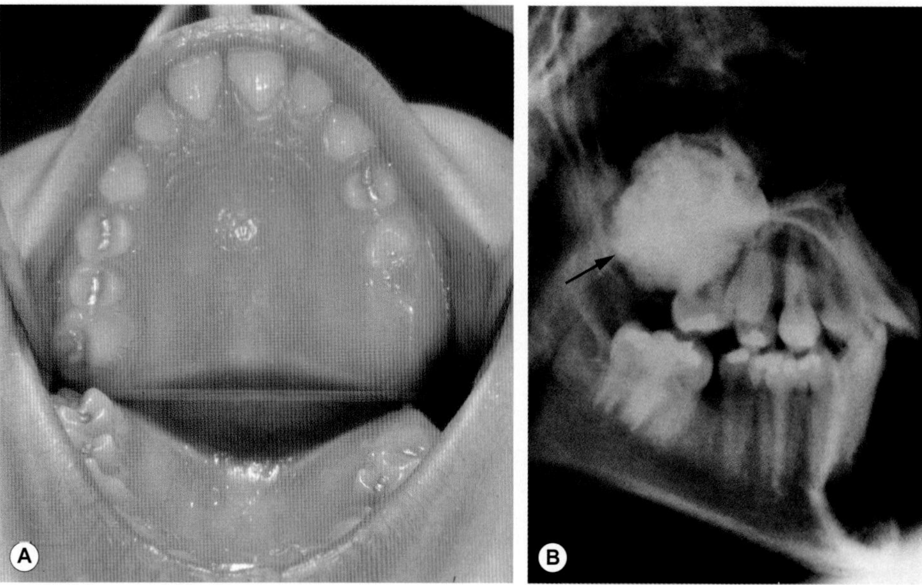

Fig. 21.51 (A) An 11-year-old patient in whom the maxillary first left permanent molar has failed to erupt because of the presence of an odontome. (B) Lateral radiograph of the patient in (A) showing the presence of a large odontome (arrow) associated with the non-eruption of the maxillary first left permanent molar. Courtesy Dr. J D Harrison.

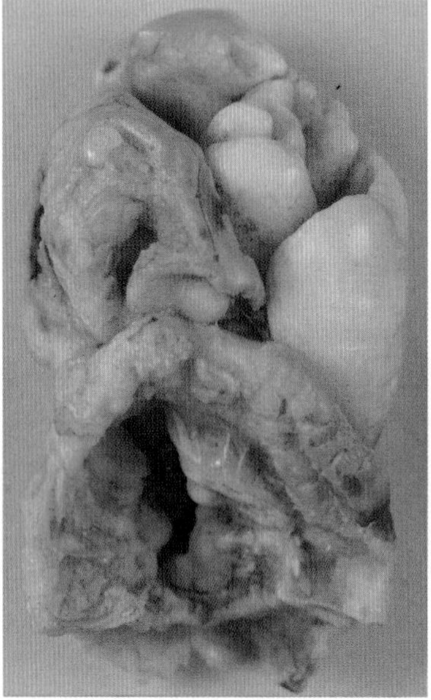

Fig. 21.52 Compound odontome removed from a patient showing several well-defined, tooth-like structures of different shapes and sizes. Copyright the Royal College of Surgeons of England.

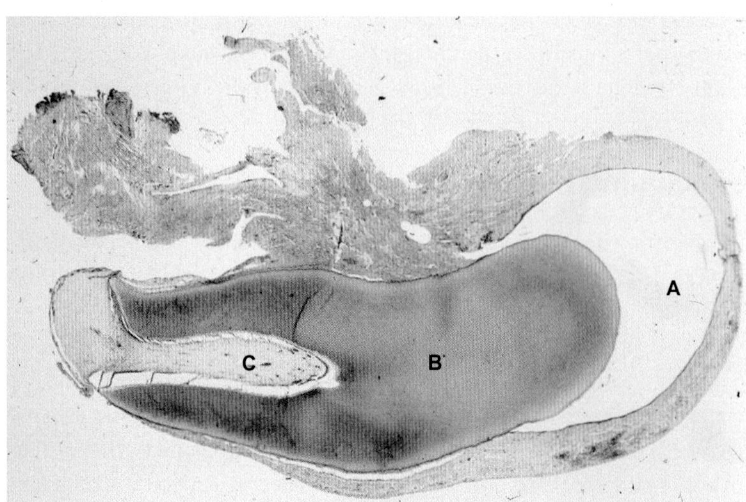

Fig. 21.53 Micrograph of a single denticle dissected from a compound odontoma showing normal distribution of dental tissues. A = enamel space; B = dentine; C = dental pulp (demineralised section; H & E; ×12). Courtesy Dr. J D Harrison.

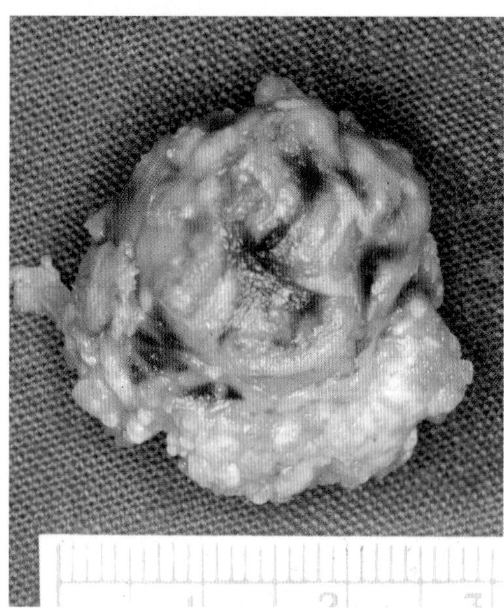

Fig. 21.54 Complex odontome removed from a patient revealed as a calcific mass. There is a low degree of morphodifferentiation compared with the compound odontome seen in Fig. 21.45. Courtesy Dr. J D Harrison.

As mentioned earlier, a considerable number of genes and growth factors are expressed during early tooth development. It has been estimated that more than 300 genes are involved with tooth development. A database has been established by the University of Helsinki (*http://bite-it.helsinki.fi/*) to allow comparisons of the expression patterns as a starting point for experimental studies. This database presently describes the expression at different stages of tooth development of growth factors, receptors, signalling molecules, transcription factors, intracellular and extracellular molecules and plasma membrane molecules. For growth factors, for example, a variety of BMPs, FGFs, Shh and TGFs are expressed at different stages of development. Epidermal growth factor (EGF) appears to be expressed only during the bell stage of development. Neurotrophins, which are growth factors promoting neuronal growth, are also expressed at various developmental stages. Recent research has suggested that the dental epithelium signals to the underlying mesenchymal cells via BMPs (particularly BMP-2 and BMP-4) and FGFs. Consequently, mesenchymal cell proliferation and condensation are stimulated, and the expression in the mesenchyme of syndecan and tenascin is upregulated (syndecan is a cell-surface heparan sulphate proteoglycan that binds to tenascin, probably

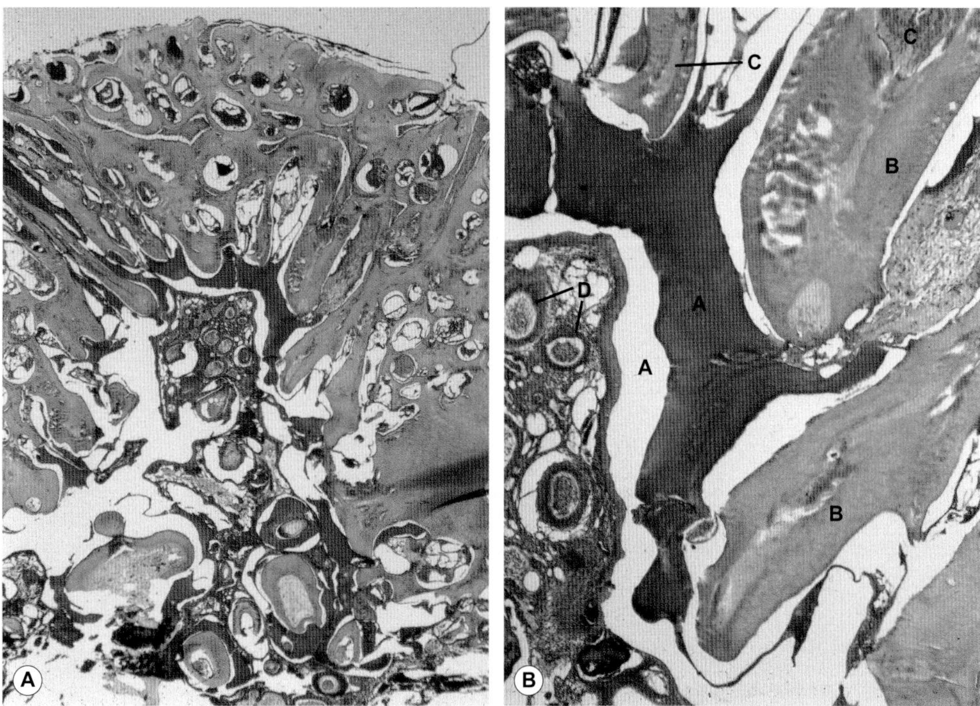

Fig. 21.55 Micrograph of complex odontome. (A) Low power (×10). (B) High power (×45). There is a lack of morphodifferentiation. Areas occupied by enamel (A) appear empty when enamel is fully calcified or contain enamel matrix (darker purple staining) when maturation is incomplete. B = dentine; C = dental pulp; D = odontogenic epithelium present as irregular proliferations in the form of sheets and trabeculae of cells and duct-like structures (H&E). Courtesy Dr. J D Harrison.

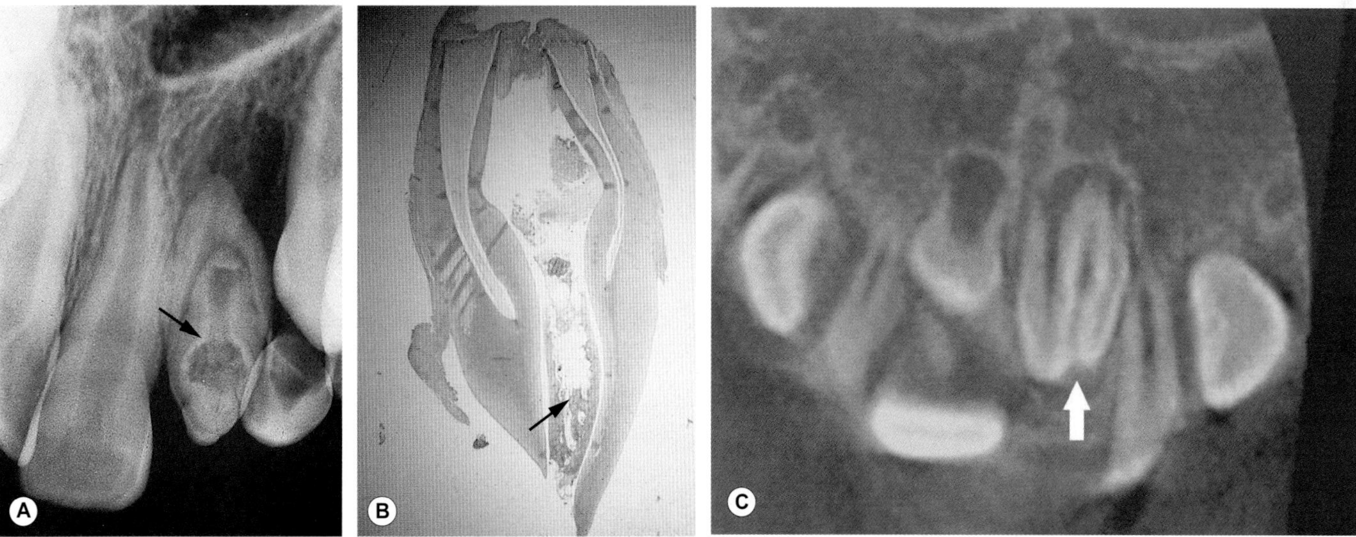

Fig. 21.56 Dens in dente (arrows) seen radiographically (A) and in a histological section (B) (H & E). (C) Cone beam CT of dens in dente (arrow) in maxillary incisor region. (A,B) Courtesy Dr J Potts. (C) Courtesy Dr. J Makdissi.

influencing cell condensation). BMPs also induce expression in the mesenchyme of *Msx1* and *Msx2* homeobox gene transcription factors.

Particular attention has been paid to the earliest stages of tooth development to help determine the biological mechanisms responsible for switching on the cascade of events. As previously mentioned, the activation of non-Hox homeobox genes is of crucial importance at this time. These genes contain DNA-binding proteins that regulate gene transcription, thus controlling the expression of other genes necessary for the development of a particular structure, in this case a tooth. To date, the precise functions of such homeobox genes are not known, but they may be assumed to regulate the production of molecules important in morphogenesis (such as growth factors, factors controlling cell division and apoptosis, cell-surface receptors, integrins and cell adhesion molecules and cytoskeletal elements). The complexity of the topic is partly indicated in Fig. 21.57, which contains just a selection of the molecules known to be present in the developing tooth, and their number is frequently being added to. Evidence to support the importance of such molecules in initiating tooth development can be seen in transgenic mice where, for example, deletion of the homeobox genes such as *Msx1* and *Pax9* results in tooth development being arrested at the bud stage. Similarly, early mesenchyme isolated from the overlying epithelium can continue to develop in tissue culture if molecules such as BMPs and FGFs are added to the medium. Consideration also needs to be given as to how forces are generated during morphogenesis.

Studies focusing on tooth regeneration and engineering *in vitro* use the current knowledge on molecular signalling, stem cell biology and physical environment (forces and scaffolds) to mimic the conditions of tooth development in the laboratory. This topic, together with that of stem cells, is discussed in Chapter 28.

Further readings for this chapter can be found in the accompanying eBook. Explore online Self-assessment quiz to test and reinforce your understanding of the material in your free ebook. Follow instructions in the Inside Front Cover to unlock your access.

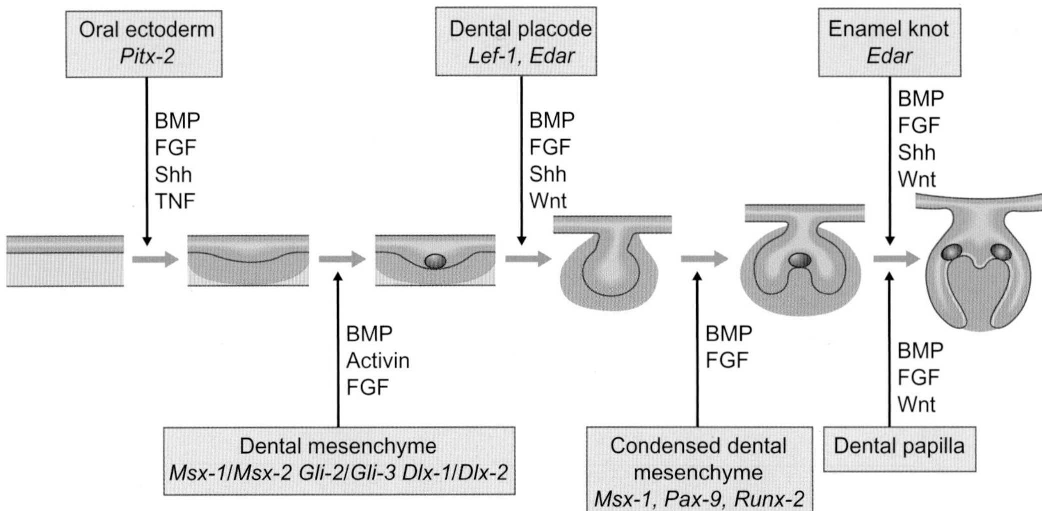

Fig. 21.57 Model of the molecular regulation of tooth development from initiation to crown morphogenesis. Interactions between epithelial (green) and mesenchymal tissues (blue) are mediated by signal molecules (BMP = bone morphogenetic proteins; FGF = fibroblast growth factors; Shh = sonic hedgehog; TNF = tumour necrosis factor). These signals operate throughout development and regulate the expression of genes in the responding tissues (shown in boxes). Signalling centres (red) appear in the epithelium reiteratively and secrete locally many different signals that regulate morphogenesis and tooth shape. Courtesy Prof. I Thesleff.

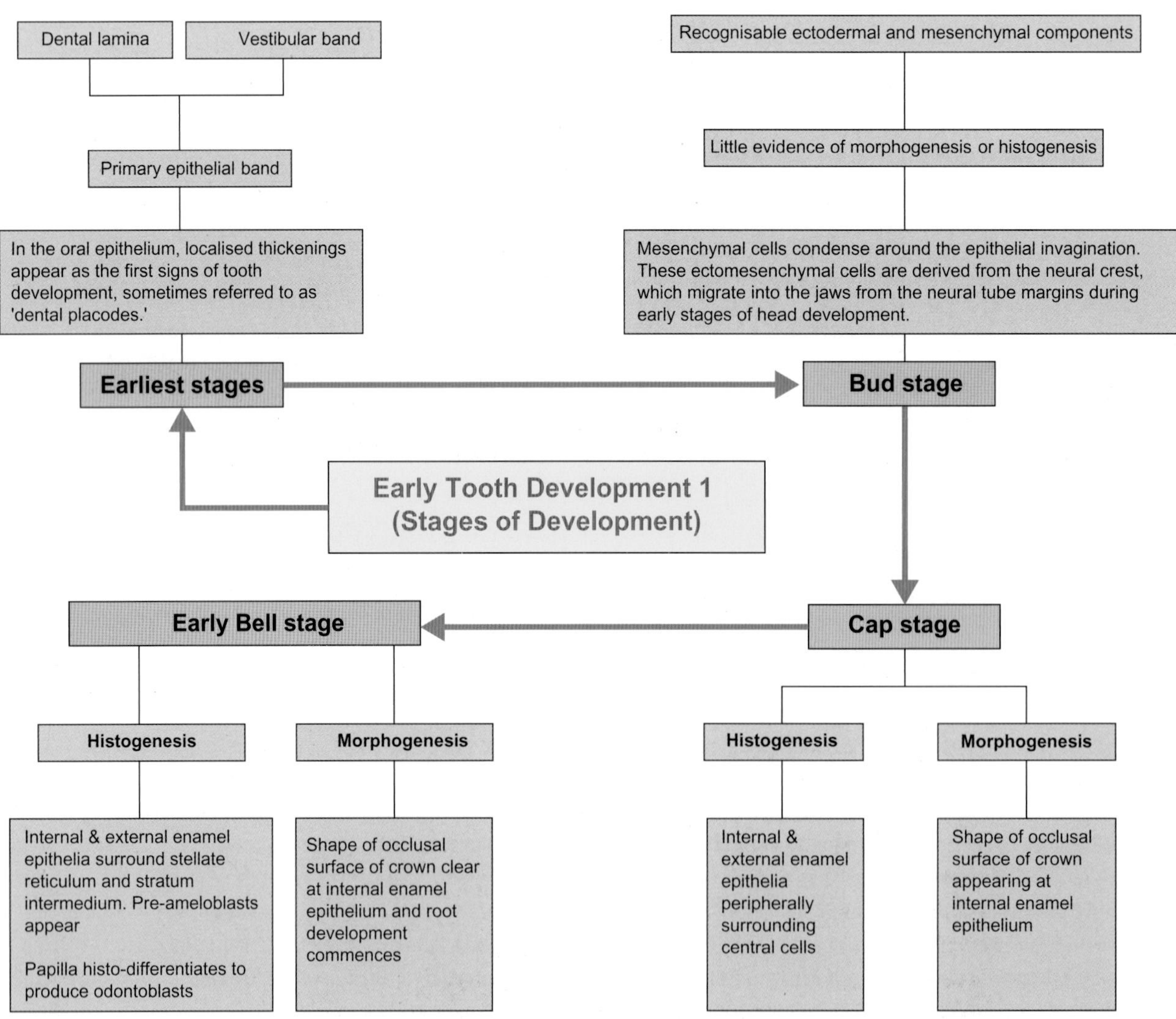

Mind Map 21.1 Early tooth development 1 (Stages of Development)

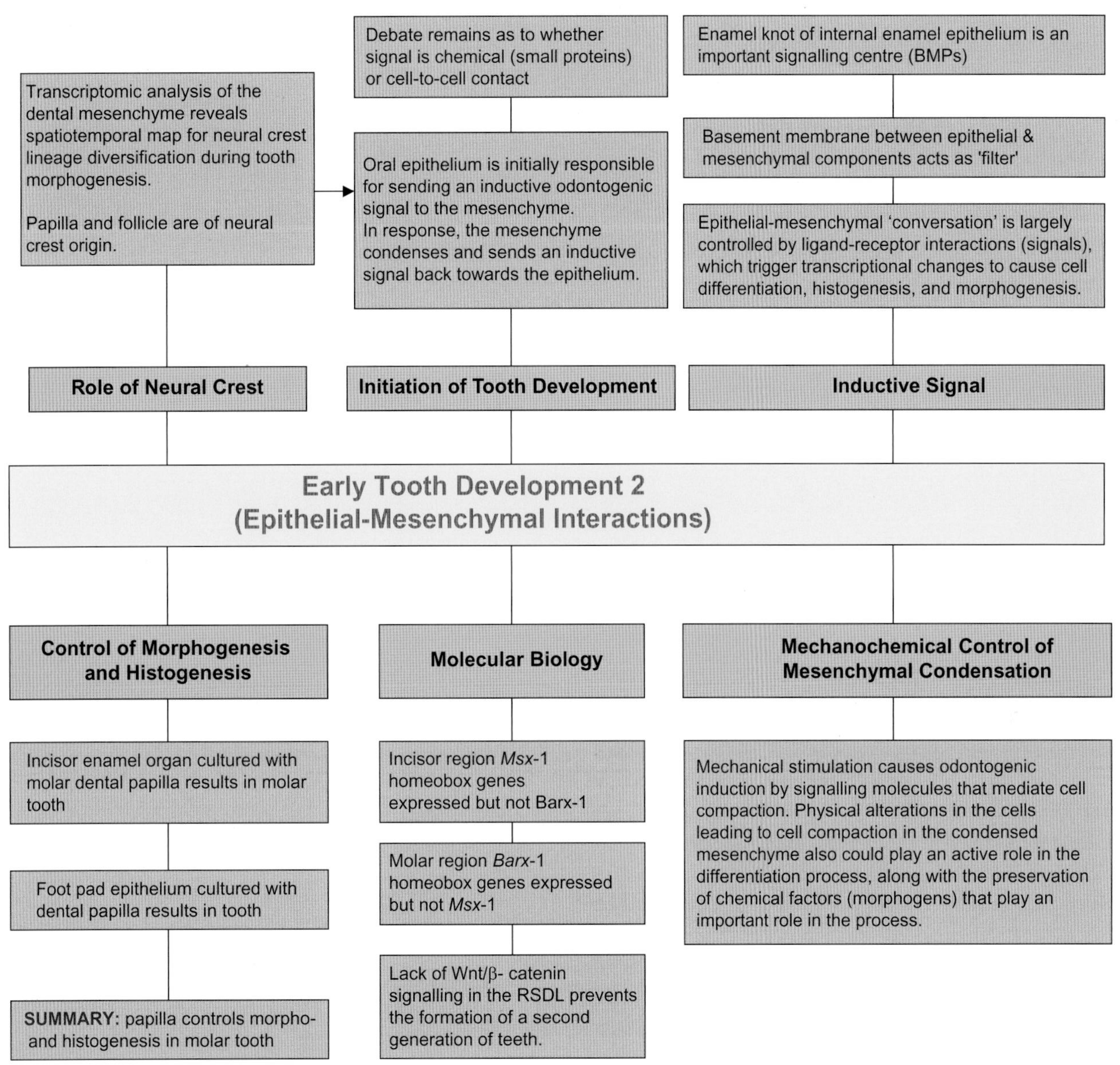

Transcriptomic analysis of the dental mesenchyme reveals spatiotemporal map for neural crest lineage diversification during tooth morphogenesis.
Papilla and follicle are of neural crest origin.
Debate remains as to whether signal is chemical (small proteins) or cell-to-cell contact
Oral epithelium is initially responsible for sending an inductive odontogenic signal to the mesenchyme.
In response, the mesenchyme condenses and sends an inductive signal back towards the epithelium.
Enamel knot of internal enamel epithelium is an important signalling centre (BMPs)
Basement membrane between epithelial & mesenchymal components acts as 'filter'
Epithelial-mesenchymal 'conversation' is largely controlled by ligand-receptor interactions (signals), which trigger transcriptional changes to cause cell differentiation, histogenesis, and morphogenesis.
Role of Neural Crest
Initiation of Tooth Development
Inductive Signal
Early Tooth Development 2
(Epithelial-Mesenchymal Interactions)
Control of Morphogenesis and Histogenesis
Molecular Biology
Mechanochemical Control of Mesenchymal Condensation
Incisor enamel organ cultured with molar dental papilla results in molar tooth
Foot pad epithelium cultured with dental papilla results in tooth
SUMMARY: papilla controls morpho- and histogenesis in molar tooth
Incisor region Msx-1 homeobox genes expressed but not Barx-1
Molar region Barx-1 homeobox genes expressed but not Msx-1
Lack of Wnt/β- catenin signalling in the RSDL prevents the formation of a second generation of teeth.
Mechanical stimulation causes odontogenic induction by signalling molecules that mediate cell compaction. Physical alterations in the cells leading to cell compaction in the condensed mesenchyme also could play an active role in the differentiation process, along with the preservation of chemical factors (morphogens) that play an important role in the process.

Mind Map 21. 2 Early tooth development 2 (Epithelial–Mesenchymal Interactions)

22 Amelogenesis

Amelogenesis (enamel formation) is under genetic control. The features that enamel confers on the tooth, such as size, shape and colour, are inherited. Even susceptibility to caries is passed on. Defects in the genes encoding enamel result in inheritable malformations such as amelogenesis imperfecta.

The tooth begins its programmed development as a localised interaction between an area of oral epithelium and underlying mesenchymal cells, many of which have been derived from the neural crest. These epithelial–mesenchymal interactions during the early stages of tooth development are discussed in Chapter 21. The process is a continuous one but is most readily described in stages that represent snapshots of the developing tooth's growth and differentiation at different points. The names for these stages – bud, cap and bell – describe the morphology of the epithelial component of the developing tooth that becomes the enamel organ. Each of these stages is described in detail in Chapter 21. The innermost cell layer of the enamel organ, the internal enamel epithelium, deposits and later modifies the enamel. The other components of the enamel organ – the stratum intermedium, the stellate reticulum and the external enamel epithelium – play important supportive roles. The original descriptions we have of the developing tooth were derived from histological studies using stains of low specificity. More precise molecular techniques have contributed detailed data that are sometimes difficult to reconcile with older hypotheses on the development of the tissue. For example, the use of the polymerase chain reaction technique, which allows the recognition of messenger RNA (mRNA) formed by transcription but present before translation, shows that the mRNA for two enamel proteins (tuftelin and amelogenin) are present in the cells of the internal enamel epithelium some time before there is any recognisable morphodifferentiation. This indicates that protein synthesis is going on at a much earlier stage than that suggested by histological studies.

In a single developing tooth, amelogenesis will be present at various stages. When enamel is being formed, the ameloblasts at different locations along the internal enamel epithelium will be at different stages of the enamel-forming process. However, by the time enamel formation finishes, each ameloblast will have completed a similar life cycle. Different tooth types form enamel at different times, at different rates and with different final morphological outcomes.

Following the epithelial–mesenchymal interactions described in Chapter 21, amelogenesis and dentinogenesis occur almost simultaneously, but as distinctly different processes. The site where they both begin is the enamel–dentine junction. Amelogenesis is a complex process, and an understanding of it is best approached by providing an initial brief overview, followed by a more focused and detailed description.

Following the epithelial–mesenchymal interactions at the future enamel–dentine junction that constitute the presecretory stage of amelogenesis, crystal formation/growth then begins on the enamel side of the enamel–dentine junction within an organic matrix formed by the ameloblasts and continues as the ameloblasts move away from the junction. The crystals become long ribbons arranged parallel to each other in bundles that, because of the presence of a Tomes process at the secretory surface of the ameloblast, form the enamel prisms (or rods). They grow primarily in length, although there is a measurable difference between inner enamel crystal width and outer enamel crystal width. The final length of the crystals, and thus the thickness of the enamel, is determined by how long the ameloblasts lay down protein matrices. This is the secretory stage. Once the full width of the immature enamel is laid down, approximately half of the ameloblasts die and the rest shorten, stop producing matrix and then begin to degrade the matrix and selectively reabsorb much of it. This is the transition stage. The face of the ameloblast that has secreted the matrix becomes ruffled and continues the degradative process and reabsorbs almost all the remaining matrix. As this is happening, more mineral is being added to the sides of the crystals (lateral growth), such that they reach their final size and the enamel achieves its final level of mineralisation. This is the maturation stage, which lasts for 3 to 4 years. The final step is the postmaturation stage, during which the enamel organ in humans degenerates and eruption begins.

Life cycle of the ameloblast

The ameloblast carries out enamel formation in five stages: presecretory, secretory, transition, maturation and postmaturation stages. Cell morphology changes at each stage, reflecting a change in function. The major changes associated with each stage are summarised in Table 22.1 and Fig. 22.1.

Presecretory stage

The odontoblasts of the developing dental pulp initiate dentine matrix formation prior to the beginning of amelogenesis. They produce collagen that is formed into bundles that point towards the cells of the internal enamel epithelium which are at this point known as *preameloblasts*.

The presecretory stage includes all activities of the future ameloblast before the secretion of the main component of the enamel matrix. This stage has two principal features: differentiation of the preameloblasts and formation and subsequent resorption of a basal lamina. The morphological changes to the enamel organ as a whole are described in detail in the section on tooth development (see Chapter 21). Here, the focus will be on the cells of the internal enamel epithelium. During the bell stage, the cells of the internal enamel epithelium (Fig. 22.2) have ceased to divide and have differentiated into committed enamel-forming cells, the ameloblasts. This differentiation begins at the future cusp tips or incisal margins and progresses cervically. During this phase, the ameloblasts differentiate from cuboidal into columnar cells over 60 μm in height and 2–4 μm in width. The cell becomes polarised as the nucleus and mitochondria stay close to the end of the cell that is in contact with the stratum intermedium. These columnar cells are preameloblasts (Figs. 22.3, 22.4).

Before any dentine is laid down, the early differentiating ameloblasts (Fig. 22.1) possess a large ovoid nucleus, several mitochondria and a small Golgi apparatus close to the stratum intermedium end of the cell. In the

Table 22.1 Features associated with the five main stages of amelogenesis

Presecretory	Secretory	Transition	Maturation	Postmaturation
Cytodifferentiation: differentiation of ameloblasts	Initial layer of aprismatic enamel formed	Ameloblasts shorten, 50% die	Cycling of ruffled and smooth-ended ameloblasts	Enamel organ degenerates
Morphodifferentiation: bell stage including formation of the enamel knot	Ameloblasts develop Tomes processes	Vascular invagination of the enamel organ	Final degradation and withdrawal of matrix	Enamel coverings established
Resorption of the basal lamina of the internal enamel epithelium	Matrix secretion to final thickness	Reformation of ameloblast basal lamina	Crystal growth continues to completion	Eruption
Epithelial–mesenchymal interactions	Initiation and continuation of mineralisation to 30% by weight	Cessation of matrix secretion	Final third of mineralisation after protein removal complete	Exposure to oral environment and posteruptive changes
	Crystallite elongation	Continued matrix degradation		
	Matrix degradation	Selective matrix withdrawal		
	Development of prismatic structure			

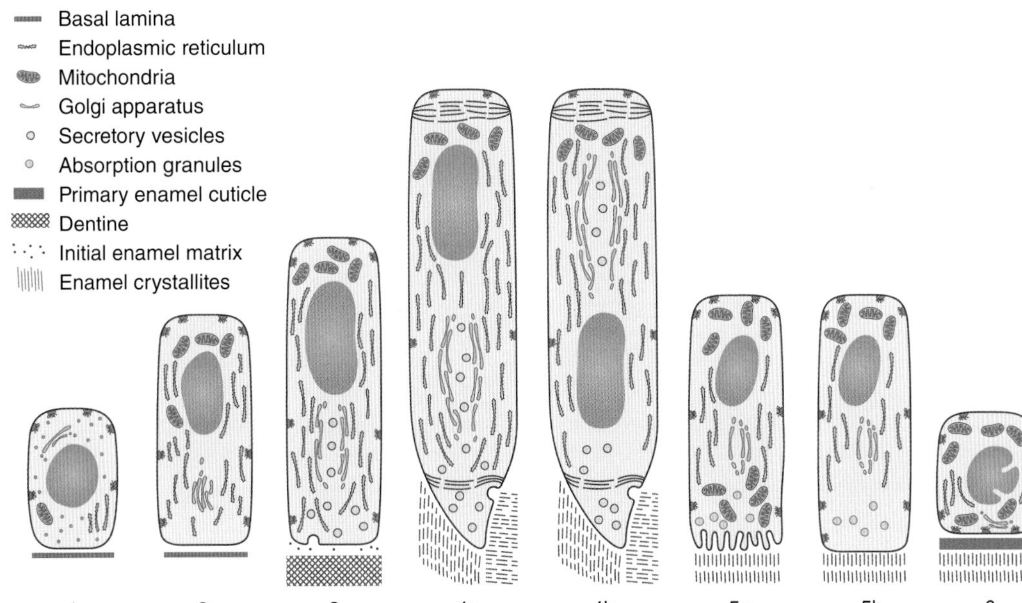

Fig. 22.1 The life cycle of an ameloblast. The cells of the internal enamel epithelium (1) start to differentiate, beginning at the future enamel–dentine junction of the cusp tip. The differentiating cell (2) is characterised by a reversed polarity; the cell becomes columnar and the nucleus moves to that part of the cell farthest from the dentine. Secreting organelles are formed, and the end of the cell adjacent to the dentine becomes the site for secretion. At the next stage (3), the cell secretes the initial enamel component of the enamel–dentine junction. This thin layer will be continuous with the inter-rod enamel of the later formed tissue. As the cell retreats, the secreting pole becomes morphologically distinct as a pyramidal Tomes process (4a). Crystallites are formed at both surfaces of the process. The proximal region between two processes, deep in the junctional regions, always secretes ahead of the more distal region so that pits surrounded by inter-rod enamel are formed. These are then filled, giving the prism configuration to the tissue. Simultaneous secretion of both organic material and mineral continues until the full thickness of the tissue is formed. In this secreting phase, two appearances of ameloblasts can be distinguished by the position of the nuclei within the cell: high (4a) and low (4b). At the beginning of secretion, half the cells are in each form. Towards the end of secretion, most of the high nuclei have moved to a low position, effectively increasing the areas of the ameloblast cells as the surface of forming enamel increases. When the full thickness of enamel has formed, ameloblasts lose the secretory extension, the Tomes process (5a). Up to 50% of them die and are phagocytosed by others in the layer. The maturation phase lasts two to three times longer than the secretory phase. During the maturation phase there is a regular, repetitive modulation of cell morphology between a ruffled (5a) and a smooth (5b) surface opposed to the enamel. Once the maturation changes are complete, the cells regress in height (6). At this stage, they serve to protect the enamel surface during eruption and later will contribute to form the junctional epithelium.

cytoplasm adjacent to the dental papilla (which will become the dental pulp), rough endoplasmic reticulum is present, with many free ribosomes, mitochondria and vesicles. Pinocytotic invaginations of the cell membrane are also found here. Adjacent cells of the internal enamel epithelium are linked by terminal bars at their proximal (near the stratum intermedium) and distal (near the dental papilla) ends. A basal lamina separates the preameloblast from the dental papilla. This lamina marks the position of the future enamel–dentine junction. Very shortly after morphological changes have begun in the internal enamel epithelium, parallel changes begin in the adjacent mesenchymal cells of the dental papilla that are differentiating into odontoblasts (Figs. 22.5, 22.6). This differentiation is controlled by the cells of the internal enamel epithelium that release growth factors (particularly members of the transforming growth factor [TGF] β family), which can be deposited in the basal lamina, from where they are released by proteolytic enzymes. Once the odontoblasts of the dental papilla have differentiated, the basal lamina separating them from the preameloblast disappears as the first layer of dentine matrix is laid down (Fig. 22.6). The preameloblasts release enzymes by exocytosis that degrade the basal lamina and then resorb the degradation products by endocytosis. For a brief period following the degradation of the basal lamina, the future

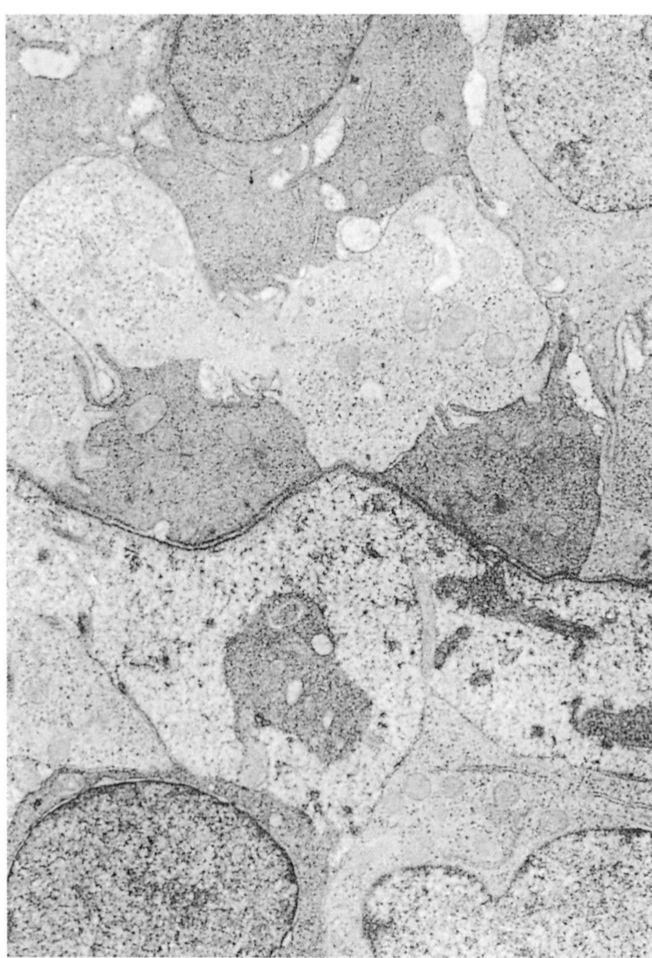

Fig. 22.2 TEM showing the undifferentiated cells of the internal enamel epithelium. No secretory specialisation is yet evident (×4,800). Courtesy Dr. T Sasaki and Karger Press.

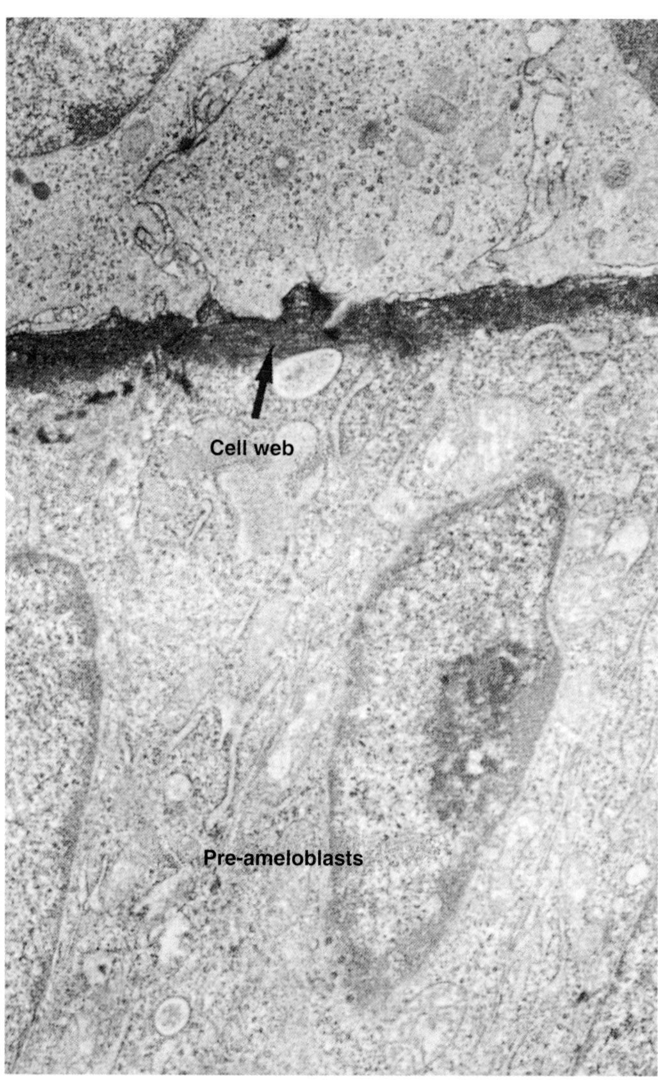

Fig. 22.3 TEM showing preameloblasts. Rough endoplasmic reticulum is evident and the terminal cell web is clearly stained (×5,350). Courtesy Dr. T Sasaki and Karger Press.

ameloblasts and odontoblasts are in intimate contact, allowing inductive signalling to occur between them. The odontoblasts are the first cells to lay down matrix, and this provides the signal for the ameloblasts to begin secretion. The odontoblasts produce non-collagenous proteins as well, dentine sialophosphoprotein (DSPP) in particular. A small amount of DSPP is also contributed by the preameloblasts. This initial matrix defines the enamel–dentine junction. Before any mineralisation begins, the preameloblasts secrete enamel proteins on top of the dentine matrix, some of which diffuses through the matrix and is taken up by the odontoblasts. Immediately after this initial enamel matrix is laid down, the basal lamina of the preameloblasts disappears and cell processes extend into irregularities on the adjacent predentine surface. Crystallites form in the enamel matrix within these irregularities in contact with the ameloblast. The processes of the preameloblast cell shrink back towards the cell body as the crystallites lengthen. The surface of the first-formed dentine, once it has mineralised, becomes covered with a very thin layer of enamel into which some odontoblast processes extend, forming enamel spindles (see page 151). This initial enamel is aprismatic, as there are no sudden changes in crystal orientation because of the absence of a Tomes process on the preameloblasts or of a specific enamel protein. In this aprismatic enamel, the crystallites appear to lie in random orientations. The final part of the enamel formed at the surface of the crown is also aprismatic, but in this region the crystallites are arranged uniformly parallel to each other.

In the terminally differentiated preameloblast, the nucleus is in the end of the cell adjacent to the stratum intermedium with mitochondria between

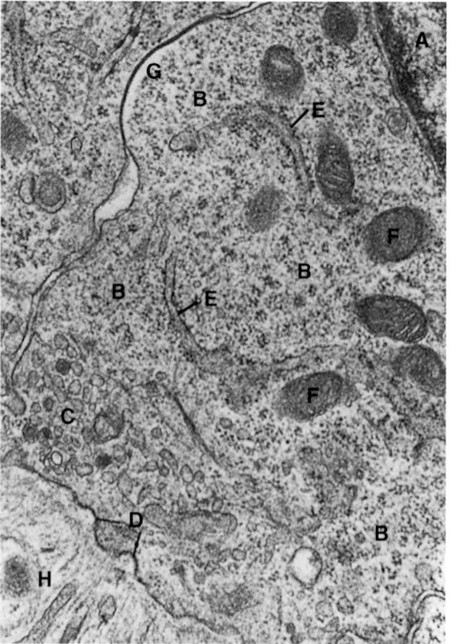

Fig. 22.4 TEM illustrating the distal cytoplasm of an early differentiating ameloblast. A = nucleus; B = free ribosomes; C = vesicles; D = pinocytotic invagination; E = rough endoplasmic reticulum; F = mitochondria; G = gap junction; H = dental papilla (×21,000). Courtesy Dr. E Katchburian.

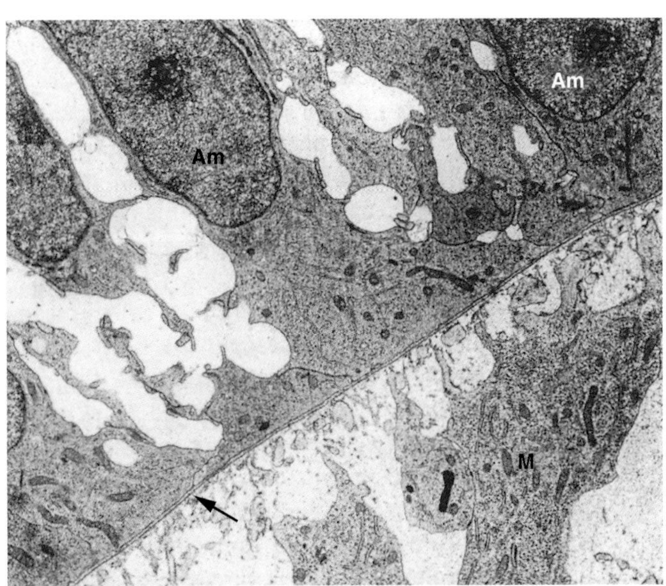

Fig. 22.5 TEM showing ameloblasts (Am) in contact with mesenchymal cells of the dental papilla (M). A basal lamina (arrow) is still present (×500). Courtesy Dr. Z Skobe and CRC Press.

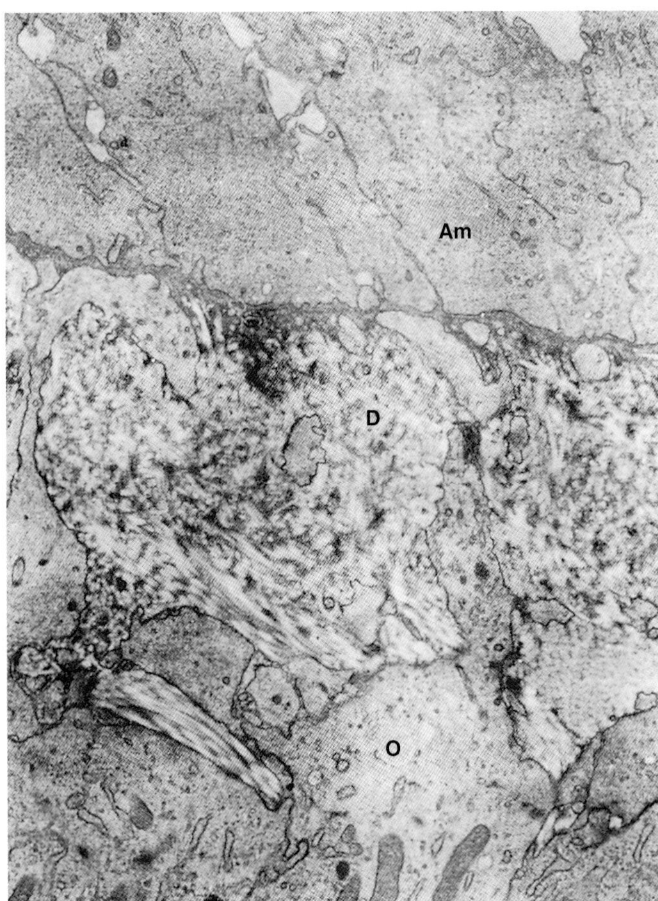

Fig. 22.6 TEM showing dentine matrix formation by odontoblasts (O) preceding the secretion of enamel by ameloblasts (Am). D = dentine matrix (×5,000). Courtesy Dr. Z Skobe and CRC Press.

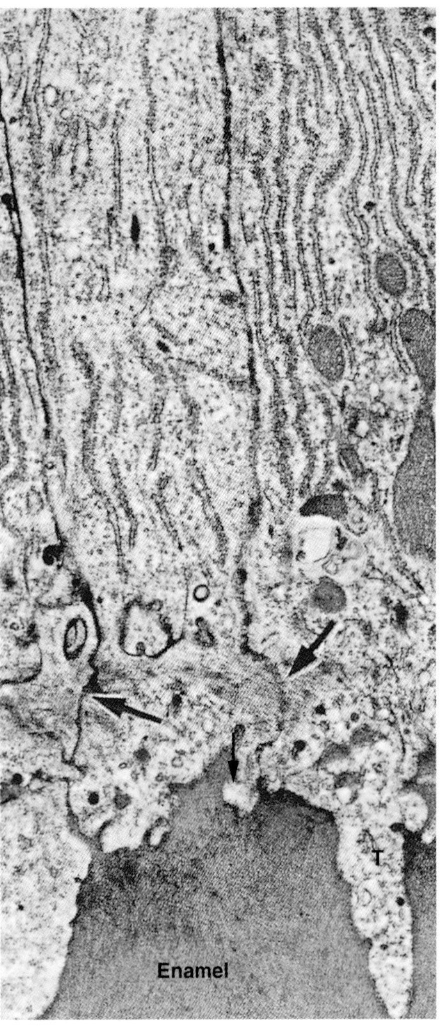

Fig. 22.7 TEM demonstrating cell junctions proximal to Tomes processes, junctional complexes (arrows) and intracellular tonofilaments. T = Tomes process (×7,500). Courtesy Dr. T Sasaki and Karger Press.

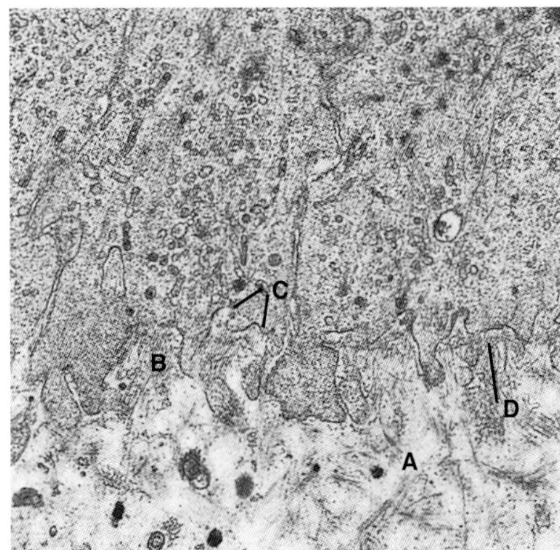

Fig. 22.8 TEM showing the distal end of a late-differentiating ameloblast. A = forming dentine; B = invagination in ameloblast; C = coated pits; D = degenerating lamina (×15,600). Courtesy Dr. E Katchburian.

it and the cell membrane. The rough endoplasmic reticulum, Golgi apparatus and secretory vesicles enlarge and come to lie between the nucleus and the end of the cell adjacent to the dental papilla, the pole from which enamel matrix will later be secreted. This redistribution of organelles is known as a *reversal of polarity*. The preameloblasts are joined to each other at the stratum intermedium end by desmosomes, forming the proximal terminal web (Fig. 22.3). A similar distal terminal web will develop a little later at the secretory end of the cells (Fig. 22.7). The preameloblasts are approximately 40 μm long and 2–4 μm wide. They bulge into the stellate reticulum, perhaps to gain the advantage of increased surface area in absorbing precursors. At their distal end following the onset of dentinogenesis, the cell membrane becomes irregular with many projections and pits (Fig. 22.8). Vesicles and vacuoles appear in the cytoplasm. These changes may, in part, be associated with the removal of the basal lamina, which allows for contact between preameloblasts and odontoblasts and possible transfer of inductive signals.

Secretory stage

At the secretory stage, enamel proteins are secreted to form an extracellular matrix that undergoes the initial stages of mineralisation. Secretory stage enamel contains 25–30% mineral by weight and is soft and translucent. Matrix secretion by the ameloblasts begins as soon as the first increment of predentine has been laid down and continues until the final thickness of the enamel layer has been reached. In addition to enamel proteins, ameloblasts express and secrete other proteins and glycoproteins (including biglycan and dentine sialoprotein) that presumably play a role in amelogenesis, including biglycan and dentine sialoprotein.

At the beginning of the secretory phase, the ameloblasts have become long, columnar cells with their nuclei at the basal end (away from the forming enamel). Following the deposition of the initial, thin, aprismatic enamel, a cone-shaped process, the Tomes process, forms at the distal, secretory end of the ameloblasts (Figs. 22.9–22.11). The Tomes process contains no organelles besides secretory granules. The shape of Tomes processes is responsible for the prismatic structure of enamel. There appears to be a relationship between ameloblast size and prism pattern (see Fig. 7.12). It is usually found that pattern three prisms are made by the largest ameloblasts and pattern two by the smallest. With the development of the Tomes processess, the shape of the mineralising surface of enamel changes to a 'picket fence' arrangement (Figs. 22.11–22.13). If the ameloblasts are pulled away from the surface, the mineralising front presents a honeycomb appearance, with the pits in the surface being occupied by the Tomes processes (Figs. 22.13, 22.14). This appearance is reminiscent of the enamel surface following etching with certain acids (e.g., Fig. 7.71). The integrity of the monolayer of ameloblasts is preserved by cell–cell connections in the form of a terminal web (terminal bar apparatus, Fig. 22.9) at the distal base of the Tomes process, junctional complexes consisting of desmosomes and tight junctions. The tonofilaments associated with the desmosomes pass for a short distance into the cell and form an incomplete septum between the Tomes process and the rest of the ameloblast. The junctions of the terminal web apparatus are zonular (encircling the cell) and effectively separate the environment of the developing enamel from the interior of the enamel organ. Thus, all secretion and modification of the matrix occur via the Tomes processes. Junctions at the basal ends of the ameloblasts, adjacent to the stratum intermedium, are macular and provide mechanical union without the same isolation of the microenvironment. There are additional isolated junctions between ameloblasts at other levels, particularly gap junctions, that may synchronise the activity of the cells. Mutations in genes encoding for cell junction proteins

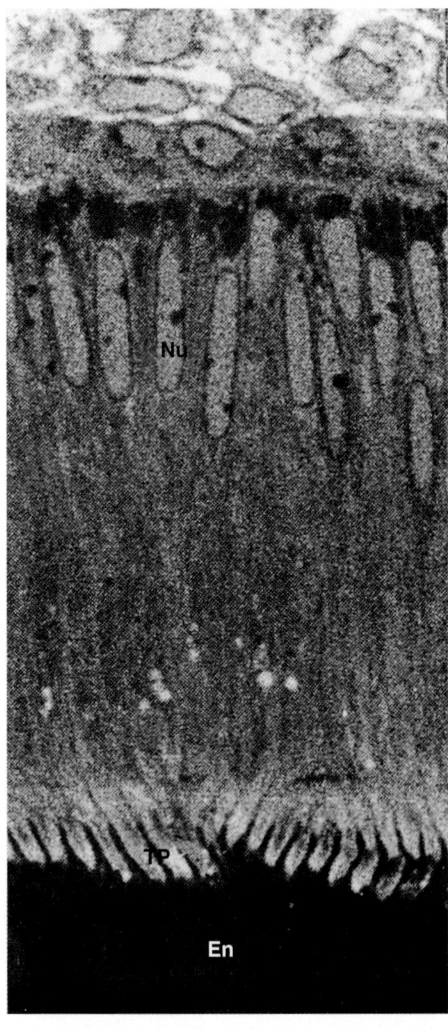

Fig. 22.10 Section showing rat secretory ameloblasts. En = forming enamel; Nu = nuclei; TP = Tomes processes (×1,000). Courtesy Dr. T Sasaki and Karger Press.

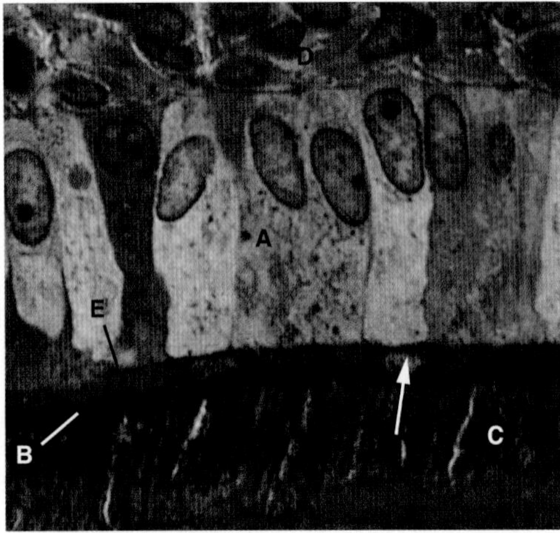

Fig. 22.9 Demineralised section of developing enamel showing the cone-shaped Tomes process (arrow) at the distal end of each ameloblast. A = ameloblast; B = enamel matrix; C = dentine; D = stratum intermedium; E = terminal bar apparatus running through the ameloblast layer (toluidine blue; ×1,000). Courtesy Dr. D W Whittaker.

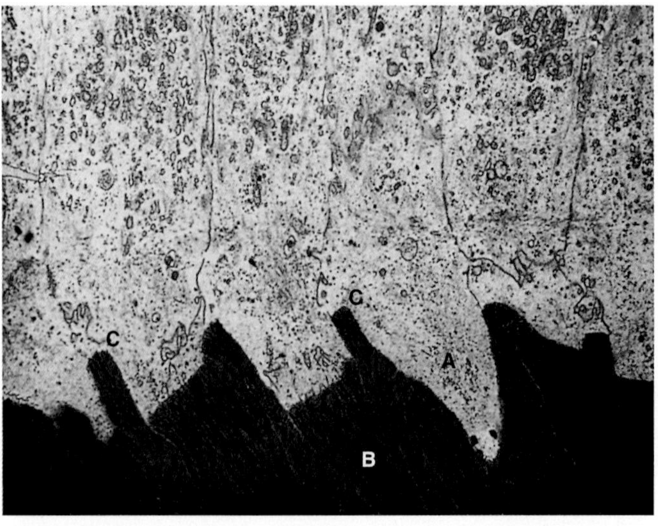

Fig. 22.11 TEM showing advanced secretory ameloblasts with their Tomes processes (A). B = developing enamel; C = interpit 'prongs' (×6,000). Courtesy Dr. A Boyde and Springer-Verlag.

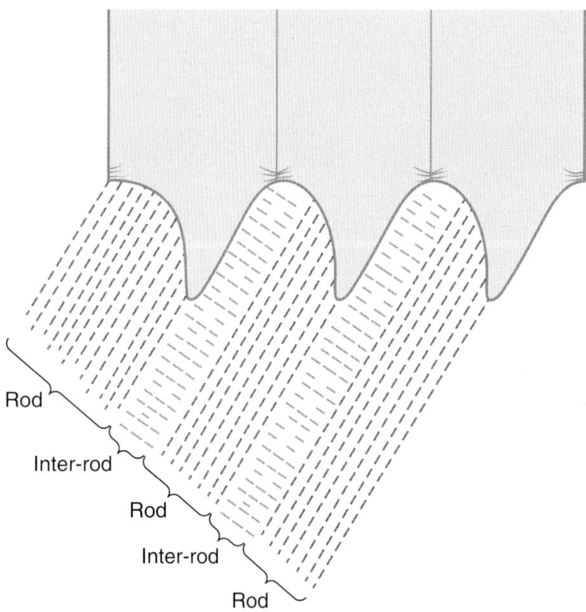

Fig. 22.12 The relationship between Tomes processes and enamel prism formation. The enamel of the core of the prism and the prism boundary/inter-rod regions differ largely in the orientation of crystallites. This is determined by the shape of the Tomes process. In human enamel, prisms are clearly seen, though at some points in the 'tail' of the prism the boundary between prismatic and interprismatic is lost (see Fig. 7.13). Each prism is formed by a single ameloblast, but four contribute to each interprismatic region. The prism boundary areas of enamel are formed first, giving the developing enamel front a pit-like surface appearance.

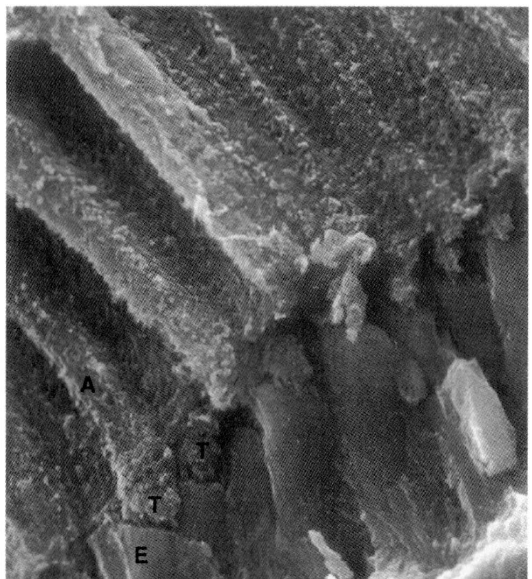

Fig. 22.13 Fractured enamel with intact secretory-stage ameloblasts (A) adhering to the forming enamel surface (E). Tomes processes (T) are clearly seen and appear triangular (×3,000). Courtesy Dr. Z Skobe.

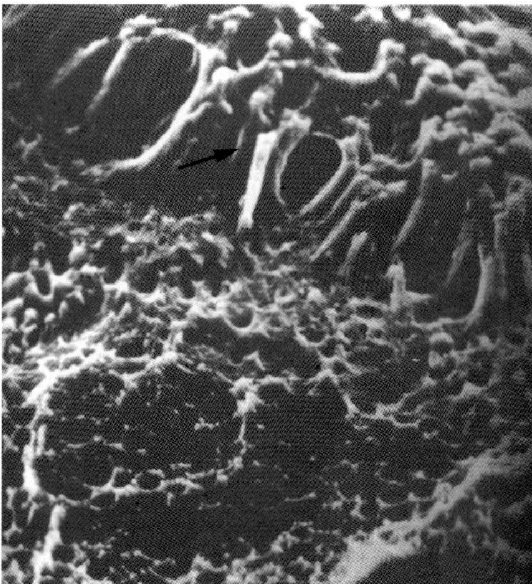

Fig. 22.14 SEM of surface of developing enamel. At the top (arrow), some ameloblasts have been retained at the surface. Below where others have been lost, the developing enamel surface shows a series of pits previously occupied by the Tomes processes of the ameloblasts (×500). Courtesy Dr. R P Shellis.

are known to cause amelogenesis imperfecta (see page 417), underlining the importance of cell–cell adhesion in amelogenesis.

Interpit 'prongs' develop between the growing and elongating Tomes processes (Figs. 22.10–22.12). The prongs between the processes deposit enamel matrix first, to form walls that represent the periphery of the prisms (and interprismatic regions) and that delineate pits or depressions in the enamel that are occupied by Tomes processes. The Tomes processes then infill the central pits as the ameloblasts retreat to form the main core of the enamel prism. The ameloblasts therefore have two main secretory sites. Each prism is formed by a single ameloblast, but four contribute to each interprismatic region. Nonetheless, there are the same number of prisms as there are ameloblasts.

The nascent enamel matrix proteins are assembled in the endoplasmic reticulum and carried by transitional vesicles to the Golgi apparatus where glycosylation, phosphorylation and sulphation take place before packaging into electron-dense secretory granules 0.25 μm in diameter (Fig. 22.15). The secretory granules are transported along microtubules towards the Tomes process of the cell.

As the ameloblasts shift from the presecretory to the secretory stage, there is a marked aggregation of vesicles (some containing stippled material) at the distal end of the ameloblast (Fig. 22.16). The material contained within the vesicles represents the organic matrix of the enamel. The contents of the vesicles are discharged into the extracellular space, both at the distal end of the cell and between the cell membranes of adjacent ameloblasts (Fig. 22.16). As the enamel matrix is secreted, the ameloblasts are pushed (or move) outwards away from the dentine surface (Fig. 22.17). Within this organic matrix, the initial hydroxyapatite crystallites of the enamel appear almost immediately, before the matrix is 50 nm thick, so that a distinct zone of unmineralised matrix analogous to predentine or osteoid is never seen in enamel (Fig. 22.16). The first-formed crystallites are thin and needle-like and much smaller than the crystallites in mature enamel. They begin as thin ribbons, 10–15 nm wide and 1–2 nm in thick. The enamel mineral is a carbonated calcium hydroxyapatite that differs from pure hydroxyapatite by including HPO_4^{2-}, CO_3^{2-}, Mg^{++}, F^- and other ions in its lattice. During development, enamel crystallites form and are aligned perpendicular to the distal surface of the ameloblasts. The mechanism (or mechanisms) responsible for this alignment is not understood, but

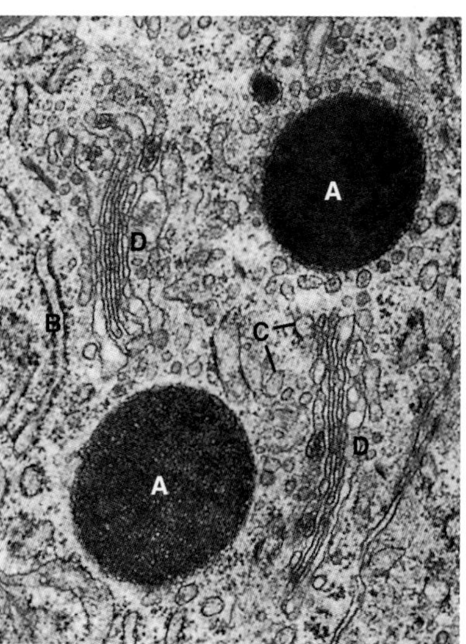

Fig. 22.15 TEM showing the synthetic and secretory apparatus in a secretory ameloblast. A = secretory granules; B = rough endoplasmic reticulum; C = Golgi vesicles; D = Golgi apparatus (×30,500). Courtesy Dr. E Katchburian.

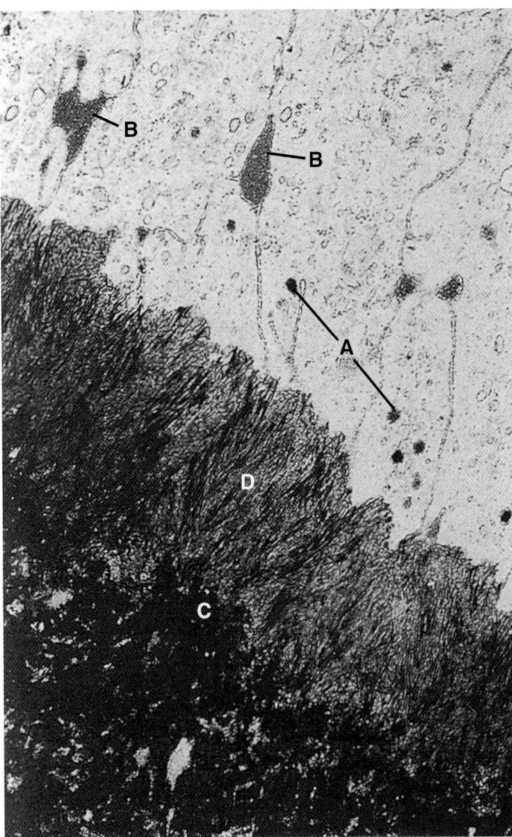

Fig. 22.16 TEM showing early enamel formation. A = secretory vesicles; B = secreted matrix between ameloblasts; C = dentine; D = early enamel (×1,500). Courtesy Dr. E Katchburian.

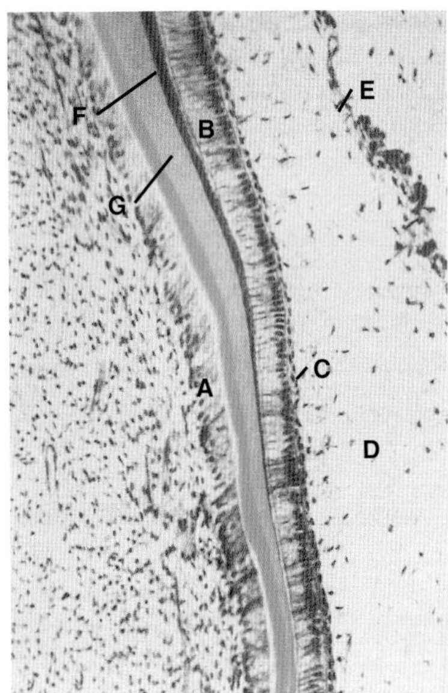

Fig. 22.17 Demineralised section showing the initial stage of enamel formation. A = odontoblasts; B = ameloblasts; C = stratum intermedium; D = stellate reticulum; E = external enamel epithelium; F = developing enamel; G = developing dentine (Masson's trichrome; ×80).

it may be a result of the organisation of the organic matrix, the concentration gradients of the crystallite ions, the presence of microvilli at the cell membrane or the contributions from ameloblast movement. In support of the contention that the organic matrix may be acting as a scaffold in this respect is the fact that mutations in certain matrix proteins result in loss of prismatic architecture, leading to amelogenesis imperfecta.

The crystallites appear as flattened hexagons when viewed in cross-section. The crystallites extend in length, still aligned perpendicular to the surface and parallel to other crystallites forming at the same cell surface. The enamel crystallites that elongate around the tip of the Tomes process form the region of the prism core. Crystallites extending from where the ameloblasts are joined to each other form the region at the prism boundary.

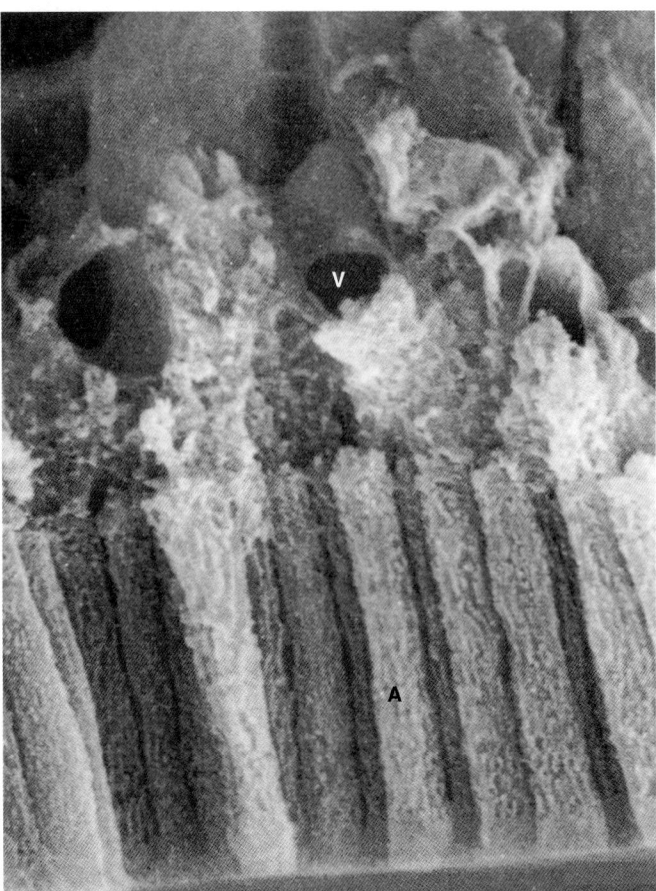

Fig. 22.18 SEM showing flat-ended ameloblasts (A) at the end of the secretory phase. V = venule (×1,000). Courtesy Dr. Z Skobe and CRC Press.

There is a clear border between the prism core and prism boundary, as part of the ameloblast is nonsecretory. Prism core and prism boundary enamel are identical except for the orientation of the crystallites. The prism core crystallites are parallel to the long axis of the prism; the prism boundary crystallites deviate from this by up to 40–65 degrees. Enamel prisms elongate incrementally. Each daily increment leads to a cross-striation (see pages 143–144). Approximately every 7 days (range 6–10), prominent cross-striations produce the appearance of an enamel stria. Apart from the initial striae over the cusps and incisal ridges, these striae end on the surface of the enamel as perikymata (see pages 145–147). The amount of enamel formed daily varies but it is approximately the same in all teeth, forming at the same time. In teeth whose enamel is mineralising at birth, there is an exaggerated incremental line, the neonatal line (see page 147).

The secretory phase ends once the full thickness of enamel matrix has been laid down. The Tomes process retracts so that the distal end becomes flat (Fig. 22.18), and a final, thin layer of aprismatic enamel is formed at the surface. However, this layer may be incomplete as prism end markings can sometimes be seen in the covering investments of newly erupted enamel or in enamel from areas that have been protected from attrition (see page 157). The crystallites in surface aprismatic enamel all run parallel to each other. The signalling mechanisms that determine when and where in the tooth the secretory process is turned on or off are unknown.

The transition stage

The enamel that is deposited initially has a high content of water and protein and a low content of mineral. It is essentially a protein-based hydrogel interspersed with long, thin mineral crystallites. Enamel maturation is carried out by the same cells that secreted the primary matrix, the ameloblasts, but in a very changed form. The period in which the ameloblasts change from a secretory to a maturation form is the transition stage. During this phase, enamel secretion stops and much of the matrix is removed. A reduction in height of the ameloblasts signals the onset of the transition. The number of ameloblasts is reduced by as much as 50% by apoptosis (programmed cell death). In those ameloblasts that remain, the organelles associated with protein synthesis (e.g., the rough endoplasmic reticulum and the Golgi apparatus) are reduced by autophagocytosis. The enamel organ becomes invaginated by blood vessels, and the cells of external enamel epithelium, stellate reticulum and stratum intermedium become covered with microvilli. However, blood vessels do not directly penetrate into the stellate reticulum, which is avascular. The blood vessels thus lie close to, but not in contact with, the proximal end (base) of the ameloblasts (Fig. 22.18).

Enamel proteins during amelogenesis

A classification of enamel proteins is shown in Fig. 22.19. As one of the main processes in the maturation of enamel is the removal and modification of the initially formed proteinaceous matrix, it is necessary here to discuss the composition of the immature enamel matrix.

Proteins and peptides account for less than 1% of the weight of mature enamel but 25–30% of early developing enamel that is soft and translucent (as compared with the opaque nature of more mineralised enamel). Developing enamel matrix during the early secretory stage is predominantly proteinaceous, and the major enamel proteins are present in much greater amounts than the traces found elsewhere. The matrix of enamel comprises several proteins, of which amelogenin (90%), ameloblastin (5%) and enamelin are the most abundant. An additional enamel protein, amelotin, has more recently been discovered and is mainly associated with the maturation stage (see page 411). These proteins are all members of the secretory calcium-binding phosphoprotein (SCPP) gene family.

In addition to enamel proteins, enamel matrix also contains two main proteases. MMP-20 (enamelysin) is mostly involved in degradation and generating specific protein fragments during secretion. KLK-4 (Kallikrein-related peptidase-4) is used to destroy any remaining protein in maturation and is much less specific than MMP-20. Knockouts of both enzymes show severe enamel defects, and human mutations in the genes encoding these enzymes lead to amelogenesis imperfecta.

During the process of maturation, much of the amelogenin proteins are degraded and removed so that, in mature enamel, the remaining 1% by weight of protein is composed mainly of the nonamelogenin proteins. Although the precise functions of the enamel proteins have yet to be determined, mutations in their genes are associated with disturbances in enamel structure. A list of some possible functions of enamel proteins is given in Table 22.2.

As enamel matrix is secreted extracellularly and away from the ameloblast surface, it must convey within its unique protein structure the necessary information to direct mineralisation to produce the complex microanatomy of human enamel. Of particular importance is the nucleation of the hydroxyapatite crystals, their controlled growth and their relative orientation to form prismatic enamel. Study of the functions of the enamel proteins is made difficult by the large number of amelogenin- and nonamelogenin-related proteins. This is a result of a combination of three features:

1) Following their initial secretion, enamel proteins undergo a series of complex degradative changes carried out by various proteolytic enzymes. This results in the accumulation of many smaller enamel proteins and peptides.
2) Amelogenin isoforms are derived from a single gene by alternate splicing (or postsecretory degradation) of full-length amelogenin. The presence of alternative RNA splicing of the mRNA transcript results in the same amino acid sequence being present at either end of the molecule but with differences occurring in the middle. Thus, there is a range of heterogeneous hydrophobic proteins.

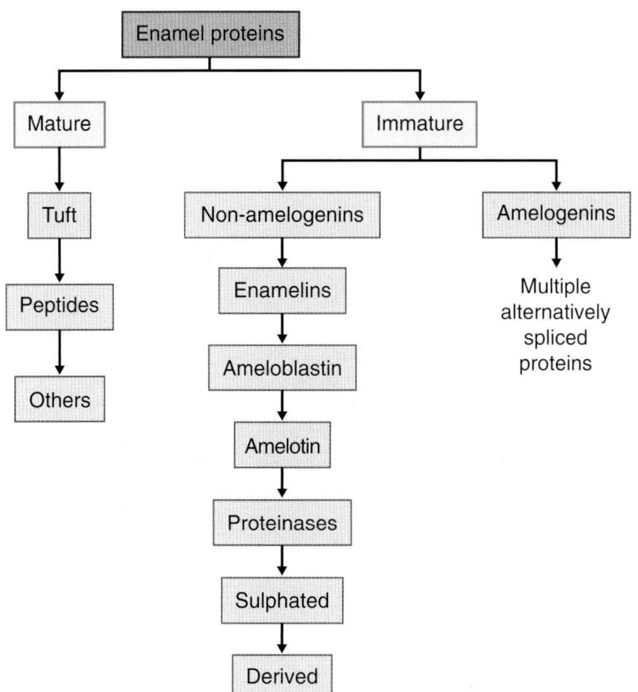

Fig. 22.19 Classification of enamel proteins. Redrawn from Fincham et al., 2000. In: Teaford et al. (Eds.), *Development, Function and Evolution of Teeth*, with permission of Cambridge University Press.

Table 22.2 Possible functions of enamel proteins and proteases

Protein	Possible functions
Amelogenin	Stabilisation of amorphous Ca-P phase
	Control of crystal morphology and organisation
	Control of enamel thickness
Ameloblastin	Cell adhesion protein
	Controls cell differentiation
	Maintains enamel rod/prism integrity
Enamelin	Control of mineral nucleation and elongated growth, possibly with amelogenin
Tuftelin	Cell signalling
Dentine sialoprotein	Initiation of mineralisation
MMP-20	Cleaves enamel proteins to produce stable intermediates with defined functions
KLK-4	Digests enamel proteins during maturation facilitating their removal
	Hardens the surface layer of enamel
Amelotin	Expressed during maturation, formation of final enamel asprismatic layer

Partly modified from Moradian-Oldak, J., 2013. Protein-mediated enamel mineralization. *Frontiers of Bioscience* 17, 1996–2021.

3) The amelogenin gene occurs on both the X and Y sex chromosomes of humans, producing slightly different proteins. However, the male-specific proteins represent only a minor proportion of the total enamel protein. The functional significance of this sexual dimorphism is not known, but it has forensic implications. The sex of an individual can be determined from viable nuclear material derived from the relatively well-protected pulps of dead individuals by detecting the nature of the amelogenin gene (see Chapter 27).

Amelogenin enamel proteins

The major structural protein in developing enamel is amelogenin. It is a hydrophobic, proline-rich molecule that also has high levels of histidine, glutamine and leucine (Fig. 22.20). It is very rapidly cleaved and only found in the newest secreted enamel. The parent 25-kDa (MDS MW) form is broken down to a 20-kDa molecule (which predominates during the secretion stage), and further processing leads to the accumulation of 13-, 11- and 5-kDa amelogenins (Fig. 22.21). The 5-kDa molecule is a tyrosine-rich amelogenin peptide (TRAP). It is relatively insoluble and builds up near the end of the secretory stage of amelogenesis. The 13- and 11-kDa moieties are relatively soluble.

The breakdown of amelogenin is enzymatic and controlled during secretion by the matrix metalloproteinase MMP-20. Degradation commences soon after secretion of the enamel matrix occurs and continues throughout the secretory stage of enamel formation. The question arises as to whether this degradation is merely to remove the matrix and allow the enamel crystallites to enlarge or whether some or all of the smaller molecules have specific functions in the development of enamel structure. For example, TRAP is thought to be important in crystal growth.

Amelogenins are hydrophobic and self-assemble, or 'clump', into oligomers, nanospheres, nanochains and other elongated assemblies in different *in vitro* situations. When added to enamel matrix, they do not form a discrete appositional band, as do the matrix proteins of dentine and bone. Instead, they spread throughout the whole, developing enamel thickness. Amelogenins are secreted and processed to generate stratified layers in increasing states of processing. One exception might be the highly soluble amelogenin fragments created by the removal of TRAP, which appears to be quite mobile in the matrix.

Folding of the molecule may permit protein–protein interactions between carboxyl and amino-terminal domains, resulting in self-assembly and the formation of minute nanospheres that have a variable diameter of between 20 and 100 nm. It has been proposed that the first crystals of enamel are formed between or within the spheres. Evidence in support of this view is that the initial thin enamel crystals are also spaced approximately 20 nm apart. Subsequently, the controlled extracellular degradation of the amelogenin proteins results in a reduction in the size and arrangement of the nanospheres (or oligomers), allowing for a later controlled increase in both the width and thickness of the enamel crystals in the deeper enamel layers.

Although originally thought to be a protein unique to enamel, amelogenin has been detected in dentine matrix and odontoblasts, in the periodontal ligament and cells associated with cementum formation, in bone cells and in non-mineralising cells such as brain and haematopoietic cells. This distribution indicates that amelogenins may have functions in a wide range of tissues.

Non-amelogenin enamel proteins

These comprise about 10% of the protein of immature enamel. Among the non-amelogenins to be considered are enamelin, ameloblastin, amelotin, proteases and sulphated enamel proteins (Fig. 22.19). Like the amelogenins, examination of the non-amelogenins is complicated by the presence of alternative splicing and their degradation to form smaller molecules. Such degradation would appear to be undertaken by the same enzymes as for the amelogenins.

Enamelin

The acidic parent molecules are the largest enamel proteins and are secreted as a 186-kDa phosphorylated precursor glycoprotein that is cleaved soon after being secreted (Fig. 22.20). They are found in the outermost

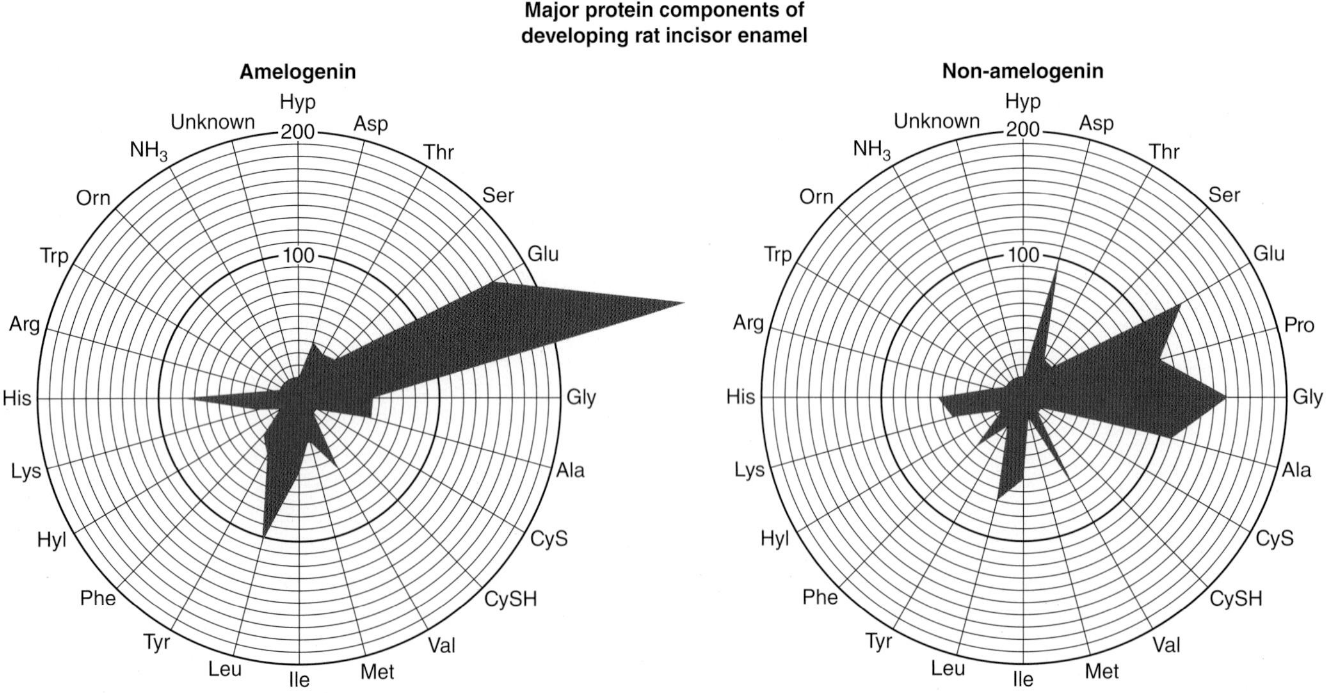

Fig. 22.20 'Rose' diagrams showing general differences in composition between amelogenin and non-amelogenin enamel proteins in developing rat incisor enamel. Courtesy Prof. C Robinson.

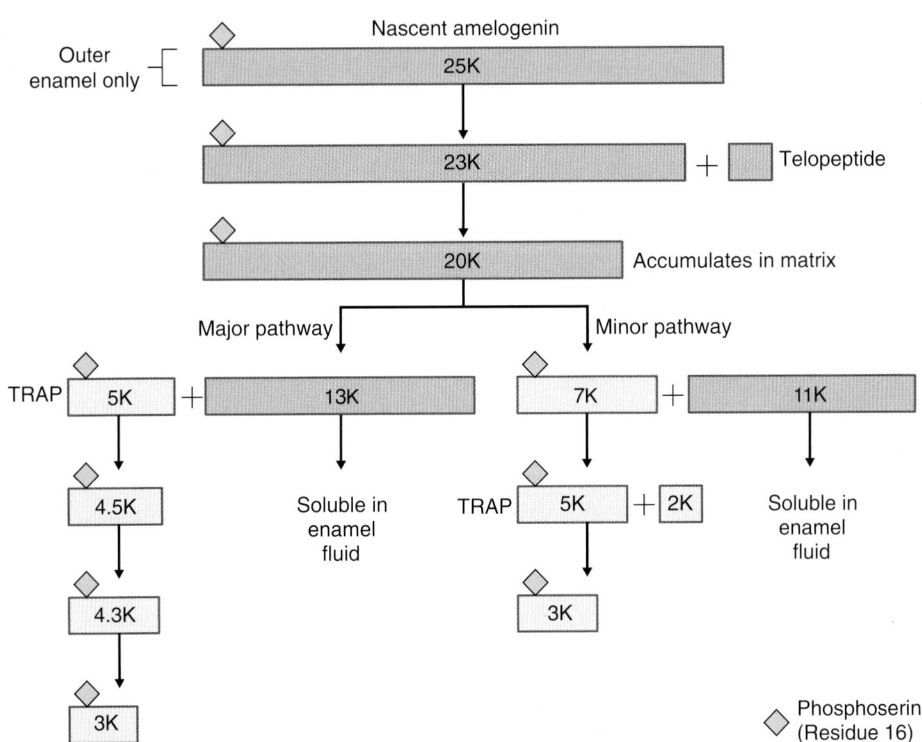

Fig. 22.21 Diagram showing various stages in the degradation of native amelogenin enamel protein. TRAP = tyrosine-rich amelogenin peptide. From Robinson, C., Brookes, S.J., Shore, R.C., Kirkham, J., 1998. The developing enamel matrix: nature and function. *European Journal of Oral Science* 106, 282–291.

layer of newly secreted enamel but are soon broken down to smaller moieties having molecular weights of 30–40 kDa. The lower-weight enamelins have been shown to be phosphorylated glycoproteins rich in proline, glycine, glutamine and aspartine. Enamelins are primarily located in the prism cores. They can form aggregates with other proteins in the organic matrix and, being seen in the region of the enamel–dentine junction, are postulated by some to control the growth of enamel crystals, perhaps in cooperation with amelogenin. Mutations in the gene encoding enamelin are a cause of amelogenesis imperfecta.

Ameloblastin (amelin, sheathlin)

Ameloblastin is almost always packaged with amelogenin in the same secretory granules, suggesting a possible functional association between the two proteins. It is the second most abundant protein expressed during amelogenesis.

This enamel protein undergoes degradation as soon as it is secreted. The two transcripts of this nascent protein produced by alternative splicing are rich in proline, glycine and leucine and have a molecular weight of 62 kDa. Following secretion, ameloblastin is cleaved into C- and N-terminus fragments by enamel matrix proteases, including MMP-20. The basic 17-kDa N-terminus fragment and its processing products are highly aggregative and can be immunolocalised to the sheath space surrounding enamel prisms. The acidic C-terminus is degraded and removed from the matrix soon after secretion. It has been suggested that the N-terminal fragments have a key role in the formation of the prism sheath.

The gene for ameloblastin is located on chromosome 4. As ameloblastin-null mice produce defective enamel and their secretory ameloblasts are seen to become separated from the developing enamel surface, losing their polarity, this suggests that ameloblastin may play a role in cell adhesion. Ameloblastin is also produced by the epithelial root sheath during root formation, and this is discussed further on page 443.

Tuftelin

The parent protein in this group is rich in glutamic and aspartic acids and has a molecular weight in the range of 58–66 kDa. Alternative splicing also occurs in the case of these proteins. The gene has been located on chromosome 1. As this is one of the earliest proteins to be produced, both before the amelogenin proteins and before the ameloblasts have differentiated, it has been suggested that one of its early functions is as a signalling molecule during epithelial–mesenchymal interactions. Its presence at the enamel–dentine junction has implicated this protein as possibly being involved as a nucleator at the commencement of initial enamel mineralisation. Although animals lacking tuftelin show deficiencies in enamel mineralisation at the lower (nanoscale) levels of enamel hierarchy, its presence in non-mineralising tissues suggests it has a broader function and may not be a true secreted enamel protein, but may become trapped within the enamel during mineralisation.

Following maturation, some protein remains in the region corresponding to the enamel tufts (see Figs. 7.63, 7.66, 7.67). Here it is referred to as *tuft protein*. Its relationship to tuftelin and/or its degraded products is unclear, although it appears to contain less proline and more leucine.

Amelotin

Amelotin is a 209–amino acid protein rich in proline, leucine, threonine, glutamine and glycine, with an N-terminal signal sequence that, once cleaved, gives rise to a mature 20.4-kDa secreted protein. Amelotin expression has been shown to be restricted to the basal lamina of maturation-stage ameloblasts, the structure that links ameloblasts with the developing enamel. Functionality studies have suggested that amelotin promotes hydroxyapatite precipitation, serving a critical role in the formation of the final compact aprismatic enamel surface layer during the maturation stage of amelogenesis. In an amelotin overexpression mouse model and an amelotin knockout, both had defective enamel. A mutation in human amelotin was found to be associated with reduced mineral density in affected teeth. Its gene occupies chromosome 4.

Sulphated enamel proteins

These represent acidic enamel proteins that are present in small amounts and appear to be degraded within about 1–2 hours after their secretion. Their function is unknown.

Proteolytic enzymes

Also present in developing enamel are low concentrations of KLK-4 and MMP-20, whose cleavage products accumulate as the hydroxyapatite crystals lengthen. The two enzymes function at different stages during amelogenesis. MMP-20 is present from the onset of secretion through to the early stages of maturation, while KLK-4 is present from the beginning of the transition stage and throughout maturation. It is thought MMP-20 processes enamel proteins into stable intermediate products, while KLK-4 degrades enamel proteins completely. MMP-20 is a tooth-specific enzyme whose gene is present on chromosome 11, while the gene for KLK-4 is found on chromosome 19.

An enamel protein that is also expressed in other tissues, odontogenic ameloblast-associated protein (ODAM), regulates MMP-20 and plays important roles in enamel mineralisation.

Serum-derived products

There are some proteins present in developing enamel that are not secreted by ameloblasts but are derived from serum. Because of their affinity for hydroxyapatite, these proteins are absorbed into the developing enamel. The major serum protein identified in developing enamel is albumin, which has the property of potentially inhibiting mineral growth.

Proteomics analyses

Recent advances in technology have allowed the identification of proteins in enamel that are present in very small quantities and that had remained unidentified in previous studies. Such proteomics analyses have revealed the presence of literally hundreds of proteins present in mature enamel matrix. Such proteins may have performed various roles in the complex process of enamel maturation, though their precise roles in amelogenesis have yet to be unravelled.

Enamel proteins in periodontal regeneration

As enamel proteins are associated with root development and cementum formation, they are being utilised clinically in periodontal regeneration (see page 452).

Maturation stage

Prior to maturation, young enamel is composed of 65% water, 20% organic material and 15% inorganic hydroxyapatite crystals by weight. Upon maturation, it consists of approximately 96% mineral, 3% water and 1% organic material. At the beginning of the maturation stage, little or none of the enamel matrix proteins are in their original form, but have been converted into smaller proteins and peptides. Secretion of the serine protease KLK-4 occurs during maturation. Enamel crystallites increase in width and thickness with a consequent reduction in intercrystalline space. Whereas amelogenin, ameloblastin and enamelin are the major secreted products of secretory-stage ameloblasts, amelotin and ODAM are secreted by maturation-stage ameloblasts

Ameloblasts move calcium, phosphate and carbonate ions into the matrix and remove water and degraded enamel matrix proteins from it. The protein content of the tissue is reduced from about 30% to about 1%. The removal of matrix occurs concurrently as the crystallites expand in width and thickness, from their early average dimensions of 1.5 nm thick to their mature thickness of 25 nm. The degradation of the enamel matrix by serine proteases released from the enamel organ seems to precede the mineral gain. At this initial stage, the space caused by enamel matrix loss is occupied by water, with the enamel becoming more porous.

The ameloblasts undergo further morphological changes. The Tomes process is lost and the organelle content reduced. The remaining organelles congregate at the distal end of the cell, where the plasma membrane infolds to form a striated border (Figs. 22.22, 22.23). The ameloblast is then described as being 'ruffle-ended'. This morphology alternates with that of the 'smooth-ended' ameloblast, in which the striated border is absent (Fig. 22.24). Ruffle-ended ameloblasts contain lysosome-like bodies, which presumably complete the degradation of the resorbed matrix, while smooth-ended ameloblasts contain smooth endoplasmic reticulum.

Modulation between the two forms occurs about five to seven times during maturation. This modulation may indicate alternation between resorptive and secretory phases of activity. The cyclical changes in ameloblast morphology seem to be linked to at least two aspects of maturation:

- The movement of calcium ions: in the ruffled-ended form, this movement may be actively controlled, whereas in the smooth-ended form, calcium ions may move only by diffusion (and hence few would enter the enamel).
- Local pH changes: physiologically normal pH favouring mineralisation (ruffle-ended) would alternate with mildly acidic conditions handicapping mineralisation (smooth-ended).

Hydrogen ions released by hydroxyapatite formation are neutralised by bicarbonate generated by the enzyme carbonic anhydrase II (CA2), which is strongly expressed by ameloblasts starting in the transition stage. Bicarbonate ion is transported out of the ameloblast by exchanging for chloride ions using anion exchanger 2 (AE2), which is highly expressed by maturation-stage ameloblasts.

The route taken by calcium into the enamel fluid varies according to the morphological stage of the ameloblast during the maturation phase. The apical location of plasma membrane Ca-ATPase in ruffle-ended ameloblasts indicates that the active transport of calcium into the enamel

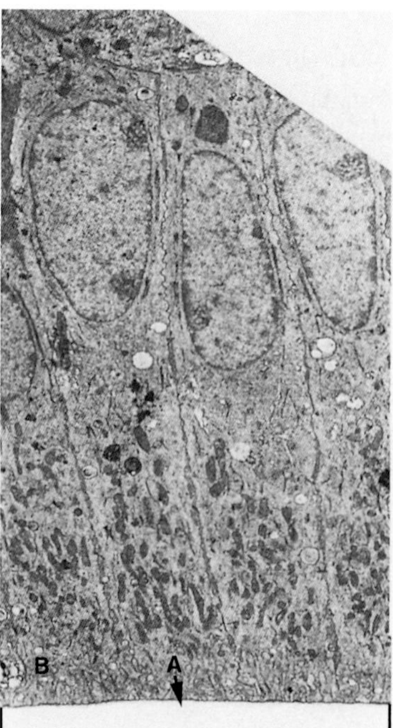

Fig. 22.22 TEM of demineralised section showing the appearance of ruffle-ended ameloblasts during maturation phase of amelogenesis. A = enamel space; B = striated border. The Tomes process has been lost. The mitochondria are grouped in a basal cluster. The rough endoplasmic reticulum is much reduced (×2,700).

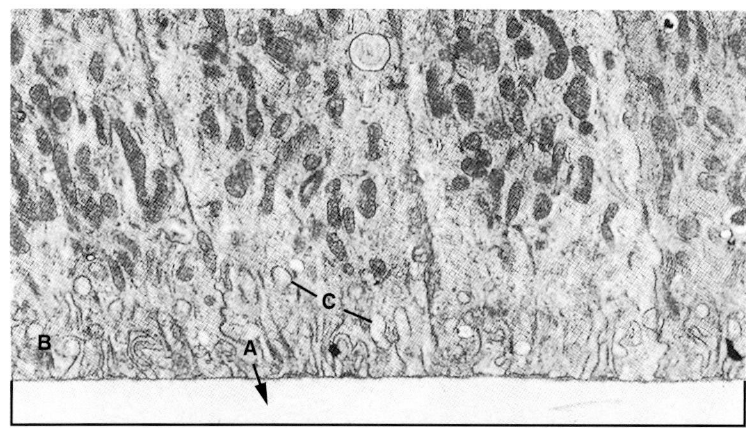

Fig. 22.23 High-power view of Fig. 22.22, showing ruffled border of ameloblast during the maturation stage. A = enamel space; B = striated (ruffled) border; C = resorptive vesicles (×6,700).

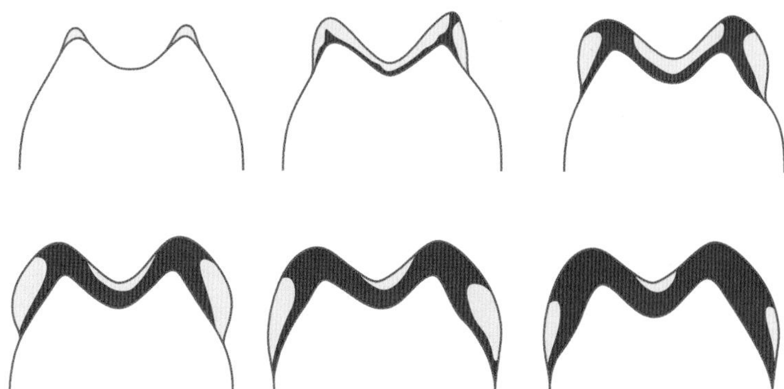

Fig. 22.25 Pattern of mineralisation during maturation, as mapped out by microradiography of ground sections. Pale yellow areas represent initial enamel deposition. Red areas show the pattern that increased mineralisation follows during maturation. Once the full thickness of enamel is formed in any area, maturation commences. Initial deposition and maturation can thus occur at the same time. Mineralisation during maturation follows a different pattern from initial deposition. Commencing at cusps, it passes to the enamel–dentine junction and along the junction before continuing throughout the more superficial regions.

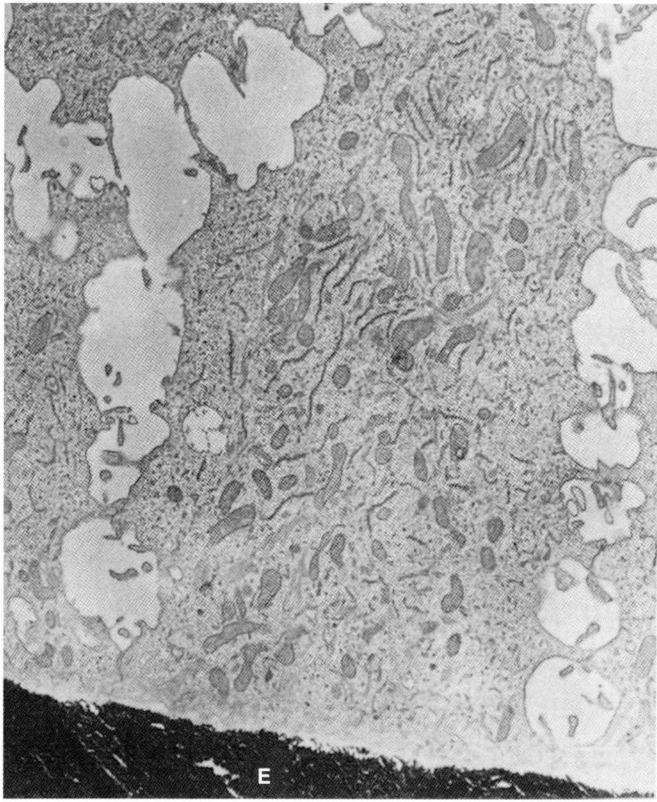

Fig. 22.24 TEM showing the appearance of a smooth-ended maturation ameloblast. At this stage the cells lack a distinct terminal web distally. E = enamel (×7,000). Courtesy Dr. Z Skobe and CRC Press.

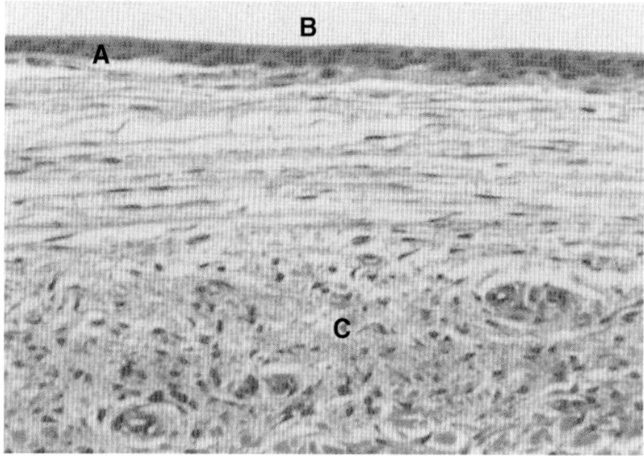

Fig. 22.26 Demineralised section showing the position and morphology of the reduced enamel epithelium (A) covering the unerupted tooth. B = enamel space; C = connective tissue of the dental follicle (H & E; ×160).

is across the cell. The major influx of calcium into the maturing enamel occurs via this route. During the smooth-ended ameloblast phase, there is a transient loss of the distal tight junctions between adjacent ameloblasts, allowing passage of material between the ameloblasts, although little calcium enters enamel via this route.

A third process in maturation, lowering the molecular weight of enamel proteins by a combination of secreting certain proteins (including amelotin and ODAM) and by the activity of proteinases resident in the enamel matrix, may be continuous rather than cyclical. The ameloblasts (which produce the enzymes) do not control the rate of this digestion, although they do resorb and degrade its end products. These protein changes may, by an unknown mechanism, affect mineralisation. Simple removal of the protein increases the relative mineral content. The final one-third of the mineralisation process goes on after virtually all protein has been removed. The increase in mineral density begins over the cusp tips and progresses cervically (Fig. 22.25).

Postmaturation stage

Once maturation of the enamel is complete, the ameloblasts become reduced further and flattened (Figs. 22.26, 22.27), except sometimes in the depths of fissures where they may remain columnar (see Fig. 8.3). A thin, amorphous layer of protein, the primary enamel cuticle, separates the cells from the enamel. At the ultrastructural level this has the appearance of a basal lamina, and it may represent either material extruded from the enamel during maturation or may be the last secretory product of the ameloblast. The cells themselves contain hemidesmosomes at their interface with the basal lamina applied to the enamel surface. The remnants of the enamel organ merge with the flattened ameloblasts to constitute the reduced enamel epithelium. The primary enamel cuticle, together with the reduced enamel epithelium, form Nasmyth's membrane (see page 157) and, during eruption, protect the enamel surface. The fluoride content of the enamel may be greater in teeth that have longer duration periods of eruption. It is not known whether the remaining cells of the enamel organ are active in this respect or not. Once the tooth has erupted into the oral cavity, the surface layer shows increasing mineralisation through interaction with saliva (posteruptive maturation).

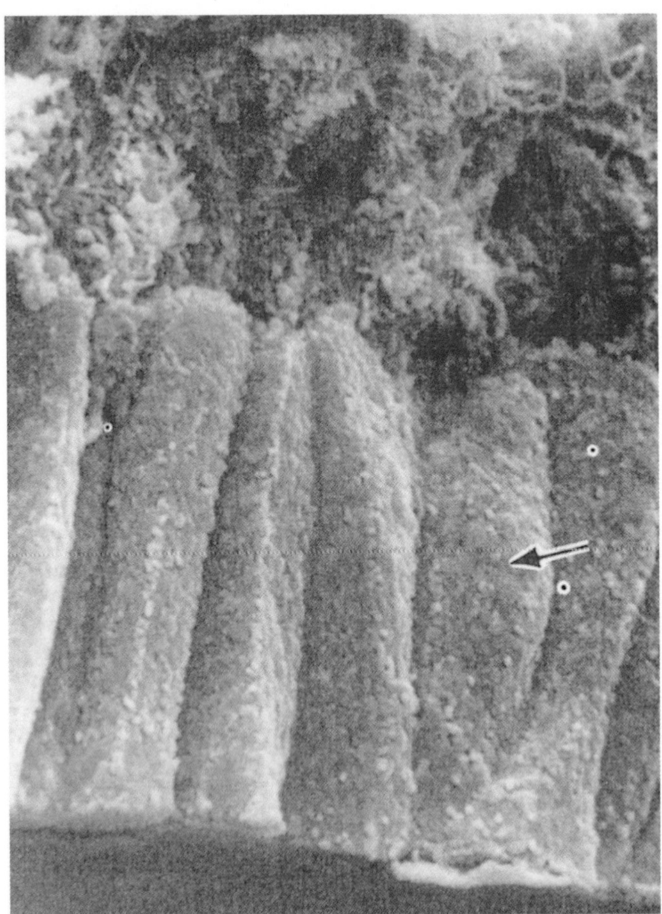

Fig. 22.27 SEM showing the appearance of reduced ameloblasts. The bulge indicated by the arrow may be the result of multiple nuclei, which are sometimes seen in these cells (×2,000). Courtesy Dr. Z Skobe and CRC Press.

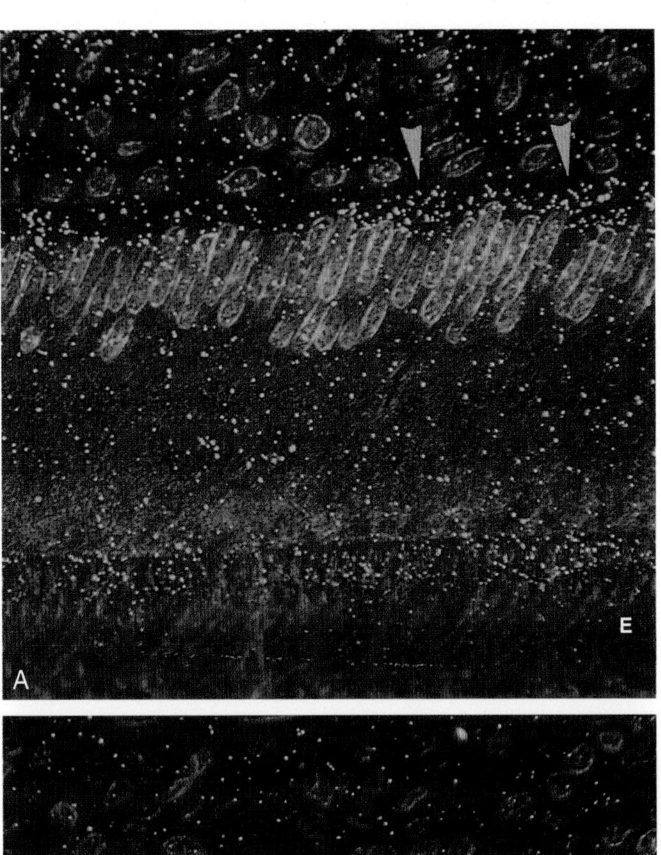

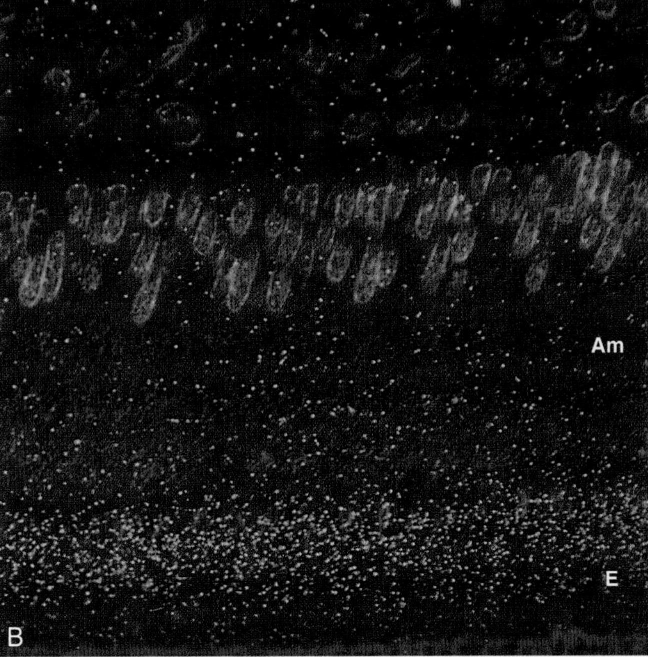

Fig. 22.28 An autoradiographically labelled histological section viewed in dark field showing the movement of calcium through the ameloblast layer. Labelled calcium-45 autoradiographs showing the movement of calcium (white dots) through ameloblasts. Am = ameloblasts; E = enamel. The tissue (rat) in (A) was taken 30 seconds after the injection of the radioactive calcium. The arrows indicate the accumulation of calcium in the proximal ameloblast adjacent to the stellate reticulum. The tissue in (B) was taken 10 minutes after injection when most of the calcium has become incorporated into the enamel (×400). Courtesy Dr. Y Takana and the editor of Connective Tissue Research.

Mineralisation

Mineralisation of enamel matrix starts very soon after secretion begins. The first crystals are initiated at the enamel–dentine junction in intimate association with the dentine crystals and grow outwards into the enamel matrix. The enamel crystals are probably nucleated mainly on organic matrix components of dentine collagen and enamel and only rarely by epitaxial growth on dentine crystals. Segments up to 100 µm long have been identified in crystals isolated from immature enamel, and it is generally considered that some crystals can eventually extend uninterruptedly from the enamel–dentine junction to the surface.

The chemistry of crystal formation in enamel awaits clarification. It has been suggested that the first mineral to form may be either octacalcium phosphate or amorphous calcium phosphate. However, as enamel mineral has a high degree of crystal perfection, it is not easy to understand how precursor calcium phosphate particles can be assembled to form highly elongated enamel crystals without introducing significant numbers of lattice defects.

There are several possible sources for the calcium that is needed for enamel matrix mineralisation. The precise pathway and transport mechanism are unclear, although some elements of the process have been determined.

Calcium reaches the matrix principally via the enamel organ (rather than the dental papilla). It travels, possibly predominantly, by an extracellular route, although there is also evidence for a transcellular route (Figs. 22.28, 22.29). There may be an active transport mechanism utilising carriers in the cell membranes of the ameloblasts, or the calcium may flow passively from high concentrations in the blood plasma to low concentrations in the enamel matrix. The ameloblast layer has a limited and variable, but controlled, permeability to ions. This property is attributed to the proximal rather than distal cell junctional complexes. It may control access not only to calcium ions but also to other significant ions, particularly fluoride.

Specific initiators of enamel mineralisation have not been convincingly identified. The first formed enamel at the enamel–dentine junction is less organised than the bulk of mature enamel in terms of crystallite size and morphology and is aprismatic. On the basis of this disordered morphology,

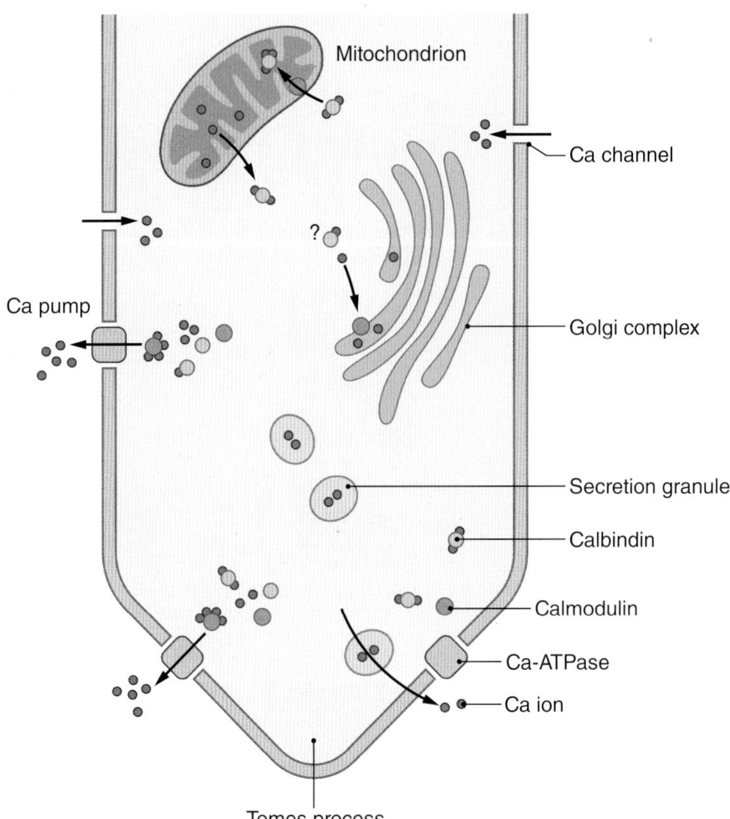

Fig. 22.29 Model showing the proposed intracellular movement of calcium in the ameloblasts. Courtesy Dr. T Sasaki and Karger Press.

it has been suggested that crystallite growth, and possibly nucleation, are directed by the enamel protein tuftelin. It has also been suggested, but not demonstrated, that initial nucleation may occur in dentine and cross the enamel–dentine junction. Matrix vesicles, which may participate in the onset of mineralisation in some parts of the dentine, have not been reported in developing enamel. It has been proposed that the amelogenins are capable of self-assembling into minute spheres (nanospheres), between which (or within) the first crystallites of enamel are formed. The initial crystallites form as a precipitate from the matrix that is supersaturated with respect to hydroxyapatite. Initially, crystallites may grow by the fusion of nucleation sites, but once the prismatic structure is established, crystallites are enlarged preferentially in length rather than in width.

The matrix can control crystallite growth by two basic mechanisms:

1) By breaking down protein in a controlled pattern to provide the space for new crystallite deposition
2) By modulating the effect of inhibitory molecules and gating mineral ion ingress

The first could be achieved by the formation in the matrix of appropriately oriented microchannels with the same dimensions as the crystallites and in which crystallites would form at the growing end of the prism. After the maturation phase, the role of the matrix proteins is largely ended, as virtually all the protein has been lost and what remains is replaced with tissue fluid. The matrix proteins are actually removed long before crystallite growth ends. The degraded matrix proteins accumulate in the extracellular space around the ameloblasts and, by inhibiting further activity, could control and limit the thickness of enamel deposited.

By understanding the role of the enamel proteins in allowing enamel crystals to seed and grow to adult form, this might allow for improvements in the development of biomimetic self-assembling peptides to assist with remineralization of enamel defects following dental caries (see pages 491–492).

Summary of development of the prismatic structure

The increase in minerals during maturation follows a different pattern from the initial deposition. The first formed enamel at what will be the enamel–dentine junction is laid against newly calcified dentine by flat-ended ameloblasts. It is aprismatic and initially contains small crystallites (10–15 nm wide, 1–2 nm thick and approximately 20 nm apart). The initial crystallites form as a precipitate within the matrix that is supersaturated with respect to hydroxyapatite. Crystallites form and grow while close to the cell membrane of the Tomes process. They grow by the deposition of ions on the crystallite faces. As the ameloblasts retreat, they form pyramidal Tomes processes at their distal ends, and the enamel produced thereafter is prismatic. As crystallites grow in length, they also increase in thickness and width, and this continues until they contact each other. Thus formed, the crystallite is a long, tapering pyramid with its apex at the enamel–dentine junction. After maturation, the crystallite is rod-shaped and of uniform size along its length (about an average of 26 nm thick × 68 nm wide) and runs from the enamel–dentine junction to the surface. Enamel matrix is deposited in a non-homogeneous form. Amelogenins become located primarily within the prism, non-amelogenins more at the periphery of the prism. The material secreted from the Tomes process forms the core of the prisms, while that secreted from the distal to the terminal web forms the peripheral parts of the prisms (prism boundaries). Enamel crystallites form at right angles to the face of the cell (see Fig. 22.12), and thus there is considerable variation in crystallite orientation within a prism. In human enamel, the crystals in the head of the prism are approximately parallel to the long axis of the prism but in the tail deviate from this direction by 60 degrees (see page 140). The path of the retreating ameloblasts determines the arrangement of prisms. Viewed longitudinally, the path of a human ameloblast seems to be in an approximately straight line from the enamel–dentine junction to the enamel surface. However, viewed transversely, the path is seen to be sinusoidal. Thus, the different directions traced out by different layers of ameloblasts are responsible for producing the appearance of Hunter–Schreger bands in mature enamel (see pages 140–141).

Towards the end of enamel formation, the Tomes process is lost such that the last formed layer of enamel, like the first, is aprismatic. In this layer, all the crystals are perpendicular to the surface and parallel to each other.

Incremental line formation

Various structural lines and patterns have been described in enamel and have been attributed to the rhythmic and incremental activity of the ameloblasts. Cross-striations appear as lines about 2.5–6 µm apart (see pages 143–144). They are formed because of a diurnal rhythm in enamel prism growth. The enamel striae (see pages 144–148) follow the contours of the developing crown and have been considered to be incremental (analogous to growth lines in trees) and may result from changes in the direction of enamel prisms. It seems more likely that the striae represent a boundary between groups of prisms formed by different cohorts of ameloblasts. In human enamel, about seven rows of ameloblasts are generated each week at the cervical loop, and the resulting prisms will extend around the crown. Each group of ameloblasts will have a somewhat different orientation from the adjacent group, and the boundary between the two could constitute a striation. The striae successively outline the position of the mineralising enamel front. They do not reach the surface over the tips of the cusps or incisal edges (see Fig. 7.37). As the daily

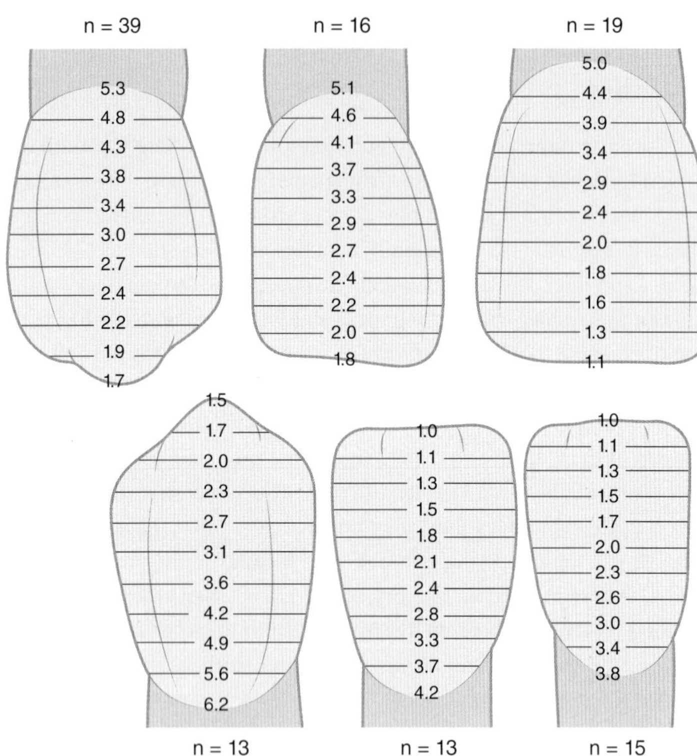

Fig. 22.30 Mean estimates for chronological ages of enamel formation in anterior teeth. The right anterior quadrant of the mouth is depicted as viewed clinically by an observer. Each height of each tooth type is divided into 10 equally spaced zones. The age of appearance of the enamel at the incisal edge is considered coincident with the completion of cuspal enamel, when the first enamel stria reaches the surface. The mean age at completion of each zone of enamel formation is shown in years rounded up or down to one decimal place. Redrawn with permission from Reid, D.J., Dean, M.C., 2000. The timing of linear hypoplasias on human anterior teeth. *American Journal of Physical Anthropology* 113, 135–139.

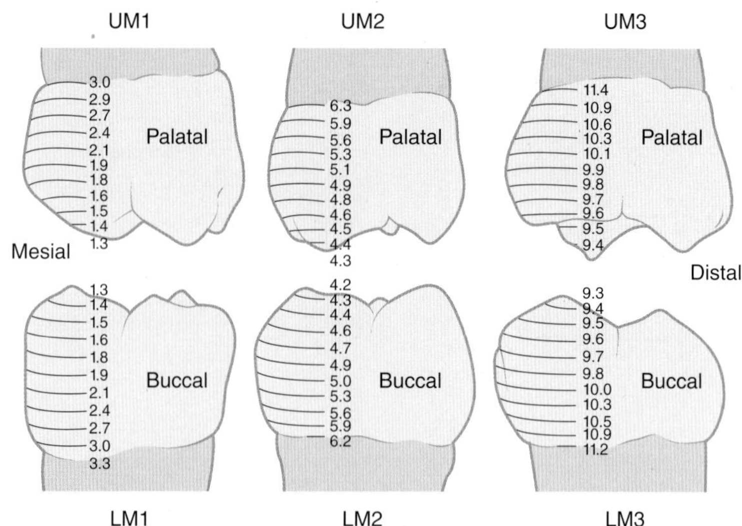

Fig. 22.31 Mean estimates for chronological ages of enamel formation in molars (UM = upper molars; LM = lower molars). Each height of each tooth type is divided into 10 equally spaced zones. The age of appearance of the enamel at the incisal edge is considered coincident with the completion of cuspal enamel, when the first enamel stria reaches the surface. The mean age at completion of each zone of enamel formation is shown in years rounded up or down to one decimal place. Redrawn with permission from Reid, D.J., Dean, M.C., 2005. Variation in modern human enamel formation times. *Journal of Human Evolution* 50, 329–346.

increments of enamel are smaller towards the end of enamel formation, the striae are closer together towards the cervical margin. There are on average about seven cross-striations between successive striae (range 6–10), so the striae are thought to represent approximately weekly incremental lines (circaseptan). One theory to account for their presence suggests that, superimposed on the normal 24-hour daily rhythm, there is another rhythm of about 27hours. The two would coincide about every 7 days, resulting in the presence of striae.

Studies based on careful quantification of incremental lines have provided information concerning the rates of enamel formation along the length of the crown. These are illustrated in Figs. 22.30 and 22.31 and show that crown formation is nonlinear and slows towards the cervix in all teeth. Also, there is no relation between tooth crown height and the total time taken to form enamel.

Molecular elements of ameloblast differentiation

As well as describing amelogenesis in morphological and biochemical terms, it is now possible, thanks to the techniques of molecular biology, to describe the patterns of expression of many regulating, inducing and signalling molecules. The expression of a certain molecule at a particular stage of development suggests, but does not establish, a role for that molecule in amelogenesis. Experimental approaches involve deleting or overexpressing the protein under investigation and documenting the changes that occur in order to define its function with conviction. Current knowledge is fragmentary and, although increasing rapidly, a coherent and comprehensive account of the molecular mechanisms of amelogenesis is some time away. What follows is a summary of the fragments that have been found to date.

Gene transcription

Virtually all cells contain genes that encode for enamel production. Gene regulation determines which genes are active and is the property of a class of DNA-binding proteins. Gene expression can be controlled at every step from the gene to the final functional protein. Much of the control is exercised at the stage of transcription when mRNA is produced on the DNA template. RNA is synthesised with an RNA polymerase acting in concert with transcription factors while binding to a promoter site on the DNA. The mRNA thus formed may be modified and edited. The final mRNA, while sliding through a ribosome and acting via translational RNA, results in the assembly of polypeptides. Multiple, often different, polypeptides are conjugated into proteins, sometimes combined with polysaccharides or phosphate groups, and given a physical configuration as they pass through the intracellular tubular pathway of the endoplasmic reticulum and Golgi apparatus. This process results most often in proteins bound in vesicles for export. The determination of which vesicles are released and when is related to intracellular signals that may be genetically programmed or may be produced in response to an external signal acting on a cell membrane receptor.

This description of protein synthesis is generic. Only some of the factors involved in gene expression in the ameloblast are known. Homeobox genes encode for transcription factors and thus regulate transcription. Msx-2 is the product of a homeobox gene expressed in the pharyngeal (branchial) arches and in the early stages (bud) in the epithelium but not at later stages in the mesenchyme. It localises in the enamel knot region and is possibly a regulator of morphogenesis (see page 386). Egr-1 is a transcription factor thought to regulate cell destiny in developing teeth. Its expression shifts back and forth between epithelium and mesenchyme, and it is briefly expressed in the polarised ameloblasts before any matrix is produced.

At the molecular level, most information relates to the gene encoding for the enamel matrix protein amelogenin. Various forms of amelogenin may be produced by post-transcriptional modification of the mRNA, and each form may have a different role in amelogenesis.

Membrane receptors

In developing tissues, cells differentiate and change their activities, usually in response to an external signal. Receptor molecules on the cell surface recognise and bind signalling molecules that may, for example, be growth factors or extracellular matrix molecules. There are several families of receptor molecules. One of the integrin family of cell surface receptors, β5, is upregulated in the internal enamel epithelium during the cap stage after being expressed in the mesenchyme during the bud stage. It is then downregulated as the ameloblast differentiates. Receptors for fibroblast growth factors (FGFs) and epidermal growth factors (EGFs) are also present in the internal enamel epithelium of the bud stage but are downregulated during the cap stage. EGF expression returns to the ameloblast in maturation.

Intracellular receptors

Some signalling molecules act on receptors that are within the cytoplasm of the cell. Cellular retinoic acid–binding proteins (CRABP) transmit the signals of retinoic acid. They are expressed in the developing tooth wherever there are high rates of cell proliferation. One of these proteins (CRABP I) appears to be expressed by secretory, but not maturation-stage, ameloblasts. Growth hormone receptor is also intracellular, but appears only on the differentiating ameloblast. It seems to be related to preameloblast proliferation. Vitamin D receptors have also been identified during differentiation.

Clinical considerations

Clinical aspects of enamel have already been considered in terms of enamel caries, enamel remineralisation and restorative dentistry in Chapter 7.

Normal enamel can be lost or damaged during life through attrition, abrasion and erosion (see pages 149–150) or through dental caries (see pages 154–155).

Structural defects to enamel during its development may result in discolouration of enamel and/or pits and grooves in the surface. If related to trauma, such enamel hypoplasia may be confined to a single tooth (Fig. 22.33). However, if related to a systemic disturbance, multiple teeth developing at the same time may be similarly affected. Defective enamel can also be produced during development because of mutations from genes synthesising enamel proteins or their associated enzymes. This condition is termed *amelogenesis imperfecta*.

Amelogenesis imperfecta

Defects in enamel formation are common. Estimates vary from 8% to 80% of the population as having at least one affected permanent tooth. Amelogenesis defects may predispose to tooth sensitivity, plaque accumulation and increased caries risk.

Over 100 different defects of amelogenesis have been identified. A group of hereditary conditions known as amelogenesis imperfecta affect only enamel and are relatively common (Fig. 22.32). Estimates of their prevalence range from 1 in every 14 people to 1.4 per 1,000, depending upon type. Three groups of amelogenesis imperfecta are recognised based on the phase of amelogenesis affected:

1) Hypoplastic, in which the enamel is of normal colour but thin and grooved or pitted

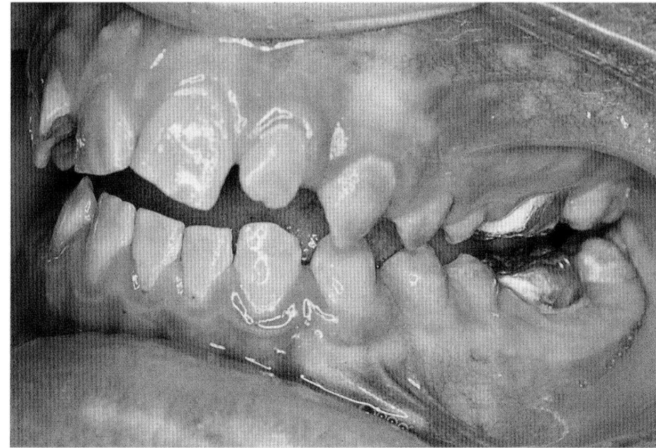

Fig. 22.32 Teeth from a patient with amelogenesis imperfecta. In this example the enamel is of apparently normal appearance in many of the teeth but seriously abnormal in the first molars, where much of the enamel has chipped off, exposing the underlying dentine. The underlying dentine is usually normal, and restorative procedures, especially crowns, can be used to maintain the dentition. Courtesy Dr. M Ignelzi.

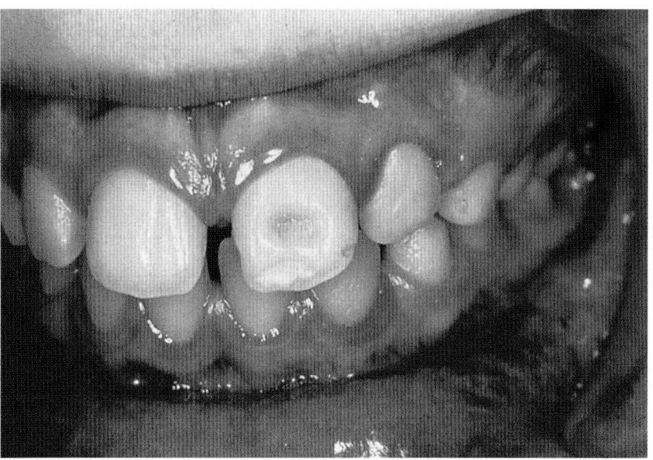

Fig. 22.33 Tooth with enamel defect caused by trauma. This child had a blow to the maxillary left first deciduous incisor that damaged the underlying developing permanent tooth sufficiently to result in a localised defect in enamel formation. This produced a pit, seen on the facial surface of the tooth when erupted. Courtesy Dr. M Ignelzi.

2) Hypocalcified, in which the mineralisation is poor and the enamel is dark and chips easily
3) Hypomaturation, in which the enamel is dark, mottled and chips easily

Other hereditary conditions (including systemic metabolic disorders) in which enamel is thin and pitted also affect other tissues (e.g., mucopolysaccharidosis), while systemic ectodermal/epidermal disorders (e.g., epidermolysis bullosa) have many subtypes (including hypoplastic enamel, among many more serious features). Localised trauma can result in disturbances in enamel formation in individual teeth (Fig. 22.33).

Fluorosis

The most obvious clinically important dietary factor that affects enamel development is fluoride (see also page 491). Ingestion of levels above 5 parts per million results in fluorosis, characterised by the presence of a diffuse white opacity of variable extent. In severe cases, the fluoritic areas may be brown and pitted (Fig. 22.34). The principal change is a subsurface hypomineralisation of varying extent.

Febrile diseases, drugs and rhesus factor

Febrile diseases can disturb amelogenesis for the term of the illness and result in a band of poorly formed enamel. Some drugs, the best known

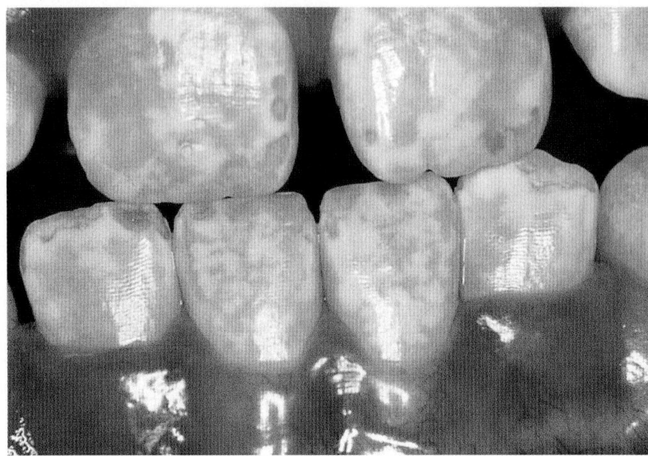

Fig. 22.34 Teeth demonstrating fluorosis. A high level of dietary fluoride has resulted in much of the enamel becoming opaque in patches, giving a 'mottled' appearance. Courtesy Dr. M Ignelzi.

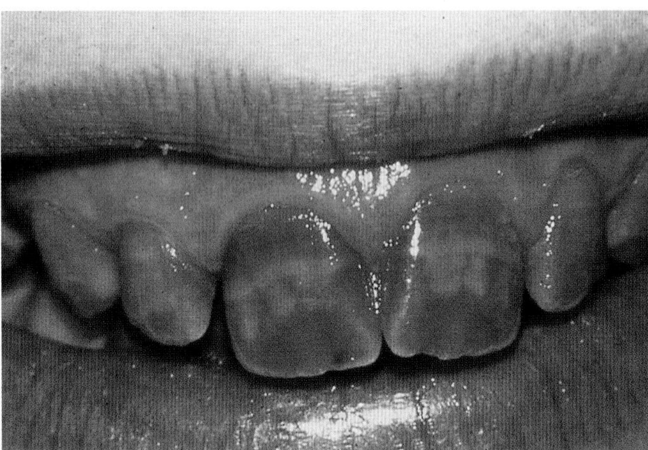

Fig. 22.35 Teeth stained as a result of tetracycline administration. This is an extreme example of tetracycline staining: the entire enamel (and dentine) has become pigmented. As the staining is built into the structure of the tooth, bleaching procedures do not usually greatly improve the appearance of these teeth. Crowns or, more conservatively, veneers, will do so. Courtesy Dr. M Ignelzi.

being the tetracyclines, may affect amelogenesis. Tetracycline is incorporated into the developing enamel and results in a band of brown enamel (Fig. 22.35). When rhesus factor incompatibility results in erythroblastosis fetalis, haemoglobin residues are incorporated into developing enamel, resulting in a brown pigmentation of the teeth (Fig. 22.36).

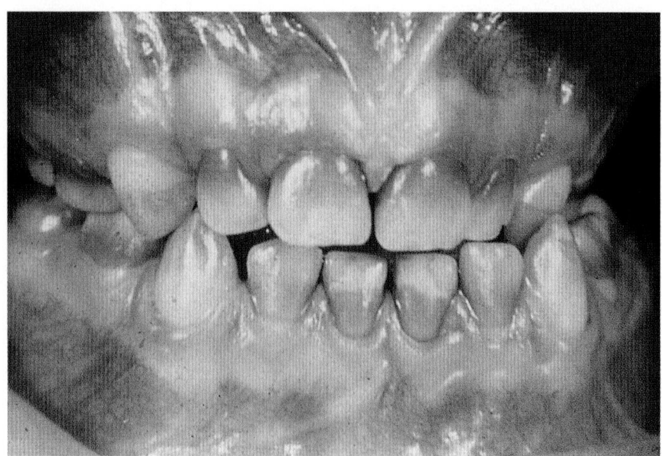

Fig. 22.36 Teeth showing haemoglobin pigmentation. Haemoglobin residues released during rhesus factor incompatibility are taken up by the developing teeth, resulting in a brown stain. Because of effective screening this is now a rare occurrence. Courtesy Dr. M Ignelzi.

Molar incisor hypoplasia

Molar incisor hypoplasia (MIH) is an increasingly common developmental enamel defect with some similarities to amelogenesis imperfecta. It is characterised by demarcated opacities in permanent molars associated with hypomineralised enamel. MIH has a frequency ranging from 2.4% to 40.2% in different populations. The hypomineralised areas are mainly located in the mesio-buccal cusps, starting at the enamel–dentine junction and continuing towards the enamel surface. The ameloblasts in the hypomineralised enamel are capable of forming an enamel of normal thickness. Chronologically, it is estimated that the timing of the disturbance is at a period during the first 6–7 months of age.

Affected teeth are prone to early clinical failure and impact adversely on the developing dental occlusion, requiring complex treatment. MIH is thought to be genetically complex, and its aetiology is poorly understood. A range of systemic and environmental factors has been implicated.

Further readings for this chapter can be found in the accompanying eBook. Explore online Self-assessment quiz to test and reinforce your understanding of the material in your free ebook. Follow instructions in the Inside Front Cover to unlock your access.

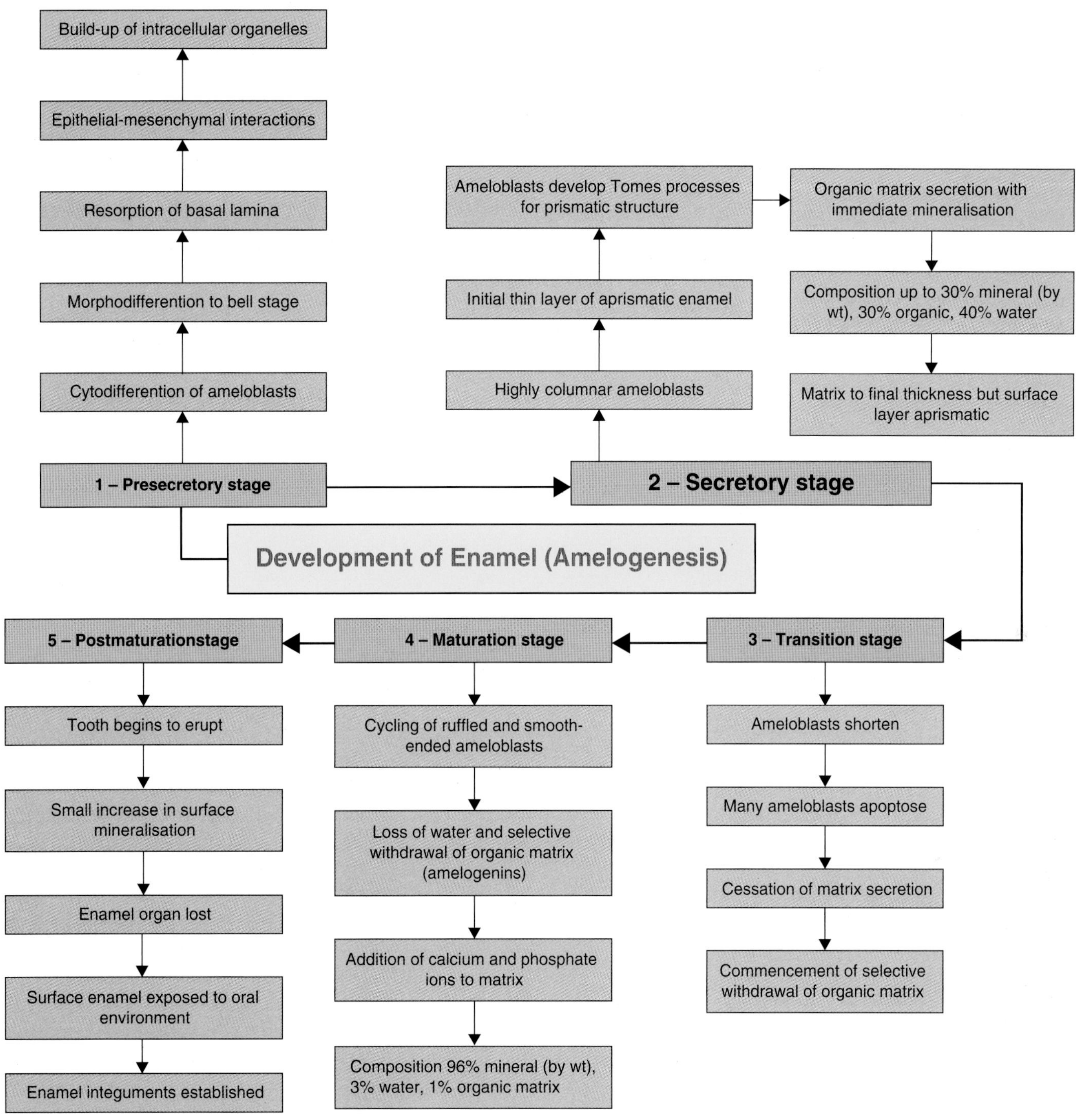

Mind Map 22.1 Development of enamel (amelogenesis).

23 Dentinogenesis

Unlike bone, dentine does not participate in the body's calcium and phosphate homeostasis. Consequently, there is usually no gross resorption of dentine by multinuclear, osteoclast-like cells except during the shedding of the deciduous teeth.

Dentine formation follows a specific anatomical pattern. It begins where cusps will later be formed and continues uniformly down the slopes of the cusps and the walls of the crown to the cervical loop. This is coronal dentine. Root dentine then forms as the root sheath extends and odontoblasts differentiate on its pulpal surface. Note that there is no distinct demarcation line between crown and root dentine. The length of the root is genetically determined and implemented, presumably by halting the extension of the root sheath. Dentinogenesis continues, and the thickness of dentine increases steadily until at a predetermined point it slows down dramatically and secondary dentine is deposited slowly. This is an age-related change, as is the simultaneous formation of peritubular dentine. Environmental factors may also affect the deposition of peritubular dentine, although this is not entirely clear.

Dentinogenesis is a continuous process but for descriptive purposes can be subdivided into five stages:

1) Differentiation of the odontoblasts
2) Deposition of organic matrix
3) Mineralisation and modification of the organic matrix
4) Peritubular and secondary dentine formation
5) Tertiary dentine formation in response to injury

Differentiation of the odontoblasts

The cells that will form the dentine differentiate from the ectomesenchyme of the dental papilla and are of neural crest origin (Fig. 23.1). The process of differentiation and the properties of the differentiated cells have been studied in detail by experiments recombining samples of dental papilla cells and cells from the oral ectoderm in co-culture. In addition, there have been extensive molecular observations describing the nature and sequence of gene expression in the differentiating cells. Odontoblasts express not only the genes responsible for production of the unique dentine matrix proteins but perhaps also those responsible for the morphology of the completed tooth, determining whether it is a molar, canine or incisor (morphogenetic genes – see pages 391–393).

Epithelial–mesenchymal interactions

The differentiation of the odontoblast does not occur in isolation. Neural crest cells from the appropriate location do not differentiate to form dentine unless they come into contact with the dental epithelium. Differentiation is initiated and controlled by a series of epithelial signals. The primary enamel knot (page 386) is a signalling centre that forms at the tip of the epithelial tooth bud. It is fully developed and recognisable in the cap stage and expresses at least 10 different signalling molecules belonging to the bone morphogenic protein (BMP), fibroblast growth factor (FGF), sonic

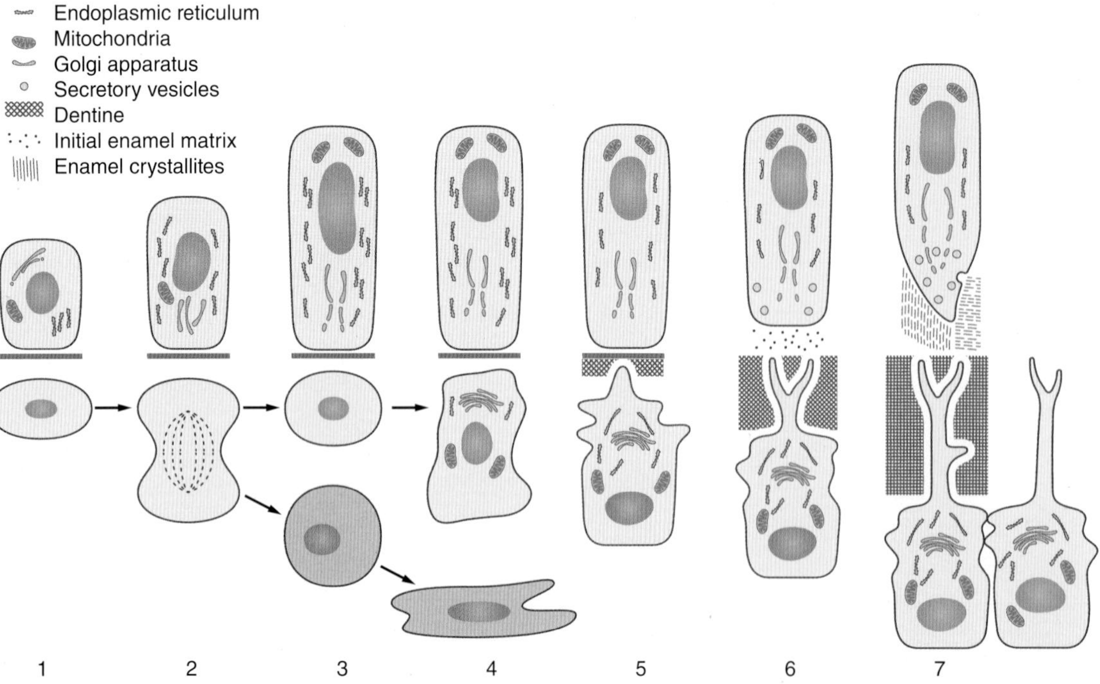

Fig. 23.1 Life cycle of the odontoblast (lower cell line) related to that of the ameloblast (upper cell line). 1 = Ameloblast begins to differentiate first. 2 = Peripheral ectomesenchymal cells divide, with some daughter cells migrating below the odontoblast layer. 3 = Acting on a signal from the ameloblast, the preodontoblasts begin to differentiate. 4 = Synthetic organelles increase in size and number, especially the Golgi apparatus and rough endoplasmic reticulum. 5 = Nucleus moves basally as the cell becomes polarised. A number of odontoblast processes begin to form. One odontoblast process becomes enlarged and begins to secrete matrix. 6 = The odontoblast retreats as matrix is laid down, leaving behind a single main process. Once a narrow layer of matrix is laid down, mineralisation commences. 7 = Once the first layer of dentine is laid down, the differentiated ameloblast begins to deposit matrix.

hedgehog (Shh) and Wnt families. In molar teeth, secondary enamel knots appear in the enamel epithelium at the sites of the future cusps. It has been suggested that they also express several signalling molecules and their formation precedes the folding and growth of the epithelium. However, the fully formed knot is only visible after there is an obvious cusp shape in the internal enamel epithelium. The differentiation of odontoblasts always starts from the tips of the cusps and therefore it is conceivable that some of the signals expressed in the enamel knots may act as inducers of odontoblast differentiation. It requires temporospatially regulated epigenetic signalling. There is also an interaction in the opposite direction. Cell-to-cell signalling pathways and their target nuclear factors have been identified as key mediators of the progressively complex exchange of information between ectoderm and ectomesenchyme. The constantly changing direction of the reciprocal signalling and cell responses between ectoderm and ectomesenchyme enables cells to monitor continuously their relative spatial positions and differentiated states. Oral ectoderm, although differentiated into enamel epithelium, does not deposit enamel matrix until dentine deposition has started.

The basement membrane of the dental epithelium plays a major role both as a substrate and as a reservoir of signalling molecules. The basement membrane is characterised by the presence of collage type IV and fibronectin. Time-limited changes in the composition of the basement membrane occur coincident with odontoblast differentiation. These changes include expression and localisation of laminin, chondroitin-containing proteoglycans and enamel proteins. Although not strictly components of the basement membrane, fibronectin and decorin also accumulate at the distal pole of the differentiating cell. It is not known which, if any, of these changes initiate or control differentiation. Other, as yet unknown, factors may pass through the membrane too quickly to have been detected.

Growth factors are signalling molecules that can control growth and repair in cells and that diffuse through the interstitial spaces between cells. Several, particularly those belonging to the transforming growth factor (TGF) family, insulin-like growth factor (IGF) and BMP, have been found in the internal enamel epithelium during the differentiation of odontoblasts. Some of these have been shown to affect, under some conditions, the development and behaviour of odontoblast-like cells maintained in culture. These cultured cells can be shown to express some of the membrane receptors for these molecules. Growth factors play an important role in the development of many tissues. While it is not currently known which of these are significant and what their precise role is in odontoblast differentiation, interesting hypotheses are being tested. These include the proposal that TGF-β family members, which are trapped and then released from the basement membrane of the internal enamel epithelium, act on the preodontoblasts and, via a series of intervening steps, modulate the expression of genes involved in the assembly of the cytoskeleton. The cytoskeleton is of pre-eminent importance in the relocation of intracellular organelles and in being associated with changes in the morphology of the cell. Members of the TGF family may also be involved in the withdrawal from the mitotic cycle of the cells that will become odontoblasts.

Morphological changes in odontoblasts during differentiation

The morphologically discernible differentiation of the odontoblast begins with the dental papilla cells adjacent to the deepest invaginations of the internal enamel epithelium, beneath what will become the cusps or incisal margins. The preodontoblast cells are those left in contact with the basement membrane of the internal enamel epithelium after the last division of the neural crest (ectomesenchyme). The preodontoblasts cells have no well-developed organelles nor a specific orientation. This changes rapidly. The cells increase in size (hypertrophy), and the nucleus comes to lie in the basal part of the cell, farthest from the internal enamel epithelium (Fig. 23.2). The Golgi complex becomes pronounced and positioned above the nucleus. The rough endoplasmic reticulum increases in size and becomes flattened parallel to what is becoming the long axis of the cell. The elongation and polarisation of the cell are accompanied by a redistribution of the intracellular skeletal proteins actin, vinculin and vimentin, as well as new expression of nestin and cytokeratin. Changes also occur in the membrane of the cell, including increased expression of the integrin receptor that binds fibronectin.

Many small cell processes extend from the differentiating odontoblast. Most of these are directed towards the basement membrane of the internal enamel epithelium. As differentiation proceeds, the number of processes is reduced and one large process will dominate, although some smaller processes will remain and link the odontoblasts to each other and to underlying cells in the pulp. Cell-to-cell junctions increase in number, particularly between odontoblasts but also linking odontoblasts to subodontoblastic cells. Tight, gap and macula adherens (desmosomes) junctions occur. It is likely that some of the signals that coordinate the activities of the odontoblasts pass through the gap junctions that allow the passage of small molecules from cell to cell, although synchrony may also (or alternatively) be achieved by response to a common external signal.

Differentiation of the odontoblasts occurs in a specific temporospatial pattern, beginning under what will become the cusp tip or incisal margin and progressing rootwards. The control of this progression may lie either in the ability of the internal enamel epithelium to induce changes sequentially or in the competence of the preodontoblasts to act on a signal that is

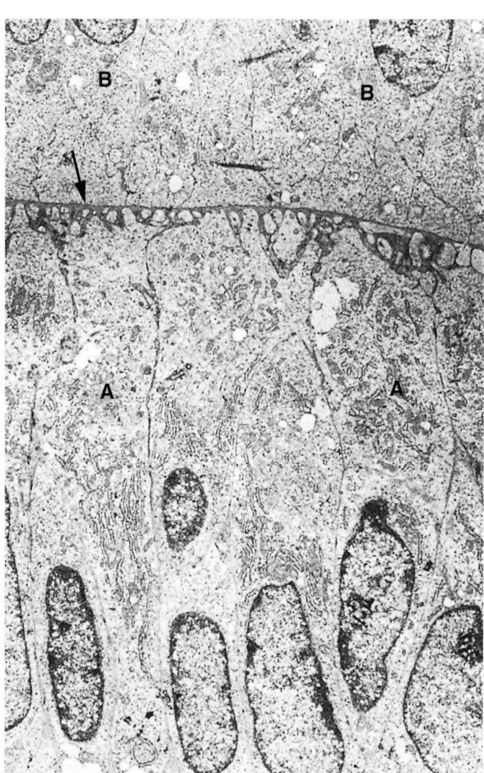

Fig. 23.2 TEM of the interface between odontoblasts (A) and ameloblasts (B) just before the deposition of matrix. The arrow indicates the basement membrane of the ameloblasts (×38,000). Courtesy Dr. P Glick.

uniformly available. Current evidence suggests the latter, although these possibilities are not mutually exclusive.

There is evidence that the transcellular flow of calcium ions through the layer of odontoblasts during dentinogenesis is of importance for the secretion of ions towards the mineralising front. The transport of calcium ions appears to be related to L-type voltage-gated channels.

Deposition of dentine matrix

Once fully differentiated, the odontoblast begins to secrete its characteristic organic matrix, the components of which are listed in Table 23.1. Both collagen type I and phosphophoryn (dentine phosphoprotein, DPP) precursors are found within the endoplasmic reticulum, the Golgi complex and secretory granules, although they are not found together within the same compartments. DPP is localised within the tubular endoplasmic reticulum, round-shaped transitional vesicles, the Golgi complex and narrow asymmetric secretory granules. These asymmetric secretory granules are abundant in the odontoblastic process boundary. Care must be taken, however, with the subcellular localisation of DPP, as producing antibodies to DPP for immunohistochemistry is notoriously difficult and unreliable. Collagen type I was localised within rosette-form endoplasmic reticulum compartments, the Golgi complex and large, distinctive secretory granules. Collagen type I is deposited at the cell–predentine boundary, with DPP deposited by the odontoblast process. The matrix thus formed consists primarily of type I collagen fibrils with DPP as the second most abundant constituent. DPP and dentine sialoprotein (DSP) are expressed not only by odontoblasts but also during the early stages of dentinogenesis by the

Table 23.1 Components of organic dentine extracellular matrix

Collagens:	Enamelysin:
Type I	
Type I trimer	
Type V	
Proteoglycans:	**Lipids:**
Decorin (PG II)	Cholesterol
Biglycan (PG I)	Cholesterol esters
Other chondroitin 4-sulphate-containing proteoglycans	Triacylglycerols
Keratan sulphate (?)	
Glycoproteins/sialoproteins:	**Serum-derived proteins:**
Osteonectin	α2HS-glycoprotein
Dentine sialoproteins (DSPs)	Albumin
Bone sialoprotein	Immunoglobulins
Osteopontin	
Bone acidic glycoprotein 75	
Syndecan 2	
Phosphoproteins:	**Growth factors:**
Dentine phosphoproteins (DPPs)	TGF-β
Dentine matrix protein 1	Chondrogenic inducing factor
γ-Carboxyglutamate-containing proteins	Bone morphogenic proteins (BMPs)
Osteocalcin	Fibroblast growth factors (FGFs)
Amelin-1 (transient expression)	Insulin-like growth factors (IGFs)
	Sonic hedgehog (SHH)

preameloblasts of the internal enamel epithelium. Note that there is a distinct difference between predentine matrix and mineralised dentine matrix. Predentine matrix has collagen and proteoglycans, and mineralised dentine matrix has collagen, DPP, a second pool of proteoglycan and other components. The absence of DPP in the predentine and its appearance at the mineralising front have been shown by dissection and chemical analysis.

Both DPP and DSP were thought to be unique to dentine and not found in bone. DSP has now been reported in alveolar bone, cellular cementum, osteocytes, cementocytes and their matrices. It has also become clear that DSP and DPP are formed from the proteolysis of a single parent molecule, dentine sialophosphoprotein (DSPP). The primary structure of DPP is characterised by aspartic acid and phosphoserine sequences: Asp–Pse, Asp–Pse–Pse and Asp–Pse–Pse–Pse.

It has been postulated that DPP has a significant role in dentine mineralisation. DSP may also have a role, although less important, in mineralisation. It has also been suggested that DPP is involved in signalling during epithelial–mesenchymal interactions. Many other proteins (such as glycoproteins and proteoglycans) are added to the matrix. In the first formed dentine (mantle dentine), some of the matrix components may be contributed by dental pulp cells beneath the odontoblasts. The odontoblast is still undergoing the late stages of differentiation as the first layer of dentine matrix is being deposited. Numerous cytoplasmic processes rapidly resolve into a single large process. As it is formed by odontoblasts that are still differentiating, and because other cells appear to contribute to its formation, mantle dentine in the crown (and possibly the hyaline and granular layers in the root) is of somewhat different structure, and probably composition, than the bulk of the matrix (Fig. 23.3).

The type I collagen fibrils that are laid down initially lie at right angles to the future enamel–dentine junction. In sections of harshly fixed tissue stained with silver, these fibres take on a 'corkscrew' appearance (Fig. 23.4).

Once the initial mantle layer has been laid down, the bulk of the primary circumpulpal dentine is laid down in a regular incremental pattern. This pattern can be followed by observing the distribution of injected radiolabelled amino acids (Fig. 23.5). The synthetic pathways followed in the cell are those well established for the production of proteins and complex molecules that include proteins. The release of the various matrix components, however, can follow differing pathways. Type I collagen is released primarily from the odontoblast cell body as it moves inwards. Thus, the odontoblast is always closely juxtaposed to the unmineralised predentine.

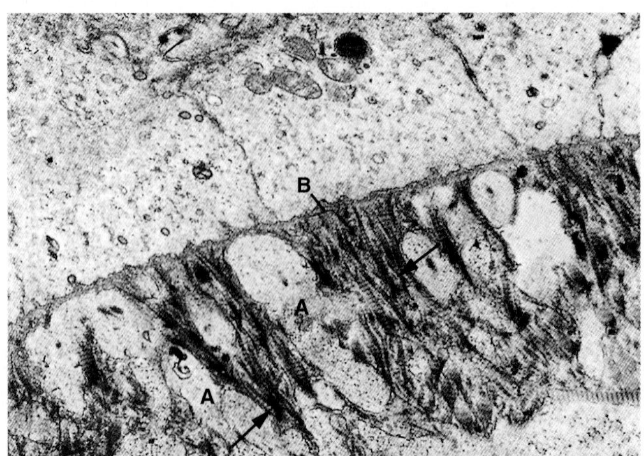

Fig. 23.3 TEM showing early dentine matrix formation. The basement membrane of the ameloblasts (B) is still present. Some components may cross the basement membrane from the ameloblasts. The odontoblasts initially have multiple processes (A). Note initial collagen fibrils are oriented perpendicular to enamel–dentine junction (arrows) (×9,500). Courtesy Dr. P Glick.

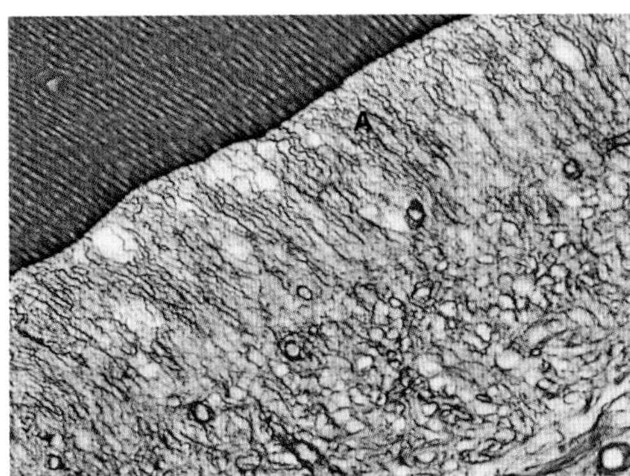

Fig. 23.4 Micrograph of a demineralised section showing 'corkscrew' fibres (of von Korff) (A). These are thought to be the first-formed type I collagen fibres whose orientation differs from those laid down later. Harsh fixation makes them curly, and the deposition of silver makes them appear thick. They are thus an artefact, but one based on a real difference between the structure of mantle and the later formed dentine (silver stain; ×200).

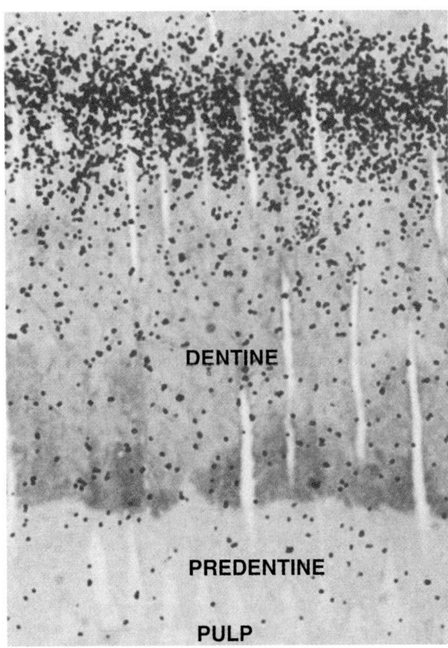

Fig. 23.5 Light microscope radioautograph of dentine formation 4 days after injection of ^{3}H-proline. A labelled band (silver grains) approximately the same width as the predentine is clearly seen, demonstrating the incremental nature of matrix deposition (iron haematoxylin stain; ×560). Courtesy Dr. H Warshawsky, Dr. K Josephsen and the editor of *Archives of Oral Biology*.

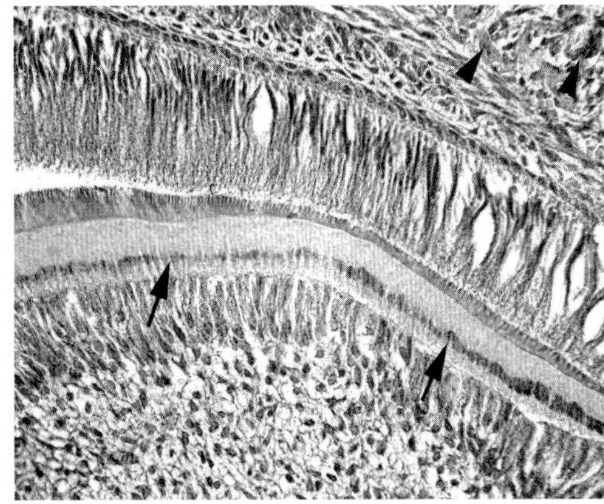

Fig. 23.6 Localisation of phosphophorin at the mineralisation front (arrows) and in the odontoblast cells. Arrowheads indicate alveolar bone (×250). Courtesy Dr. A George and the editors of *Cell Tissue Organs*.

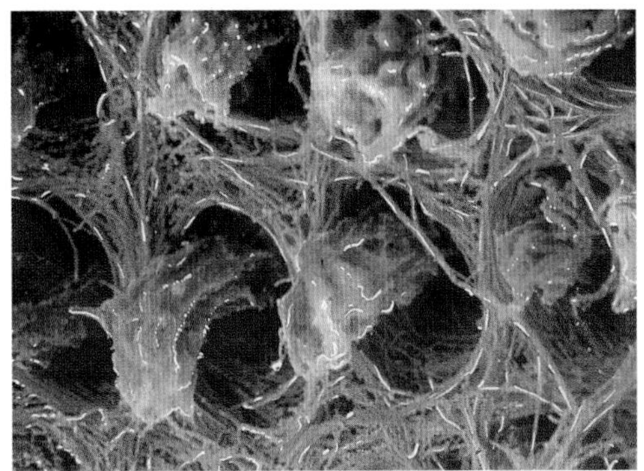

Fig. 23.7 SEM showing the surface of predentine. The collagen fibrils (brown) form an interlacing network perpendicular to the odontoblast process (blue) (×4,000). Courtesy Prof. L Fonzi.

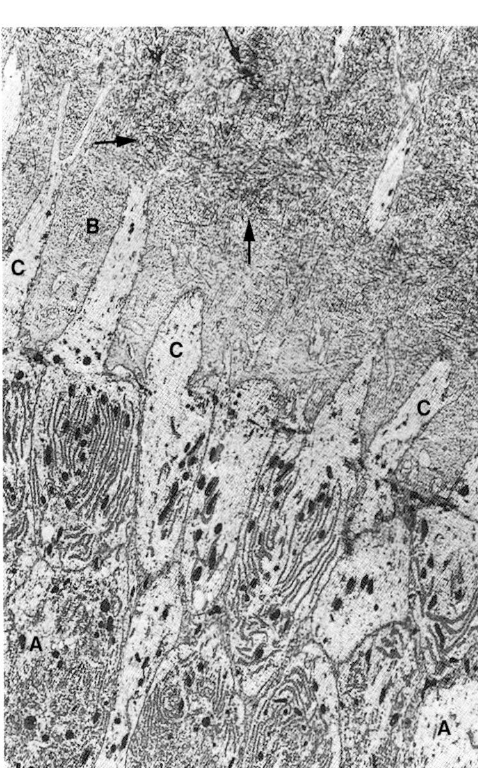

Fig. 23.8 TEM showing dentine matrix formation (B) and mineralisation. The outer matrix is mineralising (arrows), initially with small groups of crystals. The odontoblasts (A) have a single large process (C) (×6,500). Courtesy Dr. P Glick.

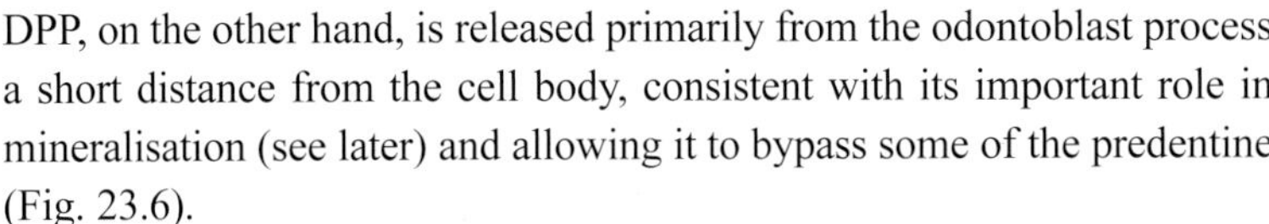

DPP, on the other hand, is released primarily from the odontoblast process a short distance from the cell body, consistent with its important role in mineralisation (see later) and allowing it to bypass some of the predentine (Fig. 23.6).

Once the mantle layer is formed, the remaining type I collagen is laid down with its fibrils approximately parallel to the pulp–dentine border (Fig. 23.7). Minor, but coincident, changes in orientation about every week (20 μm) could be responsible for the long-period incremental lines (Andresen lines – see page 179).

The deposition of new organic matrix proceeds at a pace similar to that of mineralisation, such that there is always a layer of unmineralised matrix, the predentine, on the pulpal surface of the tissue (Fig. 23.7). Collagen is secreted at the cell border, apparently primarily by the cell body of the odontoblast. The odontoblast process secretes the other non-collagenous proteins such that a complex of collagen and noncollagenous proteins is formed at the junction of the predentine and calcified dentine, the mineralisation front (Fig. 23.8). DPP and other noncollagenous proteins bind to the collagen; DPP binds in a highly specific manner at the 'e' band in the gap region of the type I fibrils.

What controls the secretory activity of the odontoblast is unclear. The rate of secretion varies, following both short-term (diurnal) and long-period rhythms. Serious systemic disturbances (such as birth and disease) can slow or stop it. Dentine seems to be less vulnerable to dietary deficiencies than bone. Presumably much of its activity is genetically predetermined. Once the odontoblast is separated from the internal enamel epithelium, the effect of other cell populations is unknown. The rate of dentine deposition can be altered (increased) by injury to the nerves supplying the pulp. Much of this effect could be explained as secondary to changes in blood flow or (in erupted teeth) as a result of a loss of sensory activity that might lead to greater wear on the teeth. However, proteins unique to synapses (synapsin

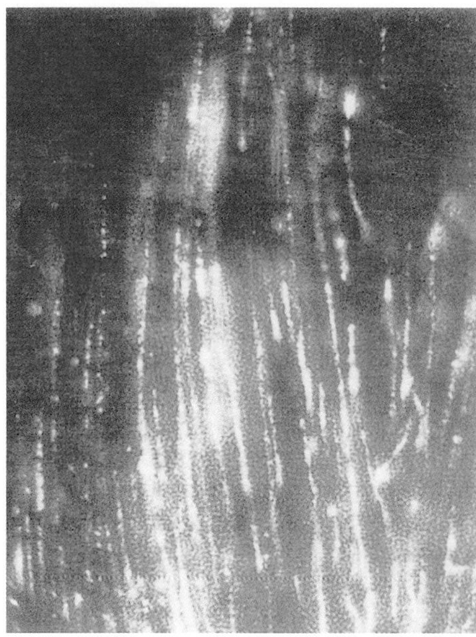

Fig. 23.9 Immunofluorescence micrograph of inner dentine close to the pulp horn stained with a labelled antibody for synaptotagmin, a protein characteristic of synapses. Its presence (white staining) and distribution in a pattern similar to nerves suggest that intradentinal nerves may be releasing a transmitter (immunohistochemistry; ×400). Courtesy T Norlin, M Hilliges, L Brodin and the editor of *Archives of Oral Biology*.

and synaptotagmin) have been detected within dentinal tubules in regions where axons enter dentinal tubules (Fig. 23.9). It is thus possible that, in some areas at least, efferent nerve activity may have an effect on matrix secretion. The effect would probably be on secretion rather than synthesis, as the synaptic proteins are absent from around the odontoblast cell body.

Mineralisation of dentine

Dentine mineralisation is a complex and controversial subject. Of the five mineralised tissues (bone, calcified cartilage, cementum, dentine and enamel), the process in enamel is unique, involving a protein matrix not found elsewhere and a two-step accumulation of mineral. In the remaining collagen-containing tissues, the process is similar but with sufficient diversity to make the structure and properties of the tissues different. The questions that are posed about mineralisation in general, and mineralisation in dentine in particular, include:

1) What initiates mineralisation? The first layers of dentine matrix are unmineralised, but when it reaches a certain width, mineralisation begins and progresses at the same rate as matrix formation.
2) Where do the ions that constitute the mineral (i.e., Ca, PO_4, carbonate, hydroxide) come from? Are they transported by odontoblasts or present in the extracellular fluid?
3) What controls the rate of mineralisation?
4) Are the dentine crystals initially deposited at their more or less final size or do they grow?
5) Are the crystals deposited in the extracellular fluid or on the fibrillar collagen of the matrix?
6) Is mineralisation merely the addition of crystals to the organic matrix, or does the matrix undergo changes during the deposition of mineral?
7) Can variations in the mineralisation process explain some of the structural features of dentine such as mantle dentine, interglobular dentine, incremental lines and peritubular dentine?
8) Does the mineralisation of secondary and tertiary dentine differ from that of primary dentine?
9) How does intrapulpal mineralisation (pulp stones) occur?
10) Does the remineralisation of dentine following exposure to acids or dental caries follow the same process as the original mineralisation of the tissue?
11) Are defects in mineralisation a component of dentine dysplasias?

Although several hypotheses have been put forward to explain dentine mineralisation and several factors may contribute to the overall process, the key element in initiating and controlling mineralisation is clearly the odontoblast. It produces the matrix that becomes mineralised. It controls the transport and release of calcium ions. It determines the presence and distribution of the matrix components that can initiate and modulate the process. Mineralisation only occurs when odontoblasts are present.

The data from which one can attempt to develop a coherent account of dentine mineralisation have been accumulated from a variety of sources: histological and histochemical studies, biochemical analyses of the tissue at various stages and *in vitro* studies either of odontoblast-like cells or pulpal tissue maintained in culture. Molecular biological (genetic expression) data directly related to mineralisation are scarce, although, as mineralisation is so closely linked to matrix formation, the body of work available from this is highly relevant. In any experimental study the data generated are obviously related to the techniques used, and no single approach can provide a complete description of a complex process. Some data from bone studies have been extrapolated to dentine.

Mineralisation of circumpulpal dentine

Odontoblasts actively transport calcium ions to the mineralisation site (Fig. 23.10). Although the precise intracellular mechanisms are not completely understood, serum calcium is taken up by the odontoblast and accumulates in the distal body and process, much of it bound to organelles rather than in the cytosol (intracellular fluid). High concentrations of calcium ions are toxic to cells but the odontoblast seems to be protected against this. Although some calcium ions reach the dentine by an extracellular pathway, this is probably not the major route. The intracellular route (Fig. 23.11) of calcium transport actively controls the level in the mineralising area and maintains calcium ion concentrations that are not in equilibrium with body fluids.

Evidence that has accumulated over the past 20 years suggests that the calcium transported by the odontoblasts becomes a crystalline mineral in the dentine by deposition onto a template formed by type I collagen fibrils. It is largely under the control of the predominant noncollagenous protein in dentine, DPP.

DPP is highly anionic and thus able to bind calcium. Changes in conformation of the protein enable it to bind increasing numbers of calcium ions, allowing the formation and growth of a crystal. In high concentrations, DPP inhibits crystal formation when free in solution, so a prerequisite for it to induce mineral formation is for it to bind to some insoluble substrate (e.g., collagen) after which it is then inductive in minute quantities. Thus, by controlling the release and level of DPP, the odontoblast can control the initiation of mineralisation and the rate of deposition.

Mineral crystals first appear in the hole zone formed by the quarter-stacking of the collagen molecules. The collagen triple helices are stacked in parallel with overlapping regions and spaces between adjacent molecules. Ultrastructurally, the bulk of the dentine mineral is on the surface of the dentine collagen.

The evidence that DPP is involved in the initiation and growth of mineral includes its distribution. DPP is absent from nonmineralised predentine matrix and concentrated at the mineralisation front (Fig. 23.6). *In vitro*, it can be shown to bind calcium, induce hydroxyapatite nucleation

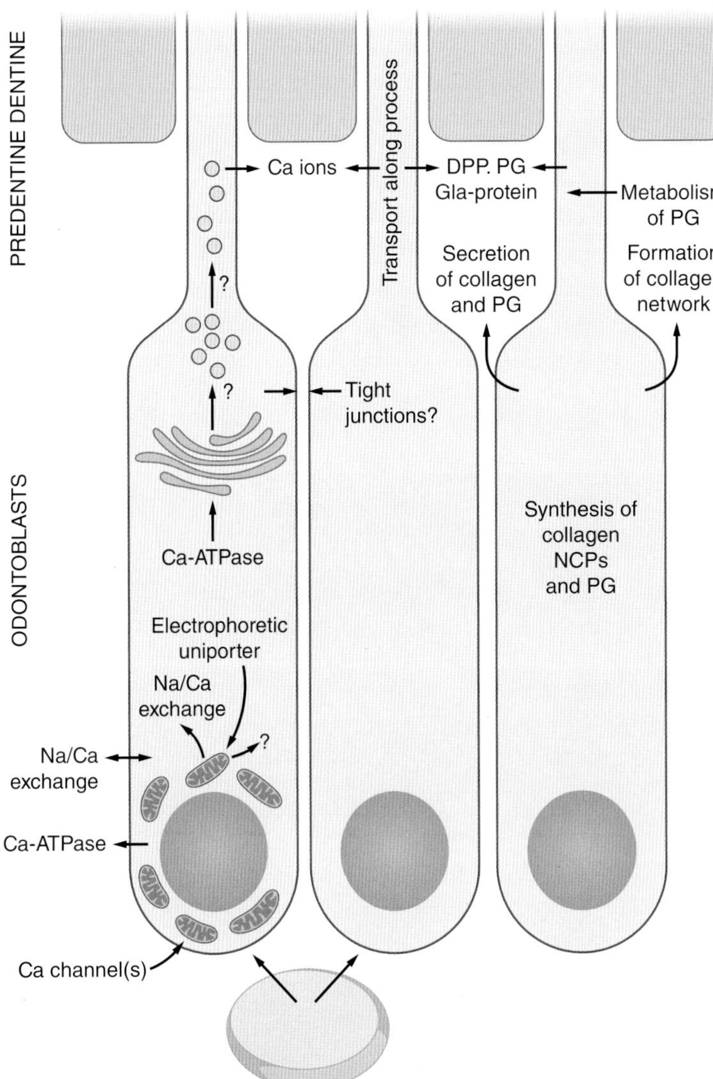

Fig. 23.10 Schematic diagram of fully differentiated active odontoblasts showing different calcium ion transport mechanisms (left side of figure) as well as putative transport routes for the dentine matrix macromolecules (right side of figure). Courtesy Dr. A Linde and the editor of *The International Journal of Developmental Biology*.

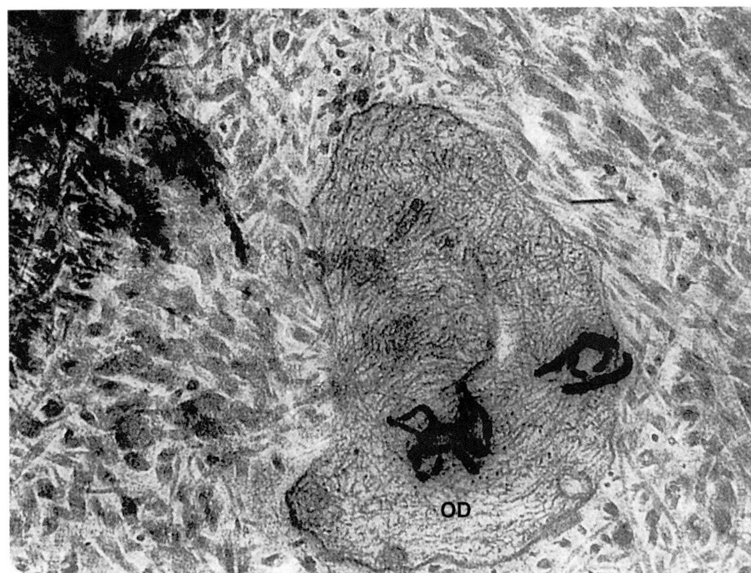

Fig. 23.11 TEM autoradiograph showing an odontoblast process (OD) near the predentine–dentine junction 30 minutes after intravenous infusion of ^{45}Ca. Note the silver grains representing this Ca over the cytoplasm of the process. The black zone at the top left corner represents mineralising dentine (×30,000). Courtesy Dr. R M Frank, Dr. N Nagai and the editor of *Cell and Tissue Research*.

and control crystal growth. It is absent from the dentine of patients with dentinogenesis imperfecta.

It has been suggested that DPP has the following roles in mineralisation:

1) Transport of ions to the mineralisation front
2) Aggregation of collagen fibres
3) Location of nucleation to specific regions of the collagen fibril surface
4) Stabilisation and orientation of the formed crystal

However, although it was once thought that DPP could transport Ca ions (because of its polyanionicity), there is no evidence to support the notion that DPP participates in ion transportation. Indeed, the capacity for Ca ion transport is much too low for the considerable amounts of Ca influx needed to build the crystals. There is also no support for the idea that DPP aids the aggregation of collagen fibres; however, small proteoglycans such as decorin may influence collagen fibrillogenesis. Furthermore, the orientation of crystals is more related to the collagen (the crystal c-axes being parallel to the collagen fibrils). There is some evidence to support the view that DPP is involved in the localisation of nucleation to specific regions of the collagen fibril, but perhaps the most important function of DPP is in the process of 'heterogeneous nucleation'.

Heterogeneous nucleation occurs where matrix components with a specific charge geometry that is similar to that of a crystal plane bind and organise the ions so that mineral induction takes place. The matrix components involved can not only induce crystal formation but may also regulate crystal type, formation rate, size and shape. Although the crystals are formed in the collagen, it is noncollagen proteins that regulate crystal formation. The polyanionic features of the noncollagenous proteins may be important, and circumstantially, the role of DPP is indicated by its absence within predentine. Experiments show that collagen alone does not induce mineralisation, whereas very small amounts of DPP can induce hydroxyapatite formation at physiological ionic concentrations. Furthermore, hydroxyapatite induction has been demonstrated on Sepharose beads that are coupled with DPP at physiological ionic concentrations (Fig. 23.12).

Although DPP gets the most attention as the 'master' of mineralisation, other proteins have mineralising characteristics *in vitro* but, given their low concentrations and more limited properties, it is difficult to say how much these other proteins may contribute to the mineralisation of dentine.

Osteonectin is a phosphorylated glycoprotein produced by the odontoblast and present in human dentine. *In vitro*, it can inhibit the growth of hydroxyapatite crystals and promote calcium and phosphate binding to collagen.

Osteopontin is a phosphorylated protein that was thought to be capable

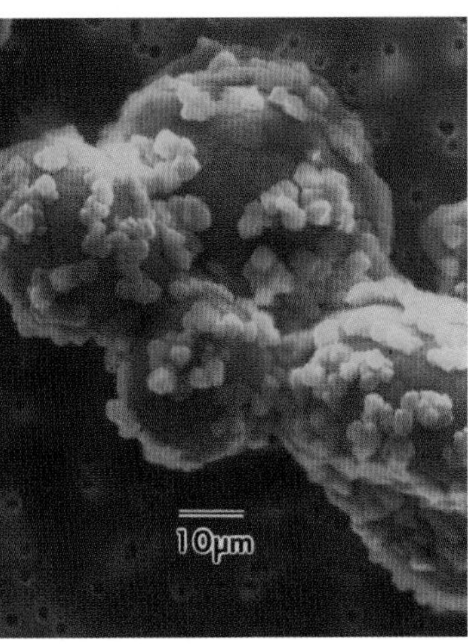

Fig. 23.12 Hydroxyapatite seeding on Sepharose beads coupled with dentine phosphoprotein (DPP) at physiological ionic concentrations. Courtesy Prof. A Linde.

of promoting mineral formation in dentine. However, experiments indicate that bone sialoprotein is a more likely candidate.

Bone sialoprotein is another phosphorylated glycoprotein found in early mineralising dentine and in peritubular dentine.

Dentine sialoprotein (DSP), the other noncollagenous protein limited mainly to dentine and the dental pulp, is a nonphosphorylated glycoprotein found predominantly in predentine and thus unlikely to be significantly involved in mineralisation.

Chondroitin sulphates 4 and 6 are present around the collagen fibrils (together with phospholipids) throughout dentine and predentine. Their properties can vary depending on whether they are in solution (as they are in the predentine) or adsorbed onto collagen (as in mineralising dentine) and/or the form they take as constituents of proteoglycans. In predentine, they may play a role in transport and diffusion and act as hydroxyapatite inhibitors, whereas in dentine they may promote hydroxyapatite initiation. The concentration of chondroitin sulphate decreases as mineralisation proceeds.

Other processes possibly involved in the initiation of mineralisation

When dentine mineralisation is initiated, two other processes have been implicated in addition to, or in place of, the DPP-mediated nucleation on collagen fibrils. Cell budding or cell fragmentation to form 'matrix vesicles' occurs in what will become mantle dentine. Membrane-bound organelles (30–200 nm) are formed, containing a variety of enzymes (including alkaline phosphatase) that lead to a concentration of phosphate ions within the vesicle. Mineral crystals develop within the vesicles (Fig. 23.13). As these are the only crystalline structures present very early in mantle dentine formation, they have been credited with an initiating role in mineralisation. Similar matrix vesicles have been implicated in the initial mineralisation of bone and calcified cartilage. Mineralising material can accumulate within cells, including the odontoblast process. As the odontoblast process retreats, cell debris may remain and form a nidus for mineralisation. The presence of matrix vesicles is limited to mantle dentine.

As matrix deposition and mineralisation continue, there will always be a zone of mineralisation discernible histologically (Fig. 23.14). The mineralising front often appears irregular: in some areas, mineralisation appears to progress linearly by apposition onto previously mineralised areas, while in others it seems to occur in spheres that eventually fuse (Figs. 23.15, 23.16). In yet other situations, mineralisation is a combination of the two

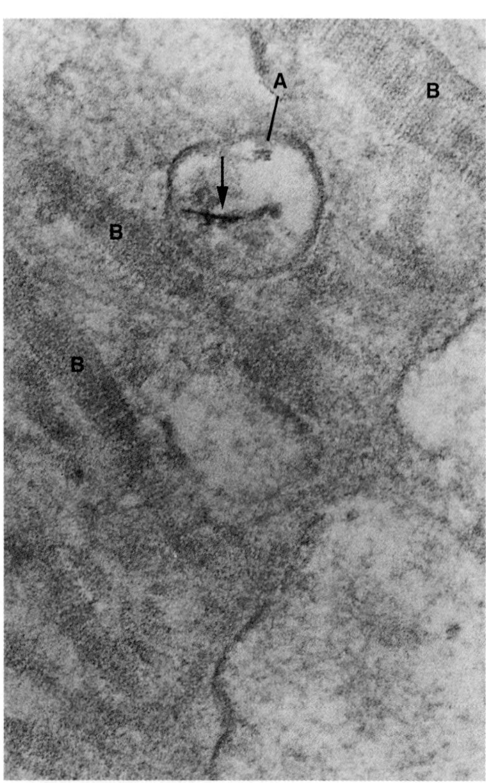

Fig. 23.13 TEM showing a matrix vesicle consisting of a membrane (A) around fluid containing a crystal (arrow) among recently deposited collagen fibrils (B) (×70,000). Courtesy Dr. P Glick.

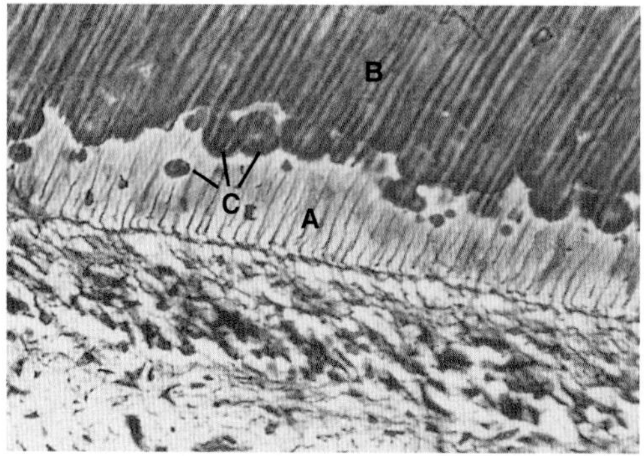

Fig. 23.14 Demineralised section showing the region of mineralising dentine. A = predentine; B = mineralised dentine; C = calcospherites (H & E; ×230).

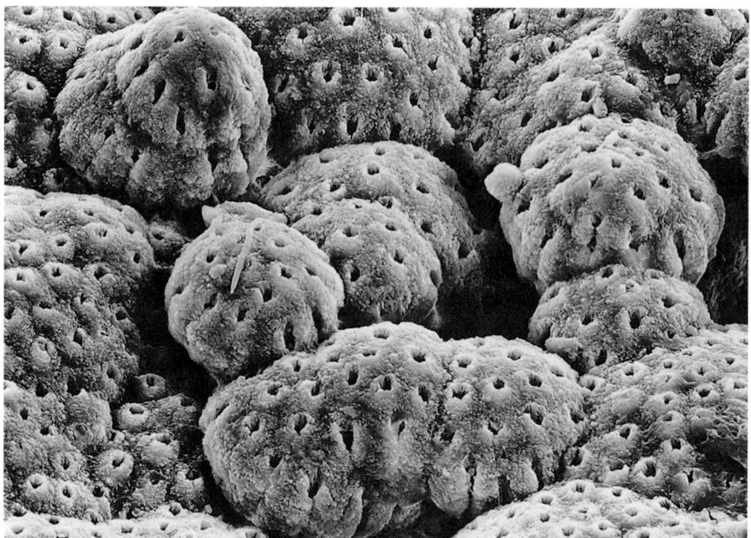

Fig. 23.15 SEM illustrating calcospherites at the mineralising front. In this preparation all the organic material (including the predentine) has been removed by hypochlorite to reveal the underlying mineralised dentine (×1,500). Courtesy Prof. M C Dean.

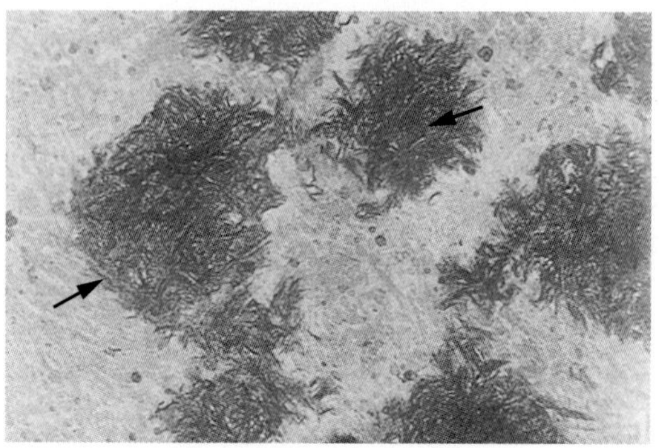

Fig. 23.16 Calcospherites (arrowed) at the mineralising front of dentine (TEM; ×1450).

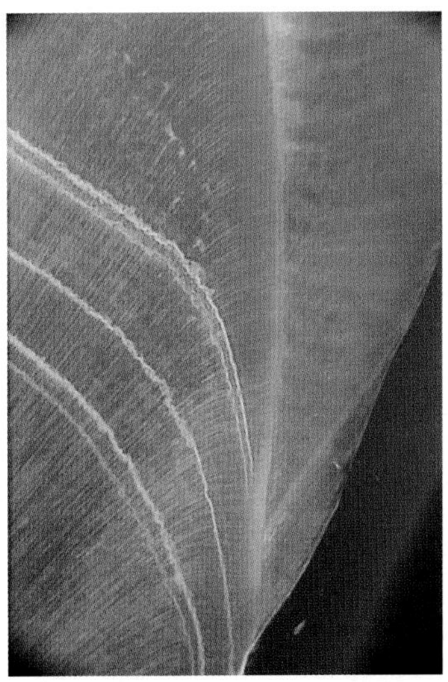

Fig. 23.17 Ground section of a tooth viewed with fluorescent light. The incremental nature of mineralisation is demonstrated in an individual who has been treated with tetracycline. Tetracycline binds to the mineral as it is deposited and is represented by the bright yellow lines, indicating that the patient has had multiple injections of the antibiotic. The irregularity of the line indicates both calcospheritic and linear patterns of mineralisation. This can lead to the discolouration of teeth, and therefore the use of tetracycline should be avoided during the period of tooth development. Tetracycline also fluoresces under ultraviolet light (ground section, fluorescent light; ×5). Courtesy Dr. B A W Brown.

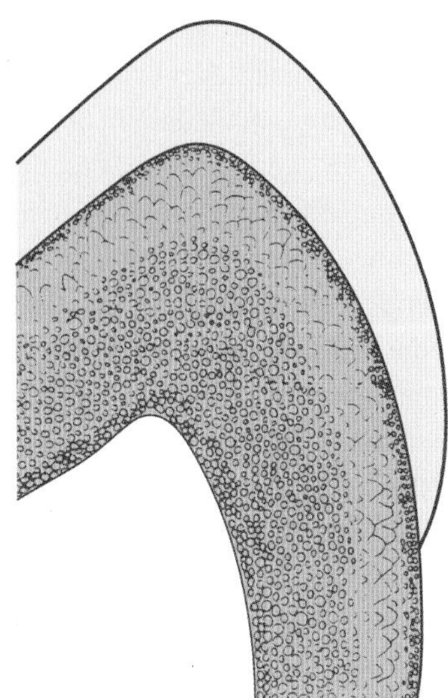

Fig. 23.19 The distribution of calcospherites in dentine. Most calcospherites are spherical. However, many have an arcade shape, such that the round apex of the arcade is directed towards the outer surface of the dentine and the opening is directed towards the pulp. The size varies considerably: the arcade variety tends to be larger than the spherical variety. The size and shape of the calcospherites seem to be governed by the rate of dentine formation and by the rate at which new calcospherites are initiated. There is a fairly consistent pattern of distribution within the tooth. In the mantle dentine of the crown, in the hyaline layer of the root and in the superficial circumpulpal dentine, the calcospherites are small, spherical and closely packed. In the middle region of the circumpulpal dentine, they are larger, more widely spaced and arcade-like in form (although the region tends to be free of calcospherites towards the root apex). The inner half to two-thirds of the circumpulpal dentine contain spherical calcospherites. Courtesy Dr. R P Shellis and the publishers of *The Companion to Dental Studies*, vol 2, Blackwell, Oxford.

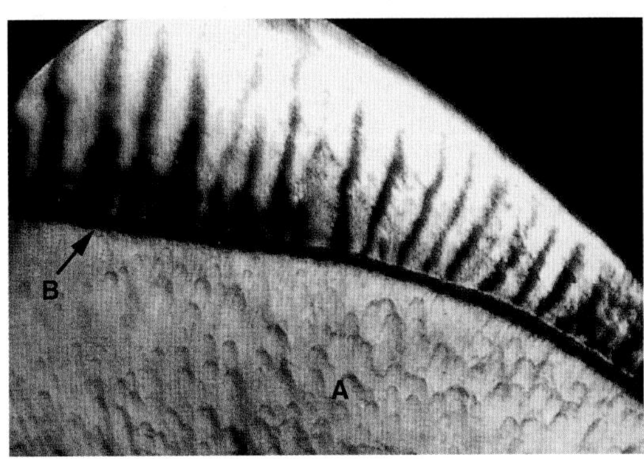

Fig. 23.18 Ground section of a tooth viewed in polarised light. Calcospherites (A) are distributed widely in circumpulpal dentine. The changes in crystal orientation at the boundary of the original crystallites differ and differentially block the polarised light. In single-phase light at this orientation, the mantle layer completely blocks transmission and thus appears black (B) (×25).

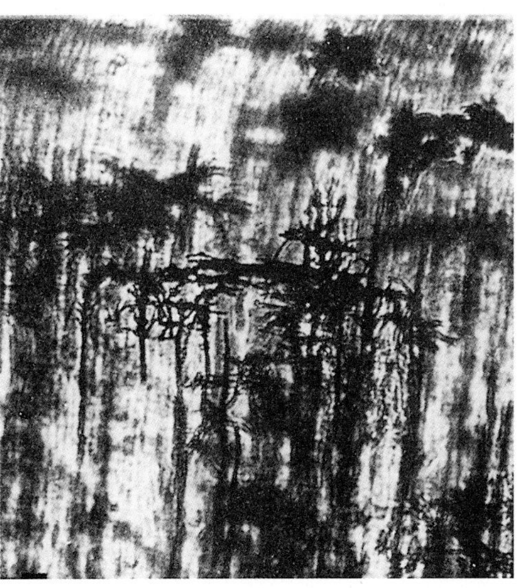

Fig. 23.20 Ground section of root showing evidence of looping and branching of dentine tubules in the granular layer of the root. In this preparation, the dentinal tubules have become filled with a silver stain and the tissue has been examined in a thicker-than-normal section. While this obscures much fine detail by superimposition, it does allow some insight into the three-dimensional arrangement. The peripheral terminations of several tubules may be seen, and a profuse branching in three dimensions can be distinguished. Above the tubules in focus are others below the plane of focus. Here, it may be seen how this arrangement could contribute to the appearance of the granular layer (silver stain; ×490).

(Fig. 23.14). These mineralisation patterns can be visualised when the mineralising front is highlighted by the antibiotic tetracycline (Fig. 23.17).

The pattern of calcospherite formation is common throughout dentine. It is possible that some form around matrix vesicles, especially in the first-formed mantle dentine, but the widespread nature of the calcospherites and the rarity of matrix vesicles suggest that such a pattern of accretion also occurs around centres of initial mineralisation that form on collagen fibrils. Failure of such calcospherites to fuse may result in the appearance of 'interglobular' dentine, often seen in peripheral dentine (see pages 176–177). In calcospherites, the crystallites are arranged in a radiating pattern, and despite complete mineralisation of the dentine, their outline can still be discerned using polarised light (Fig. 23.18). The size and shape of the calcospherites generally vary in different regions (Fig. 23.19).

Formation of root dentine

The basic process of root dentinogenesis does not differ fundamentally from coronal dentinogenesis, and neither is there any morphological difference between root and crown dentine. Such differences that occur are in the early stages so that the histological appearance of the peripheral dentine differs between crown and root. These are presumably owing to differing contributions in terms of control and content from the internal enamel epithelium of the crown (that will go on to form enamel) and the epithelial root sheath (that fragments after initiating radicular dentinogenesis and therefore does not differentiate further). Initial collagen deposition does not begin in the root immediately against the basal lamina of the epithelial cells of the root sheath. The space between the initial collagen and the epithelial cells becomes filled with an amorphous ground substance and a fine, fibrillar, noncollagenous matrix secreted by the root sheath comprising, in part, enamel-like proteins. These elements form a hyaline layer of approximately 10 μm. In the past, this has been described as a component of either dentine or cementum; it is discussed further on pages 442–444. The initial collagen fibres deposited in the root lie approximately parallel to the cementum–dentine junction. This contrasts with the mantle dentine in the crown, where the collagen fibres are deposited perpendicular to the enamel–dentine junction. Radicular odontoblasts differ slightly from those in the crown, developing several fine branches that loop in umbrella fashion (Fig. 23.20). This gives rise to the appearance of the granular layer (of Tomes), although this may be partly associated with the many small, unmineralised interglobular areas. The loss of continuity of the epithelial cells as the root sheath breaks down results in larger numbers of interglobular areas and, possibly, also in the incorporation of some epithelial remnants in the peripheral dentine. Radicular dentine forms at a slightly slower rate than coronal dentine. Its pattern of mineralisation is similar, although its initial calcospherites are smaller and its interglobular areas more numerous. In general, root mineralisation proceeds as a continuation of that in the crown, although in multirooted teeth separate isolated areas of mineralisation may occur. Unusually, there is evidence that the first-formed root dentine undergoes delayed mineralisation compared with the root dentine formed a little later; this may be related to its bonding with the cementum (see page 443).

Peritubular (intratubular) dentine

Peritubular dentine (see pages 169–170) consists of small crystals in an amorphous (nonfibrillar) matrix consisting of glycoproteins, proteoglycans, lipids, osteonectin, osteocalcin and bone sialoprotein. There is structural continuity between peritubular and intertubular dentine despite differences in composition.

The composition of the peritubular dentine suggests that it is a product of the odontoblast and plasma proteins that have diffused along the cell membrane. Evidence that it is physiological rather than a result of degeneration or retreat of the odontoblast includes:

1) The presence of small tubules where once were lateral processes of the odontoblast
2) The occasional finding of odontoblast processes surrounded by peritubular dentine
3) The occurrence in two species, the elephant and opossum, of peritubular dentine formation preceding intertubular dentine formation (Fig. 23.21)

Although much is known about the composition of peritubular dentine and a reasonable description of its origin has been established, little is known about either the signal that initiates the onset of tubular occlusion or what controls its rate of deposition. It would seem likely that age is the principal factor. The degree of tubular occlusion (as measured by the presence of translucent dentine, particularly in the root) can be used to determine the age of teeth and is applied forensically. Peritubular dentine formation does not seem to be related to outside stimuli, as it is found in unerupted teeth. The rate of tubular occlusion by peritubular dentine formation beneath dental caries is little different from that in intact teeth. Tubules directly beneath caries can become occluded, but this is thought to be related to the reprecipitation of mineral during the demineralisation process that characterises dental caries (Fig. 23.22). In older teeth, peritubular dentine formation is usually most pronounced near the root apices, remote from areas of attrition or caries. Until more detail is known about the switching of odontoblast production from intertubular to peritubular, it is best attributed to a preprogrammed genetic trigger.

Secondary dentine

As noted earlier in this chapter, the original odontoblasts form secondary dentine that, like peritubular dentine, seems to be a preprogrammed age change rather than a response to external activity. Part of this may be attributed to apoptosis (Fig. 23.23). As the pulp volume decreases with continuing dentine deposition, odontoblasts die. Over a 4-year period, the

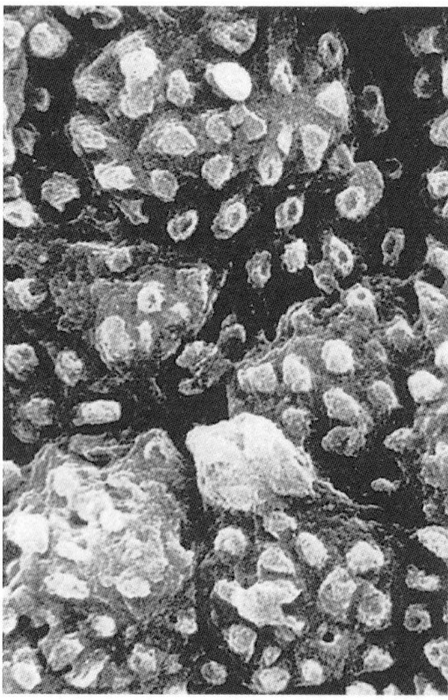

Fig. 23.21 SEM of an anorganic preparation of the surface of mineralising dentine in the opossum. Projecting localised white zones of peritubular dentine are visible, which are forming (in this species) before the adjacent intertubular dentine (×1,000). Courtesy N Azevedo and M Goldberg and the editor of *Journal de Biologie Buccale*.

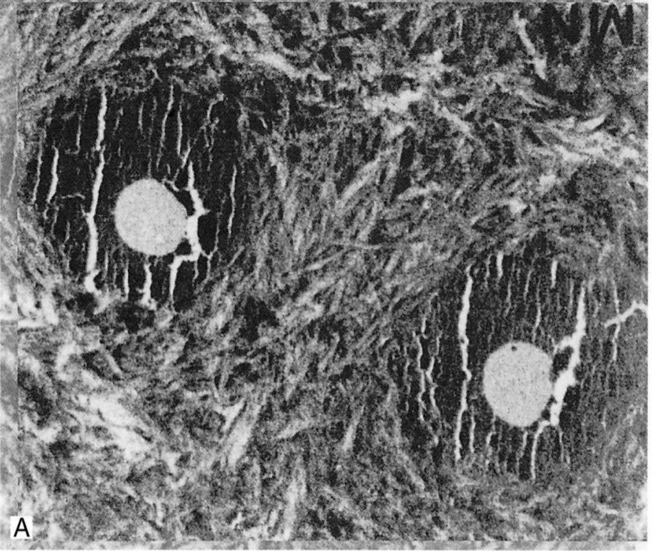

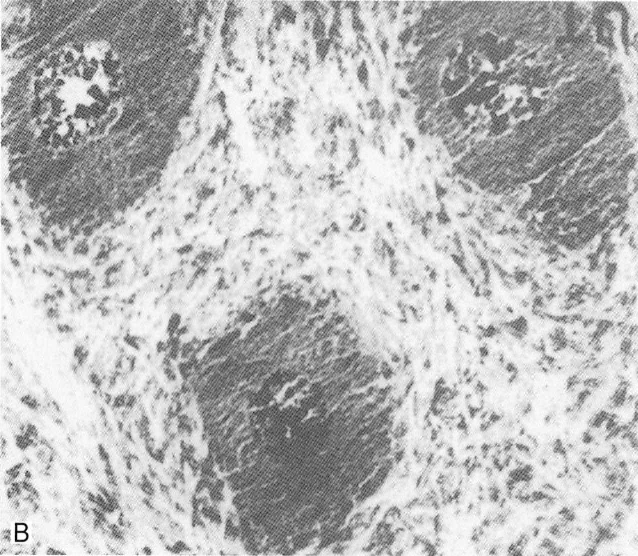

Fig. 23.22 Peritubular dentine (A) and sclerotic dentine (B). In sclerotic dentine, a second form of crystal formation, whitlockite, can fill in the tubules within, but distinct from, the peritubular dentine (TEM; ×10,000). Courtesy Dr. T Fusayama and the editor of *Journal de Biologie Buccale*.

odontoblast population may be reduced by 50%. This dramatic reduction in numbers also presumably leads to the change in direction of the tubules, establishing a contour line (see page 180).

Experimental denervation results in increased secondary dentine formation (Fig. 23.24). This may be mediated by changes in blood flow, although a direct trophic effect is possible. It is not known whether the innervation has an influence physiologically on the formation of either primary or secondary dentine.

Tertiary dentine formation in response to injury

The nature and severity of stimuli that reach the dental pulp vary over a considerable range. Dental caries will induce inflammation and may lead to necrosis. Protecting the pulp and encouraging it to recover after caries has been removed is a principal aim of restorative dentistry. Tertiary dentine is the tissue that is laid down in response to a stimulus of any kind. It is a response rather than an age change. Tertiary dentine takes one of two forms depending on the severity of the stimulus. If the stimulus is mild and the original odontoblasts remain alive, they will lay down a tubular form of tertiary dentine, *reactionary dentine*. If the stimulus is more severe and sufficient to kill the original odontoblasts, new odontoblasts will differentiate from pulpal stem cells and lay down another form of tertiary dentine, *reparative dentine*, which is atubular and bonelike (see pages 181–183).

One important difference between the activity of these new odontoblasts and those involved in primary and secondary dentine formation is that the new cells do not form dentine phosphophorin. This molecule, apparently so important to the production of primary dentine, seems to have no role in the making of tertiary dentine. The effect of signalling molecules, especially TGF-β and BMPs, may be important in tertiary dentine formation. One hypothesis suggests that members of the TGF-β family present in dentine and predentine may be released by acids produced during the progress of dental caries and diffuse through the dentine to stimulate activity in the original odontoblasts or induce the differentiation of new odontoblasts from pulpal stem cells. The difference in response could be related to differences in the nature, amount and direction of the signalling molecules.

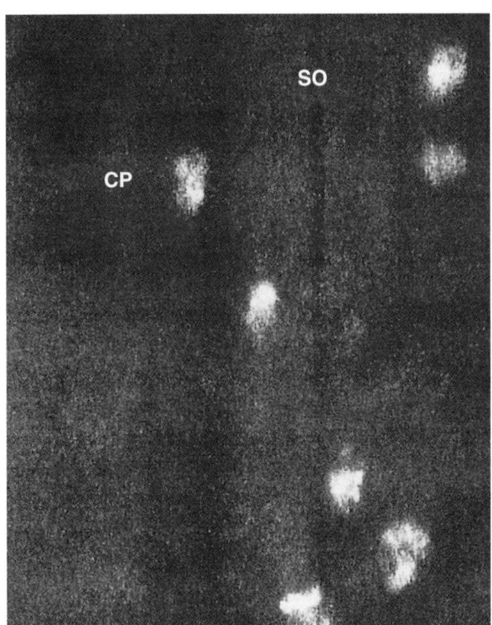

Fig. 23.23 Confocal microscope image showing apoptotic (dying) cells in the subodontoblastic region (SO) of the coronal pulp (CP). The cells have been fluorescently labelled (white) with a stain unique for dying cells (×60). Courtesy J-C Franquin and the editor of *The European Journal of Oral Science*.

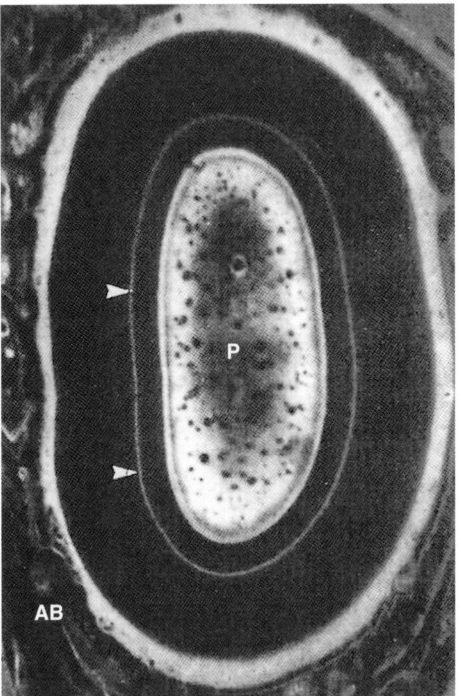

Fig. 23.24 Demineralised transverse section of a cat canine 30 days after denervation viewed with a fluorescence microscope. The animal was injected with tetracycline at the time of denervation. The arrowed line shows the dentine that has incorporated the tetracycline. Regular secondary dentine has formed after this point at a rate faster than in nondenervated teeth. The increase in rate is transient and, by 180 days postdenervation, the amount of secondary dentine deposited in control and operated teeth is the same. AB = alveolar bone; P = dental pulp (×10). Courtesy L Olgart and the editor of *The European Journal of Oral Sciences*.

Clinical considerations

Dentinogenesis imperfecta

Serious systemic disease occurring during the period of tooth development can result in the disturbance of both matrix formation and its mineralisation, which would usually be reflected in both the dentine and the enamel that were forming at the time. There are two groups of inherited defects that are limited to dentine: dentinogenesis imperfecta types I, II (Figs. 23.25, 23.26) and III and dentine dysplasia types I and II. Both dysplasias result in incomplete obliteration of the pulp chamber with histologically abnormal root dentine (dentine dysplasia type I has irregular, sparse tubules; type II has aberrantly oriented tubules). Type I but not type II causes stunted roots. Both forms of dentinogenesis imperfecta result in similar changes, but in addition the morphology of the tooth crown is bulbous. The types are distinguished by type I occurring as part of a more widespread connective tissue disease: osteogenesis imperfecta. In all these disorders the odontoblasts seem to be incompletely developed, and it is possible that the production of DPP in dentine is defective. It is known that dentinogenesis imperfecta types II and III and dentine dysplasia type II are caused by mutations in the DSPP gene, whereas dentinogenesis imperfecta type I, in

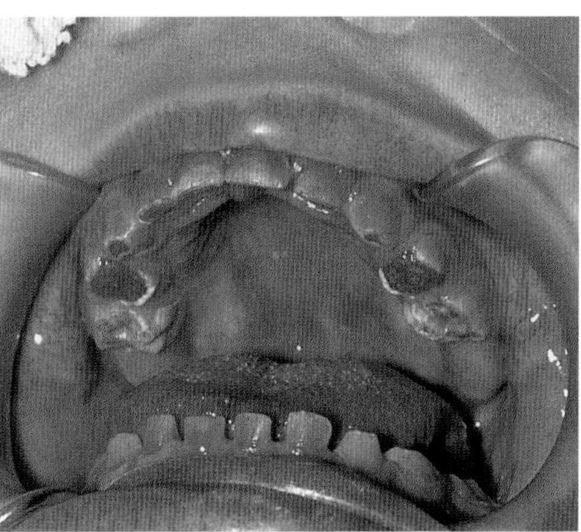

Fig. 23.25 A patient with dentinogenesis imperfecta. The teeth are malformed and are dark because of the absence of pulp chambers and the consequent loss of translucency. The enamel is normal but flakes off, as it is only weakly attached to the dentine. In this example the enamel from the first molars has been lost. Courtesy M Ignelzi.

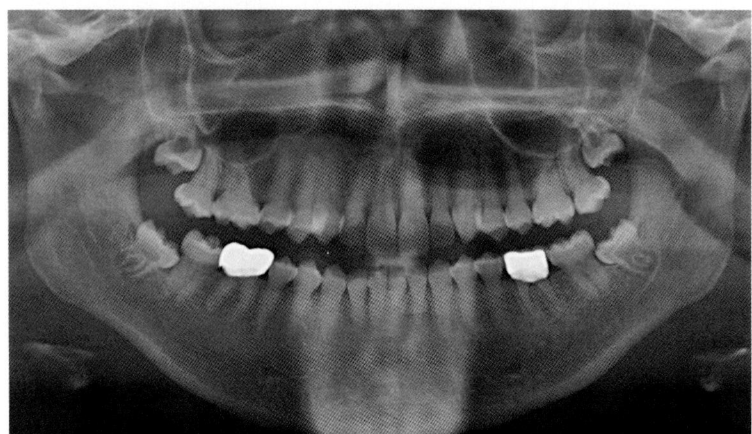

Fig. 23.26 Orthopantomogram of the teeth from a patient with dentinogenesis imperfecta. There are no pulp chambers or root canals in the teeth. Courtesy Dr. J Makdissi.

common with osteogenesis imperfecta, results from mutation in collagen type I genes.

Stem cells, regenerative dentinogenesis and tissue engineering

Aspects of tertiary dentine formation have been considered in Chapter 9 and stem cells in Chapter 10, 21 and 28.

Stem cell research suggests that DSP specifically is associated with the synthesis of dentine by dental pulp stem cells that have the properties of clonogenicity, self-renewal and plasticity. Indeed, dental pulp stem cells can synthesise *in vivo* on the surface of human dentine, a tissue that is like reparative dentine. Studies also suggest that although osteogenesis and dentinogenesis have many features in common, distinct regulatory mechanisms pertain for the activities of bone marrow stromal stem cells and dental pulp stem cells. Regeneration of dentine and pulpal tissues following damage by dental caries is a major goal arising from understanding the biology of dental pulp stem cells. It has been shown that, using 'scaffold-based tissue engineering' (e.g., gelatine scaffolds), it may be possible to replace damaged pulpodentinal tissues and restore function. Furthermore, investigations indicate that complete regeneration of the pulpodentinal tissues is possible with a high-stiffness, three-dimensional, nanofibrous gelatine scaffold containing dental pulp stem cells. It should be noted that dental pulp stem cells are localised in the perivascular regions of the dental pulp and express the specific membrane receptors TLR-2 and TLR-4. Other scaffolds, some synthetic that have the customisation of mechanical properties (including pore sizes), are being manufactured, and the inclusion of a variety of growth factors (e.g., FGF and vascular endothelial growth factor [VEGF]) is also being investigated (see Chapter 28).

Internal resorption of dentine

This is considered on page 188. However, resorption of dentine by cells of the dental pulp is usually not physiological, except during the shedding of deciduous teeth. This is because dentine is not a tissue that is involved in the body's Ca or PO_4 homeostasis.

Further readings for this chapter can be found in the accompanying eBook. Explore online Self-assessment quiz to test and reinforce your understanding of the material in your free ebook. Follow instructions in the Inside Front Cover to unlock your access.

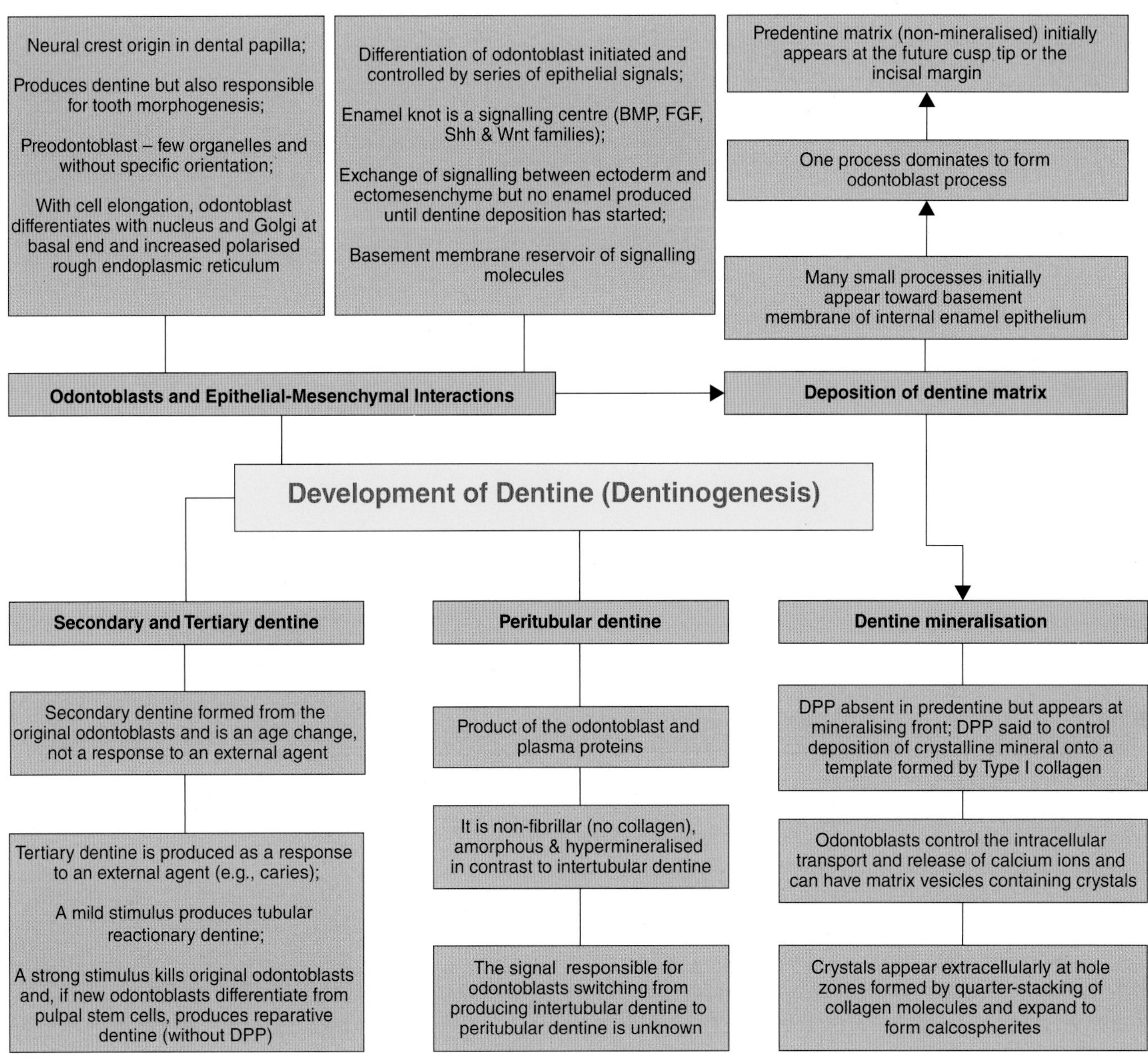

Mind Map 23.1 Development of dentine (dentinogenesis).

24

Development of the dental pulp

Early development of the dental pulp

Various aspects of the development of the dental pulp, including epithelial–mesenchymal interactions, odontoblast differentiation and ageing, are dealt with in Chapters 9, 10, and 21. At the bud stage of tooth germ development, a region of more densely packed mesenchymal cells becomes evident around the developing enamel organ (Fig. 24.1). All the cells that form the dental papilla are derived from the neural crest (ectomesenchyme) and have migrated from their position in the pharyngeal arches. Cells from other sources are not able to induce tooth formation (see Chapter 21). The first pharyngeal arch, the future mandible, is populated by neural crest cells originating near the caudal midbrain. The frontonasal process, giving rise initially to the maxillae, is colonised by neural crest cells originating near the forebrain. Neural crest cells are more densely packed than the surrounding mesenchyme, are separated by relatively little extracellular matrix and are rapidly dividing. This mass of cells expands around the tooth bud (see Fig. 21.6). Once the enamel organ at the bud stage invaginates to become the cap stage, the cells and matrix within the invagination are recognised as the dental papilla (Fig. 24.2). During growth of the tooth germ, although undifferentiated, the expansion of the dental papilla exerts a morphogenetic effect on the enamel organ (see pages 388–394). The mesenchymal cells surrounding the developing enamel organ externally form the dental follicle that will give rise to the periodontal ligament and supporting tissues of the tooth (see Chapter 25). As the enamel organ surrounding the dental papilla enlarges and enters the bell stage (Fig. 24.3), the cells within the dental papilla undergo cytodifferentiation into a peripheral layer of odontoblasts and a central mass of fibroblasts. This change is induced by signals originating in the internal enamel epithelium (see Chapter 23). Immature, dendritic antigen-presenting cells appear in, and around, the odontoblast layer at an early stage (Fig. 24.4). Once the odontoblasts have begun to lay down dentine, the dental papilla becomes, by convention, the dental pulp. The small, undifferentiated, ectomesenchymal cells of the dental papilla are packed closely together with little intercellular material relative to that in the mature tooth. They are stellate in shape with a relatively large nucleus and little cytoplasm. As the pulp develops, the cytoplasmic component of these central cells expands and synthetic organelles appear. The material

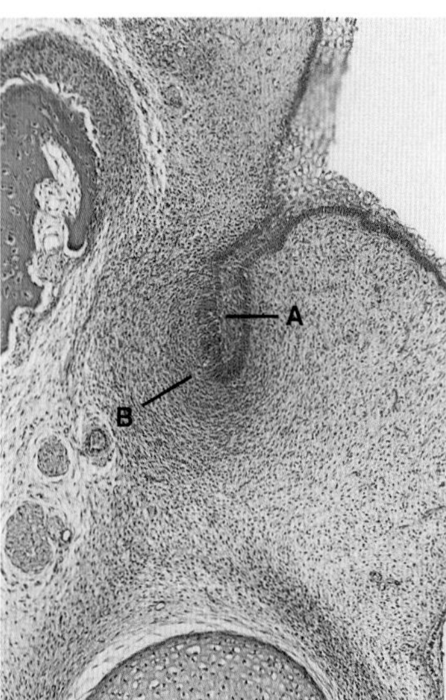

Fig. 24.1 An early developing enamel organ (A), with a condensation of mesenchymal cells (B) around it (Masson's trichrome stain; ×80).

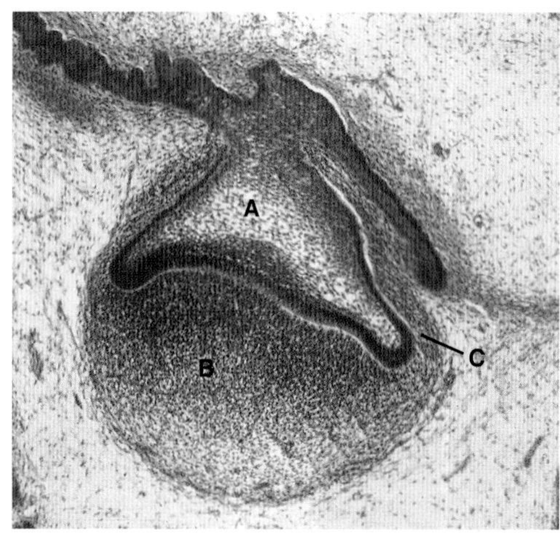

Fig. 24.2 An enamel organ at the cap stage of development (A) surrounding the mesenchymal cells of the dental papilla (B). The tooth germ is surrounded by the developing dental follicle (C) (H & E; ×80). Courtesy Prof. M M Smith.

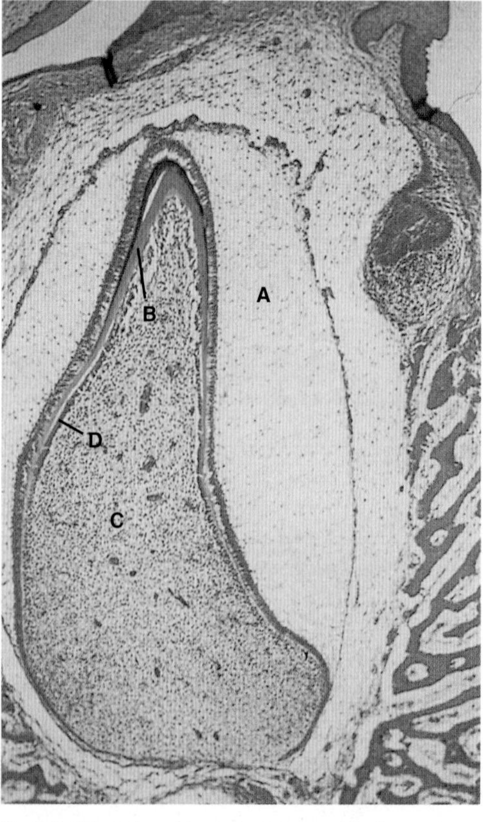

Fig. 24.3 A developing tooth at the late bell stage of development (appositional phase). A = enamel organ; B = developing dentine; C = dental papilla; D = odontoblast layer (Masson's trichrome; ×55).

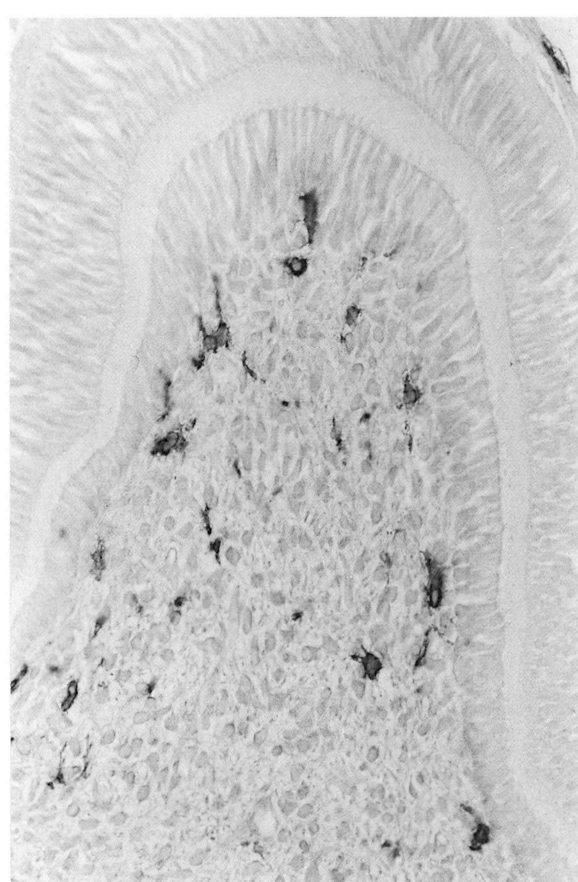

Fig. 24.4 Dark-staining dendritic cells in the periphery of the developing pulp (rat molar, postnatal day 1, immunohistochemistry; ×300). Courtesy Dr E Tsuruga, Dr Y Sakahura, Dr T Yajima, Dr N Shide and the editor of *Histochemistry and Cell Biology*.

the organelles produce is released into the extracellular space and forms fine collagen fibres that are embedded in an amorphous ground substance. Coarse fibre bundles appear only at about the time that the tooth reaches maturity. In the early stages of pulpal development, the ground substance has a high glycosaminoglycan content relative to that of the mature tooth. The level of glycosaminoglycans increases until the time of eruption and then decreases. Chondroitin sulphates are the main glycosaminoglycans present during pulp development, with only a minor quantity of hyaluronan. This composition is reversed in the mature pulp. Not all cells undergo differentiation, with a proportion remaining as undifferentiated mesenchymal cells that retain the potential to differentiate in later life.

The dental pulp at dentinogenesis

Dentinogenesis then progresses by the processes described in Chapter 23. As differentiation continues and as the enamel organ extends by means of Hertwig's epithelial root sheath to determine the final morphology of the space (pulp chamber and root canals), the final shape of the pulp is determined. The actions and interactions of the dental follicle (outside the epithelial root sheath), the epithelial root sheath and the dental papilla result in the formation of cementum (described in Chapter 25) on the surface of the developing root dentine. Once the full length of the root is established, the developmental stage of the dental pulp can be considered complete. However, dentine deposition will continue throughout life. A cell-rich zone develops beneath the odontoblast layer at the time of eruption. It arises by the migration of more central cells rather than by local cell division. A cell-free zone may be evident in the crown of the tooth at the time of eruption, although some believe this may be a fixation artefact.

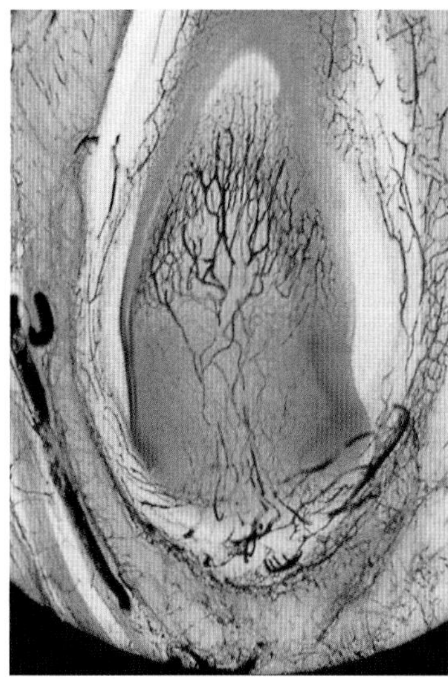

Fig. 24.5 The vascular pattern within the dental papilla at the late bell stage of development. The vascular system has been perfused with Indian ink (H & E; ×40). Courtesy Dr. D Adams.

The dental pulp retains the potential to differentiate new odontoblasts from stem cells and deposit reparative forms of dentine (see pages 492–493) in response to dental caries.

Stem cells

Throughout its life, the dental pulp retains a stem cell population, even in deciduous teeth that are about to be exfoliated. In addition to their capacity to differentiate into adipocytes, odontoblasts, osteoblasts, chondrocytes and myoblast cells, they possess the ability to induce angiogenesis and vasculogenesis during tissue repair and periodontal regeneration. They may also have a wider potential with respect to their ability to differentiate into nerve cells (see also pages 488–489).

Neurovascular development

Blood supply

Vascularisation of the developing pulp starts during the early bell stage with small branches from the principal vascular trunks of the jaws entering the base of the papilla. Of these small pioneer vessels, a few become the principal pulpal vessels. They enlarge and run through the pulp towards the cuspal regions. Here, the vessels give off numerous small branches, which form a bed of venules, arterioles and capillaries in the subodontoblast and odontoblast layers (Fig. 24.5). The vascularity of the odontoblast layer increases as dentine is progressively laid down, probably as the result of the odontoblasts migrating inwards through the vascular bed (Fig. 24.6). Eventually, some capillaries are found immediately next to the predentine surface, occasionally looping into the developing dentine (Fig. 24.7). The time and pattern of development of lymphatics in the pulp have not yet been established. The mature pulp contains macrophages, pericytes and lymphoid cells that probably enter the pulp with the blood vessels.

Nerve supply

Trigeminal nerve branches enter the mandibular and maxillary processes well before the first appearance of tooth primordia and project to future sites of tooth formation. The dental follicle becomes innervated as soon as it appears during the cap stage of tooth development. However, axons do

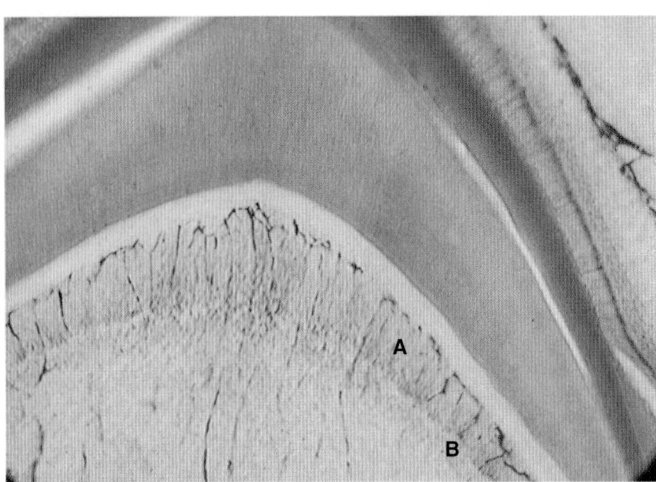

Fig. 24.6 The vascular plexuses beneath the developing cusp. A = odontoblast layer; B = subodontoblastic plexus. The vascular system has been perfused with Indian ink (H & E; ×100). Courtesy Dr. D Adams.

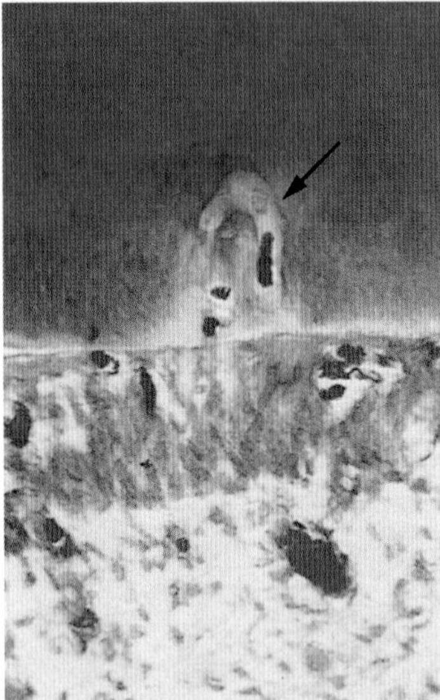

Fig. 24.7 A capillary looping (arrow) into developing dentine (Masson's trichrome; ×20).

not enter the dental pulp until dentinogenesis and amelogenesis are well under way. Thus, the innervation of the pulp is delayed in comparison to neighbouring tissues. This seems to be due to the balance between conflicting factors in the dental pulp environment, namely those that inhibit nerve growth and those that attract it. Important inhibitory neurite growth factors include the semaphorins, while neuro-attractive factors include

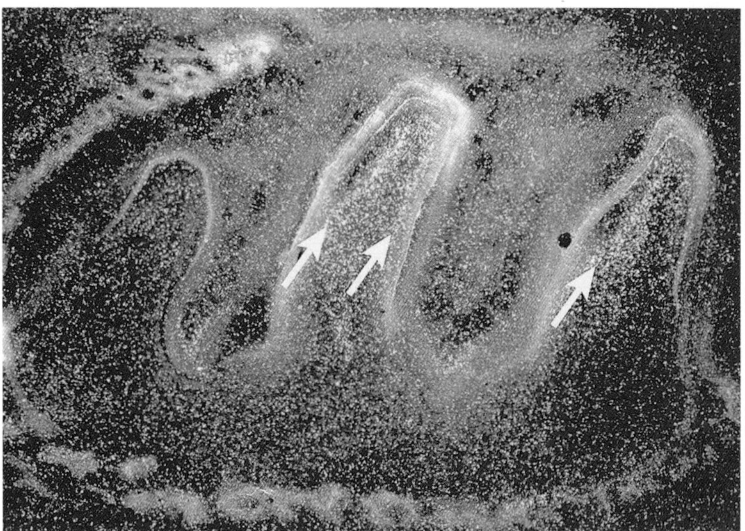

Fig. 24.8 Labelled nerve growth factor (NGF) in the periphery of the developing dental pulp (rat molars 2 days postnatal). Messenger RNA for NGF has been radioactively labelled by *in situ* hybridisation and viewed under dark field illumination. Under these conditions mineralised tissue appears as a bright solid (arrows) and NGF mRNA as bright granules (×20). Courtesy Dr. C Nosrat and the editor of the *European Journal of Oral Science*.

nerve growth factor, neurturin and artemin. In addition, local factors, such as laminin and reelins, promote neural growth.

Fig. 24.8 shows nerve growth factor being expressed in the periphery of the developing dental pulp in the odontoblast layer. However, these neurotrophins do not exert their effect in the early stages. The first fibres to enter the developing pulp become located close to the blood vessels. These nerves, although anatomically part of the sensory nervous system, play an important role via axon reflexes in controlling blood flow.

The sympathetic innervation follows later and is restricted largely to the radicular pulp as it supplies the smooth muscle of arterioles, whose presence is limited mainly to the radicular pulp. A large number of nerves enter the pulp before root formation, but the final pattern, including the formation of the subodontoblastic plexus (of Raschkow), is not established until root formation is complete. In the crown, particularly at the cusps, some sensory fibres insinuate themselves between the odontoblasts and enter dentinal tubules. This is an active process and not merely a trapping of these axons during progressive dentine deposition.

Further readings for this chapter can be found in the accompanying eBook. Explore online Self-assessment quiz to test and reinforce your understanding of the material in your free ebook. Follow instructions in the Inside Front Cover to unlock your access.

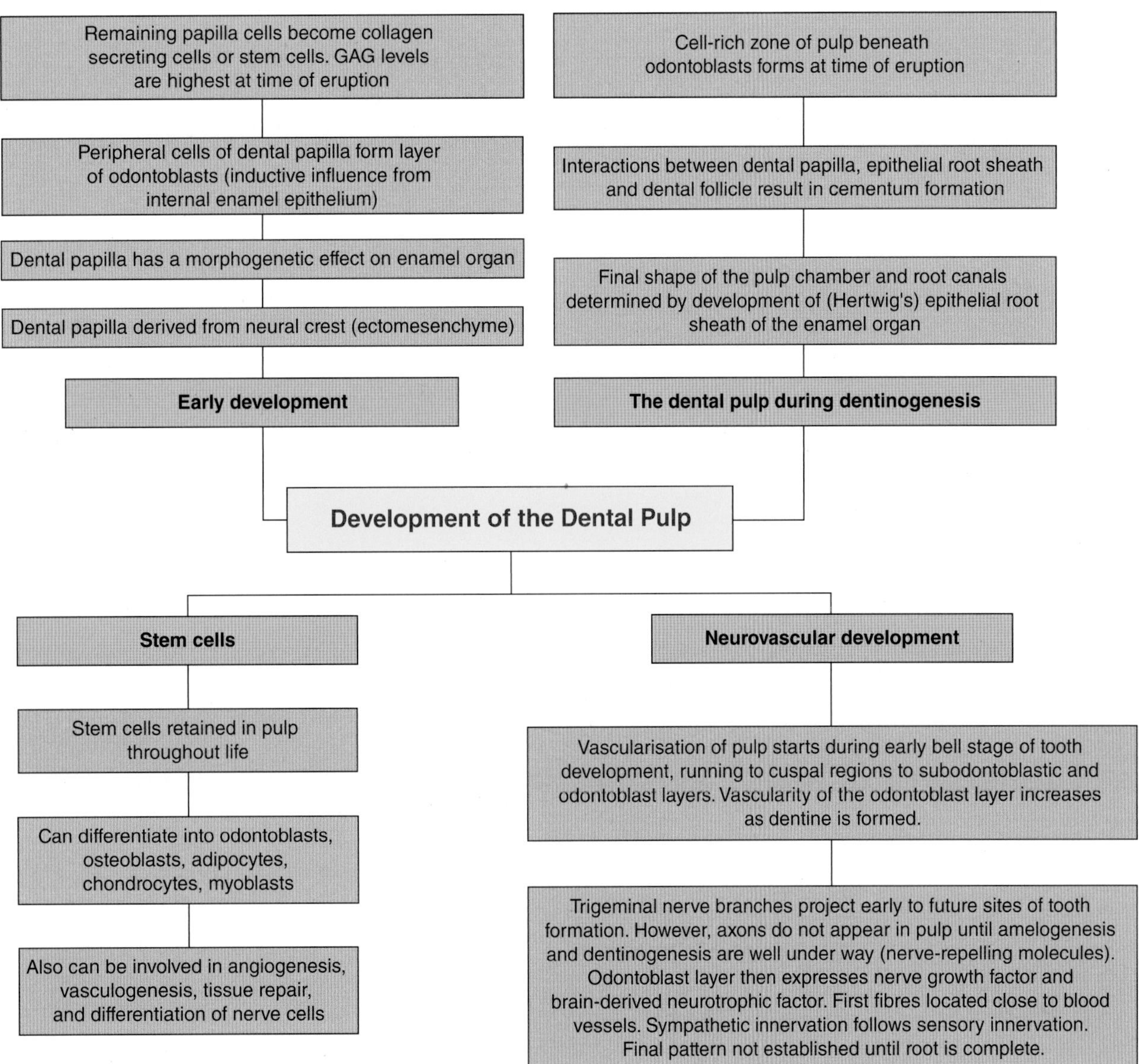

Remaining papilla cells become collagen secreting cells or stem cells. GAG levels are highest at time of eruption
Peripheral cells of dental papilla form layer of odontoblasts (inductive influence from internal enamel epithelium)
Dental papilla has a morphogenetic effect on enamel organ
Dental papilla derived from neural crest (ectomesenchyme)
Early development
Cell-rich zone of pulp beneath odontoblasts forms at time of eruption
Interactions between dental papilla, epithelial root sheath and dental follicle result in cementum formation
Final shape of the pulp chamber and root canals determined by development of (Hertwig's) epithelial root sheath of the enamel organ
The dental pulp during dentinogenesis
Development of the Dental Pulp
Stem cells
Stem cells retained in pulp throughout life
Can differentiate into odontoblasts, osteoblasts, adipocytes, chondrocytes, myoblasts
Also can be involved in angiogenesis, vasculogenesis, tissue repair, and differentiation of nerve cells
Neurovascular development
Vascularisation of pulp starts during early bell stage of tooth development, running to cuspal regions to subodontoblastic and odontoblast layers. Vascularity of the odontoblast layer increases as dentine is formed.
Trigeminal nerve branches project early to future sites of tooth formation. However, axons do not appear in pulp until amelogenesis and dentinogenesis are well under way (nerve-repelling molecules). Odontoblast layer then expresses nerve growth factor and brain-derived neurotrophic factor. First fibres located close to blood vessels. Sympathetic innervation follows sensory innervation. Final pattern not established until root is complete.

Mind Map 24.1 Development of the dental pulp.

25 Development of the root and periodontal ligament

Introduction

Root development proceeds some time after the crown has formed and involves interactions between three components:

1) The dental follicle
2) A structure derived from the cervical loop region of the enamel organ (see pages 436–439) called the epithelial root sheath (of Hertwig)
3) The dental papilla

The onset of root development coincides with the axial phase of tooth eruption.

Single and multirooted teeth are formed in the manner shown in Fig. 25.1. Soon after the crown has completed its formation, the external and internal enamel epithelia at the cervical loop of the enamel organ form a double-layered epithelial root sheath (see Fig. 25.6) that proliferates apically to map out the shape of the future root. The primary apical foramen at the growing end of the epithelial root sheath may subdivide into secondary apical foramina by the ingrowth of epithelial shelves from the margins of the root sheath (arrowed region in Fig. 25.1B and C) that subsequently fuse near the centre of the root. The number and location of these epithelial shelves correspond to the number and location of the definitive roots of the tooth and may be under the inductive control of the dental papilla. It has been suggested that the ingrowth of the epithelial shelves takes place along paths of low vascularity.

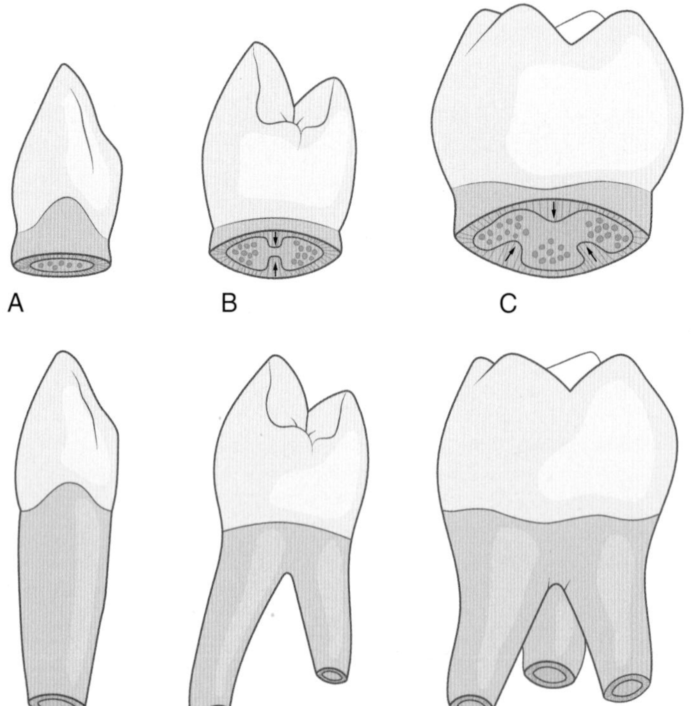

Fig. 25.1 The formation of a single-rooted tooth (A), a two-rooted tooth (B) and a three-rooted tooth (C). Small red circles indicate vascular concentrations.

When a deciduous tooth first erupts into the mouth, usually about one-half of the root is present (see Table 26.1). For permanent teeth, this figure is usually three-quarters of its final length (see Table 26.1). A wide, 'open' root apex is present in these situations, surrounded by a thin, regular knife edge of dentine (Fig. 25.2). It takes about 3 more years for root completion in a permanent tooth to occur and about 1½ years for root completion in a deciduous tooth. At this time, only a narrow pulp opening exists. The addition of root increments may result in the appearance of fine lines running transversely around the root.

Root extension rates

During root development, an average root extension rate is between 4 and 6 µm/day, but with a rise in rates to a brief peak of 6–10 µm/day about the middle of the root length. As this growth spurt does not coincide with an increase in eruption rates, this provides further evidence that root growth alone is not responsible for generating the eruptive force. That this growth spurt is a fundamental property of developing teeth independent of eruption is further supported by the observation that it can be seen in impacted teeth and teeth formed in ovarian cysts. Extension rates for permanent incisors (Fig. 25.3), canines (Fig. 25.4) and molars (Fig. 25.5) indicate that anterior teeth seem to extend slightly faster than molar root expansion rates, with permanent central incisors fastest and permanent third molars slowest.

Epithelial root sheath and tissue morphogenesis

During root development (Fig. 25.6), growth of the epithelial root sheath occurs to enclose the dental papilla, except for an opening at the base (the primary apical foramen). Beneath the dental papilla, the epithelial sheath usually appears angled to form the root diaphragm. Unlike the cervical loop region in the enamel organ of the crown, there is no stellate reticulum or stratum intermedium between the two epithelial layers of the root sheath. As the cervical loop region is the site of the stem cell niche (see page 383), its replacement by the epithelial root sheath may be related to the disappearance of Notch protein in the epithelium and growth factors (e.g., fibroblast growth factor [FGF]) in the adjacent mesenchyme. The localised retention of such factors may help explain the occasional presence of stellate reticulum and stratum intermedium in the root, giving rise to areas of enamel (enamel pearls) on the root surface (see Fig. 7.74). The dental follicle lies external to the root sheath and forms cementum, periodontal ligament and (probably) alveolar bone.

In the region of the root diaphragm, the epithelial root sheath is seen as a continuous sheet of tissue sandwiched between the undifferentiated mesenchyme of the dental papilla internally and the dental follicle externally (Figs. 25.7, 25.8) and separated from both by a basement membrane. Above the root diaphragm, towards the developing crown, the cells of the internal layer of the epithelial root sheath induce the peripheral cells of

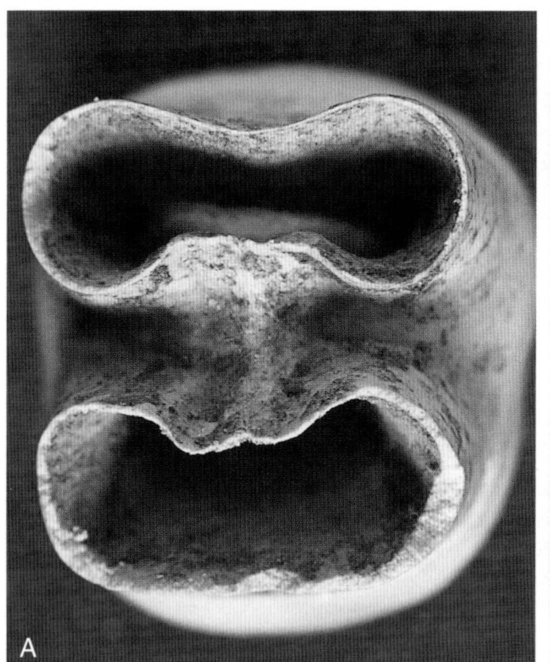

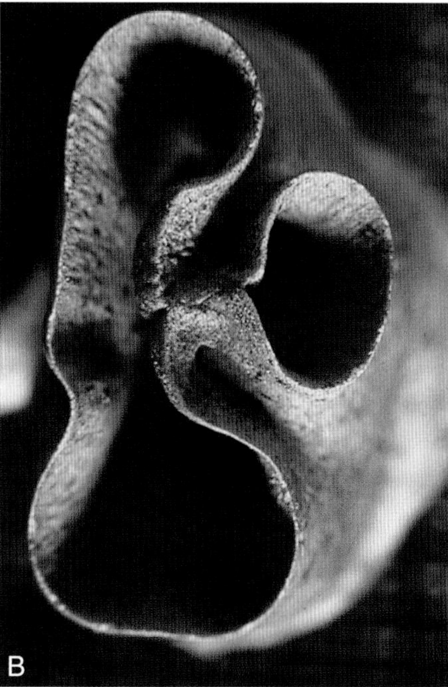

Fig. 25.2 Apices of developing roots. (A) Two-rooted tooth. (B) Three-rooted tooth.

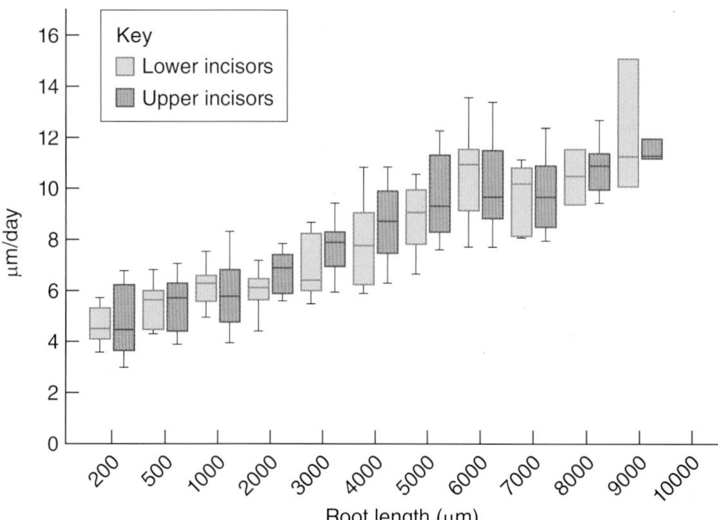

Fig. 25.3 Extension rates for permanent incisors estimated at root lengths of 200 μm, 500 μm and 1,000 μm from the mesiobuccal cervix and then at 1,000-μm intervals to 10,000 μm. From Dean, C.M., Vesey, P., 2007. Preliminary observations on increasing root length during the eruptive phase of tooth development in modern humans and great apes. *Journal of Human Evolution* 54, 258–271.

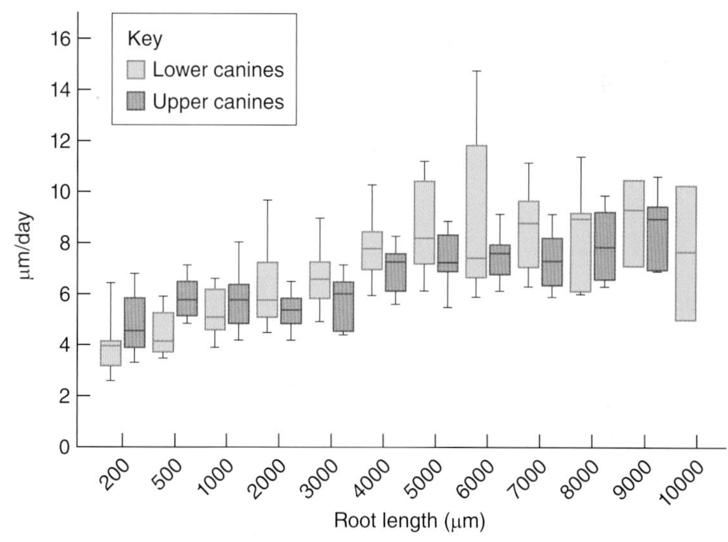

Fig. 25.4 Extension rates for permanent canines estimated at root lengths of 200 μm, 500 μm and 1,000 μm from the mesiobuccal cervix and then at 1,000-μm intervals to 10,000 μm. From Dean, C.M., Vesey, P., 2007. Preliminary observations on increasing root length during the eruptive phase of tooth development in modern humans and great apes. *Journal of Human Evolution* 54, 258–271.

the dental papilla to differentiate into odontoblasts. Following the onset of dentinogenesis in the root, the epithelial cells of the root sheath lose their continuity, becoming separated from the surface of the developing root dentine. The mesenchymal cells of the dental follicle adjacent to the root dentine now differentiate into cementoblast-like cells, and cementogenesis commences with the formation of acellular (primary) cementum. There is evidence, however, that epithelial cells of the sheath may also differentiate into the first formed cementoblast-like cells. The epithelial remnants are retained and subsequently form the epithelial rests seen in the periodontal ligament (see pages 243–245).

Fig. 25.8 shows the apical region of the developing root, periodontal ligament and alveolus. The tissues of the dental follicle in the developing root have been described as comprising three layers (see also Fig. 21.10). Adjacent to the epithelial root sheath is the inner investing layer of the dental follicle, which is thought to be derived from ectomesenchyme (neural crest). Adjacent to the developing alveolar bone is the outer layer of the dental follicle, which is separated from the inner layer by an intermediate layer. Unlike the tissues of the inner layer, the outer and intermediate layers are said to be mesodermal in origin; their cells contain few cytoplasmic organelles, and the extracellular compartment appears relatively featureless. Cells of the inner layer of the dental follicle differentiate into the cementoblasts that form an initial layer of cells on the surface of the root dentine. In primary (acellular) cementum, the collagen is of the extrinsic fibre type, being derived from the periodontal ligament and passing into the cementum roughly perpendicular to the surface (see page 446). The cementoblasts associated with acellular cementum therefore contribute little material towards the extracellular matrix of the tissue. Later, with the formation of cellular (secondary) cementum, the cementoblasts form a more distinctive layer of cuboidal cells that secrete collagen parallel to the surface, forming the matrix of the cementum (intrinsic fibre cementum).

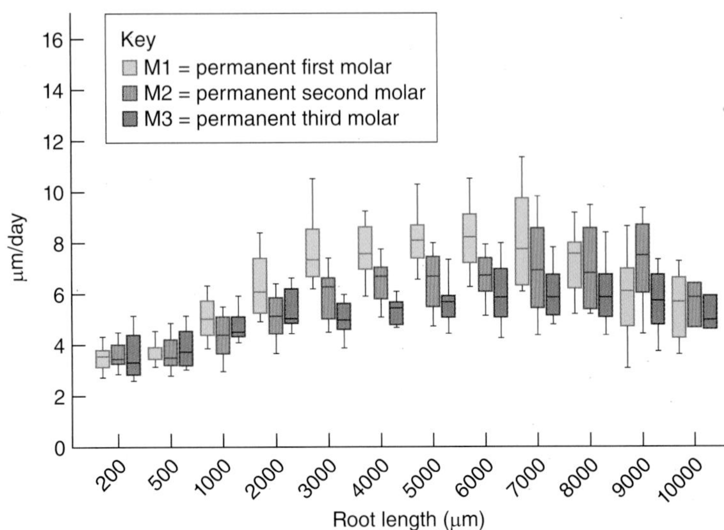

Fig. 25.5 Extension rates for permanent molars estimated at root lengths of 200 μm, 500 μm and 1,000 μm from the mesiobuccal cervix and then at 1,000-μm intervals to 10,000 μm. From Dean, C.M., Vesey, P., 2007. Preliminary observations on increasing root length during the eruptive phase of tooth development in modern humans and great apes. *Journal of Human Evolution* 54, 258–271.

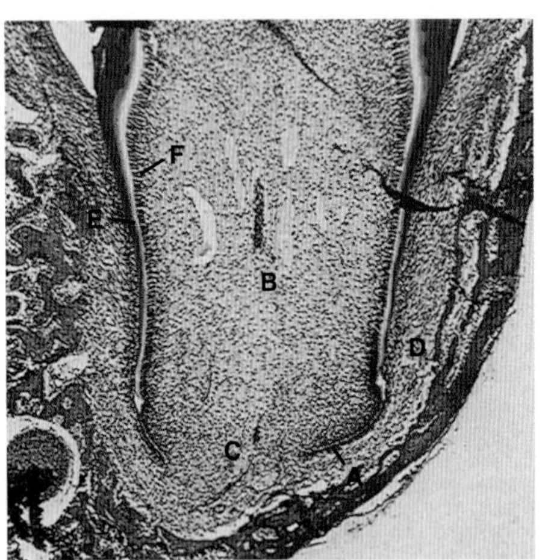

Fig. 25.6 The developing root. A = epithelial root sheath; B = dental papilla; C = primary apical foramen; D = dental follicle; E = developing root dentine; F = odontoblast layer (H & E; ×32).

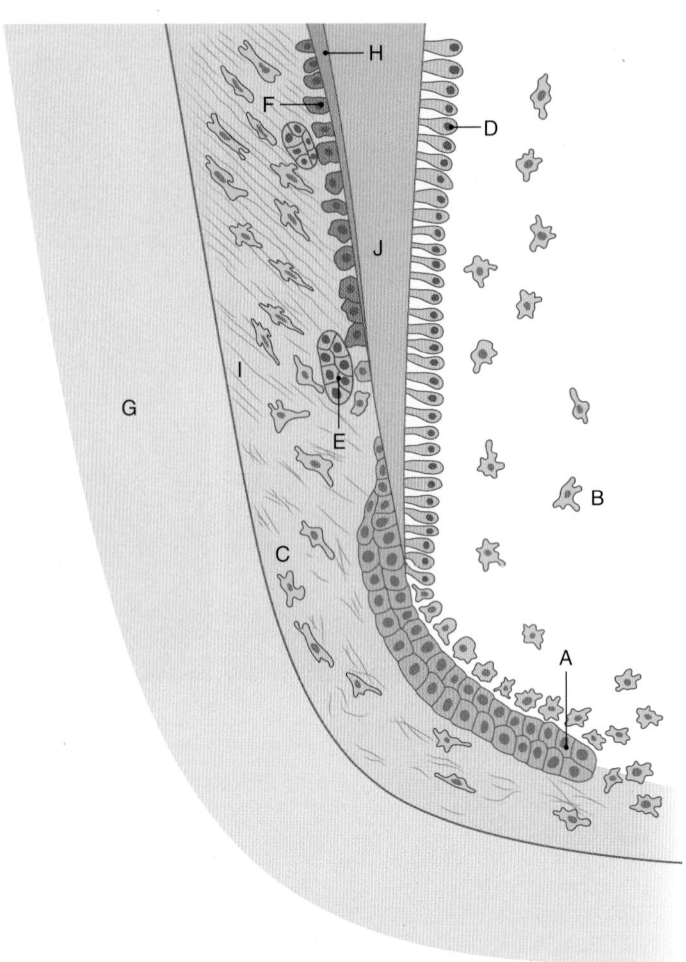

Fig. 25.7 Schematic drawing of the developing root. A = epithelial root sheath; B = dental papilla; C = dental follicle; D = odontoblasts; E = epithelial rests; F = cementoblasts; G = developing alveolar bone; H = developing cementum; I = developing periodontal ligament; J = root dentine.

Once cementogenesis has begun, cells of the remaining dental follicle become obliquely oriented along the root surface and show an increased content of intracellular organelles, becoming the fibroblasts of the periodontal ligament. These fibroblasts secrete collagen of the periodontal ligament into the extracellular compartment. This collagen will become embedded as Sharpey's fibres into the developing acellular cementum at the tooth surface and into the developing bone at the alveolar surface.

There has been controversy concerning the connective tissue immediately beneath the developing root apex. Initially called the *cushion hammock ligament*, this connective tissue was described as a fibrous network with fluid-filled interstices, with attachments on either side to the alveolar wall. It was thought to provide a resistant base so that forces produced by the growing root were prevented from causing bone resorption and were resolved into an eruptive force. This view is no longer held, as the thin fibrous membrane seen in this site is not attached to alveolar bone but merges at the sides with the fibres of the developing periodontal ligament. The structure is more correctly termed the *pulp-limiting membrane* (Fig. 25.9). It does not appear to be directly involved in tooth eruption, as its surgical removal (together with the developing root apex) does not affect tooth eruption.

It has been suggested that changes in vascular permeability in the connective tissues around the apex of the developing root can be related to

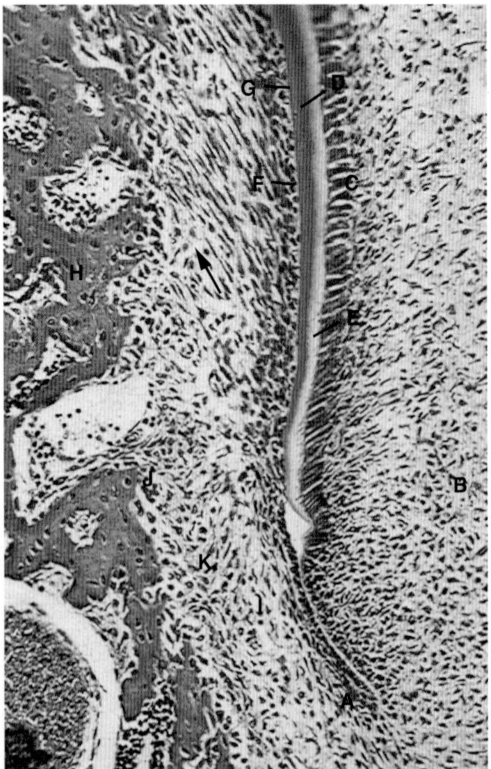

Fig. 25.8 The apical region of the developing root, periodontal ligament and alveolus. A = epithelial root sheath; B = dental papilla; C = odontoblasts; D = dentine of root; E = predentine layer; F = cementoblasts; G = developing cementum; H = developing alveolar bone; I = inner investing layer of dental follicle; J = outer layer of the dental follicle; K = intermediate layer of dental follicle. Arrow indicates oblique orientation of follicular tissue with formation of cementum (H & E; ×150).

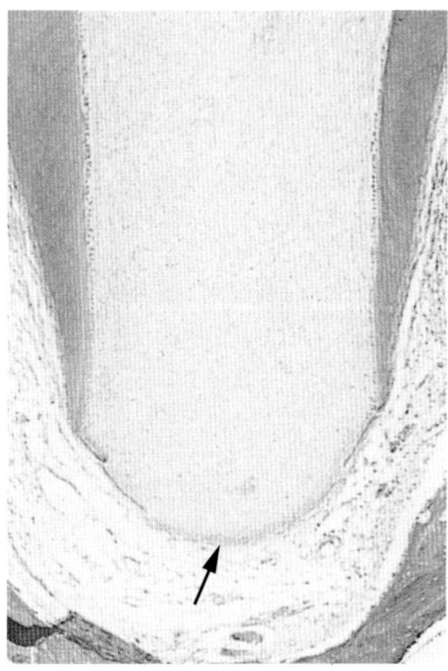

Fig. 25.9 The pulp-limiting membrane (arrowed) (Mallory's trichrome; ×30). Courtesy Dr. D Adams.

eruptive behaviour. Dense accumulations of tissue fluid (effusions) have been envisaged beneath the growing roots of erupting teeth. Furthermore, when radioactive fibrinogen is injected intravascularly, the radioactive label becomes incorporated rapidly into the effusions, supporting the view that they are vascular in origin. As effusions are seen most prominently when the growing root is situated close to the base (fundus) of the bony tooth socket/crypt, it has been suggested that they might force the root and bone apart and thereby contribute to eruption and enable further root growth. The vascular hypothesis of eruption is considered further on page 463.

Formation of collagen fibres within the periodontal ligament

A generalised view of the development of the collagen fibres of the periodontal ligament is shown in Fig. 25.10. One major difference in fibre formation exists between teeth with or without predecessors: in the latter (i.e., deciduous teeth and permanent molars) the principal fibre groups develop earlier than in the former (i.e., permanent incisors, canines and premolars). This is illustrated in Fig. 25.11. To visualise the difference, Fig. 25.12 shows an erupting permanent molar of a marmoset *(Callithrix jacchus)* just emerging into the oral cavity, where it can be seen that the coronal half of the periodontal ligament is composed of well-formed, obliquely orientated, principal collagen fibre bundles. In contrast, the bulk of the periodontal ligament of an erupting permanent premolar of a squirrel monkey *(Saimiri sciureus)* (Fig. 25.13) lacks significant numbers of organised principal collagen fibre bundles passing from tooth to alveolar bone.

It appears, therefore, that collagen fibres may not be well organised during eruption in some groups of teeth, and this is significant if it is believed that collagen fibres have an important role in the generation of tractional forces during eruption (see pages 461–462). However, there are species differences in the ontogeny of principal collagen fibres. In some animals, the fibres associated with succedaneous teeth do pass between tooth and bone as the tooth erupts into the oral cavity. For example, in a permanent canine of the ferret *(Mustela putorius)* erupting into the oral cavity, the principal collagen fibres are seen passing from tooth to bone (Fig. 25.14). This contrasts with the development of the primate periodontal ligament shown in Fig. 25.13. However, in this permanent canine tooth the collagen fibres are not as well organised in terms of thickness and orientation as those for the fully erupted tooth illustrated in Fig. 25.15.

There is some evidence of a change in the obliquity of the principal collagen fibres and in their dimensions as the tooth reaches its functional position. The inclination of the oblique fibres has been reported to decrease, while the principal fibres are said to thicken with function. However, there may again be species differences.

Qualitative differences in the type of collagen present during the development of the periodontal ligament have been reported. Thus, type VI collagen appears to be absent from the ligament during the main axial eruptive phase but present when the tooth has fully erupted. Type XII collagen similarly appears only after the tooth has erupted. It is of noteworthy that this pattern for type XII collagen is recapitulated on the pressure side of the periodontal ligament following orthodontic loading and remodelling of the ligament.

Some changes occurring in the ground substance during root formation are considered on pages 235–236.

Development of the cells of the periodontal ligament

Prior to root formation, the cells of the dental follicle have the characteristics of undifferentiated fibroblasts, containing few cytoplasmic organelles. With the onset of root formation, the cells show an increase in cytoplasmic organelles, especially those associated with protein synthesis and secretion, and extracellular spaces begin to fill with collagen and ground substance.

The cells of the dental follicle give rise to cementoblasts, fibroblasts and osteoblasts of the periodontal ligament. There is evidence that cells from the apical region of the dental papilla migrate around the epithelial root sheath and supplement the number of cells in the dental follicle. Cells may also migrate into the developing periodontal ligament from the endosteal spaces of the adjacent alveolar bone.

During the formation of the root and periodontal ligament, there is obviously a dramatic increase in the number of connective tissue–forming cells (i.e., cementoblasts, fibroblasts and osteoblasts). Stem cells exist within the region to allow for this, perhaps lying in a perivascular location. It is not clear whether the three main cell types all arise from a common stem cell or whether each type has its own specific stem cell.

There appear to be few structural differences between fibroblasts in the developing periodontal ligament of erupting teeth and those associated with fully erupted teeth. However, changes during eruption have been reported for the nonfibrous extracellular matrix elements and the vascularity of the periodontal ligament (see pages 235–236 and 463).

In addition to the main connective tissue–forming cells, osteoclasts also appear in the developing periodontal ligament at the alveolar bone surface, allowing bone to remodel in association with tooth eruption and bone growth. As the tooth erupts, there is little evidence of any significant bone deposition at the base of the socket (i.e., beneath the developing root; Fig. 25.16), with resorption often being prominent at this site. Thus, bone deposition at this site is precluded as a cause of tooth eruption. There are species differences. For example, bone deposition is found beneath the erupting permanent premolars of dogs (Fig. 25.17). The different patterns of bone activity in different species may relate to the distance a tooth has to erupt: if the distance is much greater than the length of the root, then bone deposition is clearly necessary to maintain the normal dimensions of the periodontal ligament at the root apex of the tooth. Remodelling of alveolar bone other than at the base of the socket may also be seen during eruption, and this can be related to the relocation of the teeth during jaw growth and to the establishment of occlusion.

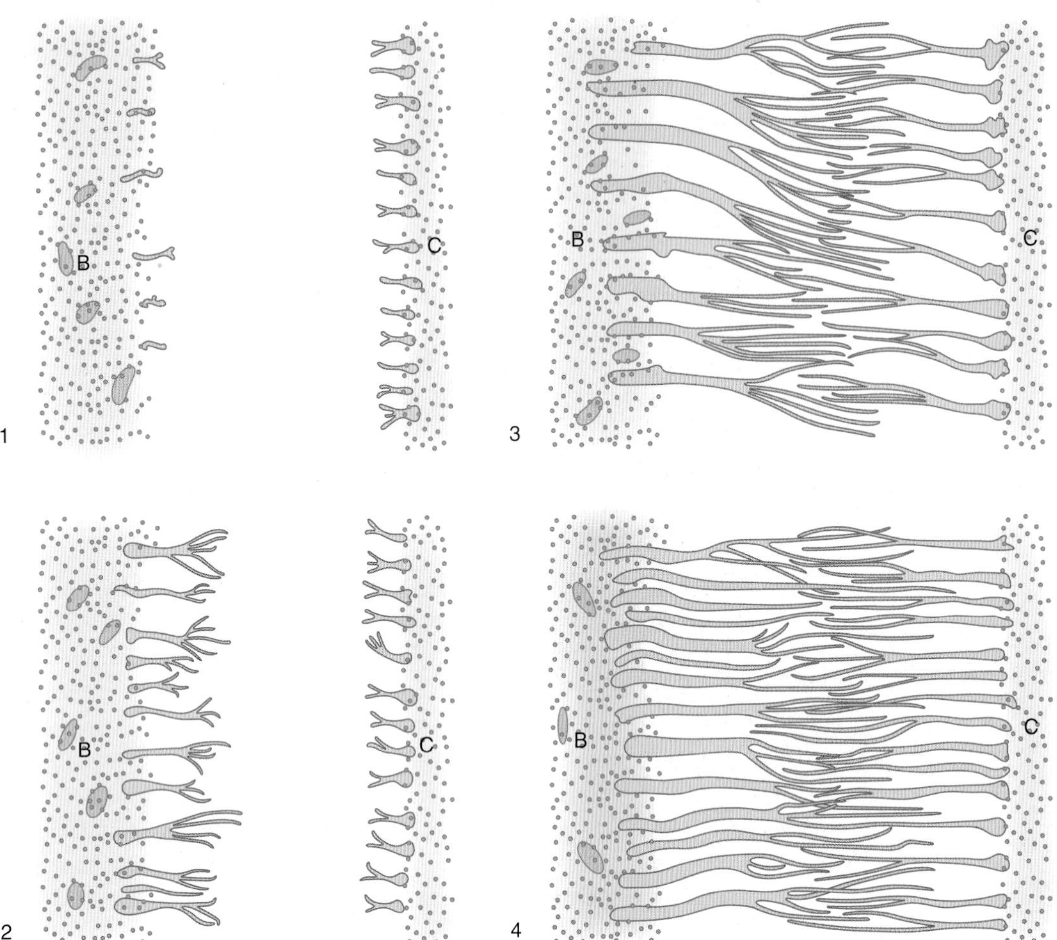

Fig. 25.10 Summary of the development of collagen fibres of the periodontal ligament. (1) Fine brush-like fibres are first seen emanating from cementum (C). Only a few fibres project from the alveolar bone (B) and extend into the unorganised collagenous elements that occupy the broad central zone of the developing periodontal ligament. (2) Sharpey's fibres, thicker and more widely spaced than those of cementum, emerge from the bone to extend towards the tooth and appear to unravel as they arborise at their ends. The closely spaced cemental fibres are still short, giving the root a brushlike appearance. (3) The alveolar fibres extend farther into the central zone to join the lengthening cemental fibres. (4) With occlusal function, the principal fibres become classically organised, thicker and continuous between bone and cementum. Redrawn with permission from Grant, D.A., Berwick, S., 1972. The formation of the periodontal ligament. *Journal of Periodontology* 43, 17–25.

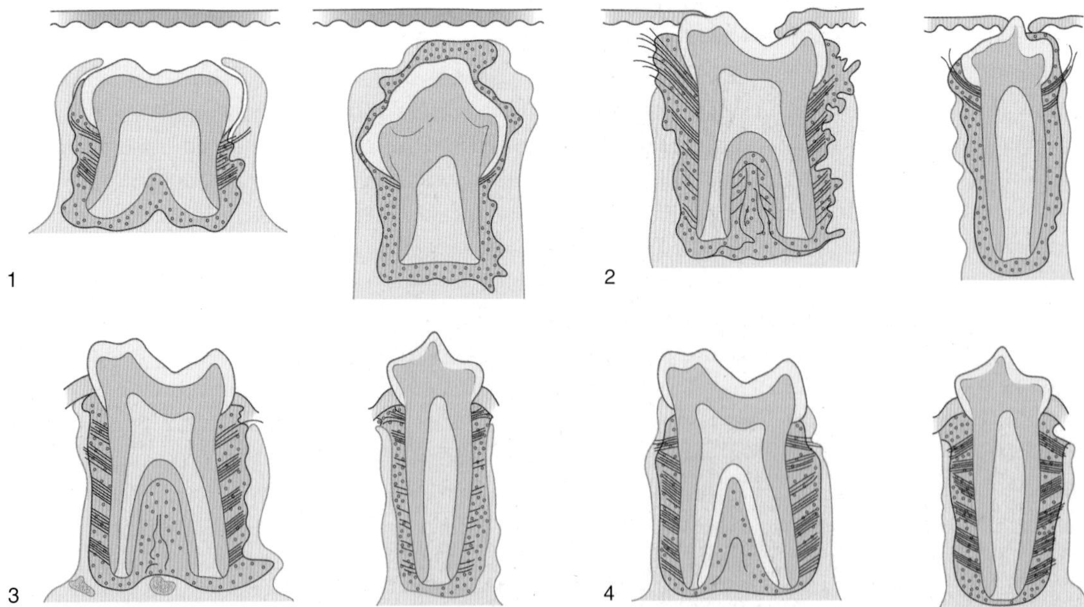

Fig. 25.11 A comparison of the development of the principal periodontal ligament collagen fibres between primary (left of each pair) and succedaneous teeth (right of each pair). (1) Before eruption, the dentogingival and oblique periodontal fibres are well developed in the permanent molar. In the permanent premolar, however, only the dentogingival fibres are organised, with the developing periodontal ligament being composed of loosely structured collagenous elements. (2) As the tooth emerges into the oral cavity, the periodontal ligament of the permanent molar is well differentiated, with the oblique fibres being the most conspicuous. However, at this stage in the permanent premolar, only the fibres in the region of the alveolar crest are becoming organised. In the periodontal ligament itself, although collagen fibres are developing, they do not yet span the periodontal space. (3) On reaching occlusion, the fibre groupings in the cervical region of the permanent molar now become organised. In the permanent premolar, while the fibre groups cervically appear prominent, those in the apical part of the root appear relatively undeveloped. (4) After a period in function, the fibres of both the permanent molar and premolar show the classical organisation of the principal fibres. Redrawn with permission from Grant, D.A., Bernick, S., Levy, B.M., Dreizen, S., 1972. A comparative study of periodontal ligament development in teeth with and without predecessors in marmosets. *Journal of Periodontology* 43, 162–169.

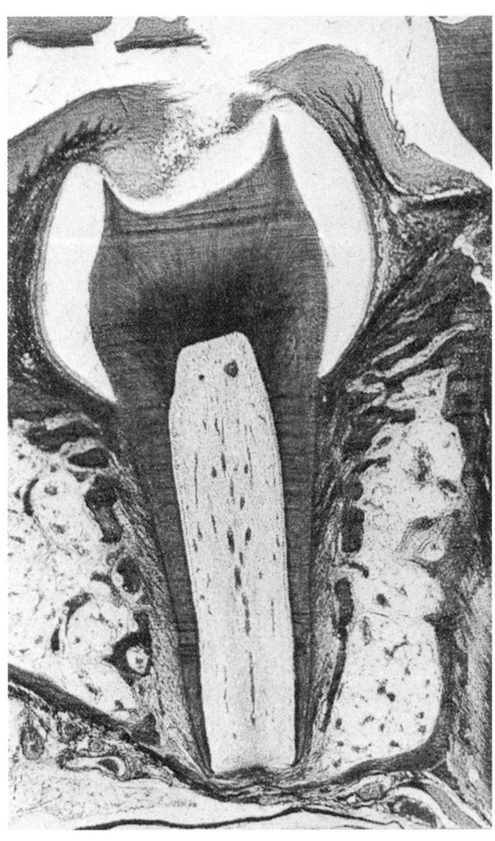

Fig. 25.12 Erupting permanent molar of a marmoset *(Callithrix jacchus)* just emerging into the oral cavity. Note the presence of periodontal ligament fibres (Mallory's trichrome; ×15). From Grant, D.A., Bernick, S., Levy, B.M., Dreizen, S., 1972. A comparative study of periodontal ligament development in teeth with and without predecessors in marmosets. *Journal of Periodontology* 43, 162–169.

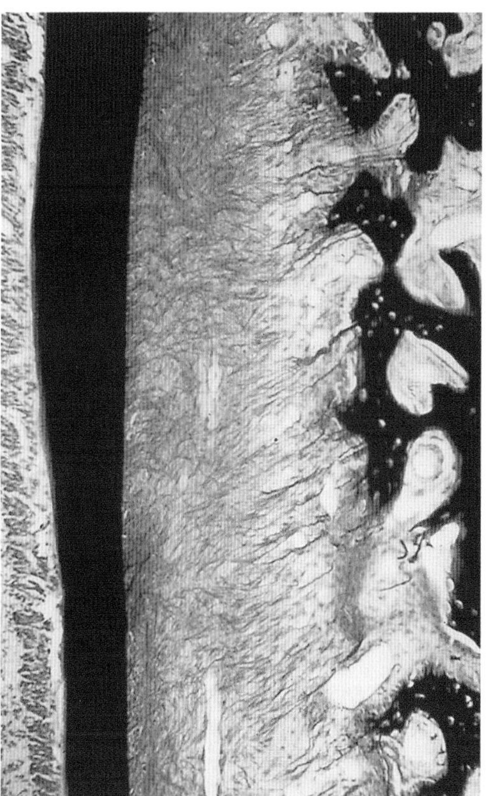

Fig. 25.14 Principal collagen fibres associated with an erupting permanent canine of the ferret *(Mustela putorius)* as it emerges into the oral cavity (aldehyde fuchsin and van Gieson; ×150).

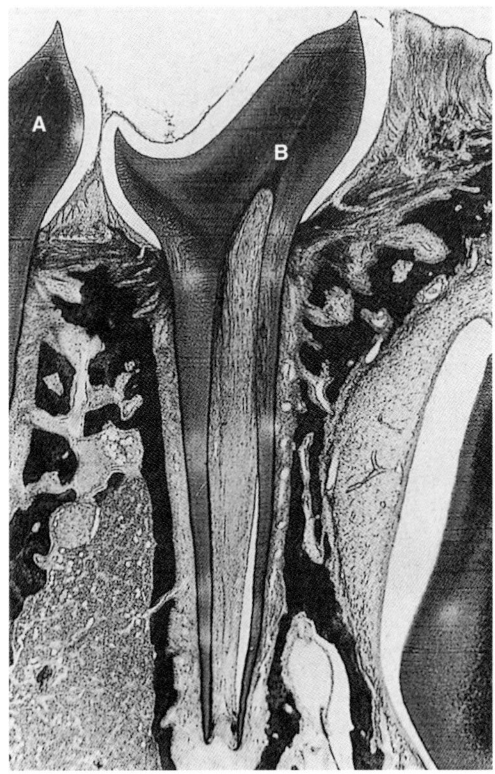

Fig. 25.13 Erupting second premolar of a squirrel monkey *(Saimiri sciureus)* just emerging into the oral cavity (B). A = erupted first premolar. Note the absence of periodontal ligament fibres (Mallory's trichrome; ×35). From Grant, D.A., Berwick, S., 1972. The formation of the periodontal ligament. *Journal of Periodontology* 43, 17–25.

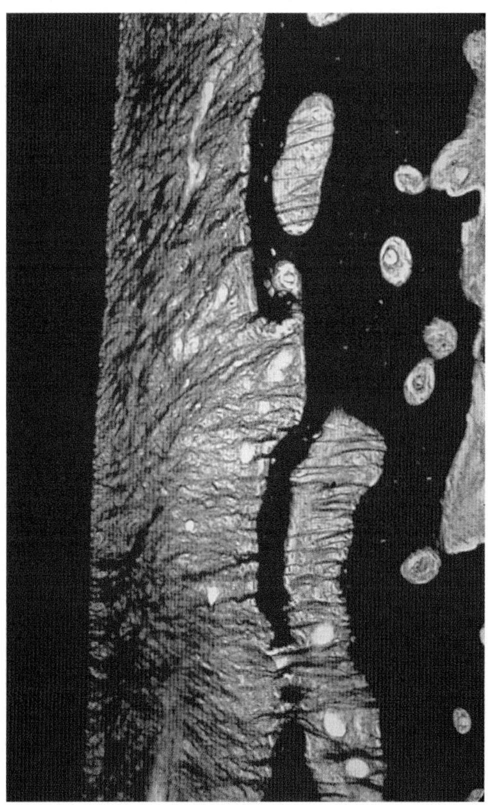

Fig. 25.15 Well-differentiated collagen fibres for the fully erupted permanent canine of the ferret *(Mustela putorius)* (aldehyde fuchsin and van Gieson; ×130).

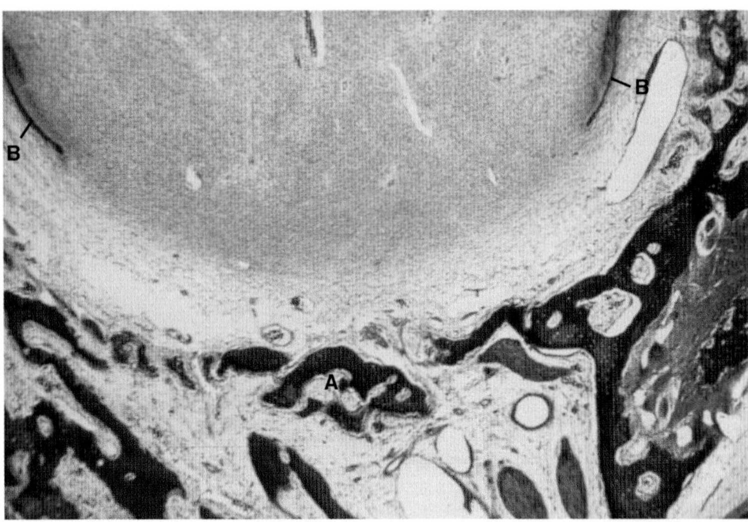

Fig. 25.16 Apical region of an erupting tooth showing little evidence of bone deposition at the base of the socket (A). B = Epithelial root sheath (Masson's blue trichrome stain; ×25).

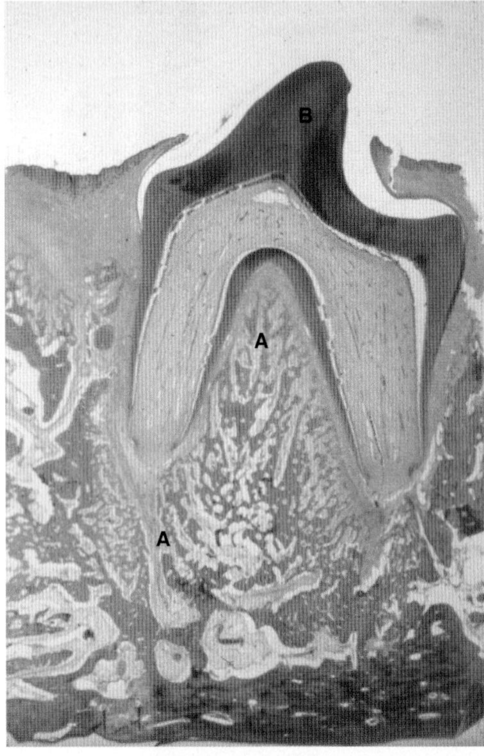

Fig. 25.17 Section of jaw of dog showing bone (A) being deposited beneath the erupting premolar tooth (B) (H & E; ×5). Courtesy Dr. S C Marks Jr.

Development of the neurovascular elements

Prior to eruption, nerve fibres can be demonstrated in the pulp, but few are present within the lower part of the dental follicle that will form the periodontal ligament. With root formation and subsequent eruption, nerves adjacent to the bone grow into the periodontal ligament, usually accompanying blood vessels, to establish its innervation. These initial nerves are autonomic. It would seem that the sensory innervation is not established until the ligament is fully organised following eruption.

Blood vessels in the forming periodontal ligament seem to be derived from two main sources. They enter from the periapical area, pass upwards within the ligament and form anastomoses with vessels entering from the adjacent developing alveolar bone. As the tooth erupts, it receives vessels from the adjacent gingiva. In the case of permanent teeth, connections also develop with the periodontal ligament of the overlying deciduous teeth. There is evidence that differences may be present in the periodontal vessels of erupting and fully erupted teeth, in that the number of fenestrated capillaries is greater in erupting teeth (see page 463).

Cementogenesis

Cementogenesis will be considered in terms of the formation of acellular (primary) cementum and then of cellular (secondary) cementum (see Chapter 11). There may be differences between the cells forming each type of cementum. Our understanding is clouded by species differences, resulting in problems of terminology, particularly with regard to structures at the cementum–dentine interface (see pages 221–222).

As for the crown, the hard tissues that comprise the root (i.e., cementum and dentine) develop under the control of epithelial–mesenchymal interactions (see pages 449–450). However, unlike that of the crown, the epithelial component involved in root formation retains a simpler morphology, rapidly loses its continuity with adjacent cells and is not evident as a conspicuous layer during initial cementum formation. Although it was once thought that its function was primarily to induce the formation of root odontoblasts, present evidence also indicates that the epithelium has an important role in cementogenesis. As the aim of periodontologists is now not only to halt the ravages of periodontal disease but also to try to regenerate the tissues lost, there has been a resurgence of interest in how cementum forms. It is only through a thorough understanding of this process that clinical strategies can be developed to encourage the regeneration of new cementum, alveolar bone and periodontal ligament.

Acellular (primary, AEFC) cementum

Once the crown has fully formed, the internal and external enamel epithelia proliferate downwards as a double-layered sheet of somewhat flattened epithelial cells: the epithelial root sheath (of Hertwig) that maps out the shape of the roots (Figs. 25.1, 25.6 and 25.18). The process of cementogenesis is initiated at the cervical margin and extends apically as the root grows downwards. The cells of the epithelial root sheath, in contrast to those of the enamel organ during enamel formation, do not enlarge during this inductive stage. The epithelial root sheath is separated by a basal lamina on both of its surfaces from the adjacent connective tissues of the dental follicle and dental papilla. The epithelial root sheath induces the adjacent cells of the dental papilla to differentiate into odontoblasts. As these odontoblasts initially retreat inwards, they synthesise and secrete the organic matrix of the first-formed root predentine, comprising ground substance and some collagen fibrils. Although some collagen fibrils are oriented perpendicular to the surface, others are aligned more obliquely. This may explain why this first-formed layer can be later distinguished from the rest of the root dentine using polarised light (see Fig. 9.38; page 177). As the odontoblasts also do not leave behind an odontoblast process in the initial few micrometres of tissue (Fig. 25.19), its structureless (and later glasslike) appearance is responsible for the term 'hyaline layer' that is given to this (approximately 10 μm) layer once it is mineralised.

The epithelial root sheath is in contact with the initial predentine layer for only a short distance before the continuity of its cells is lost. The presence within the epithelial root sheath cells of organelles, such as endoplasmic reticulum, Golgi apparatus and mitochondria, indicates that the cells are capable of the synthesis and secretion of bioactive molecules

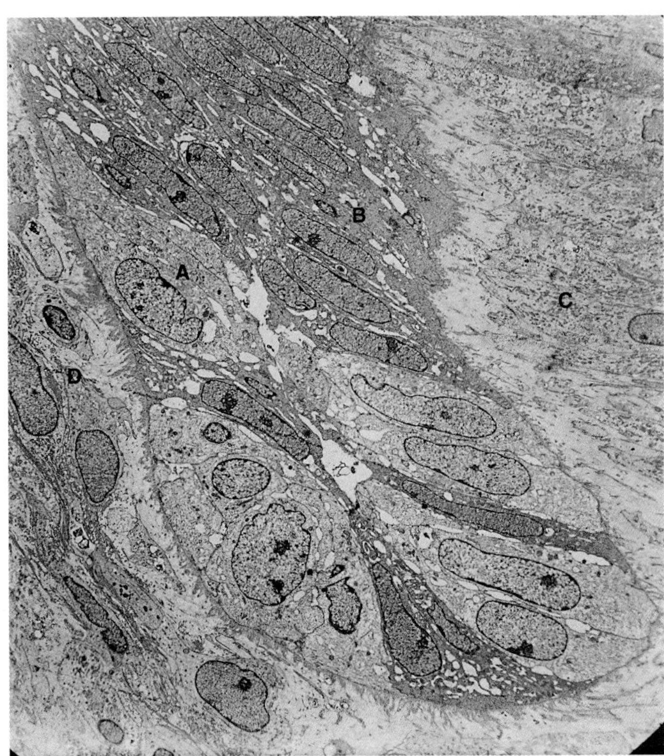

Fig. 25.18 TEM illustrating epithelial root sheath in developing root. A = outer layer of epithelial root sheath; B = inner layer of epithelial root sheath; C = differentiating odontoblasts; D = dental follicle (×2,000). From Bosshardt, D.D., Selvig, K.A., 1997. Dental cementum: the dynamic tissue covering of the root. *Periodontology 2000* 13, 41–75.

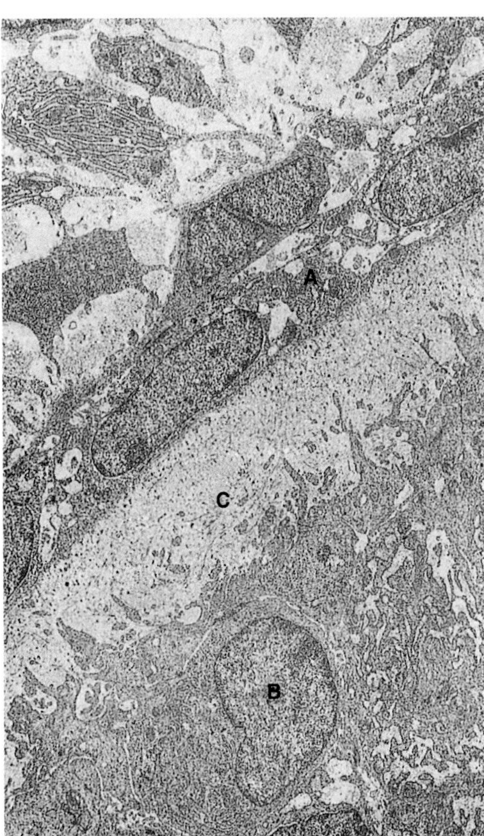

Fig. 25.19 TEM of early stage in root formation. The first-formed matrix (C) lies between the newly differentiated odontoblasts (B) and the epithelial root sheath cells (A). This matrix receives contributions from both the odontoblast and epithelial cell layers. It lacks major processes from the odontoblasts and forms the hyaline layer (×5,000). Courtesy Dr. P D A Owens.

that may play an important role in root formation. There is evidence that the epithelial root sheath cells secrete enamel-related proteins into the collagenous matrix of the hyaline layer at the cementum–dentine boundary. Thus, the hyaline layer is formed by contributions from both the odontoblast and epithelial root sheath layers. The enamel-related protein has been identified as amelogenin (Fig. 25.20), although there is some dispute as to whether another enamel-related protein, ameloblastin, is also present. Difficulties in solving this dispute relate to the small amount of protein present and to problems of cross-reactivity of antibodies. The function of such enamel-related proteins is unclear but may concern epithelial–mesenchymal interactions involving the induction of odontoblasts and cementoblasts and/or the process of mineralisation. During the subsequent mineralisation of cementum and the hyaline layer, the enamel-related protein is lost, although remnants may be retained in the granular layer of the root dentine (Fig. 25.21).

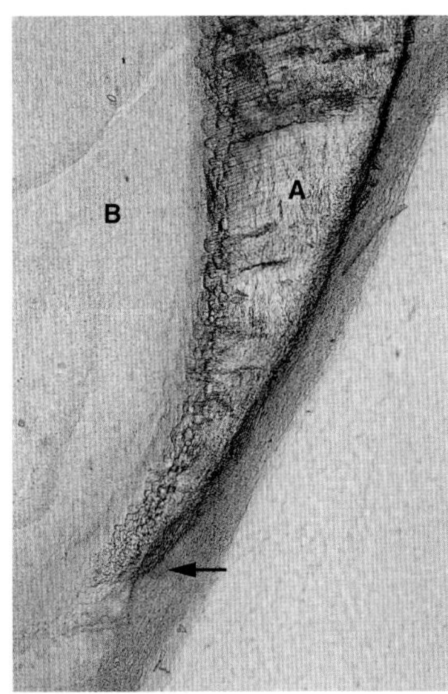

Fig. 25.20 Immunohistochemistry showing presence of enamel-like proteins (stained brown – arrow) at the surface of the developing root. This is a frozen ground section through a premolar root using an antibody against amelogenin. A = dentine; B = pulp (×100). Courtesy Prof. L Hammarström.

The cause of fenestration of the epithelial root sheath is not known, but it may not simply be related to programmed epithelial cell death (apoptosis). Fibroblast-like cells of the adjacent dental follicle pass through the fenestrations and come to lie close to the surface of the as yet unmineralised hyaline layer (Fig. 25.22). These cells, which are cementoblasts associated with the formation of acellular cementum, appear to secrete collagen fibrils. At their deep surface, these fibrils intermingle with those of the hyaline layer, with subsequent mineralisation of this zone producing a firm bond between dentine and cementum: at their superficial surface these fibrils form a 'fibrous fringe' extending perpendicularly into the periodontal space for about 10–20 μm (Fig. 25.23). These fibroblast-like cells of the dental follicle do not form a conspicuous layer at the developing root surface and may retreat and mingle with adjacent fibroblasts of the periodontal ligament.

As the newly differentiated odontoblasts at the periphery of the pulp migrate inwards (centripetally) beyond the hyaline layer, they start to trail behind them their odontoblast processes. Initially, there is much branching and looping of these processes in the future granular layer (of Tomes), after which the odontoblast processes become more regular in the region of the circumpulpal dentine.

Mineralisation of the first-formed dentine of the hyaline layer occurs within matrix vesicles. Unlike the crown, this does not initially occur at the outermost surface of the hyaline layer, but a few micrometres within it. From this initial centre, mineralisation spreads both inwards towards the pulp and outwards towards the periodontal ligament (centrifugally).

Thus, the outermost part of the hyaline layer undergoes delayed mineralisation (Fig. 25.24). This is visualised by the V-shaped configuration at the extreme apical edge of the developing root, showing continuity of the unmineralised predentine layer at the periphery of the pulp with

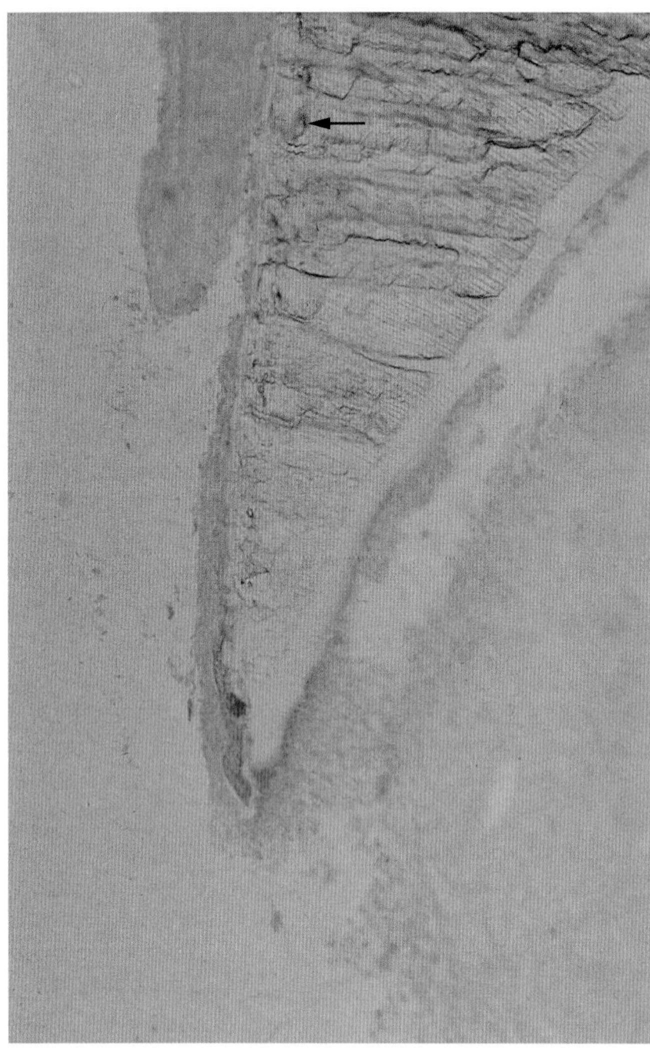

Fig. 25.21 Immunohistochemistry showing the presence of enamel-like proteins (brown staining – arrow) in interglobular dentine (×100). From Hammarstrom, L., 1997. Enamel matrix, cementum development and regeneration. *Journal of Clinical Periodontology* 24, 658–668.

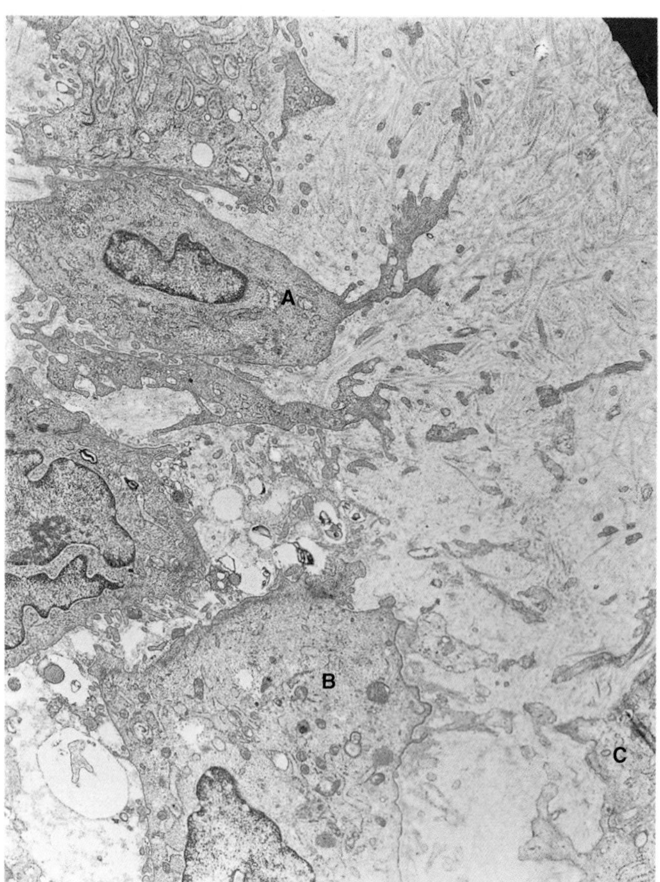

Fig. 25.22 TEM showing a fibroblast-like cell (A) from dental follicle with cytoplasmic processes lying close to the unmineralised external surface of the initial root dentine layer. B = coronal termination of intact internal enamel epithelial cell of epithelial root sheath; C = portion of odontoblast cell (×6,250). From Bosshardt, D.D., Selvig, K.A., 1997. Dental cementum: the dynamic tissue covering of the root. *Periodontology* 2000 13, 41–75.

the unmineralised part of the hyaline layer at the outer root surface (Fig. 25.25). A similar configuration is evident when the mineralising front is highlighted following administration of the antibiotic tetracycline (Fig. 25.26).

During the next phase of development in the formation of acellular cementum, the delayed mineralisation front in the hyaline layer gradually spreads outwards (centripetally) until this layer is fully mineralised and then continues on into the first few micrometres of the fibrous fringe secreted by the fibroblast-like cells of the dental follicle (Fig. 25.27). In this manner, the first few micrometres of acellular cementum are firmly attached to the root dentine. At this stage, the collagen fibres in the adjacent periodontal ligament are oriented more parallel to the root surface and have not yet gained an attachment to the fibrous fringe (Fig. 25.28). The stages in formation of acellular (AEFC) cementum are summarised in Fig. 25.29.

As with bone, the early stage of acellular cementum formation results in the secretion by the associated cementoblasts of various noncollagenous proteins (e.g., osteopontin, cementum-attachment protein, bone sialoprotein), cytokines and growth hormones (Fig. 25.30A). The precise roles of such molecules await clarification, but they may be involved in processes such as chemo-attraction, cell attachment, cell growth, cell differentiation and mineralisation. It has also been suggested that these

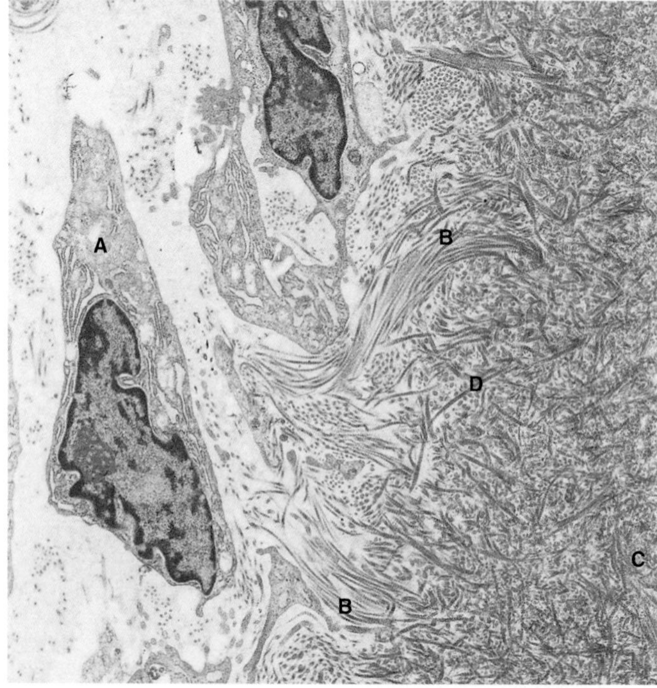

Fig. 25.23 TEM showing cementoblast (A) at the root surface secreting collagen fibrils that form a fibrous fringe (B) that intermingles with the as yet unmineralised outer region of the root predentine (C). D = site of future dentine–cementum junction and, adjacent to it, the hyaline layer (×5,800). From Bosshardt, D.D., Selvig, K.A., 1997. Dental cementum: the dynamic tissue covering of the root. *Periodontology* 2000 13, 41–75.

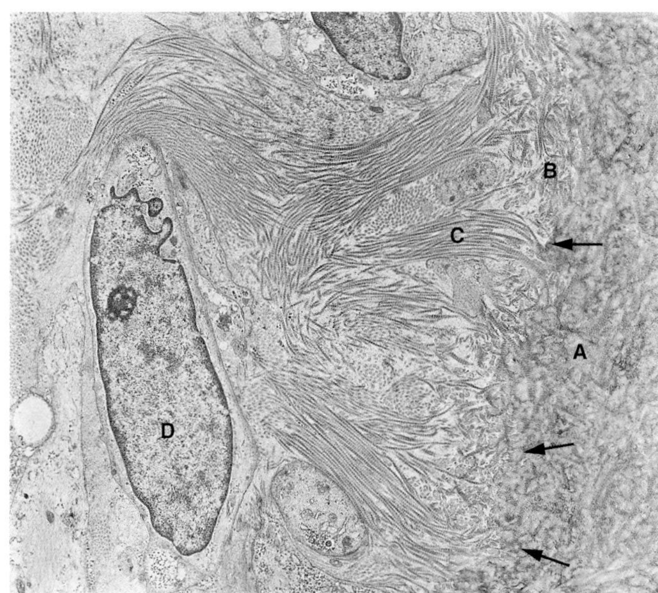

Fig. 25.24 TEM showing the external mineralisation front (arrows) of the outermost root dentine (A) has now extended outwards to reach the fibrillar dentine–cementum junction (B). The dentine is now almost completely covered by the cementum matrix in the form of a fibrous fringe (C). D = cementoblast (×5,700). From Bosshardt, D.D., Selvig, K.A., 1997. Dental cementum: the dynamic tissue covering of the root. *Periodontology* 2000 13, 41–75.

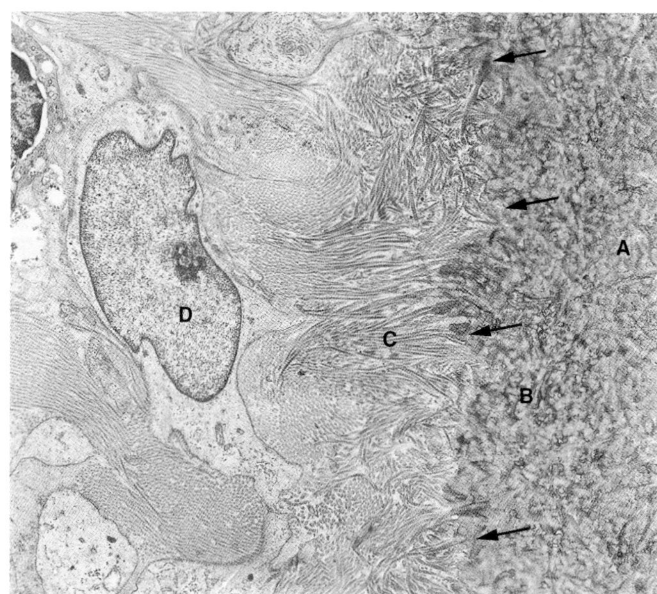

Fig. 25.27 TEM showing the mineralisation front in the developing root extending from the dentine (A) across the dentine–cementum junction (B) and into the base (arrowed) of the fibrous fringe of the cementum (C). D = cementoblast (×6,250). From Bosshardt, D.D., Selvig, K.A., 1997. Dental cementum: the dynamic tissue covering of the root. *Periodontology* 2000 13, 41–75.

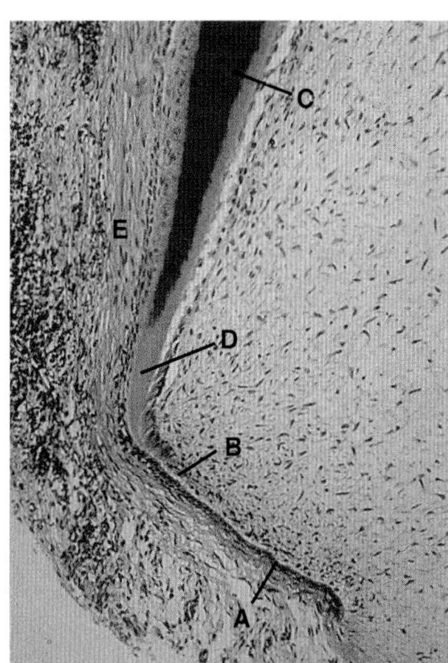

Fig. 25.25 Section of the developing root of extracted tooth. A = epithelial root sheath; B = differentiating odontoblasts at the periphery of the dental papilla; C = matrix of mineralised dentine (red); D = unmineralised predentine (pale blue) continuous around root apex with first-formed but as yet still unmineralised matrix on outer surface of dentine (corresponding to hyaline layer); E = dental follicle, which will give rise to periodontal ligament (Masson's trichrome, ×100).

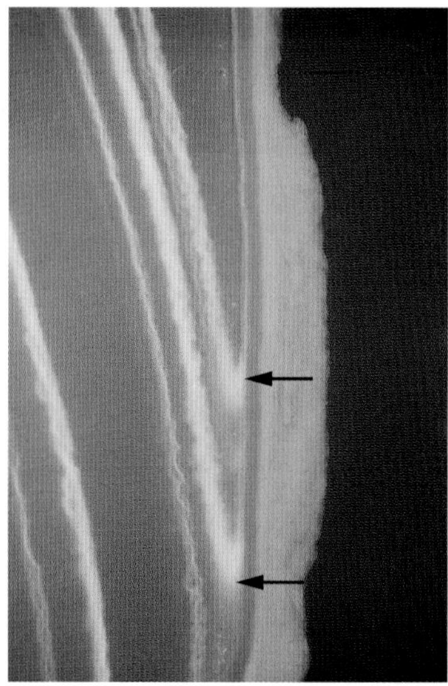

Fig. 25.26 Fluorescent micrograph of ground longitudinal section of tooth of a patient who had received multiple injections of the antibiotic tetracycline. The antibiotic is incorporated into tissues mineralising at the time of the injection. There is continuity at the edge of the section where the original predentine recurves upwards at the site of the hyaline layer (arrows), similar to the situation seen in Fig. 25.25. Courtesy Dr R O'Sullivan.

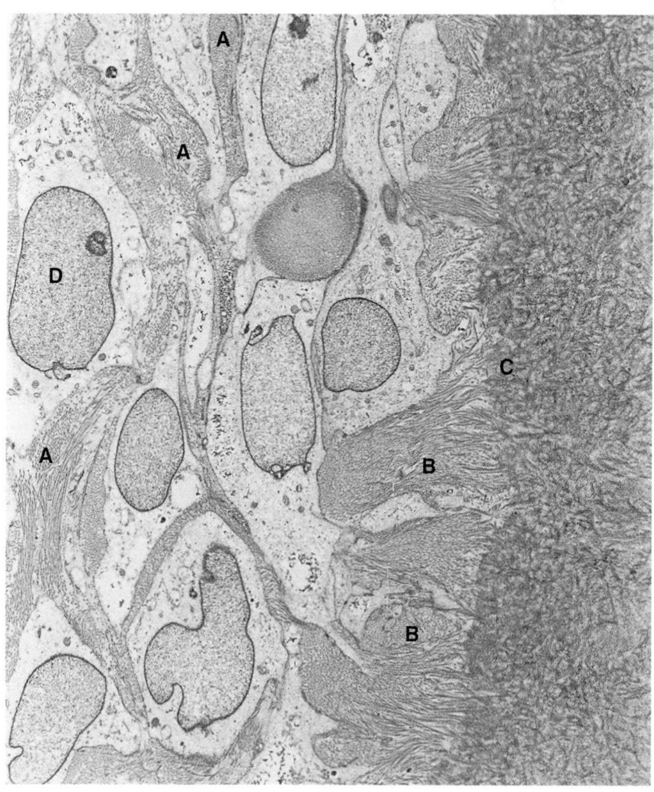

Fig. 25.28 TEM of developing root showing fibres in the developing periodontal ligament (A) running parallel to the root surface with little attachment to the cementum fibres (B), which are perpendicular to the root surface. C = dentine–cementum junction, beneath which would lie the hyaline layer; D = fibroblast of periodontal ligament. The mineralisation front extends from the dentine across the cementum-dentine junction to involve the base of the cementum fibres (×4,300). From Bosshardt, D.D., Selvig, K.A., 1997. Dental cementum: the dynamic tissue covering of the root. *Periodontology* 2000 13, 41–75.

(and other) molecules play a role in bonding the cementum to the outer surface of the root dentine. Their importance may be indicated by reference to a pathological condition in which osteoclasts are deficient. In this condition (leading to a type of osteopetrosis), where there is a failure of production of bone sialoprotein by cells at the root surface, root formation is grossly interfered with (Fig. 25.30B). As epithelial cell rests have also been shown to express a variety of bioactive molecules (e.g., glycosaminoglycans, osteopontin, cytokines, growth hormones, matrix metalloproteinases), the question arises as to whether they play an additional role in cementogenesis.

The subsequent development of acellular cementum involves:

- Its slow increase in thickness
- The establishment of continuity between the principal collagen fibres of the periodontal ligament and those of the fibrous fringe at the surface of the root dentine
- Continued slow mineralisation of the collagen at the root surface

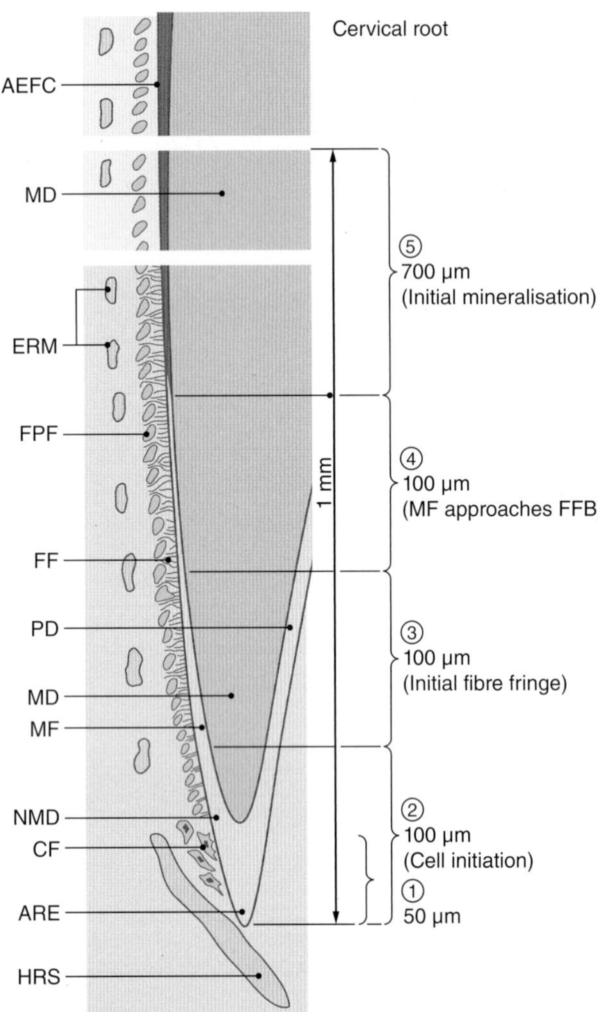

Fig. 25.29 The initial stages of root development on human premolars that have 50–60% of their final root length. 1 = Fibroblasts contact root/predentine and become committed. 2 = Fibroblasts start to form and attach collagen fibrils. 3 = Initial fibrous fringe with maximum fibre density is established. 4 = Cell/fibrous fringe meshwork is established, and the mineralisation front approaches the base of the fibrous fringe. 5 = Mineralisation front progresses into initial fibrous fringe. AEFC = acellular extrinsic fibre cementum; ARE = advancing root edge; CF = committed fibroblasts; ERM = epithelial cell rests of Malassez; FF = collagenous fibrous fringe; FPF = fibrous-fringe-producing fibroblasts; HRS = Hertwig's epithelial root sheath; MD = mineralised dentine; MF = mineralisation front; NMD = nonmineralised dentine or predentine; PD = predentine. Courtesy Prof. H E Schroeder, D D Bosshardt and the editors of *Cell and Tissue Research*.

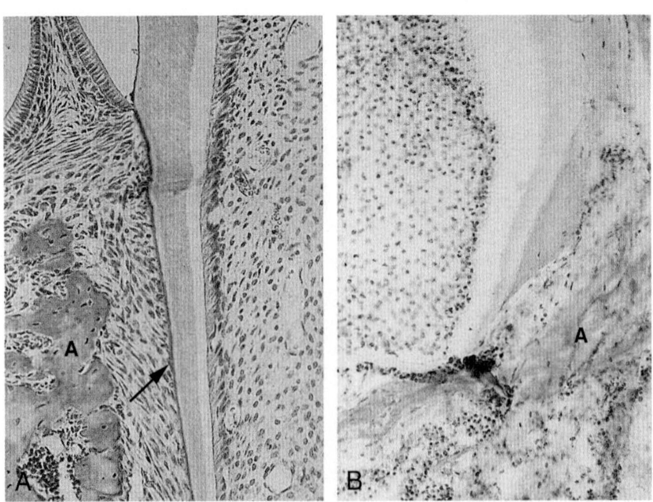

Fig. 25.30 (A) Decalcified longitudinal section of mouse molar using immunohistochemical techniques to localise the presence of bone sialoprotein (red). Positive staining is seen at the developing cementum surface (arrow) and throughout the alveolar bone (A). (H & E; ×100). (B) Similar section from an osteopetrotic mouse lacking macrophage colony-stimulating factor: the root is stunted in its development and the cementum lacks bone sialoprotein, although this molecule is still present in alveolar bone (A). From D'errico, J.A., et al., 1995. Models for the study of cementogenesis. *Connective Tissue Research* 33, 9–17.

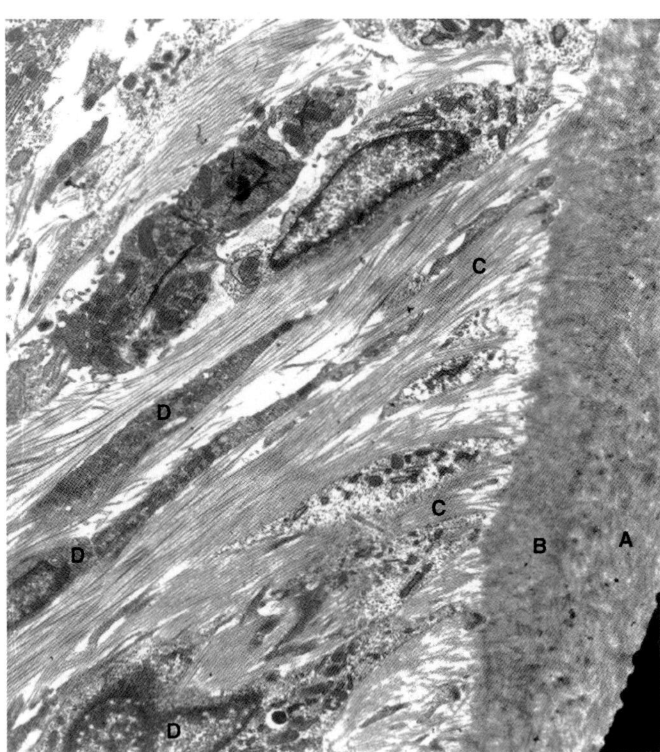

Fig. 25.31 TEM of decalcified root surface showing formation of acellular extrinsic fibre cementum. A = dentine; B = cementum; C = Sharpey's fibres; D = cells of periodontal ligament. Note the absence of a definite layer of cementoblasts (×3,500). Courtesy Prof. M M Smith.

It is only with the establishment of continuity between periodontal ligament fibres and those of the initial fibrous fringe projecting from the acellular cementum that the tooth can be properly supported within the socket. There may be a considerable difference in the timing of the establishment of this support between deciduous and succedaneous teeth (see page 439). For permanent teeth, this attachment may not occur until after the tooth has erupted into the mouth, when about two-thirds of the root has formed and the acellular cementum may only be about 10 µm thick. Thus, the acellular cementum lining the root before this time could be considered acellular intrinsic fibre cementum.

Once periodontal ligament fibres become attached to the surface of the cementum layer, the cementum may be classified as acellular extrinsic fibre cementum (Fig. 25.31). It increases slowly and evenly in thickness throughout life at a rate of about 2 µm per year. Although the cementoblasts may not form a distinctive and recognisable layer of cells that can be distinguished from adjacent cells of the periodontal ligament (Fig. 25.31), some cells lying between the perpendicularly oriented periodontal fibre bundles may become more cuboidal (Fig. 25.32). The cementoblasts contain small amounts of the intracellular organelles associated with protein synthesis and secretion and probably contribute to the formation of the ground substance surrounding the collagen. Presumably, secretion is polarised at the surface of the cells adjacent to the cementum surface and, together with the slow rate of formation, ensures that the cells are not entombed by their own secretion.

Mineralisation of the cementum matrix does not appear to be controlled by its cells, as matrix vesicles have not been observed at its surface. It may be that the presence of hydroxyapatite crystals in the adjacent dentine initiates mineralisation in cementum. The adjacent periodontal ligament fibroblasts, which are rich in alkaline phosphatase, may play a role in mineralisation, as does the presence of noncollagenous proteins, such as bone sialoprotein, in the vicinity of its surface (Fig. 25.30). Mineralisation proceeds very slowly in a linear fashion and, as with bone but unlike dentine,

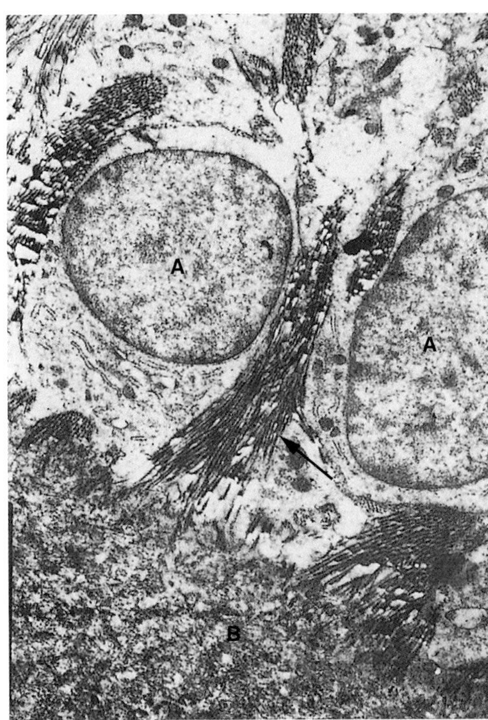

Fig. 25.32 TEM of decalcified root surface forming acellular extrinsic fibre cementum (B). Between the Sharpey's fibres (arrow), the cells (cementoblasts, A) are more cuboidal (×5,000).

calcospherites are not observed in cementum. Owing to the slow progress of mineralisation, there is usually no evidence of a layer of precementum associated with acellular cementum homologous to that in forming dentine (predentine) and bone (osteoid). When mineralisation of initial root dentine is interfered with (as following the administration of drugs known as bisphosphonates), there is inhibition of cementogenesis.

Cementogenesis occurs rhythmically, with periods of activity alternating with periods of quiescence. Structural lines may be visible within the tissue, indicating the incremental nature of its formation. The periods of decreased activity are associated with these incremental lines (see pages 216–218), which are believed to have a higher content of ground substance and mineral and a lower content of collagen than the adjacent cementum. These lines may also reflect changes in crystallite orientation. The periodicity of the incremental lines is not known, but using refined preparation techniques allied to digital graphics, it has recently been suggested that they might be annual and can be used to age individuals. As acellular cementum is formed very slowly, the incremental lines are closer together than corresponding lines seen in cellular cementum that is deposited more rapidly.

The precise origin of the fibroblast-like cells at the surface of acellular cementum is not clear. They may be derived from the cells of the investing layer of the dental follicle. However, there is also evidence suggesting that they may be derived from epithelial root sheath cells as a result of epithelial–mesenchymal transformation. This is based on some studies showing that cells having the morphological features of cementoblasts contain tonofilaments as well as the intracellular organelles for protein synthesis and secretion. Furthermore, they are linked by desmosomes and have a collagenous matrix in the intercellular spaces. Immunohistochemical studies also show that, in addition to reacting positively to vimentin as expected of mesenchymal cells, cementoblasts react positively to cytokeratins characteristic of epithelial cells. However, other studies suggest that state that epithelial cells do not undergo epithelial–mesenchymal transformations and that the cementoblasts are of direct mesenchymal origin.

Epithelial cell rests may sometimes be trapped within cementum. Cementum that contains cell inclusions near the cementum–dentine junction has been referred to as *intermediate cementum* and occurs principally in the apical half of the roots of molar teeth (see page 221). Epithelial cells may occasionally lie in the same lacunae as cementocytes, and the two types of cells may be connected by desmosome-like structures. More deeply lying epithelial cells undergo apoptosis.

Acellular afibrillar cementum

Acellular afibrillar cementum may be deposited as a thin layer overlying enamel at the cervical margin of the tooth. One explanation for this presumes that the reduced enamel epithelium overlying and protecting this cervical enamel in an unerupted tooth is damaged or lost. The adjacent connective tissue cells of the dental follicle could then come into contact with the enamel surface, where they are induced to form cementoblasts. These cells then secrete a matrix (probably consisting of noncollagenous proteins but lacking collagen fibrils) that calcifies. A similar type of layer has also been shown to occur experimentally in animals when the reduced enamel epithelium has been surgically removed from unerupted teeth. A similar layer can also be induced on top of enamel by enamel matrix alone.

Cellular (secondary, CIFC) cementum

Following the formation of acellular cementum in the cervical portion of the root, cellular cementum appears in the apical region of the root at about the time the tooth erupts. Cellular cementum is also formed in the furcation area of the cheek teeth. This type of cementum is associated with an increase in the rate of formation of the tissue. The early inductive changes associated with the development of odontoblasts and dentine appear to be similar to those described for acellular cementum. However, following the loss of continuity of the epithelial root sheath, large basophilic cells are seen to differentiate from the adjacent cells of the dental follicle against the surface of the root dentine (or acellular cementum). These cells form a more distinct cuboidal layer of cementoblasts adjacent to the root surface. They generally possess more cytoplasm and more cytoplasmic processes than the cells associated with the formation of acellular cementum. The basophilia at the light microscope level corresponds to roughened endoplasmic reticulum at the ultrastructural level (Fig. 25.33). This indicates that the cementoblasts secrete the collagen (together with ground substance) that forms the intrinsic fibres of the cellular cementum (CIFC). These fibres are oriented parallel to the root surface and do not extend into the periodontal ligament. Associated with the increased rate of formation, a thin unmineralised precementum layer (about 5 μm thick) will be present on the surface of cellular cementum (Fig. 25.34). Mineralisation in the deeper layer of the precementum occurs in a linear manner, but overall this type of cementum is less mineralised than acellular cementum. As in bone, the multipolar mode of matrix secretion by the cementoblasts and its increased rate of formation result in cells becoming incorporated into the forming matrix, and these are converted into cementocytes. Unlike bone, cementocytes lying deeply within cementum may be nonviable, and this is likely to occur when their distance from the surface exceeds that required for the diffusion of nutrients.

As the chemical composition of acellular and cellular cementum differs, it is assumed that this reflects differences in the secretory activity of the cells involved. Thus, dentine sialoprotein, fibronectin and tenascin, as well as various proteoglycans (e.g., versican, decorin and biglycan), are present in cellular cementum but not acellular cementum. This may be related to

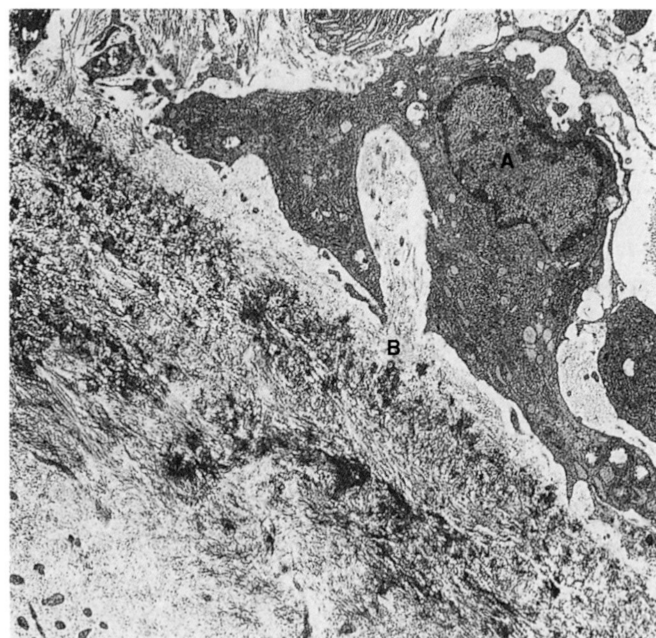

Fig. 25.33 TEM of decalcified root surface showing cementoblast (A) associated with the formation of cellular cementum. The cell is typically more irregular in morphology and contains larger amounts of the intracellular organelles associated with protein synthesis and secretion (such as endoplasmic reticulum). B = precementum (×4,000). Courtesy Dr P D A Owens.

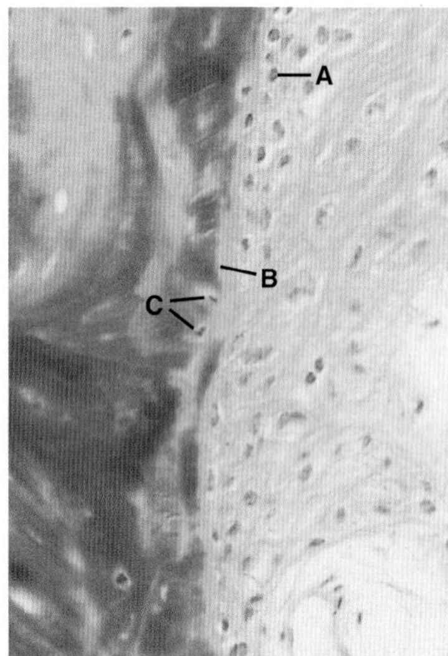

Fig. 25.34 Section of decalcified root surface showing cellular cementum formation. A = cementoblasts; B = precementum; C = cementocytes becoming incorporated into the cementum matrix (Masson's trichrome; ×230).

the presence of cementocytes, as many of the proteoglycans are located at the periphery of the lacunae and canaliculi.

The incorporation of cementocytes, as with the osteocytes of bone, necessitates the generation of new cementoblasts from stem cells/precursors within the periodontal ligament. Progenitor cells are present within the periodontal ligament, particularly around blood vessels, and must migrate through the periodontal ligament to the cementum surface. Some of these cells may represent true stem cells, having the characteristics of both self-renewal and multilineage differential potential. Other cells having the power to differentiate into cementoblasts may migrate in from the stroma of the adjacent alveolar bone.

Incremental lines will be present in cellular cementum but, because of the increased rate of formation, are more widely spaced than in acellular cementum. The stages in the formation of cellular intrinsic fibre cementum are illustrated in Fig. 25.35.

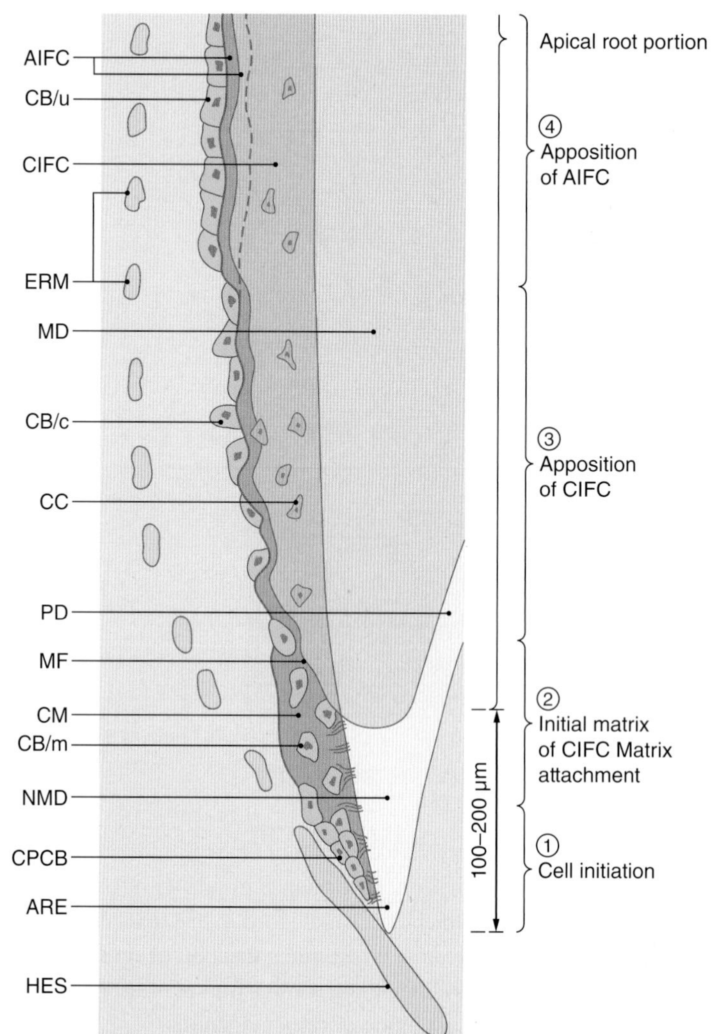

Fig. 25.35 The initial stages of the formation of cellular intrinsic fibre cementum (CIFC) for human premolars that have developed 75% of their final root length. 1 = Committed clone of precementoblasts contacts root predentine and produces first matrix fibrils. 2 = Cementoblasts form initial collagenous matrix attached to predentine. 3 = First-formed and mineralised CIFC (including cementocytes) grows by apposition. 4 = CIFC is covered with a layer of acellular intrinsic fibre cementum. AIFC = acellular intrinsic fibre cementum; CB/u = cementoblasts with unipolar matrix production; ERM = epithelial cell rests of Malassez; MD = mineralised dentine; CB/c = cementoblasts with potential to become cementocytes; CC = cementocytes; PD = predentine; MF = mineralisation front; CM = initial cementum matrix; CB/m = cementoblasts with multipolar matrix production; NMD = nonmineralised dentine or predentine; CPCB = committed precementoblasts; ARE = advancing root edge; HES = Hertwig's epithelial root sheath. Courtesy Prof. H E Schroeder, D D Bosshardt and the editors of *Cell and Tissue Research*.

Cellular cementum is usually present as the intrinsic fibre type (see Chapter 11). This type of cementum does not act in a supportive role, as no Sharpey's fibres from the periodontal ligament are inserted into it. However, most commonly in the apical and the furcation areas of human cheek teeth, this type of cementum alternates with layers of acellular extrinsic fibre cementum to form what is called *cellular mixed stratified cementum* (see Fig. 11.22A). The layers may be present in various combinations and in various thicknesses. When a layer of AEFC is covered by a layer of CIFC, there must be a functional change, as the Sharpey's fibres over the affected portion of the root will largely be detached from the root surface. Conversely, when CIFC is covered by a layer of AEFC, Sharpey's fibres will gain an attachment to the tooth.

An additional type of cementum is cellular mixed fibre cementum. In this variety, the normal cellular intrinsic cementum does give attachment to some extrinsic fibres arising from the periodontal ligament (see Fig. 11.23).

As mentioned for acellular cementum, the precise origin of the cells in the dental follicle associated with the formation of cellular cementum awaits clarification. The possibility exists that different cell populations

Table 25.1 Possible phenotypic differences between cementoblasts associated with acellular and cellular cementum

Cementoblasts from acellular cementum	Cementoblasts from cellular cementum
Identifiable for only a short time	Identifiable for longer period
Fibroblast-like morphology	Osteoblast-like morphology
Derived from epithelial root sheath	Derived from mesenchyme
Express cytokeratin	Do not express cytokeratin
Do not express osteocalcin	Express osteocalcin
Do not express receptors for parathormone	Express receptors for parathormone
Do not express TGF-β and IGF	Express TGF-β and IGF
Do not react with E11 antibody	React with E11 antibody

E11 antibody = a marker reacting with osteoblasts and young osteocytes; IGF = insulin-like growth factor; TGF = transforming growth factor.

are responsible for the formation of the two types of cementum. Evidence is building up to suggest that the cells associated with acellular and cellular cementum do show different phenotypes; some of these are listed in Table 25.1. If this suggestion is correct, then during the formation of cellular mixed stratified cementum, there is a switch from one formative cell to another. Because of the similarity between osteoblasts and cementoblasts, it has been suggested that stem/progenitor cells primarily associated with alveolar bone could migrate into the periodontal ligament and provide a source of new cementoblasts.

Alveolar bone development

The mandible and maxillae develop intramembranously. Thus, a centre of ossification appears in a fibrocellular condensation in which osteoblasts lay down first-formed embryonic or woven bone. As the teeth develop, bone extends from the developing mandible and maxillae to surround and protect the teeth, forming the alveolus (see Fig. 19.4). The alveolus is separated from the developing enamel organ by the dental follicle (see Fig. 21.10). To accommodate the growing tooth germs, the lamellae of the developing alveolar bone undergo resorption on the inner wall of the alveolus (indicated by Howship's lacunae) while, on the outer wall of the alveolus, bone is deposited (indicated by osteoblasts lining an osteoid seam). The developing teeth therefore come to lie in a trough of bone. Later, the teeth become separated from each other by the development of interdental septa. With the onset of root formation, interradicular bone develops in multirooted teeth. As in other sites, the collagen fibres in the newly formed alveolar bone have a more variable diameter and lack a preferential orientation, giving the bone a matted (basket weave) appearance when viewed in polarised light. This immature bone, termed *woven bone*, has larger and more numerous osteocytes than adult bone. It is formed more rapidly and has a higher turnover rate. Woven bone is subsequently converted to fine-fibred adult lamellar bone. The source of the cells forming alveolar bone is uncertain, although some have suggested that it may be from neural crest cells of the investing layer of the dental follicle (see Fig. 21.10).

During crown formation, relocation of the tooth germ within the growing jaws may be associated with appropriate patterns of resorption and deposition on the internal surfaces of the alveolar bone. With the onset of tooth eruption, the bone overlying the tooth undergoes resorption to provide a pathway of eruption (see pages 457–458). In addition, as the tooth erupts and the jaws increase in size, bone deposition is prominent in the region of the alveolar crest. The predominant activity in the fundus of the socket is one of bone resorption, except for teeth whose eruptive pathway is greater than the length of the root (see pages 456–457). On occasions where bone deposition is seen lining the alveolus, it may be related to relocation of the erupting tooth within the growing jaws. Sharpey's fibres from the periodontal ligament become attached to the wall of the alveolus during tooth eruption, although the timing is related to whether the tooth is of the primary or secondary dentition (see page 439). The bone of the alveolar wall may then be referred to as *bundle bone* (see page 277).

Comparison of alveolar bone and cementum

Having described aspects of the formation of cementum and alveolar bone, and with previous knowledge of their structure (see Chapters 11 and 13), it is possible to compare and contrast some of their principal features. In comparing alveolar bone and cellular cementum:

- Both tissues have a similar composition, being composed of an inorganic component of small hydroxyapatite crystals and an organic component consisting principally of type I collagen fibres and a smaller noncollagenous component. However, the noncollagenous component may be distinguished by the presence of specific components (e.g., cementum has cementum attachment protein).
- Both tissues have a lag phase in the mineralisation such that the surface is lined by a layer of unmineralised matrix: the osteoid and precementum layers.
- Both alveolar bone and cellular cementum display three similar cell types: osteocytes/cementocytes, osteoblasts/cementoblasts and osteoclasts/odontoclasts. However, compared with osteocytes, cementocytes are scattered less uniformly within cementum and their canaliculi are preferentially oriented towards the periodontal ligament (see Fig. 11.11).
- Bone remodelling is continuous throughout life, and osteoclasts are always evident. In cementum, resorption is a rarer and more localised event and the presence of odontoclasts is much less common.
- Unlike cementum, alveolar bone contains blood vessels, nerves and marrow spaces.
- Osteocytes may be arranged circumferentially as Haversian systems around central Haversian vessels. The orientation of collagen fibres in this situation is more complex than in cementum (see Fig. 13.7).
- The initial mineralisation of bone involves matrix vesicles, whereas initial mineralisation of cementum does not, and this may be the result of the prior presence of mineralised dentine.
- When exposed to similar orthodontic loading, alveolar bone will resorb preferentially.

When alveolar bone is compared with acellular cementum:

- Unlike alveolar bone, acellular cementum lacks the presence of a precementum layer and the presence of any cementocytes because of its slower rate of formation.
- Alveolar bone and acellular cementum both have Sharpey's fibres from the periodontal ligament inserted into them, providing attachment for the tooth. In acellular cementum, however, these extrinsic fibres form the sole source of collagen, there being few, if any, intrinsic fibres.

Experimental studies relating to root development

Considerable information exists concerning epithelial–mesenchymal interactions in the crown, particularly concerning the roles of transcription factors, cytokines and growth hormones (see pages 388–394).

Far less is known about the presence and functions of such molecules during root formation. However, molecules such as the transcription factors Msx2 and Dlx2, bone morphogenetic proteins (BMPs), epidermal growth factor and transforming growth factor (TGF)-β have all been identified during the epithelial–mesenchymal interactions associated with root development. Their importance can be seen from experiments in which inhibition of the activity of BMP in transgenic mice results in root abnormalities.

Experiments have shown that when a tooth germ at the early bell stage is dissected from the jaw, it is surrounded by the inner investing layer of the dental follicle (thought to be of neural crest/ectomesenchyme origin; see page 383). When the tooth germ is transplanted in this condition, the investing layer has the capacity to give rise to all the investing tissues (i.e., cementum, periodontal ligament and bone). This, however, does not preclude a contribution to the periodontium in vivo from the outer part of the dental follicle. When the dental follicle cells are excluded and the enamel organ and dental papilla alone are transplanted to an ectopic site, there is regeneration of the investing layer of the dental follicle and formation of cementum and the root-related periodontal ligament, but no formation of alveolar bone. Combined with other studies, this indicates that dental papilla mesenchymal cells in the region of the root apex, in addition to being a source of odontoblasts, provide an important reservoir of cells that migrate out into the dental follicle and may give rise to cells such as cementoblasts and periodontal fibroblasts.

The importance of the epithelial root sheath in the differentiation of root odontoblasts is indicated by experimental recombinations between isolated epithelial root sheath cells and dental papilla cells. Such studies demonstrate that root dentine will form only in the presence of the epithelial root sheath. One question that arises relates to whether the presence of root dentine alone is sufficient to induce dental follicle cells to become cementoblasts or whether the epithelial root sheath contributes to the process. This has been tested by experimental recombinations of slices of root dentine and dental follicle cells with and without the presence of epithelial root sheath cells. Although a cementum-like tissue is formed on root dentine in both cases, this tissue separates relatively easily from the dentine in the absence of epithelial root sheath cells. This supports the view that the epithelial root sheath plays an important role in early cementogenesis in firmly uniting the cement and dentine together via the presence of the hyaline layer. This may relate particularly to its secretion of enamel-related proteins.

During root formation, numerous growth factors and transcription factors, such as Shh, BMP, and Msx, are extensively expressed in the dental epithelium and mesenchyme. It is well known that Wnt/β-catenin signalling plays multiple roles in various stages of tooth morphogenesis and that during dentine formation Wnt10a is expressed in odontoblast-lineage cells. To assess the importance of Wnt during root formation, mice mutants were developed that had tissue-specific inactivation of β-catenin, an obligatory transducer of canonical Wnt signalling. In such mutants, the roots of molar teeth do not develop. At the beginning of root formation in the mutant molars, the cervical loop epithelium extends apically to form Hertwig's epithelial root sheath, but root odontoblast differentiation is disrupted and followed by the loss of some inner layer cells of the root sheath. The outer layer of the root sheath extends without the root, and the mutant molars erupt (Fig. 25.36). The periodontal tissues extensively invaded the dental pulp. These results indicate the importance of Wnt/β-catenin signalling in the dental mesenchyme for root formation.

Clinical considerations

Enamel pearls

These are small, isolated spheres of enamel that are occasionally found on the root surface, especially towards the cervical margin. They are particularly common in the root bifurcation area (Fig. 25.37, see also Fig. 7.74) but may also occur at lower levels (Fig. 25.38), usually (but not always) in interradicular regions. It is thought that in the region affected, stellate reticulum and stratum intermedium develop between the internal and external enamel epithelia of the root sheath. Enamel pearls may provide a site for the accumulation of plaque if exposed in the mouth.

Hypophosphatasia

Hypophosphatasia is a condition in which there is reduced activity of tissue-nonspecific alkaline phosphatase. It is a rare autosomal recessive disease in which there is a marked deficiency in the presence of both acellular and cellular cementum. The lack of attachment of periodontal ligament fibres to the residual cement is associated with premature loss of the deciduous teeth. In such patients, any orthodontic treatment is likely to be accompanied by the premature loss of any permanent teeth required to be moved.

Regeneration following chronic periodontal disease

The most important clinical condition affecting the periodontal ligament is chronic inflammatory periodontal disease, in which toxic products are released by dental plaque lying in the gingival crevice (see Chapter 8). Interacting with the host's defence mechanisms, including gingival crevicular fluid (see page 305), these products result in the destruction and loss of periodontal ligament tissue and adjacent alveolar bone. Such a process leads to the formation of a periodontal pocket, allowing for the accumulation of more plaque, and a vicious circle is established. The loss of attachment tissue may expose the root in the mouth and, with increasing mobility, the tooth may eventually be lost. When treating such a condition, the dental surgeon may consider two types of outcomes:

1) Repair the existing condition so that the disease progresses no further (previously involving surgical removal of diseased tissue)
2) Attempt to regenerate the lost tissues, restoring the bone, periodontal ligament and cementum to their original dimensions, including the reattachment of new periodontal ligament fibres to both the cementum and bone (see Chapter 28)

The cementum tissue needed during regeneration is acellular extrinsic fibre cementum in order to provide attachment to the periodontal fibres. To attempt to regenerate the attachment tissues, a detailed understanding of how each tissue develops normally is required, particularly the manner in which the cementum layer bonds firmly to the root dentine.

One common complication following surgery is the tendency for the junctional epithelium to proliferate rapidly downwards to cover the root surface, thereby preventing periodontal ligament fibres from fully attaching to cementum. Following periodontal surgery and the removal/cleansing of diseased tissue, a variety of methods of conditioning the root surface have been described that claim to improve the degree of reattachment of periodontal ligament fibres. Such methods include root planing and acid etching of the surface using various solutions (e.g., citric acid or ethylenediaminetetraacetic acid [EDTA]).

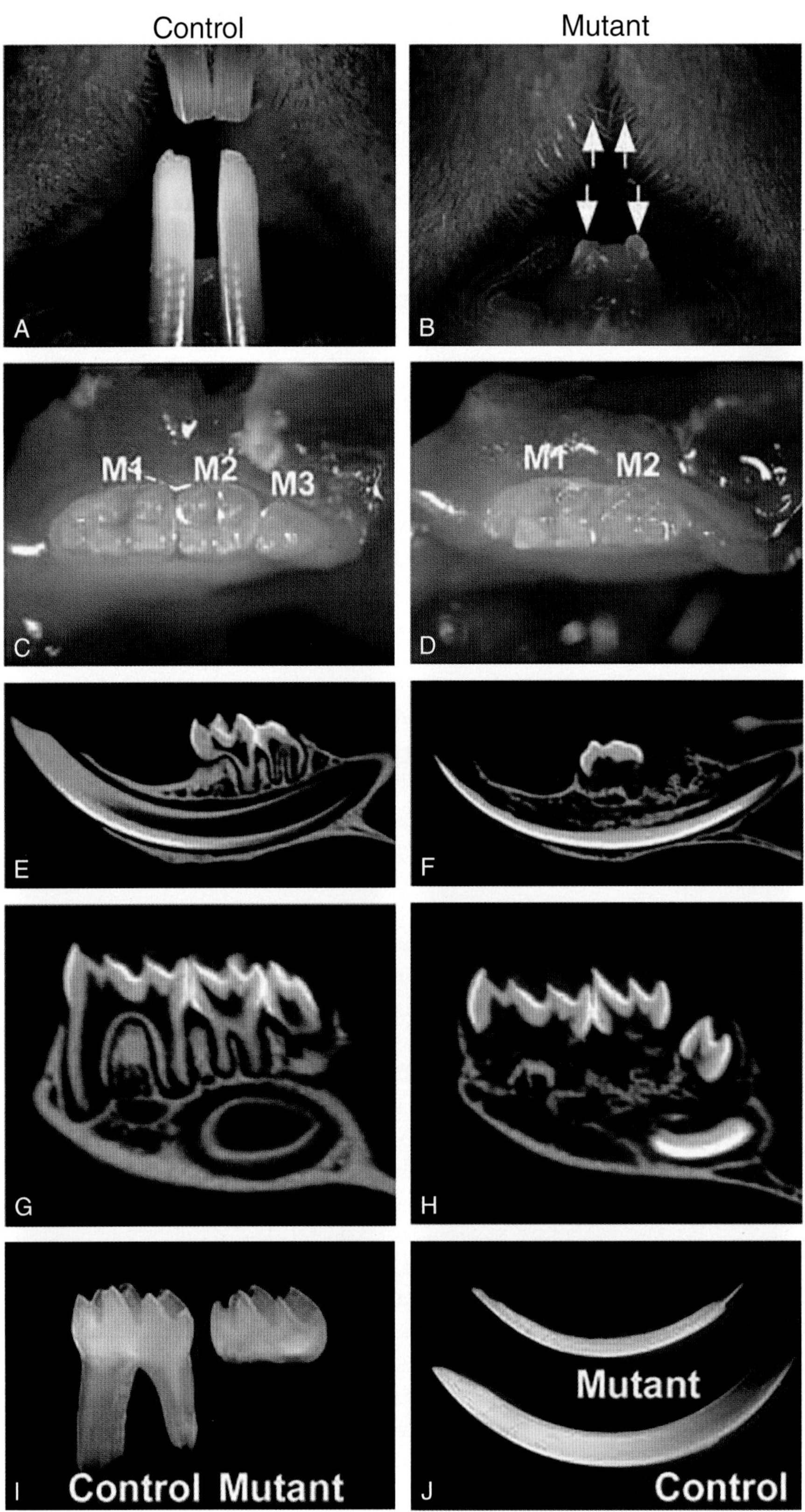

Fig. 25.36 Tomographic views of mandibles from control (G) and mutant mouse (H) with inactivation of β-catenin. Note the eruption of molars in the mutant which lack roots. (I–J) Stereoscopic appearance of the isolated mandibular first molar and incisor. From Kim, T.H., Bae, C.H., Lee, J.C., et al., 2013. β-catenin is required in odontoblasts for tooth root formation. *Journal of Dental Research* 9, 215–221.

Two surgical procedures may be used to repair or regenerate the periodontal ligament. The first is to place bone grafts or bone substitutes in a bony deficiency. The second procedure is termed 'guided tissue regeneration' and relates to the fact that, following initial periodontal surgery, the connective tissue of the wound may be repopulated by the gingiva growing down and/or by the periodontal ligament growing up. Present opinion suggests that the best result is achieved when the wound is repopulated by cells of the existing periodontal ligament. Although both connective tissues may appear to be similar, they differ in several respects, which may be important for the final outcome (Table 25.2). For this reason, the surgical technique of guided tissue regeneration has been developed to exclude the gingival tissues from the deeper part of the wound by placing a tissue barrier (resorbable or nonresorbable) over the alveolar crest. This is thought to allow the wound to be repopulated primarily by periodontal

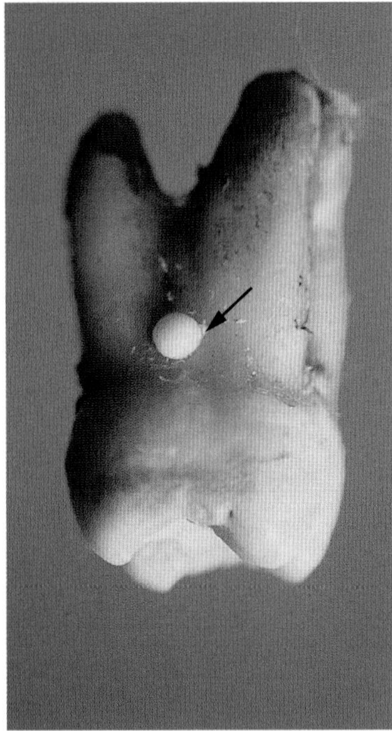

Fig. 25.37 An enamel pearl located near the root bifurcation area (arrow). Courtesy Dr. C Franklyn.

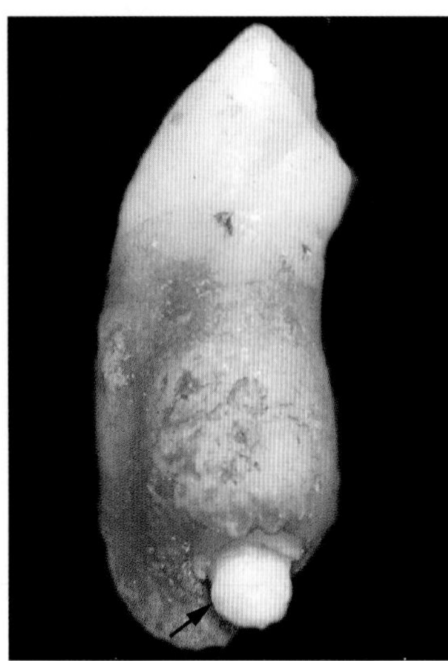

Fig. 25.38 An enamel pearl located near the root apex (arrow). Copyright the Royal College of Surgeons of England.

Table 25.2 Some features distinguishing fibroblasts from gingiva and periodontal ligament

		Gingiva	Periodontal ligament
Collagen type III		9%	20%
Collagen turnover		5 Weeks	1 Week
Cell volume		8%	40%
Ground substance		More	Less
Alkaline phosphatase		Less	More
Contractile proteins		Less	More
Prostaglandin release (in response to histamine)	*in vitro*	More	Less
Collagen production	*in vitro*	Less	More
Proliferation rates	*in vitro*	Lower	Higher
Collagen/Fibronectin positive	*in vitro*	57%	99%

ligament connective tissue. Both of these techniques do not appear to consistently provide periodontal regeneration, and they have been supplemented by the use or addition of bioactive molecules. These are agents produced by living tissue that help to induce the formation of the normal periodontal ligament.

A variety of bioactive molecules (e.g., growth factors; cytokines; and noncollagenous proteins such as bone sialoprotein, cementum-attachment protein and osteopontin) have been shown to be capable of inducing some or all of the normal components of the periodontal ligament in experimental animals. Some of these molecules (e.g., BMP) have been placed in suitable carriers within wounds and are claimed to improve the degree of periodontal ligament regeneration. However, difficulties encountered in interpreting results from such studies relate to the fact that the concentrations of the growth factor used far exceed physiological levels, and it is difficult to determine how long the factor is retained in an active form at the site. In addition, although reparative cementum may be formed, it may not be firmly attached to the root and may give little functional attachment to Sharpey's fibres.

The use of bioactive materials to improve periodontal regeneration is based on the rationale that materials found during normal development of the periodontal ligament might aid periodontal regeneration following periodontal disease. During normal development, the epithelial root sheath is important in the differentiation of root odontoblasts, as indicated by experimental recombinations between isolated epithelial root sheath cells and dental papilla cells. These studies demonstrate that root dentine will form only in the presence of the epithelial root sheath. Similar experimental recombinations of slices of root dentine and dental follicle cells, with or without epithelial root sheath cells, indicate that the epithelial root sheath cells play an important role in early cementogenesis by firmly uniting the cement and dentine via the presence of the hyaline layer. Emphasis has been placed on the findings that epithelial root sheath cells secrete enamel-related proteins that may be important in cementogenesis, although the amount secreted and their significance are in dispute. Nevertheless, it has been reported that treating the surgically cleaned root surface of periodontally affected teeth with enamel matrix derivatives (obtained from porcine enamel and commercially available, such as Emdogain®) has a positive effect on periodontal regeneration (Fig. 25.39). The main component is amelogenin (although there may be a small component containing growth factors), and there is a considerable literature suggesting good regeneration of the periodontal ligament is obtained when combining guided tissue regeneration with the application of Emdogain or other growth factors such as human platelet–derived growth factor. The principles of tissue engineering are now been applied to investigate the feasibility of assembling a construct in the laboratory that could be placed against a surgically prepared root surface and that would be able to regenerate cementum, periodontal ligament and alveolar bone in a functional setting. For this to succeed, appropriate stem/precursor cells will need to be seeded in a suitable three-dimensional scaffold, incorporating any necessary growth factors and signalling molecules. Owing to its cellular heterogeneity, tissue engineering a periodontal ligament is unlikely to be easy (see Chapter 28). Using nanotechnology, it might be possible to seed on the root surface selected precursor cells with a phenotype associated with cells forming acellular cementum, while precursor cells adjacent to the bone surface would have a phenotype associated with osteoblasts. The centrally positioned cells would have a phenotype of periodontal fibroblasts and be able to produce the necessary collagen fibre bundles. Primary cell cultures used at early passages retain the functional heterogeneity of the ligament cells, which is lost in cells at late passages. The construct would have to be immunocompatible with the patient, with the cells used being autologous stem cells derived from the patient's premolar or molar teeth. Characteristics of the stem cells may change according to the developmental/functional state of the teeth. Some of the growth factors and signalling molecules could be provided by the cells themselves if they had undergone genetic manipulation.

Assessment of clinical studies

There is extensive literature involving both animal and human studies that assesses the value of the experimental procedures outlined earlier on the outcome of periodontal surgery. For animal experimentation, an important question is how closely the 'model' resembles human chronic inflammatory periodontal disease. In particular, how are we to evaluate the conclusions reached by these studies in attempting to improve surgical outcomes? For example, there are many research papers apparently indicating that etching of the root surface improves the chances of reattaching periodontal ligament fibres to the tooth.

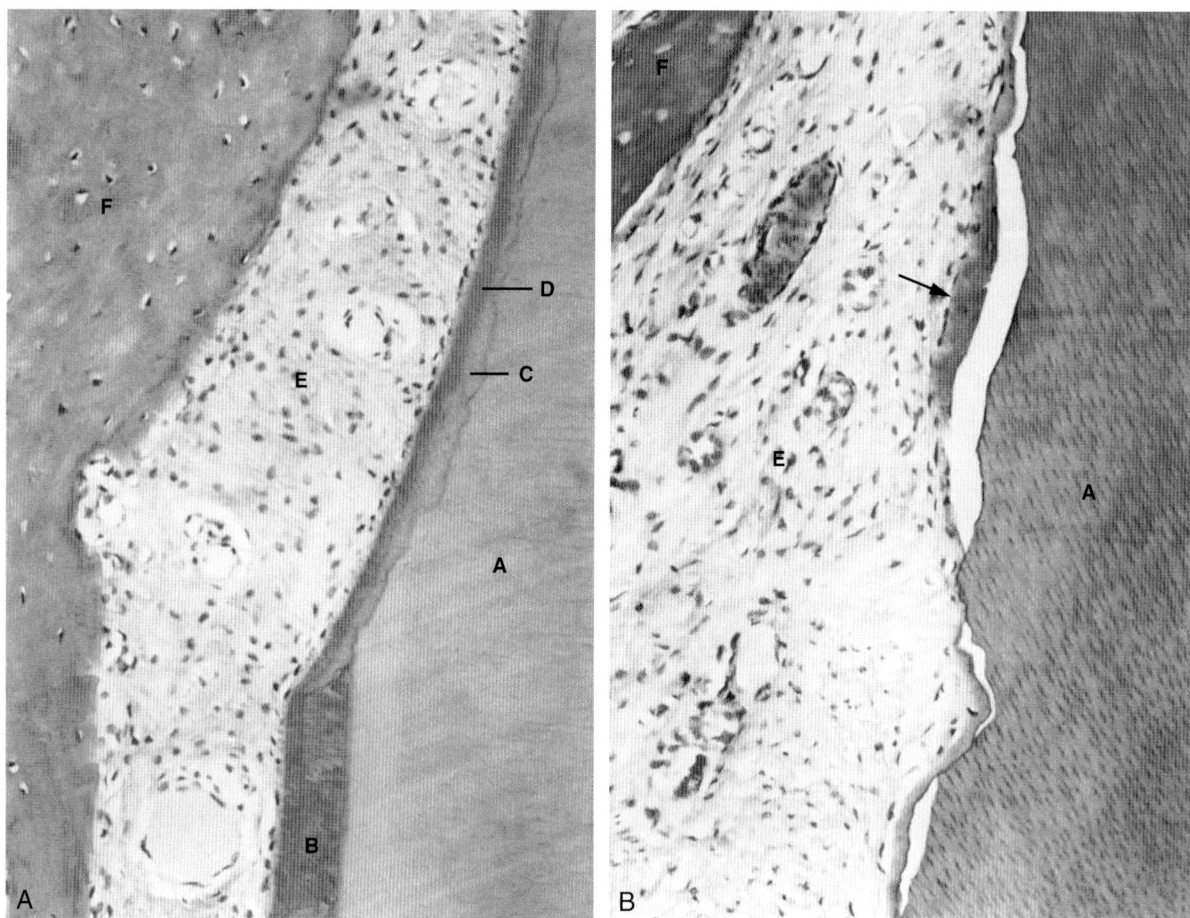

Fig. 25.39 Experimental cavities in the roots of lateral mandibular incisors of a monkey. The incisors were gently extracted, and the experimental cavities were made by means of a round burr under constant irrigation with physiological saline. Porcine enamel matrix was then applied in one of the cavities (Fig. 25.39[A]) after which the incisor was immediately replanted. The other incisor (Fig. 25.39[B]) served as control, and nothing was placed in the cavity of this tooth before it was replanted. Eight weeks after the replantation, the cavity (Fig. 25.39[A]) where enamel matrix had been placed is covered by a layer of acellular cementum. The cavity in the control tooth (Fig. 25.39[B]) is covered by a cellular hard tissue poorly attached to the dentine (arrow) (H & E; ×150). A = dentine; B = original acellular cementum; C = new regenerated acellular cementum; D = new cellular reparative cementum; E = periodontal ligament; F = bone. From Hammarstrom, L., 1997. Enamel matrix, cementum development and regeneration. *Journal of Clinical Periodontology* 24, 658–668.

Because of the complex bacteriology, the associated inflammation and the immune factors of the host response, periodontal disease is complex and multifactorial, and the combination of factors leading to disease is likely to differ among patients, making comparisons of treatment regimens difficult.

Surgical techniques are unlikely to be identical in different patients in the same study and between studies. There are patient-related factors (e.g., smoking, dental hygiene) and site-related factors (e.g., defect morphology, gingival biotype) that also complicate the interpretation of results.

Cochrane reviews

Cochrane reviews are publications aiming to provide the best available information concerning health care interventions. Their stated aim is to critically appraise the evidence for and against the effectiveness and appropriateness of treatments associated with clinical trials. Meta-analyses, in which data from studies are combined, have been used to test the assumption of similarity between studies (homogeneity) and the possible effects of bias (or other variables) on the outcome. The complete reviews are published in the Cochrane Library, available on the internet. As such, analytical methods are highly developed in Cochrane reviews, and they act as part of the quality assurance process of research. Cochrane reviews have been published in relation to aspects of periodontal regeneration.

Cochrane reviews have shown that the size of the difference between regenerative techniques and nonregenerative (conventional) surgery might be influenced in part by bias in patient selection and/or operator or examiner blinding. Indeed, the analyses show that apparently similar types of patients and procedures give rise to wider variations in treatment outcomes than would be expected by chance. Although there is some evidence suggesting the possible role of bias in this variability, it could also be related to severity of disease, presence of plaque and surgical skill, although there is a paucity of information about these factors. In consequence, care should be taken about citing only the summary meta-analysis value from systematic reviews.

Publication bias could be inflating the difference between test and control groups, with a tendency towards more frequent publication of studies with positive outcomes than those showing no difference between groups. Another limitation of the data presented in the systematic reviews is the measurement of effectiveness or success of treatment employed in the studies. This is almost always based on determining any change in features such as pocket depth (by clinical probing), clinical attachment level, tooth mobility and radiological assessment of new alveolar bone deposition. However, the relationship between such changes and true patient benefits (such as tooth retention) is not clear. It is also noteworthy that such changes may not reflect histological regeneration, and it is obvious that histological examination is not possible.

To date, the Cochrane reviews related to periodontal surgery indicate that surgery combined with guided tissue regeneration, enamel matrix proteins or bone allograft appears to result in improved clinical outcomes compared with surgery without such adjuncts. Heterogeneity between studies in these analyses is usually substantial, with a range of treatment outcomes varying from favourable to unfavourable. The degree of unpredictability is also highlighted by the calculation of the numbers needed to treat (NNT) value. This statistic indicates how many individuals would need to be treated to achieve a defined benefit. For two systematic reviews, the NNT is based upon the chance of the regenerative surgery achieving at least 2 mm more probing attachment gain than conventional surgery. This threshold is used both because it should represent a greater change than measurement error and also for convenience, as this threshold is often reported in the primary trials. The NNT for enamel matrix proteins is six. This means that for every six patients treated, one will gain this degree of advantage over conventional surgery and five will not. For guided tissue regeneration, the NNT is eight. Root conditioning with citric acid, EDTA or tetracycline is shown not to be an effective treatment.

In view of the potential impact of bias and variability on these results, it is reasonable to conclude that, comparing the benefit of surgery with adjuncts over conventional surgery, both the size and the predictability of achieving a benefit are uncertain.

Further readings for this chapter can be found in the accompanying eBook. Explore online Self-assessment quiz to test and reinforce your understanding of the material in your free ebook. Follow instructions in the Inside Front Cover to unlock your access.

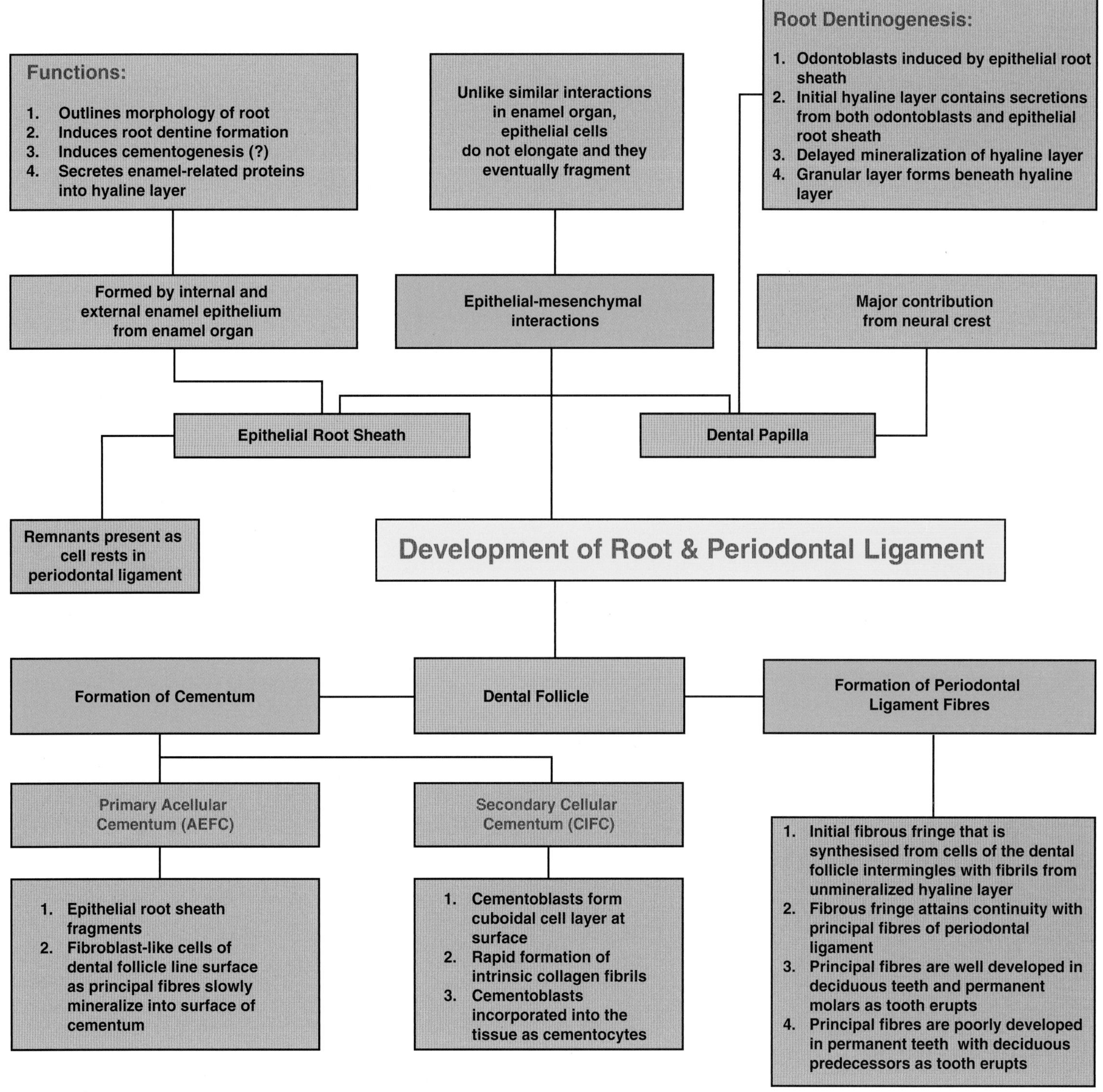
Root Dentinogenesis:
1. Odontoblasts induced by epithelial root sheath
2. Initial hyaline layer contains secretions from both odontoblasts and epithelial root sheath
3. Delayed mineralization of hyaline layer
4. Granular layer forms beneath hyaline layer
Functions:
1. Outlines morphology of root
2. Induces root dentine formation
3. Induces cementogenesis (?)
4. Secretes enamel-related proteins into hyaline layer
Unlike similar interactions in enamel organ, epithelial cells do not elongate and they eventually fragment
Formed by internal and external enamel epithelium from enamel organ
Epithelial-mesenchymal interactions
Major contribution from neural crest
Epithelial Root Sheath
Dental Papilla
Remnants present as cell rests in periodontal ligament
Development of Root & Periodontal Ligament
Formation of Cementum
Dental Follicle
Formation of Periodontal Ligament Fibres
Primary Acellular Cementum (AEFC)
Secondary Cellular Cementum (CIFC)
1. Epithelial root sheath fragments
2. Fibroblast-like cells of dental follicle line surface as principal fibres slowly mineralize into surface of cementum
1. Cementoblasts form cuboidal cell layer at surface
2. Rapid formation of intrinsic collagen fibrils
3. Cementoblasts incorporated into the tissue as cementocytes
1. Initial fibrous fringe that is synthesised from cells of the dental follicle intermingles with fibrils from unmineralized hyaline layer
2. Fibrous fringe attains continuity with principal fibres of periodontal ligament
3. Principal fibres are well developed in deciduous teeth and permanent molars as tooth erupts
4. Principal fibres are poorly developed in permanent teeth with deciduous predecessors as tooth erupts

Mind Map 25.1 Development of Root and Periodontal Ligament.

26 Development of the dentitions

Introduction

Description of the development of the dentitions requires consideration of the processes of tooth eruption and of the development of occlusion posteruptively. Three distinct phases of tooth development can be recognised that ultimately lead to the establishment of the full dentition. First, there is a phase termed the *pre-eruptive phase*, which starts with the initiation of tooth development and ends with the completion of the crown (see Chapter 21). Second, there is the phase of tooth eruption (*prefunctional phase*), which begins once the roots commence to form. Third, after the teeth have emerged into the oral cavity, there is a protracted phase concerned with the development, and maintenance, of occlusion (the *functional phase*).

Tooth eruption

Eruption is the process whereby a tooth moves axially from its developmental position within the alveolar crypt of the jaw into its functional position within the oral cavity. It is a remarkable event in that nowhere else in the body does a developing organ (in this case a tooth) leave the confines of its developing intrabony location. Although the definition of eruption suggests that eruption is entirely a developmental process, there is no evidence to suggest that eruption entirely ceases once a tooth meets its antagonist in the mouth, and outward axial movements occurring during the functional phase may also be eruptive movements (i.e., overeruption following removal of the antagonist tooth in the opposite jaw and compensatory eruption relating to attrition). It is sometimes suggested that the eruptive forces that are generated during the prefunctional (intraosseous) phase and functional (supraosseous and supragingival) phase are produced by different mechanisms. However, there is no experimental evidence to support this view, and it seems hardly likely from basic biological principles that similar axial eruptive movements would require two separate mechanisms.

Throughout the pre-eruptive phase of tooth development, there is concentric growth of the tooth within its follicle without any active bodily movement in a direction indicating eruption towards the oral cavity (Fig. 26.1). For a permanent mandibular second molar, there are two stages of active eruption (Fig. 26.2): the first stage occurs between 6 and 12 years when the tooth emerges into the mouth; a later second stage occurs at about 16 years in association with the adolescent growth spurt.

While the main direction of the eruptive force is axial (i.e., related to the long axis of the tooth), movement also occurs in other planes, accounting for tilting and drifting. Eruption rates of teeth are greatest at the time of crown emergence. Rates also differ according to tooth type. Permanent maxillary first incisors are reported to erupt at about 1 mm/month; the rates for mandibular second premolars have been determined to be about 4.5 mm in 14 weeks. For permanent third molars, where space is available, eruption rates of 1 mm in 3 months have been recorded. In crowded dentitions, however, the eruption rate may be less than 1 mm in 6 months. Following the initial appearance of the tip of the tooth into the oral cavity, it takes about 1–2 years to reach the occlusal plane.

The rate of eruption represents a balance between forces tending to move the tooth into the mouth (eruptive force) and forces tending to prevent this movement (resistive force). Resistance may be produced by overlying soft tissues and alveolar bone, the viscosity of the surrounding periodontal ligament/dental follicle and occlusal forces. Thus, changes in the rate of tooth movement may be brought about by changes in either the eruptive forces and/or the resistive forces. At present, little is known about the nature, source and magnitude of either the eruptive or resistive forces

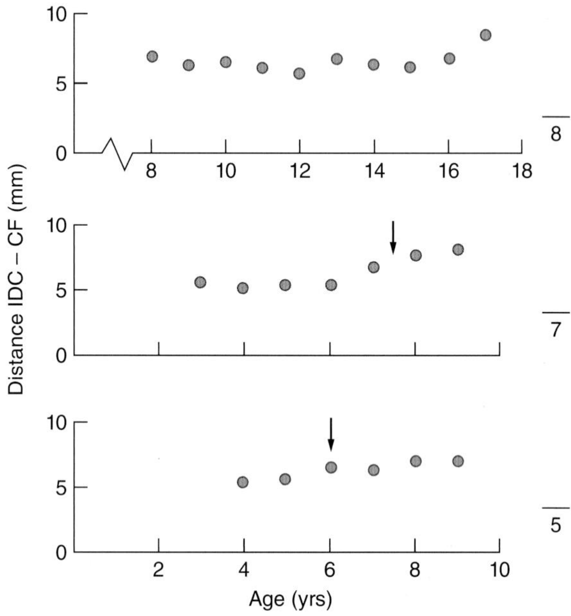

Fig. 26.1 Graphs plotting the mean distance from the mandibular canal (IDC) (regarded as a fixed point) to the centre of developing crowns of teeth during their pre-eruptive phase (CF). The upper graph is for a permanent mandibular third molar, the middle graph is for a permanent mandibular second molar, the lower graph is for a mandibular second premolar. Arrows indicate age at crown completion. Courtesy Dr. B G H Levers.

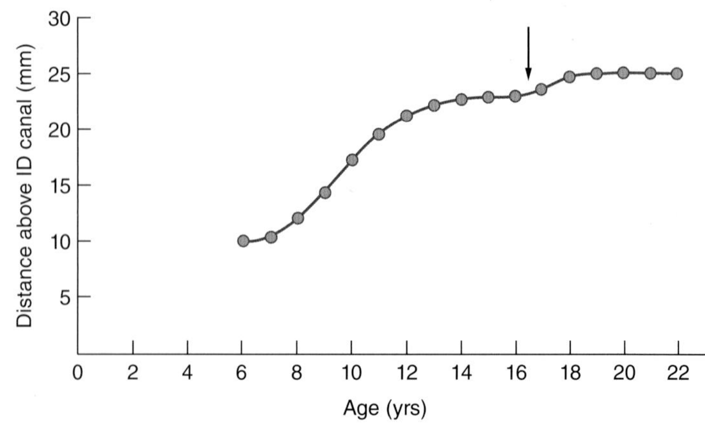

Fig. 26.2 Graph showing the mean distance from the mandibular canal (ID canal) to the occlusal surface for a permanent mandibular second molar during its eruption. Note the adolescent growth spurt (arrow). Courtesy Dr. B G H Levers.

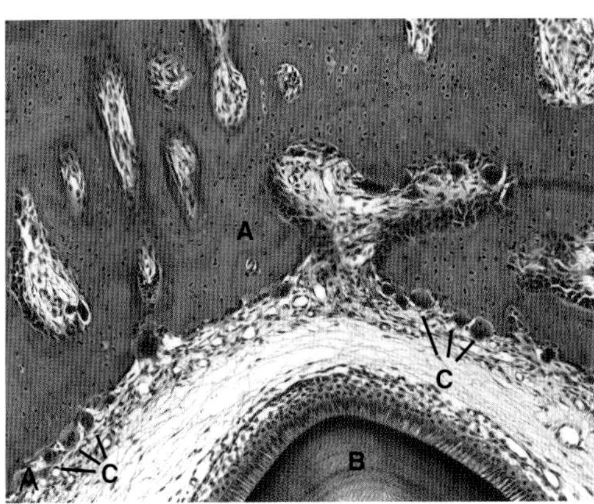

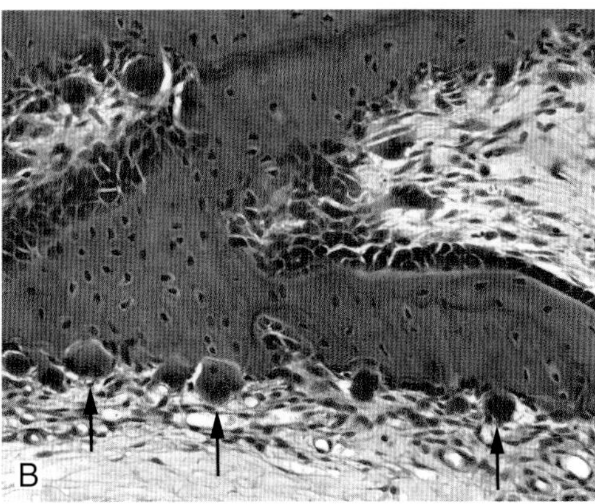

Fig. 26.3 (A) The alveolar bone (A) above the crown of an erupting tooth (B) is being resorbed by multinucleated osteoclasts (C) derived from the dental follicle. (B) High-power view of (A) showing osteoclasts (arrows) resorbing overlying alveolar bone. Courtesy Prof. T R Arnett.

(although only relatively small forces exerted by a spring are sufficient to stop a tooth erupting). Furthermore, it is not known whether the forces are of the same nature and magnitude at various stages of the eruptive cycle.

Although eruption commences at the time the root of the tooth begins to form, a growing root is not required for eruption to proceed (see page 461). The molecular events associated with the initiation of eruption are not well understood. There is evidence that epidermal growth factor (EGF) may be required and that there might also be an involvement of transforming growth factor (TGF)-α. Furthermore, macrophage colony–stimulating factor (MCSF) can induce tooth eruption. However, these growth factors can have different effects on different tooth types (incisor versus molar teeth). It has been proposed that bone deposition at the base of the developing root can initiate eruption and move the tooth axially. This is most obviously seen at the bases of erupting premolar teeth of dogs (see Fig. 25.17). However (and as mentioned on page 449), for most species there is little evidence of bone deposition beneath the base of the erupting tooth (see Fig. 25.16), with resorption often being evident. The different patterns of bone activity in different species may relate to the distance a tooth has to erupt: if the distance is much greater than the length of the root, then bone deposition is clearly necessary to maintain the normal dimensions of the periodontal ligament at the root apex of the tooth.

Undoubtedly, whatever initiates tooth eruption, and whatever generates the forces of eruption, remodelling of the alveolus is required to accommodate eruptive movements and to allow the tooth to move through the bone (via an eruptive pathway) towards the oral cavity. This will involve a complex and very well regulated process that recruits mononuclear cells that form osteoclasts for the resorption of the overlying alveolar bone (Fig. 26.3). The evidence indicates that complex signalling processes occur within and between the dental follicle and the tooth germ (Figs. 26.4, 26.5). Recruitment of mononuclear cells to the dental follicle around the erupting tooth seems to require MCSF and/or monocyte chemotactic protein (MCP)-1. The genesis of osteoclasts additionally involves inhibition of osteoprotegerin synthesis and increased receptor activator for NF-κB ligand (RANKL). From the tooth germ, signalling from the stellate reticulum of the enamel organ also appears to have a role in regulating eruption. This signalling seems to occur via parathyroid hormone–related protein and interleukin-1 (IL-1)α. EGF and TGF-β1 can also enhance the recruitment of mononuclear cells and osteoclastogenesis. Osteoblasts may influence the process of osteoclastogenesis through signalling via the RANKL/osteoprotegerin (OPG) pathway (see pages 272–275). Evidence indicates that an osteoblast transcription factor termed Cbfal (Runx2) might regulate tooth eruption and that this molecule is also expressed by the cells of the dental follicle. Note that the signalling pathways described suggest that there is a redundancy of function (e.g., both MCSF and MCP-1 act as chemokines for the recruitment of mononuclear cells to the dental follicle). Defects in bone resorption may therefore prevent eruption.

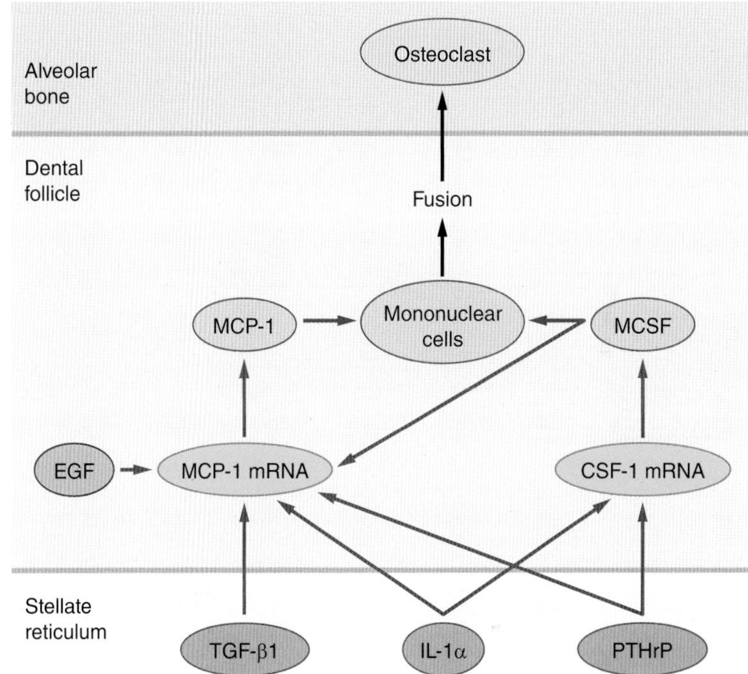

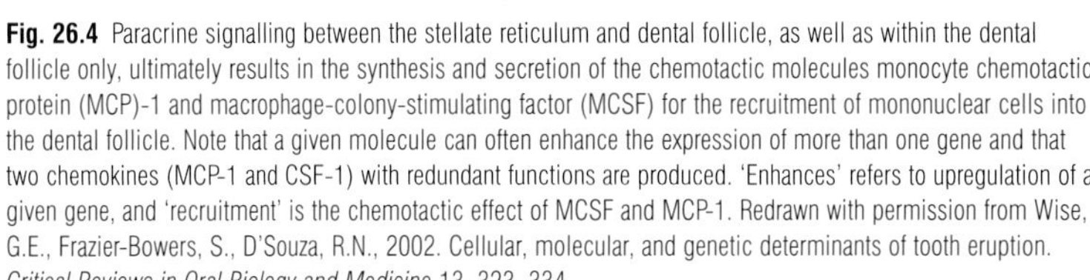

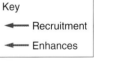

Fig. 26.4 Paracrine signalling between the stellate reticulum and dental follicle, as well as within the dental follicle only, ultimately results in the synthesis and secretion of the chemotactic molecules monocyte chemotactic protein (MCP)-1 and macrophage-colony-stimulating factor (MCSF) for the recruitment of mononuclear cells into the dental follicle. Note that a given molecule can often enhance the expression of more than one gene and that two chemokines (MCP-1 and CSF-1) with redundant functions are produced. 'Enhances' refers to upregulation of a given gene, and 'recruitment' is the chemotactic effect of MCSF and MCP-1. Redrawn with permission from Wise, G.E., Frazier-Bowers, S., D'Souza, R.N., 2002. Cellular, molecular, and genetic determinants of tooth eruption. *Critical Reviews in Oral Biology and Medicine* 13, 323–334.

As a tooth approaches the oral cavity, there are marked changes in the overlying soft tissues. The enamel surface is covered by the reduced enamel epithelium, which is a vestige of the enamel organ. Fig. 26.6 shows an erupting deciduous molar before its emergence into the oral cavity, and Fig. 26.7 is a higher-power view of the soft tissues overlying the enamel space of an erupting tooth. As the tooth erupts, the outer cells of the reduced enamel epithelium proliferate into the connective tissue between the cusp tip and the oral epithelium. It has been suggested that

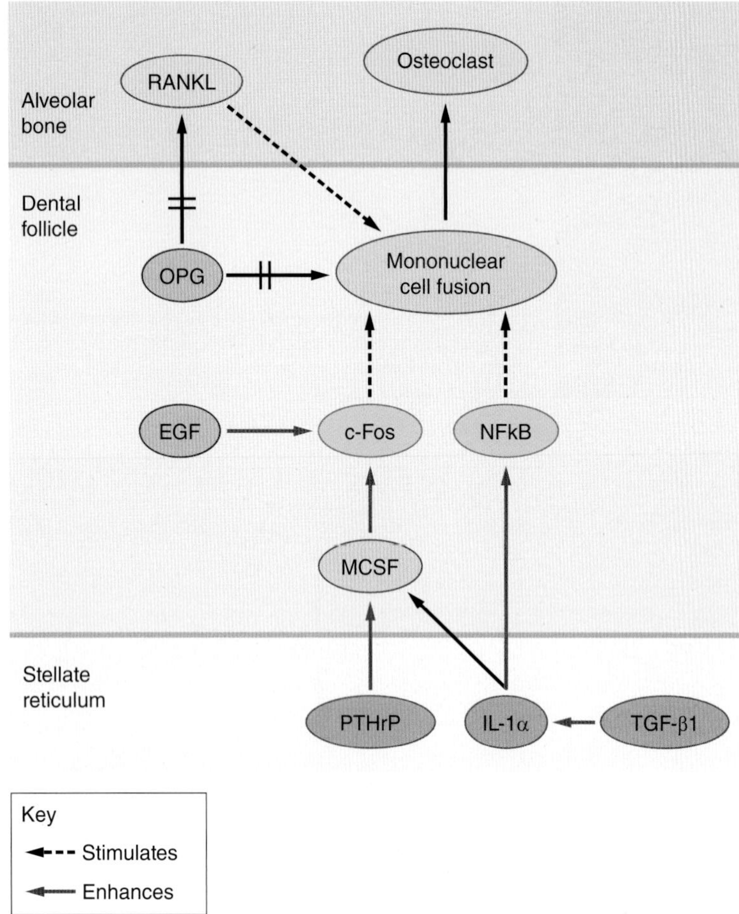

Fig. 26.5 Possible signalling cascades that may promote the fusion of the mononuclear cells recruited to the dental follicle. Both MCSF and receptor activator of nuclear factor kappa B ligand (NF-κB or RANKL) are known to promote osteoclast formation, whereas osteoprotegerin (OPG) inhibits this by preventing cell-to-cell signalling. The downstream products of the transcription factors c-Fos and NF-κB that promote osteoclast formation are not yet known. The crossed arrows with crosses (⇸) reflect inhibition of gene expression, whereas other arrows reflect enhancement of gene expression or stimulation of cell fusion. Redrawn with permission from Wise, G.E., Frazier-Bowers, S., D'Souza, R.N., 2002. Cellular, molecular, and genetic determinants of tooth eruption. *Critical Reviews in Oral Biology and Medicine* 13, 323–334.

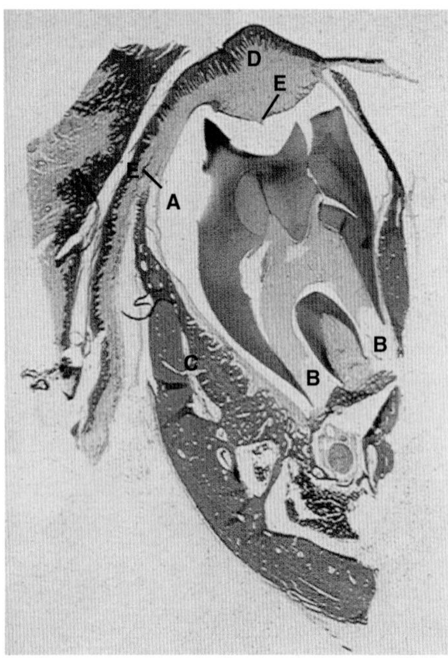

Fig. 26.6 An erupting deciduous molar before its emergence into the oral cavity. A = enamel space; B = developing roots; C = developing alveolar crypt; D = oral mucosa and overlying connective tissue; E = reduced enamel epithelium (decalcified, transverse section through the jaw; H & E; ×4).

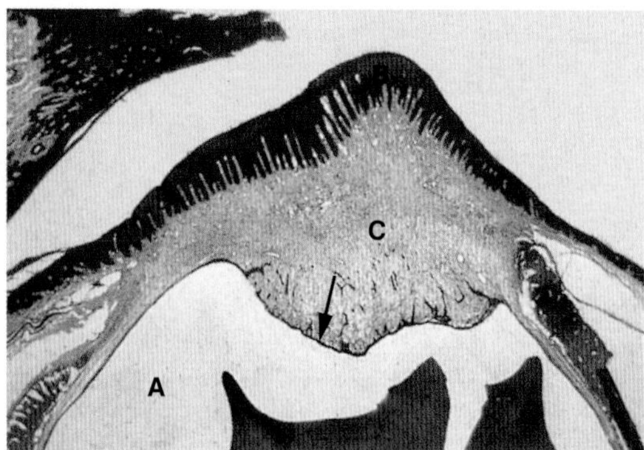

Fig. 26.7 The soft tissues overlying the enamel space (A) of an erupting tooth. B = oral epithelium; C = connective tissue between developing tooth and oral epithelium. Arrow indicates the reduced enamel epithelium (H & E; ×10).

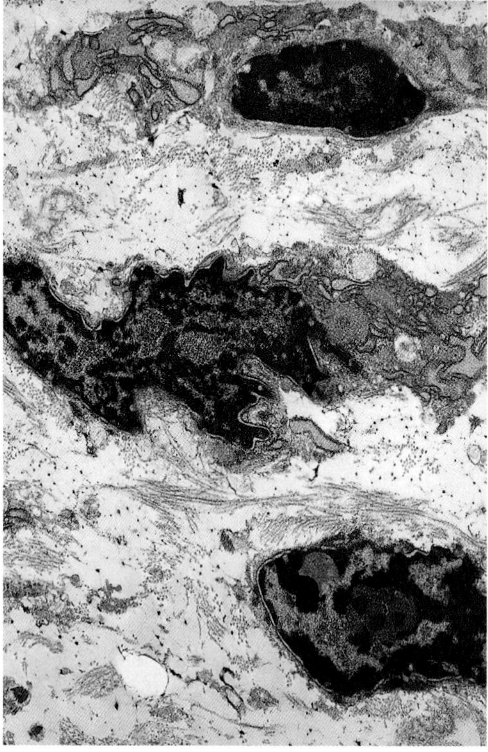

Fig. 26.8 Fibroblasts in the connective tissue overlying an erupting tooth showing evidence of degeneration (TEM; ×10,000).

these proliferating epithelial cells secrete enzymes that degrade collagen. Reduced enamel epithelial cells may also be concerned with the removal of breakdown products resulting from resorption of connective tissue. Depolymerisation of the nonfibrous components of the extracellular matrix has been detected in the connective tissue overlying erupting teeth. Although a relationship between the degeneration of the connective tissue and the pressure exerted by the underlying erupting tooth has not been established, ischaemia is thought to be a contributory factor. That pressure alone is not entirely responsible is indicated by the finding that there is always evidence of some new collagen formation in this region.

Many of the fibroblasts in the connective tissue overlying an erupting tooth cease fibrillogenesis, actively take up extracellular material (as evidenced by intracellular collagen profiles – see pages 238–239) and synthesise acid hydrolases. Eventually, the nuclei become pyknotic and the cells degenerate (Fig. 26.8).

The development of the dentogingival junction during the eruption of a tooth is shown diagrammatically in Fig. 26.9. As the tooth approaches the oral epithelium, the cells of the outer layer of the reduced enamel

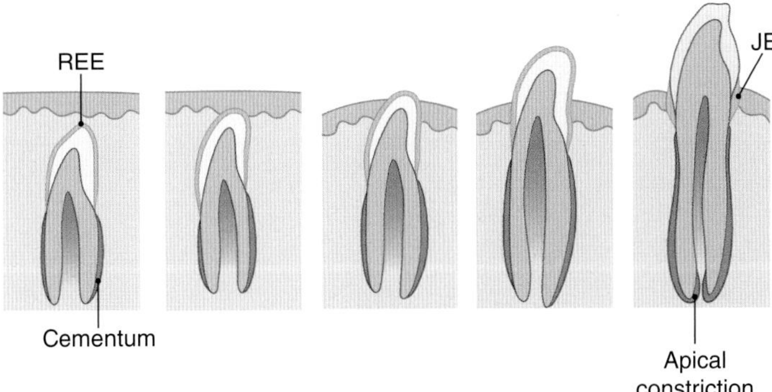

Fig. 26.9 Diagrammatic representation of the development of the dentogingival junction during the eruption of a tooth. REE = reduced enamel epithelium (blue). JE = junctional epithelium (blue). Pink outline delineates oral epithelium.

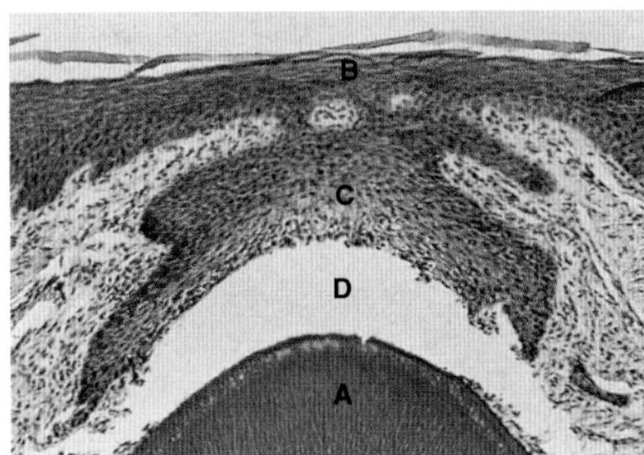

Fig. 26.10 An erupting tooth (A) about to emerge into the oral cavity through an epithelium-lined pathway as a result of fusion of the oral epithelium (B) and the reduced enamel epithelium (C). D = enamel space (H & E; ×12). Courtesy Prof. A G S Lumsden.

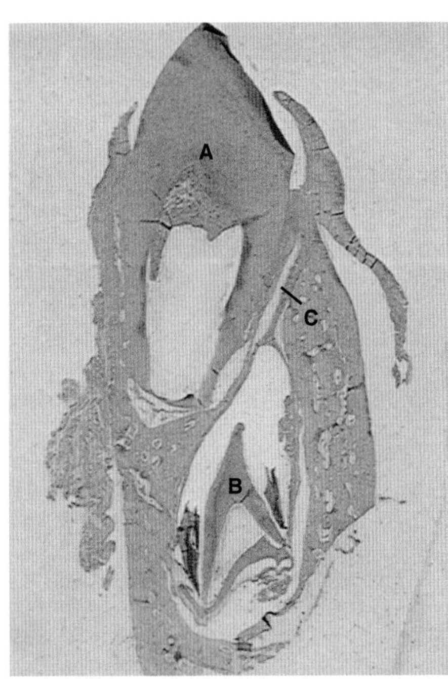

Fig. 26.11 Buccolingual section through an erupted deciduous canine (A) and its erupting successor (B). C = gubernacular canal (decalcified section; H & E; ×4).

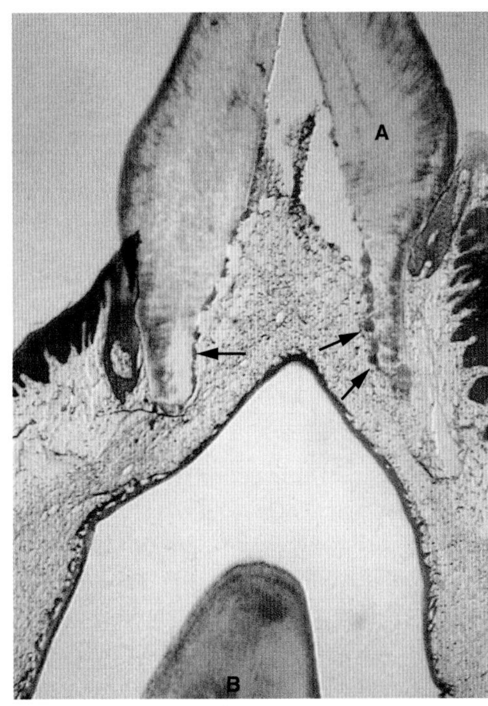

Fig. 26.12 Buccolingual section through a resorbing deciduous tooth (A) and its erupting successor (B). Arrows indicate multinucleated odontoclasts (decalcified section; Masson's trichrome; ×70).

epithelium and the basal layer of the oral epithelium actively proliferate and eventually unite. The epithelium covering the tip of the tooth then degenerates at its centre, enabling the crown to emerge through an epithelium-lined pathway into the oral cavity. Further emergence of the tooth results from active eruptive movements and passive separation of the oral epithelium from the crown surface. When the tooth first erupts into the mouth, the reduced enamel epithelium is attached to the unerupted part of the crown, thus forming an epithelial seal – the junctional epithelium (see pages 302–305). It is generally believed that the reduced enamel epithelial component of the junctional epithelium is eventually replaced by oral epithelium. With continued eruption, as more of the crown is exposed, a gingival crevice is formed. An erupting tooth about to emerge into the oral cavity through an epithelium-lined pathway as a result of fusion of the oral epithelium and the reduced enamel epithelium is shown in Fig. 26.10.

For the eruption of a permanent tooth, where there is a deciduous predecessor (i.e., excluding the permanent molars), the roots of the deciduous tooth must be resorbed to allow for shedding. Initially, each deciduous tooth and its developing permanent successor share a common alveolar crypt, with the permanent tooth germ being situated lingually to the developing deciduous tooth (see Fig. 21.16). With continued growth, this relationship changes and the permanent tooth comes to lie near the root apex of the deciduous tooth within its own bony crypt. Note that the alveolar crypt of the permanent tooth shown in Fig. 26.11 is not complete, there being the opening of a canal in its roof through which the dental follicle of the tooth germ communicates with, and is attached to, the overlying oral mucosa. This canal has been termed the *gubernacular canal* (see page 459).

The appearance of a resorbing deciduous tooth above its erupting successor is illustrated in Fig. 26.12. During the early eruptive stages of the permanent tooth, the bone separating it from its deciduous predecessor is resorbed. Following this, resorption of the hard tissues of the deciduous tooth takes place by the activity of multinucleated osteoclast-like cells termed *odontoclasts*. The vascular, resorbing tissue has been termed the *resorbing organ of Tomes*.

For a deciduous incisor or canine, root resorption initially occurs on the lingual surface adjacent to the developing permanent tooth (Fig. 26.11). With subsequent movement and relocation of the teeth in the growing jaws, the developing permanent tooth comes to lie directly beneath the deciduous tooth and further resorption occurs from the apex. For a deciduous molar, root resorption often commences on the inner surfaces where the permanent premolars initially develop. The premolars later come to lie beneath the roots of the deciduous molar, and further resorption occurs from the root apices. The shift in position of the deciduous tooth relative to the permanent successor may account for the intermittent nature of root resorption.

The initiation of root resorption may be an inherent developmental process, or it may be related to pressure from the permanent successor against the overlying bone or tooth. To assess which of these explanations

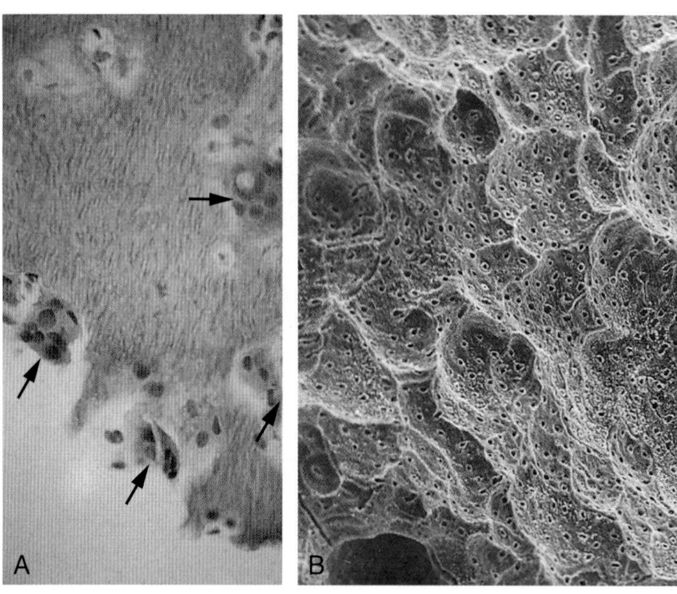

Fig. 26.13 (A) Resorbing dentine. Arrows indicate odontoclasts in Howship's lacunae (H & E; ×215). (B) SEM of the resorbing surface of a deciduous tooth showing Howship's lacunae. Within the lacunae, dentinal tubules are seen as small circular openings (anorganic specimen; ×400). Courtesy Prof. S J Jones and Springer-Verlag.

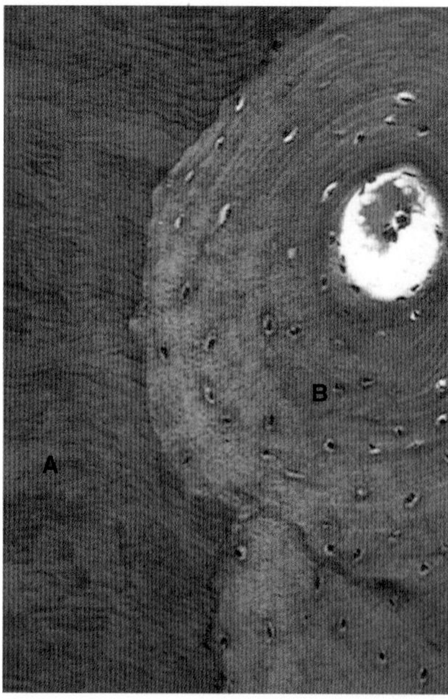

Fig. 26.14 Fusion between dentine (A) and alveolar bone (B) in an ankylosed tooth (decalcified section viewed in blue light; ×150). Courtesy Dr. B G H Levers.

is correct, when permanent tooth germs are surgically removed, resorption of the deciduous predecessors still occurs (albeit delayed). These findings are also consistent with the clinical observation that shedding of a deciduous tooth still occurs, but is retarded, where the successor is congenitally absent or occupies an abnormal position within the jaw.

It has been suggested that increased masticatory loads affect the pattern and rate of deciduous tooth resorption. Indeed, it has been shown that, if deciduous teeth are splinted following the removal of the developing permanent teeth, there is less root resorption than that seen with removal of the permanent teeth alone.

Resorbing dentine is illustrated in Fig. 26.13. Multinucleated osteoclast-like cells (odontoclasts) lie within resorption lacunae (Howship's lacunae). Odontoclasts, like osteoclasts, differentiate from circulating monocyte-like cells. They are vacuolated and have long cytoplasmic processes. In an electron micrograph, the cytoplasmic projections form a brush border with the tooth surface. The odontoclasts have an abundance of ribosomes and a large number of mitochondria. Howship's lacunae in resorbing teeth tend to be larger and more spherical than lacunae in bone.

Resorption of deciduous teeth is not a continuous process. During rest periods, reparative tissue may be formed, leading to a reattachment of the periodontal ligament. The tissue of repair is cementum-like, and the cells responsible for its formation are similar in appearance to cementoblasts (see page 447). If the repair process prevails over the resorption, the tooth may become ankylosed to the surrounding bone, with loss of the periodontal ligament (Fig. 26.14). Ankylosis may also be caused by trauma or infection of a tooth. Ankylosis is discussed further on page 474.

A specialised feature associated with the erupting permanent tooth is the presence of a gubernacular canal (Fig. 26.11). The gubernacular canal contains the gubernacular cord. The cord is composed of a central strand of epithelium (derived from the dental lamina) surrounded by connective tissue. The connective tissue is organised into inner and outer layers. Collagen fibres of the inner layer show greater organisation and run mainly parallel to the long axis of the epithelium. In the outer layer, the collagen fibres are fewer and less organised. Differences between the layers can also be discerned with respect to the vasculature, with the vessels in the outer layer being larger. During eruption, the gubernacular cords decrease in length but increase in thickness and become less dense. Surgical removal of the cord does not prevent eruption of the permanent tooth.

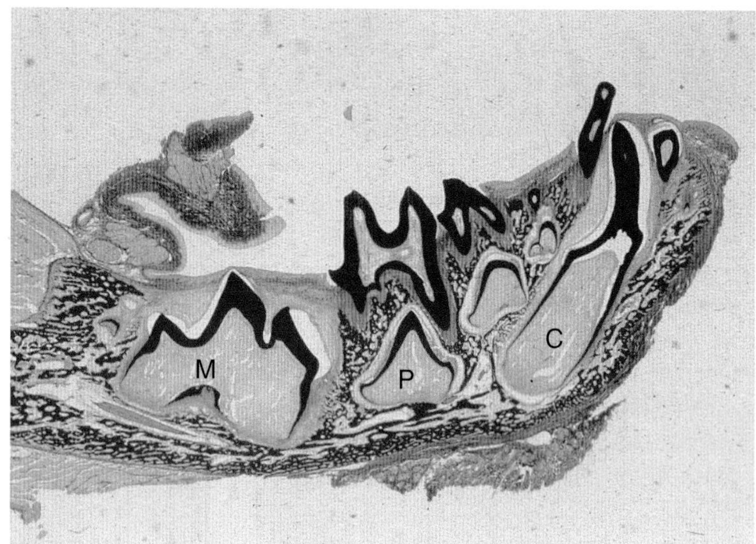

Fig. 26.15 Section of the mandible of a ferret *(Putorius putorius)* aged 42 days. Notice the absence of alveolar bone beneath the erupting first permanent molar (M), the third premolar (P) and the permanent canine tooth (C). From Berkovitz, B.K.B., Moxham, B.J., 1990. The evelopment of the periodontal ligament with special reference to collagen fibre ontogeny, *Journal de Biologie Buccale* 18, 227–238.

Mechanisms of tooth eruption

All tissues within the vicinity of the tooth thought capable of generating a force have, at one time or another, been implicated in the eruptive process. The theories advanced to explain the mechanism of tooth eruption can be divided into two main groups. One view suggests that the tooth is pushed out as a result of forces generated beneath and around it, by alveolar bone growth, root growth, blood pressure/tissue fluid pressure or cell proliferation. That alveolar bone cannot play a major role in tooth eruption is evident from the fact that no significant amounts of alveolar bone are observed being deposited beneath the root apices of erupting teeth (Fig. 26.15). Alternatively, the tooth may be pulled out as a result of tension within the connective tissue of the periodontal ligament.

Many of the experiments conducted to elucidate the eruptive mechanism have required the use of the continuously growing incisors of rats and rabbits. This is because of the ease of experimentally manipulating the teeth, the continuous eruption of the teeth and the rapid rates of eruption that can be as high as 1 mm/day. Fig. 26.16 shows the distribution of tissues in the continuously growing rat incisor. Because of what is perceived as the specialised nature of a tooth of continuous growth compared to the tooth of limited growth found in the human dentition, some researchers have questioned the use of the rodent incisor and have suggested that the results of experiments on such teeth cannot be extrapolated to human teeth. However, teeth of continuous growth evolved from teeth of limited growth, and, on basic biological principles, modification to existing systems and mechanisms would be expected rather than radically alternative mechanisms. Importantly, there are more similarities between the teeth than differences, the results of experiments and studies on the eruption of teeth of continuous and limited growth show a remarkable convergence of viewpoint (e.g., that eruption requires a force generated by the surrounding connective tissues [i.e., dental follicle or periodontal ligament] and does not require a tractional force pulling the tooth towards the oral cavity).

Although no one theory to explain the generation of eruptive forces is yet supported by sufficient experimental evidence, the brief review that follows will show that the eruptive mechanism 1) is a property of the periodontal ligament (or its precursor, the dental follicle); 2) does not require a tractional force pulling the tooth towards the mouth; 3) is multifactorial in that more than one agent makes important contributions to the overall eruptive force; and 4) could involve a combination of fibroblast activity (although the evidence to date remains poor) and vascular and/or tissue hydrostatic pressures.

Role of the periodontal ligament in eruption

Experiments involving root resection or root transection of the continuously growing incisors of rodents (or rabbits) indicate that the periodontal ligament is the probable source for the generation of the forces responsible for eruption. Root resection involves the surgical removal of the proliferative odontogenic tissues at the base of the continuously growing incisor; root transection involves cutting the incisor into proximal and distal portions. Both surgical procedures result in a situation where the tooth (or the distal segment following transection) remains merely as a fragment attached to the jaw by a periodontal ligament but without the possibility of root growth and with degeneration of the pulp. Furthermore, there can be no contribution to eruption from bone growth, as none occurs at the base (fundus) of the socket. The resected and transected incisors continue to erupt to the point where they are exfoliated from the socket. That the movement in these surgically prepared teeth is eruptive-like and not an artefactual exfoliation is indicated by experiments that show that the resected rodent incisor changes its rate of eruption in response to factors or drugs that similarly affect the rate of eruption in normal incisors.

Although the periodontal ligament is implicated in the generation of the eruptive force, experiments show that for teeth of limited growth, this property can be undertaken by its precursor, the dental follicle. When a developing unerupted premolar tooth is surgically removed and replaced with a metal replica, the replica will 'erupt', provided that the dental follicle is retained. This experiment confirms that rootless teeth (both experimentally produced and clinically observed) can erupt and that the eruptive mechanism is present in a connective tissue (periodontal ligament or dental follicle) that need not gain a direct attachment to the tooth.

Investigation into the eruptive behaviour of the continuously growing lathyritic incisor confirms that the eruptive force is unlikely to involve a tractional element that pulls the tooth towards the oral cavity. Lathyrogens are drugs that specifically inhibit the formation of collagen cross-links, thereby disrupting the fibrous network in the periodontal ligament. Compared with controls, eruption rates of lathyritic rodent incisors are unaffected, provided that occlusal forces (which could traumatise the

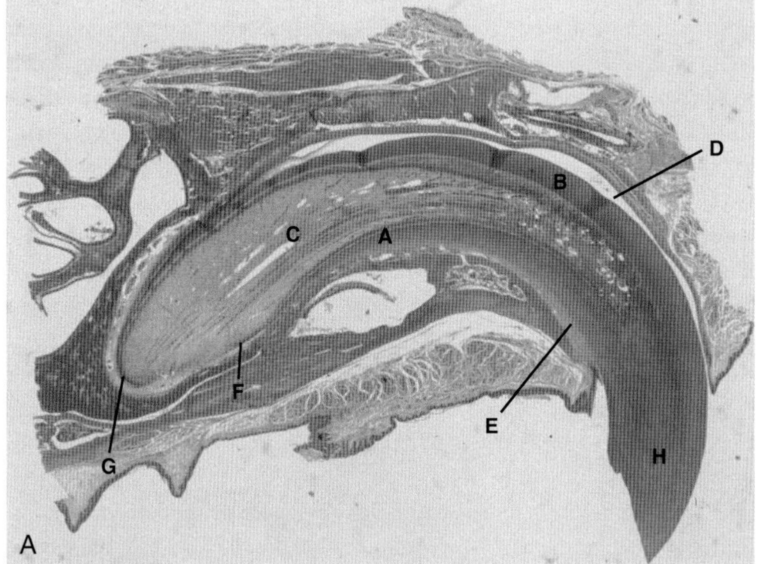

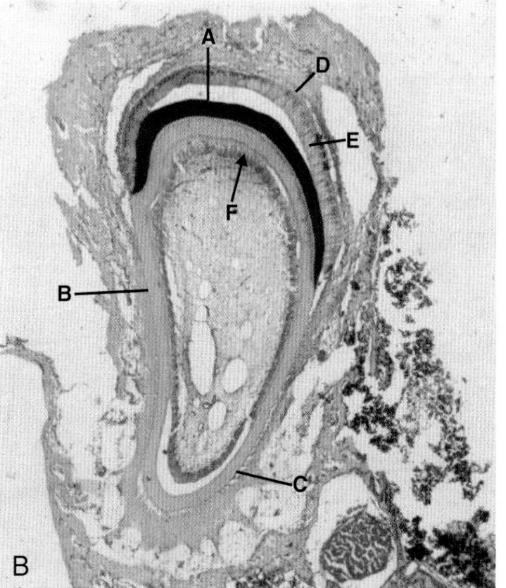

Fig. 26.16 (A) Longitudinal section of the continuously growing maxillary rat incisor, showing the distribution of tissues. In essence, this tooth presents root tissue (i.e., dentine and cementum, A) on its lingual side and crown tissue (i.e., dentine and enamel, B) on its labial side. C = dental pulp; D = enamel space. On the lingual side of the tooth, a true periodontal ligament (E) passes from the cementum to the alveolar bone, while connective tissue intervenes labially between the enamel surface and the alveolar bone (although it is not attached to the enamel). In the region of the proliferative 'root' apex, structures homologous with an epithelial root sheath (F) and an enamel organ (G) continually produce new dental tissues to compensate for attritional loss. In the laboratory rat, incisor teeth in occlusion erupt at a rate of about 400 μm/day (impeded eruption rate). If the teeth are cut out of occlusion, their eruption rate attains levels of about 1 mm/day (unimpeded eruption rate). To prevent pulp exposure during continuous incisor eruption, secondary dentine (H) is continually deposited beneath the incisal edge (H & E; ×8). (B) Cross-section of the mandibular incisor of a rat. The developing enamel matrix (A) is limited to the labial surface of the tooth. The remainder of the dentine (B) is covered by a very thin layer of cementum. A true periodontal ligament (C) is only present in association with the cementum-covered component of the tooth. A loose connective tissue (D) separates the enamel from the surrounding socket wall. E = Ameloblast layer; F = odontoblast layer. (Masson's trichrome; ×40.) A, Courtesy Dr. M Robins.

already weakened ligament) are reduced by regular trimming of the tooth to the gingival level. Thus, the lathyrogen experiments support the experiments on rootless teeth (of noncontinuous growth) and indicate that traction of collagen fibres is not required to effect eruption. Further evidence against a tractional eruptive force comes from the study of the development of the periodontal ligament (see page 439), which indicates that teeth can erupt in the absence of well-developed periodontal fibres. These studies also disprove the theory that contraction of periodontal collagen fibre is responsible for generating the eruptive force.

Although the opinion is held that the force effecting eruption is derived from a single source (i.e., a prime mover), it is conceivable that more than one agent contributes to the overall force. That the eruption is multifactorial is evident when considering the variety of processes that must be involved to produce and sustain eruption. Indeed, four processes seem to be necessary:

- First, there must be the mechanism itself that generates the eruptive forces.
- Second, there are processes whereby eruptive forces are translated into eruption by movements through the surrounding tissues (e.g., overcoming the resistance of the tissues to eruption).
- Third, eruption must be sustained by processes that enable the tooth to be supported in its new position.
- Fourth, eruption occurs alongside a process of remodelling of the periodontal tissues to maintain the functional integrity of the system.

Experiments support the view that eruption is multifactorial; on the basis of study of the interactions of various drugs or hormones known to influence eruption, they suggest at least two factors are involved – a cortisone-sensitive factor and a cortisone-insensitive factor. A study of eruption rates in rodent incisors showed that when a drug is given that severely retards eruption (in this case, the antimitotic drug cyclophosphamide), the remaining component of eruption is no longer affected by cortisone administration (which would normally produce a marked increase in eruption). Although it is possible to interpret these data in other ways, additional experiments show that the recovery of eruption following root resection (perhaps due to the removal of abnormal tissues at the base) also has both cortisone-sensitive and cortisone-insensitive phases.

Having established that the connective tissues around the developing tooth are most likely to be the source of the eruptive mechanism, two major systems have been implicated in the generation of the eruptive force. One view holds that the force is produced by the activity of periodontal fibroblasts through their contractility and/or motility, the other that vascular and/or tissue hydrostatic pressures in and around the tooth are responsible for eruption.

Whatever the system implicated in the eruptive mechanism, the evidence should be judged according to the following five criteria:

1) The proposed system must be capable of producing a force under physiological conditions that is sufficient to move a tooth in a direction favouring eruption.
2) Experimentally induced changes to the system should cause predictable changes in eruption.
3) The system requires characteristics that enable it to sustain eruptive movements over long periods of time.
4) The biochemical characteristics of the system should be consistent with the production of an eruptive force.
5) The morphological features associated with the system should be consistent with the production of an eruptive force.

Periodontal fibroblast motility/contractility hypothesis

A role for the periodontal ligament fibroblasts in eruption is based upon the notion that these cells can exert a tractional force onto the tooth through the collagen network or through cell-to-cell contacts. This is in some ways analogous to the events occurring during wound contraction, which are thought to be the result of activities of specialised cells termed *myofibroblasts*. However, the periodontal ligament differs markedly from granulation tissue, and there is considerable evidence against the requirement for a tractional eruptive force acting through the periodontal collagen network (see pages 461–462). Reviewing the evidence in terms of our prescribed criteria, there is at present nothing to indicate that the fibroblasts can exert a force under physiological conditions sufficient to move a tooth in a direction favouring eruption. Neither has it been possible to devise procedures to affect selectively periodontal fibroblast activity *in vivo* to assess whether the experimental procedures have predictable effects on eruption. It has been shown that the drug colchicine, through its known disturbance of intracellular microtubules, reduces cell motility, and this might explain the drug's significant retardatory effect on eruption. However, colchicine influences more than just cell migration (for example, it also affects connective tissue turnover). To date, the evidence relating to the fibroblast activity hypothesis relies almost entirely upon consideration of the morphology of the fibroblasts (criterion 5 earlier) and upon the possible characteristics of the system that would sustain the eruptive forces over long periods (criterion 3 earlier).

When periodontal fibroblasts are cultured on plastic, they assume the appearance and behaviour of migratory cells. They have a highly elongated shape with numerous highly polarised arrays of microtubules and microfilaments. Their motility *in vitro* ceases with colchicine. When periodontal fibroblasts are cultured in a collagen gel, they generate tension by their contractility and assume the appearance of myofibroblast-like cells (i.e., fibroblasts with some of the properties of smooth muscle cells, a feature of fibroblasts in granulation tissue). During their contractile phase, these cells possess thick cell coats, considerable amounts of microfilamentous material dispersed throughout the cytoplasm, numerous cell contacts resembling gap junctions and occasional crenulated (folded) nuclei, but little rough endoplasmic reticulum. Their contraction *in vitro* is inhibited when drugs interfering with microfilaments (e.g., cytochalasin) are added to the culture medium. *In vivo*, however, periodontal fibroblasts show features of neither migratory cells nor myofibroblasts. Instead, they tend to be rounded or flattened in outline without polarity of shape, have relatively little microfilamentous material (and then primarily as stress fibres beneath the cell membrane, a feature of cells generally exhibited after migration/contraction), have only infrequent gap junctions (but more cell contacts in the form of simplified desmosomes) and contain considerable amounts of rough endoplasmic reticulum (see page 237). Thus, the periodontal fibroblast *in vivo* shows all the characteristics of a cell actively synthesising and secreting protein rather than of a motile/contractile cell. Care must therefore be taken in extrapolating from the *in vitro* to the *in vivo* situation.

In terms of criterion 3 (earlier), there is evidence of sustained migration of periodontal fibroblasts *in vivo*. Studies where the nuclei of cells have been labelled with tritium thymidine indicate that periodontal fibroblasts move occlusally at a rate equal to that of eruption; if the eruption rate is increased, there is a concomitant increase in the rate of migration. Although providing some evidence of a shift in the position of periodontal fibroblasts, such work does not in itself indicate whether the cells are moving actively to generate the force of eruption or whether they are merely being transported passively within the ligament, with the eruptive force being generated by another mechanism.

Other morphological features of the periodontal fibroblasts argue against their involvement in the generation of the eruptive force. The presence of cell contacts (not a usual feature of fibroblasts in a mature connective tissue) might indicate that a force could be generated through cell-to-cell contacts. However, the contacts are simplified desmosomes and not the fibronexus usually seen for myofibroblasts in contracting wounds. Furthermore, many of the simplified desmosomes for periodontal fibroblasts are located at right angles to the long axes of the cells and they lack any recognisable microfilament bundles – arrangements that do not seem suited to transmit a tractional force directly through the cells themselves.

One way of assessing the contribution of the periodontal fibroblasts to eruption involves analysing quantitatively the structure of these cells in different periodontal ligaments and in teeth exhibiting different eruptive behaviours. The findings of studies using this approach also provide evidence against the periodontal fibroblast motility/contractility hypotheses. For example, there are no differences in the cells and their various organelles when periodontal fibroblasts in rapidly erupting and fully erupted teeth are compared.

Periodontal vascular/tissue hydrostatic pressure hypothesis

An eruptive force might be generated via the periodontal vasculature either directly through blood pressure or indirectly by influencing periodontal tissue (hydrostatic) pressures. Whether acting directly or indirectly, the periodontal vascular hypotheses clearly do not require a tractional mode of activity within the periodontal tissues.

That vascular pressures can alter the position of a tooth in its socket is shown by the fact that a tooth moves 0.4 μm in synchrony with the arterial pulse. Furthermore, spontaneous changes in blood pressure have been shown to influence eruptive behaviour and, at death, when the arterial blood pressure is zero, eruption ceases. Therefore, there is some evidence that without experimental intervention, vascular/tissue pressures can produce a force sufficient to move a tooth in a direction favouring eruption (criterion 1 earlier). Experimental alterations to the periodontal vasculature following the administration of vasoactive drugs or interference with the sympathetic vasomotor nerve supply also result in predictable changes in eruption-like behaviour (criterion 2 earlier). For example, using a sensitive displacement transducer, it is possible to continuously monitor eruptive behaviour. Following the administration of a hypotensive drug (e.g., hexamethonium), as a probable result of increased capillary and periodontal tissue hydrostatic pressures, there is a marked increase in the rates of extrusive, eruption-like movements. In addition, stimulation of the cervical sympathetic system results in cessation of eruption and significant intrusion of the tooth, probably as a result of vasoconstriction and decreased capillary and periodontal tissue pressures (once the stimulus is removed, eruption recommences).

To sustain eruptive movements according to the vascular hypotheses, it is necessary to postulate that periodontal tissue pressures are high, that there are pressure differentials along the periodontal ligament and that changes in such pressures alter eruptive behaviour (criterion 3 earlier). Indeed, there is evidence to support all three postulates. However, there remains debate as to whether periodontal tissue hydrostatic pressures are supraatmospheric or subatmospheric.

To assess whether the biochemical composition of the periodontal ligament is consistent with the production of an eruptive force by 'vascular' means (criterion 4 earlier), analysis of the periodontal ligament proteoglycans at different stages of tooth development has shown that a proteoglycan, with possibly significant osmotic influences on the tissue, increases in quantity during the active phase of eruption (see Fig. 12.27).

Quantitative electron microscopy of the periodontal vasculature (criterion 5 earlier) has shown that for both the degree of vasculature and the numbers of fenestrations on the capillaries, marked changes occur with different phases of eruption. For the noncontinuously growing molar of the rodent, the number of fenestrations is three times greater during eruption than after eruption. In addition, for the continuously growing incisor of the rodent, the fenestrations are relatively low in number near the alveolar crest (approximately $1 \times 10^6/mm^3$ of tissue) but are higher near the root base of the erupting tooth (approximately $4 \times 10^6/mm^3$), perhaps providing evidence for differential vascular activity along the periodontal ligament. Thus, while no single piece of evidence briefly reported here for a role in eruption of the vascular elements of the periodontal ligament is incontrovertible, the sum of the evidence does suggest that it could provide one factor in the multifactorial mechanism of eruption.

Development of the dentition and occlusion

Some observations have been made on the rate of eruption of human teeth. Initially, there is a period of slow eruption when the crown is carried towards the oral mucosa. For permanent teeth, this period may take 2–4 years. A tooth erupts most rapidly as it enters the oral cavity, at which time the length of its root is about one-half to two-thirds complete. Eruption then slows as the tooth approaches the occlusal plane. Once the tooth has emerged into the oral cavity, it may take 1–2 years to reach the occlusal plane. The emergence of the crown is partly the result of axial movement of the tooth (active eruption) and partly related to retraction of the adjacent soft tissues (passive eruption). The maximum eruption rate occurs at the time of crown emergence (further information about eruption rates are found on page 456).

Because no individuals are exactly alike, the times for tooth development shown in Table 26.1 are approximate. Variations of 6 months either way are not unusual, but the tendency is for teeth to erupt late rather than early. By and large, the development of the permanent dentition is more advanced in girls; there does not appear to be any sex difference in the development of the deciduous dentition. Ethnic differences also appear to exist.

As the sequence of development and eruption of teeth is under genetic control, and since chronological age is an unreliable guide to the progress of development of an individual child, dental age is a useful index of maturity, especially when used in conjunction with skeletal age. Dental age may be estimated clinically by a visual assessment of the stage of eruption of the dentition or, more satisfactorily, by a radiographic assessment of both the stages of development of the crowns and roots and the stages of eruption.

Orthopantomograms of the dentition at various ages are illustrated in Figs. 26.17 and 26.18, 26.19–26.25. Examples of jaws dissected to reveal the state of development of the teeth are illustrated in Figs. 26.26–26.32. A longitudinal series of models taken from the same patient show the developing dentitions from birth to 22 years of age (Figs. 26.33–26.45).

Table 26.1 Chronology of tooth development

Chronology of the deciduous dentition

Tooth	First evidence of calcification (weeks *in utero*)	Crown completed (months)	Alveolar eruption (months)	Partial eruption (months)	Root stage at PE
Maxillary					
A	15–19	4	4	9	¼
B	16–21	6	7	10	½
C	19–22	12	13	18	½
D	16–19	9	10	15	¼
E	22–26	13	16	23	½
Mandibular					
A	15–19	4	3	8	½
B	16–21	6	8	12	½
C	19–22	12	13	16	½
D	16–19	9	11½	15	¼
E	22–26	13	17	25	½

Data from Sunderland, E.P., Smith, C.J., Suwnderland, R., 1987. A histological study ofthe chronology of initial mineralisation in the human deciduous dentition. *Archives of Oral Biology* 32, 167–174. Birch, W., Dean, M.C., 2014. A method of calculating human deciduous crown formation times and of estimating the chronological ages of stressful events occurring during deciduous enamel formation. Journal of Forensic and Legal Medicine 22:,127–144. Liversidge, H.M., 2015. Tooth eruption and timing. In: Irish, J.D., Scott, G.R. (Eds.), *A Companion to Dental Anthropology*. John Wiley. Mahoney, P., 2011. Human deciduous mandibular molar incremental enamel development. American Journal of Physical Anthropology 114, 204–214. Mahoney, P., 2012. Incremental enamel development in modern human deciduous anterior teeth. American Journal of Physical Anthropology 147, 637–651.

Chronology of the permanent dentition

Tooth	First evidence of calcification	Crown completed	Alveolar eruption	Partial eruption	Root stage at PE
Maxillary					
1	3–4 months	4–5	6.9	7.1	½
2	10–12 months	4–5	7.6	8.1	¾
3	4–5 months	6–7	10.9	11.1	Complete
4	1½–1¾	5–6	10.1	10.6	¾
5	2–2½	6–7	10.8	11.1	¾
6	Birth	2½–3	5.3	6.1	¾
7	2½–3	6–7	10.4	11.6	¾
8	7–9	12–16	16.7	18.9	Complete
Mandibular					
1	3–4 months	4–5	5.7	6.3	½
2	3–4 months	4–5	6.8	7.4	½
3	4–5 months	6–7	10.1	10.5	¾
4	1¼–2	5–6	10.5	10.7	¾
5	1¼–2½	6–7	10.6	10.7	¾
6	Birth	2½–3	4.8	5.9	½
7	2½–3	7–8	10.0	11.3	¾
8	8–10	12–16	15.4	17.8	Complete

Data from Liversidge, H.M., 2015. Tooth eruption and timing. In: Irish, J.D., Scott, G.R. (Eds.), *A Companion to Dental Anthropology*. John Wiley.

Unless otherwise indicated all dates are in years and *postpartum*. The teeth are identified according to the Palmer-Zsigmondy system. Alveolar eruption describes the appearance of the cusps/incisal edges of the tooth relative to the crest of the alveolar bone. Partial eruption (PE) is when the cusp tips/incisal edges have reached the maximum bulbosity of the adjacent tooth and is slightly older than the first appearance of the tooth erupting into the mouth.

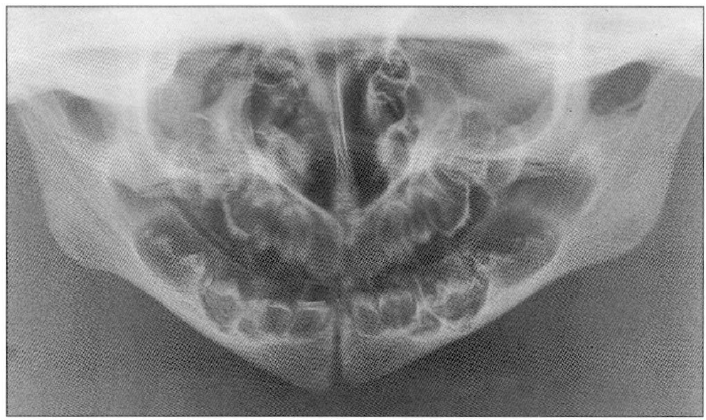

Fig. 26.17 Dental age birth. Courtesy Standring, S., ed., 2021. *Gray's Anatomy: The Anatomical Basis of Clinical Practice*, forty-second ed. Elsevier.

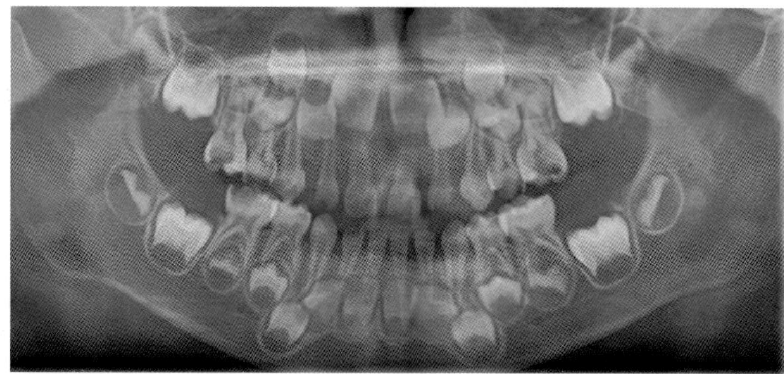

Fig. 26.19 Dental age 4 years – orthopantomogram. Courtesy Dr. J Makdissi.

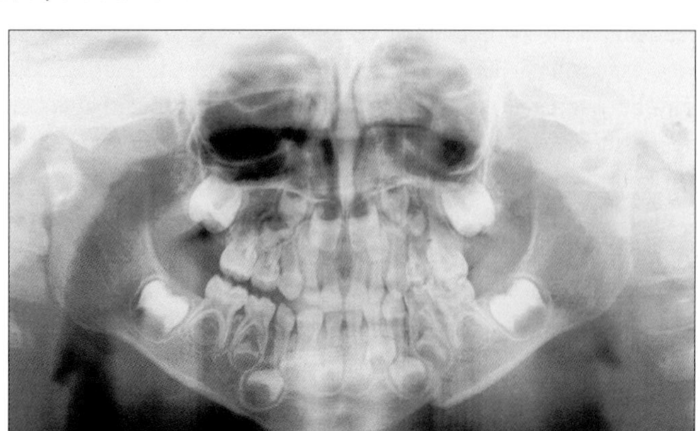

Fig. 26.18 Dental age 2½ years. Courtesy Standring, S., ed., 2021. *Gray's Anatomy: The Anatomical Basis of Clinical Practice*, forty-second ed. Elsevier.

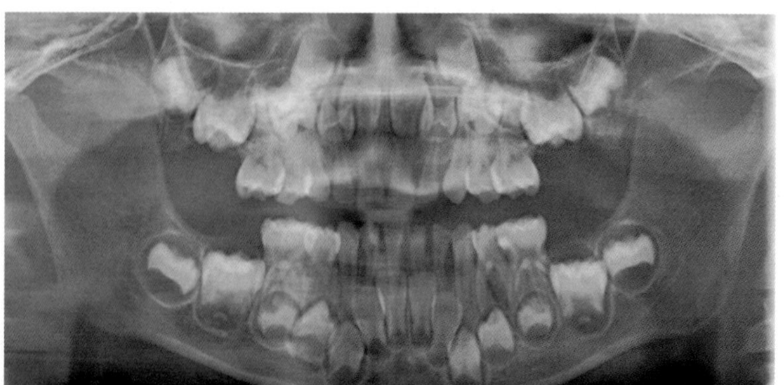

Fig. 26.20 Dental age 5 years – orthopantomogram. Courtesy Dr. J Makdissi.

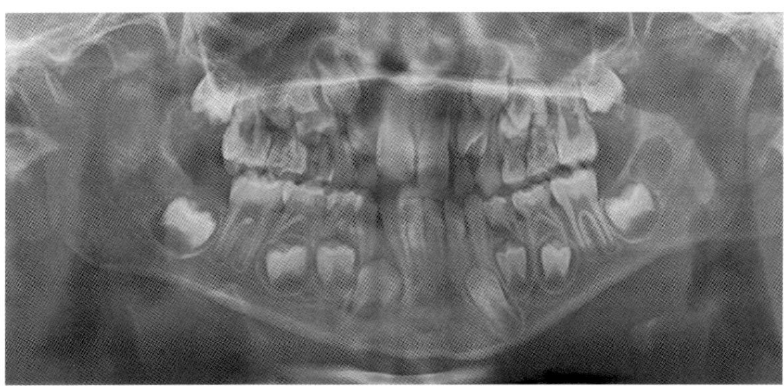

Fig. 26.21 Dental age 7 years – orthopantomogram. Courtesy Dr. J Makdissi.

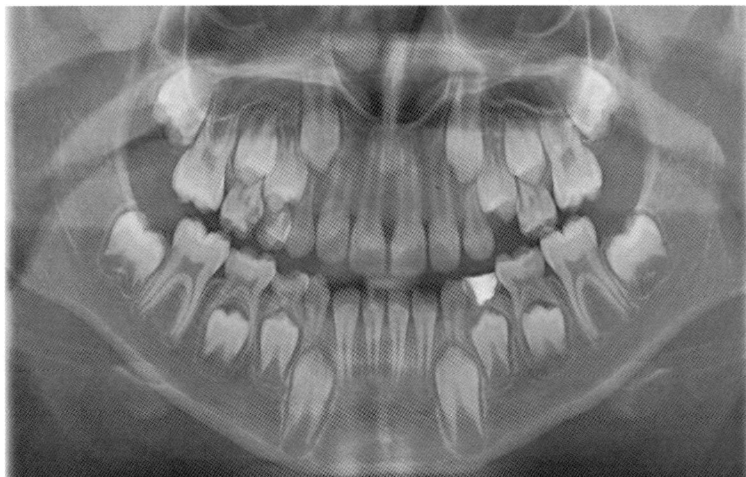

Fig. 26.22 Dental age 9 years – orthopantomogram. Courtesy Dr. J Makdissi.

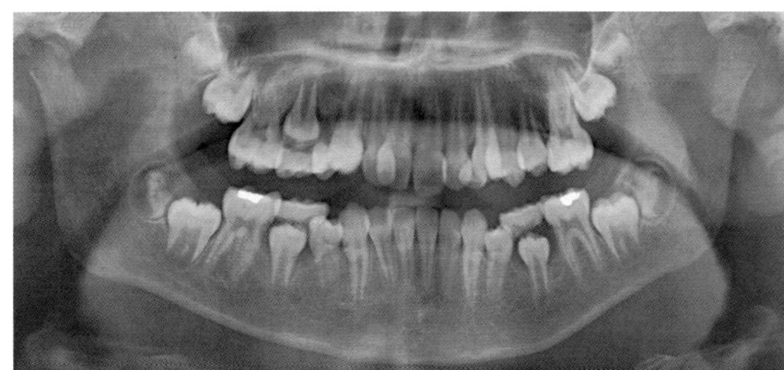

Fig. 26.23 Dental age 10 years – orthopantomogram. Courtesy Dr. J Makdissi.

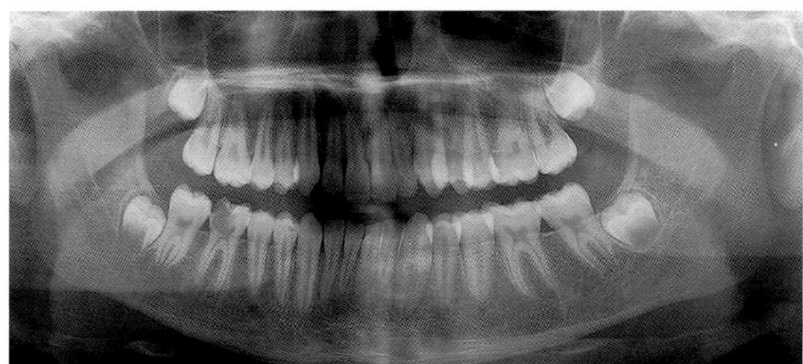

Fig. 26.24 Dental age 14 years – orthopantomogram. Courtesy Dr. J Makdissi.

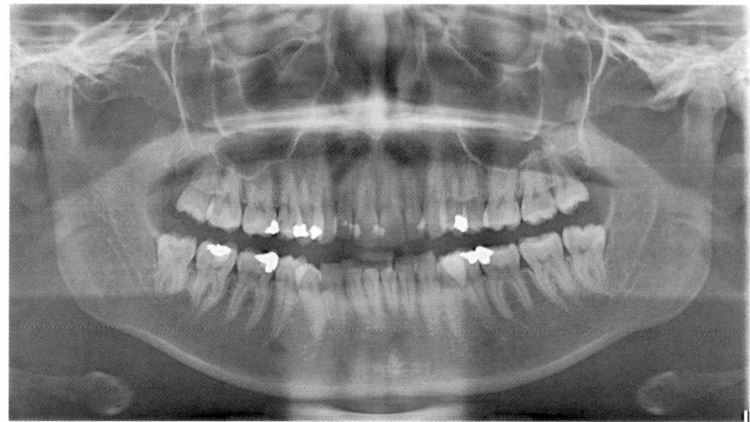

Fig. 26.25 Dental age 21 years – orthopantomogram. Courtesy Dr. J Makdissi.

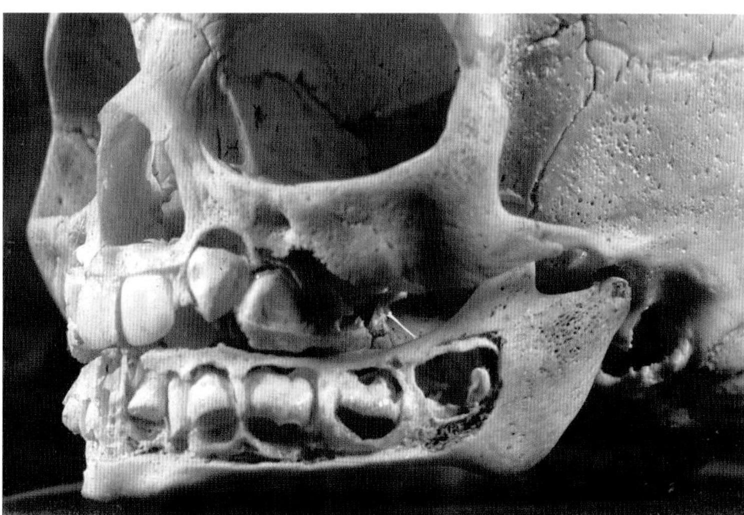

Fig. 26.26 Dissected skull showing state of development of the teeth at 4 months. Teeth erupted – none; teeth unerupted – maxilla ABCDE6; mandible ABCDE6. In this and the following six figures, the teeth are identified using the Palmer-Zsigmondy system.

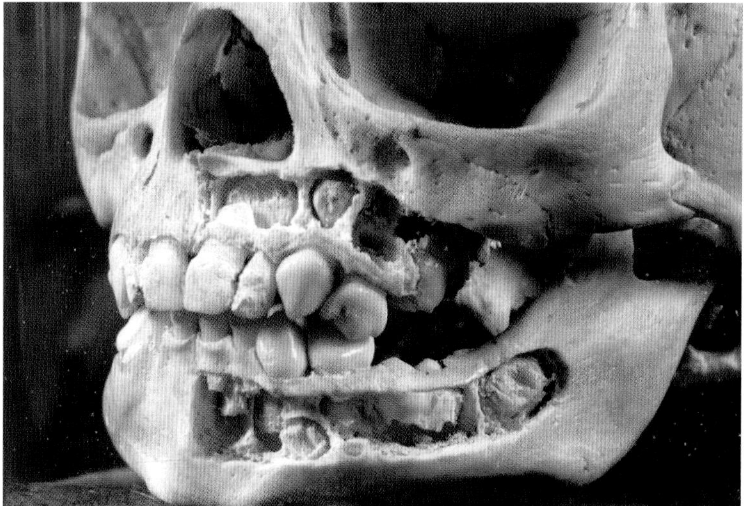

Fig. 26.27 Dissected skull showing state of development of the teeth at 18 months. Teeth erupted – maxilla ABCD, mandible ABCD; teeth unerupted – maxilla 123E6, mandible 123E6.

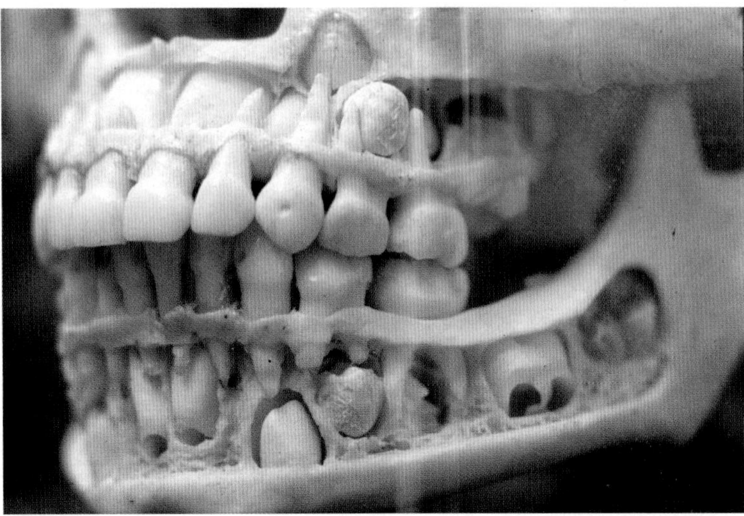

Fig. 26.28 Dissected skull showing state of development of the teeth at 4 years. Teeth erupted – maxilla ABCDE, mandible ABCDE; teeth unerupted – maxilla 1234567, mandible 1234567.

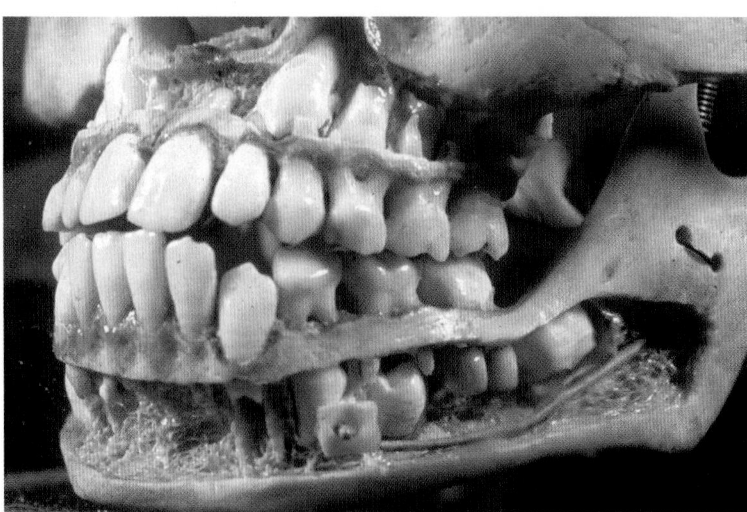

Fig. 26.30 Dissected skull showing state of development of the teeth at 9 years. Teeth erupted – maxilla 12CDE6, mandible 123DE6; teeth unerupted – maxilla 3457, mandible 4567.

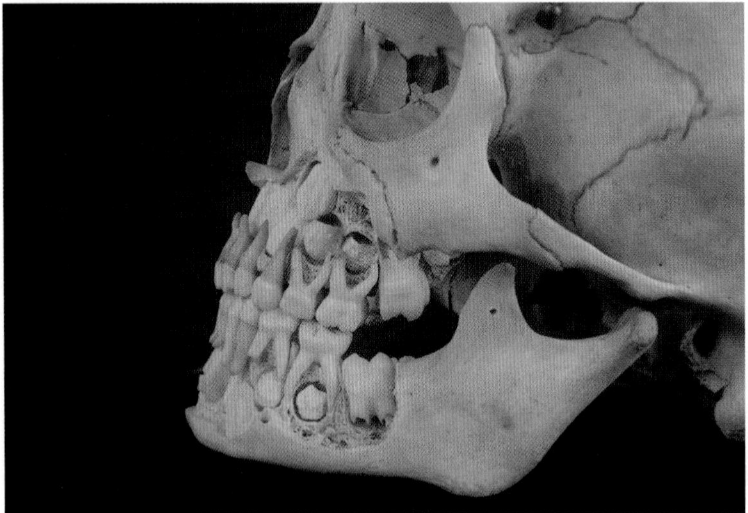

Fig. 26.29 Dissected skull showing state of development of the teeth at 5½ years. Teeth erupted – maxilla ABCDE, mandible ABCDE; teeth unerupted – maxilla 1234567, mandible 1234567. Copyright the Royal College of Surgeons of England.

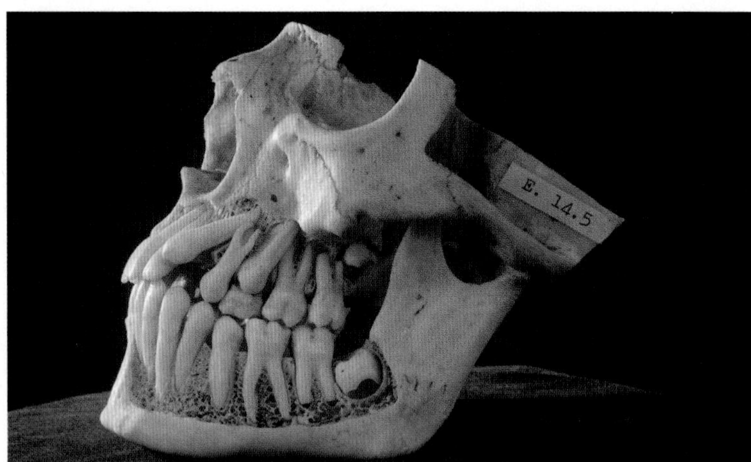

Fig. 26.31 Dissected skull showing state of development of the teeth at 11 years. Teeth erupted – maxilla 1234E67, mandible 1234567; teeth unerupted – maxilla 58, mandible 8. Copyright the Royal College of Surgeons of England.

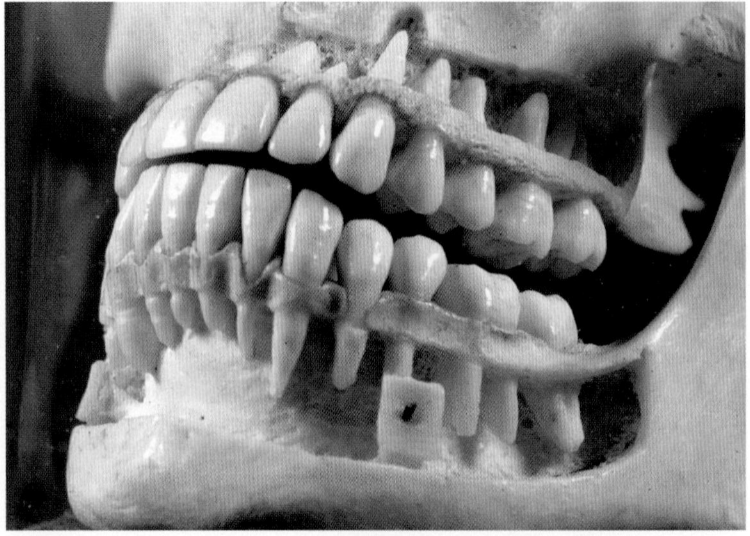

Fig. 26.32 Dissected skull showing state of development of the teeth at 15 years. Note that the permanent third molars are not present in this skull. Teeth erupted – maxilla 1234567, mandible 1234567.

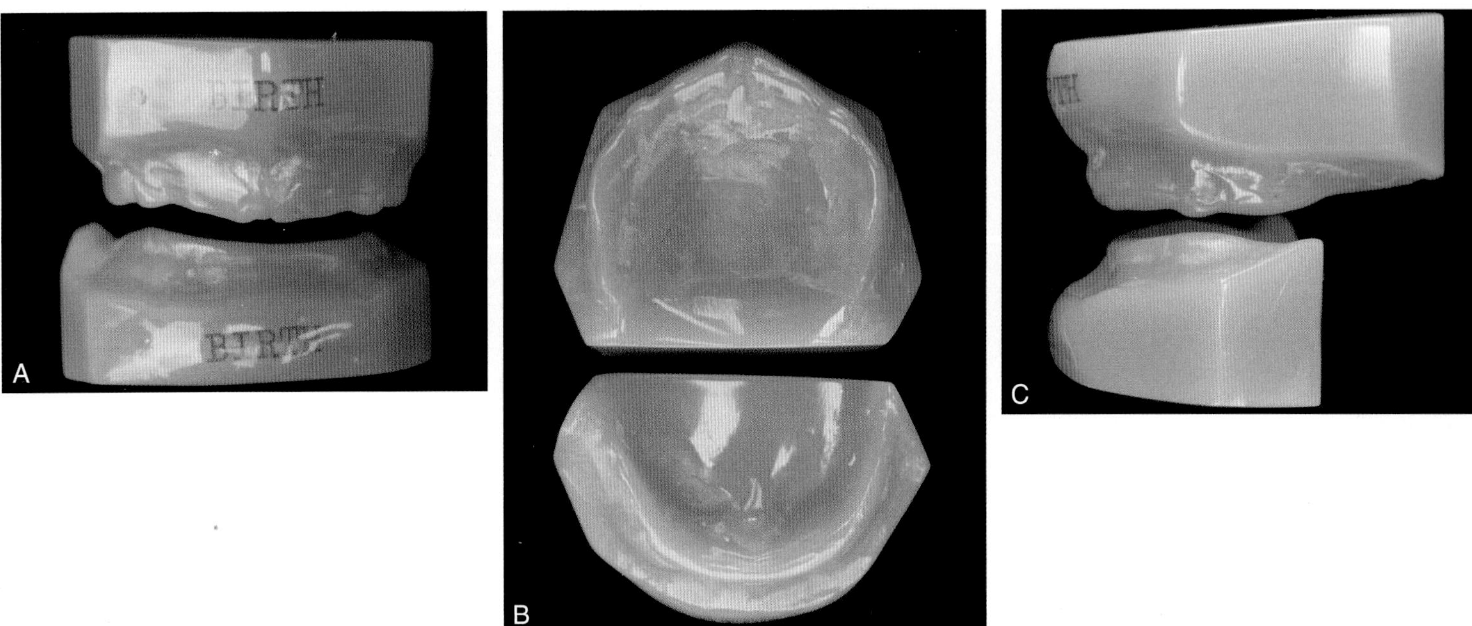

Fig. 26.33 Models of dentition at birth.

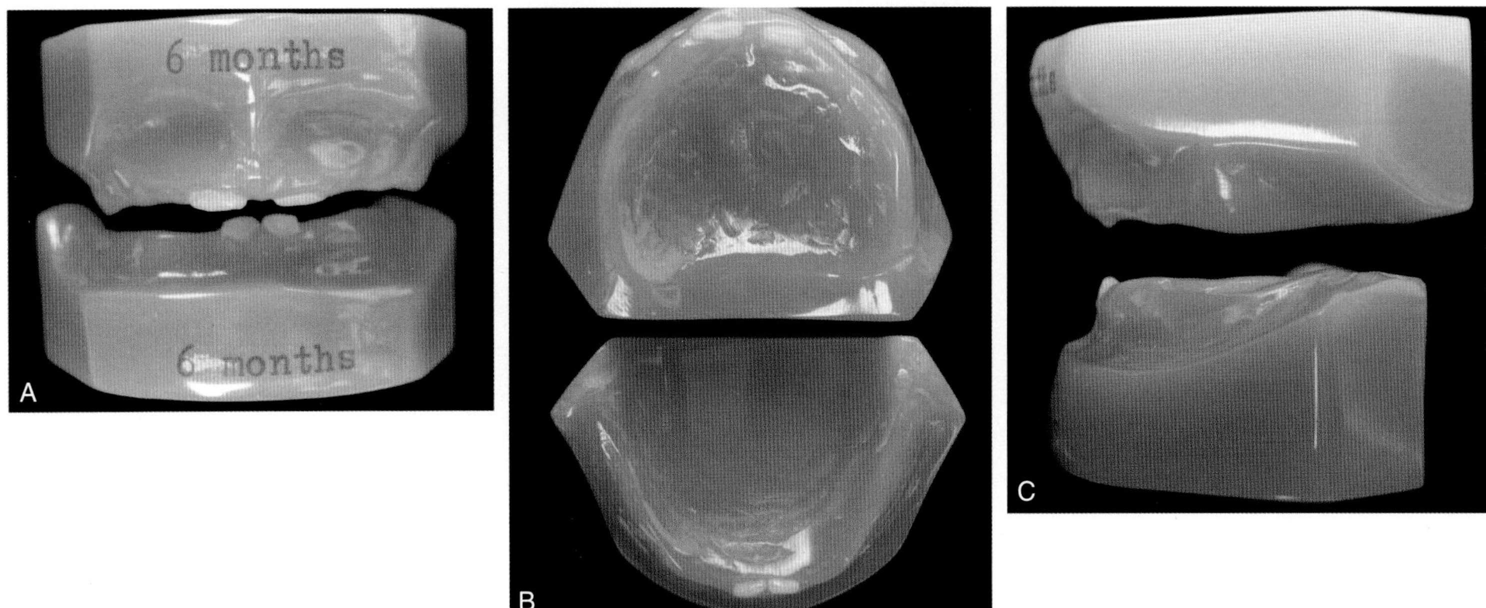

Fig. 26.34 Models of dentition at 6 months.

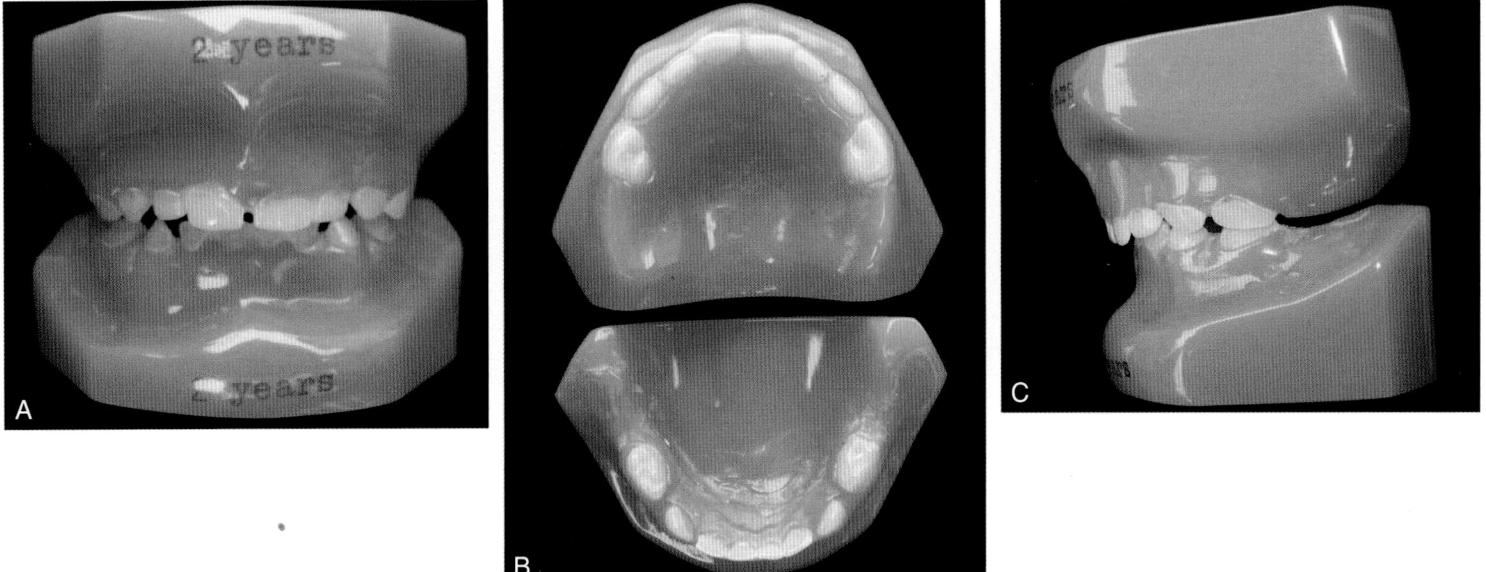

Fig. 26.35 Models of dentition at 2 years.

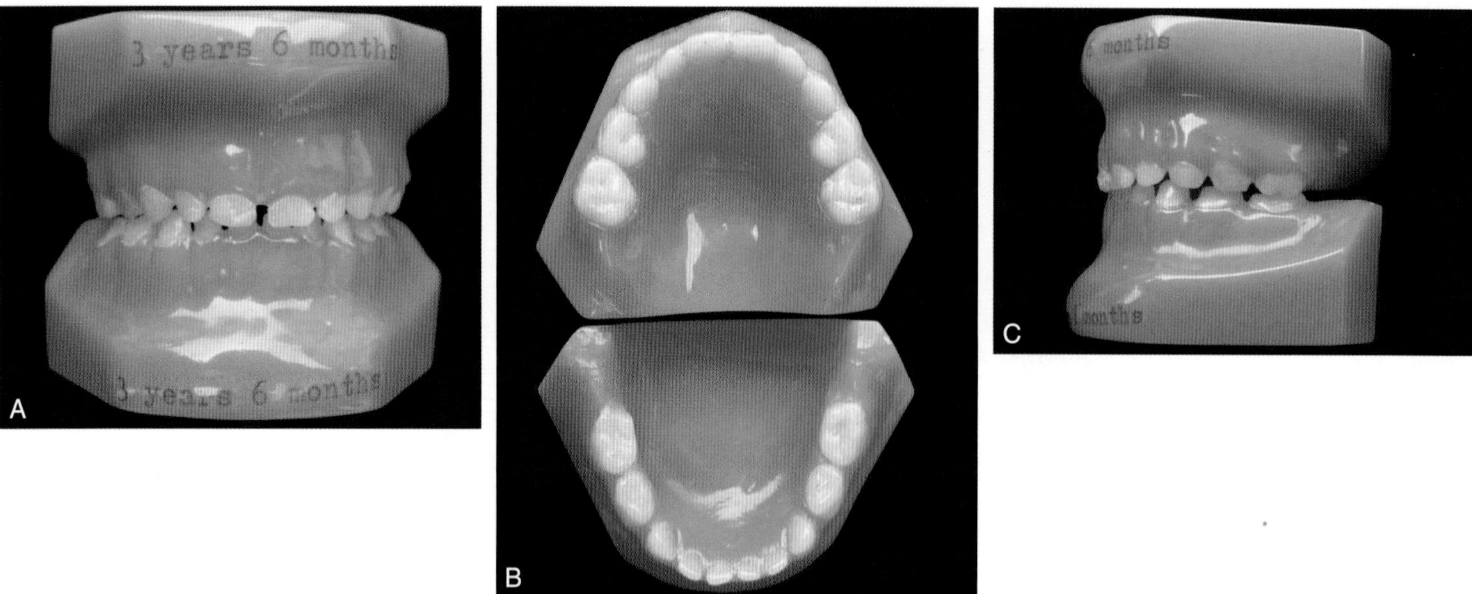

Fig. 26.36 Models of dentition at 3 years 6 months.

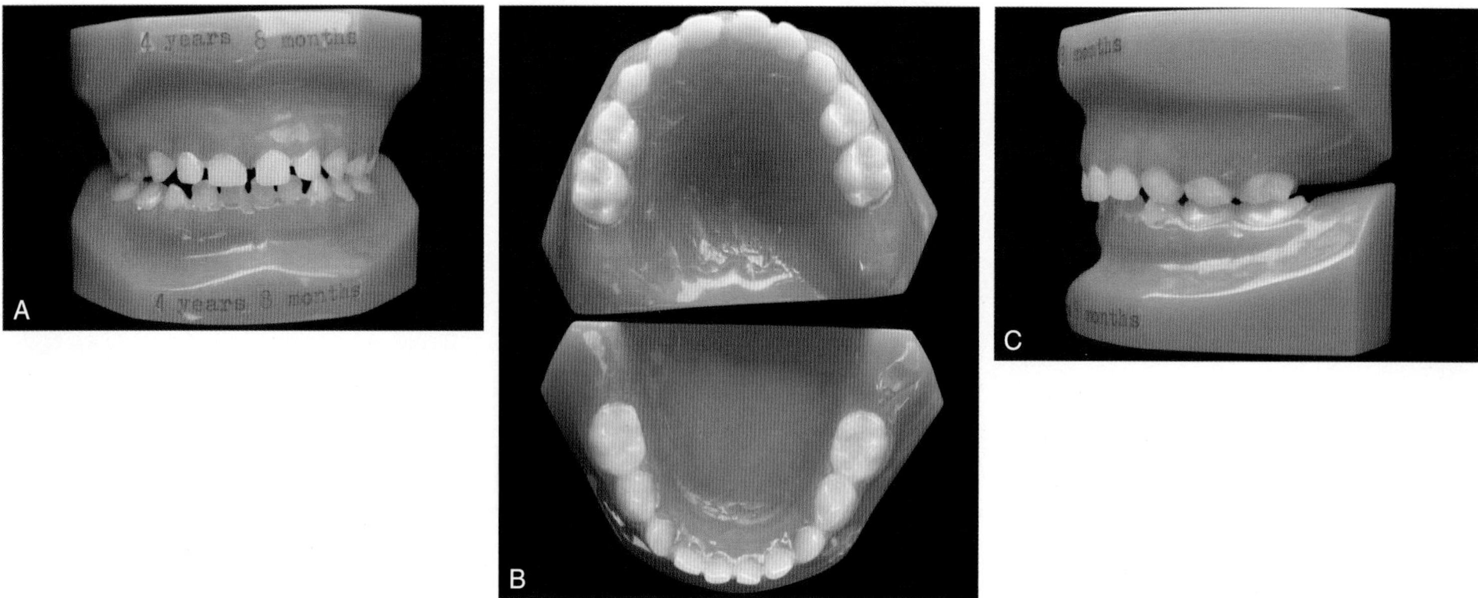

Fig. 26.37 Models of dentition at 4 years 8 months.

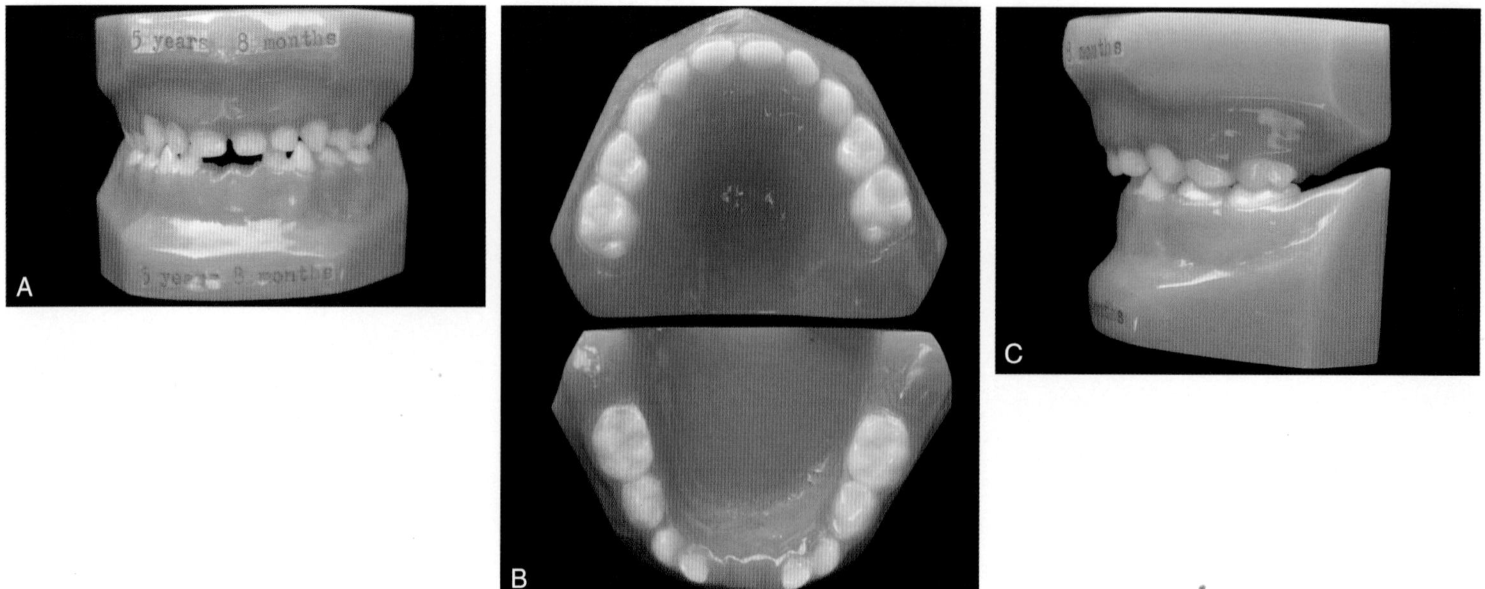

Fig. 26.38 Models of dentition at 5 years 8 months.

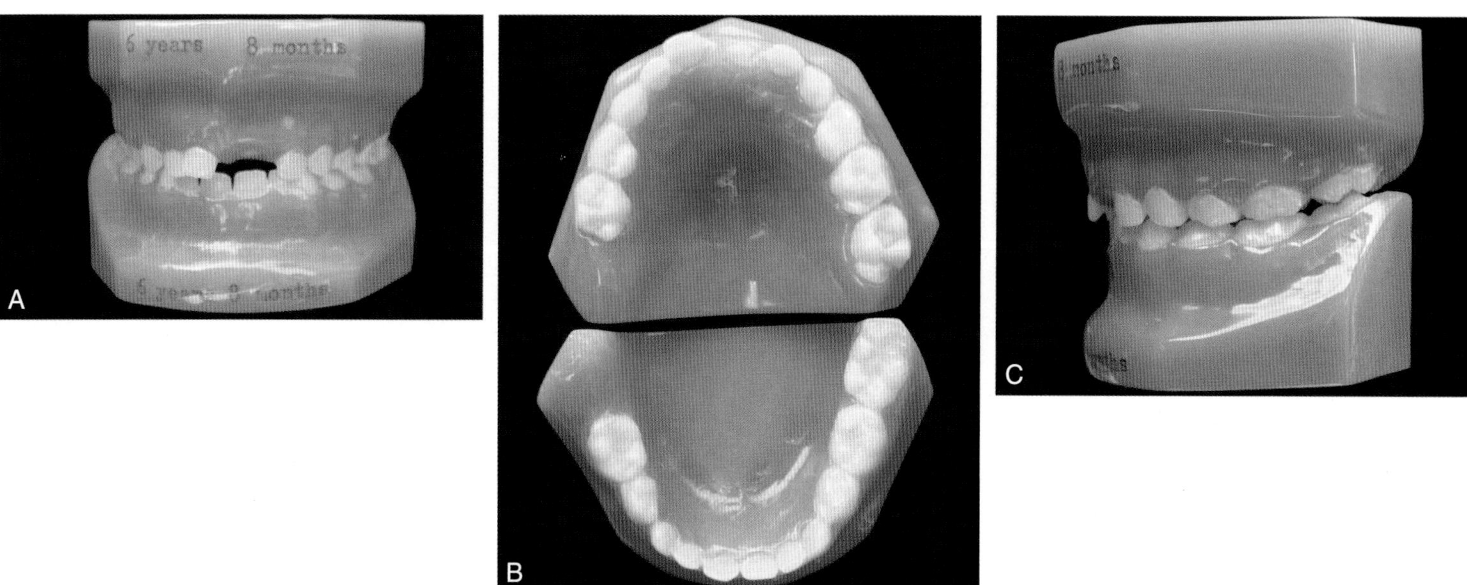

Fig. 26.39 Models of dentition at 6 years 8 months.

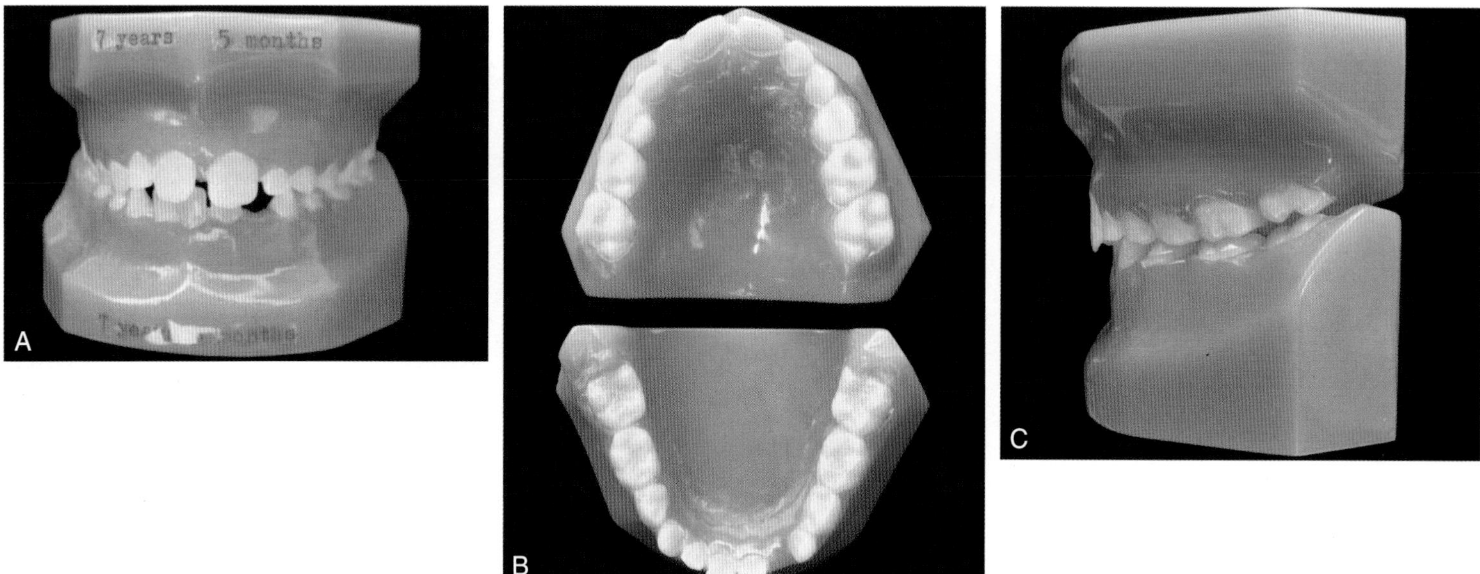

Fig. 26.40 Models of dentition at 7 years 5 months.

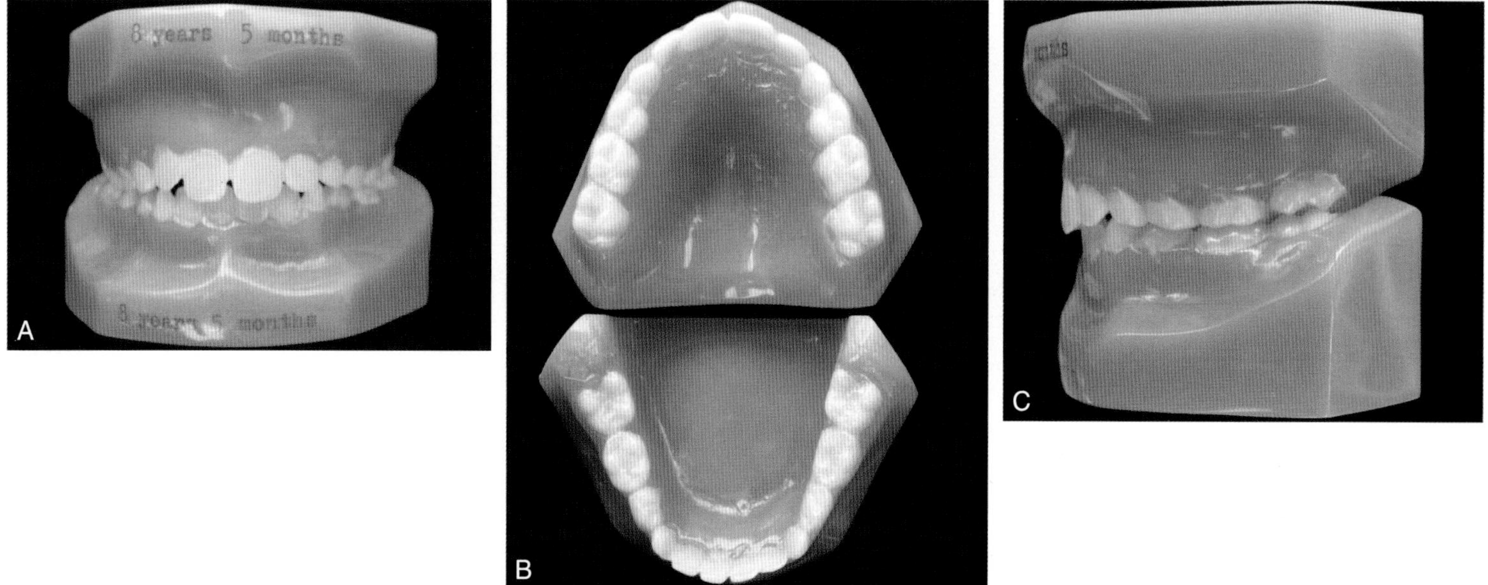

Fig. 26.41 Models of dentition at 8 years 5 months.

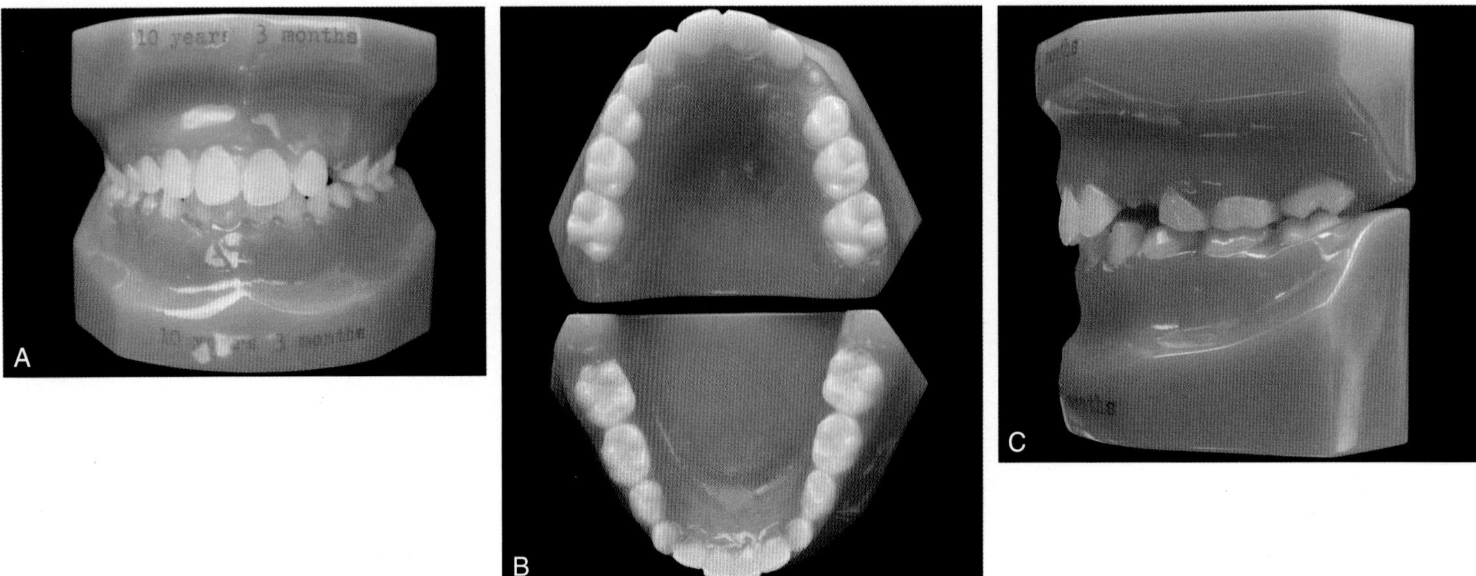

Fig. 26.42 Models of dentition at 10 years 3 months.

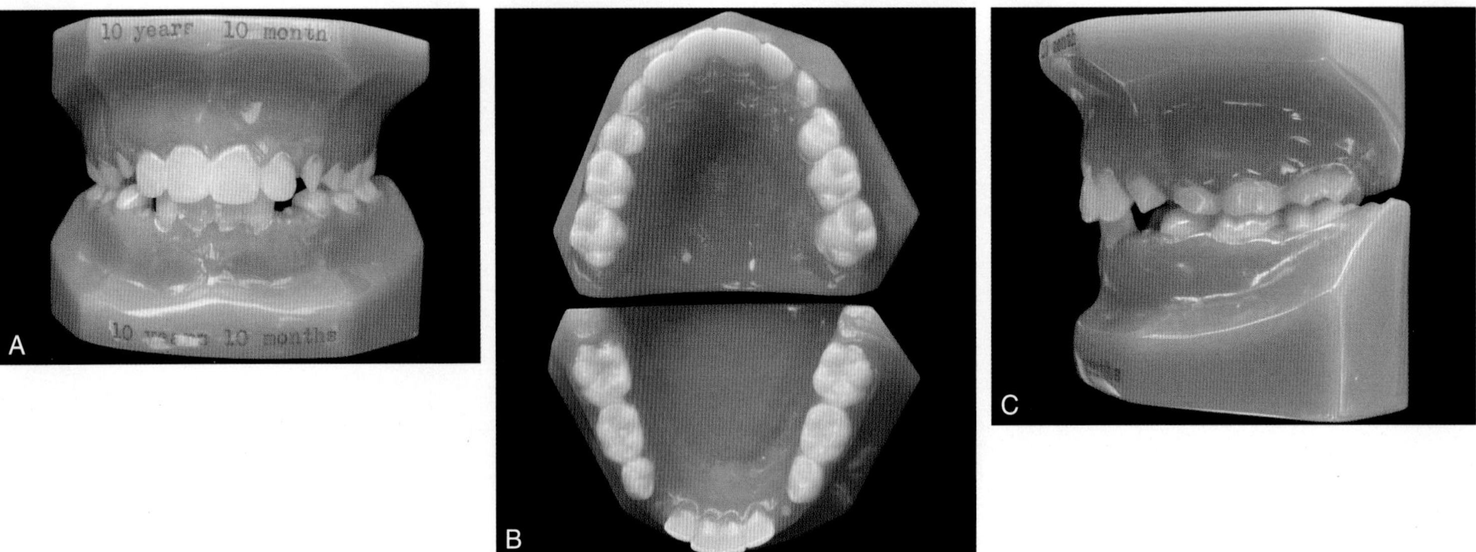

Fig. 26.43 Models of dentition at 10 years 10 months.

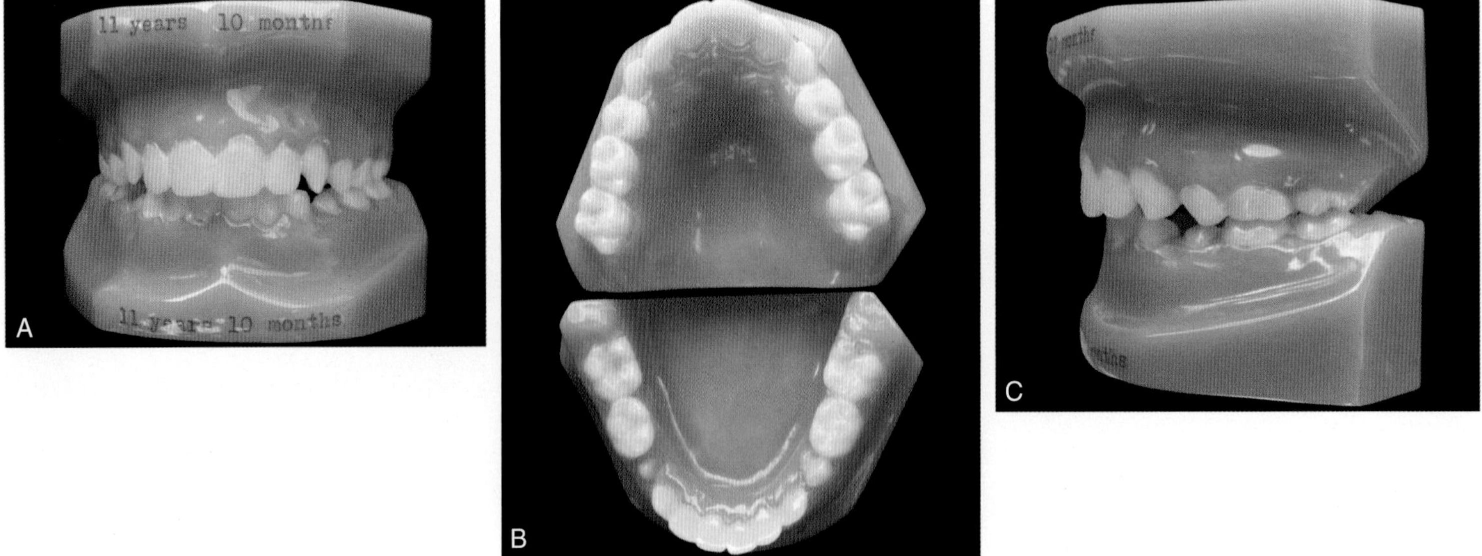

Fig. 26.44 Models of dentition at 11 years 10 months.

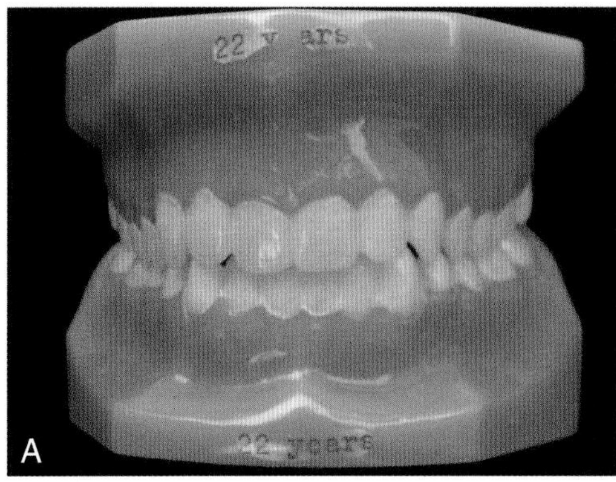

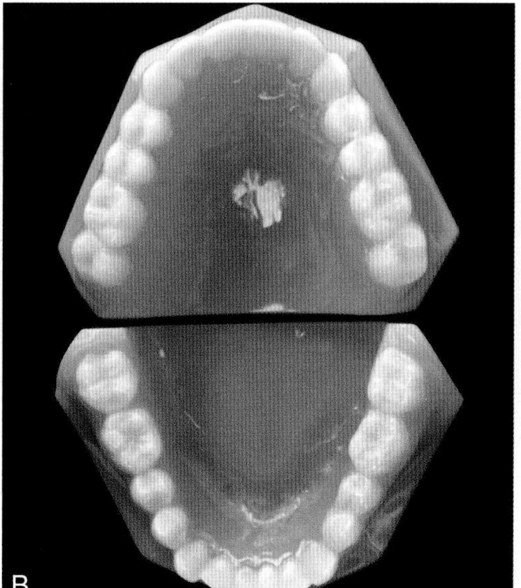

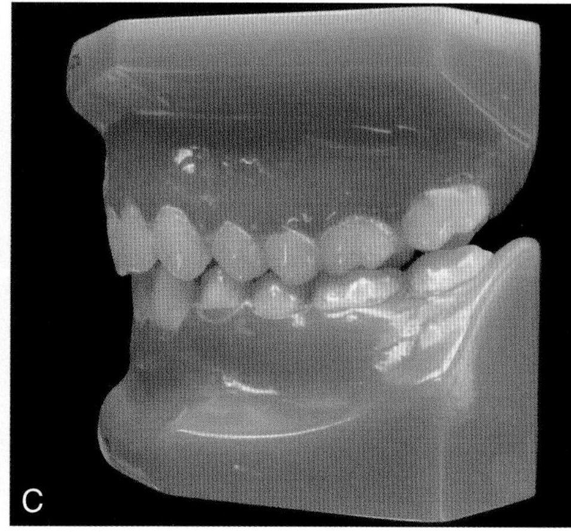

Fig. 26.45 Models of dentition at 22 years.

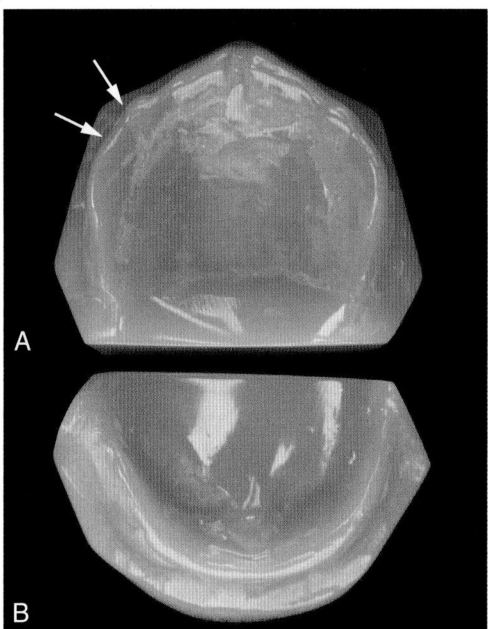

Fig. 26.46 Dentition at birth, showing gum pads with swellings (arrows) beneath which deciduous teeth are developing. A = maxilla; B = mandible.

At birth, the oral mucosa over the developing alveoli is greatly thickened to form the maxillary and mandibular gum pads. They show a series of elevations, each of which corresponds to an underlying deciduous tooth. The elevations associated with the second deciduous molars do not, however, become prominent until the age of about 6 months (Fig. 26.46). The maxillary and mandibular gum pads rarely come into occlusion, the space left between them being increased in the anterior region and being occupied by the tongue. The maxillary gum pad overlaps the mandibular gum pad both buccally and labially, with the overjet usually being considerable. This reflects the small mandible. With normal growth, the anteroposterior position of the mandible will move forward (and downward) to match that of the maxilla during the mid-teenage years. Beneath the gum pads, there is generally considerable crowding of the developing teeth, especially the incisors. During the first year of life, however, the gum pads grow rapidly, especially in lateral directions, thus providing space for the developing teeth.

The maxillary and mandibular alveolar processes are not well developed at birth. Occasionally, a 'natal tooth' is present. This tooth is usually a supernumerary tooth (see page 394), formed by an aberration in the development of the dental lamina, but occasionally it is merely a very early, but otherwise normal, deciduous first incisor (see Fig. 26.51).

The deciduous teeth start to erupt at the age of 6 months, and the deciduous dentition is complete by the age of 3 years. At this time, the occlusion of the deciduous dentition differs from that of the permanent dentition in the following respects (Fig. 26.35C):

- The incisors are more vertically positioned within the alveolus and are often spaced.
- The overbite is usually greater.
- There may be significant spacings distal to the mandibular canines and mesial to the maxillary canines (the anthropoid or primitive spaces).
- Although the anteroposterior relationships of the deciduous arches have not been adequately assessed, it appears that the distal edges of the maxillary and mandibular deciduous molars are flush and the mesiobuccal cusps of the maxillary first and second deciduous molars occlude in the buccal grooves of the mandibular first and second deciduous molars, respectively.

Several changes occur in the deciduous occlusion before the appearance of the permanent teeth. These result from changes in the dental bases. As the dental arches become wider and longer, so the deciduous teeth become more spaced. Because there is a greater forward growth of the mandible than the maxilla, the lower arch moves forwards relative to the upper, so that an edge-to-edge incisor relationship is obtained. As a further consequence, the distal surfaces of the deciduous second molars may now show a slight mesial step from maxilla to mandible, with the mesiobuccal cusp of the maxillary second deciduous molar lying distal to the buccal groove of the mandibular second deciduous molar. As the deciduous teeth approach the end of their functional life, they may show signs of considerable wear (the enamel of deciduous teeth being less mineralised and thinner than the enamel of permanent teeth – see pages 15–16).

The occlusal relationships of the deciduous and permanent molars are shown in Fig. 26.47. The flush terminal plane relationship is the usual relationship in the deciduous dentition. When the first permanent molars start to erupt, at about the age of 6 years, their relationship is determined

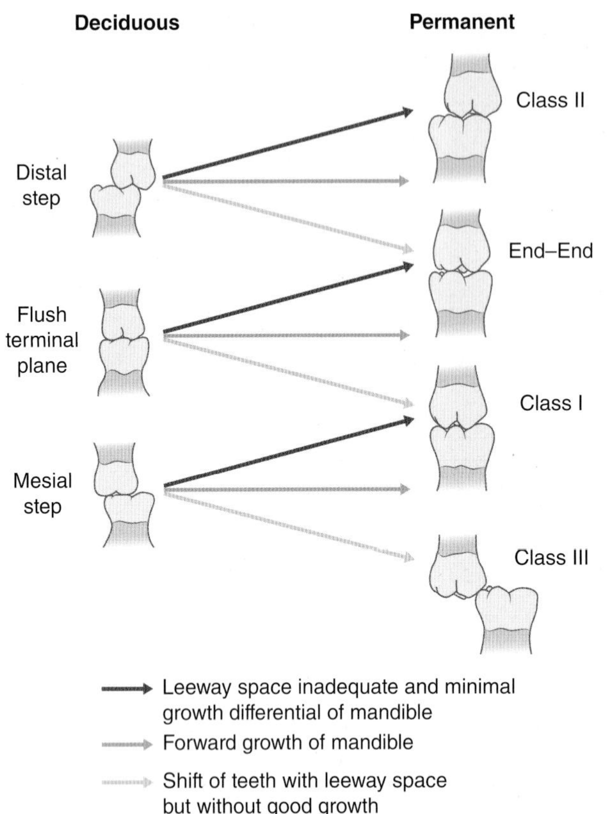

Fig. 26.47 Occlusal relationships of the deciduous and permanent molars. Modified from Moyers, R.E., 1988. *Handbook of Orthodontics*. Year Book Medical Publishers, Chicago.

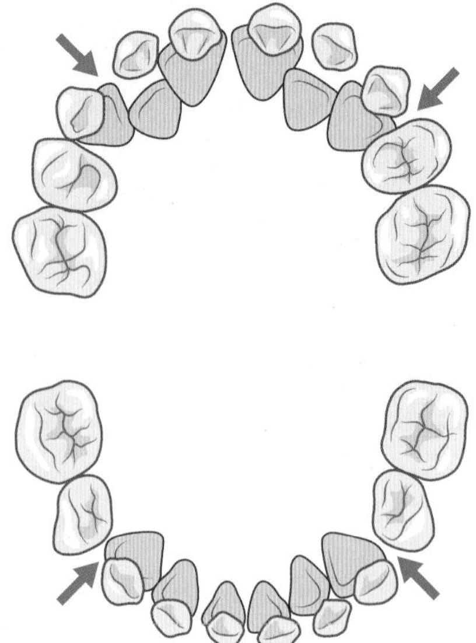

Fig. 26.48 The developmental positions of the crowns of the permanent anterior teeth (red) relative to the functional positions of the crowns of the deciduous teeth. Arrows point to the 'primate' spaces.

by that of the primary molars. The molar relationship tends to shift at the time the second deciduous molars are shed and the adolescent growth spurt occurs. As shown in Fig. 26.47, the change in molar relationship depends upon whether there is leeway space for tooth movement and upon mandibular growth.

After the age of 6 years the dentition is said to be mixed, comprising both deciduous and permanent teeth. The first molars are the first permanent teeth to erupt. Initially, they have a cusp-to-cusp relationship (the flush terminal plane; Fig. 26.47), which is governed by the position of the deciduous second molars. The first molars take up their normal adult relationship once the deciduous second molars are shed. The permanent incisors erupt between the ages of 6 and 9 years. Because the permanent incisors are much larger than their deciduous predecessors, they are accommodated into the dental arches not just by utilisation of the space left by the deciduous predecessors but also by lateral growth of the alveolar arches and the greater proclination of the permanent incisors. In their developmental positions, the lateral incisors are overlapped by the first incisors, being positioned more palatally. As a rule, space is made for the second incisors as the first incisors erupt. However, should there be insufficient growth of the alveolus, the second incisors may continue to lie in their developmental, palatal positions (Fig. 26.48). Frequently, when the permanent incisors erupt, they fan out (incline distally) so that there may be a significant space or diastema between the first incisors. This appearance has been termed the 'ugly duckling' stage and is said to result from pressure on the roots of the permanent incisors from the developing permanent canines. The diastema usually closes following eruption of the permanent canines. The canines and premolars, which usually erupt between the ages of 9 and 12 years, are readily accommodated into the dental arches because the combined mesiodistal diameters of the deciduous canines and molars are generally greater than those of their permanent successors. Any leeway space that remains is usually taken up by forward movement of the first permanent molars. By the age of 12 years, all the deciduous teeth have been shed for replacement by permanent teeth, and henceforth the occlusion appears similar to that in the adult (see pages 39–43). Space is provided for the permanent molar teeth by continued growth and remodelling of the mandible and maxilla.

In Fig. 26.48 note the lingual positioning of the permanent teeth (particularly for the maxillary lateral incisors). Spaces between the deciduous canines and the first molars for the mandible, and between the deciduous lateral incisors and canines for the maxillae, may be seen and are termed 'primate spaces', so named because they are most marked in the dentitions of primates. The primate spaces are usually seen from the time the teeth erupt. Developmental spaces between the incisors are often present at eruption but become larger as the child grows and the alveolar processes expand. Generalised spacing of the primary teeth is a requirement for proper alignment of the permanent incisors.

A graphic display of the average amount of space available within the dental arches is shown in Fig. 26.49. Note that, for both sexes, the amount of space for the mandibular incisors is negative for about 2 years after their eruption. Thus, a small degree of crowding in the mandibular arch at this time is not unusual. The teeth erupt slightly earlier in girls than in boys. In an individual, any discrepancy in eruption time greater than 6 months for a matching contralateral tooth should be investigated.

Although there is a tendency for the mandible to grow slightly farther forward than the maxilla after the age of 12 years, usually there is no appreciable occlusal change. During the later stages of facial growth there may be an accompanying uprighting of the incisors, with the result that they become more crowded. It has been suggested that mesial drift may take up any remaining space in the arches or even be responsible for some late crowding.

Once a tooth reaches its functional position, it is believed to occupy a position of equilibrium between the soft tissues of the cheeks and lips externally and the tongue internally (see Fig. 2.83).

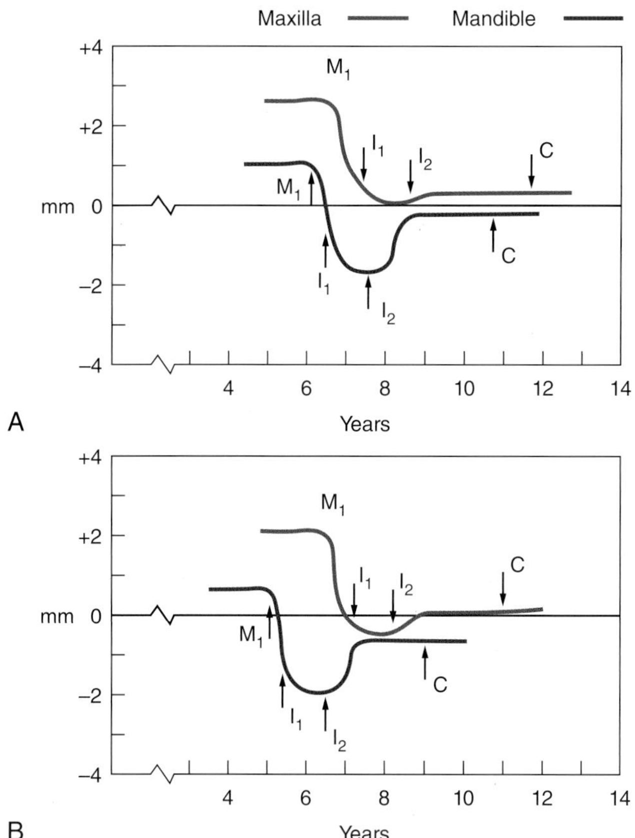

Fig. 26.49 Graphic display of the average amount of space available within the dental arches for boys (A) and for girls (B). The arrows indicate the timing of eruption of the first molars (M1), first and second incisors (I1 and I2) and canines (C). Modified after Dr. C F A Moorrees and J M Chadha and Angle Orthodontics.

Mesial drift

The interproximal contact points of newly erupted and relatively unworn teeth cover only a small area. While attrition removes hard tissues at the occlusal surfaces, it is also accompanied by wear of the interproximal surfaces of teeth. Even though this is accompanied by a reduction in the mesiodistal (anteroposterior) dimensions of the cheek teeth, the teeth maintain contact with each other because of a forward movement known as *mesial drift*. This will result in the contact points meeting over a larger area (Fig. 26.50). It has been reported that where the food is abrasive and there is considerable masticatory activity, the first permanent molar drifts approximately 4 mm in a mesial direction between the ages of 6 and 18 years. The mesial drift that occurs in these situations helps provide space for erupting mandibular third molars. The absence of an abrasive diet and the accompanying reduction in mesial drift associated with soft diets may account for the high occurrence of impacted mandibular third molars in some modern populations.

Four hypotheses have been postulated to account for mesial drift:

1) The mesial inclination of teeth produces a resultant force during biting that favours mesial drift.
2) The actions of certain jaw muscles, particularly the buccinator, 'propel' the teeth forwards.
3) Bone deposited preferentially on the distal surface of the sockets pushes the teeth mesially.
4) Contraction of the gingival connective tissues (especially the transseptal collagen fibres in the gingiva – see page 306) brings about mesial drift.

Concerning hypothesis 1, a detailed analysis of mesial drift does not suggest that there is a direct relationship with the angulation of the teeth.

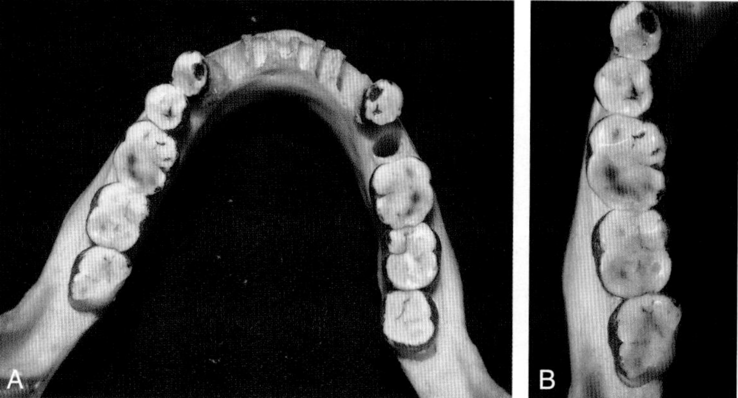

Fig. 26.50 (A) Occlusal view of mandible with teeth showing evidence of considerable attrition. Because of mesial drift, the cheek teeth have maintained contact and the interproximal contact points are broad. (B) Higher-power view of cheek teeth with interproximal attrition and broad contact points as a result of mesial drift.

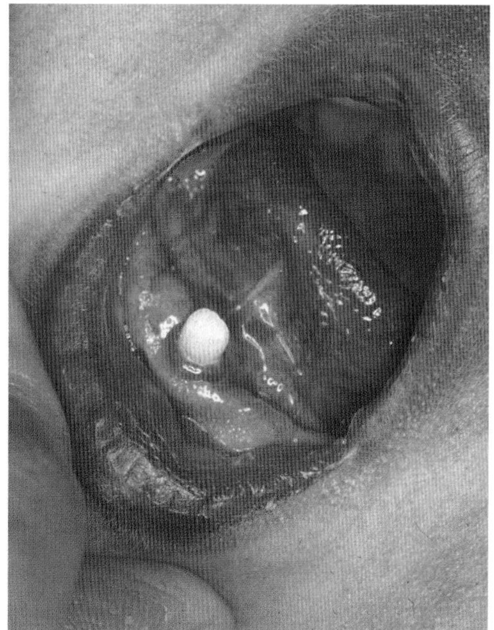

Fig. 26.51 Mandibular left deciduous incisor erupted at birth, representing a neonatal tooth.

Evidence against hypothesis 2 comes from the observation that mesial drift still occurs even when teeth are protected by an overlay that would prevent muscle contact. Bone activity is observed during mesial drift (hypothesis 3), but it is not possible to separate cause and effect. Although there is some evidence that damage to the gingiva retards mesial drift, there is little evidence that connective tissues contract *in vivo*. As with tooth eruption, the evidence might indicate that the mechanisms of mesial drift are multifactorial and involve the periodontal tissues.

Clinical considerations

Natal teeth

One or more teeth may be present at birth and are referred to as *natal teeth*. They most commonly represent deciduous mandibular incisors (85% – Fig. 26.51). If they appear during the first month of birth, they are called *neonatal teeth*. Natal teeth may be found in the anterior region of the maxilla in association with cleft lip/palate. They have only a small amount of root formed and are mobile. For this reason (together with difficulty associated with breast feeding), they are often extracted.

Premature and delayed eruption

Permanent teeth may erupt early when their deciduous predecessors have been extracted prematurely because of dental caries. Early eruption of the whole dentition may be associated with a general hormonal disturbance such as hyperpituitarism or hyperthyroidism.

The most common eruptive disorders are delayed eruption (or noneruption) of one (or more) permanent anterior maxillary teeth or the mandibular third molars. In the case of mandibular third molars, the reason is lack of space so that the tooth is impacted against the second permanent molar immediately in front (Fig. 26.52). If the crown of the impacted third molar is partially erupted, food debris may accumulate in the stagnation area between the overlying gum flap and the crown and may lead to an inflammatory reaction in the gingiva (pericoronitis). This may eventually spread to involve surrounding tissue spaces (see pages 92–95). If the tooth is malaligned, it may remain unerupted. Delayed eruption of maxillary permanent first incisors is most commonly caused by obstruction by a supernumerary tooth (Fig. 26.53) or an odontome (see Fig. 21.45). Removal of the obstruction will allow for eruption with or without the aid of orthodontic appliances. In some cases, no obstruction is present and the occlusal margins of the anterior teeth can be seen just beneath the oral mucosa and yet the teeth refuse to erupt. In such cases, surgical exposure will usually be sufficient to allow eruption. Delayed eruption may also be associated with teeth where the enamel organ has undergone a cystic change to form a dentigerous (eruption) cyst above its tooth, hence preventing its eruption (Fig. 26.54).

Because of its high developmental position within the maxilla, its malalignment and the presence of crowding within the dental arch, the maxillary permanent canine may be prevented from erupting into the dental arch, and this is reflected in the retention of its deciduous predecessor (Fig. 26.55). Assuming such impacted teeth are favourably positioned, they may be drawn into the dental arch by suitably designed orthodontic appliances.

Ankylosis

If the periodontal ligament is damaged, the root of a tooth may become fixed (ankylosed) to the adjacent alveolar bone. The deciduous tooth is then unable to move. Its position within the jaw remains constant so that, as height of the alveolar bone increases, the tooth appears to sink gradually below the level of the adjacent teeth. Such ankylosed teeth are referred to as 'submerged' teeth (Figs. 26.56, 26.57). The submergence may continue to such an extent that the teeth become completely buried within bone. The cause of this condition is not always apparent, although there may be an association with trauma or inflammation. It may also affect permanent molars.

Generalised conditions affecting eruption

There are many human syndromic conditions that can disrupt eruption, and these are shown in Table 26.2. Approximately 50% of these conditions can now be attributed to a genetic defect. Note that 'primary failure of eruption' affects mainly permanent posterior teeth and refers to a localised failure with no other systemic involvement. It has been suggested that this condition is a defect of the eruptive mechanism itself. However, the precise cause of the lack of eruption is presently unknown. As an example of a syndromic condition, Fig. 26.58 represents an orthopantomogram of a patient with cleidocranial dysplasia (dysostosis). This syndrome is caused by a mutation in the *Cbfa1* gene (see page 272). Most of the teeth are unerupted, and several supernumerary teeth may be encountered.

Further readings for this chapter can be found in the accompanying eBook. Explore online Self-assessment quiz to test and reinforce your understanding of the material in your free ebook. Follow instructions in the Inside Front Cover to unlock your access.

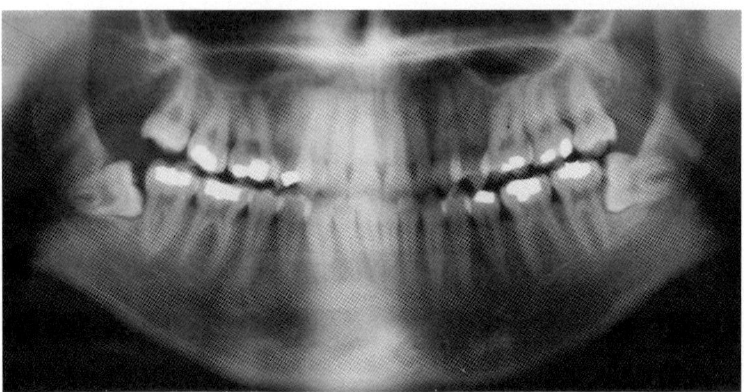

Fig. 26.52 Orthopantomogram showing impacted mandibular third permanent molars.

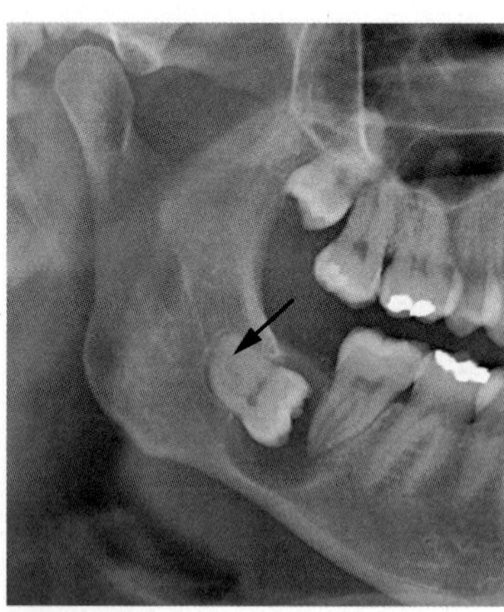

Fig. 26.54 Lateral radiograph showing an unerupted mandibular third molar (arrow) surrounded by radiolucent dentigerous cyst. Courtesy Dr. J Makdissi.

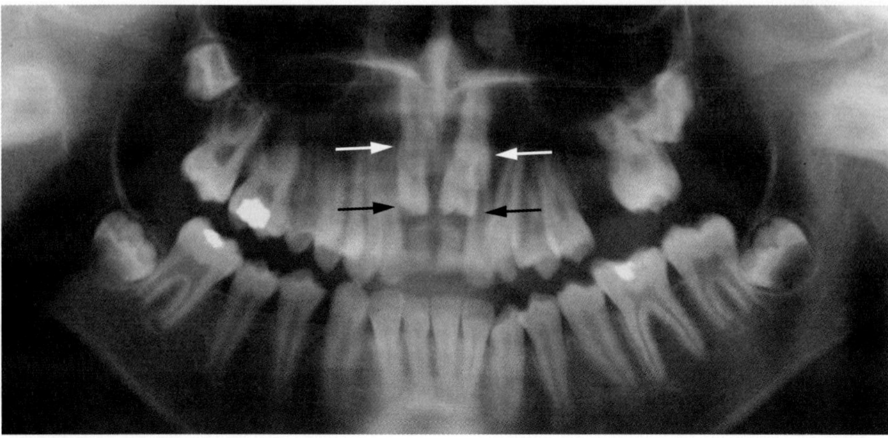

Fig. 26.53 Orthopantomogram of a 14-year-old patient with two supernumerary teeth (black arrows) preventing the eruption of the two maxillary first permanent incisors (white arrows). Note the associated retention of the two maxillary first deciduous incisors.

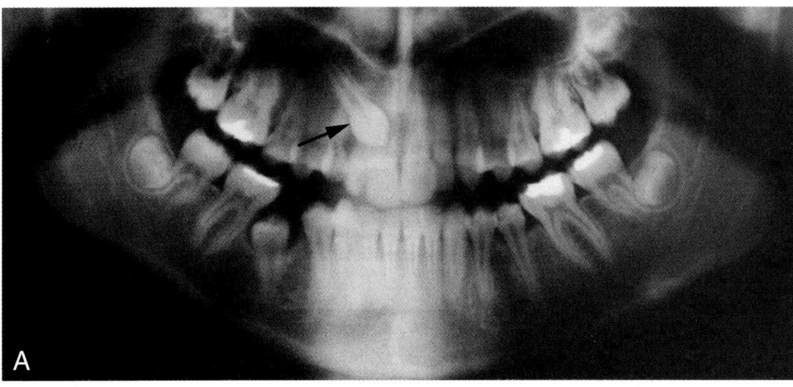

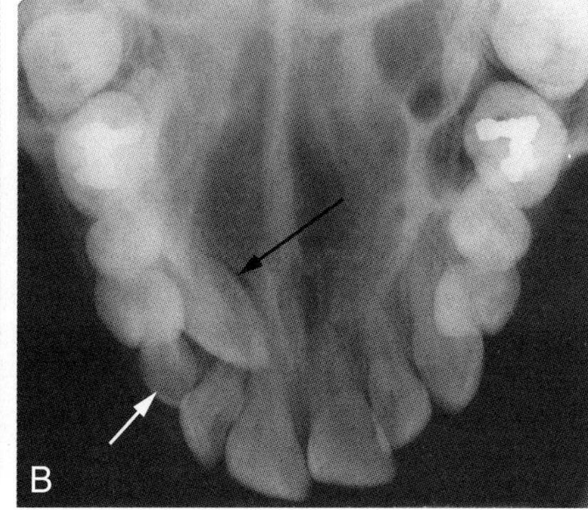

Fig. 26.55 (A) Orthopantomogram of a 15-year-old patient with an unerupted maxillary permanent canine (arrow), above which is a retained deciduous maxillary canine. (B) Maxillary occlusal radiograph showing the unerupted maxillary permanent canine (black arrow) and the retained maxillary deciduous canine (white arrow).

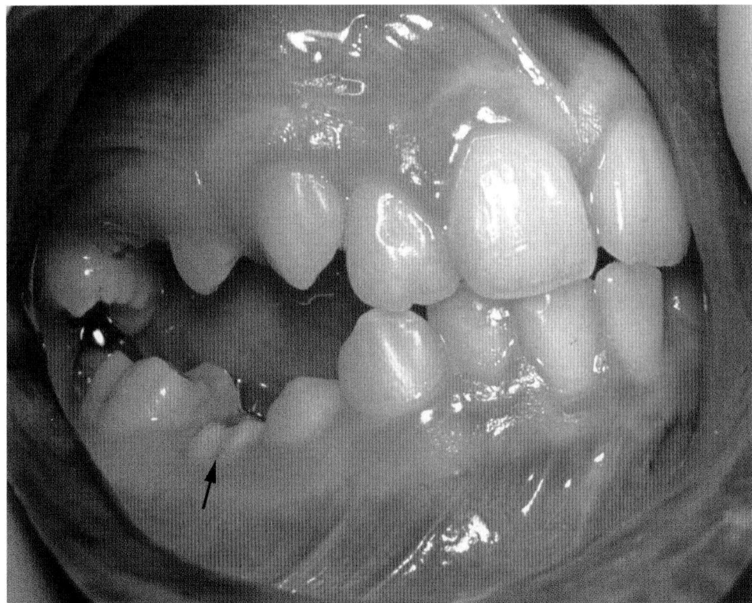

Fig. 26.56 Patient with a submerging mandibular right deciduous second molar (arrow). Courtesy Dr. P Smith.

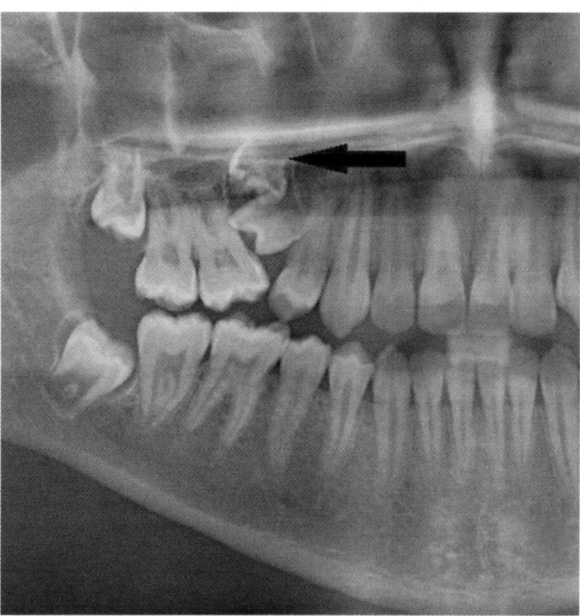

Fig. 26.57 Orthopantomogram of patient with a submerging maxillary second deciduous molar (arrow) that will prevent the eruption of the second premolar above it. Courtesy Dr. J Makdissi.

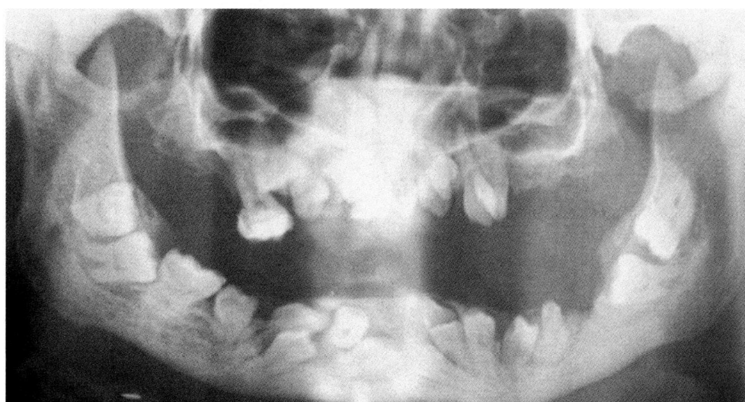

Fig. 26.58 Orthopantomogram of patient with cleidocranial dysplasia (dysostosis). The majority of teeth are unerupted and may include supernumerary teeth.

Table 26.2 Genetic disorders of eruption

Syndrome/condition	Eruption phenotype	Genetic defect	Mode of inheritance
Cleidocranial dysplasia	Delayed eruption	Six different types of mutation in *PEBP2aA/CBFA1*	Autosomal dominant
Osteopetrosis	Failure of eruption	*TRAF6*	Autosomal recessive and dominant forms
GAPO syndrome	Failure of eruption	Unknown	Autosomal recessive
Osteopathia striata with cranial sclerosis	Failure of eruption in some cases	Unknown	Autosomal dominant
Osteoglophonic dysplasia	Failure of eruption of secondary teeth	Unknown	Autosomal dominant
Singleton–Merten syndrome	Dysplastic development with delayed eruption of secondary teeth	Unknown	Possibly autosomal dominant
Aarskog's syndrome	Delayed eruption	*FGDY1* codes for Rho/Rac guanine nuclear exchange factor (involved with growth regulation)	X-linked recessive
Acrodysostosis	Delayed tooth eruption (23% of cases)	Unknown	Autosomal dominant
Albright's hereditary osteodystrophy	Delayed eruption	Variety of mutations in *GNAS1* (G, protein)	Autosomal dominant
Apert's syndrome	Delayed and ectopic eruption	Mutations in *FGFR2* gene	Autosomal dominant
Chondroectodermal dysplasia (Ellis–van Creveld syndrome)	Delayed eruption, partial anodontia	Several mutations in the *EVC* gene	Autosomal recessive
Cockayne's syndrome	Delayed eruption	*CSB* (*ERCC6*) gene (helicase)	Autosomal recessive
De Lange's syndrome	Delayed eruption	Unknown (*SHOT* is candidate gene)	Possibly autosomal dominant
Dubowitz's syndrome	Delayed eruption and hypodontia	Unknown	Possibly autosomal recessive
Frontometaphyseal dysplasia (Gorlin–Cohen syndrome)	Delayed eruption and retained deciduous teeth	Unknown	Autosomal dominant or X-linked recessive (debated)
Goltz's syndrome (focal dermal hypoplasia)	Delayed eruption and hypodontia with hypoplastic teeth	Unknown	X-linked dominant with lethality in hemizygous males
Hunter's syndrome	Delayed eruption	Variety of mutations in *IDS* (iduronate-2 sulphatase) gene	X-linked
Incontinentia pigmenti	Delayed eruption, hypodontia in 80%	Mapped to Xp11.2, rarely *IKK* gene	X-linked dominant, lethality in males
Killian's/Teschler–Nicola syndrome	Delayed eruption	Mosaic tetrasomy 12p in skin fibroblasts	Chromosomal aberration
Levy–Hollister syndrome	Delayed eruption of primary teeth	Unknown	Autosomal dominant
Maroteaux–Lamy mucopolysaccharidosis syndrome	Delayed eruption with small teeth	Variety of mutations in aryl sulphatase B (*ASB*) gene	Autosomal recessive
Osteogenesis imperfecta syndrome type I	Delayed eruption, dysplastic teeth	*COL1A1* and *COL1A2*	Autosomal dominant variable expressivity
Progeria syndrome (Hutchinson–Gilford syndrome)	Delayed eruption of primary and secondary teeth and hypodontia of secondary° teeth	DNA helicase, telomerase	Autosomal recessive
Pyknodysostosis	Delayed eruption and occasional anodontia	Cathepsin K gene	Autosomal recessive
Primary failure of eruption	Failure of secondary teeth to erupt partially or completely	Unknown	Unknown

From Wise, G.E., Frazier-Bowers, S., D'Souza, R.N., 2002. Primary and secondary refer to deciduous and permanent teeth respectively. Cellular, molecular, and genetic determinants of tooth eruption. *Critical Reviews in Oral Biology and Medicine* 13, 323–334.

Phases of development of the dentition:

Pre-eruptive phase

Eruptive (Pre-functional) phase

Functional phase

Order and Timings of Eruption:

Lower A (8.5 m), Upper A (9 m), Lower B (9 m), Upper B (11 m), Lower C (11.5 m), Upper & Lower Ds (16 m), Upper C (19 m), Upper E (24 m), Lower E (27 m)

Upper and Lower 6s (6 y), Lower 1 (6.3 y), Upper 1(7.1 y), Lower 2 (7.4 y), Upper 2 (8.1 y), Lower 3 (10.5 y), Upper 4 (10.6 y), Lower 4 & 5 (10.7 y), Upper 3 and 5 (11.1 y), Lower 7 (11.3 y), Upper 7 (11.6 y), Lower 8 (17.8 y), Upper 8 (18.9 y)

Chronology of Development

Development of the Dentition and Occlusion

Occlusion

By the age of 3 years (i.e., at the time of completion of eruption of the deciduous dentition), the occlusion of the deciduous dentition differs in the following respects to the occlusion of the permanent dentition:

1. The deciduous incisors are more vertical and spaced
2. The overbite is usually greater
3. Distal to the lower canines but mesial to the upper canines may be located 'anthropoid or primitive spaces'
4. Distal edges of upper and lower molars are flush
5. Mesiobuccal cusps of upper molars occlude in the buccal grooves of the lower molars

For the mind map related to the process and mechanism of tooth eruption, see Mind Map 26.2

Mind Map 26.1 Development of the dentition and occlusion.

The role of the periodontal ligament and dental follicle:

Root resection and transection experiments for teeth of continuous growth indicate that the source of eruptive forces resides in the PDL, and transplantation experiments for teeth of limited growth suggest that the forces are generated in the PDL's precursor, the dental follicle.

Evidence against a "tractional" eruptive force pulling the tooth via the collagen network:

From studies using lathyrogens

From tooth transplantation experiments

From studies on the development of the PDL

Eruption of rootless teeth

The fibroblast contraction/migration hypothesis

Evidence indicates that PDL fibroblasts migrate with eruption (passive or active migration to effect eruption?)

Fibroblasts *in vitro* have features of migratory or contractile cells but *in vivo* lack myofibroblast-like features, being cells rapidly turning over collagen

The vascular/tissue hydrostatic pressure hypothesis

Supported by evidence from changes in tooth position with arterial pulse, events at death, effects of vasoactive drugs and cutting or stimulating the vasomotor innervation, measurements of tissue hydrostatic pressure, the biochemistry of the ECM of the PDL, and the morphology of the PDL vasculature

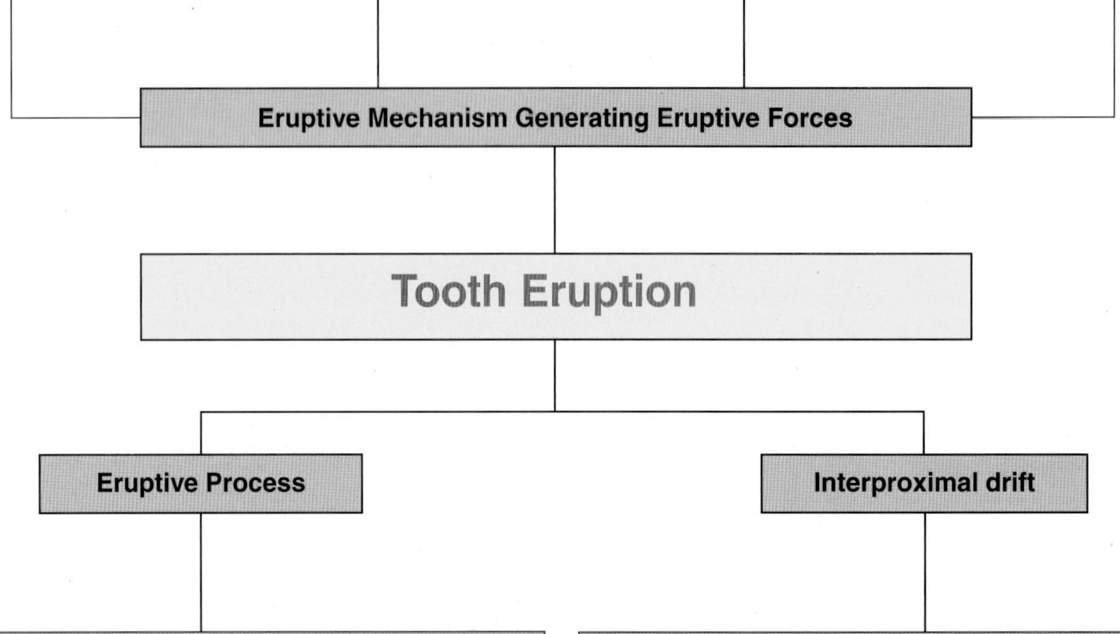

Key features: (Eruptive Process)

Pre-eruptive, eruptive/prefunctional and functional phases. Eruption commences once tooth root starts to form. Continues throughout life.

As tooth erupts, bony crypt remodels and as tooth approaches oral cavity, resorption of the connective tissues of the oral mucosa with the formation of an epithelial eruptive pathway on fusion of the reduced enamel epithelium and the oral epithelium (note formation of junctional epithelium)

Note resorption of deciduous predecessor by "odontoclasts" (phasic, with some attempts at repair)

Presence of gubernaculum for erupting permanent teeth

Key features: (Interproximal drift)

Usually mesial drift for human dentition (although distal drift possible)

Mesial drift can help provide space for eruption of third molars

Hypotheses for force generation:

- mesial inclination of teeth and direction of biting forces
- muscular activity (particularly buccinator)
- bone deposition on distal surfaces of tooth sockets
- contraction of trans-septal collagen fibres in gingiva
- vascular/tissue fluid hydrostatic pressures

Mind Map 26.2 Tooth eruption.

Archaeological applications of tooth structure

27

Because of their durability, teeth and bones are usually the only remaining traces of humans and animals from the past. For this reason, much scientific study of hard tissues has been undertaken using a variety of innovative techniques to maximise what teeth can tell us about the past.

Whereas until fairly recently if one came across a burial site, one might determine from the skeletons the approximate age of the individuals and possibly their sex, now it is possible to determine where they were born, whether and to where they have migrated to during life, the nature of the climate and considerable detail about their (e.g., whether primarily carnivorous or C3 and/or C4 plant based, whether the diet contained sea food products). Amongst any group of individuals in a burial site, it is now a simple matter to identify any 'foreigners'. Importantly, such information can be obtained from teeth that are tens and even hundreds of millions of years old.

Ageing of the human dentition

It is relatively easy to age a dentition of up to about 20 years of age from a knowledge of the dates of tooth development, eruption and root formation (see Chapter 26). However, it is less easy for dentitions in older specimens, and particularly with isolated teeth. Yet teeth may be the only parts of a body available for identifying and ageing individuals for forensic purposes (forensic odontology). All dental tissues undergo age changes (see individual chapters). Consequently, one can estimate the amount of wear in enamel and dentine and measure the amount of secondary dentine formation and the reduction in the size of the pulp cavity. One can estimate further features, such as the amount of translucent dentine and the thickness of cementum. For each of a number of such features, one can give a score and, by deriving a total score for the tooth, refer to an appropriate table to get an estimate of age. Of these variables, the single most reliable feature for age estimation appears to be the amount of translucent dentine in the root.

Ageing of skeletal material is of fundamental importance in both archaeological and forensic situations. Of all body structures, teeth are likely to provide the most accurate assessment (see earlier). An example where a knowledge of dental anatomy was important occurred when investigating skeletal material of very young babies. Some graveyards in Punic Carthage, whose peak civilisation coincided with the fourth century BCE, contained many skeletal remains of very young infants. An important question related to such material was whether it provided evidence of human sacrifice of the living new-born. Examination of the first permanent molars of such babies revealed that a large number lacked evidence of a neonatal line (see page 147), indicating that they were stillborn and therefore not ceremonially sacrificed after birth.

Childhood dependency

A critical feature in the evolution of modern humans has been the development of a large brain. This development is very expensive in terms of energy requirements and therefore food intake. It takes a prolonged period to develop a large brain and the extra skills that are consequently possible with it. All of this can only be achieved with greater dependency of an infant on its parents. For most animals, this extra cost in parental energy and attention is simply not worth it, as their lifespan is relatively short. But when mortality rates are low and animals live longer, as in the case of humans, dependency pays off because the offspring are better equipped to survive and produce more offspring of their own. During this time of dependency and protection, the infant can learn the ways of the family group and get a head start in its fight for survival. The period of increased dependency is called 'childhood', and it correlates approximately with the period between the eruption of the last deciduous molar teeth at 3 years and the eruption of the first permanent molar teeth at 6 years (see Chapter 26). Moreover, brains get bigger as childhood lengthens, and the time at which the first permanent molars erupt correlates with the time brains are almost fully grown.

In our closest living relative, the chimpanzee, the first permanent molars erupt at about 3.5 years of age, with little or no period for childhood development. It follows that if we can discover the age at which the first permanent molars erupted in extinct hominins, we can determine whether they were more like modern humans or more like living great apes. This helps identify the first fossil groups to show an extended period of childhood.

Ageing the Nariokotome boy

An example of where the importance of ageing a dentition casts light on human evolution can be seen with regard to the Nariokotome boy. He represents one of the most important *Homo erectus* specimens and comprises the almost complete skeleton of a boy, dated at 1.5 million years old, at Nariokotome, by Lake Turkana in Kenya. The very rare finding of an almost complete skeleton meant that his height and probable weight could be firmly established. In addition, because many bones initially develop as a number of separate pieces that fuse together within a specific time frame, a good estimate of age could be determined from the skeleton. Results initially indicated that the Nariokotome boy was 160 cm tall (5 feet 3 inches) with a skeletal age of about 12 years. His dentition was remarkably complete. All his permanent teeth had erupted, except for his third molars and upper canines, and comparisons with a modern human dentition would give a dental age of about 12 years (Fig. 27.1).

If correctly aged at about 12 years, this suggests he had a reasonable period of childhood, putting him close to the ancestral tree of *Homo sapiens*. It was also estimated that the Nariokotome boy would have had an adult height of over 6 feet, which would make this species very tall. However, from a detailed study using incremental lines in the teeth (see also page 147 for *Paranthrus robustus*), the age at death was re-estimated to be more correctly about 8 years, far lower than the first estimate made by analysing bone development. This would also place the growth pattern of a juvenile *H. erectus* as being similar to that of a chimpanzee and not a modern-day human. Therefore, even a fossil close to human origins as *H. erectus* lacked the slower growth phase of the human child.

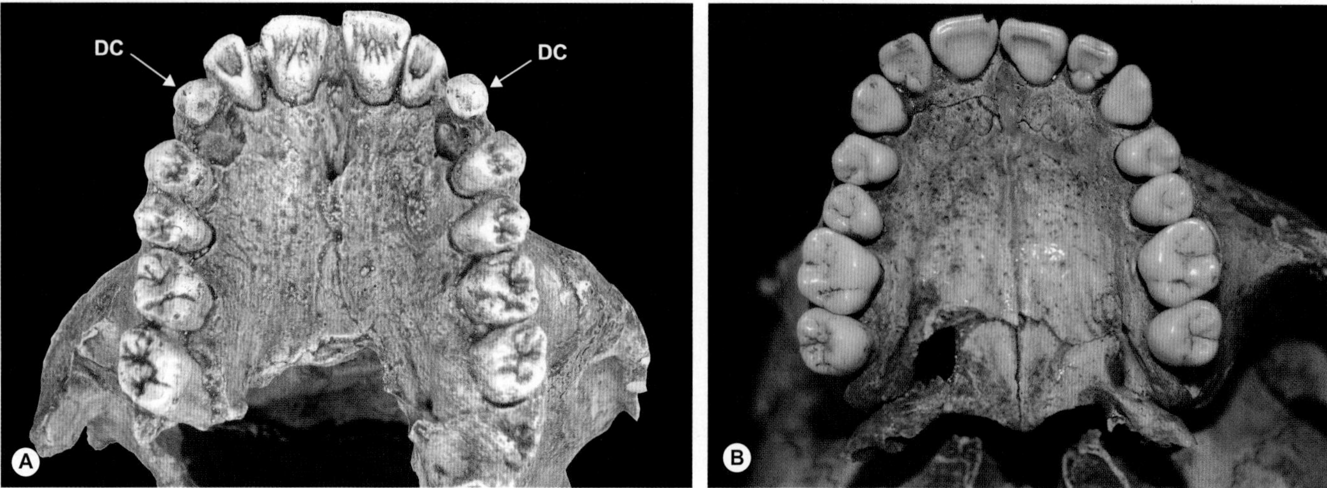

Fig. 27.1 Comparison of the upper dentition of the Nariokotome boy (A) with that of a 12- to 13-year-old modern human (B). Both are at the same stage of dental development with the second permanent molars erupted at the back (arrows). The only difference is that the permanent canines have erupted in the human, while they are just erupting in the Nariokotome boy, who still has the deciduous canine (DC) in place. Courtesy of Professor C. Dean and the Hunterian Museum at Royal College of Surgeons of England. Photographed by M. Farrell.

Wear

Teeth wear by direct contact with each other (attrition) or by contact with food (abrasion). Attrition is technically 'two-body' wear, in which material is lost from two contacting surfaces when high points are removed by shear or adhesion. Enamel particles broken off the surfaces can act as abrasive particles and can create scratch marks. Attrition facets are shiny because the surfaces are smoothed by wear and have defined edges because the wear process is limited to the area where the opposing surfaces are in contact (see pages 149–150). Abrasion is a form of 'three-body' wear in which dispersed hard particles act as abrasives and detach material from the tooth surfaces. Abraded surfaces are roughened by scratches and pits and have rounded edges because the abrasive action is not strictly limited to the contact area between the wear surfaces. The abrasive agent can be hard particles intrinsic to the food. Wear affects not only the occlusal surfaces of teeth but also the interproximal surfaces, where adjacent teeth contact each other. This approximal wear potentially creates a space between the teeth and is compensated for by mesial drift, which causes the more posterior tooth to move forward (see pages 472–473).

Microwear analysis

Microscopically, tooth enamel surfaces subjected to abrasion during food processing show a variety of pits and scratches instead of the smoother appearance typical of attrition. In microwear analysis, the depth and abundance of these features are interpreted in light of the knowledge about the physical properties of foods to provide information about the diet of an animal. Potentially, microwear analysis can discriminate between morphologically similar taxa or between different populations and can provide information on seasonal variations in diet.

It is unlikely that all components of the diet contribute to microwear patterns. The food components that seem most likely to create microwear features are plant phytoliths (particles of silica deposited in leaves), hard fruits, mollusc shells, bone and enamel particles chipped off the teeth during chewing. Dust, grit and soil ingested with the diet will also contribute to microwear.

The basis of microwear analysis is to obtain images of wear features on appropriate tooth surfaces and to quantify the images so as to obtain summary data which can be used in comparisons between taxa. To apply the method successfully, careful standardisation of such factors as choice of wear facet, cleaning method and the procedure for sampling surfaces is essential. Dental microwear patterns are short-lived, as the pattern created by one meal will be added to and 'overwritten' by the marks produced by later meals. Turnover times of microwear features are variable. They may persist for periods of from weeks down to 24 hours or less. Thus, the information relates to feeding during the last days or weeks of the animal's life. It is therefore possible that a particular microwear pattern is the result of a meal that is not typical of the animal's diet (because of opportunistic feeding or shortage of the usual food), and it is important to use large sample sizes so that anomalous patterns can be detected.

Most studies have employed scanning electron micrographs of epoxy replicas, which are then quantified manually. This method, however, is time-consuming and subject to interexaminer variability. Recently, a new and more discriminatory type of analysis – dental microwear texture analysis (DMTA) – has been developed to provide a more detailed, three-dimensional quantification of the enamel surface. This method combines scanning confocal microscopy with scale-sensitive fractal analyses to measure surface topography at different scales. Using topographic analysis software, the data are levelled, the defects are removed and the surfaces are measured using volumes, areas and vectors, resulting in a quantitative description of the surfaces at multiple scales. Five main measurements capture such features as textural complexity (or roughness), heterogeneity (variations across the field of interest) and anisotropy (the directionality of wear).

Microwear analysis has revealed, for example, significant differences between frugivorous and folivorous primates, soft-fruit diets and hard-fruit diets in primates and browsing and grazing. Typically, frugivores have higher proportions of pits relative to scratches; folivores, more scratches than pits; hard-object feeders, the most pits. Microwear analyses of modern and fossil bovids have differentiated between grazers, characterised by many scratches, and browsers, characterised by fewer scratches.

Among mammals in general, consumers of mainly hard, brittle foods tend to have higher microwear surface texture complexity, whereas those that more often shear or slice tough items have more surface anisotropy. This is illustrated by the DTMA patterns from the teeth of four pairs of related mammals with different diets.

DNA samples

DNA may be recovered from the pulp cavities of teeth and can provide significant information on the identity of the individuals concerned. Not only does this apply to modern-day individuals, but DNA has been recovered from the teeth of individuals tens of thousands of years old. Remarkably, DNA has been sequenced from three groups of hominin: Neanderthals, Denisovans and early *H. sapiens*. Present-day humans possess small traces of Neanderthal DNA, confirming that early *H. sapiens* and Neanderthals interbred.

Palaeoproteomics

This new science is dependant upon recent technical advances that to analyse ancient proteins to answer questions about the history and evolution of humans and other animals. As with DNA, proteins can be extracted from the dental tissues of ancient jaws, particularly collagen. As an example of its potential, collagen from dentine (and bone) in a more than 160,000-year-old mandible of a hominin from a location on the Tibetan Plateau was analysed. Its composition indicated a single amino acid variant that is not present in the collagen of modern humans or Neanderthals. Instead, it identified the mandible as belonging to a member of the hominin group called Denisovans. The discovery of a Denisovan outside Siberia indicated that the Denisovans had been able to live in very cold, low-oxygen environments.

The information of the numerous proteins present in the enamel matrix can be determined in material as old as the Early Pleistocene commencing about 2.8 million years ago. Analysis of the enamel proteome in an Early Pleistocene hominid, *Homo antecessor*, and that of the later *H. erectus,* demonstrate that *H. antecessor* has a close sister lineage to subsequent Middle and Late Pleistocene hominins such as modern humans, Neanderthals and Denisovans. This placement implies that the modern-like face of *H. antecessor* may have a considerably deep ancestry in the genus *Homo* and that the Neanderthal cranial morphology represents a derived form. By recovering amelogenin Y–specific peptide sequences (see later), it was also possible to conclude that the tooth fragment of the *H. antecessor* molar used from Atapuerca, Spain, belonged to a male individual.

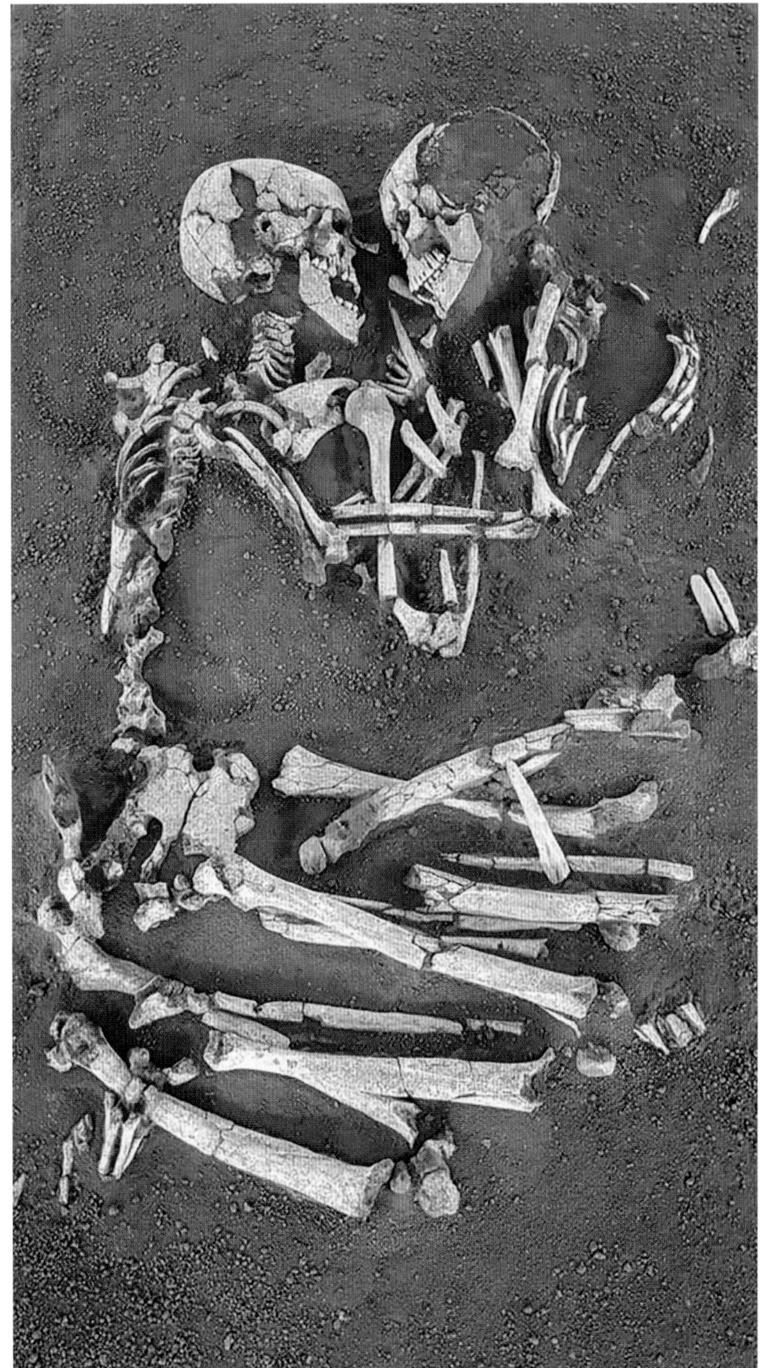

Fig. 27.2 Grave of 'lovers of Modena', shown by analysis of enamel matrix to both be males. Courtesy of Paolo Terzi and Archivio fotografico Museo Civico di Modena, and Wikipedia.

Sex determination

It is often possible to determine the sex of an adult skeleton, especially if the pelvis is preserved. However, this is more difficult if only the skull is available or if the skeleton is a juvenile, and seemingly impossible if only the teeth are present. However, it is possible to determine the sex of an individual solely from teeth by sampling the organic matrix of the enamel using acid etching. This is because there are slight differences between the X chromosome and Y chromosome versions of the amelogenin gene (*AMELX* and *AMELY*, respectively; see page 139). An example of the use of this technique relates to the burial of the 'lovers of Modena'. In a cemetery in Modena, Italy, this unusual burial site was discovered containing two adults unusually arranged so that their hands were intertwined (Fig 27.2). The burial was dated to the fourth to sixth century. Based on their intimacy (and perhaps implicitly biased), it was assumed that the skeletons represented a man and a woman in love. However, recent analysis of their enamel proteins revealed that the AMELY isoform was identified in the enamel of both of the two 'lovers', who were therefore both males.

A similar type of burial has also been discovered in Valdaro, near Mantua. Two individuals were buried face to face with their arms about each other (Fig. 27.3). Known as the 'lovers of Valdaro', they have been dated to about 6,000 years ago. They have been identified by skeletal analysis as male and female, aged about 20 years.

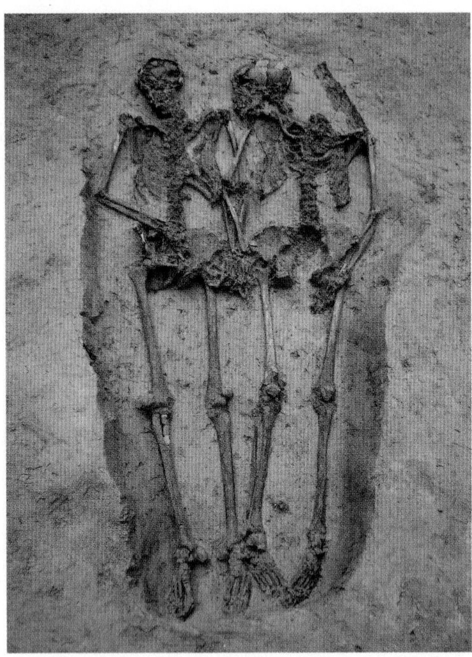

Fig. 27.3 Stable and radioactive isotopes of carbon (neutrons blue; protons green). From Berkovitz, B.K.B., 2013. *Nothing but the tooth.* Elsevier, Oxford, pp. 93–111.

Dental calculus

Examination of dental calculus around the teeth of ancient skeletal material has provided a valuable source of information regarding diet, environment and disease, not only in terms of direct visualisation of food items (e.g., phytoliths, starch granules and pollen grains) but also from recovery of DNA, which allows identification of oral bacteria. The results throw light on the diet and paleoenvironment of ancient humans, Neanderthals and even *Australopithecus sebida*. In Neanderthals, usually thought of primarily as meat eaters, examination of their dental calculus revealed the presence of diverse plant foods such as date palms, legumes and grass seeds.

In the case of the 2-million-year-old *A. sebida*, the presence of dental calculus revealed the inclusion of C3 foods (e.g., grasses and sedges) in preference to widely available C4 resources (see page 483), and they probably included bark and other fracture-resistant foods as at least as a seasonal part of their diet.

Analysis of dental calculus from the teeth of an individual dated to the end of the eighth millennium BCE revealed the presence of fish scales, flesh fragments, starch granules and other plant and animal microdebris.

Amino acid racemisation and the ageing of mineralised tissue

Amino acids comprise the bulk of the organic matrix of bone and dentine (as collagen) and of enamel (as enamel proteins). Amino acids can exist in two different forms, a left-handed form (levorotatory or L form) and a right-handed form (dextrorotatory or D form). When first formed, the amino acids are of the L form but there is a slow transformation to the D form. The changing ratio of D to L is the basis of a method for ageing archaeological and fossil material up to tens of thousands of years old. Indeed, it has also been applied on modern material to determine the age at death, although the rate of change following death is slower because of the lower temperature in the ground compared to body temperature. This chemical method of determining age is known as *amino acid racemisation* (AAR).

The two main amino acids used in AAR are aspartic acid and isoleucine. The L and D forms of aspartic acid (with one chiral centre in its structure) are known as *enantiomers*. For isoleucine, which has two chiral centres, the interconversion process is referred to as *epimerisation*. For this analysis, the amino acids in the matrix of bone, dentine and enamel are separated and quantified by gas chromatography or high-pressure liquid chromatography.

Determining age by racemisation has had somewhat limited use because of problems associated with the methodology. For example, the rate of racemisation depends on temperature, so that the thermal history of the sample needs to be known. In addition, the protein may be contaminated or may undergo denaturation depending on the surrounding pH. Thus, careful calibration must be undertaken using such methodology. Even within a dentition the D:L ratios may vary from tooth to tooth and from site to site in the same tooth. However, the method can be used in conjunction with other methods of estimating age, such as radiocarbon dating.

Diet, climate and origins

Some information concerning the diet of an animal can be obtained by studying the attrition patterns of teeth (see earlier) and, in the case of humans, by the presence of dental caries (indicating the consumption of a carbohydrate-rich diet). However, more detailed information relating to whether an animal has a mainly herbivorous or carnivorous diet, and even the type of the plant material eaten, can be determined from knowledge of the isotopes present in teeth and bones. An isotope is a variety of an element with a different number of neutrons. Interpretation of such data can additionally yield information about environmental factors, such as climate and place of origin. Because of the relative stability of the mineralised tissues, the information can be applied to specimens millions of years old. The most common isotopes studied are carbon, oxygen, nitrogen and strontium.

Stable carbon isotopes

The two stable forms of carbon are illustrated in Fig. 27.4. Although present in only very small quantities in the atmosphere, carbon-13 is incorporated into plants during photosynthesis. Herbivores eating such plants will incorporate the carbon isotopes in the amino acids of their structural proteins and in the carbonate present in hydroxyapatite crystals of their mineralised tissues. Thus, isotopic analysis of stable carbon isotopes in both the organic (collagen) and inorganic components (hydroxyapatite crystallites) of mineralised tissues will give a characteristic value that would indicate a chiefly plant-based diet. As isotope concentration is enriched by consumers as they pass between trophic levels, a carnivore feeding on herbivores will have its own distinctive isotope levels. Because collagen is derived

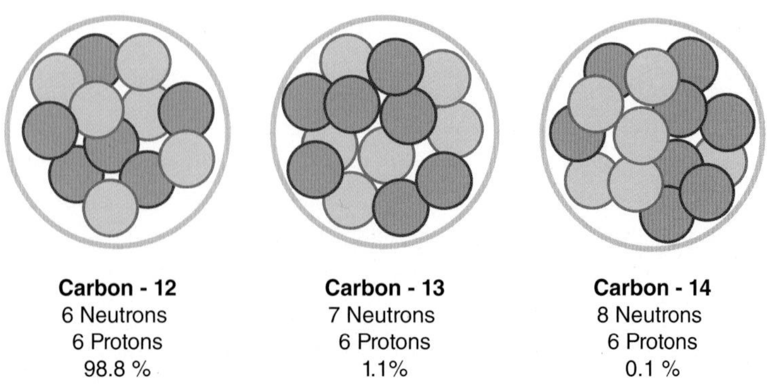

Fig. 27.4 Stable isotopes of oxygen (neutrons blue; protons green). From Berkovitz, B.K.B., 2013. *Nothing but the tooth.* Elsevier, Oxford, pp. 93–111.

only from dietary protein, the carbon present in hydroxyapatite crystals is derived from the whole diet.

Based on the manner of their photosynthesis, plants can be divided into two main groups. Most plants (95%) are known as C3 plants, as the first organic compound synthesised during photosynthesis contains three carbon atoms. C3 plants comprise trees, shrubs, flowering plants, rice, wheat, barley and potatoes and can exist in moist, colder climates. The second group constitutes C4 plants (5%), so called because the first organic compound synthesised during photosynthesis contains four carbon atoms. C4 plants are found in dry, arid regions and include maize, sugar cane and most tropical grasses. When both types of plants are available, animals may restrict themselves to C3 (browsers) or C4 (grazers) material. A key feature in the metabolism of the two groups is that they incorporate different amounts of carbon-13, with C4 plants incorporating more. Isotope levels from herbivores selectively eating either C3 or C4 will differ. Intermediate levels will indicate a herbivore with a diet composed of both types of plants. Carnivores eating the meat of land herbivores will have another distinctive isotope value.

Stable carbon isotope values for marine plants differ from those of terrestrial plants. Marine herbivores will therefore have isotope levels that distinguish them from terrestrial herbivores, while carnivores feeding on the meat of marine herbivores will have isotope levels distinguishing them from land carnivores.

Analysing the ratios of carbon-12 and carbon-13 (using a mathematical formula involving a standard) in a sample of collagen from bone or dentine or from the carbonate in the mineral phase has provided much information concerning the nature of the diet of modern and archaeological/fossil material. As bone is widely used for analysis, consideration must be given to deleterious changes such as demineralisation/remineralisation that occur within the tissue following burial (diagenesis). In this respect, the more stable enamel is especially useful to study, as the larger crystal size and the lack of porosity ensure it is more resistant to diagenesis.

As bone continually turns over, the isotope values may be considered as an overall representation of the last 10 years of the individual's life. Values associated with enamel indicate the diet at known periods in childhood, and comparisons between different teeth in the same individual can indicate a change in diet during childhood.

Archaeological application

Carbon isotope studies have provided much insight into early human evolution. The very early hominid *Ardipithecus ramadus*, from about 4.4 million years ago, retained a grasping big toe, which implies that it was arboreal. Although it existed mainly on C3 plants, carbon isotope studies of its enamel suggested that its diet was more varied than that of great apes and contained 10–25% of C4 plants such as grasses. In the later bipedal hominins, the australopithecines, isotope studies indicate a diet made up of more than 30% (up to 80%) of C4 plants.

In the robust australopithecine *Paranthropus boisei*, carbon isotope studies indicated a diet indistinguishable from that of C4 grazers This contrasts with *Australopithecus africanus, P. robustus* and *Homo habilis*, which consumed a much smaller proportion of C4 plants. Carbon isotope analysis of the enamel from the slightly earlier *A. sediba*, which belonged to a different branch from the robust australopithecines, showed that their diet was almost exclusively C3, despite the availability of C4 food. This was confirmed by the presence of phytoliths from C3 plant material in calculus retained on tooth surfaces.

Analysis of stable carbon and nitrogen isotopes indicated that Neanderthals were top predators, hunting mainly large herbivores such as mammoths, whereas contemporaneous, early modern humans probably had a broader diet, including aquatic (freshwater and marine) resources. This dietary flexibility could have been important in the competition between the two groups.

Carbon isotope studies have also been applied to determine the date at which early human populations in America first introduced the agriculture of maize, the only significant C4 crop grown by Native Americans. Maize (corn) was domesticated about 10,000 years ago in Mexico. It appears to have been selected, cultivated and enormously improved nutritionally from the wild grass, teosinte. The change from small populations of mobile, hunter–gatherers to a sedentary, agricultural society was a major event in the history of the American continent. Once agriculture was firmly established, it produced an increasing supply of food that allowed for the development of greater populations and eventually civilisations, such as the Maya in Mexico. The establishment and spread of maize throughout America have been traced by studying stable carbon isotopes in the teeth and bones found at burial sites. This has shown that maize production spread from Mexico over the whole of the American continent, both North and South. When the Spanish conquistadors arrived in the New World at the beginning of the 16th century, they transported maize back to Europe. Moreover, knowing the status of an individual skeleton from the presence and nature of burial goods, it has been possible to show that there were differences in the consumption of maize within the social hierarchy.

Radioactive carbon

In addition to its stable isotopes, ^{12}C and ^{13}C, carbon is present in a third form, namely the radioactive isotope ^{14}C. This isotope contains six protons and eight neutrons (Fig. 27.4) and it is unstable, eventually decaying into nitrogen-14 (^{14}N). It comprises an infinitesimal amount of carbon (one part in a trillion), but this is measurable using a very sensitive apparatus. As its decay rate in organic material is known, it is used in radiocarbon dating whereby the age of any archaeological material containing carbon can be accurately assessed up to about 60,000 years ago.

The main source of ^{14}C is cosmic ray action on nitrogen in our atmosphere. Additional contributions also appear as a by-product from the explosion of atomic bombs. Although only two bombs were dropped on Japan at the end of the Second World War in 1945, many bombs were exploded during the testing of nuclear weapons between 1955 and 1963 and before a nuclear test ban treaty was signed. Radioactive carbon, like normal stable carbon isotopes, is taken up by plants in carbon dioxide and, through this pathway, is incorporated into developing enamel when people (and animals) eat the plants. The level of ^{14}C present in enamel reflects the level in the atmosphere at that time. By measuring the ^{14}C levels in enamel and comparing them with the known records of ^{14}C in the atmosphere, it is possible to age a person born after 1953 to within about 1.6 years, just from an isolated tooth. This method is more accurate than other methods for ageing adults. An absence of any significant radioactive ^{14}C isotope would indicate a person born before 1945. The technique has been used to help in the identification of some victims of the tsunami in Southeast Asia in 2004.

Stable nitrogen isotopes

As with carbon, the ratios of two stable nitrogen isotopes, nitrogen-15 and nitrogen-14, in the collagen of bone can be used to reveal dietary information, as nitrogen is absorbed by land plants from the soil. When these plants are eaten by land herbivores, the nitrogen is incorporated into the collagen protein making up a considerable component of bone and dentine (and other soft tissues). Like carbon, the $^{15}N/^{14}N$ ratio increases as it passes up the food chain (fractionation or trophic enrichment).

Nitrogen's trophic enrichment is even greater than carbon's. Nitrogen isotope studies are particularly informative where the diet includes fish, as animals eating fish or marine mammals will have even higher values than those preying on terrestrial sources.

Herbivores feeding on legumes will have a different nitrogen-15 fingerprint from animals eating plants that derive their nitrogen from the soil. Stable nitrogen isotope values from bone collagen will also help differentiate carnivores from herbivores and marine from terrestrial feeders. Individuals consuming a mixture of terrestrial and marine foods will have intermediate nitrogen isotope values.

Archaeological applications

Stable isotope values for nitrogen (as well as for carbon) have been determined from collagen in the bones of Neanderthals living between 120,000 and 27,000 years ago. These values have then been compared with those obtained for the bones of early modern humans living between 40,000 and 27,000 years ago. The results indicate that Neanderthals obtained all or most of their protein by consuming the flesh of herbivores. On the other hand, early modern humans showed more variety in their diet, also eating fish and other marine species. This adaptability to utilise other food sources could have been important in the struggle for survival between the groups.

There are four distinct stages of nutritional intake during early life: gestation, exclusive breastfeeding, a transitional or weaning stage and fully weaned. The trace element and stable isotope composition of developing and infant tissues differs during each of these stages owing to differences in the source of nutrients and changes in metabolic parameters. Nitrogen-15 values in the collagen of teeth and bones from birth onwards have been investigated in an attempt to determine the approximate time of weaning. This is based on the observation that breastfed children have slightly higher nitrogen-15 levels in their collagen than their mothers. By observing a fall in nitrogen-15 values, weaning in a medieval population was found to occur at less than 1 year of age and to be terminated relatively abruptly.

It has been observed that levels of barium in tooth enamel rise while a child is breastfed but drop off when they are weaned. Barium levels have been measured in a 100,000-year-old first molar from a Neanderthal child, from which it was concluded that it had been weaned at 14 months, which is far quicker than a human, where weaning normally occurs at 2 or more years.

Stable oxygen isotopes

Oxygen has two stable isotopes, oxygen-16 and the rarer oxygen-18 (Fig. 27.5). Water vapour evaporated from the ocean in clouds will fall as rain over the land, with the heavier isotope, oxygen-18, falling sooner and therefore being more common in the drinking water associated with a warmer tropical climate nearer the ocean. The lighter oxygen-16 will be given off later at a farther distance from the ocean and in colder climates towards the poles. Thus, the ratio of stable oxygen isotopes in water will vary according to latitude, water temperature and weather patterns. During the Ice Age, with so much water incorporated in the polar ice, rain everywhere would have had a higher concentration of oxygen-18. Reference isotope levels for most regions of the Earth are known and are relatively stable with time, although corrective factors can be applied to take account of climatic changes.

The oxygen incorporated into the structure of the hydroxyapatite crystallite is ultimately derived from drinking water. Crystallites from enamel, being the most stable, would give precise information about the environment during the period of crown formation. Comparisons between the isotope values from different teeth in the same individual would also indicate any migration to areas with different isotope values. Indeed, sampling across a section of enamel from a single tooth might provide considerable information about an individual's movement during childhood. Dentine and bone, being slowly deposited throughout life, would provide information particularly concerning an individual's environment after the age of about 20 years. Similar information may also be extracted from mineral crystals in any dental calculus present around the teeth.

Archaeological applications

Analysis of stable oxygen isotopes has provided important information for assessing collections of bodies at burial sites, it being possible to distinguish 'locals' from 'foreigners'. An important example of the use of isotopic analysis in shedding light on human archaeology relates to the 'Iceman', who was estimated to have died about 5,200 years ago. His well-preserved, mummified remains were found in 1991 high up on an alpine glacier in the Otztal Alps (hence his nickname, Otzi), between Italy and Austria. His body was accompanied by various clothes, tools and weapons, including a copper axe and a quiver of 14 arrows. Because of the discovery of an arrowhead embedded in his left shoulder and other wounds, it is believed he was murdered. Although initially taken to Innsbruck for study, his body was later determined to have been found just inside Italian territory and returned to Italy. The presence of the mountain results in distinct isotopic oxygen profiles for water occurring north and south of it. Analysis of the stable oxygen isotopes from both enamel and bone samples indicated that the 'Iceman' had lived on the south side in Italy (having more of the heavier isotope). In addition, isotopic values also indicated that, having spent his childhood at a lower altitude, he had later migrated to higher ground.

Stonehenge is one of the largest and most important Neolithic (New Stone Age) monuments in the world. Its circular arrangement of standing stones is sited in dramatic isolation on Salisbury Plain in Wiltshire, Southern England (Fig. 27.6). Considerable interest therefore attaches to any burials in the region. The richest burial to date was discovered in

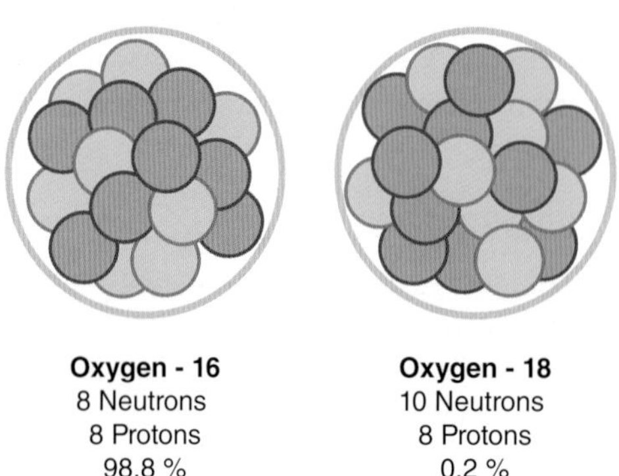

Fig. 27.5 Grave of 'lovers of Valdaro' near Mantua. Courtesy of Dangmar Hollmann and Wikipedia.

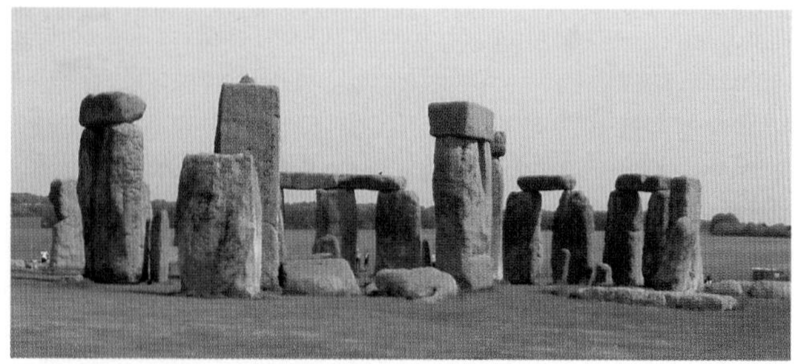

Fig. 27.6 View of Stonehenge, Wiltshire.

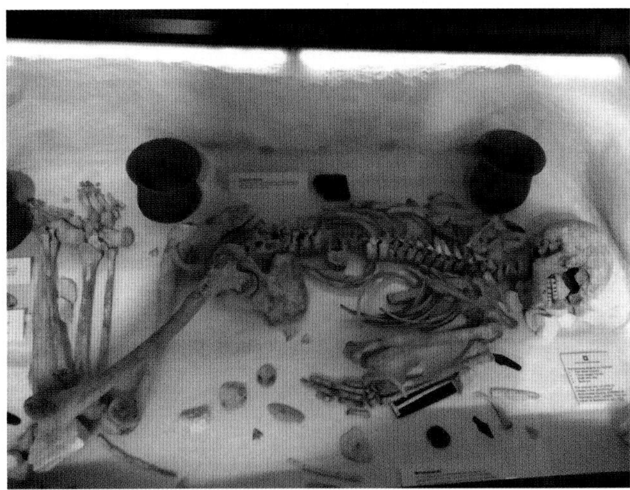

Fig. 27.7 Grave of the Amesbury archer. Note the richness of the grave goods. Courtesy Pasicles and Wikipedia.

the village of Amesbury, about 5 km from Stonehenge. Dated to between 2400 and 2200 BC, the grave contained the skeleton of a man about 40 years of age. Among the many valuable grave goods were 15 beautiful flint arrowheads (hence the nickname the 'Amesbury archer'), boar tusks, copper knives and gold hair decorations (hence the alternative name 'King of Stonehenge'; Fig. 27.7). Of great interest would be knowledge of where he came from. Was he a local chieftain?

When the enamel of the teeth of the 'Amesbury archer' was analysed for oxygen isotopes, he was found not to be a local. In fact, his origin was much farther afield, from an alpine region in central Europe that could be Switzerland, Germany or Austria. Although one mystery was solved, the information raised a host of new questions that may never be answered, such as why did he undertake so long journey and why was he buried so close to such an important monument?

A second burial near Stonehenge, on Boscombe Down, contained the skeleton of a 14- or 15-year-old boy, dated at about 800 years after the 'Amesbury archer'. The grave contained a remarkable amber necklace with 90 beads (hence the nickname 'boy with the amber necklace'). However, no evidence was forthcoming as to where he came from. Oxygen isotope analysis from his teeth indicated that the boy with the amber necklace, like the archer, was not local but also originated from a considerable distance away. Unlike the 'Amesbury archer', who came from a cold, mountainous region, the boy came from a warmer, Mediterranean climate.

A third important burial near Stonehenge occurred at Boscombe Down. This burial was unearthed in 2003 when workmen were digging a trench for a new water pipe. Although most Neolithic burials contain a single individual, this site was unusual as it contained the remains of seven individuals: three male adults, one male teenager and three children. There were also grave goods, including pottery, a boar's tooth and five flint arrowheads, giving the group the nickname the 'Boscombe Bowmen'. To obtain more information about the origin and movements of the adults, combined strontium and oxygen isotope analyses were undertaken on the enamel of premolar teeth and third permanent molars. The premolars provided information as to their whereabouts between the ages of 3 and 6 years and the third molars their whereabouts between 9 and 13 years. The results provided three findings of interest. First, there was a difference between the readings taken from the two teeth, indicating that they had lived in two different areas during the two time periods. Second, that the region which best matched the isotope values was the region in Wales from which the bluestones of Stonehenge were quarried. Third, the values also differed from the site of their burial at Stonehenge, indicating that they moved between at least three different areas during their lives. Isotope levels in two of the children buried in the same grave indicated that they did not share the same homeland as the adults.

The teeth of human skeletons found in the spectacular Iron Age 'chariot' burials of East Yorkshire, which also contained the skeletons of horses, have been subjected to stable isotope analysis. Radiocarbon tests dated the burials to the fourth to second century BCE, while isotope studies indicated the individuals to have been born and to have lived locally.

Stable strontium isotopes

As with carbon and nitrogen, strontium passes from the soil into plants and thence up the food chain. Strontium readily substitutes for calcium in the hydroxyapatite crystallite and is therefore present in relatively high amounts (100 ppm). It can provide information concerning aspects of the diet (for example, carnivores show a lower strontium:calcium ratio than herbivores). However, perhaps a more important application concerning strontium levels is to suggest the place of origin of a bone/tooth sample and possibly indicate any significant movement away from this site. The two stable isotopes of strontium used in such studies are strontium-87 and strontium-86. As the former isotope is created by the radioactive decay of rubidium, it can also be used for ageing specimens.

Strontium-87:strontium-86 ratios provide a unique 'fingerprint' of the geology of an area. By matching such values locked up in the mineralised tissue of an individual with those of the surrounding land, information can be gleaned on her or his origin. Data from enamel crystallites provide information as to the whereabouts of an individual during early childhood, while those of adult bone and dentine, because of their continual formation, reflect their more recent location. Unlike the more resistant enamel, allowance must be made when examining bone and dentine from archaeological/fossil specimens to account for diagenesis associated with possible crystal dissolution and absorption of strontium from the surrounding soil.

Archaeological applications

As for oxygen values, strontium levels in teeth reflect the origin of a person during enamel development and therefore can also separate locals from strangers or foreigners in a graveyard.

An example of the use of strontium isotope analysis in human archaeology again relates to the 'Iceman' (see earlier). Oxygen isotope studies showed him to have originated on the Italian side of the Alps, and stable strontium isotope analysis of tooth and bone samples pinpointed his origin to just a few valleys about 60 km from the site of the body.

Slave burial grounds have been unearthed in Campeche, Mexico (dating from between the mid-16th and late 17th centuries) and in Rio de Janeiro in Brazil (dating from between 1760 and 1830). Because of the limited documentation of the early slave trade, could any information be found as to where the slaves originated? Had they been captured in Africa and transported to Mexico and Brazil, or had they been born in these two latter countries? Enamel from the permanent teeth of ten of the specimens at the Mexican site was analysed for strontium isotopes, and results showed that, while six had been born locally, four of the subjects had been born in Africa and transported to Mexico. In the case of the specimens from Brazil, however, strontium isotope analysis showed that they were all born in Africa. Furthermore, instead of being limited to the western coastal region of Africa, as once thought, they reflected a much wider origin involving the east coast and the central regions. Isotope analysis of teeth has the power to illuminate great historical events, one of which was the discovery (rediscovery?) of the New World by Christopher Columbus in 1492. This discovery led to the establishment of the slave trade between America and Africa. The skeletons of 20 individuals were recently unearthed at La Isabela, in the Dominican Republic, a place thought to be the first European town founded in the New World. Remarkably, there is strong evidence that these remains represent part of the original crew of Columbus' second visit to the New World (1493–1496). Historical records of the crew are incomplete, but it is known that Columbus had a personal African slave on his voyages of discovery. Isotope analysis of the enamel of the teeth, studying carbon, oxygen, strontium and nitrogen values, helps indicate the birthplace and diet of the crew and has provided a totally unexpected result. There was strong evidence that not one but three of the skeletons were of individuals born in Africa. This view was further supported by the findings that some of the teeth showed intentional dental modifications whereby the teeth had their shape deliberately altered by filing typical of West Africa. These new findings indicate that more native Africans were involved in the first documented explorations of America than previously suspected.

Normal trace elements

The amount of trace elements occurring in enamel can also be used to provide answers to archaeological questions.

The presence of lead in mineralised teeth can be used to provide data similar to that of strontium when considering premetallurgical societies. However, once lead-containing artefacts were manufactured, such as drinking utensils and lead pipes, lead values rose and were a reflection of cultural habits. They could also be interpreted as an indication of class as, for example, only the rich in Roman society could afford to drink from pewter vessels (and therefore risk dying from lead poisoning!).

Analysis of calcium-normalised strontium levels in teeth provide information reflecting the onset and duration of breastfeeding and the introduction of non-maternal sources of food.

From this account, it can be seen that analysis of mineralised tissues supports the contention that 'you are what you eat and you were what you ate'.

Clinical considerations of age changes

A different clinical approach is taken when treating old patients compared with young ones. The chief reason relates to changes that have taken place in the dentine–pulp complex. The continued deposition throughout life of secondary (and tertiary) dentine means there is a reduction in the size of the pulp cavity. When treating a carious young tooth, care must be taken not to open into the comparatively large pulp. When carrying out the same procedure in an old tooth, there is far less likelihood of entering the pulp. Indeed, root canal therapy is complicated by the small size of the tooth. The increased thickness of the dentine, as well as the formation of peritubular dentine, means the resulting permeability of old teeth is less than that of young teeth. This may explain the reduced sensitivity of an old tooth, as may the reduced innervation. Consequently, some conservative treatment in old patients may not require local anaesthesia. This reduced sensitivity may also complicate vitality testing of the tooth, resulting in false negatives. The presence of pulp stones may also complicate root canal treatment in old teeth. Older teeth may be more resistant to dental caries. However, they may also be less able to respond to healing following clinical procedures. This could be an effect of a reduced blood supply and/or a reduction in the amount of stem cells in the pulp.

Further readings for this chapter can be found in the accompanying eBook. Explore online Self-assessment quiz to test and reinforce your understanding of the material in your free ebook. Follow instructions in the Inside Front Cover to unlock your access.

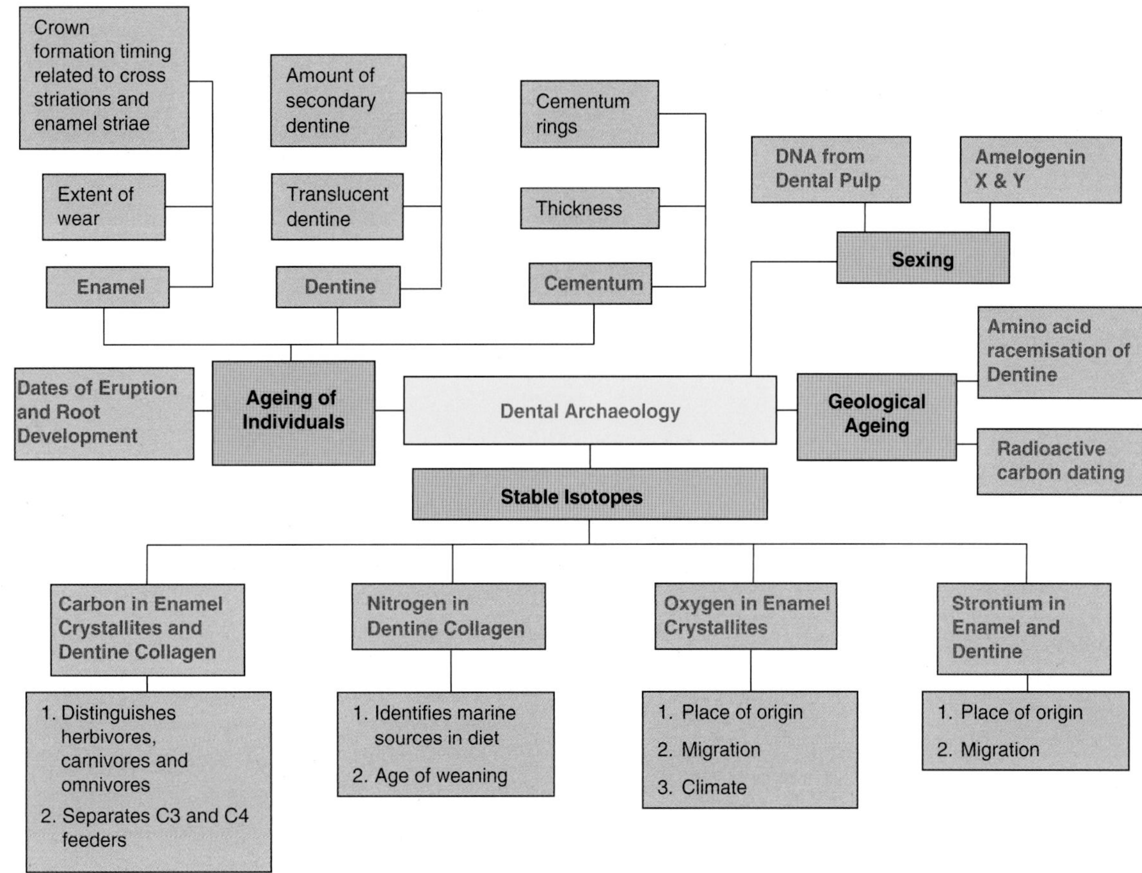

Mind Map 27.1 Dental Archaeology.

28 Regenerative dentistry

RRegenerative dentistry is a new concept, based on cell and molecular biology, that is designed to provide therapies to repair and regenerate oral tissues. Biomedical research has led to advances in the understanding of the mechanisms driving development and repair. These provide the basis for understanding how oral tissues might be restored clinically. Because of advances in stem cell biology, genetics, epigenetics and new generations of biomaterials, regenerative dentistry explores cell-based therapies, gene therapies and the use of scaffolds for stimulating repair mechanisms. Thus, repair and regeneration employs a variety of tissue and organ engineering techniques to deliver cells and genes. Owing to the considerable number of abbreviations generally available for the understanding of cell and molecular biology, to aid the reader a glossary for these abbreviations is supplied on pages 506.

Tissue engineering

In regenerative dentistry, tissue engineering is one of the main approaches. It uses principles in developing biological substitutes to improve oral health and quality of life for millions of people globally by restoring, maintaining or enhancing the functions of oral tissues.

For the successful outcome of a tissue engineering approach, several factors are significant:

- Appropriate **cells** (source of new tissue growth and differentiation)
- **Signals** (growth factors and other bioactive molecules that modulate cellular activity and provide stimuli for cells to differentiate, support the formation of a specific tissue, and stimulate an endogenous regeneration process)
- **3D environment** (various scaffolds made of biomaterials to support and facilitate cellular processes that are critical for tissue formation)
- **Vascularisation** (angiogenic signals to provide the nutritional base for tissue growth and homeostasis)

The functional biology of the oro-dental tissues also requires consideration of some additional factors, including:

- **Mechanical loading** (for tissues such as the periodontal ligament [PDL] and bone where appropriate mechanical loading is essential for the development of highly organised, functional PDL fibres)
- **Infection control** (owing to the microbial load in the oral cavity, pathogen control and host response are required to optimise periodontal regeneration)

The main approaches in regenerative medicine and dentistry that are used as 'tools' in tissue engineering are:

- Cell-based approaches, where **cells are used as**:
  - Carriers/vehicles to deliver growth or cellular signals
  - A source able to differentiate into multiple cell types to promote regeneration
- The **use of signalling molecules and gene therapy** to mobilise and direct the proliferation and differentiation of cells, enhancing the ability of tissues and organs to heal
- **Biomaterials and scaffold fabrication technologies** for delivering cells and appropriate signalling at sites in need of repair or regeneration

Organ engineering

By exploring the mechanisms that govern cell proliferation, differentiation and histogenesis, organ engineering integrates knowledge of how certain organs develop from an embryological perspective while incorporating technologies that can mimic the developmental environment spatio-temporally under laboratory conditions. Among these approaches are the development of organoids and the use of 3D biomaterials for scaffolding and biofabrication.

Stem cells

Any organ needs continuous replenishment of new cells during development, growth and differentiation. To achieve this, stem cells exist in both embryos and adults. Human stem cells are unspecialised cells that can differentiate into specialised cells and can self-renew.

There are three main types of stem cells:

- **Embryonic stem cells** (ESCs; isolated from the inner mass of a blastocyst)
- **Adult stem cells** (ASCs; existing within stem cell niches in different tissues and organs throughout life)
- **Induced pluripotent stem cells** (iPSCs; *in vitro* reprogrammed adult cells that exhibit properties similar to ESCs)

ESCs were generated from mouse blastocysts in 1981. In 1998, human embryonic cells were subsequently derived and grown in the laboratory. ESCs are pluripotent and, when given the appropriate stimuli, can give rise to every type of cell in a fully formed body. They also divide indefinitely into daughter cells. Nanog, Oct3/4 and Sox2 are transcription factors that identify ESCs. It is thought that specific growth factors and bone morphogenetic proteins (BMPs) support the 'stemness' and pluripotency of ESCs.

ASCs, also called *somatic stem cells* or *tissue-specific stem cells*, reside in stem cell niches within adult tissues and organs. They maintain homeostasis and contribute to tissue and organ repair. They are characterised as multipotent because they can generate different kinds of cells for the specific tissue or organ in which they reside. ASCs are slow-cycling and take up labelled thymidine. It is also possible to identify them by their transcription factors and by pulse chase labelling experiments. This is where their initial label remains for an extended period. Despite their low numbers within tissues, they can be isolated, grown and amplified by 'cell culture' in well-controlled laboratory conditions.

iPSCs are cells that have been engineered in the laboratory by reprogramming ASCs (such as skin fibroblasts) into cells that behave like ESCs. Pluripotency (the ability to give rise to all types of cells in the body) is a characteristic that iPSC cells share with ESCs.

Currently, stem cell biology focuses on understanding stem cell behaviour and niches (environments where stem cells reside) and applying this knowledge to effect repair and regeneration. The use of ESCs raises several ethical concerns. Therefore, targeting tissue repair and regeneration using ASCs is the most viable option in designing future therapeutic approaches.

iPSCs have been used to study normal development and disease onset and progression. Additionally, they can be used to develop and test new drugs and therapies. Although iPSCs possess pluripotent abilities, their safety for use in clinical therapeutic approaches is still being investigated. This is because the first iPSCs were produced by inserting genes into ASCs through viruses. Research is currently being conducted to develop virus-free methods for producing iPSCs so that they can be considered a safe cell source in the future.

Progenitor cells are cells that may be multipotent but can divide only a limited number of time, compared to the stem cells. They may be considered to be a stage between stem cells and fully differentiated cells.

The oral cavity is a 'treasure chest' of stem cells

Oral tissues and teeth have been described as a 'treasure chest' of ASCs. Several parts of the tooth contain mesenchymal and/or epithelial cells with stem cell properties. Under laboratory conditions, these cells are characterised by the expression of stem cell markers and the ability to differentiate into a variety of specialised cells.

Mesenchymal stem cells can be isolated from different dental tissues, such as the dental pulp of deciduous teeth (known as *stem cells of human exfoliating dentition* [SHEDs]); dental pulp of adult/permanent teeth (known as *dental pulp stem cells* [DPSCs]); the PDL (known as *periodontal ligament stem cells* [PDLSCs]); from the apical papilla of developing roots (known as *stem cells of the apical papilla* [SCAPs]); bone chip mass populations derived from implant surgery sites (BCMPs); the gingiva (known as *gingival stem cells* [GSCs]); and the dental follicle (known as *dental follicle stem cells* [DFSCs]) (Fig. 28.1).

A variety of cell types can be differentiated from the dental stem cells (DSCs), including neural cells, adipocytes, osteoblasts and odontoblasts. After being isolated and expanded *in vitro*, DSCs can be cryopreserved long-term.

Research indicates that it is possible to restore damaged dental tissues using DSCs and to use them for tissue engineering in novel ways, such as generating a dental pulp, regenerating the periodontium lost in periodontal disease or generating complete or partial tooth structures for biologically repairing and/or replacing lost teeth. Under laboratory conditions and during osteogenic differentiation, different DSC populations produce materials with dissimilar mineral and matrix compositions. The *in vitro*–produced materials differ from native dental mineralised tissues, such as enamel and dentine. As a result of these variations in mineral compositions, different DSC populations may have significantly different clinical applications for future therapeutic approaches.

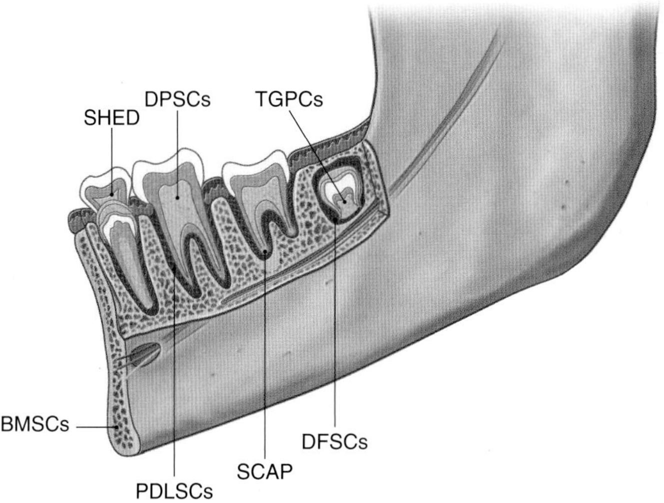

Fig. 28.1 Diagram showing source of stem cells in the regions of the jaws and teeth. Sites of various populations of dental stem cells. BMSCs = bone marrow stem cells; DFSCs = dental follicle stem cells; DPSCs = dental pulp stem cells; PDLSCs = periodontal ligament stem cells; SCAP = stem cells of the apical papilla; SHED = stem cells from the pulp of human exfoliate deciduous teeth; TGPCs = stem cells of the tooth germ's papilla cells. Redrawn from Fouad, S.A.A., 2015. Dental stem cells: a perspective area in dentistry. *International Journal of Dental Sciences and Research* 3, 15–25.

The application of oral stem cells in regenerative medicine

Dental mesenchymal stem cells (MSCs) have many of the same properties as bone marrow MSCs, which makes them an excellent source of cells for different stem cell therapies. Because the tooth is so accessible for a variety of stem cells, along with the attached gingival tissue (which is usually discarded in clinics), it is a great source of autologous and/or allogeneic stem cells that can be used in the treatment of a wide range of dental and medical conditions.

It has been shown that MSCs modulate and regulate T and B lymphocytes, dendritic cells and natural killer cells. In culture, mesenchymal cells do not express major histocompatibility class (MHC) class II antigens, indicating that they can be used to treat graft-versus-host disease (GVHD). Immunosuppressive and immunomodulatory properties have also been demonstrated for mesenchymal DSCs. The immunomodulatory properties of dental MSCs are largely mediated by inflammatory cytokines produced by immune cells.

Regenerative medicine approaches can utilise DSCs for bone regeneration, muscle repair and nerve regeneration, opening doors to their broader application.

In animals that model muscular dystrophy, such as murine dystrophic mice and golden retriever muscular dystrophy dogs, DSCs have been shown to promote wound healing and muscle regeneration. When cultured under steady flow conditions *in vitro*, PDLSCs commit to the heart valve cell lineage, namely the concomitant differentiation of endothelial cells (ECs) and smooth muscle cells (SMCs). This makes them useful for tissue engineering of heart valves.

As stem cells derived from the cranial neural crest, dental MSCs have inherent advantages in terms of neural repair and neurogenesis. Neurotrophic and neuroprotective properties of these cells have been demonstrated in various experimental models, suggesting they are an ideal source for regenerating neural tissues.

As well as the possibility of using mesenchymal DSCs in regenerative medicine, epithelial cells isolated from the oral mucosa also possess stem cell properties, and their usage has been explored for the treatment of severe ocular surface disorders. Cell sheets have been grown *in vitro* and applied to the eye surface, showing promising results in long-term clinical trials.

Studying dental stem cells

To translate the knowledge of oro-dental stem cells into reliable and relevant clinical treatments, scientists focus on studying the *in vivo* microenvironment where these cells reside, as well as their behaviour *in vitro* once these cells are isolated and propagated under laboratory conditions. To maintain the homeostasis of tissues and trigger repair and healing, these stem cells reside in stem cell niches and respond to cellular, chemical and physical stimuli. Cell behaviour is affected by shear stress, stiffness and intercellular communication with stromal cells, blood vessels, neural cells and immune cells.

One of the most established models for studying DSCs is the mouse incisor. It is also a good model for studying MSC development and repair. At the apical end of the incisor, continuous cell turnover compensates for the loss of cells at the incisal tip. There, MSCs and epithelial stem cells reside in distinct niches, providing a source of cells for continuous growth of the incisor (see also Fig. 26.16).

In vitro studies of DSCs, where cells are isolated and grown in laboratory conditions, have been extensive, and their behaviour and gene expressions have been well documented. However, *in vitro* studies fail to capture the significant '*in vivo* microenvironment' that aids cell clonogenicity and differentiation within tissue-specific stem cell niches. These obstacles are being overcome by the introduction of single-cell RNA sequencing and various transcriptome analysis methods, and as a result, new insights into tissue architecture and cell interactions are being gained.

Building the 'Human Cell Atlas' cell by cell

Decoding the oral tissues

To map the different cell populations within a tissue, single-cell and spatial multiomics assays (genomics, epigenomics, transcriptomics, proteomics and metabolomics) provide powerful tools. Different transcriptomic technologies are employed to study an organism's transcriptome, which is the sum of all of the RNA transcripts that are found in the genome. In recent years, single-cell RNA sequencing has proven to be a state-of-the-art approach to uncovering the heterogeneity and complexity of individual RNA transcripts within individual cells. Several methods for visualising and interpreting gene expression data can be used. Heat maps and cluster analysis are two of the most common methods for analysing data (Fig. 28.2).

To understand how stem cells interact with their environment and drive regeneration based on data from studies using transcriptomics, transcriptomics a 'Human Cell Atlas' of cellular and molecular mechanisms is being created. These studies reveal cell heterogeneity between tissues both within and between species.

The human body contains approximately 40 trillion cells, of which about 2 trillion are found in oral and craniofacial tissues. There has been significant progress in the field of research on oral tissues, using transcriptomics as an approach. Atlases of the buccal mucosa, tongue, gingiva, major and minor salivary glands, dental pulp, PDL, tonsils and saliva have been published. Additionally, the temporomandibular joint and skeletal muscles are being mapped as craniofacial niches.

Enamel repair

Enamel provides protection against external damage to a tooth (see Chapter 7). It is the hardest substance in the human body and contains 96% minerals. The remaining 4% is water and organic material. When enamel is fully formed, it does not contain any blood vessels, nerves or cells. Therefore, once enamel is lost, unlike bone or dentine, it lacks the capacity to regenerate itself. As a result of its multilevel structure of directional hydroxyapatite crystals, enamel has a high mechanical performance. Any 'regrowth' of enamel structure would need to re-establish these properties to sustain functionality.

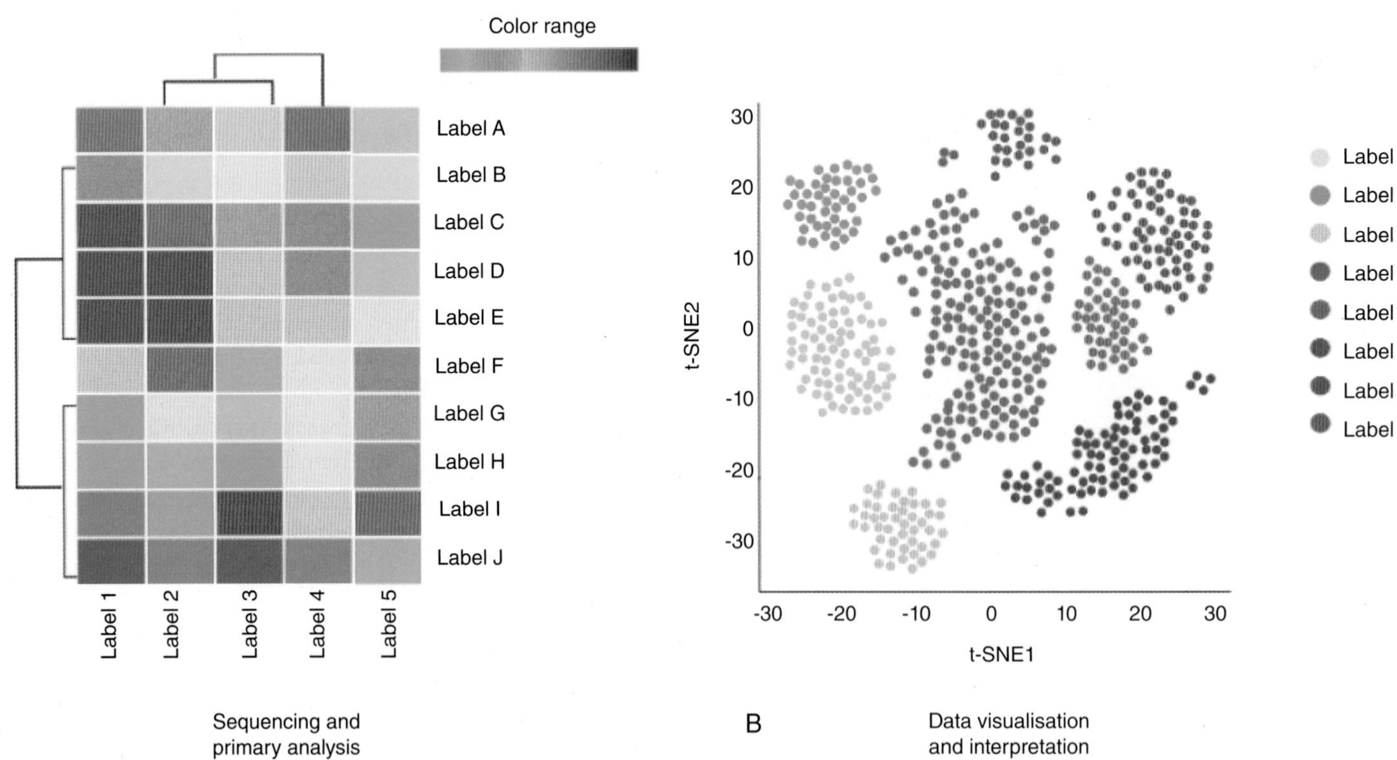

Fig. 28.2 The heatmap (A) is a common method of visualising gene expression data. In heat maps the data are displayed in a grid. Heatmaps are used to show relationships between two variables, one plotted on each axis. By noting how cell colours change across each axis, it is possible to observe if there are any patterns in value for one or both variables. The colour and intensity of the boxes are used to represent changes (not absolute values) of gene expression. In the example (A), red represents upregulated genes and green represents downregulated genes. The heatmap may also be combined with clustering methods, which group genes and/or samples together based on their gene expression pattern similarity. A different colour is displayed for each cluster (B). This can help identify genes regulated in a similar manner or biological signatures associated with certain diseases. *Adapted from Zhang, X., Caetano, A.J., Sharpe, P.T., Volponi, A., 2022. Oral stem cells, decoding and mapping the resident cells populations. Biomaterials Translational 3, 24–30.*

The highly specialised cells that form enamel (ameloblasts) are lost after tooth eruption. In the absence of enamel's forming cells, an endogenous biological regeneration of enamel is not feasible. This contrasts with dentine, cementum and bone, which all retain their forming cells (odontoblasts, cementoblasts and osteoblasts, respectively). Another significant difference between enamel and bone is that enamel does not remodel over a lifetime, unlike bone that is continuously remodelling. (see Chapter 13). As enamel cannot be biologically regenerated or repaired, the concept of 'healing' damaged enamel consists of acellular remineralisation processes.

Demineralisation/remineralisation equilibrium

At the surface of enamel, hydroxyapatite crystals are constantly in dynamic equilibrium with saliva and dental plaque. During acidic attacks (and low pH of saliva), enamel can lose most of its ionic content, leading to dental caries or erosion. Cariogenic bacteria and carbohydrates in the diet produce acids that damage enamel by demineralisation it. Depending on the pH and on the amount of calcium and phosphate ions, dissolution will occur at a particular rate and amount.

An early dental caries lesion has a porous mineral surface and is characterised by subsurface demineralisation (see Fig. 7.70). Remineralisation occurs when calcium phosphate–supersaturated saliva either deposits minerals on crystallites already present or triggers *de novo* crystallisation. Demineralisation and remineralisation alternate, and remineralisation can successfully reverse and stop the initial lesion. Alternatively, the lesion may grow in size, damaging hard dental tissues (enamel and dentine) and causing irreversible inflammation of the dental pulp (pulpitis). The equilibrium can be pushed toward remineralisation by using additives. Several products contain fluoride, calcium and phosphates, which are well-established approaches for preventing demineralisation and promoting remineralisation.

Fluoride

Fluoride acts by its incorporation into the crystal lattice, resulting in lower solubility of the enamel by substitution of some hydroxyl (OH^-) ions with fluor (F^-) ions to create areas of fluorapatite. Nevertheless, this protective product only forms on the surface of the enamel within ~30 μm. In the subsurface, regeneration and repair of hydroxyapatite crystals still present challenges.

Fluoride can be provided through drinking water, toothpastes, mouthwashes or topically applied fluoride products. Approximately 50% of the hydroxyl groups need to be replaced with fluoride for fluoride to have its maximum effect. Fluoride levels on enamel surfaces can reach 3,000 parts per million in areas where the water is fluoridated. It is most effective when added to the drinking water or given in tablet form during the time of enamel formation.

During toothbrushing, fluoride added in the toothpaste reaches its highest concentration in saliva. This allows it to pass into the biofilm, where it can remain for a long period, preventing demineralisation and promoting remineralisation.

By remineralising early caries lesions, topical fluoride application is a major advance in non-invasive clinical management. Calcium and phosphate ions must also be available at sufficient levels for net remineralisation to take place. To form one unit cell of fluorapatite ($Ca_{10}(PO_4)_6F_2$), 10 calcium ions and 6 phosphate ions are required. Consequently, calcium and phosphate ions are limiting factors for remineralisation, especially when salivary flow or content changes.

When fluoride is present at high concentrations in drinking water, fluorosis and enamel discoloration can occur. (see Fig. 22.34). During the maturation phase of amelogenesis, excessive fluoride levels affect the activity of ameloblasts, resulting in enamel matrix with higher protein levels.

Calcium and phosphate

Calcium and phosphate levels in saliva (and dental plaque) are critical for the remineralisation of surface enamel. Several calcium-phosphate–based remineralisation systems have been developed in recent years. Dental products, such as toothpastes, mouthwashes and chewing gums containing suitable levels of these systems have been shown to promote remineralisation.

Casein phosphopeptides

The anticariogenic properties of dairy products have been known for a long time. The observed properties might be because casein, the predominant protein in milk, stabilises calcium and phosphate ions. As a result, casein phosphopeptide–stabilised amorphous calcium phosphate complexes (CPP-ACP) and casein phosphopeptide–stabilised amorphous calcium fluoride phosphate complexes (CPP-ACFP) have been developed as remineralising technologies. Several of these complexes have been incorporated into topically applied dental products with the goal of remineralising subsurface lesions more effectively.

Bioactive materials

The bioactivity of a material is determined by its ability to interact with living tissue or cause a reaction. Although initially used for bone regeneration (see Fig. 13.53), bioglass has the remarkable bioactive capacity to form hydroxycarbonate when submerged in simulated body fluid solutions. Consequently, it has been proposed that it may be used to remineralise dental tissues, being particularly relevant for enamel remineralisation. There are four main ingredients in bioglass: calcium, sodium, silicate and phosphate. Continuous ion exchange occurs in the oral cavity. Sodium ions exchange with hydrogen ions, which raises pH, releasing calcium and phosphate ions, forming silanol (Si-OH) and a silica-rich layer. Afterwards, calcium phosphate is deposited on the surface, which gradually transforms into crystalline hydroxyapatite that mimics the mineral phase naturally found in vertebrates. As a result, bioactive glass and related materials (e.g., calcium silicate) are being evaluated for their potential as remineralising agents.

Biomimetics and synthetic biomineralisation platforms

Using biomimetic approaches inspired by natural processes, artificial enamel has been developed using synthetic hierarchical materials that enhance functionality. Molecular building blocks can be controlled at precise length scales in materials science to produce bioinspired functional materials that resemble native enamel structure (Fig. 28.3). Using membranes containing cell-binding domains Arg–Gly–Asp (RGD) and elastin-like recombinamers, a protein-mediated mineralisation process can take advantage of the disorder–order interplay to program organic–inorganic interactions into hierarchically ordered mineralised structures. The materials consist of elongated apatite nanocrystals, which have been aligned and arranged into microscopic prisms to provide the desired effects. These structures are studied for use in dentine hypersensitivity as a mineralising bandage to occlude exposed dentinal tubules.

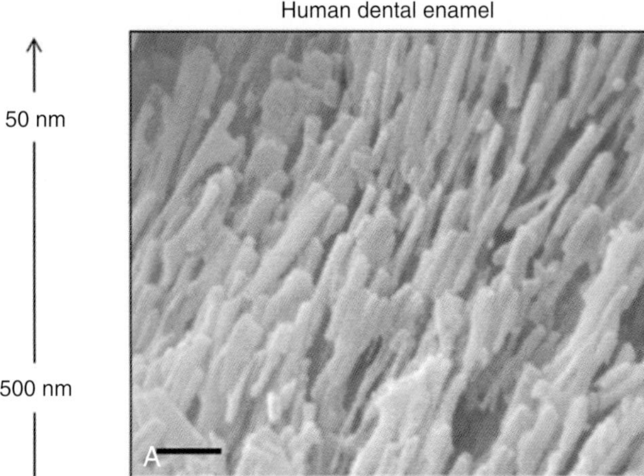

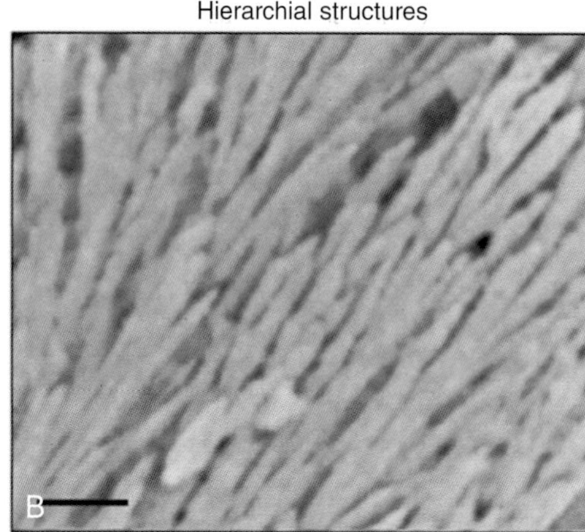

Fig. 28.3 SEM images illustrating the close resemblance of human dental enamel (A) to the hierarchically ordered mineralized structures (B) grown on membranes containing cell-binding domains (RGDs) and elastin-like recombinamers (ELRs). Scale bars: 200 nm. In dentine hypersensitivity, these structures (B) may provide a mineralising bandage to occlude exposed dentinal tubules. *From Elsharkawy, S., Al-Jawad, M., Pantano, M.F., et al., 2018. Protein disorder–order interplay to guide the growth of hierarchical mineralized structures. Nature Communications 9, 2145.*

There are several alternative materials that facilitate the subsurface mineralisation of enamel in carious lesions, including amelogenins, self-assembling peptides and polypeptides that are similar to elastin. Research has been focused on programming organic–inorganic interactions into hierarchically ordered mineralised structures using protein-mediated mineralisation.

Amelogenins

Studies have been conducted using shorter amelogenin sequences, retaining the N-terminal, mid-section and C-terminal domains of amelogenins that have been shown to play a key role in hydroxyapatite crystal growth. Using chitosan hydrogels containing amelogenin, an innovative way has been developed to reconstruct enamel by stabilising Ca-P clusters and guiding their arrangement into linear chains. A cluster group process is observed that anchors these enamel-like co-aligned crystals to the natural enamel substrate after their fusion with enamel crystals. As a pH-responsive and antimicrobial hydrogel, this chitosan hydrogel could also help prevent secondary dental caries if used in new therapeutic approaches.

Self-assembling peptide scaffolds

Using environmentally responsive beta-sheet–forming peptides that mimic extracellular matrix (ECM) proteins found in mineralised tissues, a new biomimetic approach is being used to promote remineralisation of carious lesions. By triggering anionic charge domains on the fibril surfaces, these peptides form a three-dimensional fibrillar scaffold inside the lesion that induces hydroxyapatite nucleation and growth. As a result, lesion repair is promoted through 'filling without drilling'. Alternatively, an artificial material composed of calcium–phosphate clusters that mimics the biomineralisation frontier of crystalline-amorphous hard tissue formation in nature has been proposed to create a precursor layer to induce enamel apatite epitaxial growth.

A self-assembling peptide known as P_{11}-4 is now available in a commercial product named Curolox Technology. Known as CurodontTM repair it has been tested on white spot lesions, where it filled the entire volume of the lesion, resulting in a significant increase in mineral density within subsurface carious lesions and supported the nucleation of *de novo* hydroxyapatite nanocrystals.

There are two key components of enamel with different acid-resistant properties: prismatic and interprismatic enamel. As a result, synthesising these directly onto the surface of damaged enamel and within the dynamic oral environment remains challenging.

Reviewing the literature to date, the following characteristics might be expected from successful enamel remineralisation products:

- **The ability to self-assemble**. This provides a scaffold that will encourage hydroxyapatite crystal formation similar to natural enamel formation as carried out by native amelogenin protein.
- **A calcium-binding motif at the N terminus**. This will enhance the ability to bind calcium ions.
- **A C-terminal domain motif**. This highly charged tail region will facilitate hydroxyapatite crystal formation.
- **Polyproline motifs**. Eleven or more of these polyproline repeats are stated as being required to aid hydroxyapatite crystal formation.
- **Glutamine residues**. These are crucial to the composition of the polyproline motifs.

Biological repair of the dentine–pulp complex

The tooth has an ability for limited repair by production of a newly formed layer of dentine that is deposited by specialised odontoblast-like cells located at the dentine–pulp border. Despite decreases in cell division and secretory activity of odontoblasts in the fully developed dental pulp, these processes are reactivated following dentine/pulp damage. Whenever enamel or dentine is compromised by a shallow dental carious lesion, the pulp's primary odontoblasts perform repair by forming reactionary dentine. A cascade of events may be triggered if primary odontoblasts cannot cope with further injury and damage, resulting in the recruitment, activation, proliferation and differentiation of new odontoblast-like cells, which will then secrete reparative dentine (see also pages 167–168).

The dental pulp is a soft connective tissue that consists of many different cell populations, some of which have stem cell properties. Research has revealed that DPSCs originate from a population of pericytes, which differentiate into odontoblast-like cells during tooth growth and development and in response to damage *in vivo*. Additionally, an MSC-like population has been identified as part of the dental pulp resident cell population. This type of cell migrates toward areas of tissue damage and differentiates into odontoblasts when stimulated. Some of these cells may come from peripheral nerve–associated glial cells.

DPSCs can be derived from the dental pulp tissue and can be expanded *in vitro*. Having properties similar to bone marrow stem cells, they are MSCs. When grown and expanded *in vitro* under controlled conditions, these cells produce dentine-like structures.

Tertiary dentine

Tertiary dentine (see Chapter 9) is dentine produced as a reaction to external stimuli or injuries such as heat, chemicals, bacteria or mechanical forces. Although clinically and histologically it is difficult to discriminate between reactionary dentine secreted by primary odontoblasts and tertiary dentine formed by a new population of pulp-derived, odontoblast-like cells, the cascade of events and features determine these two types of tertiary dentine as a response to injury. In more accurate terms, tertiary dentine beneath a carious lesion may consist of both reactionary and reparative dentine.

Reactionary dentine (see page 168)

Primary odontoblasts deposit growth factors and proteins into the dentine matrix when primary and secondary dentine are formed. Whenever there is limited damage and odontoblasts survive, these 'fossilised' growth factors are released, stimulating the cells and activating the immune system, leading to the formation of reactionary dentine. Reactionary dentine secretion is affected by Wnt activation. Wnt signalling can be activated in damaged tooth models with GSK-3 inhibitors, resulting in increased production of reactionary dentine. The inhibition of Wnt, however, does not impair reactionary dentine secretion. Cements made from hydraulic silicates, such as mineral trioxide aggregate (MTA), calcium-enriched cements and tricalcium silicates, are currently used in clinical treatment to stimulate production of reactionary dentine. In addition to promoting mineralisation, these biocompatible and bioactive materials increase factors such as tumour growth factor (TGF)-β1, TGF-β and BMP (implicated in the tubular organisation of reactionary dentine secretion).

Reparative dentine (see page 168)

A progressive injury of the dentine with odontoblast death causes a cascade of events that results in recruitment of new odontoblast-like cells and leads to formation of reparative dentine. During ECM breakdown, the breakdown products and immune response events attract progenitor cells that differentiate into odontoblast-like cells and produce reparative dentine.

When pulp exposure is limited, a mineral apposition layer forms, called a 'dentine bridge', because reparative dentine production is upregulated. This 'dentine bridge' protects the pulp from further bacterial infection.

Considerable knowledge is emerging about the underlying mechanisms of tertiary dentine formation from studies that investigate the activation of reparative dentine formation with pharmacological triggers. One of those investigations has focused on the activation of Wnt/β-catenin signalling as an initial response to tissue damage. Using biodegradable collagen sponges, small molecules that act as antagonists of glycogen synthase kinase (GSK-3) have been applied, causing activation of Wnt/β-catenin signalling. Activated Wnt induces odontoblast-like cells to form reparative dentine that effectively repairs deep dental lesions (Fig. 28.4). This biomimetic approach opens new opportunities for translational studies. Using bioactive molecules in combination with biomaterials can further promote repair of dental tissues. This is because these biomaterials will be able to interact with living tissue, stimulate cell growth, promote tissue regeneration and modulate the body's inflammatory response. A successful dental repair requires all these factors.

De novo regeneration of the dental pulp

Regeneration aims to restore and regain the tissue's original architecture and function. Micro-organisms, or their endotoxins, can cause irreversible pulpitis when they reach the dental pulp through a dental carious lesion. Current treatment options include removing all dental pulp tissue and then performing root canal therapy, which involves disinfecting the pulp chamber and filling it with artificial, inorganic materials. In regenerative dentistry (regenerative endodontics), novel approaches aiming at *de novo* formation of dental pulp tissue have been investigated based on biological repair/regeneration principles (Fig. 28.4).

Some clinical approaches that are established to treat infected teeth with incomplete root formation and open root apices have shown that successful revascularisation contributes to achieving full root length development and dentine thickness leading to apexification (see page 210).

Dental pulp tissue is lost after a root canal treatment on a fully developed tooth. Therefore, regeneration of dental pulp tissue using tissue engineering to produce the tissue from scratch is being investigated. It is often possible to engineer tissue by combining stem cells with biomaterials and scaffolds. Growth factors and bioactive molecules can sometimes be used in conjunction with these approaches.

When grown on collagen scaffolds and co-cultured with human endothelial cells, SHEDs have been shown to generate pulp tissue in human tooth slices (Fig. 28.5 A–C). Furthermore, the resulting pulp-like tissues share similar structural characteristics with physiological dental pulp (Fig. 28.5 D and E). Promising results from such studies have been obtained where there is regeneration of the dental pulp that is well-vascularised with an odontoblast-like layer forming on existing dental walls of the root canal. Thus, a continuous layer of mineralised tissue resembling dentine is established (Fig. 28.5E).

The use of scaffolds that can be loaded with bioactive factors has also been explored in dental pulp tissue engineering. An example of pulp regeneration in a full-length human tooth root involves nanofibrous microspheres that encapsulate vascular endothelial growth factor (VEGF) with heparin. Hierarchical microsphere systems offer good protection against denaturation and degradation of bioactive molecules (such as VEGF) as well as good control over their sustained release, resulting in new blood vessels within the regenerated tissue. This new generation of injectable microspheres mimics collagen structures found in the natural ECM and can act as carriers for pulp-forming stem cells.

In a pilot study, mobilised dental pulp stem cells (MDPSCs) have been assessed for their therapeutic potential and safety in the regeneration of the dental pulp. Autologous DPSCs are isolated from discarded teeth that have irreversible pulpitis without periapical lesions for the study. Granulocyte colony-stimulating factor (G-CSF) is used to treat DPSCs and then these treated cells are implanted into previously disinfected, emptied root canals. To evaluate the feasibility of the approach, magnetic resonance imaging (MRI) and cone beam computed tomography (CBCT) are performed. After 24 weeks, pulp-like regenerated tissue and new dentine are evident in most cases. In addition, electrical pulp testing reveals positive results.

A three-dimensional, controlled environment combined with stem cells and growth factors emphasises the regenerative concept in which the biological system is re-created in all its complexity.

Biological repair of the periodontium

There is a significant economic and social burden associated with periodontal disease around the world. Periodontal disease is chronic, progressive, inflammatory and multifactorial. It is characterised by host–microbiome disruption (dysbiosis) and an immunomodulatory response that irreversibly destroys the complex of tissues supporting the teeth (periodontium).

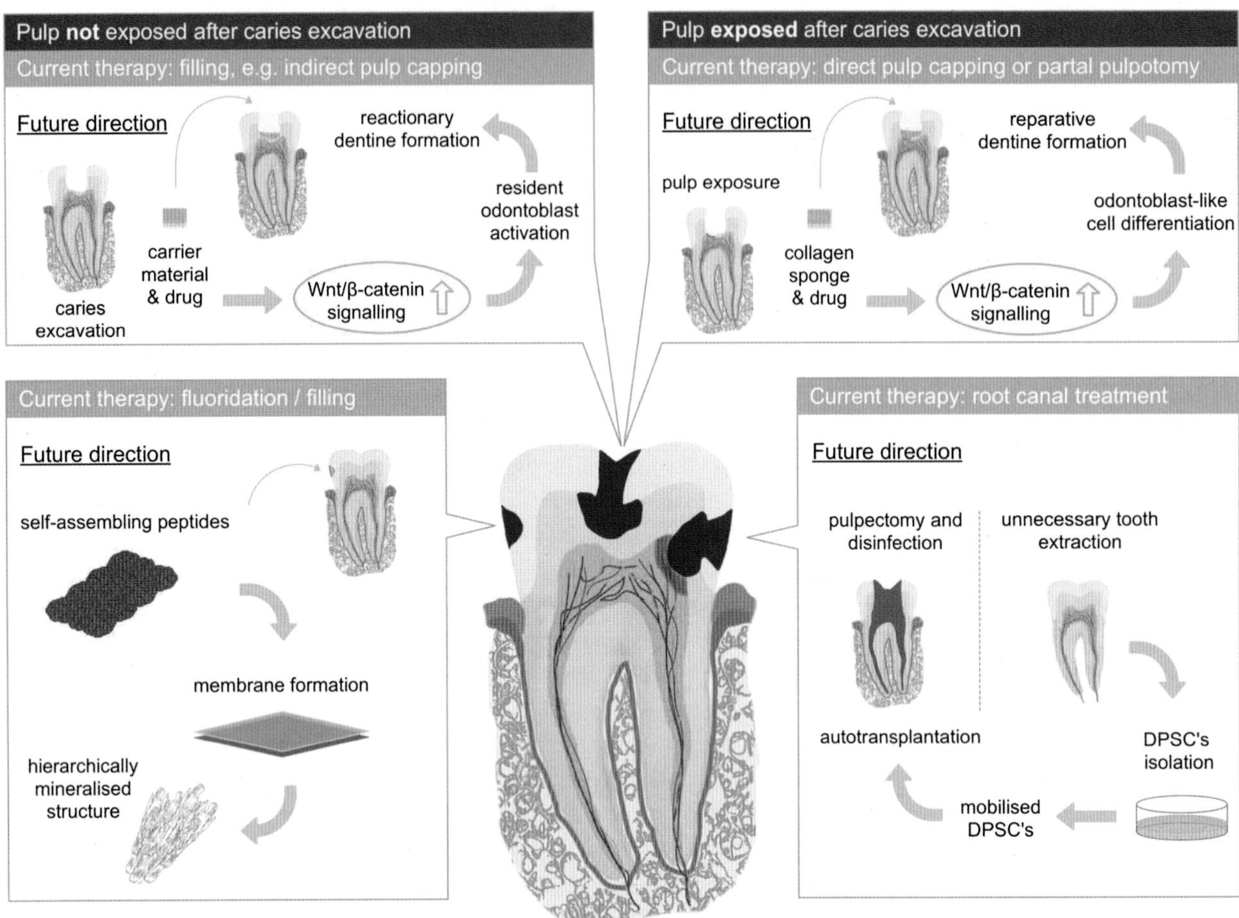

Fig. 28.4 A schematic representation of the different approaches for repairing and regenerating dentine–pulp complexes. Modulating the Wnt/β-catenin signalling pathway shows natural dentine apposition in both deep cavitation without pulp exposure (reactionary dentine, upper left box) and cavitation with exposed pulp tissue (reparative dentine, upper right box), if the underlying pulp tissue is vital and harbours resident odontoblasts and dental pulp stem cells (DPSCs), respectively. Current treatment options for pulp infection and necrosis (lower right box) include orthograde root canal therapy or, if there is incomplete root development, revascularisation. Recent cell-based approaches show that autologous isolated, expanded and mobilised DPSCs have the capacity to re-innervate (positive response on pulp testing) a pulpectomised and disinfected tooth after auto-transplantation. Non–cell-based approaches for mimicking lost enamel structure exists (lower left box), yet the mineralisation potential of self-assembling peptides needs to be further evolved and clinically tested. Adapted from Angelova Volponi, A., Zaugg, L.K., Neves, V., et al., 2018. Tooth repair and regeneration. *Current Oral Health Reports 5, 295–303.*

Loss of teeth eventually occurs. Periodontal disease damages (or destroys) both hard and soft tissues within the periodontium, and this complexity poses a challenge to repairing and regenerating them. In the field of periodontology, advanced bioengineering and stem cell biology knowledge may be employed to restore the structure and function of alveolar bone, PDL, cementum and gingival tissue to re-create the periodontal interface complex that is characterised by a high degree of integration and proper orientation of tissues.

Several studies have demonstrated the ability of periodontal tissues to repair and regenerate, directed by multipotent stem cells resident within the tissues.

Gingival stem cells

As one of the body's most rapidly dividing tissues, the oral mucosa heals quickly and with minimal scarring. Indeed, in comparison with cutaneous wounds, the oral mucosa has a remarkable abilility to heal wounds with negligible complications. Located around the cervical the cervical portion of the tooth, gingiva is part of the oral mucosa and a part of the periodontal complex, protecting the PDL from mechanical forces and microbes. Histologically, it consists of a keratinised, stratified squamous epithelium and an underlying connective tissue (see Chapter 14).

It has been suggested that gingival wound healing capabilities and homeostasis depend on several mechanisms, such as proliferative and differentiation cell programmes, epithelial remodelling, reduced inflammation and a distinct population of ASCs residing in the gingival tissue. The epithelial stem cell niche appears to play an important role in healing according to studies using single-cell RNA sequencing. These studies suggest that the transition from mild periodontitis to severe periodontitis is related to changes in the interactions between epithelial, mesenchymal and immune cells.

Because the gingiva is highly accessible during routine dental procedures, it can be used as a source to obtain both mesenchymal and epithelial stem cells. The cells derived from human gingival connective tissues are characterised by the expression of MSC markers, such as octamer-binding transcription factor 4 (Oct-4), stage-specific embryonic antigen-4 (SSEA-4) and STRO-1 (the first isolated monoclonal antibody to identify stromal/mesenchymal stem cells). Under controlled *in vitro* conditions, these cells can differentiate into osteocytes, adipocytes and neural types of cells. The ability of gingival cells to generate bone-like tissues and connective tissue has been demonstrated *in vivo* through ectopic subcutaneous transplantation. *In vitro* and *in vivo*, GSCs exhibit less pro-inflammatory cytokine-induced impairment of osteogenic potential and osteogenic activity than PDLSCs. Moreover, the cells isolated from inflamed gingival tissue retain the capacity to differentiate into adipogenic, osteogenic and chondrogenic identities. These cells express the same stem cell markers as the ones isolated from healthy gingival tissue. The GSCs, like other MSCs, modulate innate immune cells such as macrophages, dendritic cells (DCs) and mast cells.

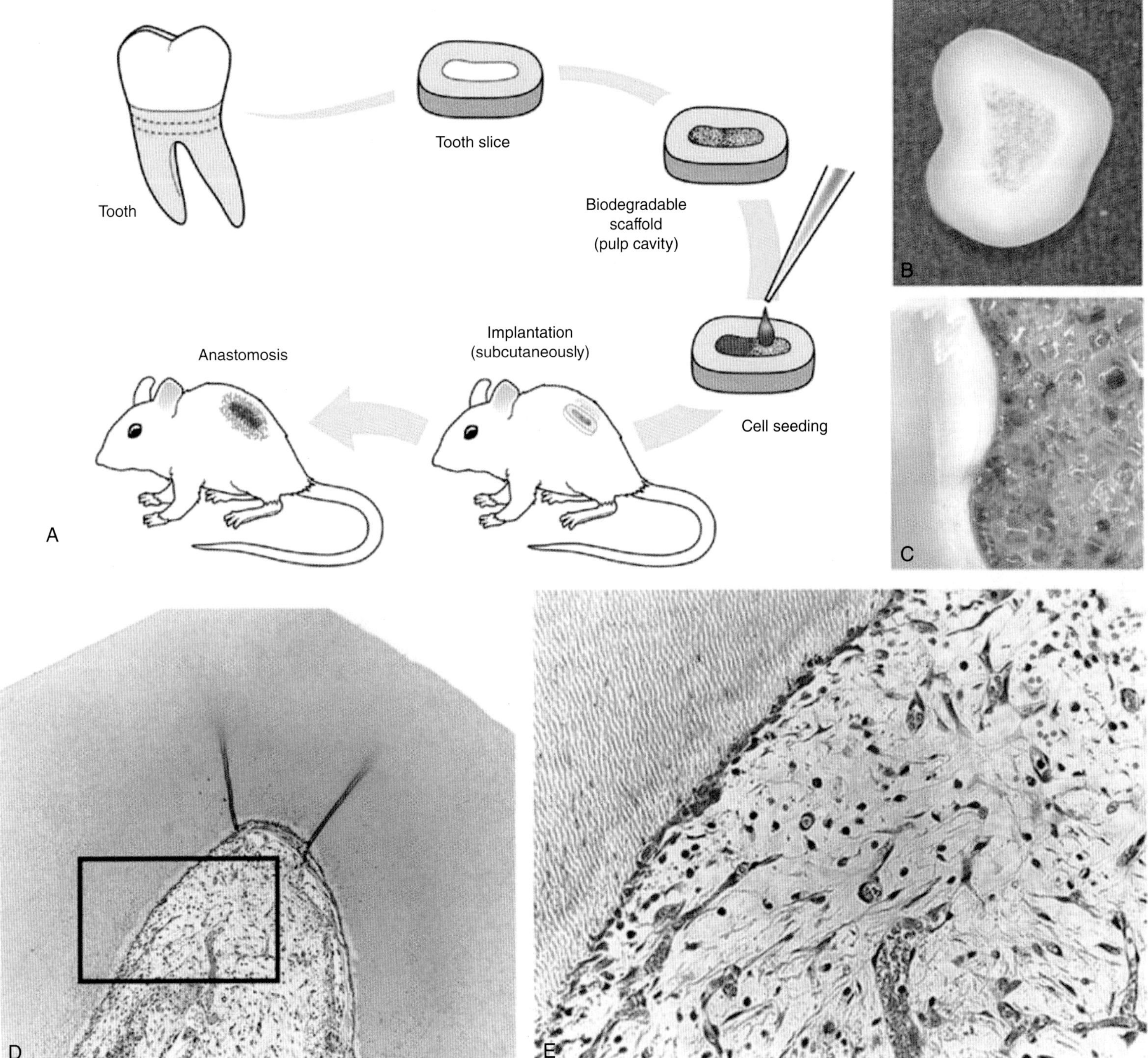

Fig. 28.5 Stem cells from human deciduous teeth (SHED) are seeded on biodegradable scaffolds (A, C) prepared within human tooth slices (A, B) and transplanted into immunodeficient mice (A). The resulting bioengineered tissue exhibits histological features that closely resemble those of a physiologic dental pulp (D, E). From Cordeiro, M.M., Dong, Z., Kaneko, T., Zhang, Z., et al., 2008. Dental pulp tissue engineering with stem cells from exfoliated deciduous teeth. *Journal of Endodontology 34, 962–969.*

Periodontal regeneration and treatment of peri-implantitis with gingival mesenchymal stem cells

Gingival mesenchymal stem cells (GMSCs) have been shown to promote periodontal tissue regeneration by increasing alveolar bone height in established periodontitis models. Additionally, an infusion of human GMSCs lowers the systemic inflammatory response and facilitates the regeneration of periodontal tissues. As shown in a randomised clinical trial study, implanting autologous GMSCs loaded on calcium triphosphate into intrabony periodontal defects covered with collagen membrane can reduce vertical pocket depth and clinical attachment loss. Moreover, six months after surgery, enhanced bone gain is observed when compared with a control group.

A major challenge in contemporary clinical practice is treating peri-implantitis, the destructive inflammatory process affecting the soft and hard tissues surrounding dental implants. New approaches using GMSCs have been explored. Advanced biomaterials, such as adhesive hydrogels (AdhHGs), are being used to encapsulate and introduce human GMSCs into bony defects around implants. After these experiments, significant bone formation is found that rescues the implants, accompanied by a reduction in inflammation around the peri-implantitis sites. These results demonstrate the potential of GMSCs for helping to treat this challenging condition.

Periodontal ligament stem cells

Several studies have identified cells nearby PDL blood vessels (pericytes) that are slow-dividing and exhibit stem cell characteristics. After injury, these PDLSCs are activated: they proliferate and migrate toward the cementum and bone.

Using perivascular markers, such as alpha-smooth muscle actin (α-SMA), it has been shown that these PDL stem cells differentiate into osteoblasts and cementoblasts during growth and development. Additionally, α-SMA–lineage PDL cells have been shown to be involved in repair by proliferating and differentiating to form new periodontal tissues after injury.

A population of progenitor cells has also been identified around neurovascular bundles. This population expresses Gli1 that is a target of the sonic hedgehog signalling (Shh) pathway and plays a role in tissue homeostasis. The previously discussed α-SMA–lineage cells also co-express Gli1, suggesting that they may be a subset of Gli 1 cells. During cementogenesis, a gradual decrease in Gli1-lineage cells and a progressive increase in their progeny can be observed. These cells respond to Wnt signalling, playing an important role in homeostasis and repair. In lineage tracing studies, it has been found that Axin2-lineage cells remain in the residual PDL after tooth extraction, then migrate into the alveolar socket, contributing to new bone matrix formation (confirmed by osteoblast marker co-expression). These Axin2-lineage cells are also important during development of the PDL.

In PDL-resident progenitor cells, a common MSC marker such as CD90 (Thy1) has a high level of expression. However, it was found that this marker is active only during PDL development, and its activity decreases with age.

Periodontal ligament stem cells *in vitro*

The stem cells from the PDL are easily accessible and can be obtained from extracted teeth or by exposing the root surface during clinical procedures. Under controlled culturing conditions, they can be easily expanded *in vitro*.

Once isolated and expanded *in vitro*, these cells have been shown to express common MSC markers, including STRO-1, STRO-4, CD29, CD73, CD90 (Thy1), CD106 (VCAM-1) and CD146 (MUC18). Cells that express these markers *in vitro* have the capacity to differentiate into a variety of specialised cells such as osteogenic, adipogenic and chondrogenic cells. When derived from both healthy and inflamed tissue, PDLSCs retain similar immunophenotypic characteristics, suggesting that inflamed tissue could also be used as a source to isolate cells with MSC properties during routine periodontal surgery.

Extracellular vesicles in regeneration

A cell's ability to maintain homeostasis depends on the continuous exchange of extracellular vesicles with its surrounding environment. The extracellular vesicles (EVs) are a group of membrane-derived vesicles of varying origin, size and features, and they play a crucial role in the exchange of information between cells.

According to the size and route of synthesis of the EVs, they can be classified as either exosomes, microvesicles or apoptotic bodies.

Cell-free therapies utilising EVs have attracted considerable scientific attention, along with cell therapies and tissue engineering in regenerative medicine and dentistry. There is a lower risk of infection or rejection with cell-free therapies compared with cell-based therapies, as EVs are unable to replicate. In this case, the uncontrolled differentiation associated with cell treatments is not present.

EVs carry nucleic acids, proteins, lipids and signalling molecules in the form of bilayer lipid membrane vesicles. Most eukaryotic cells secrete EVs that act as a means of communication between cells. Having the capacity to transmit active signals to nearby or distant recipients, they play an important role in maintaining homeostasis and preventing disease development. Based on their function, EVs can serve as prognostic biomarkers for cancer and neurodegenerative diseases, and therefore could serve as diagnostic tools for these diseases in the future. The use of EVs as drug vectors has also been reported.

Numerous studies suggest that EVs can play an important role in controlling the paracrine activity of MSCs. Accordingly, current research focuses on exploring whether MSC-derived EVs can complement the physiological functions of MSCs in repair. The secretome of the MSC-derived EVs shows potential, like the cells, and can therefore be an attractive target for cell-free tissue regeneration approaches.

Extracellular vesicles from gingival mesenchymal stem cells

EVs derived from human gingival mesenchymal stem cells (hGMSCs) have been found to have similar regenerative potential to hGMSCs themselves. Transcriptomic analyses of hGMSC-EVs revealed that these properties are related to the cargo present within the EVs, which contains proteins involved in inflammatory responses, bone regeneration, neuronal differentiation processes and angiogenesis (e.g., interleukins, TGF-β, BMPs, growth differentiation factors [GDFs], Wnt, VEGF, fibroblast growth factor [FGF], and neurotrophins).

Cell-based periodontal tissue regeneration

The use of extraoral and intraoral MSCs for tissue engineering of the periodontium has been explored. MSCs from bone marrow have been used and are seen to differentiate into osteoblasts and cementoblasts, promoting bone regeneration up to 20%.

Expansion of bone marrow mesenchymal stem cells (BMSCs) and application of platelet-rich plasma (PRP) as an autologous scaffold have been shown to promote bone healing and osseo-integration of dental implants. Other extraoral MSCs, such as the adipose-derived MSCs, have also been used in combination with PRP and showed promising results for periodontal regeneration.

A culturing technique that uses temperature-responsive cell culture dishes has been developed and used to culture PDLSCs that have been isolated and expanded *in vitro*. Using this culturing system, the cells are grown as cell sheets that can then be applied to promote repair and regeneration. A significant amount of cementum is formed after transplantation of these cell sheets on the root surface, where PDL fibres are also formed and anchored in the cementum.

Dental implants create a direct bond with bone, lacking the PDL (see pages 281–282). As the absence of a PDL can hinder the biological function of implants, ways are being found to embed a PDL tissue onto the implant surface and create a so-called 'ligaplant'. For this purpose, autologous PDLSCs derived from extracted teeth are expanded *in vitro* using tissue bioreactors and then transplanted onto titanium implants. Although these engineered 'ligaplants' have demonstrated functional loading for long periods, more research is needed before implementing this approach into clinical practice.

Similarly, a 'bio-root' structure encircled with PDL tissue has been engineered when PDLSCs (grown on a gel-foam carrier) is combined with SCAPs and seeded on an hydroxyapatite carrier shaped as a root. In an experiment where an engineered 'bio-root' capped with a dental crown was transplanted into the alveolar socket of a mini-pig, promising results were obtained when the tooth was tested by applying occlusal loads.

Periodontal wound healing and guided tissue regeneration

Endogenous cell recruitment

The use of chemokines on periodontal defects to stimulate the recruitment of endogenous cells is one of the approaches used to promote host wound healing. Among these chemokines is stromal derived factor-1 (SDF-1), also known as CXCL12, which helps recruit bone marrow stromal cells. Some PDL cells also express the receptor for SDF-1: CXCR4.

When SDF-1 is loaded on a collagen sponge into a periodontal defect, the number of MSCs and hematopoietic cells increases, while there is a reduction in immune cells. The application of SDF-1 leads to an increase in osteoclast activity at the wound margins, followed by an increase in bone formation. Biomaterials based on self-assembling peptides (e.g., hydrogels) are also used with SDF-1 and BMP-2 as an approach to increasing bone formation.

Guided tissue regeneration (see also pages 451–454)

Autologous bone grafts have initially been used for periodontal tissue regeneration. Despite promising results, attachment of the PDL does not always accompany new bone growth and, instead of cementum and PDL being formed, epithelium grows between the root surface and bone. The hypothesis that the type of cell that first reaches the root surface during wound healing determines what type of new tissue will be formed is based on the knowledge that the PDL, gingival tissue and alveolar bone harbour progenitor cells. To promote periodontal tissue regeneration, studies focus on targeted and selective cell repopulation using cells from both the PDL and bone or gingival connective tissue.

Although PDL cells can form new cementum and PDL, alveolar bone cells or gingival fibroblasts are incapable of doing so when PDL cells are absent. Furthermore, rapidly proliferating gingival cells (epithelial and fibroblasts) can interfere with the regenerative process of cementum and PDL if not excluded from the root surface.

As part of the guided tissue regeneration (GTR) technique, an occlusive barrier membrane is secured around the roots to allow cells to migrate from bone and the PDL into the defect while preventing epithelial downgrowth and gingival connective tissue from contacting the root. Even though this approach is well received and used in clinical procedures, the complete regeneration of the PDL complex is often inconsistent, and the results depend on the bone and PDL regenerative capacity, as well as the defect size and surface characteristics. Currently, GTR uses new biomaterials (e.g., titanium-reinforced expanded polytetrafluoroethylene [ePTFE]) (Fig. 28.6), but finding a biomaterial that is stiff enough to maintain space while adaptable to a wide range of defects remains a significant challenge. A minimal inflammatory reaction and a timely resorption of the biomaterial are also essential for the success of the treatment.

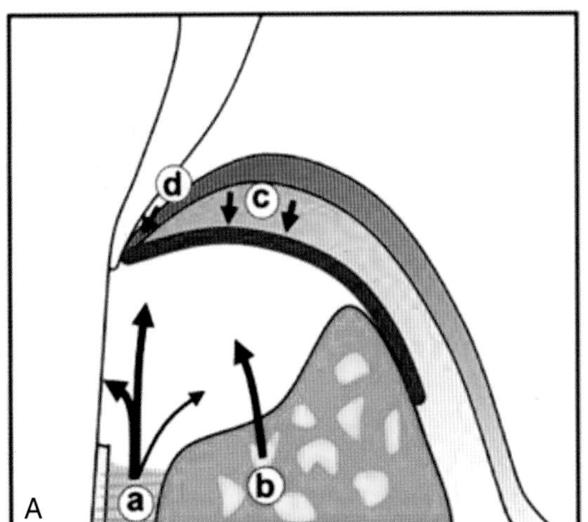

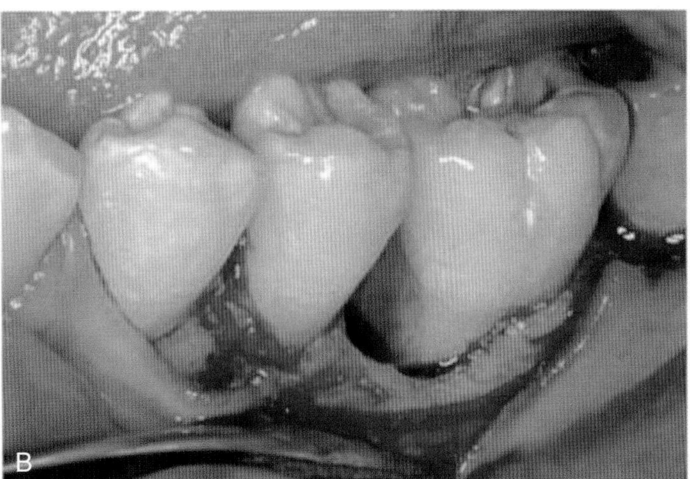

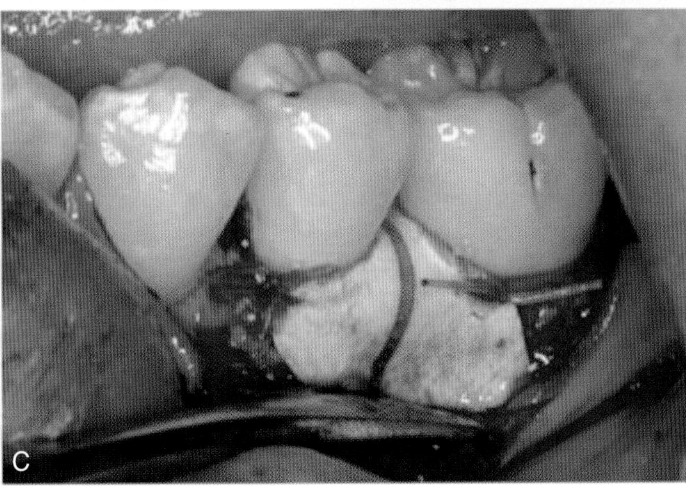

Fig. 28.6 (A) Illustration of guided tissue regeneration with a barrier membrane (blue line) which allows cells from the PDL (a) and alveolar bone (b) to fill the wound space while excluding cells from the gingival connective tissue (c) and gingival epithelium (d). (B) Clinical photographs of a periodontal defect after reflection of the gingiva and debridement of the bone defect and root surface and (C) after placement of a titanium-reinforced expanded polytetrafluoroethylene (ePTFE) guided tissue regeneration barrier. From Fraser, D., Caton, J., Benoit, D.S.W., 2022. Periodontal wound healing and regeneration: insights for engineering new therapeutic approaches. *Frontiers in Dental Medicine* 3, Article 815810.

Growth factors in periodontal tissue repair

Different cell populations of mature PDL tissues, such as fibroblasts, cementoblasts and osteoblasts, express TGF-β1 and TGF-β receptors and TGFβR-II and -III, while other receptors are predominantly found in newly regenerated tissues (underneath GTR barriers).

During early wound healing of gingival connective tissue, an increase in platelet-derived growth factor (PDGF) expression is observed. Nevertheless, this decreases by the time granulation tissue replaces the fibrin clot. As a result of these findings, soluble factors that are released during the first stages of wound healing – PDGFs, transforming growth factors (TGFs), FGFs, epidermal growth factors (EGFs) and insulin-like growth factors (IGFs) – are highlighted as important factors for the repair process. PDL cells migrate, proliferate and synthesise ECM proteins in response to these soluble factors.

Bone morphogenetic proteins

BMPs, which are part of the TGF-β superfamily, are well established as powerful inducers of cell differentiation. When periodontal defects heal, BMP-2, -4 and -7 are found within newly formed cementum, suggesting a complex role for BMPs not only in PDL development but also homeostasis and repair. In periodontal defects, BMP-2 promotes osteogenesis and can be used to drive the process. Nevertheless, as cementogenesis occurs at a slower rate than bone formation, the application of BMPs can also increase the incidence of ankylosis and root resorption.

Platelet-derived growth factor

As a multifunctional polypeptide growth factor, PDGF plays an important role in the initiation of the repair process. To achieve cell recruitment, proliferation and differentiation, PDGF is used in combination with other growth factors, such as BMPs. It is important to note that the time of application, the dosage and the anatomical site of application can play a role in whether a mitogen combined with growth factors has additive, synergistic or even inhibitive effects on bone healing. To promote vascularisation and aid the healing process and repair, adding angiogenic factors, such as VEGF, may be beneficial.

Autologous platelet concentrates

In comparison to recombinant growth factors, autologous platelet concentrates (APCs), including PRP and platelet-rich fibrin (PRF), are thought to have a similar function to trigger wound healing by releasing factors such as TGF-β, FGF, and IGF.

However, PRF and PDL cells alone are unable to promote bone and cementum formation in the context of a bone fenestration defect. Nevertheless, a combination of the two treatments results in an increase in bone density and cementum density.

Even though APCs are widely accessible and easily obtainable, their preparation is not standardised, leading to differences in composition, growth factor concentrations and release profiles, making it difficult to compare their effectiveness.

Wingless (Wnt)

Proliferation, differentiation and apoptosis of cells are all regulated by Wnts, a family of 19 secreted glycoproteins.

Cells that are responsive to Wnt are found in the PDL, and on the surface of alveolar bone and cementum. As a result of Wnt signalling, periodontal tissues can grow and maintain their structures. Several studies have confirmed this by showing that deleting Wnt signalling leads to the loss of cementum and bone, widening of the PDL and disorganisation of the PDL fibres. A smaller PDL space can be observed in the presence of overexpressed Wnt receptors, such as LRP5. There is also evidence to suggest that knocking out a Wnt inhibitor, sclerostin, results in thicker cementum and better alveolar bone formation.

Sclerostin is present in the PDL at sites adjacent to active physiological root resorption of deciduous teeth. Additionally, PDL cells, which are Wnt-responsive, are also responsible for depositing reparative cement at resorption sites.

Because Wnts play such an important role in bone development, homeostasis and repair, translational research has been initiated to find pharmaceutical targets in this pathway to treat skeletal and dental diseases (see page 268).

Enamel matrix derivatives

One of the widely used biological factors for clinical periodontal tissue regeneration is the enamel matrix derivative (EMD). Purified enamel matrix proteins are available commercially as Emdogain®, suspensions that precipitate and enable adhesion of enamel matrix proteins (EMPs) to the root surface. Hertwig's epithelial root sheath cells might also secrete EMPs, or structurally similar proteins, to direct cementum formation (see pages 442–443).

As a result of the application of EMP or EMD, new cementum and bone are formed, epithelial downgrowth is inhibited and bacterial activity is inhibited, while angiogenesis is improved and immune cell signalling is altered.

EMD is suggested to be more effective in narrow intrabony defects than wide ones. To overcome the obstacles of space maintenance and wound stability, a combination of EMD with various bone grafts should be explored.

Modified formulations of EMD are being tested in conjunction with various biomaterials, such as loading EMD onto electrospun hollow fibres, loading EMD onto collagen membranes and loading EMD onto decellularised dermal matrix.

Biomaterials and scaffolds used in periodontal regeneration

To facilitate osteogenesis, scaffolds must be biocompatible and have a specific configuration to facilitate cell migration, differentiation and mineralisation.

Diverse biomaterials are often used as carriers of bioactive molecules and as factors to stimulate recruitment of cells and to promote healing and periodontal/bone regeneration. Some of these include organic compounds such as collagen matrices and synthetic polymers (polylactic/polyglycolic acid fibres), inorganic osteoconductive ceramic materials (such as deproteinated corals and synthetic hydroxyapatites) and soluble bioactive glasses (see Fig. 13.53). With the latter, the ionic dissolution products (including silicon) and their gel-like surface accrete hydroxyapatite, accelerate mature functioning osteoblast production within a wound and provide an osteoconductive surface for the growth of new bone.

Several different forms of biomaterials are used to promote early or sustained release of growth factors, directing wound healing and periodontal regeneration. PDGF can be loaded into polymer microspheres (shells) for early release, and simvastatin can be loaded into their cores for more sustained release. The controlled release of IGF-I and BMP-2 has also been achieved using microsphere systems containing two different materials (dextran and gelatine).

PLGA-PLLA composite electrospun meshes have been engineered with a similar core–shell structure to facilitate a burst release of FGF-2 from the shell and sustained delivery of BMP-2 from the core to fenestration defects (an isolated area that is denuded of bone). Likewise, a tri-layer chitosan membrane has been developed for the rapid release of epigallocatechin-3-gallate, an anti-inflammatory compound, and for the sustained release of lovastatin, an osteogenic drug.

To assess their application in tissue engineering of craniofacial defects, a new generation of nanomaterials is being developed in the form of nanoparticles, nanofibres, nanotubes and nanosheets. In addition to promoting cell invasion and proliferation, nanofibres resemble ECM components, while nanotubes and nanoparticles enhance mechanical and chemical properties of scaffolds, promote cell attachment and facilitate tissue regeneration.

PDL fibre-guiding scaffolds

One of the greatest challenges in tissue engineering of the PDL is the direction of the collagen fibres that anchor the cementum to the bundle bone. Their correct and complex orientation is crucial for tooth support and function. By introducing a new concept of fibre-guiding scaffolds, efforts are being made to overcome this challenge. These innovative scaffolds can induce a spontaneous alignment of PDL fibres.

Polymeric scaffolds with 'pillars' have been made that run perpendicularly against the tooth roots *in vivo*. This allows PDL cells and fibres (such as Sharpey's fibres) to grow in a directed manner and attach to cementum and bundle bone. Further development of the concept has been achieved by creating pillars with micro-grooves containing specific depths and widths. Furthermore, CT scans might be used presurgically to ensure high customisation of the scaffold to fit anatomical defects, thus providing a personalised treatment approach in the future.

Personalised scaffolding technologies for periodontal regeneration

With the advent of new technologies, such as 3D bioprinting, customised scaffolds can be produced based on anatomical data that are specific to each individual. Multiple steps are involved in this tissue engineering approach, including:

1) Image acquisition: Using CT or MRI, patients' image datasets are created. These data are then used for scaffold production that is based on computer-aided design/computer-aided manufacture (CAD/CAM).
2) Image processing with DICOM **(a file format produced by MRI and CT scanners)** conversion and STL file **(a format accepted by 3D printers)** generation: This enables the creation of porous scaffolds using an image-based hierarchical design method.
3) Image post-processing and scaffold fabrication: A solid freeform fabrication (SFF) method that produces individual-specific scaffolds using 3D printing and materials or parameters based on CAD/CAM.

To treat periodontal defects, especially those at the root furcation area, a variety of models are being developed which use personalised scaffolding approaches. Using a 3D-printed scaffold made of PCL and PLGA that have been formulated in an equitable ratio, researchers have presented new ways to deliver genes to the periodontal tissue for healing and tissue engineering purposes. Implementing these technologies, we are rapidly advancing the field of personalising scaffolds, enabling better clinical application of these scaffolds in the case of large bone defects.

Biological repair and tissue engineering of the temporomandibular joint

There are a variety of disorders that affect the temporomandibular joint (termed TMJDs) that are clinical conditions associated with the TMJ and related structures of the masticatory system. Several factors can cause these conditions, including traumatic, inflammatory and congenital. Besides having a deficient wound healing process, TMJD patients also suffer from continuous and irreversible injuries that result in fibrosis. In many cases, patients experience considerable pain during basic oral activities such that their quality of life is diminished (see also page 329).

As for other synovial joints, breakdown of the bony surface of the TMJ condyle results in osteoarthritis and degenerative joint disease, which can also result in severe pain. Understanding the basic structure and development of the joint has led to novel approaches to potentially treat the disease. As seen in Chapter 15, a reservoir of stem cells is present in the superficial layer of the condyle that gives rise to chondrocytes and osteoblasts critical for TMJ development and homeostasis.

The limited therapeutic options to treat TMJ diseases have led to an increased interest in regenerative strategies that utilise stem cells, implantable scaffolds and bioactive molecules that are well targeted to accelerate the healing process. It is very challenging to succeed in functional and structural regeneration of the TMJ because of its complex nature. As a result of its limited healing capacity, its unique histological and structural properties and the necessity of long-term prevention of ossified or fibrous adhesions, it is extremely important to develop innovative strategies and biomaterials for regeneration of the TMJ. Indeed, its tissues are amongst the most difficult to regenerate.

Because of a lack of detailed characterisation of the cellular network, it is extremely difficult to develop targeted therapies for TMJD. Single-cell transcriptome analysis of disc cells at different postnatal stages has revealed chondrogenic and non-chondrogenic clusters of fibroblasts. It has been suggested that disc progenitors are characterised by ubiquitous expression of Notch3 and Thy1 pathways in the resident mural cell population.

Strategies that are used for cartilage and bone engineering in TMJ repair and regeneration approaches include:

- Introducing an acellular scaffold matrix into the environment to attract and stimulate resident cells ('cell homing')
- *Ex vivo* tissue engineering, where competent cells are seeded into scaffolds and then implanted within the TMJ
- Intra-articular drug and/or stem cell delivery methods applied to the TMJ (for both pain management and regenerative strategies)

Stem cell sources for TMJ regeneration strategies

The multilineage differentiation capacities and high proliferation rates of BMSCs make them an excellent source of MSCs for regenerative therapies of various craniofacial tissues and organs. However, the BMSCs have a tendency for endochondral ossification, which can hinder their use in TMJ repair.

Adipose-derived stem cells (ADSCs) are another potential source of stem cells with MSC properties for TMJ regeneration. When considering the environmental conditions within the TMJ, these cells are ideally suited for performing their functions under low-oxygen conditions.

The regeneration of fibrocartilage in the TMJ disc could also be achieved using dermal fibroblasts as a source of stem cells, as they have high chondrogenic potential when treated with IGF-1.

Owing to their well-documented osteogenic and chondrogenic differentiation abilities, dental tissue–derived MSCs, including PDLSCs, SCAPs, DFSCs, and DPSCs, are also being considered as potential cell sources for TMJ repair.

Scaffolds for TMJ cartilage regeneration

A variety of scaffolds have been used in research studies to address the TMJ's specific anatomical and histological conditions and to promote regeneration and repair.

It is important to note that hyaluronan is a polysaccharide found in abundance in cartilage matrices. Taking advantage of its ability to promote differentiation of stem cells into chondrocytes, it is one of the most ideal scaffolds for cartilage regeneration. Despite its obvious advantages, its downside is its mechanical properties, which is why other molecules have been added to improve them and render hyaluronan more suitable. To be used as a scaffold, the hyaluronan needs to be chemically modified and cross-linked to form a hydrogel.

Poly-vinyl alcohol (PVA) is a scaffold material that supports cartilage repair. Due to its high water content and elastic properties, PVA can be an ideal polymer for cartilage regeneration.

Another scaffold material that promotes cartilage repair is poly-L-lactic-co-glycolic acid (PLGA). Owing to its versatility, its ability to promote MSCs differentiation *in vivo*, and Food and Drug Administration (FDA) approval for use in clinical settings, this scaffold material is a good option for regenerating cartilage in the TMJ.

Fibrocartilage regeneration (TMJ disc)

Different scaffolds have shown their efficacy in both *in vitro* and *in vivo* experiments when it comes to the regeneration of the TMJ disc. Polyglycolique acid (PGA), which is a biodegradable polyester, is used to engineer a disc in which cells are enclosed in PGA mesh scaffolds. These scaffolds of PGA have the capability to support the culture of stem cells from human umbilical cords and to differentiate and expand them into chondrogenic cells. Poly-L-lactic acid (PLLA) has also been used owing to its slow degradation rate. A PLLA scaffold seeded with porcine TMJ cells and treated with TGF-1 shows improved mechanical properties as well as a higher level of collagen and glycosaminoglycan (GAG) deposition as compared to PGA scaffolds. GAGs are native components of the ECM that drive cell behaviour and regulate the microenvironment.

The use of porcine-derived ECM has been studied as an acellular regenerative template for reconstruction of TMJ discs. The results of implanting this scaffold after 6 months are promising.

Osteochondral regeneration

Regeneration of the TMJ presents several challenges, including the need for both bone regeneration and cartilage regeneration to happen simultaneously, while respecting the very different competing constraints that accompany these two processes.

When a large osteochondral defect in the condyle has been treated with PLGA composite implants seeded with Nel-related protein 1 (NRP1) and modified-autologous BMSCs to repair the defect, both bone and cartilage are regenerated following the procedure.

Combining scaffolds and growth factors

In vitro investigations show the effectiveness of 'compartmental implants' containing alginate hydrogels at the cartilaginous ends and collagen membranes at the bony ends. These strategies are used to differentiate human MSC populations into osteogenic and chondrogenic cell lineages. Six weeks after implantation of PLGA microsphere scaffolds containing TGF-1 at the cartilaginous end and BMP-2 at the bony end, newly formed osteochondral tissue has been observed in rabbit mandibular condylar experimental defects.

A Wnt approach to treat osteoarthritis of the TMJ

As with other differentiating systems, it is likely that Wnt signalling is involved in TMJ stem cell fate specification toward chondrocytes. It is seen that suppression of Wnt signals promotes fibrocartilage stem cells to differentiate into chondrocytes, while, conversely, overactive Wnt signals disrupt fibrocartilage homoeostasis by enhancing chondrocyte maturation, depleting the stem cell pool and eventually causing degeneration of the condyle. Such considerations have generated a possible non-surgical treatment by injecting small-molecule Wnt inhibitors, such as sclerostin (SOST), into the joint to maintain the stem cell pool and repair cartilage.

3D approaches and personalised scaffolding technologies for TMJ regeneration

Technology that is enabling the production of customised 3D scaffolds according to the specific anatomy of the patient is attracting the interest of many research groups that work on the regeneration of TMJs. The reason for this is that, when the TMJ is being rebuilt, it must reflect the unique anatomical, structural and functional characteristics of the mandibular condyle and its disc if they are to function properly. Therefore, it is very important to provide an environment that can be guided in 3D.

TMJ-shaped polyethylene glycol–based hydrogel implants seeded with MSCs and capable of differentiation into chondrogenic and osteogenic cells are some of the first attempts in building a 3D scaffold following the anatomical features of TMJs. There have also been attempts to mimic the size and shape of the TMJ by using scaffolds made from porcine ECM. These scaffolds have led to regeneration of a functional TMJ following implantation in a canine model of TMJ discectomy.

With the advances in manufacturing personalised 3D prostheses and the usage of bio-reactors, the field of regenerative dentistry is now able to use these technologies for the manufacture of computer-designed nanofibrous and microporous scaffolds that can be loaded with cells for the application of customised regenerative treatments.

For the replacement of the mandibular condyle, the use of a customised 3D polyamide implant manufactured and coated with nanoscale hydroxyapatite has been shown to provide positive clinical outcomes.

To deliver growth factors directly to the targeted cells via a spatiotemporal delivery system, 3D printed scaffolds with anatomical shapes that mimic the TMJ discs of rabbits have been engineered, where the growth factors are encapsulated in microparticles. After 3D-printed scaffolds are functionalised with microparticles of connective tissue growth factor (CTGF) and colonised over 6 weeks by human MSCs, a heterogeneous fibrocartilaginous matrix mimicking that of a human TMJ disc is observed.

Through these approaches, reproducible matrix heterogeneity and viscoelastic properties can be achieved in 3D implants. It is crucial to translate these aspects into future clinical applications.

Salivary gland biological repair and regeneration

Salivary glands are imperative for oral health, and their dysfunction negatively affects the quality of life. In autoimmune diseases such as Sjögren's syndrome (SjS) (see also page 348) and patients with head and neck salivary gland cancer, irreversible damage to the glands occurs. Insufficient salivation causes xerostomia (dry mouth, see page 348), which interferes with oral functions such as chewing, speaking and tasting. Xerostomia can be treated palliatively (relieving symptoms) with artificial saliva for moisturising the mucous membranes of the mouth or with sialagogues to stimulate residual secretary cells within the salivary glands. There is a limited effect of these treatments, however, which has motivated the search for new regenerative treatments that can restore tissue and organ function. To repair and regenerate salivary glands, tissue engineering approaches use stem cells, gene therapy, bioactive factors and biomaterials. A summary of the current approaches is shown in Fig. 28.7.

Stem and progenitor cell populations in the salivary glands

Multiple populations of stem/progenitor cells can be found in the salivary glands (see Fig. 16.24). In response to the micro-environment, salivary gland stem cells can differentiate into acinar, ductal or myoepithelial cells.

Salivary progenitor cells that are resident within the tissues divide and differentiate into specific cell types, and their presence is crucial to tissue regeneration. Different populations of salivary gland progenitor cells are identified, based on the markers they express. Cell migration, proliferation and differentiation of salivary gland stem cells are closely related to the activation of c-Kit receptor tyrosine kinase (stem cell factor receptor). Keratin 14 (K14) is another significant marker (see Fig. 16.24D). The K14+ cells represent a multipotent population of salivary gland epithelial stem cells (SMGs) that give rise to acinar, myoepithelial and ductal tissue. During cellular self-renewal and pluripotency, Sox2 plays a critical role in adult salivary gland tissue.

Gene therapy approaches

Cells can be modified with genes to stimulate the proliferation of acinar cells, the number of endothelial cells and the flow of saliva. The loss of functional water channels in the salivary gland epithelium is one of the major disruptive processes that characterise gland dysfunction. One of the first gene therapies for salivary glands involved targeting the aquaporin-1

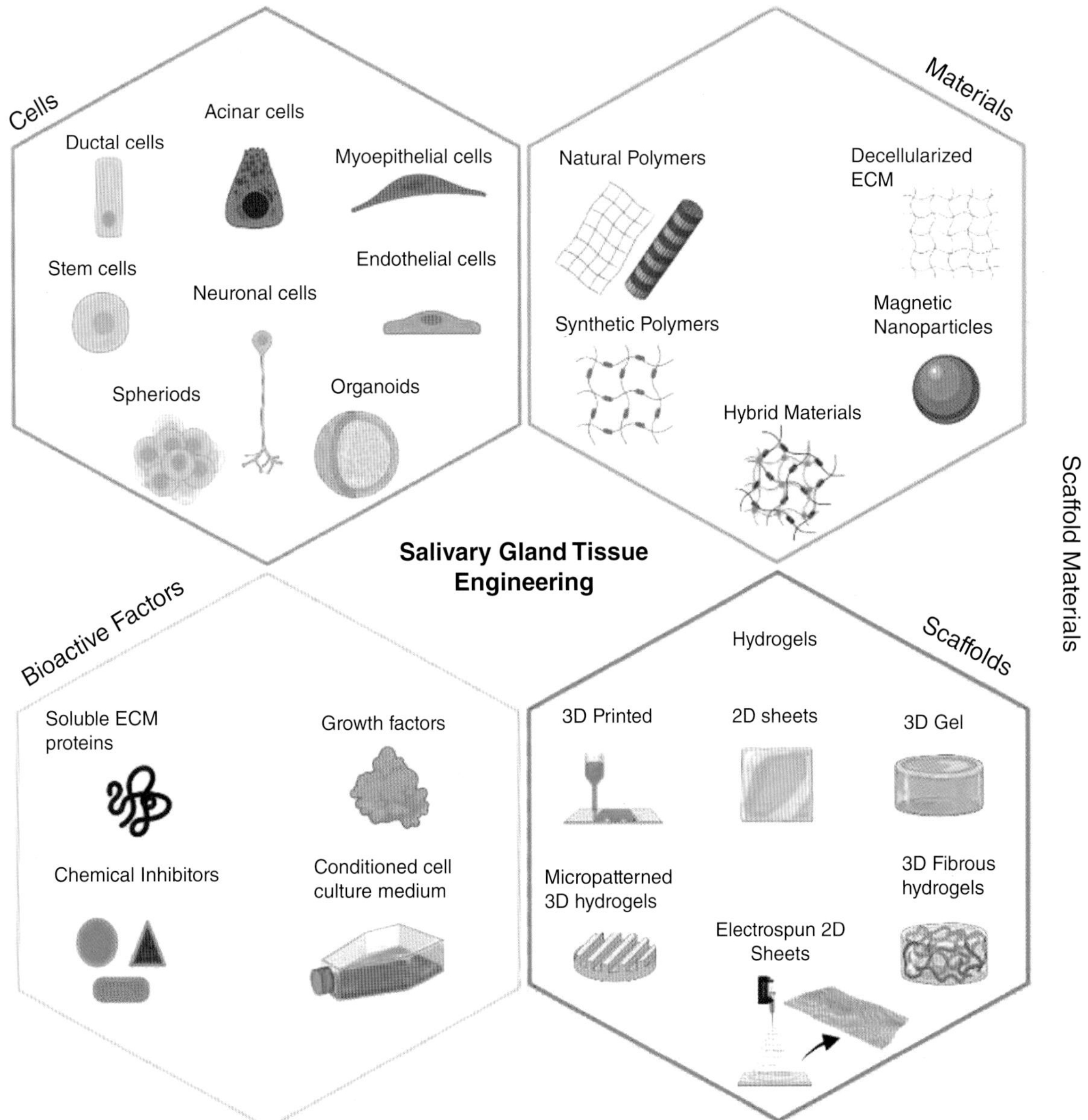

Fig. 28.7 Summary of the current approaches for salivary gland tissue engineering. To repair and regenerate salivary glands, approaches focus on stem and progenitor cells, bioactive factors (growth factors, soluble ECM, chemical inhibitors), biomaterials and fabrication of innovative scaffolds. From Hajiabbas, M., D'Agostino, C., Siminska-Stanny, J., et al., 2022. Bioengineering in salivary gland regeneration. *Journal of Biomedical Science* 29, 35.

(AQP1) gene, which encodes an integral membrane protein associated with the passive transport of water along osmotic gradients. This salivary gland gene therapy study demonstrated that recombinant adenovirus vector (AdhAQP1) is an effective method for delivering the human AQP1 gene into the salivary glands of donor Wistar rats. Further studies supported the development of clinical trials. Preliminary results indicate high tolerability of vector administration, with only mild to moderate side effects. Five out of 11 radiation therapy patients who participated in the study had improved symptoms of xerostomia and parotid gland discharge 3 to 4,7 years after treatment. The improved symptoms are observed for ~2 to 3 years following the treatment.

In SjS patients, neutralisation of inflammatory mediators may also be a possible therapeutic approach based on gene therapy. Despite encouraging results, gene therapy still faces challenges, such as host immune response and control of off-target effects and mutagenesis.

Cell therapy and tissue engineering

Research is being conducted on how salivary gland cells can maintain their 3D spatial organisation *in vivo* after they have been dissociated from the gland tissue. *In vitro* expansion of rare salivary gland stem cells (SGSCs) is possible through the development of three-dimensional 'salispheres' as viable salivary gland-derived organoids. Compared with non-transplanted irradiated mice, salisphere transplantation significantly increases saliva production by 42% in treated irradiated mice. Selecting and enriching salivary gland-derived cells expressing stem cell–specific markers (CD24+ CD29+) yields even more promising results. In comparison to the control group, these enriched grafts rescue up to 70% of normal gland function in the irradiated group.

The development of salivary gland organoid systems offers another important aspect focusing on characterisation of key niche signalling components necessary for salivary gland homeostasis and regeneration. In mouse models, Wnt-stimulated salivary gland organoids contain heterogeneous populations of differentiated salivary gland cells and stem/progenitor cells. Significant improvement in salivary flow is also observed when these salivary gland organoids are transplanted into irradiated recipients. Moreover, more uniform acinar spheroids can be grown *in vitro* with the use of micropatterns and nanofibrous hydrogel structures that are being developed. The use of hydrogel materials as the 3D culturing environment promotes the formation of spheroids derived from adult salivary gland cells into acinar structures.

Other approaches include the use of non-salivary gland cells with predominantly MSC properties, such as bone marrow–derived MSCs, MSCs of human adipose origin and ESCs and iPSCs. These approaches use non-salivary gland stem cells as sources to activate repair and regeneration mechanisms irradiated salivary glands. The observed effects suggest that the cells might play a role through their pro-survival/proliferative paracrine effects on nearby stem/progenitor cells. The paracrine effects of cells derived from adipose tissue and bone marrow are supported by the release of bioactive components with anti-apoptotic and proliferative actions. However, MSCs have limitations, such as their heterogeneous nature and donor-dependent efficacy, and concerns about their safety (potential for metastasis to other tissues or organs) prevent their widespread adoption as stem cell therapy. The long-term safety of MSC cells in salivary gland cell therapy has not yet been reported.

Scaffolding materials

Salivary gland tissue's properties (mechanical, physicochemical and biological) properties can be replicated using a variety of scaffolds. These are employed in assembling implantable and secretory tissue models by providing an environment for stem/progenitor cells from adult salivary glands. There are three main categories of biocompatible materials used in salivary gland tissue engineering research: biomaterials of natural origin, synthetic polymers and hybrid scaffolds.

Salivary gland bioengineering

Salivary gland organoids created *in vitro* can develop into fully functional glands when transplanted *in vivo*. The salivary gland organoid is engineered by mimicking the cascade of events that happen during salivary gland development and enabling previously dissociated embryonic mesenchymal and epithelial cells to interact *in vitro*. The bioengineered germ undergoes acinar formation with a myoepithelium and innervation. After being transplanted into a salivary gland defective mouse model, it produces saliva in response to pilocarpine and gustatory stimulation and restores swallowing. Despite this approach providing support for the concept of bioengineered salivary gland regeneration, it is still challenging to obtain non-embryonic epithelial and mesenchymal cells in sufficient numbers that retain their genetic profile *in vitro* and use them in the process of bioengineering salivary gland germs.

Organ engineering

The holy grail of regenerative dentistry

Engineering a bio-tooth

Regenerative dentistry's 'holy grail' has always been whole-tooth bioengineering. To engineer a 'bio-tooth', scientists must understand the underlying mechanisms that govern tooth development and re-create these conditions *in vitro* to mimic the natural cascade of events (Fig. 28.8).

Chapter 21, described how teeth are formed by sequential, reciprocal interactions between oral epithelial cells (ectoderm) and neural crest–derived mesenchymal cells. To direct and drive tooth development and organ engineering in laboratory conditions, two-way 'conversations' between epithelium and mesenchyme must take place under well-controlled spatiotemporal conditions. Laboratory conditions must establish the following:

- Presence of active cells/tissues, where there is tissue capable of producing the inductive signal (odontogenic) and tissue capable of receiving and responding to the inductive signal
- Complex signalling network composed of signalling molecules, receptors and transcription control systems
- Controlled spatiotemporal conditions, such as controlled 3D environments with physical properties that enable cell-to-cell communication, signal exchange, cell proliferation, differentiation and growth

Through bio-tooth engineering, new knowledge could be gained and applied to repair and regenerate other organs whose morphogenesis depends on reciprocal interactions between epithelial and mesenchymal tissues through distinct stages (e.g., hair follicles, mammary, sweat and salivary exocrine glands).

In classical tissue recombination experiments (see Chapter 21), the dental epithelium and the mesenchyme signal sequentially to form teeth. These reciprocal responses between epithelium and mesenchyme during tooth development are the basis of whole-tooth engineering approaches. *In vitro* growth of a tooth organoid (tooth primordia) is the first step toward implantation *in vivo*, leading to the full formation of a tooth.

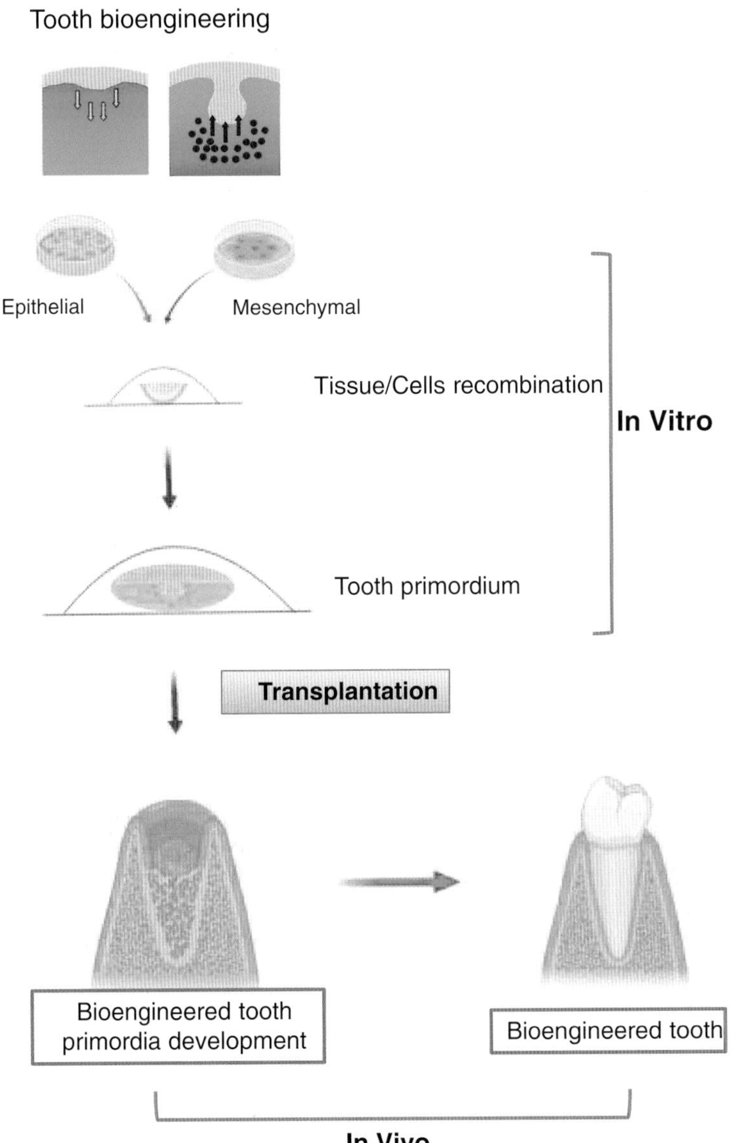

Fig. 28.8 Schematic representation of bio-tooth engineering. Patients with missing teeth can provide suitable epithelial and mesenchymal cells that can be expanded *in vitro*. Cell populations of either epithelial or mesenchymal origin are made odontogenic (capable of initiating *de novo* odontogenesis) and recombined with their counterparts. Through epithelial–mesenchymal cell recombination, an early-stage tooth primordium (organoid) can be generated, which can then be transplanted at the location of the missing tooth or cultured *ex vivo* to form a whole tooth. Courtesy of Dr. Ana Angelova Volponi.

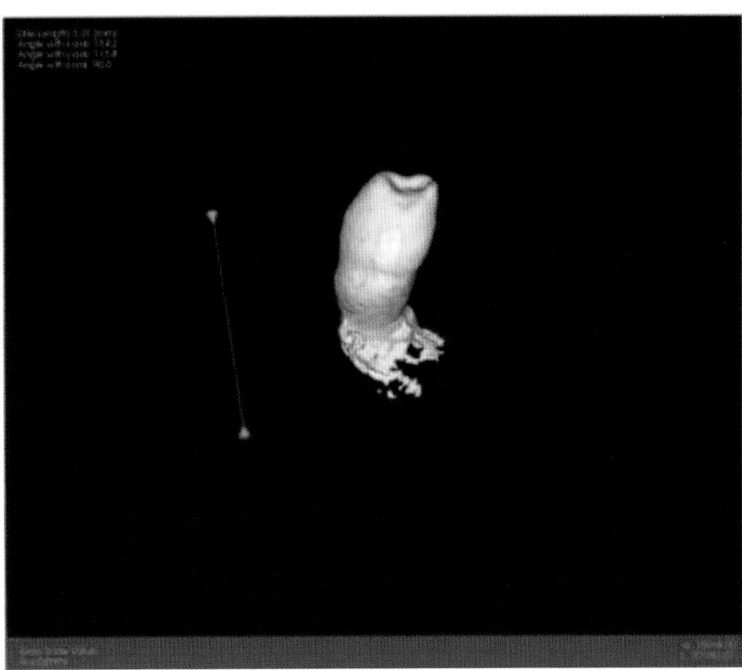

Fig. 28.9 MicroCT analysis of 'bio-tooth' engineered by using adult human gingival cells and mouse odontogenic mesenchyme to form tooth organoid (tooth primordium) *in vitro*. After 6 weeks of *in vivo* transplantation under the kidney capsule of immunosuppressed mice as a host, a whole tooth has developed. Hard tissue formation is evident, and 3D reconstructions show a bio-tooth with well-developed crown and roots. From Angelova Volponi, A., Kawasaki, M., Sharpe, P.T., 2013. Adult human gingival epithelial cells as a source for whole-tooth bioengineering. *Journal of Dental Research* 92, 329–334.

It has been established that when the tissues of a tooth germ are dissociated and the resulting cells allowed to re-associate in an ECM (scaffold), they reassemble and re-sort to form tooth organoids. These organoids develop into a fully functional tooth when transplanted into the alveolar bone in the lost tooth region. The bioengineered tooth subsequently erupts, occludes and is functional in terms of mastication. It exhibits the correct tooth structure and hardness of mineralised tissues and responds to noxious stimulations such as mechanical stress and pain. Nevertheless, these experiments have always used at least one source of cells obtained from fresh embryonic tooth primordial tissue (epithelium or mesenchyme), which has demonstrated odontogenic (inductive, tooth-forming) characteristics at certain developmental stages.

A significant advance has been made when adult bone marrow mesenchyme cells were is combined with early, inductive, embryonic dental epithelium. As a result, adult mesenchymal cells respond to the odontogenic (inductive) signal from the early epithelium and fully contributes to tooth development. Even though mesenchymal cells can be derived from several sources, the challenges with tissue-engineering teeth relate to locating suitable odontogenic epithelial sources. A further breakthrough has been achieved when human adult gingival epithelial cells are exposed to an inductive (odontogenic) signal derived from (mouse) embryonic mesenchyme. As a consequence, ameloblasts and epithelial root sheath cells are found to be of human origin (derived from human gingival epithelial cells) during the formation of fully formed teeth (Fig. 28.9), while the rest of the fully formed tooth is of mouse mesenchymal origin. ASCs can respond to an inductive odontogenic signal and form teeth, but the inductive signal has always to come from fresh cells (non-cultured) derived from embryonic tooth–primordium tissue (epithelium or mesenchyme), and this presents one of the challenges in bio-tooth engineering research.

It has been established that tooth initiation *in vitro* requires a high number of cells, and to obtain odontogenic (inducing) cells, multiple embryos must be harvested – an approach not feasible in humans. Additionally, it has been found that these odontogenic cells lose their inductive capacity after 24–48 hours of culturing. Thus, *in vitro* expansion of embryonic inductive dental cells using standard culture methods might not be an appropriate approach for bioengineering human teeth. In the embryonic tooth primordium, dental mesenchymal cells line up condensed together with significant cell-to-cell contact, but this arrangement of dental mesenchymal cells and the tight contacts between the cells is lost when these cells are cultured using conventional methods and grown as monolayers.

Creating odontogenic cell lines that can be stored long-term and available in large numbers is the greatest challenge in the field of bio-tooth engineering. Several methods of three-dimensional microenvironmental reprogramming have been explored to solve these problems. Studies have shown that mechanical stimulation can modulate and control cell lineage commitment during development. The shape of the cells and the contact and communication between them can also be altered mechanically to control and direct cell fate.

Based on studies on hair regeneration, hanging drops have been used to promote cell condensation in 3D cell culture conditions. This approach has also been applied to preserving the odontogenic signal in cells that have been expanded *in vitro*. An *in vitro* 'hanging drop' culture system has been proposed for reorganising epithelial–mesenchymal cells to produce the micro-environment for tooth histogenesis and organogenesis. Moreover, gene expressions assays have been used to identify signalling factors whose expression would be lost in two-dimensional *in vitro* cell culture to study the type of cell signalling that drives tooth development.

Studies focusing on cell communication have identified the 'cell community effect' during embryonic development as a process that enables mixtures of different cells to differentiate along the same pathway because of cell communication–driven changes. As a result of mixing freshly derived mesenchymal cells from embryonic tooth germs (odontogenic/inducing) with cultured cells that had lost their odontogenic capacity, it has been observed that the cultured cells are able to regain their odontogenic capacity. As a result, these cells could fully participate in the bioengineered development of teeth, giving rise to dental pulp cells and odontoblasts.

These studies, seen in a context of obtaining an atlas of different cell populations within the tissues and during development, pave the way for gathering data on cell communication and behaviour that could then be tailored, and directed, *in vitro*.

Establishing proper vascularisation and innervation of the bioengineered teeth is crucial in generating fully integrated and functional organs as a biological replacement. In bioengineered tooth primordia cultured *in vitro*, blood vessel–like structures remain in the peri-dental mesenchyme and never develop into the dental tissues. However, when these *in vitro*–generated primordia are implanted *in vivo*, they became revascularised.

There is evidence that the newly-formed blood vessels originate from the host, which permits their survival, as well as providing a favourable environment for organ growth, mineralisation and full integration within the implanted site. It has also been found that exogenous innervation-promoting agents can enhance the innervation of bioengineered teeth, such as semaphorin 3A inhibitors (Sema3a inhibitors). Also, cells from bone marrow can promote the innervation of bioengineered teeth.

Despite all the remarkable progress in developing different bioengineering approaches that produce tooth organoids that develop into fully functional teeth *in vivo*, challenges remain. The quest is on to discover how to preserve, or gain, inductive (odontogenic) properties within accessible human cell sources that can be isolated from patients.

Further readings for this chapter can be found in the accompanying eBook. Explore online Self-assessment quiz to test and reinforce your understanding of the material in your free ebook. Follow instructions in the Inside Front Cover to unlock your access.

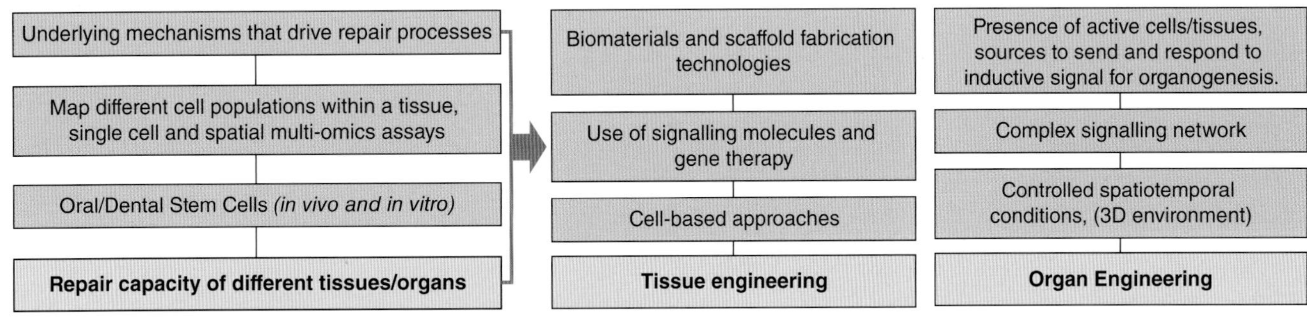
Underlying mechanisms that drive repair processes
Map different cell populations within a tissue, single cell and spatial multi-omics assays
Oral/Dental Stem Cells (in vivo and in vitro)
Repair capacity of different tissues/organs
Biomaterials and scaffold fabrication technologies
Use of signalling molecules and gene therapy
Cell-based approaches
Tissue engineering
Presence of active cells/tissues, sources to send and respond to inductive signal for organogenesis.
Complex signalling network
Controlled spatiotemporal conditions, (3D environment)
Organ Engineering

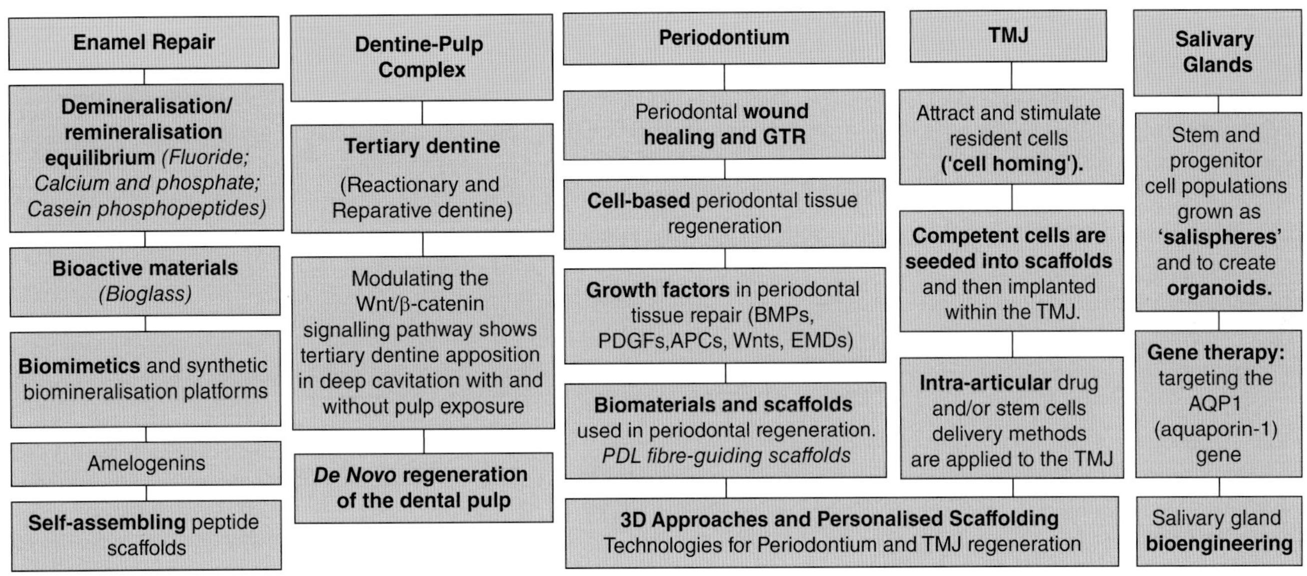
BIOLOGICAL REPAIR AND REGENERATION (REGENERATIVE DENTISTRY)
Enamel Repair
Demineralisation/ remineralisation equilibrium (Fluoride; Calcium and phosphate; Casein phosphopeptides)
Bioactive materials (Bioglass)
Biomimetics and synthetic biomineralisation platforms
Amelogenins
Self-assembling peptide scaffolds
Dentine-Pulp Complex
Tertiary dentine (Reactionary and Reparative dentine)
Modulating the Wnt/β-catenin signalling pathway shows tertiary dentine apposition in deep cavitation with and without pulp exposure
De Novo regeneration of the dental pulp
Periodontium
Periodontal wound healing and GTR
Cell-based periodontal tissue regeneration
Growth factors in periodontal tissue repair (BMPs, PDGFs,APCs, Wnts, EMDs)
Biomaterials and scaffolds used in periodontal regeneration. PDL fibre-guiding scaffolds
TMJ
Attract and stimulate resident cells ('cell homing').
Competent cells are seeded into scaffolds and then implanted within the TMJ.
Intra-articular drug and/or stem cells delivery methods are applied to the TMJ
3D Approaches and Personalised Scaffolding Technologies for Periodontium and TMJ regeneration
Salivary Glands
Stem and progenitor cell populations grown as 'salispheres' and to create organoids.
Gene therapy: targeting the AQP1 (aquaporin-1) gene
Salivary gland bioengineering

Mind Map 28.1

Glossary of abbreviations

ADhAQP1 Adenoviral vector encoding human aquaporin-1 (hAQP1)
AdhHGs Adhesive hydrogels
ADSCs Adipose-derived stem cells
AE2 Anion exchanger 2
AEFC Acellular extrinsic fibre cementum
AgNOR Silver-binding nucleolar organiser region
AIDS Acquired immunodeficiency syndrome
Alpha-SMA Alpha-smooth muscle actin
APC Autologous platelet concentrates
APC gene Adenomatous polyposis coli gene is a key tumor suppressor gene and regulator of Wnt signalling.
APCs Autologous platelet concentrates
AQP1 Aquaporin-1 gene
ASCs Adult stem cells (somatic stem cells)
Axin-2 Axis inhibition protein 2
Barx1 This gene encodes a member of the Bar subclass of homeobox transcription factors.
BCMPs bone chip mass populations (derived from implant surgery sites)
Beta (β) catenin β-catenin is a core component of the cadherin
BMPs Bone morphogenetic proteins
BMSCs Bone marrow stem cells
c-Fos Member of the AP (Activator protein-1) family of inducible transcription factors
c-Myc Cellular Myc (the Myc family of human transcription factors was identified after discovering homology between an oncogene carried by the Avian virus, Myelocytomatosis).
Ca-P clusters Calcium -Phosphate clusters
CA2 Carbonic anhydrase II
CAD Computer-aided design
CAM Computer-aided manufacture
cAMP Cyclic adenosine monophosphate
CAP Cementum-derived attachment protein
CBCT Cone beam computed tomography
Cbfa1 Core binding factor 1
CCL Chemokine (C-C motif) ligand
CD Computer design
CD90 Cluster Differentiation 90
CGRP Calcitonin gene–related peptide
CHLR Chlorcyclizine
CIFC Cellular intrinsic fibre cementum
CK Cytokeratins
Claudin6 A protein coding gene expressed in the dental epithelium during early developmental stages
CMSC Cellular mixed stratified cementum
CPG Central pattern generator
CPP-ACFP Casein phosphopeptide-stabilised amorphous calcium fluoride phosphate complexes
CPP-ACP Casein phosphopeptide-stabilised amorphous calcium phosphate complexes
Crym Crystallin mu (thyroid-binding protein)
CSph Calcospheric
CT scan Computerised Tomography scan
CTGF Connective tissue growth factor
CTGF Connective tissue growth factor
CXCL Chemokine (CXC motif) ligand
DCN Decorin
DFSCs Dental follicle stem cells
DHLNL Dehydro-hydroxylysino-norleucine cross-link
DICOM Digital Imaging and Communications in Medicine
Dlx1 Distal-Less Homeobox 1 gene
Dlx2 Distal-Less Homeobox 2 gene. Diseases associated with Dlx2 include Syngnathia and Tooth Agenesis.
DMP1 Dentine matrix protein 1
DNA Deoxyribonucleic acid
DPP Dentine phosphoprotein
DPSCs Dental pulp stem cells of permanent teeth
DSCs Dental stem cells
DSP Dentine sialoprotein
DSPP Dentine sialophosphoprotein
ECM Extracellular matrix
ECs Endothelial cells
EDA Ectodysplasin A
EDJ Enamel–dentine junction
EDTA Ethylenediaminetetraacetic acid
EGF Epidermal growth factor
EGFR Epidermal growth factor receptor
Egr3 Early growth response gene 3
EK Enamel knot
ELRs Elastin-like recombinamers
EMD Enamel matrix derivative
EMPs Enamel matrix proteins
Epha3 EPH receptor 3. This gene belongs to the ephrin receptor subfamily of the protein-tyrosine kinase family. EPH and EPH-related receptors have been implicated in mediating developmental events, particularly in the nervous system.
ePTFE Expanded polytetrafluoroethylene
ESCs Embryonic stem cells
EVs Extracellular vesicles
F- Fluor ions
FAP Familial adenomatous polyposis
FDA Food and Drug Administration
FGF Fibroblast growth factor
Foxp4 Forkhead Box P4 is a protein coding gene. Diseases associated with Foxp4 include ventricular septal defect and sensorineural hearing loss.
Fxyd7 Fxyd domain containing ion transport regulator 7
G-CSF Granulocyte colony-stimulating factor
GAGs glycosaminoglycans

GCF Gingival crevicular fluid
GDFs Growth differentiation factors
GF Growth factor
GLA carboxylation/gamma-carboxyglutamic (GLA) protein domain
Gli 1 Glioma-associated oncogene 1
GMSCs Gingival mesenchymal stem cells
GSCs Gingival stem cells
GSK-3 Glycogen synthase kinase 3
GTR Guided tissue regeneration
GVHD Graft-versus-host disease
HA Hyaluronan acid
HA/TCP Hydroxyapatite and tricalcium phosphate
HERS Hertwig's epithelial root sheath
hGMSCs Human gingival mesenchymal stem cells
Hnf3-β Helix transcription factor hepatocyte nuclear factor 3β (known also as Foxa2) is essential for multiple stages of embryonic development.
ICAM-1 Intercellular adhesion molecule
Ig (A; G; M) Immunoglobulins (A; G; M)
IGF Insulin-like growth factor
IL Interleukin
iPSCs Induced pluripotent stem cells
K14 Keratin 14
KLK-4 Kallikrein-related peptidase-4
Lef1 Lymphoid enhancer binding factor 1
LRP5 Low-density lipoprotein receptor-related protein 5
LUM Lumican
M-CSF Macrophage colony-stimulating factor
MCPs Matricellular proteins
MDPSCs Mobilised dental pulp stem cells
MEPE Matrix extracellular phosphoglycoprotein
MHC Major histocompatibility complex
MIH Molar incisor hypoplasia
MMP Metalloproteinases
MRI Magnetic resonance imaging
MSCs Mesenchymal stem cells
MSX1 Protein Coding gene -Msh Homeobox 1
MSX2 Protein Coding gene -Msh Homeobox 2
MTA Mineral trioxide aggregate
Nanog DNA binding homeobox transcription factor involved in embryonic stem (ES) cell proliferation, renewal, and pluripotency
NCPs Non-collagenous proteins
NFATc1 Nuclear factor of activated T cells 1
NFkB Nuclear factor kappa beta
NGF Nerve growth factor
Notch protein Family of type 1 transmembrane proteins that form a core component of the Notch signaling pathway, which is highly conserved in animals. Notch signaling promotes proliferative signaling during neurogenesis.
Notch3 Transmembrane protein 3 that is a component of the Notch signaling pathway
NRP1 Nel-related protein 1
OCN Osteocalcin
Oct-4 Octamer-binding transcription factor 4
ODAM Odontogenic ameloblast-associated gene
OH- Hydroxyl ions
OMD Osteomodulin
ON Osteonectin
OPG Osteoprotegerin
OPGL Osteoprotegerin ligand
OPN Osteopontin
Pax9 Paired box 9. RNA polymerase II transcription factor, regulates human ribosome biogenesis and craniofacial development
PCL Polycaprolactone
PCLA Poly(ε-caprolactone-co-lactide)
PDGF Platelet-derived growth factor (AA/BB isoforms)
PDL Periodontal ligament
PDLSCs Periodontal ligament stem cells
PGA Polyglycolique acid
pH Quantitative measure of the acidity or basicity of aqueous or other liquid solutions
PHEX Phosphate-regulating neutral endopeptidase
Pitx2 Paired-like homeodomain transcription factor 2 also known as pituitary homeobox 2
PLGA Poly-L-lactic-coglycolic acid
PLGA-PLLA Poly(lactic-co-glycolic acid) - poly(L-lactide)
PLLA Poly-L-lactic acid
POSTN Periostin
PRF Platelet-rich fibrin
PRP Platelet-rich plasma
PRPs Proline-rich proteins
Ptch1 Member of the patched gene family and is the receptor for sonic hedgehog, a secreted molecule implicated in the formation of embryonic structures and in tumorigenesis
PTH Parathyroid hormone
PTH1R Parathyroid hormone receptor-1
PTHrP Parathyroid hormone-related protein
PU 1 DNA-binding transcription factor
PVA Poly-vinyl alcohol
RAII Rapidly adapting type II
RANK Receptor activator of nuclear factor kappa beta (NFkB)
RANKL Receptor activator of nuclear factor kappa beta (NFkB) ligand
Rbm35a RNA binding motif protein 35A
RGD (Arg-Gly-Asp) motif in the transferrin receptor is required for binding to transferrin
RGSs Cell-binding domains
RHAMM Hyaluronan-mediated motility receptor, also known as HMMR
RNA Ribonucleic acid
RSDL Rudimentary successional dental laminae
RUNX2 Runt-related transcription factor 2
SARS-CoV-2 Severe-acute-respiratory-syndrome-related coronavirus 2
SCAPs Stem cells of apical papilla
SCPP Secretory calcium-binding phosphoprotein
SDF-1 Stromal derived factor-1 (also known as CXCL12)
SEK Secondary enamel knot
SEM Scanning electron microscope
SFF Solid freeform fabrication
SHEDs Stem cells of human exfoliating dentition
Shh Sonic hedgehog signalling
Si-OH Silanol
SIBLING Small Integrin-Binding Ligand N-linked Glycoprotein
SjS Sjögren's syndrome
SLRPs Small leucine-rich proteoglycans
SMCs Smooth muscle cells
SMGs Salivary gland epithelial stem cells

SOST Sclerostin

Sox2 also known as SRY (sex determining region Y)-box 2 is transcription factor that is essential for maintaining self-renewal, or pluripotency of undifferentiated embryonic stem cells

SPARC Secreted protein acidic and rich in cysteine

SSCS Skeletal stem cells

SSEA-4 Stage-specific embryonic antigen-4

STL file File format native to the stereolithography computer-aided design software

STRO 'Stro' means 'mesenchyme'

STRO-1 A monoclonal antibody for identifying stromal/mesenchymal stem cells

Syndecan1 Protein which in humans is encoded by the SDC1 gene. The protein is a transmembrane (type I) heparan sulfate proteoglycan and is a member of the syndecan proteoglycan family. Participates in cell proliferation, cell migration and cell-matrix interactions

TGF Tumour growth factor

TGF beta (TGFβ) Transforming growth factor-beta

TGFA Transforming Growth Factor Alpha

TGPC Tooth germ papilla stem cells

Thy 1 Thymocyte antigen 1

TIMPs Tissue inhibitors of matrix metalloproteinases

TLR Toll-like receptor

TMJ Temporomandibular joint

TMJDs Temporomandibular joint disorders

TN Tenascin

TNF-α Tumour necrosis factor alpha

TRAP Tartrate-resistant acid phosphatase

UDPGD Uridine 5'-diphospho-glucuronosyltransferase (UDP-glucuronosyltransferase, UGT) is a microsomal glycosyltransferase

VEGF Vascular endothelial growth factor

Wnt Wingless-related integration site (secreted factors that regulate cell growth, motility, and differentiation during embryonic development

α-fetoprotein Alpha-fetoprotein (AFP) is the main component of mammalian fetal serum

α-SMA Alpha-smooth muscle actin

Index

Page numbers followed by "*f*" indicate figures, "*t*" indicate tables, and "*b*" indicate boxes.

Q

R

S

T